Desk Reference for
Critical Care Nursing

The Jones and Bartlett Series in Nursing

Desk Reference for Critical Care Nursing

Jonelle E. Wright, PhD, RN

Assistant Professor
The Johns Hopkins School of Medicine
Baltimore, Maryland

Director of Nursing Research
The Francis Scott Key Medical Center
Baltimore, Maryland

Brenda K. Shelton, MS, RN, CCRN, OCN

Critical Care Clinical Nurse Specialist
The Johns Hopkins Oncology Center
Baltimore, Maryland

JONES AND BARTLETT PUBLISHERS

Boston   *London*

Editorial, Sales, and Customer Service Offices
Jones and Bartlett Publishers
One Exeter Plaza
Boston, MA 02116

Jones and Bartlett Publishers International
PO Box 1498
London W6 7RS
England

Library of Congress Cataloging-in-Publication Data

Wright, Jonelle Evangeline.
    Desk reference for critical care nursing / Jonelle E. Wright,
Brenda K. Shelton.
      p. cm.
    Includes bibliographical references and index.
    ISBN 0-86720-325-0
    1. Intensive care nursing—Outlines, syllabi, etc. 2. Intensive
care nursing—Examinations, questions, etc. I. Shelton, Brenda K.
(Brenda Kurtz) II. Title.
    [DNLM: 1. Critical Care. 2. Nursing Care. WY 154 W951d 1993]
RT120.I5W76 1993
610.73'61—dc20
DNLM/DLC   93-18291
for Library of Congress   CIP

Sponsoring Editor: Jim Keating
Production Editor: Judy Songdahl
Editorial Production Service: Lifland et al., Bookmakers
Cover Design: Hannus Design Associates
Typesetting: ATLIS Graphics & Design, Inc.
Printing and Binding: Rand McNally

The selection and dosage of drugs presented in this book are in accord with standards accepted at the time of publication. The authors and publisher have made every effort to provide accurate information. However, research, clinical practice, and government regulations often change the accepted standards in this field. Before administering any drug, the reader is advised to check the manufacturer's product information sheet for the most up-to-date recommendations on dosage, precautions, and contraindications. This is especially important in the case of drugs that are new or seldom used.

Printed in the United States of America
97 96 95 94 93   10 9 8 7 6 5 4 3 2 1

*To strengthen the hands
caring for those in critical need,
we offer this book.*

*In celebration of
The memory of that one in our lives
who wanted so to live to this day
but could not,*

and

*The presence of those whom we love,
who continue to fill our lives daily
with inspiration, fortitude, and joy.*

CONTENTS

4   *The Cardiovascular System*   **467**

7 The Endocrine System 990

8 The Hematologic and Immune Systems 1073

9 Multisystem Problems 1248

NURSING CARE PLANS

MEDICATIONS COMMONLY USED

FOREWORD

Critical care nursing has evolved into an important specialty based on extensive clinical expertise and a broad and important body of knowledge. This new reference text provides the critical care nurse with a detailed, scholarly, yet usable reference book. The authors have consistently written clinically useful and authoritative chapters using a very well-balanced approach that includes the scientific basis for clinical decision making. The database for critical care nursing is so extensive that no single text can be encyclopedic. The editors of this book have clearly chosen to emphasize the areas of most common concern to the critical care nurse (the respiratory, nervous, cardiovascular, gastrointestinal, endocrine, hematologic, and immunologic systems). The pre-test and post-test included with each chapter make this book useful as a working handbook in addition to a reference source. As a longtime supporter of critical care nursing, I am proud to recommend to my colleagues in the nursing field this important new contribution to the critical care literature. The editors are to be congratulated for the development of this unique reference source, and my hope is that the important information contained herein will provide nurses with a broader basis for extending the wonderful work they do in the intensive care unit.

Bart Chernow, MD, FACP, FCCP, FCCM
Professor of Medicine, Anesthesia, and Critical Care
The Johns Hopkins University School of Medicine
Physician-in-Chief
Sinai Hospital of Baltimore
Editor-in-Chief, *Critical Care Medicine*
Baltimore, Maryland

PREFACE

Many nurses preparing for critical care practice or the critical care certification examination find that reviewing an extensive body of scientific knowledge and making the appropriate clinical applications necessitates a very difficult study of numerous sources, which then must be synthesized to provide a base of information for practice. The purpose of this desk reference is to provide a succinct yet comprehensive source of core information necessary for critical care certified nursing practice. We developed this desk reference to prepare nurses for critical care certification and assist them in practicing effectively in the critical care setting. To achieve these goals, this text material reflects the principles and practice of adult education within the framework of critical care concept analysis. The *Desk Reference for Critical Care Nursing* incorporates in one book the resource material needed to carry out present-day critical care nursing practice. By integrating the sciences of anatomy, physiology, and pathophysiology, the knowledge of individual risk factors and precipitating factors, the practices of clinical diagnostics, and nursing standards in the application of the nursing process, we have made this text relevant to all facets of critical care nursing.

Desk Reference Format

The desk reference was developed using a systems approach, reflecting knowledge and skills required in the care of individuals experiencing illness in any of the physical systems outlined in the American Association of Critical Care Nurses' core curriculum. Each system chapter incorporates the various components of clinical concept analysis:

1. Pre-Test (sample CCRN questions)
2. Overview of system anatomy and physiology (normal processes)
3. System assessment (both physical assessment and diagnostics)
4. Nursing interventions and evaluation measures for care of individuals with specific disease processes. These interventions focus on
   a. Clinical antecedents (risk factors and precipitating factors leading to the event)
   b. Critical referents (specific pathophysiological processes of the event)
   c. Resulting signs and symptoms
   d. Nursing care plans for managing individuals experiencing the event. Nursing care plans provide:
      1. review of medical management
      2. nursing diagnosis
      3. signs and symptoms indicating the nursing diagnosis
      4. intervention measures specific to the nursing diagnosis
      5. rationale for each nursing intervention
      6. table of medications detailing actions and side effects
5. Post-Test (sample CCRN questions)

Desk Reference for Critical Care Nursing may be used in a number of ways:

- as a critical care resource for clinical problem solving and practice review;
- as an orientation to the practice of critical care nursing;
- as a text in a structured course of study of critical care nursing practice;
- for individual and group preparation for critical care nursing certification testing;
- as a self-paced study desk reference for certified critical care nursing practice;
- as a resource and self-evaluation desk reference throughout one's career in critical care nursing practice.

Functioning successfully in the critical care setting requires expertise in, and an in-depth understanding of, the care practices and technical procedures performed in the care of the critically ill patient. All too often nurses are oriented to the ICU setting and the critical care nursing role through short-term clinical educational offerings and hands-on training. To fully integrate clinical information and knowledge into practice, however, one must understand the basic physiologic and pathophysiologic principles underlying the condition being manifested. This knowledge must then be synthesized systematically into a comprehensive plan of care specific to the biological, spiritual, and psychosocial needs of the patient. This reference book provides the information needed to accomplish such an effort in the clinical nursing setting.

ACKNOWLEDGMENTS

We, the authors, wish to acknowledge . . .

. . . the family members and co-workers who spent endless hours enduring our commitment to this project, encouraged us during difficult times, and rose to the challenges of deadlines and frequent chaos. Among these stellar individuals are Rachel Rachis, Patricia Knighton, Dawn Bishop, Lawrence Jewell, Christina Bennett, Sandra Oldaker, and Carol Gogel (who helped with photocopying and preparing illustrations and tables), Rich Shelton, Anna Bond, Martha Kennedy, Sharon Krumm, and Joan Franks. Jonelle wishes to extend special gratitude to Dr. Jay R. Shapiro for his support when, two weeks before the entire manuscript was due, Jonelle broke her right index finger. Dr. Shapiro provided secretarial services to finish the job. Ms. Lisa Philips also deserves special recognition for her work in preparing the manuscript;

. . . the sponsoring editor, Jim Keating, who in his infinite wisdom predicted the difficulties we encountered in producing this manuscript and demonstrated patience, tolerance, and humor throughout the entire process; and

. . . Quica Ostrander, who even in the most stressed times maintained a positive attitude (albeit one tinged with a sense of urgency) when working on the manuscript. She had a way of strongly encouraging us to meet our deadlines in the face of multiple revisions and was so very good at putting up with us.

CONTRIBUTORS

Mary Angela Allen, MS, RN
Clinical Nurse Specialist
Warren Grant Magnusson Clinical Center
National Institutes of Health
Bethesda, Maryland

Mary Michael Brown, MS, RN, CCRN
Nurse Manager, Cardiac Surgery ICU
Georgetown University Hospital
Washington, DC

Mary Elizabeth Clark, RN
Nurse Educator IV
The Francis Scott Key Medical Center Regional
    Burn Center
Baltimore, Maryland

Christina Cunningham, MS, RN, CCRN
Shock Trauma Unit
Maryland Institute of Emergency Medicine
Baltimore, Maryland

Sandra Dearholt, MS, RN, CCRN
Nurse Manager, Solid Tumor
The Johns Hopkins Oncology Center
Baltimore, Maryland

Susan R. Feldman, MS, RN, CDE
District Manager
Caremark, Healthcare Services Division
Baltimore, Maryland

Andrea R. Fisher, MS, RN, CNS
Ottowa Civic Hospital
Ottowa, Ontario, Canada

Vici Heineman, MS, RN, CCRN
The Johns Hopkins Asthma and Allergy Clinics
Baltimore, Maryland

Mary Jo Holechek, MS, RN, CNN
Clinical Nurse Specialist in Nephrology
Department of Medical Nursing—Nephrology
The Johns Hopkins Hospital
Baltimore, Maryland

Sarah Kaplan, MS, RN, CCRN
Private Practice
Chambersburg, Pennsylvania

Martha M. Kennedy, BSN, RN, CCRN
Critical Care Instructor
The Johns Hopkins Oncology Center
Baltimore, Maryland

Lori J. Kozlowski, MS, RN, CCRN
Clinical Nurse Specialist in Pediatrics
The Johns Hopkins Hospital—Pediatrics
Baltimore, Maryland

Marilyn A. Leherr, BSN, RN, OCN, CCRN
Clinical Nurse Specialist
St. Anthony's Medical Center
Louisville, Kentucky

Barbara Griffith Lubejko, MS, RN, CCRN
Research Nurse
The Johns Hopkins Oncology Center
Baltimore, Maryland

David F. Matuszak, PhD, RRT
Respiratory Therapy
Good Samaritan Hospital
Baltimore, Maryland

Ann Medinger, MD, FACP
Associate Professor of Medicine
George Washington University
Washington, DC

Mary Lou Mullen-Monakil, MS, RN, CDE
Research Nurse Coordinator
Division of Endocrinology and Metabolism
The Johns Hopkins University
Baltimore, Maryland

Kathy Robey-Williams, MS, RN, CCRN, NREMT-P
The Advanced Life Support Program Coordinator
The Johns Hopkins Hospital
Baltimore, Maryland

Kathleen S. Rohrer, MS, RN
Instructor, Surgical Nursing
The Johns Hopkins Hospital
Baltimore, Maryland

Jane Shivnan, BSc, RN, CCRN
Nurse Manager, Bone Marrow Transplant Unit
The Johns Hopkins Oncology Center
Baltimore, Maryland

Steve Wilson, MS, RN
Clinical Nurse Specialist, Spinal Cord Injury
Sinai Hospital of Baltimore
Baltimore, Maryland

Frances B. Wimbush, PhD, RN
Assistant Professor
Medical College of Ohio School of Nursing
Toledo, Ohio

Terri Smith Zemel, MS, RN, CCRN
Nephrology Private Practice
Baltimore, Maryland

REVIEWERS

Christina Bennett, BSN, RN
Research Nurse IV
Francis Scott Key Medical Center
Baltimore, Maryland

Michael Bloom, RRT
Director, Respiratory Therapy
Francis Scott Key Medical Center
Baltimore, Maryland

Michael Donohoe, MD
Private Cardiology Practice
Chambersburg, Pennsylvania

Dorrie Fontaine, DNSc, RN, CCRN
Associate Professor
University of Maryland Graduate School of
    Nursing
Baltimore, Maryland

Angeliki Georgopoulos, MD
Associate Professor
The Johns Hopkins School of Medicine
Baltimore, Maryland

Donna J. Huffer, BSN, RN, OCN
Senior Partner, Educator Oncology ICU
University of Maryland Cancer Center
Baltimore, Maryland

Lawrence Jewell, RN
Research Nurse
Francis Scott Key Medical Center
Baltimore, Maryland

Patricia A. Knighton, RN
Research Nurse, Asthma and Allergy
Francis Scott Key Medical Center
Baltimore, Maryland

Claire Lewellyn, BSN, RN
Neonatal Intensive Care Unit
University of California at San Francisco Medical
    Center
San Francisco, California

Sandra Oldaker, BSN, RN
Research Nurse
Francis Scott Key Medical Center
Baltimore, Maryland

David Pearse, MD
Assistant Professor
Division of Pulmonary Medicine
The Johns Hopkins School of Medicine
Baltimore, Maryland

Rachel Rachis, BSN, RN
Research Nurse
Francis Scott Key Medical Center
Baltimore, Maryland

Robin A. Remsberg, PhD, RN
Research Coordinator
Chesapeake Physicians' Practice Association
Baltimore, Maryland

Ann Scheve, MS, RNC
Clinical Nurse Specialist
Francis Scott Key Medical Center
Baltimore, Maryland

Jay R. Shapiro, MD
Professor
The Johns Hopkins School of Medicine
Baltimore, Maryland

Vivian Sheidler, MS, RN
Clinical Nurse Specialist, Neuro-Oncology and
    Pain
The Johns Hopkins Oncology Center
Baltimore, Maryland

Stephanie Walter-Coleman, RN, CCRN
Clinical Nurse
University of Maryland Cancer Center
Baltimore, Maryland

Alan J. Watson, MD
Associate Professor, Department of Medicine
Division of Nephrology
The Johns Hopkins Hospital
Baltimore, Maryland

Stephen M. Zemel, MD
Board Certified Internal Medicine and Nephrology
Private Practice
Baltimore, Maryland

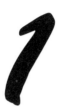

Preparing for the CCRN Examination

Introduction

Since the 1960s, the science and practice of nursing have developed rapidly in tandem with the technological and service progress that has been realized in health care. Lives that only last year would have been considered lost are being saved through complex and spectacular means as the various members of the health care team work to overcome the effects of disease and ill-health. Extremely sophisticated techniques for the diagnosis and treatment of health disorders have become commonplace, and the demand for nurses expert in the bedside care of patients undergoing such interventions has increased at even greater rates than the strides being made. A good proportion of the technology for today's health care is found in critical care units, where intense utilization of personnel, equipment, and facilities occur.

Because of the above trends, critical care nursing has become the largest specialty group within the nursing profession. Its members are noted for their strong clinical base and leadership activities. Moreover, with the advent of fiscal and economic constraints on the health care delivery system during this time of "quicker and sicker," the professional nurse embarking on a career in critical care nursing faces unprecedented challenges and opportunities. To aid critical care nurses in meeting fully both the explicit and the implicit demands being placed on them, the American Association of Critical Care Nurses (AACN) became one of the first organizations to develop a certification program for clinicians, establishing a standard for excellence in practice that many other organizations have since emulated.

The AACN established its critical care certification program to "promote the health and welfare of those experiencing critical illness by advancing the science and art of critical care nursing through certification processes" (*CCRN News*, 1988, p. 6). Furthermore, the American Association of Critical Care Nurses addressed the priorities of furthering the educational development of its members and maintaining a national reputation for excellence in practice. These goals are met through the administration of the core curriculum and certifying exam for critical care nurses (the CCRN exam). By this means, critical care nurses are identified and recognized as individuals who emulate the current state of the art in critical care nursing and demonstrate a scientific knowledge base that enhances critical care outcomes. Based on practice delineation surveys conducted by the AACN, the CCRN exam is designed to reflect current and common general practice in critical care and to provide the public with a measure of accountability.

Since the AACN has used the certification process to establish the professional competency of its members, the credential has come to symbolize expertise in critical care nursing and to be held in high esteem by all in the institutional health care delivery system.

Content of the CCRN Exam

The AACN's *Core Curriculum for Critical Care Nursing* describes the knowledge base required for nurses who care for the critically ill and highlights content areas that have been addressed in past CCRN exams. Many critical care nurses who are preparing to take the exam find it beneficial to use the core curriculum when studying, but others realize the need for independent study materials that provide greater detail and are reflective of the most current content of the exam. This desk reference will help the CCRN candidate or clinician to focus on knowledge important to the delivery of quality critical care nursing. Prior to beginning study, the CCRN candidate should become familiar with available information about the content of the current exam and suggestions about how to improve test-taking ability.

In 1984 the AACN's certification corporation presented "Role Delineation/CCRN Validation Study," the findings of a landmark research project defining the practice of critical care nursing. As a result of this important research, the CCRN exam blueprint was changed from its original version to one that was considered to provide a more valid assessment of clinical practice in critical care. The revised version was put into effect in February 1985. In 1990 the CCRN exam development committee again evaluated the validity of the exam and implemented a new blueprint for institution in February 1992. Revisions included changes in the numbers of questions within system content areas, elimination or addition of specific disease processes, and a redistribution of cognitive levels addressed by items on the exam. Changes regarding specific system content are outlined in Table 1-1.

The content of the CCRN exam is determined by the blueprint and addresses practices involved in the care of individuals experiencing serious illness in the physical systems listed in Table 1-1. Within each of these eight systemic divisions, focus is placed on three major content areas:

1. Anatomy and physiology
2. Assessment and identification of the problem
3. Devising, providing, and evaluating a plan of care for specific pathophysiologies

Table 1-1 Overview of Changes in the Content of the CCRN Exam

System	Exam Content 1984	Exam Content 1992
Neurological system	19% of total exam	8% of total exam
	Altered level of consciousness Increased intracranial pressure Head trauma Skull fracture Aneurysm/Arteriovenous malformation Seizures and status epilepticus Spinal cord injury Hydrocephalus Neurologic tumors Craniotomy CVA/Stroke/Transient ischemic attack Intracranial/Neurologic bleeds/Hematomas Neurologic infectious disease Neuromuscular disease	Encephalopathy Head trauma Aneurysm Acute spinal cord injury Space-occupying lesions Cerebral embolic events Intracranial hemorrhage Neurologic infectious disease Seizure disorder
Pulmonary system	19% of total exam	22% of total exam
	Acute respiratory failure Adult respiratory distress syndrome Pulmonary embolus Chronic obstructive pulmonary disease Neoplastic lung disease Status asthmaticus Chest trauma	Acute respiratory failure Adult respiratory distress syndrome Acute respiratory infections Status asthmaticus Acute pulmonary embolus Thoracic trauma Pulmonary aspirations Airleak syndromes
Cardiovascular system	19% of total exam	39% of total exam
	Myocardial infarction Angina/Atherosclerosis Myocardial conduction system defects Hypertensive crisis Dysrhythmia Cardiogenic shock Cardiac surgery Vascular surgery Hemorrhagic shock Pericarditis	Acute myocardial infarction/ischemia Unstable angina Myocardial conduction system defects Acute congestive heart failure/Pulmonary edema Hypertensive crisis Cardiogenic shock Structural heart defects Ruptured or dissecting aortic aneurysm Hypovolemic shock Acute inflammatory disease Dysrhythmias Cardiomyopathies Cardiac trauma Acute peripheral vascular insufficiency
Renal system	14% of total exam	5% of total exam
	Acute renal failure Hyperkalemia Hypokalemia Hypernatremia Hyponatremia Hypercalcemia Hypocalcemia Hyperphosphatemia Hypophosphatemia Chronic renal failure	Acute renal failure Life-threatening electrolyte imbalances Renal trauma

(continued)

Table 1-1 Overview of Changes in the Content of the CCRN Exam (*continued*)

System	Exam Content 1984	Exam Content 1992
Gastrointestinal system	13% of total exam	8% of total exam
	Peptic ulcers Gastrointestinal malignancies Esophageal varices Cirrhosis Hepatic failure Acute pancreatitis Inflammatory bowel disorders Bowel infarction Gastrointestinal trauma	Acute GI hemorrhage Hepatic failure/Coma Acute pancreatitis Bowel infarction/Obstruction/Perforation Acute abdominal trauma
Endocrine system	7% of total exam	4% of total exam
	Diabetes insipidus Inappropriate secretion of ADH Thyrotoxic crisis Hypoparathyroidism Acute adrenal insufficiency Hyperglycemic ketoacidotic crisis Hyperglycemic nonketotic hyperosmolar coma Hypoglycemia/Insulin shock Myxedema coma	Diabetes insipidus Syndrome of inappropriate secretion of ADH Diabetic ketoacidosis Hyperglycemic hyperosmolar nonketotic coma Acute hypoglycemia
Hematology immunology system	7% of total exam	4% of total exam
	Anemia Anaphylaxis Disseminated intravascular coagulation Multiple myeloma Hemophilia Lymphoma	Organ transplantation Life-threatening coagulopathies Immunosuppression
Multisystem problems	Not included	10% of total exam Sepsis/Septic shock Toxic ingestions Asphyxia Burns

Specific task statements addressing these focal areas have been developed by the AACN certification corporation and are used as the guide for writers of test items.

Test Items

Test item writers are practicing CCRNs who are nominated and endorsed by their local chapters as content experts in particular topical areas. An application process involving submission of a curriculum vitae is required prior to endorsement. After selecting the item writers, the certification corporation launches item-writing drives, asking specific writers to address particular task statements. Test questions are written to address particular objectives, such as anatomy and physiology of the renal system or psychosocial implications of acute pancreatitis. Each test item writer may be asked to develop questions at one cognitive level or simply to identify the cognitive level at which questions are posed.

All test items submitted are referenced. Item writers are cautioned to use routine current practice as a standard and to test general knowledge rather than greatly specialized and trivial details.

The test evaluation committee reviews each test item submitted to further evaluate it for appropriateness, accuracy, educational soundness, and compliance with the following guidelines:

1. Multiple-multiple questions are discouraged.
2. Questions have only one correct answer.
3. Question stems address only one subject.
4. Abbreviations are not used.
5. Options are relatively short and equal in length.
6. Options "all of the above" or "none of the above" are avoided.

7. Use of "all" or "never" or other absolutes in the stem is avoided.
8. Use of negative stems ("except" or "not") is discouraged.
9. Universally accepted concepts and procedures are tested rather than trivial, obscure, or esoteric information.

Cognitive Levels of Exam Questions

In early CCRN exams, about 85% of the questions were based at the knowledge recall level of cognition. However, the validation study found that critical care decision making required higher levels of thought processing than the ability to recall facts. With the 1985 test revision, a higher level of cognitive functioning was required of CCRN candidates by distributing test questions across three levels: knowledge recall, application and analysis of information, and synthesis and evaluation of information for practice. As of 1989, the distribution of questions was further revised as follows:

	1985	1989
Knowledge recall (I)	39%	36%
Application and analysis (II)	36%	39%
Synthesis and evaluation (III)	25%	25%

Although the overall level of difficulty of the questions is now somewhat higher, the questions more closely reflect clinical decision making and may actually seem easier to the practicing clinician. In any case, when studying, CCRN candidates can now emphasize the cognitive level they personally find most difficult.

Knowledge Recall

Questions requiring knowledge recall may test the recall of specific or isolated information or ways and means of dealing with specific situations. Some words that clue the test taker that the item is of the recall type are *know, list, state, name, identify,* and *recognize.* The following are examples of this type of question.

Recall of specific information
1. Identify the three cranial nerves responsible for eye movement:
   a. trochlear, accessory, and optic nerves.
   b. oculomotor, trochlear, and abducens nerves.
   c. optic, oculomotor, and trochlear nerves.
   d. optic, trigeminal, and facial nerves.

Recall of ways of dealing with situations
2. Before transfusing a unit of packed red cells, the nurse should be certain that:
   a. the patient has never had a transfusion reaction previously.
   b. the patient has not febrile in the past 12 hours.
   c. the blood has been warmed to room temperature.
   d. the blood is compatible to that specific patient's blood type.

Application and Analysis

Questions requiring application and analysis address the ability to use information in practice. This involves the use of principles or theories in concrete situations as well as the identification of conceptual relationships. Words that signal a question posed at this cognitive level are *calculate, complete, analyze, explain, relate, detect, apply,* and *utilize.* Examples of these questions are as follows:

Application of specific knowledge or principles
1. Patients receiving diuretics should be taught the importance of all of the following behaviors *except:*
   a. weighing themselves regularly.
   b. taking potassium supplements as ordered.
   c. ensuring adequate carbohydrate intake to offset hypoglycemia.
   d. reporting swelling of ankles or fingers.

Identification and use of the relationship among conceptual parts
2. M.S. is a postcraniotomy patient with an intraventricular catheter. His blood pressure is 102/50, and his intracranial pressure is 18 mm Hg. Calculate his cerebral perfusion pressure.
   a. 84 mm Hg
   b. 49 mm Hg
   c. 35 mm Hg
   d. 32 mm Hg.

Synthesis and Evaluation

Synthesis and evaluation, the highest level of cognition, requires that the individual compile information and explain relationships or make judgments about the information. To do this, the critical care clinician must have an adequate foundation in physiology and knowledge of normal critical care problems and therapeutics. Frequently, this cognitive domain is tested with small case study questions. Words often used in synthesis and evaluation questions are *evaluate, judge, assess, interpret, propose,* and *plan.* These are examples of such questions:

The synthesis of informational elements to form a complex interrelationship as found in practice

1. A 29-year-old female presents to the emergency room with evidence of acute respiratory distress evidenced by stridor, central cyanosis, tachypnea, tachycardia, and diaphoresis. The patient has a recent history of bee sting, but has not previously noted such symptoms. ABGs are drawn, and the results are pH 7.12, pO_2 52, pCO_2 60, HCO_3 22, and O_2 saturation 80%. The nurse's interpretation of the blood gas report would lead to the conclusion that this patient's primary problem is:
   a. respiratory acidosis with hypoxemia.
   b. respiratory alkalosis with hypoxemia.
   c. metabolic acidosis with hypoxemia.
   d. metabolic alkalosis with hypoxemia.

The evaluation of how well criteria for practice are met by methods of practice

2. A 67-year-old female is admitted after several syncopal attacks and complaints of chest pain. She presents with pitting edema, moist rales, puffy eyelids, and a history of rapid weight gain. V.S.: BP 178/98, P 132, R 28 and labored, and T 98.8°F. A thermodilution catheter is inserted, and the pulmonary artery wedge pressure is 25 mm Hg. The nurse's evaluation of these data is that the patient is experiencing:
   a. left ventricular failure.
   b. normal variation.
   c. low blood volume.
   d. profound dehydration.

Test Taking

Testing is a measure of competency. Therefore, the words *test* and *examination* cause both emotional and physical changes in the individual to be tested. The emotions evoked often result in stress and anxiety. The body reacts to stress and anxiety with defense or coping mechanisms. Physiologically, the general adaptation system becomes dominant (a response also called *fight or flight*), with the sympathetic nervous system overriding the parasympathetic division. Norepinephrine is secreted, causing blood pressure to increase. Epinephrine is also secreted, and the central nervous system is activated, resulting in increased cardiac output, increased oxygen exchange, and dilated pupils (which enhance vision). The release of ACTH contributes to higher energy levels.

These physiological responses to stress and anxiety may have a positive or negative effect, depending on the individual's ability to harness stress levels. In moderate amounts, stress and anxiety can increase concentration and mobilize energy, thereby benefiting a test taker. However, high levels of stress can cripple a test taker by increasing anxiety levels and decreasing concentration. In this case, energy is not productively harnessed, and energy reserves are depleted. Therefore, each test taker must be aware of his or her individual tolerance level in order to put the body's general adaptation system to efficient use when preparing for an examination and taking it.

To successfully take an exam, the individual must organize. The CCRN candidate should familiarize himself or herself with all aspects of the certification exam by reviewing the blueprint, assessing his or her learning ability at various cognitive levels, and understanding the unique circumstances surrounding the CCRN examination. The candidate should begin studying early so that normal work and sleep habits are not interrupted. Normal, unhurried schedules help lessen anxiety and stress. An established study routine that includes scheduled breaks for both exercise and nourishment will help to pace study periods. During any extended study session, the candidate should stand and stretch for 5 minutes every hour.

A written timetable that includes all of the material to be covered, daily study times, regular self-tests, and reviews of unmastered material should be developed. More specifically, review of the content outlined in this desk reference will help in formulating a picture of all that must be covered in study sessions. With this picture in mind, the candidate can decide what content areas to concentrate on. Summary outlines of each area should be prepared and read daily. These outlines may be used to place concepts and facts in perspective and to highlight specific information to be studied in depth.

The day before the exam should be used for review and relaxation. If previous study time has been used wisely, the material should be familiar; if not, it will be too late to remedy the deficit. Regardless, the candidate should eat well, relax, and get a good night's sleep.

The examination day should begin with a well-balanced meal. Studying on the morning of the examination can only increase anxiety and instill doubt. Upon arrival at the examination site, the test taker should not panic or get drawn into the paranoia of frenzied colleagues. The confidence developed from being familiar with the content of the exam and from effort put into studying will be the best defense.

The CCRN exam consists of 200 questions, which the candidates are given four hours to complete. Test answers are marked with No. 2 pencils on an answer sheet separate from the test booklet. Candidates are allowed to write in the test booklet, and scrap paper is also provided. It may be beneficial to use this paper for doing computations or to note unanswered items, since a later question may either reveal the answer needed or trigger a correct response to the earlier question. The test taker may even wish to use the scrap paper as soon as the test period begins to note formulas or normal values that may be difficult to remember later. Such complex information will then be readily available later in the period when the individual is tired and perhaps less able to recall specific and detailed facts.

The scoring mechanism used counts all correct answers without penalty for incorrect ones. Thus, it is beneficial for the test taker to answer all questions even when uncertain of the response.

Exam questions are randomly selected (by an independent testing agency) from a large pool of questions submitted by item writers. The questions are then distributed throughout the exam in no particular order. Because the exam is not organized into systemic subdivisions as most study materials are, individuals should be prepared to answer questions in an erratic order.

The test taker must be sure to *read the directions carefully*. Skipping or misreading important directions could cost points. After reading the directions, it is a good idea to quickly skim the test and plan time accordingly. The test taker at this point should answer two questions: "How many questions are there?" and "How much time should be spent on each question?" Some questions can be answered quickly, others will require a few minutes. Then the time should be checked, a watch set on the desk top, and the test begun.

Each question should be carefully read, and it may be beneficial to highlight key terms and important words and phrases. The ability to supply an answer before the choices are read is evidence that the answer is correct. When the correct response is selected, the answer sheet should not be marked. The question should first be actively read again, and the test taker should think carefully about what the test item is addressing. For example, there is a big difference between the most common side effect and the most life-threatening. It is only after such deliberation that an answer should be marked.

The test taker should remain calm, even when one or more questions cannot be answered. During moments like these, it is best to take a deep breath and resort to the use of common sense. Since incorrect answers are not penalized, it is best to guess at the answer, but only after increasing the chance of choosing the correct answer by eliminating the choices known to be incorrect. It is also good to remember not to spend too much time on questions that seem difficult. Go on to other questions, and return to them later, for all questions should be answered, someway, before the finish of the exam.

Upon completion of the test, the test taker should return to the beginning and review as many of the items as possible. A test taker should think *very* carefully before changing an answer, however, for the initial response is usually the best response. Also, the answer sheet should be checked for stray marks, incorrect placement of answers, and blanks.

Finally, the test taker should not participate in postmortems. It is best to forget the test until the results arrive, approximately 6–8 weeks later. A passing score is determined by the group means, and items may be eliminated due to questions of validity. A candidate must achieve a passing score on each system division as well as a total score of at least 135 points. Those recertifying usually score the highest, followed by first-time candidates. Those who have previously failed the exam experience the most difficulty, and poor preparation and study habits are thought to be the major contributing factors to test-taking problems. Developing an organized, methodical approach to studying is recommended by all experts.

The following sample exam simulates the CCRN exam. The content of the questions reflects the various subsystems and knowledge levels in the actual exam. Each question has been labeled to indicate the cognitive level it addresses: I, Knowledge recall, II, Application and analysis, and III, Synthesis and evaluation. The learner can use this sample exam to identify topics requiring further study and to assess individual strengths and weaknesses of learning style. This 100-question exam should take 1½ to 2 hours to complete.

SAMPLE EXAM

Please refer to the following clinical vignette in answering questions 1 through 3.

L. J. is a 28-year-old male brought to the emergency room after a motor vehicle accident in which he suffered a head injury and steering wheel injury to the chest. He was initially unconscious, but has begun to move his extremities and moan. The nurse notes a sudden onset of agitation and labored breathing with retraction of the intercostal muscles. Frank cyanosis is present and the trachea is deviated to the right.

1. The complication that has most likely occurred is (III):
   a. right hemothorax.
   b. right tension pneumothorax.
   c. left tension pneumothorax.
   d. adult respiratory distress syndrome.

2. Another assessment finding is likely to be (II):
   a. severe hypertension.
   b. absent chest wall movement on the left.
   c. tympanic left chest.
   d. severe jugular venous pulsations.

3. The medical treatment of choice at this time would be (II):
   a. transfer to the OR for thoracotomy.
   b. needle insertion into the left fifth intercostal space.
   c. needle insertion into the right second intercostal space.
   d. right lower lobe chest tube insertion.

4. The hallmarks of adult respiratory distress syndrome are (I):
   a. hypoxemia and poor compliance.
   b. hypercapnea and high pulmonary artery pressures.
   c. diffuse fluffy infiltrates on chest x-ray and wheezing.
   d. hypoxemia and high pulmonary capillary wedge pressure.

5. Severe and refractory adult respiratory distress syndrome may be treated with (II):
   a. low PEEP levels, high tidal volumes, and paralysis.
   b. inverse inspiratory/expiratory ratio and semi-prone positioning.
   c. high-frequency jet ventilation and pressure-support ventilation.
   d. a rotating bed, ventilation with an inspiratory pause, and high peak flow rates.

6. The normal breath sounds with the longest inspiratory phase are (I):
   a. tracheal.
   b. bronchial.
   c. bronchovesicular.
   d. vesicular.

7. Pleural friction rubs have all the following characteristics *except* (I):
   a. they are most prominent in the anterior-lateral lung field.
   b. they disappear after coughing.
   c. they are caused by the grinding of inflamed parietal and visceral pleural linings.
   d. they have a high squeaking or grating quality upon auscultation.

8. While auscultating a patient's lung fields, a nurse hears light crackles bilaterally in the bases. Even after forceful coughing, the sounds persist. The following is suspected (II):
   a. asthma
   b. atelectasis
   c. pneumothorax
   d. heart failure

9. Hemodynamic effects of vasodilators can include (II):
   a. significantly decreased right atrial and wedge pressures with no change in cardiac output.
   b. significantly increased right atrial and wedge pressures and cardiac output.
   c. significantly decreased right atrial and wedge pressures accompanied by a significant increase in cardiac output.
   d. significantly increased right atrial and wedge pressures with no change in cardiac output.

Please refer to the clinical vignettes to answer questions 10 through 20.

An 80-year-old female was admitted after a syncopal episode following two previous episodes of dizziness and "nearly passing out." A prior admission 2 months ago was to evaluate possible episodes of cardiac dysrhythmias, which at that time were diagnosed from Holter monitoring to be asymptomatic ventricular tachycardia and supraventricular tachycardia. She was stabilized, treated with Quinidine and digoxin, and discharged.

History: Two weeks of diarrhea and 4 days of intermittent nausea, which prompted her to stop taking her prescribed Quinidine

Lab: Digoxin level is pending; electrolytes were normal except for $K^+ = 3.8$

ECG: Sinus bradycardia with a complete right bundle branch block and a left anterior hemiblock

Physical assessment: Unremarkable

VS: T = 98.6°F(o); P = 50 bpm; R = 18/min; BP = 104/50

10. The most likely cause of the syncope is (III):
    a. sinus pauses.
    b. complete heart block.
    c. ventricular tachycardia.
    d. transient ischemic attacks.

11. The most important factor to include in a teaching plan for this patient is (II):
    a. checking pulse rate prior to taking medications.
    b. need to maintain dietary balance of potassium.
    c. The danger of orthostatic changes that may resemble the original episode of syncope.
    d. risk of life-threatening dysrythmias if medication is not taken.

12. Signs of digoxin toxicity include all of the following *except* (I):
    a. halos around visual images.
    b. photophobia.
    c. hallucinations.
    d. night blindness.

13. This patient should be closely monitored for complete heart block because (III):
    a. her heart rate is very low.
    b. the recent events may have caused a myocardial infarction.
    c. it is still unknown if the patient is digoxin-toxic.
    d. cause of the syncope is still unconfirmed.

The patient then developed short episodes of ventricular tachycardia with return to sinus bradycardia. One occurrence of R on T phenomenon was evidenced, followed by coarse ventricular fibrillation. After defibrillation, a junctional rhythm of 40 bpm was apparent on the ECG. Because of poor perfusion, atropine 0.5 mg was administered twice, with no increase in heart rate.

14. What is the mechanism by which R on T phenomenon causes ventricular tachycardia? (I):
    a. The irritable focus overrides the heart's depolarization potential.
    b. A new stimulus to the heart during the relative refractory period can lead to aberrant conduction.
    c. A new stimulus to the heart during the absolute refractory period can lead to aberrant conduction.

d. An irritable stimulus from the ventricle can override the normal conduction pathways.

15. The mechanism by which atropine works to increase heart rate is (I):
    a. sympathetic nervous system stimulation.
    b. interruption of impulses from the vagus nerve.
    c. parasympathetic nervous system stimulation.
    d. direct stimulation of the heart to increase intrinsic rate.

16. Nursing preparation for initial defibrillation includes all of the following *except* (I):
    a. confirmation of ventricular fibrillation by ECG.
    b. clearing bed of conduction pathways to health care providers.
    c. use of saline or conduction gel to diffuse current and reduce electrical burns.
    d. defibrillator voltage set at 360 mV in preparation for defibrillation.

17. If defibrillation for ventricular fibrillation is unsuccessful after 3 attempts, which of the following drugs would most likely be administered? (II)
    a. sodium bicarbonate
    b. xylocaine
    c. epinephrine
    d. calcium

At a heart rate of 40 bpm, the patient's BP and level of consciousness began to decrease. A temporary transvenous pacemaker was inserted, after which the patient's BP returned to 104/58, and she once again became alert and oriented. Her ECG showed 100% paced rhythm at 75 bpm.

18. The type of pacemaker that was inserted was (II):
    a. an atrial pacemaker.
    b. an A-V sequential pacemaker.
    c. a ventricular demand pacemaker.
    d. an automatic implantable cardioverter-defibrillator.

19. Signs that the pacemaker is no longer properly placed include all of the following *except* (II):
    a. runs of ventricular tachycardia within the paced rhythm.
    b. pacemaker spikes not coinciding with QRS complexes at a heart rate of 90 bpm.
    c. a visible heart rate of 50 bpm.
    d. 2-second pauses between complexes with occasional ventricular escape beats.

20. Nursing interventions for the patient with a temporary pacemaker would not necessarily include (II):
    a. restraints as ordered in the case of confusion accompanied by agitation.
    b. avoiding vigorous movements to decrease the risk of dislodgement.
    c. sterile dressing changes with the use of gloves, as with central lines.
    d. stabilization of the pacemaker box on the patient's chest to reduce risk of altering the catheter position.

21. The most likely psychosocial response of a patient suffering an acute myocardial infarction is (II):
    a. anger.
    b. denial.
    c. depression.
    d. fear.

Please refer to the following clinical vignette to answer questions 22 and 23.

M. B. is a 17-year-old white male who is admitted to the Intensive Care Unit after being thrown from the passenger side of a car during a collision with another car at a stoplight. He has bilateral femur fractures and a right flank bruise. He is awake, moaning in pain, and guarding his abdomen.

22. The most common method of immediately assessing these injuries is (II):
    a. paracentesis with lavage.
    b. serum amylase level.
    c. exploratory laparotomy.
    d. continued observation in the Intensive Care Unit.

23. A poor prognostic factor in this patient may be the presence of which of the following? (III)
    a. concomitant fractures
    b. flank bruising
    c. erratic glucose and electrolytes
    d. guarding of the abdomen

Please refer to the following clinical vignette to answer questions 24 through 26.

L. L. is a 78-year-old woman admitted from a nursing home with a diagnosis of "altered level of consciousness and hypotension." She has been chronically debilitated with arthritis and has required complete care for two years. Two years ago, L. L. had a right hemispheric stroke, which left her with residual left-sided weakness, incontinence, and erratic behavior. Until the last few days, L. L. was transferred to the wheelchair for several hours daily and used adult diapers. L. L. had an in-dwelling catheter placed at the nursing home approximately 7 days ago. Upon admission to this institution 3 days ago, she

had a fever of 103°F and was started on broad-spectrum antibiotics. Last night L. L. maintained a temperature of 101°F for 4 hours, and her antibiotics were changed. This morning a fluid challenge of 500 cc NS was given for a blood pressure of 80/50. During the fluid challenge, she was transferred to your unit, and her blood pressure is now 90/50. Upon initial assessment, you note occult blood in the urine and scattered petichiae across the trunk. After drawing blood, you notice some difficulty achieving hemostasis.

24. The most likely etiology of L. L.'s bleeding is (III):
    a. thrombocytopenia.
    b. antibiotic-induced coagulopathy.
    c. poor platelet quality.
    d. consumptive coagulopathy.

25. If the patient continues to bleed after replacement of RBCs, FFP, and platelets, which of the following is likely to be done? (II)
    a. recheck for DIC
    b. administer cryoprecipitate
    c. warm all blood products to enhance effectiveness and reduce bleeding
    d. test the patient for hemolytic anemia

26. The most common transfusion reaction is (I):
    a. hemolytic.
    b. anaphylactic.
    c. febrile.
    d. volume overload.

27. Complications of massive transfusions may include (II):
    a. hyperkalemia, alkalosis.
    b. hypothermia, increased 2,3-DPG.
    c. hypermagnesemia, circulatory overload.
    d. hypocalcemia, ammonia intoxication.

28. A patient in the intensive care unit is found to suffer high blood pressure and elevated blood levels of aldosterone. Which of the following is considered an antecedent to this condition? (II)
    a. partial occlusion of renal arteries
    b. an increase in sympathetic stimulation caused by anxiety
    c. depressed renin release
    d. a cerebral tumor

29. Laboratory findings indicative of SIADH include (II):
    a. increased urinary specific gravity, decreased urinary sodium.
    b. increased urinary sodium, increased urine osmolality.
    c. increased HCT, decreased serum osmolality.

d. normal urine specific gravity, decreased HCT.

30. A patient in the intensive care unit has the following hemodynamic values: cardiac index = 2.2, wedge pressure = 24, and systemic vascular resistance = 2400. Which of the following should be administered? (III)
    a. nitroglycerin
    b. Apresoline
    c. Nipride
    d. digitalis

31. In the event of a myocardial infarction from coronary heart disease, which of the following statements about treatment objectives is true? (II)
    a. Positive inotropic agents should be given to help maintain sufficient cardiac output.
    b. The primary goal should be to attain a balance between myocardial oxygen consumption and oxygen supply.
    c. It is advantageous to increase the viscosity of the blood.
    d. Prothrombin and vitamin K should be administered to promote coagulation, thus preventing unexpected blood loss.

32. Pain with injection of epidural medications is most likely caused by (II):
    a. a misplaced catheter.
    b. an infected catheter.
    c. the effect of the medication entering the epidural space.
    d. too rapid injection of medication.

33. A patient presents with severe headache, convulsions, transitory focal neurologic compromises, a sudden rise in blood pressure, and nausea and vomiting. The probable cause is (II):
    a. hypertensive encephalopathy.
    b. thyroid storm.
    c. acute renal insufficiency.
    d. carotid occlusion.

34. The most appropriate management strategy for pain in a patient with pancreatitis is (II):
    a. high fat diet.
    b. morphine.
    c. epidural analgesia.
    d. Demerol.

35. Hypercalcemia can cause (I):
    a. hypotension.
    b. cardiac arhythmias.
    c. hemorrhage.
    d. seizures.

Please refer to the following clinical vignette to answer questions 36 through 39.

A 19-year-old male suffered multiple injuries in a motor vehicle accident and was admitted unconscious, with responses only to deep pain and the following baseline.

V.S.: Temperature: 99.8 axillary; BP: 90/50; pulse: 56, regular; resp.: 24, regular

HEENT: Pupils: 5 mm, bilaterally reacting sluggishly to light; no drainage from ears or nose; 5-cm laceration across right parietal region with moderate bleeding

Chest: Normal heart sounds; ECG: sinus brady without ectopy; normal chest excursions with shallow respiratory effort; normal breath sounds without respiratory distress

Abdomen: Vomited undigested food; bowel sounds hypoactive in all four quadrants; no abdominal distention or tenderness

GU: Incontinent of moderate amount of clear yellow urine

Extremities: Upper extremities with intact reflexes, lower are without

X-ray: Fractured C7

CBC: Hct: 40; Hgb: 13

36. In the face of this cord injury, the most functional, yet realistic, rehabilitative goal for the patient is (III):
    a. writing.
    b. feeding himself.
    c. walking.
    d. learning communication techniques with his tongue.

37. The patient's incontinence is most likely due to the (II):
    a. unconscious state.
    b. inability to communicate the need to void.
    c. loss of sphincter control.
    d. forced fluids while still out in the field.

38. The spinal cord injured patient who cannot grasp but can flex and extend the arms is most likely suffering a lesion at approximately the level of (I):
    a. C3 or C4.
    b. C7 or C8.
    c. T4 or T5.
    d. L1 or L2.

39. In the ER, the patient displayed symptoms of all of the following complications of spinal trauma *except* (III):
    a. autonomic dysreflexia.
    b. increased intracranial pressure.
    c. neurogenic shock.
    d. respiratory compromise.

40. The most frequent manifestations of autonomic dysreflexia are alterations in (I):

a. temperature.
b. blood pressure and heart rate.
c. level of consciousness.
d. cranial nerve function.

41. A spinal cord disorder typified by motor losses that are more pronounced in the upper than the lower extremities is the (I):
a. central cord syndrome.
b. Brown-Sequard syndrome.
c. anterior cord syndrome.
d. Guillain-Barre syndrome.

42. Signs and symptoms of spinal shock include (I):
a. subnormal temperature.
b. narrow pulse pressure.
c. bradycardia.
d. fixed and small pupils.

43. A sign that spinal shock is subsiding in the patient with acute spinal cord injury is (II):
a. flaccid paralysis.
b. response to plantar stimulation.
c. lack of sacral nerve reflex.
d. decreased deep tendon reflex.

Please refer to the following clinical vignette to answer questions 44 through 46.

A 24-year-old female with a 10-year history of insulin-dependent diabetes was brought to the emergency room after becoming increasingly unarousable. The family reported a recent history of an upper respiratory infection, frequent urination, and nausea. Clinical signs include Kussmaul respirations; fruity breath; warm, dry skin with poor turgor; BP 80/50; and P 120/min. Laboratory findings are as follows:

Glucose: 750 mg%

K: 6.0

Na: 150

Positive urine ketostix

ABG: pH 7.2
pCO$_2$ 20
paO$_2$ 96
O$_2$ sat 97%
HCO$_3$ 12.2

44. The primary cause of this patient's neurological disorder is (III):
a. hyperglycemia.
b. hyperosmolarity.
c. ketosis.
d. acidosis.

45. The patient is exhibiting what medical complication of diabetes mellitus? (III)
a. acute hypoglycemic crisis
b. secretion of inappropriate antidiuretic hormone

c. diabetic ketoacidosis
d. hyperosmolar hyperglycemic nonketotic coma

46. Which of the following sequences indicates the appropriate priority of treatment within the first 2 hours of therapy? (III)
a. rapid correction of acidosis, continuous IV of regular insulin, intake equals output infusions with 0.45% normal saline, bicarbonate added.
b. rapid correction of acidosis, intermittent IV injections of regular insulin, minimal IV fluids until urinary output slows
c. rapid rehydration with normal saline, continuous IV of regular insulin, gradual correction of acidosis
d. intravenous insulin infusion, correction of acidosis, rehydration with ½ NS

47. Risk of a hypertensive crisis is high in all of the following *except* (II):
a. renal vascular disease.
b. hyperosmolar coma.
c. polycythemia.
d. adrenocortical disease.

48. Hyperkalemia can cause the following ECG changes (I):
a. peaked and elevated T wave, ST depression, widened QRS, and prolonged PR.
b. inverted and prolonged T wave, widened QRS, and shortened PR.
c. peaked and elevated T wave, ST depression, shortened QRS, and shortened PR.
d. peaked and elevated T wave, ST elevation, widened QRS, and shortened PR.

49. Increasing the heart rate by using an artificial pacemaker (I):
a. shortens filling time more than does sympathetic stimulation.
b. increases strength of contraction.
c. causes cardiac output to increase as the rate rises between 30 and 40 bpm.
d. mimics sympathetic stimulation.

50. The major complication of status epilepticus is (I):
a. alkalosis.
b. hyperglycemia.
c. respiratory distress.
d. hypothermia.

51. Circulatory effects of stimulation of alpha and beta receptors are (I):
a. alpha receptors sense changes in blood

pressure, beta receptors can sense heart rate changes.
b. alpha receptors are only excited by norepinephrine, beta receptors only by epinephrine.
c. alpha receptors influence only vascular smooth muscle, beta receptors can directly influence the heart.
d. alpha receptors may excite the heart, beta receptors affect only vessels.

52. The presence of gurgles (rhonchi) upon auscultation may indicate any of the following *except* (II):
a. lung consolidation.
b. emphysema.
c. atelectasis.
d. bronchitis.

53. Critical care problems or medications known to cause SIADH include (II):
a. diabetic ketoacidosis.
b. nitroprusside.
c. positive pressure ventilation.
d. Parkinson's disease.

54. Cardiac output is determined by (I):
a. stroke volume and contractility.
b. stroke volume and heart rate.
c. afterload and stroke volume.
d. heart rate and contractility.

55. The action potential for a pacemaker cell in the heart can be altered by (II):
a. an increase in core temperature, which slows the rate.
b. an increase in afterload, which speeds the rate.
c. norepinephrine, which increases Na^+ influx.
d. acetylcholine, which increases K^+ influx.

56. In teaching an acute MI patient about cardiovascular disorders and risk factors, the nurse should place special emphasis on (II):
a. stress factors and their control.
b. low cholesterol and sodium diets.
c. family history.
d. control of hypertension.

57. The primary objective for the care of a patient suffering an acute myocardial infarction is to provide care in such a manner as to (II):
a. alleviate discomfort.
b. reduce risk of further myocardial damage.
c. prevent heart failure from developing.
d. prevent dysrhythmias from occurring.

58. In carbon monoxide poisoning, which inhibits cellular respiration, the gas binds with which of the following? (I)

a. lymphocytes
b. iron-containing proteins
c. IgG
d. phagocytes

59. Important criteria for ensuring that the aritificial kidney functions properly during renal replacement therapy include all of the following *except* (II):
a. the same size arterial and venous access devices should be used.
b. intravenous pumps should be used to ensure consistent fluid circulation and removal of ultrafiltrate.
c. heparinization of removed arterial blood prevents filter occlusion.
d. filters should be changed every day to prevent infection.

60. Nursing care for the ventilator patient should include all of the following *except* (II):
a. hyperinflation and hyperventilation prior to suctioning.
b. providing alternate means of communication.
c. checking ETT cuff pressures every 4 hours; maintaining less that 15 mm Hg.
d. maintaining alarms at 10–15 millimeters above patient settings.

61. Depolarization through the heart (I):
a. is slowest through the Purkinje system.
b. travels slowest through the AV node.
c. is faster with vagal stimulation.
d. follows a specialized conduction pathway in the atria.

62. If a patient suffers a 30% loss in blood volume, cardiovascular compensatory mechanisms will cause (II):
a. an increase in capillary fluid filtration.
b. a decrease in vasomotor tone.
c. an increase in heart rate and contractility.
d. an increase in skin blood flow.

63. Alpha receptors in the circulatory system (I):
a. are primarily sensitive to vessel wall distension.
b. produce cardiac vasodilation with sympathetic nerve stimulation.
c. can cause a rise in cardiac contractility.
d. produce peripheral vasoconstriction with sympathetic nerve stimulation.

64. An ectopic pacemaker (I):
a. has the same effect as a preventricular contraction.
b. can be life-threatening.
c. serves as an indication of pathological damage to the SA node.

d. is rarely of concern to the physician.

65. Dialysis disequilibrium syndrome is (I):
    a. hypotension related to the large volume of blood required to prime the artificial kidney.
    b. hemoconcentration of solutes due to excessive fluid removal during hemodialysis.
    c. rebound hypokalemia and hypernatremia that occurs after the removal of the artificial kidney.
    d. cerebral edema resulting from intracellular fluid shifts and serum abnormalities that occur as serum solutes are removed.

66. Oliguria is a 24-hour urine output of (I):
    a. nothing.
    b. less than 400 mL.
    c. 400–700 mL.
    d. less than 70 mL.

67. Altered mental status in a patient with known HIV infection may represent any of the following *except* (II):
    a. primary brain lymphoma.
    b. neurologic HIV (AIDS dementia).
    c. cryptosporidium.
    d. toxoplasma infection.

68. Early signs of oxygen toxicity may include (II):
    a. decreased compliance, paresthesia in extremities.
    b. cyanosis, retrosternal distress.
    c. sense of impending doom, agitation.
    d. restlessness, lethargy, cough.

Please refer to the following clinical vignette to answer questions 69 and 70.

M. S. is a 40-year-old female brought to the ED after hitting the dashboard of the passenger side of a car during a motor vehicle accident. She incurred a blunt trauma to the abdomen and is suspected of having a ruptured spleen and/or lacerated liver. Upon admission she is awake and moaning with severe abdominal and flank pain, with radiation to the upper back and shoulder. She soon complains of nausea as well. A chest x-ray shows fractures of the right 10th and 11th ribs, but no pneumothorax. A Foley catheter is inserted with bloody urine returns. Her abdomen is tender; she has flank tenderness and a palpable mass in the laparotomy area. Her blood pressure is 80/60. A mini-laparotomy is performed with bloody returns, and she goes to the operating room for exploratory surgery.

69. Renal trauma is most common when (II):
    a. the trauma is a penetrating wound.
    b. an acceleration-deceleration injury has occurred.

c. injuries are incurred to the pelvic area.
d. blunt abdominal trauma has occurred.

70. The most definitive diagnostic tool for evaluating a patient with potential renal injury is (I):
    a. urinalysis.
    b. mini-laparotomy.
    c. abdominal CT scan.
    d. intravenous pyelogram.

71. Red blood cells are ordinarily produced (I):
    a. nearly exclusively in the liver of elderly people.
    b. nearly exclusively in bone.
    c. primarily in the liver, spleen, and lymph nodes until puberty.
    d. primarily in the liver and spleen.

72. A patient's red blood cell count can be increased by (I):
    a. a chronic elevated level of lactic acid in muscle.
    b. a rise in renal erythropoietic factors.
    c. an increase in absorbed iron.
    d. a decrease in renal erythropoietic factors.

73. Risk of which of the following is highest after mitral valve replacement? (II)
    a. hypovolemic shock
    b. pulmonary edema
    c. cardiac tamponade
    d. cardiogenic shock

74. The hormone gastrin is secreted (I):
    a. in response to protein ingestion.
    b. by the pancreas.
    c. by the stomach's cardiac area.
    d. when the body is under physical stress.

75. The signs or symptoms most likely to indicate the progression of sepsis into irreversible shock are (II):
    a. low diastolic BP and confusion.
    b. mottling of extremities and lactic acid of 5.0.
    c. hypoxemia and weak and thready pulses.
    d. hyperkalemia and oliguria.

76. G. I., aged 50 years, was admitted after an episode of hematemesis. She has a previous history of a peptic ulcer (15 years ago) that was resolved with medical management. Prior to admission today, she was performing household chores when suddenly overcome with dizziness and profuse sweating accompanied by abdominal cramps. She claimed she had a large loose black stool and vomited coffee ground material. Upon arrival at the Emergency Department, the

patient fainted. Her lying blood pressure was 90/60, and her heart rate was 139/minute without ectopy. The priorities for this patient's care are (III):
a. transfuse blood, gastric lavage, IV fluids.
b. IV fluids, gastric lavage, transfuse blood.
c. gastric lavage, antacids, transfuse blood.
d. gastric lavage, transfuse blood, histamine blocker administration.

77. Which of the following serves as a major predictor of survival after myocardial infarction? (II)
a. left ventricular function
b. amount and degree of chest pain experienced
c. amount of ST elevation
d. incidence of arrhythmias

78. Conditions that might cause prerenal failure include (I):
a. high doses of nephrotoxins.
b. beta-hemolytic streptococcus infections.
c. nephron degeneration.
d. decreased cardiac output.

Please refer to the following clinical vignette to answer questions 79 and 80.

A post-MI patient exhibits a new episode of severe chest pain, bilateral crackles (rales) accompanied by severe shortness of breath and a respiratory rate of 36 bpm, and severe JVD. His pulse rate increased to 120 bpm, and his BP dropped to 70/54. His hemodynamic status mirrored his symptoms: right atrial pressure = 6 mm Hg; right ventricular pressure = 70/2 mm Hg; pulmonary artery pressure = 70/40 mm Hg; and pulmonary capillary wedge = 40 mm Hg.

79. The patient has probably developed (III):
a. cardiogenic shock.
b. hypervolemia.
c. cardiac tamponade.
d. pulmonary edema related to COPD.

80. Dopamine and nitroprusside are administered to the patient to (II):
a. increase BP and increase afterload.
b. maintain BP while improving cardiac contractibility.
c. increase both heart rate and preload.
d. improve coronary artery perfusion and increase systemic vascular resistance.

81. One etiology of vasodilation in sepsis is (II):
a. Thromboxane.
b. histamine.
c. sympathetic hormone-induced increased vascular tone.
d. gram-positive endotoxins.

82. The most common location for a stress ulcer is the (I):
a. stomach.
b. fundus.
c. pylorus.
d. duodenum.

83. In peritoneal dialysis, inadequately warmed dialysate could cause the patient to experience (II):
a. abdominal cramping, sweating, vasoconstriction.
b. sweating, decreased creatinine clearance rates.
c. chills, sweating, decreased clearance rates.
d. increased clearance rates, sweating.

84. In the event of an acute anterolateral myocardial infarction, which of the following coronary arteries will most likely be affected? (I)
a. the right coronary artery
b. the left anterior descending and circumflex arteries
c. the circumflex artery
d. the left anterior descending artery

85. Prolongation of the QT segment can be a side effect of which of the following drugs? (I)
a. Inderal
b. Dilantin
c. Quinidine
d. Lidocaine

86. The classic triad of symptoms for opioid intoxication include (I):
a. coma, pinpoint pupils, and seizures.
b. pinpoint pupils, agitation, and seizures.
c. coma, pinpoint pupils, and respiratory depression.
d. respiratory depression, seizures, and pinpoint pupils.

87. Evidence of hypomagnesemia in a patient with chronic renal failure may include (II):
a. irritability, premature ventricular contractions.
b. sedated appearance, hyporeflexia.
c. hyperactive bowel sounds, nausea, vomiting, diarrhea.
d. edema, hypertension.

88. All of the following may lead to hypophosphatemia in a burn patient *except* (II):
a. antacids.
b. metabolic acidosis.
c. respiratory alkalosis.
d. renal failure.

89. One of the most significant effects of hypoxia on the respiratory system is (I):
    a. vasodilation.
    b. vasoconstriction.
    c. bronchoconstriction.
    d. bronchodilation.

90. A shift of the oxyhemoglobin dissociation curve to the left is caused by (I):
    a. hyperthermia.
    b. acidosis.
    c. a decrease in alveolar oxygen tension.
    d. alkalosis.

91. Dimensions of pain experienced can include all of the following *except* (I):
    a. behavioral.
    b. ethnic.
    c. emotional.
    d. sociocultural.

92. Routes by which poisons may enter the body include all of the following *except* (I):
    a. inhalation.
    b. skin.
    c. ingestion.
    d. conduction.

Please refer to the following clinical vignette to answer questions 93 through 98.

A 66-year-old alert and oriented male was admitted in moderate respiratory distress for COPD exacerbation, which started with an upper respiratory tract infection a week ago. In the past week, the patient progressively became more dyspneic and unable to cough productively of sputum. V.S.: T = 100.4(o); P = 118/min; R = 38/min, accompanied by nasal flaring and use of accessory muscles; BP = 138/94. Physical assessment revealed the following:

  mild equilateral muscle weakness

  barrel chested, with even excursion upon respiration

  coarse gurgles (rhonchi) throughout both lung fields; greatly diminished breath sounds in the right middle lobe, posteriorly

  JVD 6 cm above clavicle while in semi-Fowler's position

  Bounding PMI; holosystolic ejection murmur at apex

  palpable and bounding pulses; slightly decreased pedal pulses

  clubbed fingers with cyanotic nailbeds

  cyanotic lips; mottled chest and extremities

93. The presenting respiratory distress is most likely a result of (III):
    a. asthma.

    b. emphysema.
    c. bronchitis.
    d. pneumonia.

94. The patient's arterial blood gas values would most likely be which of the following? (III)
    a. pH = 7.34; pCO_2 = 58; pO_2 = 60; HCO_3 = 26; O_2 sat. = 99%
    b. pH = 7.31; pCO_2 = 42; pO_2 = 68; HCO_3 = 20; O_2 sat. = 98%
    c. pH = 7.44; pCO_2 = 32; pO_2 = 62; HCO_3 = 24; O_2 sat. = 100%
    d. pH = 7.43; pCO_2 = 49; pO_2 = 58; HCO_3 = 28; O_2 sat. = 86%

95. Therapeutic interventions for the patient would probably include (II):
    a. humidified oxygen, restricted fluids.
    b. intermittent positive pressure breathing (IPPB), sedation.
    c. chest physiotherapy, cholinergic agents, steroids.
    d. bronchodilators, nasopharyngeal airway for suctioning.

96. If the patient were to develop pulmonary hypertension, all of the following signs would be exhibited *except* (II):
    a. JVD.
    b. bounding pulses.
    c. cyanosis.
    d. systolic murmur.

97. Nursing interventions to prevent long-term complications should include (III):
    a. skin care for the immobilized
    b. aggressive pulmonary hygiene, periodic sputum culture to monitor for infection.
    c. fluid restriction, diversional and recreational therapy.
    d. sedation for adequate rest at night.

98. The patient worsens, developing severe gurgles (rhonchi) and bibasilar crackles (rales), increased respiratory distress and labored breathing, tachycardia, and ABG values of pH = 7.30; pCO_2 = 50; pO_2 = 58; HCO_3 = 26; O_2 sat. = 96%. Which of the following actions would be most appropriate in the care of the patient? (III)
    a. changing antibiotics and assessing improvements in respiratory status
    b. intubation and mechanical ventilation
    c. administration of bronchodilators and diuretics and IPPB treatments
    d. administration of oxygen at 100% via face mask

99. Signs of tension pneumothorax include (II):
    a. absent breath sounds, tracheal displacement to affected side.

b. acute hypoxemia, tracheal displacement to unaffected side.
c. hyperresonance on affected side and decreased PCWP.
d. increased RAP, PAP, PAD, and PCWP.

100. Emergency interventions for the care of a patient suffering tension pneumothorax include (II):

a. inserting a large-bore needle into the second anterior interspace on the affected side.
b. inserting a large-bore needle into the second anterior interspace on the unaffected side.
c. adding/increasing PEEP on ventilator.
d. mechanically "ambuing" the patient until surgery can be performed.

2 The Respiratory System

CHAPTER 2 PRE-TEST

1. All of the following clinical signs are associated with adult respiratory distress syndrome *except*:
   a. bilateral crackles (rales):
   b. falling pO_2 with increasing FIO_2.
   c. PCWP greater than 25 mm Hg.
   d. x-ray evidence of pulmonary congestion.

2. The severity of an oxygenation defect is determined by the magnitude of the:
   a. oxygen diffusability.
   b. alveolar-capillary membrane diffusability.
   c. intrapulmonary shunt volume.
   d. oxygen deficit.

3. The patient suffering adult respiratory distress syndrome may manifest complications of:
   a. cardiac arrhythmias.
   b. acid-base disturbances.
   c. infection.
   d. all of the above.

4. All of the following are optimal treatments for adult respiratory distress syndrome *except*:
   a. high tidal volumes.
   b. high FIO_2.
   c. fluid restrictions.
   d. PEEP.

5. PEEP aids in restoring acceptable pO_2 levels by:
   a. increasing FRC.
   b. decreasing shunting.
   c. opening small airways and alveoli.
   d. all of the above.

6. The most common dysrhythmia seen in association with pulmonary emboli is:
   a. multifocal atrial tachycardia.
   b. paroxysmal atrial tachycardia.
   c. sinus tachycardia.
   d. atrial fibrillation.

7. The most reliable diagnostic tool for pulmonary emboli is:
   a. the physical examination.
   b. the chest x-ray.
   c. the lung scan.
   d. the pulmonary angiogram.

8. A pulmonary embolus is in which of the following respiratory disease classes?
   a. obstructive
   b. restrictive
   c. hypoxic
   d. ataxic

9. All of the following are signs that an endotracheal tube may be improperly placed or occluded *except*:
   a. difficulty experienced by the nurse when attempting to introduce a suction catheter.
   b. the presence of a localized inspiratory wheeze.
   c. the presence of a localized expiratory wheeze.
   d. excessive coughing.

10. The best way to position a patient for auscultating the respiratory system is:
    a. erect in bed with legs dangling over the side.
    b. leaning over the bedside table.
    c. prone, flat in bed.
    d. in the semi-Fowler's position, propped up with pillows.

11. An intravenous infusion of $NaHCO_3$ produces a transient increase in blood pCO_2. During this transient phase:
    a. blood pH decreases.
    b. CSF pH increases.
    c. breathing decreases.
    d. breathing increases.

12. The amount of oxygen and carbon dioxide in the blood would rise and fall markedly with each respiration if it were not for the:
    a. inspiratory reserve volume.
    b. functional residual volume.
    c. expiratory reserve volume.
    d. tracheal dead space.

13. Intrathoracic pressure is normally:
    a. positive throughout the respiratory cycle.
    b. highest (least negative) at the end of inspiration.
    c. positive when expiratory efforts are made with a closed/obstructed glottis.
    d. positive, which aids in right heart filling.

14. A lung lacking in surfactant would be unstable, and as a result:
    a. the large alveoli would collapse and overinflate the small alveoli.
    b. the small alveoli would tend to collapse.
    c. a pressure gradient would build up between large and small alveoli.
    d. surface tension would decrease uniformly throughout the lung.

15. Inelasticity of lung tissue leads to:
    a. increased risk of air trapping.
    b. collapsing of airways during expiration.
    c. expiration becoming active rather than passive.
    d. all of the above.

16. A spirometer can provide accurate measures of all of the following *except*:
    a. tidal volume.
    b. functional residual capacity.
    c. vital capacity.
    d. inspiratory reserve volume.

17. In the event of a spontaneous pneumothorax, a nurse would expect to see:
    a. a decrease in intrathoracic pressure on the affected side.
    b. a decrease in pulmonary blood flow on the affected side.
    c. a decrease in pulmonary blood flow on the intact side.
    d. an increase in intrathoracic pressure on the intact side.

18. Work of breathing in the adult is normally minimal:
    a. at the slowest rate that can be maintained by the patient.
    b. at a respiratory rate of 14 to 16.
    c. at a respiratory rate of 20 to 28.
    d. when functional residual volume is decreased.

19. The oxyhemoglobin dissociation curve is displaced to the left by:
    a. a decrease in hemoglobin concentration.
    b. an increase in temperature.
    c. an increase in blood pH.
    d. all of the above.

20. The PaO_2 of a patient is 70 mm Hg. You would expect that the corresponding oxygen saturation would be approximately:
    a. 70%.
    b. 40%.
    c. 90%.
    d. 100%.

21. A patient suffering obstructive lung disease might be expected to exhibit:
    a. a reduced FEV_1 (1-second forced expiratory volume).
    b. an elevated total lung volume.
    c. a slightly low arterial pH.
    d. all of the above.

22. If a patient is placed on 100% oxygen after being on room air and experiences no change of respiratory rate or tidal volume, the patient's alveolar CO_2 tension can be expected to:
    a. remain unchanged.
    b. decrease significantly.
    c. first decrease, then increase.
    d. first increase, then decrease.

Overview of the Respiratory System

The respiratory system is composed of the lungs, the conducting air passages, the central control system for the muscles of ventilation, which are attached to the thoracic cage, and the alveoli. Figure 2-1 depicts the components of the respiratory system.

The main function of the respiratory system is to allow for the interchange of gases between the atmosphere and the bloodstream. Oxygen is transported into the lungs during inspiration and carbon dioxide is expelled during exhalation (see Figure 2-2). Functions of the respiratory system include promoting the gas exchange necessary for survival, maintaining acid-base balance, and contributing to phonation, pulmonary defense, and metabolism. The primary function of the respiratory apparatus is, however, the bulk movement of gases into and out of the lung system. To generate the mechanical energy necessary for bulk gas movement into and out of the lungs and circulation between the lungs and the rest of the body, active work takes place in a subtle and harmonious interplay between the respiratory muscles and the heart.

Anatomy of the Respiratory System

An appreciation of pulmonary anatomy is germane to the study of clinical medicine and the practice of competent professional nursing. A knowledge of this anatomy is essential to diagnosis, airway management and maintenance, and the rational and safe performance of respiratory care procedures for the patient's benefit and safety.

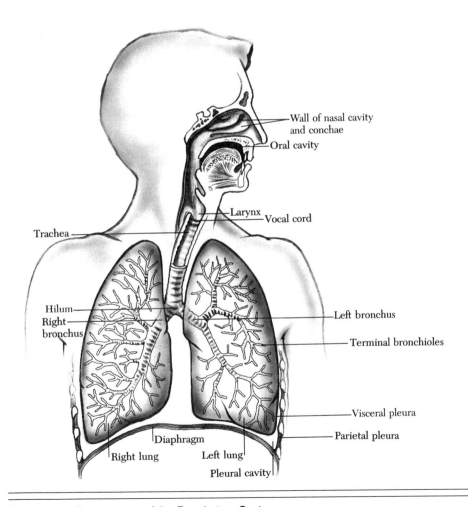

Figure 2-1 Components of the Respiratory System

The Upper Airway

Air normally enters the respiratory system through the mouth or nose. This entrance is considered the beginning of the upper airway, whose boundaries are from the anterior nares to the true vocal cord (Figure 2-2).

The Nose

Functions of the nose are (1) filtration of inspired gases, (2) olfaction (the work of smelling), (3) humidification of inspired gases to a relative humidity of approximately 100% at body temperature, (4) heating of inspired gases to body temperature (37°C), (5) assisting in the production of sound in phonation, and (6) acting as a beginning conduction passageway for ventilation.

Structurally, the nose consists of both internal and external components. The external portion, located on the face, is a rigid structure composed of bone and cartilage, which prevent its collapse during a rapid and forceful inspiratory effort. The two external openings are called nostrils, external nares, or anterior nares. Their lateral margins are called alae. Inside the nares (commonly referred to as the vestibule of the nose) are coarse nasal hair projections (vibrissae) that project anteriorly and inferiorly. These help protect the pulmonary system by filtering dust and other large (aerosolized) particles (5 μ and larger). The nasal hairs are the first line of defense for the upper airway. Also located within this vestibular region are sebaceous glands that secrete sebum, a greasy material that keeps the nasal hair soft and pliable.

The interior portion of the nose is a hollow cavity that is separated into right and left portions by a perpendicular structure composed of the nasal septal cartilage and the ethmoid and vomer bones. Each side of the nose is constructed of a floor, a roof, and lateral walls, which form a structural framework; attached to the lateral walls are three bony projections referred to as conchae or turbinates. The three turbinates (superior, middle, and inferior) overhang and comprise three corresponding passageways through each nasal cavity, known as the superior, middle, and inferior meati, respectively.

The nasal sinuses are hollow cavities, filled with air, in the bones of the cranium. Their function is to give the voice resonance through prolongation and intensification of the manufactured sound. The four pairs of sinuses are located in the forehead and are designated the frontal, the maxillary, the sphenoidal, and the ethmoidal. All of these sinuses may be involved in allergic or respiratory infections, and fluids collecting in them drain through openings into the upper nasal passages. The frontal sinuses drain into the anterior portion of the middle meati; the maxillary sinuses, the largest of all the air sinuses, drain into the middle meati; the sphenoidal sinuses drain into the superior meati; and the ethmoidal sinuses drain into the superior and middle meati. When any of the sinuses fail to drain properly, pressure builds, causing headaches and pain in the region of the sinus.

The turbinates increase the surface area of the nasal structure because of their design and the overfolded mucous membrane covering them. The nose

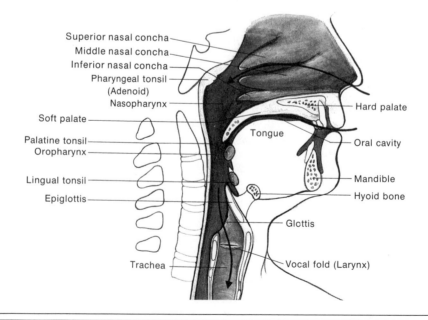

Figure 2-2 Movement of Gases During Inspiration and Expiration

has an approximate volume of 20 cc and a surface area of approximately 150 cm^2. The mucosal lining of the respiratory region of the nose is covered by pseudostratified ciliated columnar epithelium and by squamous nonciliated mucous cells with serous and mucosal glands. The mucosal tissue is heavily perfused by blood vessels very close to the surface. The combination of the shallowly placed capillary mucosal structure and the anatomical structuring of the turbinates makes the nose an excellent heat and moisture exchanger (humidifier). Another significant characteristic of the nose is that resistance to airflow through the nose is approximately two to three times the total resistance to airflow through the mouth. It is for this reason that the individual experiencing dyspnea will breathe through the mouth as well as the nose.

When air is inspired through the nose, a turbulent gas flow is created. This turbulent flow enhances the probability that each gas molecule will come into contact with the surface area of the vascular mucosal membrane that heats inspired gases to body temperature (37°C or 98.6°F). The mucosal membrane also ensures that the relative humidity of the inspired gas reaches about 80% before leaving the nose and entering the nasopharynx. The clinical importance of the structural characteristics of the nose cannot be understated. The nose plays a very important role in the process of breathing, and this is especially evident when tubes placed in the nose to assist breathing bypass the natural heating, humidification, and protection functions of the nose.

The olfactory region within each nasal cavity is bordered by the superior concha laterally, by the nasal septal cartilage in the medial region, and by the roof of the nasal cavity above. This region contains specialized cellular epithelia responsible for the sense of smell. Due to the architecture of the nasal cavity, inspired gases drawn to the olfactory region by sniffing are not disseminated much further along the nasal passage; the nasal cavity thus provides a protective mechanism against inspiring potentially dangerous environmental gases.

The nose ends with the outlet of the nasal cavity into the nasopharynx through the internal nares (posterior nares, or choanae).

The Pharynx

The pharynx is a hollow muscular structure that forms the upper portion of the throat, beginning at the opening of the posterior nares (or choanae) and extending inferiorly to the esophagus. The pharynx is about 5 inches long and is lined with a mucous membrane. It serves as a passageway for foods and inspired gases. In the normal and conscious patient,

the gag reflex may be elicited by stimulating the posterior pharyngeal wall. This reflex is mediated by the glossopharyngeal (IX) and vagus (X) nerves.

Generally, for identification purposes the pharynx is subdivided into three parts: the nasopharynx, the oropharynx, and the laryngopharynx.

Nasopharynx The functions of the nasopharynx include (1) the humidification of air, (2) the conduction of air, and (3) the containment of the tonsillar defense mechanism of the body. The nasopharynx is behind the nasal cavity and extends to the tip of the uvula. It is located between the soft palate and the tongue. During swallowing, the uvula and soft palate move posteriorly and superiorly to keep food or liquid from entering the nasopharynx and nasal cavity. The epithelial structure of the nasopharynx is continuous with the epithelial structure of the respiratory region and is composed of pseudostratified ciliated columnar epithelia. The pharynx serves to filter and humidify inspired gases.

The adenoids, or pharyngeal tonsils, are located in the posterior portion of the nose at the beginning of the nasopharynx. The pharyngeal tonsils consist of dense concentrations of lymphoid tissue, which surrounds and guards the entranceway into the respiratory and gastrointestinal tracts. This tissue frequently becomes enlarged, usually along with the tonsils. When this occurs, the individual may become febrile and experience obstructed ventilation. The right and left eustachian tubes also open into the nasopharynx on the lateral walls and communicate with the tympanic cavity, or middle ear. This connection allows for the equalization of pressure on both sides of the eardrum in the presence of environmental pressure differences. Infection or closure of these tubes prevents the equalization of pressure in the middle ear and causes discomfort to the eardrum, the result of which is an earache. Mucosal congestion, excessive sinus drainage, and overgrown adenoidal tissue all impair the function of the normal eustachian tube. Nasal intubation frequently blocks the eustachian tube openings and, if left uncorrected, may lead to otitis media. A lack of humidity in the inspired gases can also cause the eustachian tube to block.

Oropharynx The functions of the oropharynx are fourfold: (1) the movement of gas, (2) the movement of food and fluid, (3) the containment of defense mechanisms of the body, and (4) the humidification of inspired gas. The oropharynx extends from below the nasopharynx to the epiglottis, forming the posterior portion of the mouth. It is located behind the oral, or buccal, cavity and is commonly referred to as

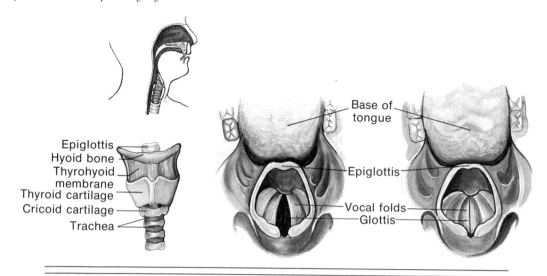

Figure 2-3 The Larynx

the throat. The oropharynx is lined with nonciliated squamous epitheliated mucosa. It is the junction of the respiratory and digestive systems.

The palatine (facial) and lingual tonsils are located in the oropharynx. The palatine tonsils are located laterally to the uvula on the lateral and anterior aspects of the oropharynx. It is the palatine tonsils that are most frequently removed by tonsillectomy. The lingual tonsils are located at the base of the tongue.

The tongue is formed of skeletal muscle covered by mucous membranes and is used for speech, taste, and deglutition (swallowing). The sensory nerve supply to the tongue has multiple sources: the lingual nerve, the chord tympani branch supplying taste fibers, the glossopharyngeal nerve (IX), and the superior laryngeal nerve. The tongue receives its major motor supply from the hypoglossal nerve (XII), which is very superficial at the angle of the mandible and is prone to injury during vigorous mechanical manipulation of the airway.

In the unconscious patient, the oropharyngeal musculature tends to relax. The tongue displaces posteriorly, causing occlusion to the airway. Thus, the tongue is one of the major causes of partial or complete airway obstruction and must be a critical anatomical consideration in airway management.

Laryngopharynx The functions of the laryngopharynx (or hypopharynx) are (1) food and fluid movement and (2) movement of gas. The laryngopharynx is located below the oropharynx, extending from the tip of the epiglottis to the point where it splits into the larynx and esophagus. The larynx lies anteriorly, and the esophagus lies posteriorly. The laryngopharynx contains the arytenoid cartilage (aryepiglottic folds). It is lined with stratified squamous epithelium without cilia. The laryngopharynx also contains the anatomical landmarks for intubation: the epiglottis and the vallecula.

The Larynx

The functions of the larynx are (1) protection of airways from foreign substances, (2) involvement in the production of sound (phonation), and (3) involvement in coughing, with the vocal cords and the epiglottis functioning together to allow for increases in intrathoracic pressures.

Some basic knowledge of the anatomy of the larynx is essential for understanding and using airway management techniques. The larynx, or the voice box, is located below the pharynx and at the most proximal end of the trachea. It is important to understand that the larynx is the connection between the upper and lower airways; it connects the pharynx with the trachea and supplies the structural matrix for the vocal cords and the upper trachea, as illustrated in Figure 2-3.

The larynx is located at the level of the fourth, fifth, and sixth cervical vertebrae; the superior portion is considered part of the upper airway, and the inferior portion part of the lower. The superior part of the larynx is the hyoid bone, which is the only bone in the larynx. It is a box-like structure forming a major part of the airway. The larynx is the major organ of speech as well as the most powerful sphincter in the human body. The larynx has a volume of approximately 4 cc and is composed of cartilages, ligaments, muscles, and mucous membranes. It is lined with stratified squamous epithelium above the vocal cords and with pseudostratified columnar epithelial cells below the vocal cords. The opening into the larynx (the glottis) is the narrowest point of the adult's upper airway.

The intrinsic laryngeal musculature is innervated by the recurrent laryngeal nerves, which are branches of the vagus nerve located on each side of the neck. Injury to these nerves (such as may occur with tracheostomy) will cause a loss of speech and the destruction of the protective mechanisms of the larynx.

The larynx consists of three single cartilages (the epiglottic, the thyroid, and the cricoid) and three paired cartilages (the arytenoid, the corniculate, and the cuneiform). The thyroid and cricoid cartilages, along with the hyoid bone, form the primary skeletal structure of the larynx and can be palpated in the anterior portion of the neck.

The thyroid cartilage is the largest laryngeal cartilage. Its anterior aspect is known as the Adam's apple, a shieldlike structure whose notched formation is more prominent in men than in women. The thyroid cartilage is triangularly shaped and serves as the anterior attachment of the vocal cords. The thyroid cartilage is attached superiorly to the thyroid bone by the thyroid membrane and is attached inferiorly to the cricoid cartilage by the cricothyroid membrane. The thyrohyoid membrane may be punctured in an emergency in order to provide an airway; this procedure is known as a cricothyroid stab. Such emergencies usually occur when a patient presents with a critical upper airway obstruction resulting from tumor, trauma, foreign body, tissue swelling, or infection. (The membrane can be identified by hyperextending the head backward, extending the neck forward, and feeling for a transverse indentation located about a half inch below the Adam's apple.)

The cricoid cartilage is located just below the thyroid cartilage and is the only cartilage in the respiratory tract that completely encircles the airway (it is shaped like a signet ring). The first cartilaginous tracheal ring is attached to the cricoid cartilage by a ligament. Since the cricoid cartilage lies anteriorly to the esophagus, external pressure exerted on the cricoid cartilage (cricoid pressure) may facilitate the viewing of the glottis during tracheal intubation and can, at the same time, prevent reflux of stomach contents by direct compression of the esophagus.

The epiglottic cartilage provides the structural support for the epiglottis and is attached to the thyroid cartilage and to the folds of mucous membrane, called aryepiglottic folds. The epiglottic cartilage is a leaf-shaped structure whose upper aspect is not attached to any anatomical structure; thus, it can freely move to cover either the esophagus during breathing or the larynx during swallowing. The lateral borders of the epiglottis attach to the arytenoid folds, causing the posterior portion of the epiglottis

to be in a fixed position. Upon swallowing, the epiglottis is compressed between the thyroid cartilage and the base of the muscular tongue; the compression causes the epiglottis to move posteriorly and inferiorly to cover the laryngeal outlet.

As mentioned above, there are three paired laryngeal cartilages: the arytenoid, the corniculate, and the cuneiform. The cuneiform cartilages are small and club-shaped, and are attached to the arytenoid cartilages. They can be found in the aryepiglottic folds. The corniculate cartilages are apical projections of the arytenoid cartilages and are the smallest cartilages of the larynx. They supply the structural support for the arytenoid cartilages. The arytenoid cartilages are pyramid-shaped; the base of each articulates with the posterior portions of the cricoid cartilage. The arytenoid cartilages and the cricoid cartilage comprise the posterior surface of the larynx. The fine muscles of voice control are attached to the arytenoid cartilages, which are also the posterior site for the attachment of the vocal cords.

The true vocal cords mark the true division between the upper and lower airways. The true vocal cords consist of muscles, ligaments, mucous membrane, and submucosal soft tissue. They stretch between the arytenoid cartilages posteriorly and the thyroid cartilage anteriorly. The arrangement of the vocal cords between these two points creates a triangular opening called the rima glottidis (glottis). It is the smallest opening of the adult airway, and it is essential to accommodate its size when choosing an endotracheal tube. Since this space is the narrowest in the adult airway, it experiences the greatest airflow during expiration. The glottis is smaller in the female than in the male, and its size is variable, depending on the state of the vocal cords.

The false vocal cords are similar in appearance to the true vocal cords, but are not as fully developed or as functional in voice production. They do, however, serve an important protective function for the trachea by contracting and closing the airway against foreign objects. Aspirated foods may frequently be found lodged between these cords.

The epithelial lining of the larynx above the true vocal cords is continuous with the laryngopharynx and consists of stratified squamous epithelia. Below the true cords, the epithelial lining changes in nature, becoming ciliated pseudostratified columnar epithelia.

The Lower Airway

The lower airway is composed of the trachea and the conducting airways, as illustrated in Figure 2-4.

The Trachea

The functions of the trachea are threefold: (1) to complete humidification of inspired gases to a relative humidity of 100% at body temperature, (2) to serve as the largest gas conduit to the lungs, and (3) to provide protective functions. The trachea is a membranous tubular structure between 10 and 15 cm (about 4 in.) in length, depending on the height of the individual. It has an outer diameter of about 2.0 to 2.5 cm in the adult. It extends from the cricoid cartilage at the fifth or sixth cervical vertebra to about the level of the fifth thoracic vertebra, where it bifurcates into the right and left mainstem bronchi. This bifurcation is known as the carina. The trachea has the shape of the letter D, with the flat segment positioned posteriorly. Structurally, the trachea is composed of 16 to 20 C-shaped cartilages that are close anteriorly and connected posteriorly by the smooth trachealis muscle. Because of this smooth muscle, the trachea is able to dilate and elongate during breathing. Major blood vessels located in close proximity to the trachea are the anterior jugular veins, the interior jugular veins, the innominate artery, the carotid arteries, and the inferior thyroid veins.

The trachea is lined with several different types of cells, the most numerous of which are the ciliated pseudostratified columnar epithelial cells. The next most frequently occurring cell type is the goblet cell.

Goblet cells and mucosal glandular cells are interspersed throughout the lung epithelium and are responsible for the production in the normal lung of about 100 mL/day of clear, watery, odorless mucus. The mucous glands are found primarily in the submucosa near the supporting cartilage of the larger airways. The mucus is a complex mucopolysaccharide composed of approximately 95% water, 1% glycoprotein, and 4% cellular debris and foreign materials. The mucus exists in two layers: the sol layer, a watery bottom layer, which covers specialized hairlike projections emanating from the mucosal surface; and the gel layer, a viscous layer on the surface of the water.

The columnar pseudostratified epithelial cells lining the trachea have a unique function, for it is from luminal surfaces of these cells that the 200 to 250 ciliated (hairlike) projections emanate. The cilia of adjacent cells beat in an energetic, coordinated, and sequential fashion, producing what can be described as a wavelike motion. This wavelike activity is directed cephalad and promotes the unidirectional flow of mucus. The wavelike activity occurs throughout all lung tissue, from the upper airways down to the terminal bronchioles. It is an especially important defense mechanism that allows for the removal of trapped inhaled particles and mucus that come to rest in the airways.

On the forward stroke, the cilia become rigid.

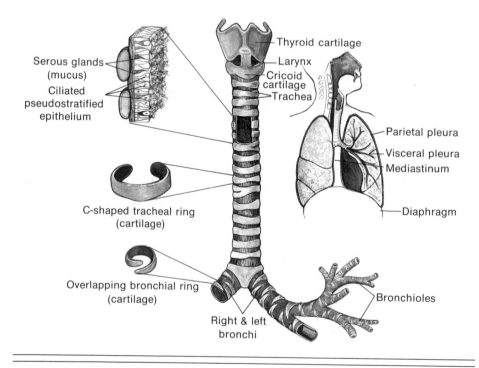

Figure 2-4   The Lower Airway

The tips of the cilia just touch the underside of the gel layer and propel the gel layer of the mucus in a forward direction toward the oropharynx. During the backstroke, the cilia are flaccid and fold upon themselves, so as to slide entirely though the sol layer without creating a retrograde, or backward, flow of mucus in the gel layer. The cilia beat about 1000 to 1300 times per minute and are capable of propelling the gel layer about 2 cm a minute.

This process is known as the mucociliary escalator. Mucus that reaches the pharynx in this manner is usually swallowed, but can be expectorated or removed by blowing one's nose. Studies have found that ciliary function is inhibited or impaired by smoking, poor nutrition, various drugs, and anesthesia. It is important for the nurse to understand that the patient who cannot clear tracheobronchial secretions (such as the intubated patient or one with depressed cough mechanisms) nonetheless continues to produce mucoidal secretions. If the secretions cannot be removed from the airway, either by suctioning or other means, airway obstruction may develop. In contrast, it is helpful to know that beta-adrenergics, cholinergics, and methylxanthines increase mucus production, ciliary beating, and the mucociliary transport functions.[1]

The goblet cells located throughout the trachea synthesize the mucus and secrete it to the epithelial surface. Secretion is facilitated by stimulation or irritation, resulting in increases in mucus production. In pathological states such as chronic bronchitis, the number of goblet cells may increase while the mucosal glands hypertrophy, resulting in a greatly increased mucous gland secretion as well as an increase in the viscosity of the mucus. It is important, though, to remember that hydration of the mucous layers is essential for the maintenance of adequate bronchopulmonary toilet.

The Conducting Airways

When inspired gases are fully conditioned (filtered, heated, and humidified), they are at the carina at about the level of the fifth thoracic vertebra, the point where the trachea ends. It is here that the airway divides into the right and left mainstem bronchi, also referred to as the primary bronchi. Histologically, the mainstem bronchi are similar to the trachea, and like the trachea, the mainstem bronchi are surrounded by C-shaped cartilaginous rings.

The right mainstem bronchus is wider and shorter than the left. It forms approximately a 25-degree angle with the vertical axis of the body. It appears to be a vertical extension of the trachea.

Clinically, this fact is significant because the right bronchus is a more direct (straight) passage into the lungs; foreign objects, aspirated substances (food or fluid), and endotracheal tubes will more often than not find their way into the right mainstem from the carina. The left mainstem forms an angle of 45–55 degrees with the vertical axis. A portion of the mainstem bronchi exists outside the lung (extrapulmonarily), in the mediastinum. However, the majority of the mainstem bronchi are within the lung.

There is one real structural difference between the trachea and the mainstem bronchi: the intrapulmonary mainstem bronchi are covered by the peribronchiolar connective tissue. The function of this tissue is to cover the large nerves, lymph nodes, and bronchial blood vessels as they course through the branchings of the subdividing airways. This tissue extends until it reaches the bronchioles, where it usually terminates. The mainstem bronchi divide and subdivide into smaller and smaller bronchi, which serve the lungs and their various lobes and segments (see Figure 2-5).

Bronchi continue further into the three right and two left lobes of the lungs; each lobe of the lung is supplied by corresponding lobar bronchi. Histologically, they are similar to the trachea and the mainstem bronchi. The right mainstem bronchi trifurcates into the right upper, middle, and lower lobar bronchi; the left mainstem bifurcates into the left upper and lower lobar bronchi. The lowest part of the left upper lobe serves as the lingular segment.

After subdividing into lobar bronchi, the conducting airways divide into the segmental bronchi corresponding to the 18 segments of the lungs. The right lung contains 10 segments, and the left, 8 segments. Within these 18 segments, the lungs further subdivide into the subsegmental parenchymal regions, which possess corresponding subsegmental bronchi. Although these regions are histologically similar to the previously mentioned conducting sections, they are somewhat different in that the epithelial lining is more cuboidal in structure than columnar. There is also a significant decrease in the number of submucosal glands and goblet cells.

By the time the conducting airway is 1 mm in diameter, there is no longer any cartilage present. At this level the lung is made up of noncartilaginous airways whose patency is dependent on the fibrous, elastic, and smooth muscle tissue of which they are composed. (These are still only conducting airways to the area of gas exchange.) Eventually the terminal bronchioles are reached, and these mark the end of the conducting airways.

The terminal bronchioles have an average diameter of about 0.5 mm. There are no goblet cells or

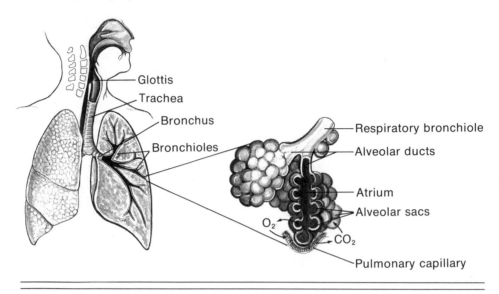

Figure 2-5 Subdivisions of Mainstem Bronchi

submucosal cells. Mucus is still present, however. Cilia can no longer be identified in the epithelium, and the cuboidal cellular structure gives way to a squamous epithelium. Within these terminal bronchioles are found Clara cells, bulging columnar cells that are invasive into the lumen of the terminal bronchioles and appear to function as secretory cells (probably responsible for the mucus and surfactant found in this region). The secretions produced by the Clara cells contribute to the extracellular liquid lining of the bronchioles and contain enzymes that detoxify inhaled substances. The portion of the lung distal to the terminal bronchioles forms the terminal respiratory unit called the acinus.

The terminal bronchioles are subdivided into the respiratory bronchioles. This is the area where actual pulmonary gas exchange begins to occur. Up to this point, no gas exchange has occurred; the gas has simply been conducted through a series of bifurcating and increasingly smaller airways. Some of the actual gas exchange units of the lung, the alveoli, appear within the respiratory bronchioles, although only a very small portion of gas exchange actually takes place at this point.

Alveolar ducts arise from the respiratory bronchioles and are composed of simple squamous epithelia. The only real structural difference between the respiratory bronchioles and the alveolar ducts is that the walls of these ducts are totally constructed of alveoli. Smooth lung muscle continues as small fibers in the openings of the alveolar ducts. About half the total number of alveoli are found in the alveolar ducts; the remaining alveoli are in the alveolar sacs. The alveolar ducts lead into alveolar sacs, which appear functionally similar to the alveolar ducts but

are grapelike clusters of 15 to 20 alveoli sharing common walls.

It should be noted that the cartilaginous rings of the airway gradually give way to cartilaginous plates of irregular shapes. The rings surround the intrapulmonary bronchi and give them their cylindrical shape. The cartilaginous plates help support the larger airways but diminish until they disappear in the airways that are 1 mm in diameter. Airways that possess no structural cartilage are termed bronchioles and are subject to collapse when compressed. Appreciation of this basic fact of respiratory anatomy is important, for it serves as the foundation for developing appropriate pulmonary interventions in the care of the respiratory patient.

The Alveoli

The alveoli represent the terminal anatomical units of the structure of the lung. There are approximately 300 million alveoli in the two lungs. In adults, approximately 90 to 95% of the pulmonary epithelial surface is covered by Type 1 alveolar cells, which are responsible for the maintenance of the integumentary air-blood barrier (usually considered the epithelial basement membrane). The cytoplasmic junctions (squamous pneumocytes) between alveolar cells are usually very tight and are impermeable to water. The Type 1 cell line is so sensitive to cellular injury yet so highly differentiated and metabolically controlled that some cell biologists believe it is impossible to ever replicate.

Between the alveoli in the intraalveolar septa are openings known as the pores of Kohn (or alveolar septal pores). Their purpose and function remain controversial, but for the most part they are believed to contribute to collateral ventilation between the alveoli. However, some cytoplasm of the Type 1 cells also fills these pores, so it may be that their role in ventilation is minimal.

Type 2 alveolar cells comprise about 5% of the alveolar surface area. These cells are cuboidal and highly active metabolically. Surfactant is believed to be produced by the Type 2 cells. When Type 1 cells are destroyed, Type 2 cells increase their mitotic activity and replicate to form a cuboidal cell line. After another mitotic period, some of these progeny develop into Type 1 cell lines.

Type 3 cells are pulmonary macrophages, mononuclear phagocytes that originate in the bone marrow as monocytes and are distributed throughout the body. These mononuclear cells migrate into the pulmonary interstitial space, where they mature and develop their own idiosyncratic biochemical nature, which distinguishes them from other mononuclear cell lines. Type 3 cells are extremely important in lung defense in that they serve as the main mechanism for clearing bacteria and other particles from the terminal airways. Finally, they also appear to function as synthesizers of interferon and tumor-inhibiting factors.

Among other specialized cells located in the respiratory system are mast cells, found in the respiratory submucosa, connective tissue, and parenchyma. When these cells are stimulated by antigen-antibody reactions or through cholinergic stimulation, they release chemical mediators of inflammation: heparin, histamine, slow-reacting substance of anaphylaxis (SRA-A), platelet activating factor (PAF), serotonin, and eosinophilic chemotactic factors. Each mast cell contains approximately 1000 secretory granules, which contain potent chemical inflammatory agents. When the cell is stimulated (causing degranulation), these secretory granules are released. The chemicals contained in the granules increase vascular permeability, cause contraction of smooth muscle, increase mucus production, and trigger vasodilation (resulting in edema). This reaction produces the airway obstruction of asthma, manifested by bronchospasm, mucous plugging, and mucosal edema.

Degranulation of the mast cells is partly controlled by the autonomic nervous system. Beta-adrenergic (sympathomimetic) agents are potent inhibitors of degranulation. Also, parasympatholytic agents can block cholinergic reflex stimulation and reduce this mediator release. Cromolyn sodium with appropriate treatment can result in inhibition of mast cell degranulation. This substance is considered a mast cell stabilizer but must be used prophylactically, as there is no evidence that it is effective in acute attacks. The protective effect of cromolyn sodium is dose-dependent; the usual dose is 20 mg four times daily for about six to eight weeks and thereafter 40 to 60 mg per day.

The Thoraco-Abdominal Structure

The body wall of the central trunk surrounds the thoracic and abdominal cavities, and it is the diaphragm that separates the two. The thorax (shown in Figure 2-6) is cone-shaped. It must be rigid to protect the vital organs of the heart, lungs, great vessels, liver, and spleen and at the same time resilient (compliant) to accommodate the expansion and reduction of lung volume that occurs with ventilation. The thorax serves as the mechanical pump that moves air in and out of the lungs. To keep the thorax from collapsing, muscular walls are reinforced by bones: the sternum anteriorly, the ribs bilaterally, and the thoracic vertebrae posteriorly.

The sternum (also known as the breastbone) has three parts: the manubrium, the body, and the xiphoid process. The small depression in the top of the manubrium is the suprasternal notch. The lateral edges of the sternum supply the articulation points for the upper seven ribs (known as the true ribs), which are joined to the sternum by costal cartilages. Each of the false ribs (8 through 10) articulates with the rib directly above and is not attached to the sternum. The articulation point of these ribs is the costochondral joint. The last two ribs (11 and 12) are called floating ribs, for they have no cartilaginous attachments either to the sternum or to other ribs anteriorly. Posteriorly, each rib attaches to a thoracic vertebra. Between adjacent ribs are the internal and external intercostal muscles, which are situated in the intercostal space. During inspiration and expiration, the size of the thoracic cavity changes as the ribs move about the anteroposterior axis and the transverse diameters simultaneously.

The thoracic cavity contains the heart, the lungs, the esophagus, and other structures previously mentioned. The center of this cavity is the mediastinum, which is a very complicated structure that contains parts of the trachea and esophagus, the phrenic and vagus nerves, components of blood vessels that enter and leave the heart, lymph nodes, nerves, and other anatomical components such as the thoracic duct.

On each side of the mediastinum are two cavities called pleural cavities, which contain serous fluid. The lungs are compressed into the medial walls of the pleural cavities in a way that has been compared

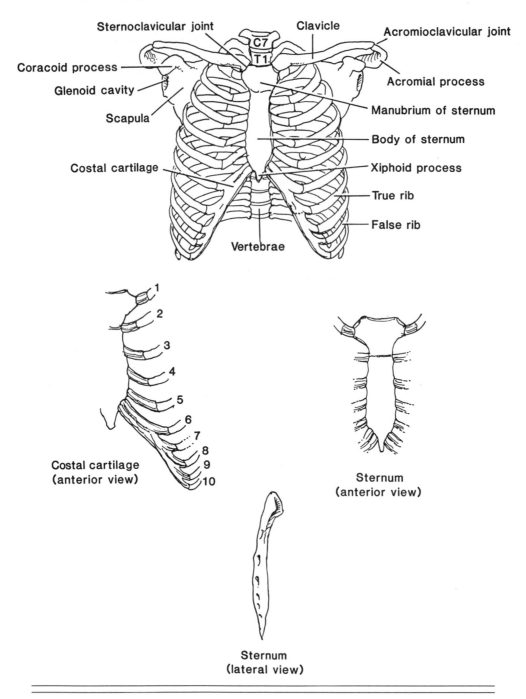

Figure 2-6 The Thorax

to a fist in a balloon. When the thorax expands during inspiration, the pleural cavities become larger. Each pleural cavity is lined by two membranous regions: the outer parietal layer lines the chest wall, and the inner visceral layer lines the lungs. Between these two layers of protective tissue is a layer of serous fluid (about one molecule thick) that serves as both a lubricant and an adhesive between the visceral pleura and the parietal pleura as they slide along

each other with each ventilatory cycle. For this movement of the two pleural surfaces (which accomplishes the expansion of the thoracic cavity) to occur, a mechanical force needs to be applied to the thoracic cavity. The locus of this force is muscular contraction by both inspiratory and expiratory muscles of ventilation.

The respiratory muscles possess no inherent rhythm but generate tension from a rhythmic pattern of neurally induced action potentials from the autonomic nervous system. (Acetylcholine serves as the primary neurotransmitter.) The most important muscle of ventilation is the diaphragm, which is responsible for 80 to 85% of ventilation action during quiet breathing. The dome-shaped diaphragm is about 250 cm^2 in surface area and is responsible for moving about two-thirds of the air that enters the lungs. It is innervated by two phrenic nerves, which originate from the spinal cord at the third through the fifth cervical vertebrae. The diaphragm is composed of two hemidiaphragms connected by a central membranous tendon that is contiguous with the pericardium. At rest the right hemidiaphragm is slightly higher than the left because the liver rests under the right hemidiaphragm, lifting it slightly. Also, the heart tends to push down on the left side of the diaphragm.

During normal quiet breathing this dome-shaped muscular organ contracts and descends 1–2 cm into the abdominal cavity. This movement causes an increase in the vertical diameter of the chest and an increase in the transverse diameter of the lower chest. Diaphragmatic descension increases to 3–8 cm during a deep breath.

When the external intercostals contract, they raise the ribs and simultaneously prevent bulging or "sucking in" of the intercostal spaces. These muscles are innervated by spinal motor nerves T1 through T11.

The accessory muscles of inspiration are not usually involved in quiet breathing but are activated during play, exercise, or the inspiratory phase of coughing or sneezing or in the presence of pathology. The origins and actions of these muscles are listed in Table 2-1.

Upon expiration during normal quiet breathing, muscular activity is absent. Healthy normal expiratory effort requires no active effort at all; expiration is usually passive and no respiratory muscles contract. As the inspiratory muscles relax, inherent pressures and the natural tendency of the alveoli to close are sufficient to decrease alveolar volume. Thus, the diaphragm is also considered to be completely relaxed during expiration, but recent evidence suggests diaphragmatic muscular tone is maintained even during expiration (especially during horizontal positioning and in the case of obesity). It is also thought that this maintenance of muscular tone may hold some transitional function during inspiration and expiration and may in part be responsible for phonation.

During normal inspiration, as the diaphragm descends into the abdominal cavity, it compresses abdominal contents and gas, raising abdominal pressure. On normal exhalation, this increased abdominal pressure assists in pushing the diaphragm back into the thoracic cavity and in the passive expulsion of air from the lungs.

In contrast, the muscles of the anterior abdominal wall (the internal oblique, external oblique, rectus abdominis, internal intercostal, and transverse abdominis, shown in Figure 2-7) are involved in active expiration. Innervation of this musculature is found to originate in the spinal nerves T7 to L1. During active expiration, these abdominal muscles contract even more forcefully, increasing the pressure in the abdominal cavity by compressing the abdominal viscera up against the diaphragm. This action permits a more forceful pressure to be exerted against the diaphragm to expel air from the lungs. At the same time these active abdominal muscles are also involved in depressing the lower ribs and pulling down the anterior portion of the lower chest.

Physiology of the Respiratory System

The principle functions of the respiratory system are the provision of oxygen and the elimination of carbon dioxide commensurate with the body's metabolic needs. These functions are accomplished by

Table 2-1 Accessory Muscles of Inspiration

Accessory Muscle	Origins	Actions
Scalenes	Lower five cervical vertebrae; attached to first and second ribs	Enlargement of the upper rib cage, supports the apex of the lung
Sternocleidomastoid	The manubrium and clavicle; attached to mastoid process and occipital bone	Elevates the sternum and helps to increase the anterioposterior and transverse diameters of the chest; believed recruited after three-fourths of vital capacity has been inspired

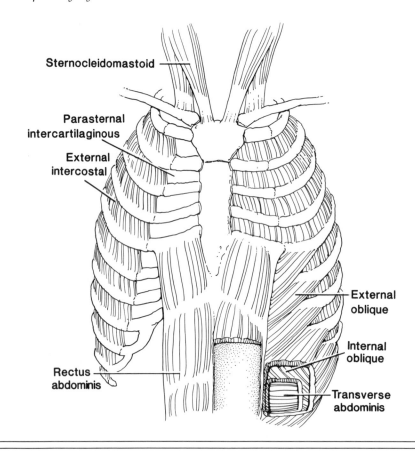

Figure 2-7   Thoracic and Abdominal Muscles

ventilation, perfusion, diffusion, and gas transport from lungs to tissues and regulated by a control mechanism that matches ventilation to metabolic needs. Normal resting values of the various components of respiratory function are detailed in Table 2-2.

Ventilation

Ventilation is the bulk movement of air between the atmosphere and the alveoli.

Muscles of Respiration

[Note: To promote consistency in the use of terms and equations in discussions of respiratory physiology, the Joint Committee on Pulmonary Nomenclature of the American College of Chest Physicians and the American Thoracic Society compiled a list of symbols and terms. The following information incorporates the terminology set forth by the committee. Readers may also find helpful an article entitled "Pulmonary Terms and Symbols," which appeared on pages 583–593 of *Chest, 67* (5), published in 1975.]

Inhalation is the intake of atmospheric air. It is achieved when negative intrathoracic pressure causes the thorax to expand and allow the atmo-

spheric air to flow in. The diaphragm contracts, becoming shorter and pushing down on the abdominal contents. Simultaneously the external intercostal muscles contract, lifting the ribs up and outward. The muscles of the pharynx and the genioglossus also contract during inspiration to prevent the narrow upper airway from collapsing under the negative pressure generated by the thoracic muscles, maintaining an open upper airway between atmosphere and alveoli (see Figure 2-8). When the work of breathing is increased, the anterior and posterior serratus and the strap muscles of the neck (especially the sternocleidomastoid and scalene muscles) are recruited to assist inspiration by lifting the ribs and enlarging the thorax.

Exhalation is the movement of air from alveoli to the atmosphere. During quiet breathing exhalation is achieved when the inspiratory muscles relax and the stretched elastic tissues of the lung recoil, returning the thorax to its resting equilibrium volume. During forced exhalation, positive pressure exceeding the relaxation force of the muscles and the recoil force of the lungs is provided by the rectus abdominus, internal and external oblique, and transverse abdominal muscles, which press the abdominal contents against the diaphragm, forcing air out of the chest.

Table 2-2 Normal Resting Values of Respiratory Function

Component	Value
Ventilation	
VE (L/min)*	6–10
VA (L/min)*	4–7.5
Lung Volumes	
TLC (L)*	4.8
VC (L)*	3.5
FRC (L)*	2.5
RV (L)*	1.3
V_T (L)*	0.6
Air Flow	
FEV1 (L/min)*	3.0
FEV1/FVC (%)*	>69
PF (L/sec)*	10
Maximum Pressure	
Inspiratory (cm H_2O)*	120
Lung Resistance	
Airway (cm H_2O/L/sec)	0.5–2.5
Total (cm H_2O/L/sec)	1.3–4.4
Compliance, Cst (L/cm H_2O)*	0.1–0.4

	Pressure (mm Hg)	Sat (%)	Other
Hemodynamic Measurements			
SVC	0–5	70–75	
IVC	0–5	75–80	
RA	0–5	70–75	
RV	25/0–5	70–75	
PA	25/10	70–75	
Ppcw	5–10	98–100	
LA	5–10	95–98	
LV	120/0–5	95–98	
Aorta	120/80	95–97	
Q (L/min)			5
CI (L/min/m²)			2.8–4.2
SV (mL/beat)			50–80
PVR (mm Hg/L/min)			1.5–3
SVR (mm Hg/L/min)			11–18

	Arterial	Mixed venous	Other
Gas Exchange			
PO_2 (mm Hg)*	95	40	
PCO_2 (mm Hg)	40	45	
pH	7.40	7.36	
HCO_3 (plasma)	26	27	
Hb (gm/100 mL)*	15		
SO_2 (%)*	97	75	
CO_2 (vol %)*	19.4	14.4	
$PA\text{-}aO_2$ (mm Hg)*			10
VD/VT			0.33
Q_{VA}/Q_T			0.04
Q_S/Q_T			0.02
DLCO (mL/min/ mm Hg)*			28
VO_2 (mL/min)*			200
VCO_2 (mL/min)*			250
R			0.8

*Values apply to a normal Caucasian man, age 40, height 150 cm. Values may vary with specific individual characteristics (including age, height, race, and gender).

Internal intercostal muscles also contract, lowering the ribs and drawing them inward.

Conditions that alter the normal function of these muscles impair ventilation. Four classes of condition and examples of each are listed in Table 2-3. When the diaphragm is paralyzed and other inspiratory muscles are intact, the diaphragm moves paradoxically, rising in the chest on inspiration. Diaphragmatic paralysis can be detected fluoroscopically with a sniff test.

Lung Volumes

The volume of air in normal lungs fluctuates with the respiratory cycle, which is controlled by the respiratory muscles. The various volume compartments of the lung are as follows:

Tidal volume (V_T): The volume of air exhaled per breath during quiet breathing

Functional residual capacity (FRC): The volume of air remaining in the lungs at the end of a quiet exhalation

Residual volume (RV): The volume of air remaining in the lungs after forced exhalation; it is the volume of air that cannot be exhaled.

Vital capacity (VC): The largest volume a person can exhale from full inflation

Total lung capacity (TLC): The volume of air in the lungs at total inflation, equal to the sum of residual volume and vital capacity.

Lung volumes are graphed in Figure 2-9.

By convention, all determinations of lung volume, except residual volume, are made with exhalation measurements. There are no universal normal values for lung volume measurements; the normal lung volume and capacity measurements vary with age, height, gender, and race.

Measurement of Ventilatory Function

To assess ventilation, measurements of minute ventilation, lung volume, air flow, maximal inspiratory and mouth occlusion pressures, resistance, compliance, and arterial blood gases are taken.

The arterial blood gas carbon dioxide tension (P_aCO_2) serves as the most accurate indication of the success of overall ventilation. Normal P_aCO_2 is 40 mm Hg at normal $\dot{V}_E$ of 5 L/min. P_aCO_2 rises with alveolar hypoventilation ($\dot{V}_A < 2$–4 L/min) and falls with alveolar hyperventilation ($\dot{V}_A > 6$–8 L/min).

Minute ventilation ($\dot{V}_E$) is the volume of air exhaled per minute; it can be determined by measuring the total volume of air exhaled in one minute

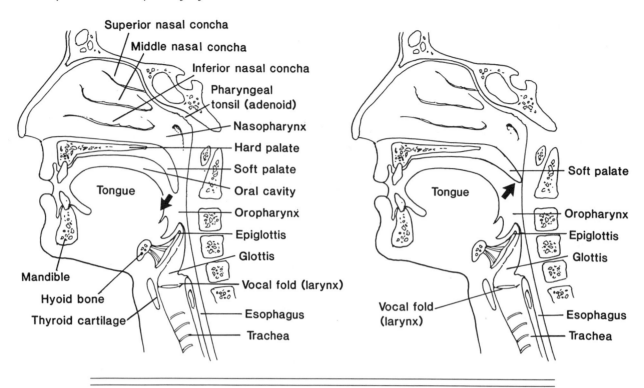

Figure 2-8 Upper Airway Muscle Contraction to Prevent Soft Palate Tissue Collapse During Inspiration

Table 2-3 Conditions Altering Respiratory Muscle Function

Class	Example
Primary muscle diseases	Myotonic dystrophy
Myoneural disease	Myasthenia gravis Anticholinesterase insecticide poisoning
Peripheral neuropathy	Poliomyelitis Guillaine-Barre syndrome
Spinal cord disruption	Cervical cord transection above C5

or by measuring tidal volume (V_T) and respiratory rate (F_R):

$$\dot{V}_E = V_T \times F_R$$

Alveolar ventilation ($\dot{V}_A$) is the most important portion of the $\dot{V}_E$; it is the volume of air coming from the alveoli that has participated in gas exchange. $\dot{V}_A$

is reduced when $\dot{V}_E$ is low, but it may be low even when $\dot{V}_E$ is normal if deadspace ventilation is increased. $\dot{V}_A$ is assessed indirectly by subtracting deadspace from total minute ventilation (normal $\dot{V}_A \approx 4$ L/min):

$$\dot{V}_A = \dot{V}_E - \dot{V}_D$$

Deadspace ventilation ($\dot{V}_D$) is the volume of air exhaled per minute that has not participated in gas exchange. Normal anatomic deadspace is the volume of the conducting airways; it is about equal in milliliters to the ideal body weight in pounds. Anatomic deadspace is assessed in the pulmonary function lab by measuring nitrogen concentration as a function of exhaled volume after a single breath of 100% oxygen. Physiologic deadspace includes anatomic deadspace plus some alveolar volume from poorly perfused alveoli; it is calculated as a fraction of tidal volume by measuring arterial carbon dioxide gas (P_aCO_2) and mixed exhaled carbon dioxide gas (P_ECO_2) tensions and applying the Bohr equation:

$$\frac{\dot{V}_D}{\dot{V}_T} = \frac{P_aCO_2 - P_ECO_2}{P_aCO_2}$$

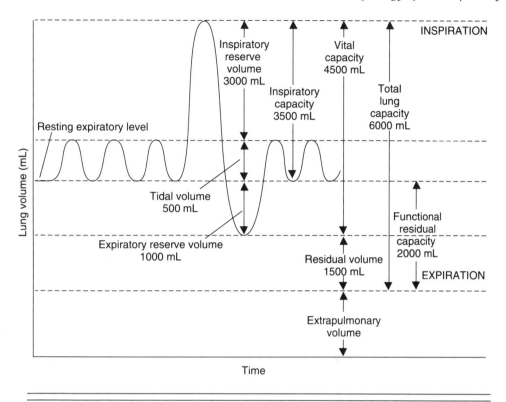

Figure 2-9 Normal Lung Volumes and Capacities

(See the section on Ventilation-Perfusion Matching, pages 44–47, for further discussion of deadspace.)

Lung volumes are measured by direct and indirect methods. Vital capacity and tidal volume are measured by collecting exhaled air into a volume displacement device such as a Douglas bag or a water-seal spirometer or by deriving volume from continuous flow measurements. Determining the volume of air remaining in the lungs after full exhalation and at full inflation requires a measurement of residual volume, functional residual capacity, and total lung capacity, which must be acquired using an indirect method such as nitrogen washout, inert gas dilution, body plethysmography, or chest radiographic planimetry.

Lung volumes are altered by disease conditions. *Obstructive* pulmonary conditions (asthma, emphysema, chronic bronchitis, vocal cord paralysis) create narrow conducting airways; vital capacity is low and functional residual capacity and residual volume are high. Air is trapped in the lung behind weakened or narrow peripheral airways which close on exhalation, limiting the exhalation volume. In patients with such conditions, the total lung capacity (TLC) is normal or increased, and the ratio of residual volume to total lung capacity (RV/TLC) is high. (Normal RV/TLC < 0.3.) Hence they have smaller movable lung volumes. Their larger resting inflation volumes give them increased work of breathing. *Restrictive* pulmonary conditions (interstitial fibrosis, kyphoscoliosis, myotonic dystrophy) result from small lungs; the volume compartments of the lungs are uniformly small (TLC, VC, RV), leaving RV/TLC normal. Some obstructive, restrictive, and vascular lung disorders are listed in Table 2-4.

The P_{Imax} is helpful in distinguishing muscle impairment from other causes of restrictive ventilatory impairment. It measures the maximum negative pressure generated by the inspiratory muscles as the patient inhales from RV against an occluded mouthpiece. (Normal $P_{Imax} > 100$ cm H_2O.) This measurement is low in those with muscle weakness. This test is particularly useful in evaluating mechanically ventilated patients who have small spontaneous VC and weaning difficulties.

Mechanics of Breathing

The muscles of respiration generate positive and negative pressures within the thorax, causing the bulk flow of air in and out of the lung. The effect of the positive and negative forces on the volume of air moved is determined by the elastic characteristics of the lung and chest wall and by the resistance properties of the thoracic tissues and the conducting airways. Figure 2-10 illustrates changes in pressure, volume, and flow during a single breath.

Table 2-4 Functional Classification of Lung Disease

Obstructive	Restrictive	Vascular
Asthma	Chest-wall deformity or scar	Pulmonary arteritis
Emphysema	Pleural disease	Thromboembolism
Bronchitis	Massive obesity	Veno-occlusive disease
Tracheal stenosis	Interstitial disease	Plexogenic arteriopathy
Tracheal malacia	Neuromuscular disease	
Vocal cord paralysis	Diaphragm paralysis	
Epiglottitis	Chest trauma	
Parkinson's disease	Pulmonary edema	
Upper airway tumor	Pneumonia	
Cystic fibrosis	Atelectasis or lobar collapse	
Foreign body		
Sarcoidosis		

Compliance The elastic properties of both the lung and the chest wall are defined by pressure and volume, that is, by how much pressure is required to change a unit volume of the thorax.

The pressure-volume characteristics of the lung, independent of the chest wall, are determined by two physical features:

1. The matrix of elastin and collagen fibers that surrounds the alveoli, airways, and vessels in the lung, which opposes inflation; and
2. The surface tension of the surfactant liquid lining the alveoli, which facilitates inflation.

Plotting pressure across the lung vs. volume makes it clear that at very low and very high inflation volumes (where the curve is flat), the work (or pressure) required to change lung volume is much greater than at mid-lung volumes. Figure 2-11 illustrates the relationship.

Mid-lung inflation volumes are the most efficient and minimize the work of breathing. The slope of the pressure-volume curve in Figure 2-11 represents lung compliance (C_L), a measure of the elastic recoil of the lung. (Normal C_L at FRC is 200 mL/cm H_2O.)

$$C_L = \frac{\Delta \text{ volume}}{\Delta \text{ pressure}}$$

There are regional compliance differences in the lung that are gravity-dependent. The apex of the upright lung is less compliant and receives less ventilation than the base.

Compliance of the lung is altered in certain conditions. In left heart failure, the lung is engorged with blood from the high left atrial pressure; it becomes stiff and less compliant, requiring higher pressure and more work to inflate. In pulmonary fibrosis (asbestosis, sarcoidosis), the lung is stiffened by increased interstitial collagen. Surfactant deficiency, such as occurs in infant respiratory distress syndrome and may occur with excessive distention of alveoli (as with high-pressure mechanical ventilation), reduces compliance and increases the work of breathing. Compliance increases with normal aging; it is also increased in patients with emphysema.

The chest wall has a network of elastic tissues that give it compliance properties as well. Pressure must be applied to stretch and inflate the chest wall up to total lung capacity. However, at the mid-to-low lung inflation of FRC, the chest wall's elastic network is like a compressed spring, assisting inhalation.

The compliance of the chest wall is decreased in patients with such conditions as extreme obesity, kyphoscoliosis, chest-wall burns, or progressive systemic sclerois. Chest-wall compliance may be increased when traumatic rib fractures cause flail chest.

Under the equilibrium conditions of quiet breathing, the chest wall tends to be pulled outward by the tension of its elastic network; at FRC this outward pressure is evenly balanced by the inward tension of the lung's elastic network of collagen and elastin. This relationship is illustrated in Figure 2-12.

The chest wall's lining of parietal pleura and the visceral pleura lining the lung are separated only by a thin layer of pleural fluid. This fluid serves to lubricate the movement of lung and chest wall as they slide over each other. (See the section on Perfusion, pages 40–44, for further discussion of fluid dynam-

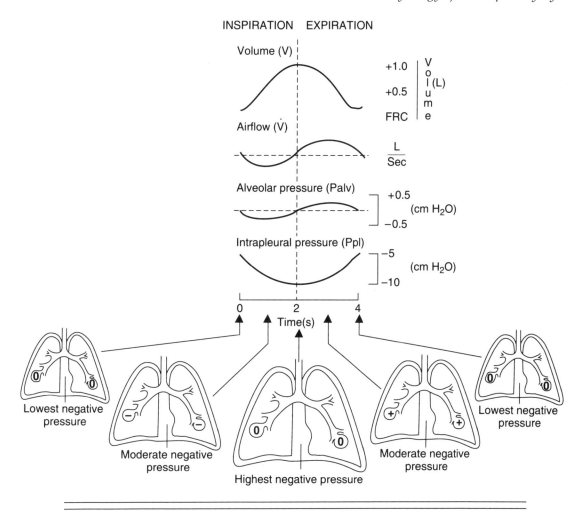

INSPIRATION   EXPIRATION

Figure 2-10   Changes in Pressure, Volume, and Flow During a Single Breath
Source: Martin, L. (1987). *Pulmonary Physiology in Clinical Practice: The Essentials for Patient Care and Evaluation.* St. Louis: The C. V. Mosby Company, p. 45.

ics.) When air is introduced into the pleural space (pneumothorax), the lung recoils to a much smaller size while the chest wall expands in response to released elastic forces.

Measurements of compliance of lung and thorax identify changes in the elastic characteristics that affect the work of breathing. Compliance measurements can identify and further characterize restrictive ventilatory impairment. The pressure across the lung is the difference between pleural and alveolar pressures. Pleural pressure is approximated by an esophageal measurement, and alveolar pressure is equivalent to mouth pressure, since the glottis is open and the airway unobstructed. Figure 2-13 indicates the various pressure measurements that determine compliance. By measuring these pressures at changing lung volumes, a calculation of lung compliance as the change in volume over change in pressure can be made. For thoracic compliance deter-

minations, the pressure difference between the atmosphere and the alveoli is measured at the mouth. Thoracic compliance in the mechanically ventilated patient can be measured in the ICU by occluding the airway at end inspiration and measuring airway pressure. Inflation volume divided by end-inspiratory airway pressure reflects thoracic compliance. Lung compliance is likewise measured by inserting an esophageal pressure transducer to estimate alveolar pressure. These bedside compliance measurements are not comparable to those determined in the pulmonary function lab, because lung inflation volumes are higher and compliance of the ventilator apparatus plays a role. However, serial measurements are useful for detecting changes in the patient's status. Decreasing compliance in a mechanically ventilated patient may signify fluid overload, onset of adult respiratory distress syndrome, progressive air trapping, or pneumothorax. Bedside

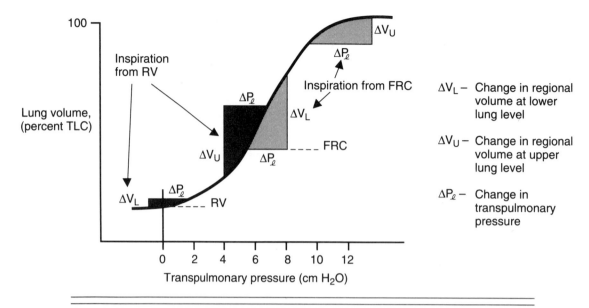

Figure 2-11   Relationship of Lung Volume Upon Initiation of Inspiration to Regional Lung Compliance
Source: Slonim, N. B., and Hamilton, L. H. (1981). *Respiratory Physiology* (4th Edition). St. Louis: The C. V. Mosby Company, p. 110.

compliance measurements are also useful in adjusting positive end expiratory pressure (PEEP) to an optimal level. Generally PEEP increases the compliance of fluid-filled lungs. However, excessive PEEP reduces the left ventricular return, stiffens the lung, and paradoxically reduces lung compliance.

Resistance   In addition to the elastic properties of the lung and the chest wall, resistance of tissues (viscosity) and resistance to airflow also determine the impact of respiratory muscle contractions on air movement in and out of the lungs.

The resistance to airflow (R) of a rigid tube is directly proportional to its length (l) and the viscosity of the gas flowing (n); it is inversely proportional to the fourth power of its radius (r):

$$R = \frac{8nl}{r^4}$$

Small changes in airway caliber have a profound effect on airway resistance. The airways are not a single tube but a circuit of many branching tubes, whose length and radius decrease from mouth to the alveolus, but whose combined radius increases geometrically (illustrated in Figure 2-14). There are seventeen divisions of conducting airways; the total resistance of the circuit is:

$$\frac{1}{R_T} = \frac{1}{R_1} + \frac{1}{R_2} + \frac{1}{R_3} + \ldots$$

Because the peripheral airways are short and because collectively they have a large radius, they contribute relatively little to the overall airway resistance. Eighty percent of the total resistance of the tracheobronchial tree is in the trachea and its first seven divisions.

Airway resistance (R_{aw}) is normally determined by lung inflation volume, bronchomotor tone, and the density of the ventilating gases. At large lung inflation volumes, airways are stretched open and total airway resistance is lowest.

Contraction of the bronchial smooth muscle causes bronchoconstriction, airway narrowing, and increased resistance to airflow. Bronchoconstriction is triggered by parasympathetic stimulation, humoral factors, and stimulation by irritants.

Although airway resistance (R_{aw}) can be measured directly, it is more commonly assessed indirectly by measuring airflow. The equipment required for such flow measurement is more accessible. Resistance and flow measurements identify obstructive ventilatory impairment.

Direct measurement of airway resistance requires a body plethysmograph, which simultaneously quantifies measures of flow ($\dot{V}$), volume (V), and mouth pressure (P_M) as the patient pants into the mouthpiece. Volume measurements are used to calculate alveolar pressure (P_A) by applying Boyle's law. Resistance is computed by applying Ohm's law:

$$R_{aw} = \frac{(P_A - P_M)}{\dot{V}}$$

The resistance measurement must be normalized for lung volume and it is usually measured at FRC

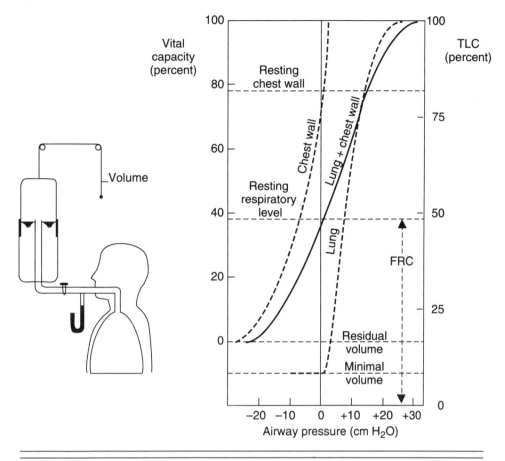

Figure 2-12 Pressure-Volume Curves for Lung and Chest Wall, and Sum of Both
Source: West, J. B. (1989). *Respiratory Physiology: The Essentials* (4th Edition). Baltimore, MD: Williams & Wilkins, p. 100.

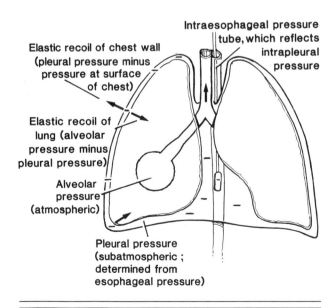

Figure 2-13 Pressure Measurements for Determination of Compliance

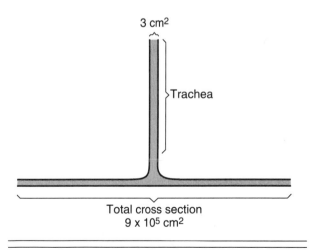

Figure 2-14 Cross-Sectional Area of Conducting Airways
Source: Martin, L. (1987). *Pulmonary Physiology in Clinical Practice: The Essentials for Patient Care and Evaluation.* St. Louis: The C. V. Mosby Company, p. 37.

(normal R_{aw} = 0.5–2.5 cm H_2O/L/sec). In the mechanically ventilated patient, significant differences between peak and relaxation airway pressures (made when the airway is occluded at end inspiration) indicate airflow obstruction. Measurements of trends in the individual patient are more useful than single measurements.

Airflow is inversely proportional to the airway resistance:

$$\dot{V} = \frac{(P_A - P_M)}{R_{aw}}$$

Airflow assessment is made by measuring the rate of change in exhaled volume over time as the patient forcibly exhales full vital capacity. This breathing maneuver is more effort-dependent than the airway resistance measurement. Key flow measurements include peak flow (PF), forced vital capacity (FVC), forced one-second expiratory volume (FEV_1), and FEV_1 as a percent of FVC (normal FEV_1/FVC > 0.69). The peak flow (PF) measurement is the most effort-dependent of the flow measurements and is simple to measure, but FEV_1 is a more accurate measure for monitoring the more critically ill patient.

Conditions obstructing airflow   Under normal conditions of breathing at rest, air moves so easily through the conducting airways that 1 cm of water pressure is enough to overcome the airway resistance and cause air to be exchanged between alveoli and atmosphere. Any conditions that reduce airway diameter increase airway resistance: breathing at low lung volumes, bronchoconstriction (such as with asthma), excessive mucus secretions (such as with chronic bronchitis), airway inflammation (as in angioedema), loss of the elastic matrix supporting the airways (as in emphysema), or upper airway obstruction (as in vocal cord paralysis).

Asthmatic individuals have increased airway resistance from bronchoconstriction, mucous gland hypertrophy, and bronchial inflammation. Breathing a mixture of helium and oxygen reduces resistance and improves airflow in patients suffering respiratory failure due to severe airflow obstruction. Flow is inversely proportional to density in narrow airways, and helium is less dense than nitrogen. Sympathetic stimulation (such as by beta adrenergic medication) reduces airway resistance by relaxing bronchial smooth muscle. Antiinflammatory agents (corticosteroids) reduce airway edema. Endotracheal intubation narrows the upper airway and increases its resistance. Resistance is further increased if the tube becomes kinked or obstructed with mucus.

Work of breathing   Work of breathing is measured by multiplying pressure times volume and has three components: compliance work, which is required to overcome the elastic forces of lung and chest wall; tissue resistance work, which is required to overcome the viscosity of the lung and chest wall; and airway resistance work. The three components are represented graphically in Figure 2-15.

Normally ventilation consumes only 3 to 5% of the body's total oxygen uptake, but this may increase fiftyfold with disease. Patients with lung disease spontaneously develop patterns of breathing that minimize their work of breathing. For example, those with stiff lungs (interstitial fibrosis) develop shallow rapid breathing to minimize the compliance work, whereas those with increased airflow resistance (asthma) develop slow deep breathing to minimize airway resistance work. These patterns should be considered when controlling ventilation mechanically.

Perfusion

Pulmonary perfusion is the process by which respiratory gases are conveyed between the alveoli and the systemic tissues. The right ventricle pumps 500–750 mL of blood through the pulmonary circulation (10–15% of the total blood volume). The volume of capillary blood in the lungs is 100 mL, and it flows in a sort of sheet around the alveoli (50–100 square meters of surface). Overall pulmonary perfusion is determined by the force of contraction of the right ventricle, the resistance of the pulmonic valve, the pulmonary vascular resistance, and the hydrostatic pressure in the left atrium.

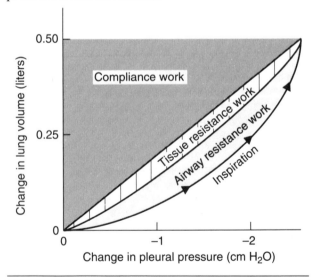

Figure 2-15   The Three Components of the Work of Breathing
Source: Guyton, A. C. (1991). *Textbook of Medical Physiology* (8th Edition). Philadelphia: W. B. Saunders Company, p. 406.

Characteristics of Pulmonary Perfusion

The right ventricle is a low-pressure pump, generating a mean pressure of only 15 mm Hg to pump blood through the low-resistance pulmonary vascular circuit. Features of the pulmonary vascular circuit that keep right heart work low include:

1. Thin-walled, compliant arterioles, which dilate under increasing pressure. (There is little arteriolar smooth muscle because there is little need to regulate regional blood flow within the normal lung.)
2. The proximity of the pulmonary vascular tree to the heart, requiring blood to be pumped only 15 to 20 cm against gravity to the top of the lung.
3. The fact that the main pulmonary artery extends only a short way before it branches. (Vascular resistance is directly proportional to the length of the conduit and inversely proportional to the collective diameter of parallel branches.)
4. Pulmonary vascular channels that are closed at rest and recruited when right ventricular or left atrial pressure increases. Hence pulmonary vascular resistance (PVR) initially decreases when pressure across the lung increases.

The right heart and pulmonary circulation contrast sharply with the left heart and systemic circulation. The left heart must generate a high pressure (mean pressure is 100 mm Hg) in order to distribute blood to distant regions (up to 80–100 cm along an arm stretched above the level of the heart). In the systemic circulation, blood flows long distances from the heart before arteries branch. The arterioles are rigid and muscular and can constrict to regulate flow as needed by a wide array of organs. Resistance in the systemic circulation is six to ten times that in the lungs. Hence, the work of the left heart is much greater than that of the right heart. When the left ventricle fails (as in acute myocardial infarction), intravascular blood volume increases (in fluid overload), or the left atrium is obstructed (as in mitral stenosis) and hydrostatic pressure in the pulmonary veins doubles (8–10 mm Hg), the capacity of the pulmonary circulation for dilation and recruitment is exceeded. Beyond this point, the increased hydrostatic pressure is transmitted to the pulmonary artery and increases the work of the right heart. When left atrial pressure triples, water begins to leak out of the capillaries into the interstitial space, impairing gas exchange. Pulmonary and systemic circulatory pressures are depicted in Figure 2-16.

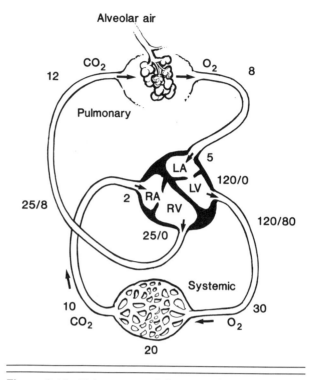

Figure 2-16 Pulmonary and Systemic Circulatory Pressures (mm Hg)

Intrathoracic Pressure

The pulmonary circulation is affected by the intrathoracic pressure changes occurring over the respiratory cycle. The capillaries are surrounded by gas. During spontaneous inspiration alveolar pressure is negative and the capillaries expand in response to expansile transmural pressure, which reverses during expiration. Positive pressure mechanical ventilation imposes positive pressure across the lung on inspiration, compressing vessels and increasing resistance in the pulmonary capillary bed.

Lung Inflation

Pulmonary blood flow is also affected by the volume of lung inflation. Very large inflation volumes stretch and compress the pulmonary capillaries but stretch and enlarge pulmonary arteries and veins. The net effect of lung volume on pulmonary vascular resistance (PVR) is that resistance increases at very high and very low lung volumes; PVR is lowest in the mid-volume range of normal quiet breathing (see Figure 2-17).

Regional distribution The distribution of blood flow to the lung is not uniform. Gravity is the primary determinant of the uneven distribution; alveoli in the dependent portions of the lung are better perfused than those uppermost. There is a normal hydrostatic pressure difference of 23 mm Hg from

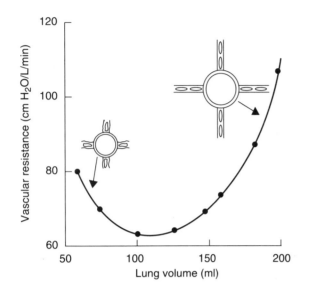

Figure 2-17 Relationship of Pulmonary Vascular Resistance to Lung Inflation Volume
Source: West, J. B. (1989). *Respiratory Physiology: The Essentials* (4th Edition). Baltimore, MD: Williams & Wilkins, p. 38.

the apex to the base of the lung of a person standing upright. The lung can be divided into three perfusion zones which are defined by the pressure relationships between the pulmonary artery (P_a), the alveoli (P_A), and the pulmonary vein (P_v). Figure 2-18 illustrates these relationships. As shown in the figure, in zone 1, P_A exceeds P_a and there is no forward flow of blood. This condition does not normally occur but may be present in the uppermost lung under conditions of low blood pressure, intravascular volume depletion, or positive pressure mechanical ventilation. In zone 2, $P_a > P_A > P_v$; flow is driven by the difference between arterial and alveolar pressure. This region is the principle area for recruitment and distention of vessels during high output states, as when flow increases with exercise. In zone 3, $P_a > P_v > P_A$; there is continuous forward flow of blood, independent of alveolar pressures.

Pulmonary Vascular Tone

In addition to being affected by right ventricular and left atrial hydrostatic pressure, lung inflation volume, the respiratory cycle, and gravity, pulmonary perfusion is affected by active vasoconstriction. The most powerful stimulus for vasoconstriction is alveolar hypoxia. When $P_A O_2$ falls below 70 mm Hg, the vasoconstrictive response to hypoxia is marked and blood is diverted away from poorly ventilated alveoli, so that the best ventilated alveoli are the ones that become most perfused. Acidemia, hypercapnea,

histamine (H_1 receptors), serotonin, angiotensin II, and prostaglandin also vasoconstrict the pulmonary circulation. Sympathetic stimulation and pharmacologic doses of alpha adrenergic agonists vasoconstrict. Acetylcholine, histamine (H_2 receptors), bradykinin, and prostaglandin I_2 and E_1 vasodilate the pulmonary circulation. Administration of theophylline, beta adrenergic agonists, calcium channel blockers, and other antihypertensives may also cause vasodilation. Administration of these agents may worsen hypoxemia by inducing vasodilation in poorly ventilated lung units.

Pulmonary Perfusion Measurements

Assessment of overall pulmonary perfusion requires measurement of pressures in the right ventricle, pulmonary artery, and left atrium and measurement of cardiac output. A balloon-tipped right heart catheter (Swan-Ganz catheter) measures right heart pressures directly; the pulmonary capillary wedge pressure measurement reflects left atrial pressure. (Note that the balloon tip must be placed in perfusion zone 3 of the lung to accurately reflect left atrial pressure.) Pulmonary vascular resistance (PVR) is calculated by taking the pressure difference between the right ventricle (P_{rv}) and the left atrium (P_{la}) and dividing by cardiac output ($\dot{Q}$):

$$PVR = \frac{(P_{rv} - P_{la})}{\dot{Q}}$$

Normal PVR is 1.5–3 mm Hg/L/min. Cardiac output is the same for right and left heart. It is calculated using either the Fick oxygen uptake or the dye dilution method.

In addition to measuring overall PVR, one can assess regional perfusion problems (thromboembolism) using ventilation-perfusion lung scanning and radiocontrast arteriography.

Pulmonary hypertension Pulmonary hypertension is increased pulmonary vascular resistance. It may be caused by elevated left atrial pressure associated with impairment of the left heart, left atrial obstruction, or left ventricular failure. It may also be caused by elevation of right ventricular pressure with a normal left heart as a result of pulmonic valve obstruction or, more commonly, pulmonary vascular obstruction. Pulmonary vascular obstruction is usually due to thromboembolism or severe chronic vasoconstriction from alveolar hypoxia. Giving supplemental oxygen therapy to raise alveolar oxygen tension has been shown to lower PVR and prolong life in patients with pulmonary hypertension from alveolar hypoxia and severe chronic lung disease.

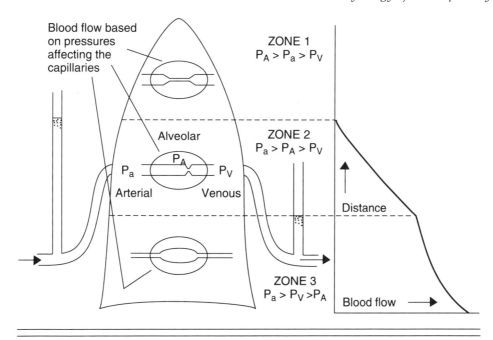

Blood flow based on pressures affecting the capillaries

ZONE 1
$P_A > P_a > P_V$

Alveolar

ZONE 2
$P_a > P_A > P_V$

P_a P_A P_V

Arterial   Venous

Distance

ZONE 3
$P_a > P_V > P_A$

Blood flow

Figure 2-18 Regional Differences in Pulmonary Blood Flow Related to Gravity, Alveolar Pressure, and Hydrostatic Pressure in Pulmonary Artery and Left Atrium
Source: West, J. B. (1989). *Respiratory Physiology: The Essentials* (4th Edition). Baltimore, MD: Williams and Wilkins, p. 41.

Primary and secondary causes of pulmonary hypertension are listed in Table 2-5.

Water balance The flow of interstitial fluid in the lung (F_L) is determined by the balance of intravascular (P_c) and interstitial (P_t) hydrostatic pressures and colloid osmotic (π_P, π_t) pressures,

Table 2-5 Causes of Pulmonary Hypertension

Primary Causes	Secondary Causes
Plexogenic arteriopathy	Alveolar hypoxia:
Veno-occlusive disease	Restrictive or obstructive lung disease
	Chest-wall deformity
	Hypoventilation
	High altitudes
	Pulmonary vascular obstruction:
	Pulmonary thromboembolism
	Pulmonary arteritis
	High-pressure mechanical ventilation
	Cardiogenic increased hydrostatic pressures:
	Left ventricular failure
	Mitral stenosis
	Left atrial myxoma
	Pulmonic stenosis
	Congenital heart disease with L-to-R cardiac shunt

$$F_L = k[(P_c - P_t) - (\pi_P - k\,\pi_t)]$$

where k is a permeability factor. Normally there is a low, continuous flow of fluid from pulmonary capillaries into the interstitium. This fluid returns to the circulation by way of the pulmonary lymphatics.

Increased interstitial water impairs respiration by increasing the distance for gas diffusion across the alveolar capillary surface.

Pulmonary Edema

Conditions that alter the normal filtration balance in the lung cause pulmonary edema. At first the fluid accumulates in the interstitium, but if the process continues unabated and the interstitial fluid volume increases by more than 50%, fluid ruptures into the alveoli. Physiological conditions causing pulmonary edema include:

1. Increased capillary hydrostatic pressure (left ventricular failure, fluid overload)
2. Reduced plasma colloid oncotic pressure (cirrhosis, nephrotic syndrome)
3. Lymphatic obstruction (lymphangitic carcinomatosis)
4. Reduced interstitial hydrostatic pressure (re-expansion pulmonary edema)
5. Increased capillary permeability (adult respiratory distress syndrome)

Hydrostatic pulmonary edema Normal left atrial pressure (P_{la}) is 3–5 mm Hg. If P_{la} exceeds 7–8 mm

Hg, the normally closed pulmonary vascular channels open and compliant arterioles dilate so that further increases in pressure are transmitted directly to the pulmonary artery and the work of the right ventricle is increased. When left atrial pressure exceeds 25–30 mm Hg, hydrostatic pressure begins to exceed the colloid osmotic pressure of the capillaries, and there is an increased flow of water into the interstitium; in the acute stage this flow exceeds the capacity of the lymphatic drainage. To effectively decrease hydrostatic pulmonary edema, left atrial pressure must be decreased.

Permeability pulmonary edema Pulmonary edema is also caused by compromises in the pulmonary capillary filtration barrier, which allow fluid rich in plasma protein to flow out of the capillaries into the interstitium. This permeability pulmonary edema occurs with adult respiratory distress syndrome, inhalational toxic injury, oxygen toxicity, radiation injury, and certain infections. Although keeping left atrial pressure low minimizes the hydrostatic component in such cases, permeability pulmonary edema is resolved by treating the cause of capillary compromise.

Pleural Effusion

There is also a continuous flow of fluid through the pleural space of the thorax. The fluid flows from the parietal pleura of the chest wall to the visceral pleura and is absorbed by the pulmonary lymphatics. The direction of this flow is principally determined by the higher hydrostatic pressure in the systemic capillary bed that perfuses the parietal pleura compared to that of the pulmonary capillary bed of the lung. Figure 2-19 illustrates normal pleural fluid dynamics.

Pleural effusion is the accumulation of fluid in the pleural space, which occurs when the balance of filtration forces between parietal and visceral pleura is altered.

Transudative pleural effusion Transudative pleural effusions are characterized by pleural fluid low in protein. The causes of transudative pleural effusion are the same as those of hydrostatic pulmonary edema: lymphatic obstruction (tumor), increased pulmonary capillary hydrostatic pressure (left ventricular failure), or reduced colloid oncotic pressure (nephrotic syndrome).

Exudative pleural effusion Inflammation of pleural surfaces promotes increased movement of water plus protein into the pleural space. Exudative pleural effusions have high protein concentrations. The fluid

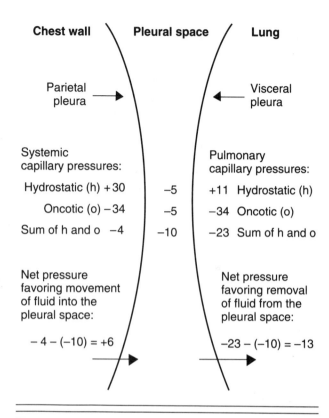

Figure 2-19 Normal Pleural Fluid Dynamics
Source: Martin, L. (1987). *Pulmonary Physiology in Clinical Practice.* St. Louis: The C. V. Mosby Company, p. 261.

may also have increased cellularity and alterations in chemistry (LDH, glucose, amylase, hyaluronic acid) and pH, depending upon the etiology. Causes of exudative pleural effusions include infection, malignancy, collagen vascular disease, thromboembolism, and benign asbestos pleural disease.

Ventilation-Perfusion Matching

The success of gas exchange between the atmosphere and the arterial blood depends not only on the total ventilation, total pulmonary perfusion, and free diffusion of the respiratory gases, but also on the ratio of ventilation to perfusion in the various regions of the lungs as well as over the entire lung surface.

John West's lung mixer model (Figure 2-20) illustrates the importance of matching ventilation with perfusion for setting the concentration of oxygen in the alveoli (P_AO_2) and hence in the arterial blood (P_aO_2). Powdered dye (representing oxygen, O_2) pours into the lung mixer (representing ventilation, $\dot{V}$) and water flows continuously through (representing perfusion, resulting from cardiac output, $\dot{Q}$), carrying off the dye (representing PO_2). The concentration of dye in the lung mixer (P_AO_2 and P_aO_2) is

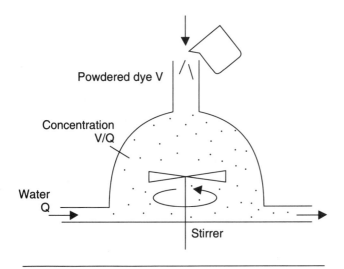

Figure 2-20 West Model Illustrating the Ventilation-Perfusion Ratio Determining PO_2
Source: West, J. B. (1989). *Respiratory Physiology: The Essentials* (4th Edition). Baltimore, MD: Williams and Wilkins, p. 58.

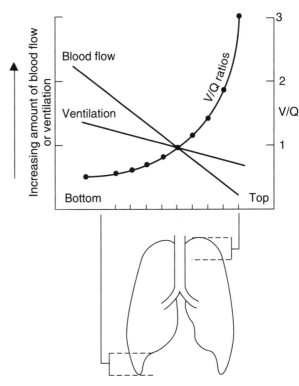

Figure 2-21 Regional Variation in Ventilation-Perfusion Matching in the Normal Upright Lung
Source: Martin, L. (1987). *Pulmonary Physiology in Clinical Practice: The Essentials for Patient Care and Evaluation.* St. Louis: The C. V. Mosby Company, p. 100.

determined not by the absolute quantity pouring in ($\dot{V}$), or by the flow carrying the dye away ($\dot{Q}$), but rather by the ratio of the two:

$$\frac{\dot{V}}{\dot{Q}}$$

V/Q imbalance is the cause of most pulmonary hypoxemia in clinical medicine. P_aO_2 may be reduced if ventilation is reduced relative to perfusion (as with asthma) or if perfusion is increased relative to ventilation (as with arteriovenous malformation). Both represent low V/Q states.

Regional V/Q Matching

The normal lung has regional differences in perfusion and ventilation, which are principally determined by gravity. Both ventilation and perfusion are greater in the dependent portions of the lung than in the uppermost lung. (In a person in the upright position, most blood and ventilation flow to the bases of the lung; in a person in the supine position the dependent regions are dorsal.) The gradient is steeper for perfusion. Hence, there is a normal imbalance of regional ventilation and perfusion in the lung. Figure 2-21 illustrates this imbalance: in the base of the lung perfusion is greater than ventilation (low V/Q) and in the apex the opposite is true (high V/Q). The mid-lung regions are evenly matched. Normal overall V/Q is 0.8. During exercise and other high output states, the match between ventilation and perfusion normally improves over the whole lung.

Physiologic Deadspace

Regions of lung in which perfusion is poor or absent relative to the ventilation received (high V/Q) are termed physiologic deadspace. The air ventilating these regions does not contribute normally to gas exchange; it has gas tensions approaching or equal to those of tracheal air. Most of the volume of deadspace in the normal lung is in the conducting airways (the anatomic deadspace); however, the uppermost portions of the resting lung also contribute to physiologic deadspace.

Venous Admixture

Regions of pulmonary perfusion in which ventilation is poor or absent relative to perfusion (low V/Q) are termed venous admixture regions. The pulmonary venous blood returning to the left heart from these regions has respiratory gas tensions that approach or are equal to those of mixed venous blood entering the lung in the pulmonary artery. The most dependent portions of the normal lung contribute some venous admixture blood to the pulmonary venous return. In the normal cardiopulmonary circulation, most venous admixture blood comes from normally occurring right-to-left shunts.

Right-to-left shunt   Right-to-left shunts are vascular channels that convey blood from the right heart into the left ventricle, thus preventing it from participating in gas exchange. Normally occurring right-to-left shunts are listed below.

1. Bronchial arteries to pulmonary veins
2. Lower esophageal veins to pulmonary veins
3. Coronary arteries to thebesian veins and left ventricle
4. Pulmonary arteriovenous connections

Two to four percent of cardiac output bypasses the alveoli in these normally occurring right-to-left shunts. In pathologic conditions, right-to-left shunts are found in the lung parenchyma (pneumonia) or vessels (arteriovenous malformation, cirrhosis) or in the heart (atrial septal defect with reverse flow).

V/Q and Gas Tensions

John West's V/Q diagram (Figure 2-22) helps explain the impact of ventilation-perfusion inequality on the concentration of respiratory gases in the lung. Regions of deadspace (high V/Q) are best identified by their impact on PCO_2. Regions of venous admixture and right-to-left shunt are best identified by their impact on PO_2. The extreme ends of this V/Q curve represent right heart and tracheal gas tensions.

Measurement of V/Q   In the research laboratory overall ventilation-perfusion matching is assessed

with a technique that measures the pulmonary distribution of multiple inert gases of various solubilities, administered simultaneously and correlated with cardiac output and minute ventilation. At the bedside overall V/Q matching is identified by analyzing gas exchange outcome and determining deadspace, venous admixture, and shunt fractions.

Physiologic deadspace (high V/Q) is determined as a fraction of tidal volume, $\frac{V_D}{V_T}$, by collecting arterial blood and mixed expired gas samples, measuring carbon dioxide tension, and applying the Bohr equation.

$$\frac{V_D}{V_T} = \frac{P_aCO_2 - P_ECO_2}{P_aCO_2}$$

P_aCO_2 is arterial carbon dioxide tension. P_ECO_2 is mixed expired carbon dioxide tension. Normal resting $\frac{V_D}{V_T} \leq 0.30$.

Venous admixture ($\dot{Q}_{va}/\dot{Q}_T$) is determined as a fraction of total blood flow by collecting arterial blood and mixed venous blood samples (mixed venous blood from the pulmonary artery), measuring or calculating oxygen content and applying the venous admixture equation:

$$\frac{\dot{Q}_{va}}{\dot{Q}_T} = \frac{C_{c'}O_2 - C_aO_2}{C_{c'}O_2 - C_{\bar{v}}O_2}$$

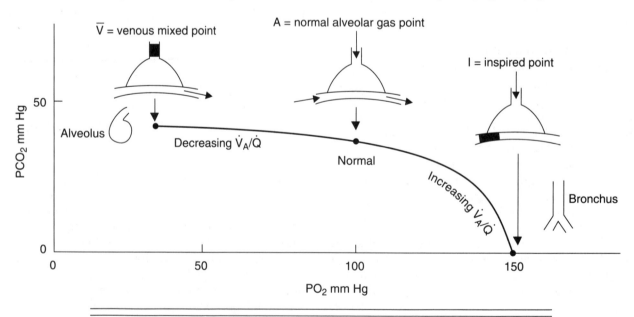

Figure 2-22   West O_2-CO_2 Diagram
Source: West, J. B. (1989). *Respiratory Physiology: The Essentials* (4th Edition). Baltimore, MD: Williams and Wilkins, p. 60.

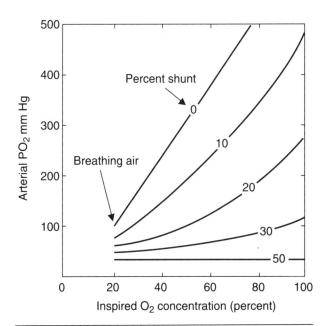

Figure 2-23 Response of P_aO_2 to Supplemental Oxygen in Right-to-Left Shunting
Source: West, J. B. (1991). *Pulmonary Pathophysiology: The Essentials.* Baltimore, MD: Williams and Wilkins, p. 174.

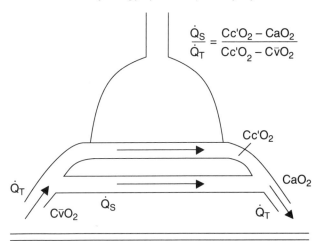

Figure 2-24 Right-to-Left Shunt
Source: West, J. B. (1989). *Respiratory Physiology: The Essentials* (4th Edition). Baltimore, MD: Williams and Wilkins, p. 56.

C_aO_2 is arterial content of oxygen:

$$C_aO_2 = .003 \cdot P_aO_2 + 1.34 \cdot Hb \cdot S_aO_2$$

$C_{c'}O_2$ is capillary content of oxygen:

$$C_{c'}O_2 = .003 \cdot P_AO_2 + 1.34 \cdot Hb \cdot S_AO_2$$

$C_{\bar{v}}O_2$ is mixed venous content of oxygen:

$$C_{\bar{v}}O_2 = .003 \cdot P_{\bar{v}}O_2 + 1.34 \cdot Hb \cdot S_{\bar{v}}O_2$$

Normal $\dot{Q}_{va}/\dot{Q}_T < 0.04$. (See the section on Gas Transport, pages 50–54, for further discussion of blood oxygen content.)

Right-to-left shunt ($\dot{Q}_s/\dot{Q}_T$) can be distinguished from venous admixture by measuring arterial and mixed venous blood gases after the patient has been breathing 100% oxygen for 20 minutes. Breathing 100% oxygen raises the alveolar oxygen tension of low V/Q (venous admixture) lung regions sufficiently to normalize the oxygen content of their capillary beds and remove their venous admixture effect on the arterial oxygen tension. Right-to-left shunts result in no ventilation of the blood flow and cannot be corrected with 100% oxygen (see Figure 2-23). As illustrated in Figure 2-24, the following

equation applies for the patient breathing 100% oxygen (normal $\dot{Q}_s/\dot{Q}_T < 0.03$):

$$\frac{\dot{Q}_s}{\dot{Q}_T} = \frac{C_{c'}O_2 - C_aO_2}{C_{c'}O_2 - C_{\bar{v}}O_2}$$

Some of the physiological conditions that can alter V/Q balance are listed in Table 2-6. Regional abnormalities in ventilation-perfusion matching can be caused by the presence of bullae, which are high V/Q regions of increased deadspace accompanying emphysema, or by pulmonary arteriovenous malformations, which create regions of right-to-left shunt.

Diffusion

Diffusion is the movement of molecules from a region of higher concentration to one of lower concentration. It occurs by the random kinetic motion of the molecules.

Driven by muscular work, the process of ventilation delivers a mass of conditioned air to the terminal

Table 2-6 Conditions That Alter V/Q Balance

Low V/Q, High $Q_{VA}/\dot{Q}_T$	High V/Q, High V_D/V_T
Asthma	Emphysema
Chronic bronchitis	Pulmonary thromboembolism
Pneumonia	Pulmonic stenosis
Pulmonary edema	High pressure mechanical ventilation
Interstitial fibrosis	
Pulmonary arteriovenous malformation	

bronchioles. From this point bulk movement ceases and further gas exchange of oxygen and carbon dioxide between the terminal bronchioles and the capillary blood occurs by the process of diffusion.

In discussing diffusion, consideration is given to the specific gas constituents of the air mixture rather than to the mass movement of air (ventilation). The atmosphere is a mixture of several gases, principally oxygen and nitrogen. The pressure and volume relationships of these gases are defined by the ideal gas law:

$$PV = nRT$$

where

P = pressure of the gas
V = volume of the gas
T = temperature of the gas
n = number of moles of the gas
R = the gas constant

Hence, the pressure of a gas varies directly with the number of moles and the temperature of the gas and inversely with the volume of the gas.

Atmospheric Pressures

Each gas in the atmospheric mixture contributes to the total pressure of the atmosphere in direct proportion to its concentration. Barometric pressure, the pressure of the atmospheric gases bombarding earth's surface, is the total pressure of the gases we breathe; it is the sum of the partial pressures of the individual gases:

$$P_T = PN_2 + PO_2 + PCO_2 + PH_2O + \ldots$$

At sea level the average total atmospheric pressure is 760 mm Hg. The concentration of nitrogen is approx-imately 78.62%; hence, PN_2, the average partial pressure of nitrogen at sea level, is 597 mm Hg (.7862 × 760). The concentration of oxygen is approximately 20.84%; hence, PO_2, the average partial pressure of oxygen at sea level, is 159 mm Hg (.2084 × 760). Atmospheric pressure is lower above sea level (at high altitude) and higher below sea level (in deep-sea diving). (For example, the pressure of oxygen drops from 109 mm Hg at 10,000 feet to 47 mm Hg at 30,000 feet.)

When atmospheric air enters the trachea, it is conditioned by the upper airway, warmed to 37°C, and humidified. The PH_2O rises to 47 mm Hg, which causes the concentration of the other gases to fall slightly, since the total pressure remains equivalent to atmospheric pressure (760 mm Hg at sea level). Changes in partial pressures of respiratory gases during breathing are listed in Table 2-7.

Alveolar Gas Equation

As the conditioned oxygen mixture diffuses into the alveoli, the partial pressure of oxygen (PO_2) falls again as carbon dioxide and oxygen are exchanged across the alveolar-capillary membrane. The alveolar oxygen tension can be calculated by using the alveolar gas equation:

$$P_AO_2 = F_IO_2 (P_B - PH_2O) - P_aCO_2/R$$

where

P_AO_2 = partial pressure of alveolar oxygen
F_IO_2 = fraction of inhaled oxygen
P_B = barometric pressure
PH_2O = water vapor pressure
P_aCO_2 = partial pressure of arterial carbon dioxide
R = the respiratory quotient

Table 2-7   Partial Pressures of Respiratory Gases as They Enter and Leave the Lungs (at sea level)

	Atmospheric Air* (mm Hg)	Humidified Air (mm Hg)	Alveolar Air (mm Hg)	Expired Air (mm Hg)
N_2	597.0 (78.62%)	563.4 (74.09%)	569.0 (74.9%)	566.0 (74.5%)
O_2	159.0 (20.84%)	149.3 (19.67%)	104.0 (13.6%)	120.0 (15.7%)
CO_2	0.3 (0.04%)	0.3 (0.04%)	40.0 (5.3%)	27.0 (3.6%)
H_2O	3.7 (0.50%)	47.0 (6.20%)	47.0 (6.2%)	47.0 (6.2%)
TOTAL	760.0 (100.00%)	760.0 (100.00%)	760.0 (100.0%)	760.0 (100.0%)

*On an average cool, clear day.
Source: Guyton, A. C. (1991). *Textbook of Medical Physiology* (8th Edition). Philadelphia: W. B. Saunders Company, p. 424.

P_aCO_2 is assumed to equal alveolar CO_2 tension because of the rapid diffusion of this gas between capillary and alveolus. F_IO_2 is 0.208 when a person is breathing atmospheric air; supplemental oxygen therapy increases F_IO_2 from 0.208 to 1.00. The respiratory quotient, R, is the ratio of carbon dioxide output ($\dot{V}CO_2$) to oxygen uptake ($\dot{V}O_2$) at the lungs:

$$R = \frac{\dot{V}CO_2}{\dot{V}O_2}$$

Normal R = 0.8.

Respiratory Quotient

The respiratory quotient (R) is determined by three things:

1. The metabolic substrate (carbohydrate, fat, protein) used to fuel oxidative phosphorylation
2. The proportion of anaerobic metabolism contributing to energy needs (i.e., the adequacy of the oxygen supply to the tissues)
3. The bicarbonate buffer state of the individual

In steady-state conditions R reflects the metabolic respiratory exchange ratio in the tissues. A healthy individual who consumes a typical American diet with moderate to high fat content has an R value of 0.8. In the hospital a patient receiving only carbohydrate nutrition may have R as high as 1.0. R exceeds 1.0 in individuals who are exercising above their anaerobic thresholds. The critically ill, who have metabolic requirements exceeding tissue oxygen delivery (lactic acidosis), also may have R values greater than 1.0. When the means of measuring oxygen and carbon dioxide uptake and release are not available and R is needed to calculate alveolar oxygen tension in the alveolar gas equation, it is estimated from knowledge of the metabolic status of the patient.

Alveolar-Capillary Interface

Oxygen diffuses from the alveolus across the alveolar-capillary interface into the capillary blood down a concentration gradient. Partial pressure of oxygen in the alveolus (P_AO_2) is normally 100 mm Hg; normal mixed venous oxygen ($P_{\bar{v}}O_2$) entering the capillary bed is 40 mm Hg. The diffusion of oxygen from gas into liquid is determined by the area and thickness of the membrane interface, the pressure differential across the membrane, the molecular weight of oxygen, and its solubility. Although oxygen is highly soluble, carbon dioxide is much more soluble; it diffuses twenty times more rapidly than does oxygen.

Although the alveolar capillary surface is vast (70 m²) it is very thin (0.5 micron). These characteristics greatly facilitate gas exchange. The layers of the alveolar capillary interface are as follows:

1. The surfactant fluid lining the alveoli
2. The alveolar cell epithelium
3. The epithelial basement membrane
4. The interstitial space
5. The capillary basement membrane
6. The capillary endothelial cell membrane

Once oxygen has diffused through the alveolar capillary membrane, it moves through the plasma to the red cell and across its membrane. In the red cell it combines with hemoglobin. It is in this combined form that 98% of the oxygen is carried to the tissues.

The resistance to movement of oxygen from the gas phase into its hemoglobin combined state is described by the equation

$$\frac{1}{D_L} = \frac{1}{D_M} + \frac{1}{\Theta V_c}$$

where

$\frac{1}{D_L}$ = the total diffusion resistance

$\frac{1}{D_M}$ = the resistance attributable to diffusion through the alveolar-capillary membrane

Θ = the rate of reaction of oxygen with hemoglobin

V_c = the volume of capillary blood

Pulmonary Capillary Transit

Normally, the transit time of red cells through the pulmonary capillary bed is long enough to allow diffusion to saturate the hemoglobin. However, during vigorous exercise (when transit time shortens) or in disease states (when diffusion is slowed by a thickened alveolar-capillary membrane), full saturation of hemoglobin does not occur.

Measurement of Diffusion

Diffusion is assessed by measuring the alveolar-arterial oxygen tension difference and the diffusing capacity.

Alveolar-Arterial Oxygen Difference The alveolar-arterial oxygen difference ($P_{(A-a)}O_2$) is the difference in oxygen tension between alveolar and arterial blood. It is calculated by subtracting arterial oxygen tension (PaO_2, measured directly from arterial blood) from PAO_2 (determined from the alveolar gas equation):

$$P_{(A-a)}O_2 = (P_B - 47)\,F_IO_2 - (P_aCO_2/R) - P_aO_2$$

Normal $P_{(A-a)}O_2 < 18$. P_aO_2 decreases normally with hypothermia (each degree centigrade causes a 3% change in P_aO_2), with increasing age (3–4 mm Hg per decade over thirty years), and at high altitudes. The expected P_aO_2 when a patient is receiving supplemental oxygen can be estimated by multiplying the oxygen percentage by 6. $P_{(A-a)}O_2$ normally increases with increasing age and with increasing F_IO_2.

When disease thickens the alveolar-capillary interface, obstructing normal diffusion of alveolar oxygen, $P_{(A-a)}O_2$ rises. (Because of its greater solubility, carbon dioxide is little affected.) However, $P_{(A-a)}O_2$ also rises when overall ventilation or perfusion is impaired, particularly when there is significant venous admixture or right-to-left shunt. (Such conditions are described further in the section on Ventilation-Perfusion Matching, pages 44–47)

Diffusing capacity   The diffusion (or transfer) factor is normally assessed by measuring the rate of uptake of carbon monoxide (CO) by the lung after inhalation of a single breath of 0.3% CO. Carbon monoxide is preferred to oxygen when measuring because the rate of reaction of carbon monoxide with hemoglobin is so fast that its uptake across the lung primarily reflects the alveolar-capillary membrane resistance, $\frac{1}{D_M}$.

Like increases in $P_{(A-a)}O_2$, reduction in the carbon monoxide diffusing capacity (D_{LCO}) may be due either to abnormalities in the alveolar-capillary membrane or to impairment of overall ventilation or perfusion (especially increased deadspace). Conditions that specifically impair membrane transfer include those that (1) increase the thickness of the membrane (pulmonary edema, interstitial fibrosis), (2) decrease its surface area (emphysema), or (3) decrease its hemoglobin uptake (carbon monoxide). In critically ill patients, diffusion is most often acutely altered by increased interstitial and alveolar fluids (pulmonary edema).

Gas Transport

Respiration is the exchange of oxygen and carbon dioxide between tissues and the atmosphere. Once oxygen has been provided to the capillary blood by ventilation, gas diffusion, and matched perfusion, the oxygen must be transported to the tissues, where it is taken up by the tissue mitochondria (in exchange for CO_2) to contribute to oxidative phosphorylation. Respiration is complete when this final process of delivery and uptake has occurred. Figure 2-25 provides a diagram of this process.

Oxygen Content of Blood

Oxygen diffuses across the alveolar capillary membrane and dissolves in the pulmonary capillary blood. Its concentration in solution is proportional to its partial pressure in the gas phase in the alveolus, but its content in solution is indirectly related to partial pressure. Oxygen is carried by the blood in two forms: as dissolved oxygen (3–8%) and as oxygen combined with hemoglobin (92–97%).

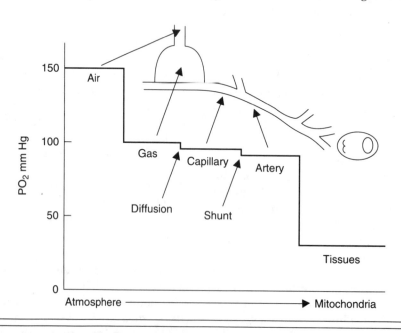

Figure 2-25   Movement of O_2 from Atmosphere to Mitochondria
Source: West, J. B. (1989). *Respiratory Physiology: The Essentials* (4th Edition). Baltimore, MD: Williams and Wilkins, p. 55.

Oxygen combines reversibly with hemoglobin and is primarily transported in this combined form. (The proportion of oxygen in solution to hemoglobin-combined oxygen depends on the F_IO_2 and the fraction of venous admixture.) The total oxygen content of blood (C_aO_2) is determined by the oxygen tension (P_aO_2), the hemoglobin concentration (Hb), and the fraction of the hemoglobin in the arteries that is saturated with oxygen (S_aO_2).

$$C_aO_2 = 0.003\ P_aO_2 + 1.34 \cdot Hb \cdot S_aO_2$$

where

0.003 = the oxygen solubility coefficient
1.34 = the number of mL of oxygen that can combine with one gram of hemoglobin

(Normal CaO_2 = 19.4 volume %.) Hemoglobin concentration and oxyhemoglobin saturation are the key determinants of blood oxygen content.

Oxyhemoglobin dissociation curve Oxygen tension (PO_2) is directly proportional to oxyhemoglobin

saturation (SO_2); the relationship is described by the sigmoidal oxyhemoglobin dissociation curve (Figure 2-26). In the range of normal sea level P_aO_2, 80–100 mm Hg, the S_aO_2 is 0.95–0.97 and the oxyhemoglobin curve is relatively flat. In this range, large changes in the P_aO_2 have little impact on the S_aO_2 and oxygen content of the blood. When the P_aO_2 is 60 mm Hg and the S_aO_2 is 0.9, the curve begins to drop off, and further decreases in P_aO_2 have a big impact on the S_aO_2 and oxygen content of the blood. Hence, when the P_aO_2 is over 65–70 mm Hg, a patient is in a zone of safety; small fluctuations in the P_aO_2 will do little harm to the patient's oxygen content. A P_aO_2 of 40 mm Hg yields an S_aO_2 of 0.75, the normal value for mixed venous blood entering the lungs to be oxygenated. A P_aO_2 of 27 mm Hg is the tension at which normal hemoglobin is 50% saturated.

The exact position of the oxyhemoglobin dissociation curve along the horizontal axis depends upon blood pH, $PaCO_2$, body temperature, variations in the structure of the hemoglobin molecule, and the 2,3 DPG content of the red cell. Shifting the curve to the right has the effect of reducing the affinity of

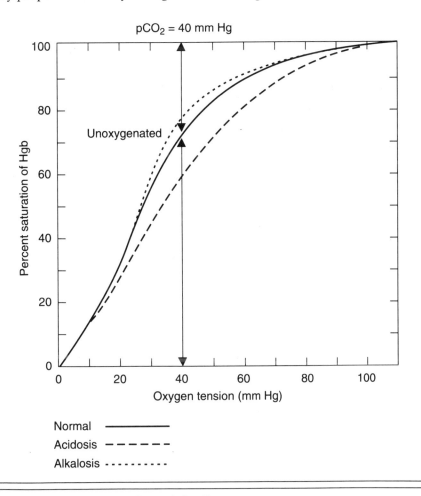

Figure 2-26 Oxyhemoglobin Dissociation Curve

hemoglobin for oxygen at a given PO_2; shifts to the left increase oxyhemoglobin affinity. Factors affecting oxygen affinity and oxygen dissociation curve shifts are listed in Table 2-8.

The Bohr effect (illustrated in Figure 2-27), is the right shift of the oxyhemoglobin dissociation curve caused by increased CO_2 tension in the blood. This shift facilitates unloading of oxygen from hemoglobin in the periphery as CO_2 diffuses into the capillary blood. The converse is the Haldane effect, which occurs in the pulmonary capillary bed. CO_2 tension falls as ventilation removes CO_2 from the lung, increasing hemoglobin's affinity for oxygen and facilitating oxygen loading in the lung.

Hypoxemia and hypoxia Hypoxemia is a state of inadequate oxygenation of the arterial blood, or low C_aO_2. Oxygen content is reduced by a low hemoglobin concentration (anemia) and reduced arterial oxyhemoglobin saturation (S_aO_2). Low S_aO_2 may be due to a shift in the oxyhemoglobin dissociation curve (as with hemoglobinopathy, MetHb, etc.), but it is most often due to respiratory system impairment resulting from one of the following:

1. Hypoventilation (normal $P_{(A-a)}O_2$; normal $\dot{Q}_s/\dot{Q}_T$), which is treated by increasing ventilation
2. Diffusion impairment (increased $P_{(A-a)}O_2$; normal $\dot{Q}_s/\dot{Q}_T$), which is treated by increasing F_IO_2

3. Ventilation-perfusion imbalance (increased $P_{(A-a)}O_2$; normal $\dot{Q}_s/\dot{Q}_T$), which is the most common cause of pulmonary hypoxemia and is treated by increasing F_IO_2
4. Right-to-left shunt (increased $P_{(A-a)}O_2$; increased $\dot{Q}_s/\dot{Q}_T$), which is treated with F_IO_2 and PEEP or with procedures specific to the site of the shunt

Hypoxia is a state that develops when oxygen supplies are inadequate to meet the metabolic needs of the individual. Hypoxia is often due to hypoxemia, but it can occur with a normal C_aO_2, when the delivery of oxygen is impaired by cardiac insufficiency or tissue uptake of oxygen is prevented by maldistribution of blood flow or metabolic poisons. Physiological factors causing hypoxia are listed in Table 2-9.

Oxygen uptake Oxygen delivery to the periphery, $\dot{D}O_2$, is determined by the oxygen content of the blood and by cardiac output.

$$\dot{D}O_2 = \dot{Q} \cdot C_aO_2$$

(Normal $\dot{D}O_2$ is 1020 mL/min.) Tissue uptake of oxygen from the capillary blood and release of carbon dioxide occur by diffusion, along the concentration gradient for each gas. The arteriovenous oxygen difference across each organ depends upon that organ's rate of metabolism and blood flow. (The normal average of $C_{a-\bar{v}}O_2 = 5$ vol %; $P_{a-\bar{v}}O_2 = 60$ mm Hg.) The utilization coefficient is the fraction of blood that releases oxygen as it passes through the tissue capillary bed. During vigorous exercise or in other hypermetabolic states, the utilization coefficient may triple. During sepsis syndromes, when blood is inappropriately diverted away from hypermetabolic tissues, it falls. (The normal resting average utilization coefficient is 25%.)

Total oxygen uptake is measured directly by collecting a sample of exhaled air and finding the difference between inhaled and exhaled oxygen volume per minute (normal resting $VO_2 = 250$ ml/min):

$$\dot{V}O_2 = \dot{V}_I \cdot F_IO_2 - \dot{V}_E \cdot F_EO_2$$

It can also be determined indirectly by using a modification of Fick's equation, measuring cardiac output ($\dot{Q}$) in liters per minute, hemoglobin concentration (Hb) in gm per 100 mL, and the oxyhemoglobin saturations of arterial (S_aO_2) and mixed venous ($S_{\bar{v}}O_2$) blood:

$$\dot{V}O_2 = 13.4 \cdot \dot{Q} \cdot Hb (S_aO_2 - S_{\bar{v}}O_2)$$

Table 2-8 Factors Affecting Oxygen Affinity and Oxygen Dissociation Curve Shifts

Left Shift	Right Shift
Decreased H^+	Increased H^+
Acidosis	Alkalosis
Polycythemia	Anemia
Decreased temperature	Increased temperature
Decreased $PaCO_2$	Increased $PaCO_2$
Decreased PO_4	Increased PO_4
Stored blood (2,3 DPG)	
Increased CO	
Fetal hemoglobin	
Methemoglobin	
Abnormal hemoglobins:	Abnormal hemoglobins:
Hb (Chesapeake)	Hb (Kansas)
Hb (Little Rock)	Hb (Bristol)
Hb (Ranier)	Hb (Seattle)

Source: J. Wright et al.

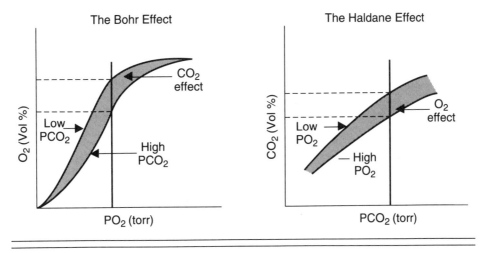

Figure 2-27 The Bohr and Haldane Effects
Source: Slonim, N. B., and Hamilton, L. H. (1981). *Respiratory Physiology* (4th Edition). St. Louis: The C. V. Mosby Company, p. 136.

13.4 is a constant factor representing the oxyhemo-globin combining coefficient and a unit conversion factor.

Normal individuals can rapidly increase oxygen uptake ninefold by tripling both cardiac output and tissue oxygen extraction (the factors in the system that can be readily changed). Each of these factors can also provide compensation if the other is im-paired. Hence patients with chronic heart failure, for example, exhibit increased tissue oxygen extraction reflected in a low $S_{\bar{v}}O_2$ when their bodies' oxygen demands exceed their cardiac capacity. Increases in oxygen demand beyond this adaptive capacity cause metabolic acidosis from anaerobic metabolism. Con-versely, patients suffering chronic lung disease or other causes of persistently low oxyhemoglobin

Table 2-9 Physiological Causes of Hypoxia

Condition	Indication	Possible Etiology

Hypoxemia	Reduced PaO_2	Nonrespiratory:
		   R-to-L cardiac shunt
		   Low mixed venous PO_2
		   Low PIO_2
		Respiratory:
		   Hypoventilation
		   Diffusion defect
		   V/Q imbalance
		   R-to-L pulmonary shunt
		Artifact:
		   Extremely high WBC
		   Hyperthermia

	Reduced SaO_2	COHb MetHB SuHb Congenital hemoglobinopathy Plasma factors: temperature, pH, 2,3 DPG
	Reduced Hb content	
Reduced oxygen delivery	Reduced cardiac output (Q) L-to-R systemic shunt	
Decreased tissue oxygen uptake	Displaced oxyhemoglobin dissociation curve (left shift) Mitochondrial poison	

saturations develop chronic compensatory polycythemia to maintain adequate oxygen content and tissue delivery.

Lactic Acidosis The hallmark of hypoxia is increased lactic acid production, as cells resort to anaerobic metabolism to supplement ATP production for energy needs. Although normal individuals develop lactic acidosis at the highest levels of exercise, the condition is abnormal at low levels of exercise or at rest. Pathologic lactic acidosis is usually due to low cardiac output or an inability to raise cardiac output to meet increasing metabolic needs. However, it can be caused by impairment of any of the systems that determine oxygen uptake: cardiac output ($\dot{Q}$), hemoglobin concentration (Hb), arterial oxyhemoglobin saturation (S_aO_2), or tissue oxygen extraction ($S_aO_2 - S_{\bar{v}}O_2$). Normal $S_{\bar{v}}O_2 = 0.75$; normal $S_aO_2 - S_{\bar{v}}O_2 = 0.22$. Low tissue oxygen extraction is reflected in an inappropriately high $S_{\bar{v}}O_2$ or low $S_aO_2 - S_{\bar{v}}O_2$ difference; it can be caused by inappropriate regulation of perfusion (sepsis) or by metabolic poisons such as cyanide.

Carbon dioxide output Carbon dioxide is transported in blood in three major forms: as dissolved carbon dioxide (5%), as bicarbonate (90%), and as carbamino compounds (5%). Bicarbonate is formed when CO_2 enters the red cell; intracellular carbonic anhydrase promotes the reaction of CO_2 with water to form hydrogen ion and bicarbonate. Bicarbonate diffuses out of the red cell as the concentration increases and chloride enters to maintain electrical neutrality. The hydrogen ion binds to hemoglobin, shifting the oxyhemoglobin dissociation curve to the right, facilitating the unloading of oxygen. The Haldane effect (Figure 2-27) is the increased bicarbonate capacity of blood resulting from deoxygenation of hemoglobin. It is a reciprocal of the Bohr effect. Carbamino compounds are formed by the reaction of CO_2 with the terminal amino acids of blood proteins, principally the globin of hemoglobin.

The CO_2 dissociation curve depicts the relationship of PCO_2 to total blood CO_2 content; it is relatively linear over the normal range of CO_2 tensions (35–45 mm Hg).

Although CO_2 output ($\dot{V}CO_2$) increases nine to tenfold under hypermetabolic conditions such as vigorous exercise, increased production does not cause elevated blood CO_2 tensions. (Normal resting $\dot{V}CO_2 = 200$ mL/min.) Conditions that alter carbon dioxide clearance cause elevated P_aCO_2 and respiratory acidosis and include hypoventilation, as in the case of sedative overdose, and severe ventilation-perfusion imbalance, which accompanies severe chronic airflow obstruction.

Respiratory exchange quotient The respiratory exchange quotient (R) is the ratio of carbon dioxide output ($\dot{V}CO_2$) to oxygen uptake ($\dot{V}O_2$) at the mouth.

$$R = \dot{V}CO_2/\dot{V}O_2$$

Normal R = 0.8. (See the section on Diffusion, pages 47–50, for further discussion of R.)

Control of Breathing

The mechanism that synchronizes ventilation and metabolic needs is critical to respiratory function. Ventilation must match carbon dioxide production so that carbon dioxide tension does not increase or decline in the blood, causing acidosis or alkalosis by altering the Henderson-Hasselbach balance:

$$pH = \frac{6.1 + \log [HCO_3]}{0.03 \cdot PCO_2}$$

Ventilation must also meet oxygen demands so that anaerobic metabolism does not occur, causing metabolic acidosis.

The respiratory control system has three parts, as diagrammed in Figure 2-28: sensors, central control, and effectors. The effectors are the muscles of respiration (described in the section on ventilation). The sensors gather information and deliver it to the central controllers, where the information is coordinated, needs are assessed, and impulses are transmitted to the effectors. The respiratory sensors are shown in Figure 2-29 and include central chemoreceptors, peripheral chemoreceptors, and mechanoreceptors.

Central Chemoreceptors

The most important sensors determining minute-to-minute control are in the brain stem, near the ventral surface of the medulla. These sensors respond to hydrogen ion concentrations. They are bathed in cerebral interstitial fluid; the pH of the fluid is determined by brain metabolism, cerebral blood flow, and most importantly, the constituents of the cerebrospinal fluid (CSF). The CSF is impermeable to the charged hydrogen and bicarbonate ions in the arterial blood, but carbon dioxide diffuses freely between blood and CSF. When PCO_2 rises in the arterial blood, it diffuses into the CSF. Catalyzed by carbonic anhydrase, the PCO_2 reacts with water and releases hydrogen ion, which stimulates the medullary receptors. Hence blood PCO_2 regulates ventilation by changing the pH of the CSF. Rising P_aCO_2 decreases the pH of the CSF, stimulating ventilation, which in turn decreases the P_aCO_2 (see Figure 2-30).

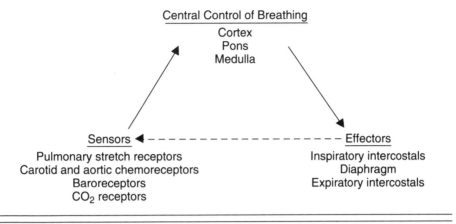

Figure 2-28 Elements of Respiratory Control

This central regulation is so well tuned that no fluctuation in arterial blood PCO_2 can be detected, even when tissue CO_2 production increases ninefold, as during exercise. CSF does not have the buffering capacity of blood; hence the pH of the CSF deviates more than arterial pH with changes in PCO_2 (normal CSF pH = 7.32). When the arterial PCO_2 is chronically elevated (as in chronic obstructive pulmonary disease, neuromuscular diseases, and severe kyphoscoliosis), there is an increase in bicarbon-ate transport into the CSF (within hours); however, the pH does not completely normalize. The central chemoreceptors are affected only by extreme changes in arterial blood pH in which the blood-brain barrier becomes partially permeable to hydrogen ion.

Peripheral Chemoreceptors

The peripheral chemoreceptors are located in carotid bodies at the bifurcation of the common carotids and in the aortic arch. Carotid bodies are

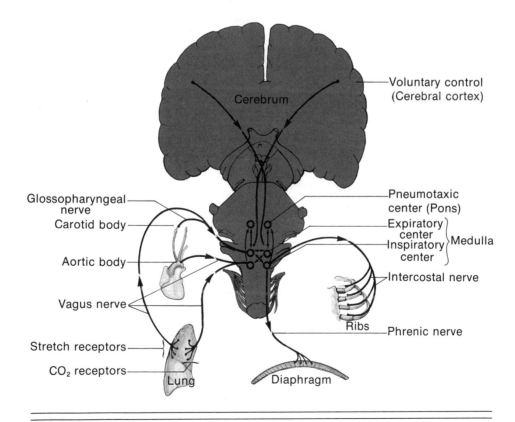

Figure 2-29 Chemical and Nervous Control of Respiration

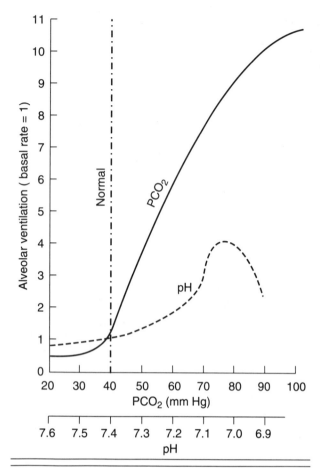

Figure 2-30   Relationship of Arterial PCO_2 and pH to Alveolar Ventilation
Source: Guyton, A. (1991). *Textbook of Medical Physiology* (8th Edition). Philadelphia: W. B. Saunders Company, p. 447.

2. Airway irritant receptors, which are found in airway epithelial cells and may cause bronchoconstriction and hyperpnea
3. J receptors, which are found adjacent to capillaries in alveoli and respond to distention of pulmonary capillaries and to increases in interstitial fluid to trigger rapid shallow breathing
4. Upper airway receptors
5. Muscle and joint stretch receptors
6. Peripheral pain and temperature sensors
7. Systemic artery receptors

Coughing, sneezing, and the Hering-Breuer reflex (switching off inspiration after a fixed volume of inflation) are all mediated by the mechanoreceptors.

Respiratory Control Center

The central control of rhythmic spontaneous breathing is achieved by the coordinated function of the three sites of specialized respiratory neurons in the brain stem: the medullary respiratory center, the lower pontine apneustic center, and the upper pontine pneumotaxic center. Respiratory components of the upper and lower pontine centers are illustrated in more detail in Figure 2-31. Sensory impulses from the peripheral receptors travel to the medullary center primarily by way of the vagus and glossopharyngeal nerves. The medullary center is in the reticular for-

most important, for these are the chemoreceptors that respond to changes in PO_2, PCO_2, and pH.

The unique function of the peripheral sensors is sensing oxygen tension in arterial blood. The ventilatory response to hypoxia is nonlinear. That is, ventilation increases slightly when P_aO_2 falls below 100 mm Hg and greatly when P_aO_2 is less than 60 mm Hg. Since normal arterial oxygen tension is 90 to 100 mm Hg, oxygen does not play a significant part in the control of normal breathing.

Mechanoreceptors

The peripheral mechanoreceptors deliver information to the respiratory control center. There are several types of mechanoreceptors:

1. Airway stretch receptors, which are smooth muscle stretch receptors that function to slow breathing frequency

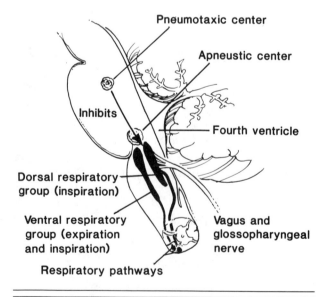

Figure 2-31   Organization of the Respiratory Center
Source: Guyton, A. C. (1991). *Textbook of Medical Physiology* (8th Edition). Philadelphia: W. B. Saunders Company, p. 445.

mation, adjacent to but separate from the medullary chemosensor. It includes a dorsal respiratory group (DRG) that controls inspiration and a ventral respiratory group (VRG) for expiration, which normally remains inactive during quiet breathing. The apneustic center generates impulses that stimulate the DRG, prolonging inspiration. The pneumotaxic center inhibits or turns off inspiration initiated by the DRG; hence it regulates breathing volume and rate.

The cerebral cortex also controls the medullary respiratory centers and can temporarily override medullary control (as during vocal expression). Supratentorial emotions, especially fear and anger, increase ventilation. There are breaking points for cerebral breath control, determined by pH and PCO_2, beyond which the automatic function prevails.

Impulses travel from central controllers to the diaphragm through the lateral corticospinal tracts, anterior horn cells, and phrenic nerve through the cervical plexus. The cervical level of phrenic origin is C4, with some contributions from C3 and C5. Impulses to the accessory muscles (including the scalene and sternocleidomastoids) travel through cranial nerves X through XII and cervical roots 1 through 3; impulses to intercostal muscles travel through thoracic nerves.

Measurement of Respiratory Drive

Assessment of control of breathing is made by measuring ventilatory responses to altered arterial oxygen and carbon dioxide tensions. Inhalation of 5% CO_2 normally doubles ventilation. Complete loss of respiratory control can be assessed in the mechanically ventilated patient by observing spontaneous respiratory effort when mechanical inflations are withheld. The patient is first administered 100% oxygen to assure adequate oxyhemoglobin saturation as PCO_2 is allowed to rise in the unventilated blood to stimulate breathing.

Disease conditions may impair this respiratory control system by altering any one of the three components of the system. Alteration of the central chemoreceptors is seen in patients with severe airflow obstruction (COPD) who chronically retain carbon dioxide because of ventilation-perfusion imbalance and increased work of breathing. Such patients often have medical histories of chronic airflow obstruction, elevated serum HCO_3^-, and polycythemia. They accumulate bicarbonate in their CSF, which results in a resetting of their medullary sensors. When acute or chronic ventilatory failure further increases P_aCO_2, respiratory drive does not respond in the normal way. In such cases the peripheral chemoreceptors, sensing hypoxia, are the primary source of sensory input for respiratory drive. Care

must be taken not to remove this hypoxic respiratory drive by administering a high dose of oxygen, raising P_aO_2 above 60–70 mm Hg, unless the patient's blunted respiratory drive is assisted with mechanical ventilation.

Alteration in the neuromuscular apparatus of the effectors also impairs control of breathing. Transection of the cervical spine above C4 eradicates most intercostal function and severely reduces or eliminates the diaphragm's contribution to ventilation. Some of these patients are able to ventilate with rapid shallow breaths using accessory muscles innervated by cranial nerves C1 and C2, which allows them to live without mechanical ventilatory support. Anterior horn cell diseases (poliomyelitis), nerve diseases (Guillain-Barré syndrome), neuromuscular junction disease (anticholinesterase insecticide poisoning and myasthenia gravis), and muscular dystrophy all can reduce ventilation by impairing the respiratory effectors.

Nonrespiratory Functions of the Respiratory System

In addition to gas exchange, the lung serves a number of nonrespiratory functions. Its defenses against foreign material include:

1. Cough and sneeze reflexes
2. Mucociliary escalator
3. Tissue and alveolar macrophages
4. Lymphatic drainage
5. Immunoglobins
6. Lymphocytes

The pulmonary circulation serves as a water and heat exchanger and a blood reservoir. It filters circulating particulate material and undissolved gas, protecting the brain and other vital organs from embolic infarction. The lung contributes to fibrinolysis and anticoagulation. It releases, removes, and transforms vital humoral substances, such as angiotensin 1.

Finally, the respiratory system contains the instrument of and provides the power for vocal communication, which has been key to the evolution of homo sapiens.

Assessment of the Respiratory System

It is necessary to understand that a patient's respiratory complaints will not always be straightforward, nor will the pathophysiology responsible for the production of these complaints be obvious. With experience and alertness, the responsible critical care nurse will develop the facility and intuitiveness necessary for valid clinical intervention strategies.

The evidence of pulmonary illness may be circumscribed in a vast psychophysiological process that compounds diagnostic efforts. The patient experiencing the stress of pain or dyspnea has a difficult time attending to the content and process of the clinical assessment until some relief is achieved. The patient will communicate discomfort nonverbally, exhibiting signs such as sighing, restlessness, spontaneous trance, or avoidance of eye contact and/or interpersonal interaction.

It is essential for all members of the health care team to have achieved the skills and knowledge that permit strategic assessment of a respiratory patient. The goal of strategic assessment is to provide the team with sufficient clinical data for ongoing assessment, diagnosis, and intervention. Physical examination and diagnostic study provide the objective information; the subjective data can only be described by the patient.

History

Since there is such a strong correlation between smoking and chronic pulmonary disease, heart disease, respiratory infections, and lung cancer, the need for an assessment of smoking history is obvious. Cigarette smoking history is recorded in pack years, or the number of packs per day the patient smoked multiplied by the number of years the smoking continued. If the patient smoked 2 packs a day for the last 5 years, the smoking history would be recorded as 10 pack years.

When taking a history from the patient who presents with pulmonary complaints, it is also important to determine the frequency and treatment success of the following diseases or conditions:

Pneumonia
Fungal disease
Colds
Bronchiectasis
Allergies
Pneumothorax
Heart disease
Heart failure
Heart or chest surgery
Occupationally related lung diseases
Pleural disease
Tuberculosis

Sinus infections
Asthma
Bronchitis
Emphysema
Hypertension
Congenital heart disease
Cancer
Toxic exposures

Furthermore, it is reasonable to assume that some abnormalities of the pulmonary system are manifestations of other pulmonary systemic disease processes. For this reason, assessment of the chest alone is insufficient, and a comprehensive evaluation of the patient's entire health status is important. Systemic diseases with accompanying pulmonary symptoms include:

Neoplastic diseases and their treatments
Congenital diseases, both treated and untreated
Thrombic and embolic phenomena resulting in pulmonary embolism
Acquired infectious disease processes
Pulmonary edema and associated processes
Connective tissue diseases

Physical Assessment

A thorough respiratory physical assessment is performed using all the senses in inspection, palpation, percussion, and auscultation. The physical examination of the patient should be performed in a multidimensional matrix of diagnostic, therapeutic, and caring perspectives.

Inspection

Inspection is the process of patient observation. Inspection can provide information regarding the following:

1. Level of consciousness
2. Thoracic configuration
3. Characteristics of breathing: rate and pattern, symmetry of chest movement, accessory muscle activity, presence of intercostal or sternal retractions
4. Characteristics of skin: color (cyanosis, flushing), diaphoresis
5. Characteristics of extremities: presence of edema, clubbing, capillary refill, venous distention, muscle wasting
6. Evidence of disorder: characteristic of cough, characteristic of sputum

An initial impression can be gained by observing the patient's level of consciousness and competency in interacting with the nurse, general state of health, current physical and emotional presentation, and vital signs. The following specific inspections should also be conducted.

Inspection of the skin The color of the patient's skin can suggest some clinical interpretations; for example, a yellow appearance may indicate the presence of bilirubin, a brown coloration of the skin may mean that excessive melanin is present, a bluish-gray discoloration may indicate argyria (silver ingestion), and a bright, rosy, pinkish color may lead one to suspect carbon monoxide poisoning. The clinical appearance of cyanosis should always be evaluated carefully. Cyanosis indicates an above-normal level of deoxyhemoglobin in the blood. The presence or absence of cyanosis is usually determined subjectively; the nurse's impressions may be influenced by such factors as thickness of skin, color of skin, environmental lighting, and the status of the superficial capillary bed. Special conditions may also mimic a cyanotic appearance. Argyria is not a true cyanosis. The discoloration of argyria does not blanch when pressure is delivered to the skin as does the discoloration with cyanosis. Methemoglobin should be suspected if the oxygen capacity is low in the presence of a normal total hemoglobin or if oximetry measurements are low in the presence of normal oxygen tension in the arterial blood. This clinical condition, if suspected, can be confirmed through spectroscopic analysis of the blood.

It should be noted that cyanosis is not always considered a reliable indicator of hypoxemia. Cyanosis is usually noted only when hypoxemia is severe, and often the observation of clinical cyanosis results from impaired blood flow rather than low PaO_2 concentrations. The level of unsaturated hemoglobin must reach at least 5 gm % before cyanosis can be observed. It can be evaluated centrally or peripherally, and it is considered best to assess for cyanosis by inspecting and observing the skin of the entire body, placing emphasis on the periphery, earlobes, lips, gums, and nail beds. Such inspection can lead to differential diagnosis. Peripheral cyanosis (acrocyanosis) is commonly found in conditions of reduced cardiac output, local reduction of blood flow, increased venous pressure, or local vasomotor disturbances. It does not usually affect the lips or gums. In contrast, central cyanosis is common in patients suffering advanced pulmonary disease, airway obstruction, pneumonia, chronic bronchitis, pulmonary edema, and cardiac defects. This cyanosis is representative of alveolar hypoventilation, physio-logic and anatomic shunting, the rare diffusion defect, and ventilation-perfusion abnormalities. It is important to note that decreased saturation of hemoglobin with the above antecedents can be life-threatening.

Signs of cyanosis must be considered in light of other clinical events. For example, since cyanosis is hemoglobin-dependent, the anemic patient may not show visible clinical cyanosis until significant hypoxemia exists. In contrast, polycythemic patients are likely to exhibit cyanosis but may not be hypoxic. When methemoglobinemia or sulfhemoglobinemia is documented, the presence of cyanosis is assessed as well. If a pathological function of the oxygen-hemoglobin mechanism is suspected, actual analysis of hemoglobin using co-oximetry is performed. This analysis provides information on actual hemoglobin content, saturation, methemoglobin, carboxyhemoglobin, and oxygen content.

Further assessment of the skin includes examining the extremities for clubbing, pedal edema, capillary refill, peripheral skin temperature, and scars of trauma or past surgeries. Clubbing is most commonly found with bronchogenic carcinoma, chronic obstructive lung diseases, and chronic cardiovascular disease. The pedal edema of chronic respiratory disease is usually associated with right-sided heart failure (cor pulmonale). Capillary refill of less than 3 seconds suggests a reduced cardiac output and that digital perfusion is poor. Changes in peripheral skin temperature may suggest peripheral vasoconstriction; the reduction in perfusion results in a loss of warmth in the extremities. Cool extremities indicate inadequate perfusion.

Inspection of the chest If at all possible, inspection of the chest should be performed with the patient sitting. Physical landmarks that can serve as references for thoracic components are presented in Figure 2-32. The normal adult thorax is longer laterally than it is anteroposteriorly. The thorax is normally symmetrical when viewed from most aspects. With advancing age some increase in the anteroposterior diameter occurs.

Certain bony abnormalities of the thorax significantly alter pulmonary function. All thoracic spine deformities can cause restricted ventilation. Pressure-volume loops demonstrate an inordinate work load and energy use in the effort to breathe because of the severe limitations imposed on chest distensibility. The patient with thoracic cage or spinal deformity who demonstrates substantial decreases in total lung capacity, vital capacity, tidal volume, and corresponding increased respiratory rates is at risk for cor pulmonale and other serious complications. Likewise, pneumonias in the structurally abnormal patient can prove to be especially disastrous.

Observation of Respiratory Rate and Pattern   Observing the various characteristics of breathing aids the nurse in assessing the patient's status. The normal adult respiratory rate is 12 to 20 breaths per minute, depending on age, weight, and metabolism. In the critical care environment, a more generous upper frequency of 30 breaths per minute is used as a standard. However, current clinical thought suggests that the patient whose spontaneous ventilatory rate exceeds 30 will not tolerate ventilatory weaning. The patient on mechanical ventilation during the acute phase of disease onset is done a disservice if kept at rates nearing 30 breaths per minute unless clinical necessity dictates. In the longer-term supportive or maintenance phase, respiratory rates can vary within the 25–30 breaths per minute range according to patient need, institutional protocol, and individual physician's experience. The judicious and appropriate use of pharmacological agents, when necessary, can benefit the patient substantially, both physiologically and psychologically. The ventilator must be adjusted for the patient's benefit—not just according to set protocol. To accomplish this, the flow settings, rate settings, sensitivity settings, tidal volume settings, I:E ratio times, and pressure settings must be determined individually for each patient according to current state of pathology, response to pathology, and the mechanical ventilation device used.

The normal individual of whatever age or metabolic status offers no positional preference for breathing. In contrast, patients who adopt specific body positions in an effort to reduce dyspnea or the work of breathing are providing evidence of their pathology, as detailed in Table 2-10.

Not only does patient positioning indicate clinical pathology, other signs serve as indicators as well. Rapid respiratory rates (tachypnea) may occur as a result of exercise, fever, reduced arterial oxygen content, acidosis, low pH, anxiety, and pain. Respiratory rates slower than 10 breaths per minute (bradypnea) may occur with head injuries (open or closed), hypothermia, or drug overdose, or as a side effect of narcotics. An increase in the depth of a respiration greater than normal is called hyperpnea. Hyperpnea may exist with or without hyperventilation and is caused by decreased $PaCO_2$ in the circulating blood as a result of increased ventilation.

Monitoring of respiratory pattern   Variations in respiratory rate and rhythm (respiratory pattern) also serve as indicators of underlying clinical conditions; these are delineated in Table 2-11.

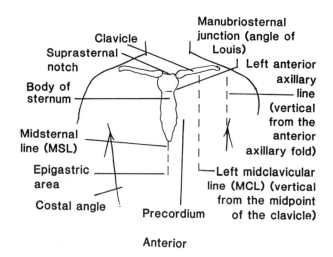

Anterior

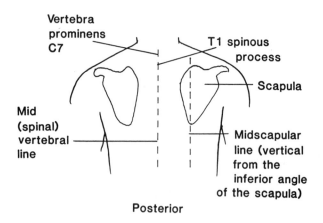

Posterior

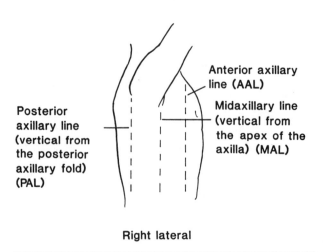

Right lateral

Figure 2-32   Physical Landmarks on the Chest

Table 2-10 Body Positioning Relating to Pulmonary Disorders

Position	Clinical Cause
Orthopnea (pillow)	Conjestive heart failure
Emphysematous habitus (pillow)	COPD
Obstructive sleep apnea (decreases when patient sleeps on side)	Obesity Obstructive sleep apnea syndromes
Orthodeoxia (relieved when patient lies supine)	Pulmonary fibrosis
Platypnea (pathology-specific)	Associated with various body positions, probably related to active pathology

Respiratory pattern monitoring is an old technique of monitoring a patient's ventilatory pattern using a variety of noninvasive technology methods. Most acute pulmonary deterioration is preceded by changes in the breathing pattern. Developing failure in the respiratory system is marked by changes in the ventilatory frequency, changes in normal abdominal and thoracic patterns for inspiration and expiration, decreasing tidal volume (V_T), and respiratory alternans. Real-time continuous monitoring of these parameters allows health care workers to carry out successful strategic interventions before severe ventilatory muscular failure and ventilatory deterioration occur. Ventilatory pattern monitoring may be useful in diagnosing diaphragmatic flutter or paralysis, upper airway obstruction, excessive work of breathing due to inappropriate ventilator methods and settings, central apneas, and failed thoracic cage. It is particularly useful when monitoring the difficult-to-wean patient. When used in conjunction with electrocardiographic monitoring, respiratory pattern monitoring can clarify the distinction between cardiac arrest and pulmonary cause of cardiac decompensation.

Palpation

Palpation is the process of using touch to determine physical signs. Generally, palpation techniques are used to determine the density of tissue and movement of the thorax. A number of other conditions can be determined by palpation:

Skin temperature
Skin moisture
Skin turgor
Symmetry of chest wall motion

Respiratory muscular use
Quality of pulmonary vibrations
Crepitus (subcutaneous emphysema)
Tracheal position
Chest wall tenderness

If a patient complains of chest wall pain or discomfort and distress, palpation of the spine and bony thorax is likely to reveal tenderness over the specified area.

Palpation of the thoracic cage may be particularly effective in differential diagnosis. It is accomplished by placing both hands on the posterior chest (or the anterior chest) with the thumbs contacting at the midspinal (or midsternal) line. The chest should move symmetrically and evenly. Asymmetrical chest movements may indicate:

Pulmonary parenchymal conditions
Massive unilateral atelectasis
Displaced endotracheal tube
Pneumothorax
Massive pleural effusion
Deformities of chest/spine
Flail chest (rib injuries)
Diseases of the pleura
Decreased hemidiaphragmatic excursion
Postoperative splinting

Palpation of the trachea reveals the placement of the trachea and serves as a sensitive indicator of the position of the mediastinum. The index finger is placed between the trachea and sternocleidomastoid muscle, and the space between these landmarks is assessed. Obviously, both lateral margins of the trachea need to be assessed to determine if tracheal deviation is present. In the older patient the otherwise normal trachea may be shifted to the right because of the pressure of an elongated atherosclerotic arch of the aorta.

The trachea can be shifted either toward the affected side or away from the affected side. The shift in the trachea toward the affected side is caused by a lack of mechanical/muscular ability, which decreases the distending forces of the lung in that area, causing the trachea to be pulled to the affected side from the lack of opposing air pressure. The shift to the unaffected side can be considered a compression of the good lateral side by the mass and extent of the mechanical and pressure forces being exerted by the pathological site. Pathological states indicated by tracheal shifts are listed below.

Shift Toward Affected Side:
Atelectasis

Table 2-11   Respiratory Patterns and Corresponding Clinical Conditions

Pattern	Condition
Eupnea: respiratory rate of 10–20 breaths per minute in adults, up to 44/min in infants	Normal
Hypopnea: shallow respirations, with possible increase in rate	Deep sleep CNS depression Circulatory failure Unconsciousness Meningitis
Hyperpnea: deep respirations with some rate increase; even, regular pattern	Exercise Anxiety Metabolic acidosis Midbrain and pons insult Acute infarction, hypoxia, or hypoglycemia
Bradypnea: slow respirations	Diabetic coma Drug-induced respiratory depression (alcohol or narcotics) Increased intracranial pressure Sleep Metabolic alkalosis Brain tumors Uremia
Tachypnea: rate > 20 breaths per minute; depth same or less than normal tidal breath	Restrictive lung disease Pleuritic chest pain Chest pain Elevated diaphragm Exercise Fever Hypoxia Anxiety Metabolic acidosis Obesity Brain lesions Drugs (aspirin)
Cheyne-Stokes respiration: Waxing and waning with periods of apnea between repetitive patterns; related to decreased cerebral oxygen caused by decreased cardiac performance or absent or diminished cerebral perfusion	Heart failure Renal failure (uremia) Drugs (morphine) Bilateral cerebral hemisphere or diencephalon brain damage Increased cerebral spinal fluid pressure Aortic valve lesions Meningitis
Biot's breathing (ataxic breathing): irregular and unpredictable ventilatory pattern with periods of apnea; impaired respiratory control centers	Respiratory depression Brain damage (medullary level) Meningitis Basal encephalitis Head trauma
Kussmaul breathing: hyperpneic respirations; fast, normal, or slow rate	Metabolic acidosis Diabetic ketoacidosis (pH 7.20–6.95) Renal failure Peritonitis
Sighing Occasional Frequent	 Normal Possible hyperventilation syndrome
Obstructive breathing	Prolonged expiration (I:E ratio of 1:4 considered indicative of obstruction)

Table 2-11   *(continued)*

Pattern	Condition
Paradoxical abdominal breathing: reversal of normal abdominal-thoracic sequence; discoordinated motion of chest wall and abdomen	Ventilatory muscular fatigue Acute respiratory failure Impending ventilatory failure Inappropriate ventilator settings (flow, timing, pressure) for patient's ventilatory drive needs Less than mechanically efficient body position
Apneustic breathing: sustained maximal inhalatory pause	Brain stem infarct Abnormal function of cerebral inspiratory/expiratory centers Pneumotaxis lesions
Apnea (absence of breathing)	Respiratory arrest Respiratory and cardiac arrest
Sustained exhalatory pause	
Sleep	>10 seconds and occurring >30 periods during sleep
Obstructive	Upper airway
Increased airway resistance	Tongue, facial defects, heavy alcohol use, increased upper airway gland size (tonsils)
Centrally controlled	Encephalitis
No initiation of inspiration	Brainstem infarct

Fibrosis
Pneumonectomy
Phrenic nerve paralysis
Partial closed pneumothorax
Shift Away from Affected Side:
  Pleural effusion
  Consolidation
  Mediastinal tumor
  Thyroid enlargement
  Pneumothorax
  Hemothorax

Palpation is also used in the determination of fremitus (vibrations of the chest wall created during speech or breathing). Vibrations during these activities are conducted through the bronchi and the pulmonary parenchyma to the skin surface, where the oscillations are felt as vibrations of the chest wall. To assess fremitus in the clinical situation, the nurse should ask the patient to speak phrases ("ninety-nine") or words ("one") repeatedly until the examination is finished. Bilateral fremitus should be checked and compared, over both the posterior and the anterior chest.

Increases in fremitus are usually associated with conditions that increase the density of the underlying tissue. Solid or liquid materials in these tissues transmit vibrations better than air; increased fremi-

tus is found in conditions where the ratio of solid or liquid matter to air is increased. Decreases in fremitus occur when there is an abnormal amount of air in the lung or the pleural space. Specific pathologies causing increased and decreased fremitus are listed in Table 2-12.

Percussion

Percussion is a technique of striking the thorax or body and interpreting the resulting audible vibrations. It is essential to perform percussion in a systematic manner and to compare a percussive finding with that on the corresponding location on the oppo-

Table 2-12   Fremitus in Pulmonary Disorders

Increased Fremitus	Decreased Fremitus
Pneumonia (consolidation)	Pleural effusion
Atelectasis	Pneumothorax
Fibrosis	Emphysema
Pulmonary edema	Pleural thickening
Abnormal tissue masses	Decreased air flow (obstruction)
Bronchitis	
Pleural inflammation	

site side of both posterior and anterior planes. The sequence of positions to be used in thoracic percussion is illustrated in Figure 2-33. It is important to realize that information gained by the use of percussion may be limited. Only very large lesions or pathological processes (pleural effusions exceeding 500 cc, lobar consolidation, or severe air trapping) can be determined by this technique. It is probably useless in the diagnosis and localization of small infiltrates, a small pneumothorax, or small pleural effusions.

There are two basic techniques of percussing the chest: direct (or immediate) percussion, and indirect (or mediate) percussion. Mediate percussion is the most frequently used technique, and it involves placing a finger firmly against the chest and tapping that finger with another. Usually the third or middle finger of the left hand (the pleximeter) is placed on the chest surface and tapped by the third finger of the right hand (the plexor). Direct percussion is performed directly onto the chest without the use of a pleximeter. The chest wall is struck directly with the pads of one or two fingers. This type of percussive technique can be used to assess abnormalities in the upper lobes by tapping the clavicles.

The pitch of the note produced is determined by the ratio of tissue containing air to solid tissue directly beneath the percussing finger. Normal percussion notes are presented in Figure 2-34. Appropriately aerated lung parenchyma produces a low-pitched sound that may be likened to a muffled drum. A sound higher in pitch but with a dull or flat note suggests an increased amount of tissue beneath the percussing finger. A percussion note that resonates will resonate at different pitches depending on the amount of air present. Below are descriptions of percussive notes and pathologies associated with them.

1. *Resonant*   Resonance is the sound produced when percussing normal lung tissue. It is low-pitched and nonmusical in character.

2. *Hyperresonant*   This is definitely an abnormal percussive note over the chest. It is a loud, low-pitched sound of long duration, possessing a slightly musical note. This percussive note is produced as sound passes through areas of tissue that have a greater proportion of air in relation to tissue (high air-to-tissue ratio). One may hear a hyperresonant sound in adults or children with thin chest walls. It is also characteristically heard over an air-filled stomach. The presence of hyperresonance indicates hyperinflation. Causes include

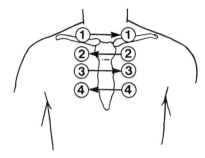

Anterior

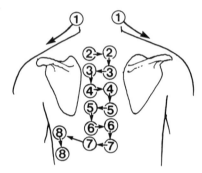

Posterior

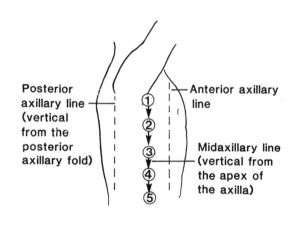

Right lateral

Figure 2-33   Sequence of Positions for Thoracic Percussion

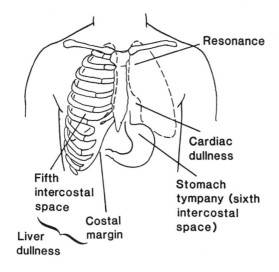

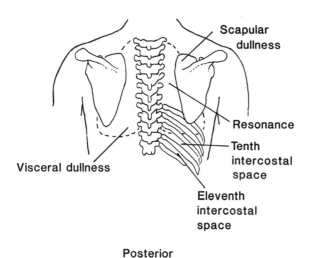

Figure 2-34 Normal Percussion Notes

a. air trapping of emphysema
b. asthmatic episode
c. pneumothorax

3. *Tympanic* A tympanic percussion note is produced by the presence of air in an enclosed chamber. It is a very high-pitched musical note of long duration. It may be described as "drum-like." Normally it can be heard only over a stomach bubble. It it always abnormal if heard in the chest. Causes include:

a. tension pneumothorax,
b. pulmonary cavities due to neoplastic or fungal processes.

4. *Dull* This is a sound of medium intensity and pitch and short duration. It is nonmusical and muffled. The presence of dull percussive notes indicates a decreased amount of air in the underlying structure. (*Note:* The same abnormal conditions responsible for an increased fremitus are usually responsible for dullness of percussive notes.) Normal areas of dullness in the chest include the chambers of the heart, liver, spleen, spine, diaphragm, and bony structures. It is not a normal sound over the lung fields. Causes include:

a. the presence of fluid in the pleural space,
b. pneumonia (consolidation),
c. atelectasis,
d. pulmonary fibrosis,
e. pulmonary edema,
f. neoplasm,
g. pleural thickening.

5. *Flat* A flat percussive note is an extreme example of the dull percussive note. It is a sound of low amplitude and pitch and resembles a "thud." It is characteristically heard over areas with no air content, such as the liver. Causes include:

a. pneumonectomy,
b. *large* pleural effusion,
c. massive atelectasis.

Diaphragmatic movement or mobility can be determined by percussion of the posterior chest wall, which should be performed while the patient is sitting upright. The patient should be instructed to take a deep breath and hold it while the posterior chest is percussed from top to bottom until the point where a dull note is heard. Then the patient is instructed to exhale as much as possible and to hold exhalation while percussion is performed again to determine the expiratory level of the diaphragm. Both hemidiaphragmatic regions should be examined in the above fashion. There should be a difference in diaphragmatic levels of 3–5 cm between inspiration and expiration. Causes of limited diaphragmatic excursion include (1) neuromuscular diseases, (2) emphysema, (3) restrictive disorders, and (4) chest-wall deformities. Causes of asymmetrical diphragmatic excursion include (1) phrenic nerve paralysis, (2) unilateral lung processes, and (3) unilateral pleural processes. (It is important to note that if the diaphragm is paralyzed unilaterally, diaphragmatic movement is paradoxical: rather than descending, the diaphragm ascends above resting level on inspiration.)

Auscultation

Auscultation involves the use of a stethoscope to listen to breath sounds to ascertain indicators of normal air flow, obstructed or pathological processes, or endotracheal placement and ventilator effectiveness. The order in which various points around the lungs should be auscultated is illustrated in Figure 2-35. Normal breath sounds can be auscultated in the selected thoracic regions indicated in Figure 2-36.

Breath sounds are reflective of the manner in which air swirls through the pulmonary passageways. Normal breath sounds are described below.

1. *Vesicular* Heard over most of the lung fields, these are soft, low-pitched sounds similar to the sound of wind rustling through trees. Inspiration is longer, higher-pitched, and louder than expiration.

2. *Bronchial* Heard near the manubrium, these are high-pitched and louder than vesicular sounds. In contrast to vesicular sounds, expiratory time is longer than inspiratory for bronchial sounds.

3. *Tracheal* Heard below the larynx and over the trachea, these are loud raspy sounds with a long inspiratory time followed by a pause, then a long expiratory time. If these sounds are heard directly over a lung field, they indicate some sort of pulmonary pathology.

4. *Bronchovesicular* These are heard over the bronchi on either side of the sternum and posteriorly between the scapulae. Inspiratory and expiratory times are equal.

Breath sounds indicating some sort of pulmonary pathology include the following.

1. *Crackles (rales)* Sounding like hair strands being rubbed between one's thumb and fingers, crackles indicate movement of air through fluidous tissue. Some crackles will clear with coughing, and these are considered benign. Crackles grow more coarse in sound

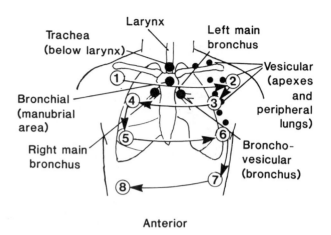

Anterior

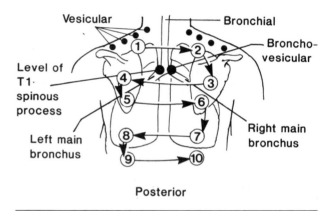

Posterior

Figure 2-35   Order of Sites for Auscultation

(gurgles) as more fluid accumulates. Medium and coarse crackles indicate congestive heart failure, pulmonary edema, bronchitis, and other bronchial inflammations.

2. *Wheezes* Wheezes are heard primarily during expiration. A wheeze is a high-pitched sound heard when air is being sucked past partially collapsed or obstructed airways. These sounds are heard with chronic bronchitis, asthma, aspiration of a foreign body, and cystic fibrosis.

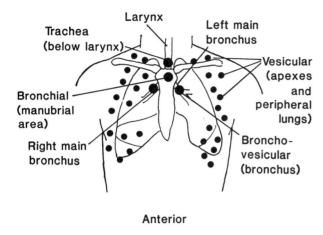

Anterior

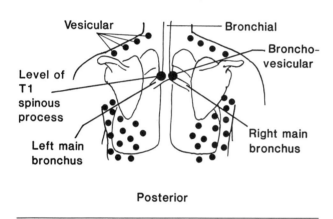

Posterior

Figure 2-36 Regions for Auscultation

3. *Pleural friction rub* A pleural friction rub is a grating sound caused by the viscera and parietal pleura rubbing against each other (they normally do so easily and smoothly). This sound worsens upon deep inspiration and is heard best in the lower anterior and lateral regions of the chest, for that is where thoracic movement is greatest. To differentiate this sound from a pericardial friction rub, the nurse should ask the patient to hold a breath; if the sound continues, it is pericardial in nature.[2]

Table 2-13 provides an overview of the results of inspection, palpation, percussion, and auscultation with various disease states.

Arterial Blood Gas Analysis

The interaction of states occurring in the cardiovascular and pulmonary systems is reflected in the arterial blood gases. The total gas exchange occurring in the body is reflected in the blood leaving the right side of the heart. Blood leaving the left ventricle reflects the degree of oxygen exchange and mechanical ventilating ability.

Any change in cardiopulmonary status results in changes in arterial blood gas values, and these, in turn, lead to changes in pulmonary and renal systems as they attempt to compensate for the imbalance. The degree of a physiological abnormality is determined broadly by the severity and acuteness of the disease process and the degree of increased compensatory work by the cardiopulmonary system. Arterial blood gas analysis provides very essential and critical data: the patient's acid-base state, the ventilatory status, and the oxygen status. (It should be noted that normal arterial blood gases do not mean that cardiopulmonary disease is absent. Abnormal arterial blood gases, however, do mean that an uncompensated disease is present.)

When sampling arterial blood for laboratory analysis, the nurse must keep certain key factors in mind. First, arterial puncture may cause vascular spasm, intraluminal clotting of the vessel, or bleeding that results in an extravascular hematoma and vascular compression. It is important when choosing an arterial puncture site to make sure that adequate collateral blood flow is available in the event some untoward arterial complication occurs. Good sites for arterial puncture include the radial, brachial, and dorsalis pedis arteries, for they possess appropriate collateral blood flow. Second, it is less difficult to palpate, stabilize, and puncture a superficial artery than a more deeply placed one. Superficial arteries are readily accessible at the distal ends of the extremities. Third, arteries that are surrounded by insensitive body tissues such as muscle, tendon, and fat are desirable for arterial puncture to reduce or minimize pain. Major arteries in the upper extremity are illustrated in Figure 2-37.

The risks associated with arterial puncture are usually low for single sticks, but increase rapidly with persistent cannulation of the same vascular access. Infection of the puncture site rarely occurs. Occult bleeding into adjacent tissues has been noted

Table 2-13 Inspection, Palpation, Percussion, and Auscultation Findings of Respiratory Problems

Process	Inspection	Palpation	Percussion	Auscultation
Pneumonia	Coryza symptoms; pyrexia, chills; productive cough; rapid, shallow, grunting respirations (dyspnea); pleuritic pain (splinting of chest); occasional cyanosis	Limited motion of chest on affected side; increased fremitus when consolidation fully established	Dullness; decreased diaphragmatic excursion	Early: decreased breath sounds Later: bronchial sounds; bronchophony; whispered pectoriloquy; fine crepitant crackles (rales); occasional pleural friction rub
Chronic obstructive lung disease	Increased respiratory rate; pursed lip breathing; increased AP diameter (barrel chest); use of accessory muscles and intercostal retraction; leaning forward to assist breathing; cyanosis or hyperemia (depends on type); increased JVP	Decreased fremitus; diminished chest expansion; possible crepitus; rhonchal fremitus	Decreased diaphragmatic excursion; hyperresonance; lowered hepatic dullness	Decreased breath sounds; prolonged expirations; crackles (rales), wheezes, or gurgles (rhonchi); in some instances no adventitious sounds present
Bronchitis	Cough with sputum production; sore throat; fever; malaise; occasional dyspnea with use of accessory muscles	Normal fremitus	Resonance	May have prolonged expirations with vesicular breath sounds; wheezes, crackles (rales), and gurgles (rhonchi) may be heard
Pleural effusion	Pain; dyspnea; pallor	Prominence of interspaces; tracheal deviation from side of effusion; decreased fremitus	Increasing dullness with the increase in amount of fluid	Decreased breath sounds; egophony and whispered pectoriloquy
Neoplasm	Asymptomatic or mild cough; fever; chills; sputum	Mass may be palpated if on chest wall; absent fremitus	Dull over area of lesion	Decreased breath sounds if airway is occluded; egophony and whispered pectoriloquy if airway is not occluded; often fine crackles (rales) and localized wheezes; occasional pleural friction rub
Atelectasis	Increased respiratory rate; increased pulse; often cyanosis	Tracheal shift to side of involvement; decreased fremitus; decreased chest expansion on affected side	Dullness	Diminished breath sounds; occasional crackles (rales)

Table 2-13 (*continued*)

Process	Inspection	Palpation	Percussion	Auscultation
Pulmonary edema	Increased respiratory rate; cyanosis; sitting upright; use of accessory muscles; apprehension	Increased fremitus	Dullness	Bronchovesicular breath sounds, often obscured later by crackles (rales), gurgles (rhonchi), and wheezing
Pneumothorax	Pain; dyspnea and cyanosis; apprehension; increased respiratory rate	Possible tracheal shift to side of pneumothorax; absent fremitus on affected side	Hyperresonance; decreased diaphragmatic excursion on affected side	Absent breath sounds on affected side
Emphysema	Dyspnea; wheezing; cough with sputum; increased use of accessory muscles of the neck; exhaustion	Normal fremitus or decreased; occasional palpable rhonchi	Hyperresonance; decreased diaphragmatic excursion	Vesicular or bronchovesicular sounds; wheezes/gurgles (rhonchi) throughout chest

in femoral and brachial arteriotomies. Trauma to surrounding nerve tissue is usually related to inexperience or carelessness.

Decisions to undertake invasive arterial monitoring for the purpose of continuous blood pressure measurement and as an access for frequent blood sampling should be made cautiously. Patients experiencing hemodynamic problems, shock, severe oxygenation and ventilation problems, and malignant hypertension are good candidates for arterial cannulation. Care should be exercised when placing and maintaining arterial lines, for serious complications related to hemorrhage, infection, and thrombosis are possible.

Infrequently, arterial catheters may erode the vascular wall to cause aneurysm, hematoma, or a-v fistula. Generally, radial site infection rates are low as long as sterile procedures and practices are followed meticulously. Femoral catheterization and cutdown procedures create the highest risk of infection.

Generally, injections of pharmacologic agents are contraindicated for lines into the radial artery. Calcium compounds and vasopressors can cause serious hand injuries if ischemia and necrosis occur as a result of injecting drugs through the arterial line. Likewise, aggressive flushing of saline or other fluids in the catheter and vessel could possibly dislodge clot or gas emboli to the brain.

In preparing for arterial puncture (particularly radial puncture, as that site is considered the most accessible and safe), a simple clinical maneuver for assessing collateral circulation prior to puncture is mandatory. This is the Allen's test (or a modified version of it), which was devised for confirming the presence of radial artery occlusion. (A positive test indicates the presence of such occlusion.) The test most frequently performed, however, is the modified Allen's test; a positive result on this test indicates the presence of ulnar collateral flow, allowing a degree of safety in using the radial artery for punc-

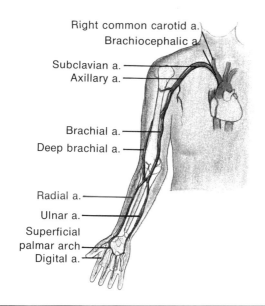

Right common carotid a.
Brachiocephalic a.
Subclavian a.
Axillary a.
Brachial a.
Deep brachial a.
Radial a.
Ulnar a.
Superficial palmar arch
Digital a.

Figure 2-37 Major Arteries of the Upper Extremity

ture. The steps of the modified Allen's test are as follows:

1. The patient's hand is closed tightly so as to form a fist.
2. Pressure is applied to the wrist to compress and obstruct both the ulnar and radial arteries.
3. The hand is then relaxed, revealing a blanched palm and fingers.
4. The obstructing pressure at the wrist is removed from the ulnar artery only.
5. The hand, if normal, should flush within 15 seconds.

The flushing of the entire hand suggests that the ulnar artery is capable of supplying adequate blood flow to the hand if the radial artery is compromised. If the ulnar artery does not adequately supply the hand with collateral circulation (a negative modified Allen's test), the radial artery should not be cannulated and an alternative site should be found if possible. When necessary, the ulnar artery may be chosen as the arteriotomy site, although it is not the vessel of choice because of its size, smaller vascular diameter, and the difficulty of stabilizing it, all of which place it at increased risk for thrombosis. The use of the modified Allen's test is limited for the following reasons:

It is not easily performed on the unconscious patient.

It is difficult to evaluate reperfusion in the patient experiencing hypoperfusion states.

Frequent previous radial cannulation often obliterates the pulse.

Jaundiced patients are difficult to evaluate for reperfusion.

The test is inconclusive if reperfusion takes longer than 15 seconds.

When the dorsalis pedis is to be used for arteriotomy, a similar test can be conducted by occluding the dorsalis pedis artery with the hand and blanching the great toe by compressing the toenail. A rapid return to color in the great toe suggests that lateral plantar flow is present. However, in extremities that are cold or with poor circulation, flushing may be difficult to evaluate. Major arteries of the lower extremity are illustrated in Figure 2-38.

Two to three milliliters of blood are usually needed for blood gas analysis. After the arteriotomy is performed and the needle is withdrawn, pressure should be applied to the arterial site for at least 3 to 5 minutes. If needle entry is more oblique than perpendicular, the incidence of hematoma lessens.

The blood sample is collected in a heparinized tube. If too much heparin is added, changes in the pH, $PaCO_2$, and PaO_2 values may occur. In preheparinized blood gas packages the anticoagulant is in either liquid or powder form. A heparinized syringe is prepared by flushing a syringe with about 1 cc of heparin and discarding the heparin from the syringe; the deadspace of the syringe in the hub will contain 0.15–0.25 mL of sodium heparin. This volume will safely and adequately anticoagulate the desired 2–3 cc of blood.

Air bubbles should be kept from entering the blood sample as room air may lower $PaCO_2$ values, increase the pH, and cause PaO_2 to reach 150 mm Hg. The syringe should not be aspirated to withdraw blood. The arterial blood pressure should be allowed to fill the syringe. The filled syringe should be capped immediately after removal from the site and placed in ice and water mixed to form an ice slush. The temperature of the blood sample will fall rapidly and variances in $PaCO_2$ and pH levels will be minimized. If the sample is not chilled immediately, there can be significant errors in the test results.

Table 2-14 lists selected normal values based on laboratory, statistical, and clinical experience that can be used in the interpretation of arterial blood gas values. Interpretation must take into consideration ventilatory and acid-base information, tissue oxygenation status, and supporting clinical presentation.

An arterial blood gas report gives information about three factors:

1. pH value (yields the acid-base status of the blood—normal, acidosis, or alkalosis)
2. $PaCO_2$ value (yields direct information regarding ventilation and provides an analysis of the expected acid-base status)
3. HCO_3 (yields information regarding the condition of the acid-base status of the blood).

Below are listed parameters of acid-base status and an indication of the pathological process involved.

pH	7.35–7.45	Normal
	<7.35	Acidosis/emia
	>7.45	Alkalosis/emia
$PaCO_2$	35–45 mm Hg	Normal
	>45	Acidosis/emia
	<35	Alkalosis/emia
HCO_3	22–26 mEq/L	Normal
	<22	Acidosis/emia
	>26	Alkalosis/emia

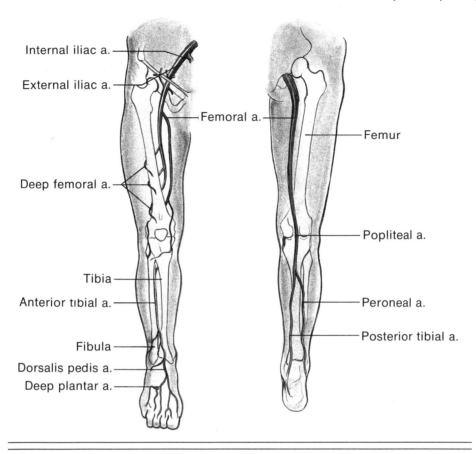

Internal iliac a.
External iliac a.
Femoral a.
Deep femoral a.
Tibia
Anterior tibial a.
Fibula
Dorsalis pedis a.
Deep plantar a.

Femur
Popliteal a.
Peroneal a.
Posterior tibial a.

Figure 2-38 Major Arteries of the Lower Extremity

The critical care nurse presented with these three values may make comprehensive and informed interpretations that allow for the evaluation of the patient's ventilatory status and metabolic acid-base relationships. A respiratory abnormality is identified from the $PaCO_2$ level, and an abnormal HCO_3 level indicates metabolic disturbances.

Table 2-14 Normal Arterial Blood Gas Values

Value	Normal Mean	Normal Range
pH	7.40	7.35–7.45
$PaCO_2$	40 mm Hg	35–45 mm Hg
HCO_3^-	24 mEq/L	22–26 mEq/L
BE	0	+/− 2
TCO_2	25	23–27
PaO_2	100 mm Hg	80–100 mm Hg
SaO_2	97%	>95%
Hb	14 gm %	12–15 gm %
O_2 Content	20 vol %	19–22 vol %
pyO_2	60 torr	>40–75 torr

To interpret the acid-base status, the nurse examines the pH value first, then checks the other two parameters to see if they support the diagnosis of the disorder suggested by the pH value. The parameters are graphically illustrated in Figure 2-39. A list of primary disorders and etiologies is provided in Table 2-15. Any parameter that is not in the expected direction of the acid-base status represents the compensatory system's attempt to reverse the underlying problem. Compensatory mechanisms are detailed in Table 2-16. As the compensatory mechanism attempts to restore physiologic equilibrium to the body, patterns of acid-base disorders and parameter changes begin to emerge; these patterns can suggest the stage of compensation, as detailed in Table 2-17.

The metabolic rate of the body and the mechanical efficiency of the pulmonary system are reflected in the $PaCO_2$ level. An increase in the $PaCO_2$ level (hypercapnia) is associated with alveolar hypoventilation. A decrease in the $PaCO_2$ level (hypocapnia) is consistent with alveolar hyperventilation. When acute changes in ventilation occur, there is a predictable change in the relationship between pH and plasma carbonic acid. This change is related to the level of $PaCO_2$. The plasma carbonic acid level for a

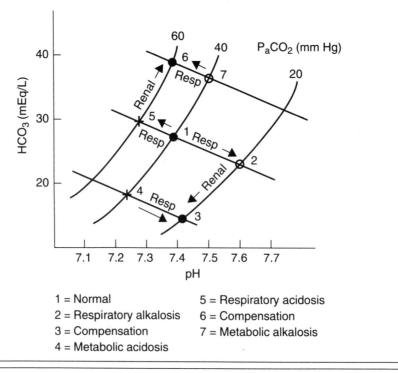

Figure 2-39 pH, HCO₃, and PₐCO₂ in Respiratory and Metabolic Acidosis and Alkalosis

1 = Normal
2 = Respiratory alkalosis
3 = Compensation
4 = Metabolic acidosis

5 = Respiratory acidosis
6 = Compensation
7 = Metabolic alkalosis

patient is calculated by multiplying the individual's known $PaCO_2$ level (in mm Hg) by the factor 0.03. This change represents the change in pH due to alterations in alveolar ventilation ($PaCO_2$). The relationship is not perfectly accurate, but within clinical range. For every 20 mm Hg increase in $PaCO_2$ above 40 mm Hg, the pH is expected to decrease by 0.10 pH unit. For every 10 mm Hg decrease in $PaCO_2$ below 40 mm Hg, the pH will increase by 0.10 pH unit. This rule of thumb may help the nurse to quickly estimate the degree of abnormality that can be attributable to acute ventilatory change. The table below illustrates the principle.

PaCO₂ (mm Hg)	pH	HCO₃ (mEq/L)
80	7.20	28
60	7.30	26
40	7.40	24
30	7.50	22
20	7.60	20

Assessment of the relationship between arterial carbon dioxide and arterial pH (the Henderson-Hasselbach relationship) allows one to determine whether the presenting problem is of a ventilatory nature or of a metabolic acid-base origin, according to the following.

Alveolar hyperventilation ($PaCO_2 < 30$ mm Hg)
1. pH > 7.50: acute alveolar hyperventilation
2. pH 7.40–7.50: chronic alveolar hyperventilation
3. pH 7.30–7.40: compensated metabolic acidosis
4. pH < 7.30: partially compensated metabolic acidosis

Acceptable alveolar ventilation ($PaCO_2 = 30–50$ mm Hg)
1. pH > 7.50: metabolic alkalosis
2. pH 7.30–7.50: acceptable ventilatory and metabolic acid-base status
3. pH < 7.30: metabolic acidosis

Ventilatory failure ($PaCO_2 > 50$ mm Hg)
1. pH > 7.50: partially compensated metabolic alkalosis
2. pH 7.30–7.50: chronic ventilatory failure
3. pH < 7.30: acute ventilatory failure

When deficits in arterial oxygen levels are encountered, the presence of hypoxemia is indicated; hypoxemia is confirmed by reduced oxygen-related values: the partial pressure of oxygen (PaO_2), the saturation of arterial hemoglobin (SaO_2), and the combined dissolved and transported content of oxygen within the arterial blood system (CaO_2). The

Table 2-15 Acid-Base Abnormalities and Some Etiologies

Condition	Possible Etiologies
Respiratory acidosis	Acute/chronic ventilatory failure Obstructive diseases Restrictive diseases Respiratory depression Neuromuscular depression/fatigue Cerebral ischemia/infarct Increased intracranial pressure CSF alkalosis Pickwickian syndrome Alcohol, anesthetic, barbituate, narcotic, or morphine overdose Botulism Guillain-Landry-Barre syndrome
Metabolic acidosis	Diarrhea Renal failure Lactic acidosis Ketoacidosis Increased anion gap Cardiac arrest Hyperchloremia (increased Cl^-) Hyperkalemia (increased K^+) Liver failure Diamox usage CO poisoning Paraldehyde
Respiratory alkalosis	Hypoxia Emotional stress response syndromes: anxiety, neurosis, pain Fever CNS trauma Gram-negative infections Metabolic acidosis Pulmonary emboli Anemia Early COPD Obesity Abdominal distension Pregnancy (third trimester) Mechanical ventilation
Metabolic alkalosis	Vomiting Continuous nasogastric drainage Hypokalemia Corticosteroids Diuretics (Lasix, thiazides) Hypernatremia Massive blood replacement Aldosteronism

Table 2-16 Acid-Base Disorders and Compensatory Mechanisms

Acid-Base Disorder	Compensatory Mechanism
Respiratory acidosis ($PaCO_2$ and pH)	Increased renal retention of bicarbonate to reduce excessive acid loads
Metabolic acidosis (HCO_3 and pH)	Pulmonary hyperventilation to lower $PaCO_2$ and increase pH
Respiratory alkalosis ($PaCO_2$ and pH)	Increased renal excretion of bicarbonate to increase systemic physiologic acid loads
Metabolic alkalosis (HCO_3 and pH)	Pulmonary hypoventilation to increase $PaCO_2$ and systemic physiologic acid loads

the diagnosis of hypoxemia must be made presumptively in such cases. A general principle by which to determine if a patient would have become hypoxemic on room air is to note the patient's current FIO_2. The PaO_2 that is expected is usually five times greater than the FIO_2. If the current PaO_2 is not at least equal to $5 \times FIO_2$, then the patient would have been hypoxemic on room air.

Hypoxia, on the other hand, is defined as inadequate supply of oxygen (less than what is necessary for normal cellular function). Hypoxemia and hypoxia are clearly two distinctly different phenomena. However, in the clinical environment, since one cannot accurately predict when hypoxemia is sufficient to produce hypoxia or accurately measure tissue hypoxia, it is assumed that some degree of hypoxemia reflects the presence of inadequate tissue oxygenation. It is quite possible, though, for cellular hypoxia to exist even in the face of apparently normal arterial oxygen levels, such as in the case of anemia or hypotensive states.

It is generally useful to characterize four clinical presentations of hypoxia.

1. Anoxic (hypoxic) hypoxia: This condition is secondary to a problem in gas exchange (oxygenation) in the lung. Causes may include:
   a. abnormal ventilation-perfusion relationships
   b. decreases in the alveolar pressure of oxygen
   c. alterations in the a-c membrane due to interstitial processes or fibrosis
2. Anemic hypoxia: This condition is secondary to reduced oxygen-carrying capacity of the blood. Causes may include:
   a. blood loss

pathophysiological process present in hypoxemia is outlined in Table 2-18.

Since the diagnosis of hypoxemia can only be made while the patient is on room air (21% oxygen), and there is no sound indication for withholding oxygen therapy from a patient in respiratory crisis,

Table 2-17   Stages of Compensation of Acidosis and Alkalosis

Disorder	pH	PCO$_2$	HCO$_3$	BE
Metabolic acidosis				
Acute (uncompensated)	Decreased	Normal	Decreased	Decreased
Subacute (partially compensated)	Decreased	Decreased	Decreased	Decreased
Chronic (fully compensated)	Normal	Decreased	Decreased	Decreased
Metabolic alkalosis				
Acute (uncompensated)	Increased	Normal	Increased	Increased
Subacute (partially compensated)	Increased	Increased	Increased	Increased
Chronic (fully compensated)	Normal	Increased	Increased	Increased
Respiratory acidosis				
Acute (uncompensated)	Decreased	Increased	Normal	Normal
Subacute (partially compensated)	Decreased	Increased	Increased	Increased
Chronic (fully compensated)	Normal	Increased	Increased	Increased
Respiratory alkalosis				
Acute (uncompensated)	Increased	Decreased	Normal	Normal
Subacute (partially compensated)	Increased	Decreased	Decreased	Decreased
Chronic (fully compensated)	Normal	Decreased	Decreased	Decreased

   b. abnormal hemoglobin
   c. reductions in red blood cell production
   d. carbon monoxide poisoning
3. Circulatory hypoxia: This condition is secondary to a reduced blood flow in the body or a (stagnant) reduction in cardiac output. Causes may include:
   a. shock
   b. cardiac arrest
   c. congestive heart failure
4. Histotoxic hypoxia: This condition is secondary to the inability of the cells to utilize oxygen. Causes include cyanide poisoning.

Table 2-18   Pathophysiology of Hypoxemia

Condition	Possible Etiologies
Ventilation-perfusion mismatching	
Decreased mixed venous oxygen content	Increased temperature Increased metabolic activity Anemia Decreased arterial oxygen content Cardiac embarrassment
Decreased PaO$_2$	Hypoventilation CNS depression High altitudes Breathing less than 21% oxygen Airway obstruction Underventilated alveoli

The effects of the types of hypoxia on PaO$_2$, SaO$_2$, and SvO$_2$ are listed below (D = decreased, I = increased, N = normal).

Type	PaO$_2$	SaO$_2$	SvO$_2$
Anoxic	D	D	D
Anemic	N	N	D
Circulatory	D	D	D
Histotoxic	N	N	I

Responses to decreasing PaO$_2$ are as follows:

PaO$_2$ < 55 mm Hg
   Oxyhemoglobin dissociation curve shifts to right: decreased affinity for oxygen
   Increased erythropoietin stimulates red blood cell production to increase oxygen-carrying capacity
   Short-term memory impairment
PaO$_2$ = 30 mm Hg to 55 mm Hg
   Cognitive and motor function deterioration
   Slowing heart rate
   Vasoconstriction
   Bronchoconstriction
PaO$_2$ < 30 mm Hg
   Loss of consciousness
   Circulatory failure
   Shock
   Cardiac arrest
   Decrease in renal blood flow

Atropine-refractory bradycardia
Respiratory depression
Impaired autonomic control

Signs and symptoms of hypoxia are listed below.

Acute Hypoxia	*Chronic Hypoxia*
Tachycardia	Tachycardia
Increased respiratory rate	Increased respiratory rate
Arrhythmias	Arrhythmias
Decreased $PaCO_2$	Decreased/increased $PaCO_2$
Hypertension	Pulmonary hypertension
Dyspnea	Dyspnea
Anxiety	Irritability
Impaired judgment	Impaired judgment
Euphoria	Tiredness
Blurred vision	Papilledema
Tremors/hyperactive reflexes	Myoclonic jerking
	Trancelike behavior
Stupor	Polycythemia
Coma	Clubbing
Death	

Clinical conditions for which there is increased incidence of hypoxia include:

Myocardial infarction
Acute pulmonary disorders
Sepsis
Drug overdose
Liver failure
Head trauma
Congestive heart failure
Hypovolemic shock
Blunt chest trauma
Acute neuromuscular disease
Acute abdomen (splinting)
Acute pancreatitis
Spinal cord injury

In the face of hypoxemia or hypoxia, the pharmacologic agent of choice is controlled, precisely monitored oxygen therapy. The goals of oxygen therapy include (1) treating or preventing hypoxia; (2) preventing or reducing the physiologic compensatory mechanisms initiated by hypoxia; and (3) providing adequate amounts of oxygen to the tissues without causing the adverse effects of oxygen toxicity or oxygen-induced hypoventilation (COPD, bronchitis, hypoxic drive). Administering supplemental oxygen serves to increase PaO_2, decrease the work of breathing, and decrease myocardial work. Indications for oxygen therapy include the following:

Tachycardia
Cyanosis
Restlessness
Disorientation
Cardiac arrhythmias
Slow bounding pulse
Tachypnea
Hypertension
Dyspnea
Coma
Labored breathing (use of accessory muscles; nasal flaring)
Lethargy
Tremors/seizure activity

Clinical indications for oxygen therapy in the absence of hypoxemia include:

Suspected myocardial infarction
Myocardial infarction
Carbon monoxide poisoning
Sickle cell crisis
Massive burns
Hemorrhagic shock
Anaphylactic shock
Hypotension
Anemia

Finally, there are three major hazards of oxygen therapy.

1. Oxygen-induced hypoventilation, with the following risk criteria:
   a. Patient's baseline $PaCO_2 > 50$ mm Hg
   b. Baseline saturation $< 90\%$
   c. With supplemental O_2, PaO_2 doesn't exceed 60 mm Hg
2. Absorption atelectasis with the following risk criteria:
   a. $FIO_2 > 50\%$
   b. Decreasing alveolar volumes
   c. Airway obstruction
3. Retrolental fibroplasia with the following risk criteria:
   a. High PaO_2
   b. Level of maturity of preterm infant
   c. Oxygen exposure length

Clinical signs and symptoms of oxygen toxicity are as follows:

Substernal pain

Cough

Dyspnea

Anxiety

Paresthesia

Fatigue

Pulmonary infiltrates

Decreased PaO_2

Decreased compliance

Pulmonary edema

Atelectasis

Decreased vital capacity

Increased shunting

The onset of oxygen toxicity can vary in different clinical circumstances. Conditions or substances that can potentiate oxygen toxicity include CO_2 inhalation or retention, vitamin D deficiency, adrenocortical hormones, thyroid hormones, amphetamines, epinephrine, insulin, and norepinephrine. In contrast, factors that can inhibit the occurrence of oxygen toxicity include vitamin E, anesthesia, adrenergic blockers, ganglionic blockers, hypothermia, hypothyroidism, intermittent O_2 therapy, and acclimatization to hypoxia.[3]

Finally, the nurse must ascertain the presence of classic symptoms most commonly associated with problems of the respiratory system, including coughing (with or without production of sputum), dyspnea (breathlessness), hemoptysis, chest pain (of cardiac, pleural, or thoracic-muscular origins), wheezing of lower airway or upper airway, cyanosis, hoarseness or other vocal changes, syncopal episodes, heart failure, fever and chills, exercise intolerance, weight loss, nausea and vomiting, long bone and joint pain, and altered sleep patterns.

Coughing and dyspnea account for at least 90% of the respiratory complaints offered by patients. A cough is a coordinated, forceful expiratory effort in which accessory muscles contract while the glottis is still partially closed, thus creating high intrapulmonary and intrathoracic pressures. When the glottic closure relaxes suddenly, an explosive rush of gas exits the airways, clearing them of foreign substances and/or secretions.

There are multiple etiologies for the stimulation of cough receptors, but the basic concept of a vagally-mediated reflex bronchoconstriction elucidates the cough mechanism. The airways contain subepithelial receptors. Stimuli, whether chemical or mechanical, cause impulses to travel from these receptors via an afferent pathway of the vagus nerve to reflexive efferent vagal receptors, which release acetylcholine at the neuroeffector muscular junctions. Mucus production and coughing both result from the stimulation of these receptors.

Changes in the airway itself may alter the threshold sensitivity of the epithelial cough receptors. This can be demonstrated clinically in respiratory processes that are marked by lung congestion. Inflation of the lung during passive activity (sleeping) can stimulate the lung receptors, resulting not only in cough but also in increased bronchomotor tone. Coughing alone may be the presenting clinical symptom for asthma without the presence of wheezing, such as in the case of exercise-induced asthma.

The major types of cough receptor stimulation are listed below.

1. Inflammatory stimulation resulting from infection, abscess, drug or radiation assault, edema, hyperemia, collagen vascular diseases, allergy, or tuberculosis
2. Chemical or temperature stimulation by inhalation of hot or cold air, gases, fumes, or smoke
3. Mechanical forms of stimulation such as foreign bodies aspirated during the breathing cycle, high flow rates of inspiratory activity whether spontaneous or mechanical, a tumor mass or granuloma within the thoracic cavity, and pathological mechanical changes (decreased compliance) such as atelectasis, fibrosis, interstitial pneumonitis, and pulmonary edema
4. Some neural stimulation has been identified such as stimulation arising from tactile pressure in the ear canal (Arnold's response) and otitis media

If cough is clinically present, its approximate time of onset and progress should be documented. Frequent, annoying, painful, and persistent cough or throat clearing are not normal phenomena, especially when productive. In the intubated and mechanically ventilated patient, coughing assumes particular significance. This reflexive protective response may indicate endotracheal tube movement downward toward the carina, cuff herniation, pneumothorax, airway obstruction, or the presence of airway secretions. Hacking, frequent coughing, or clearing of the throat may be the byproducts of smoking, early viral infection, postnasal drip, bronchospasm, or nervous habit. Chronic productive cough is generally indicative of significant bronchopulmonary disease. The frequency of the chronic cough may demonstrate some pattern that can suggest diagnosis. Table 2-19 details the significance of some cough patterns.

Table 2-19 Indications of Cough Timing and Pattern

Cough Frequency	Significance
Fairly constant	Effects of smoking, seasonal weather change, dust, fumes, and other such factors
Episodic	Possible bronchitis or hyperreactive airways
Acute/severe (frequent)	Probable acute infection
Chronic	Chronic recurring cough that persists for months and is not associated with any localized bronchopulmonary disease is a feature of chronic bronchitis

Coughing characterized by seal-like barking, brassiness, or hoarseness, and the cough associated with inspiratory stridor are usually heard when there is an upper airway problem. Hay fever, allergies, acute sinusitis, postnasal discharge, and frequent cold and flu episodes are upper-respiratory symptoms usually associated with the presence of pulmonary disease.

A hallmark of pulmonary compromise is the presence of secretions, whether from the alveoli, trachea, or pharynx. This sputum may contain a variety of materials including mucus, cellular debris, pus, blood, microorganisms, and foreign aerosolized particulate substances inhaled from the environment. (Sputum should not be confused with saliva.) Clinical assessment of a productive cough and its secretions should include collection and inspection of a sputum sample. Sputum is generally described according to color, odor, consistency, quantity, time of day produced, and the presence of blood or other identifiable materials.

It is important that sputum be collected properly. The ideal time to collect sputum is shortly after the patient awakens. The nurse should be sure that the secretions obtained are tracheobronchial in origin. When obtaining the sample, the nurse should exercise care to reduce contamination by organisms that normally colonize the pharynx. Good daily oral care by the patient and gargling with sterile water solution before sputum expectoration may help to reduce contaminants. Sputum samples sitting in open containers are subject to colonization and infection by saprophytic organism such as fungi; all samples should be stored in closed containers.

Presumptive diagnoses can be accomplished based on the examination of sputum. Table 2-20 provides descriptions of sputum and possible etiologies.

Streaks and specks of blood in the sputum occur frequently in acute respiratory infection and bronchitis. The expectoration of pure blood is obviously a serious symptom. One should immediately ascertain if the bleeding is from a nonpulmonary source such as the gums, nose, or stomach. In the intubated patient, the presence of small amounts of blood in either the endotracheal sample or the buccal sample may suggest destabilization of the endotracheal tube and possible laceration of pharyngeal, laryngeal, tracheal, or oral/nasal mucosa.

Pulmonary Function Tests

Pulmonary function studies include a wide variety of tests that evaluate many respiratory functions, including mechanics (lung volumes, lung capacities, and gas flows), gas exchange across the alveolar capillary membrane, and ventilatory drive.

The lung system can be described by four basic lung volumes and four lung capacities (which are combinations of at least two or more volumes).

Lung Volumes
1. Tidal volume: the amount of gas inspired during a normal inspiration
2. Inspiratory reserve volume: the amount of gas that can be inspired over and above a normal inspiration
3. Expiratory reserve volume: the amount of gas that can be exhaled after a normal exhalation
4. Residual volume: the amount of gas that remains in the lung after a maximal exhalatory effort

Lung Capacities
1. Inspiratory capacity: the maximum volume of gas that can be inhaled after a normal exhalation
2. Vital capacity: the maximum volume of gas that can be exhaled either forcefully (FVC) or slowly (SVC) after a maximal inspiration
3. Functional residual capacity: the volume of gas that remains in the lung after a normal exhalation
4. Total lung capacity: the total volume of gas that is contained in the lung after a maximal inspiration

Lung volumes and capacities are based on statistical normalization of data derived from specific groups of individuals differentiated by height, age,

Table 2-20   Descriptors and Possible Etiological
Causes of Sputum Change

Appearance of Sputum	Possible Etiology
Mucoid (clear or white)	Bronchial asthma Early chronic bronchitis Early airway irritating processes Legionnaire's disease Neoplasms
Mucopurulent	Pulmonary tuberculosis Acute bronchitis or chronic bronchitis Pseudomonas pneumonia Cystic fibrosis Infections Tuberculosis
Purulent: Copious green or yellow	Bronchiectasis Advanced chronic bronchitis Pseudomonas pneumonia
Thick green	Hemophilus influenza pneumonia
Thin pink or blood-streaked	Streptococcal pneumonia Staphylococcal pneumonia
Red, like currant jelly	Klebsiella pneumonia
Rusty	Pneumococcal pneumonia Lung abscess Aspiration Anaerobic infections Bronchiectasis
Fetid, dark yellow or green	Lung abscess Bronchiectasis Anaerobic infections Cystic fibrosis Aspiration
Black	Smoke/coal dust inhalations
Frothy pink	Pulmonary edema

Bloody (hemoptic)	Pulmonary:
	  Embolism with infarction
	  Pneumonia
	  Tuberculosis
	  Bronchiectasis
	  Trauma
	  Neoplasms
	  Abscess
	  Pulmonary hypertension
	Cardiac:
	  Pulmonary edema
	  Mitral valve disease
	Systemic:
	  Sarcoidosis
	  Goodpasture's syndrome
	  Coagulation disorders

and sex. Thus, predicted normal values are found to vary on the basis of race, environmental relationships, occupational exposures, residency (rural or urban), socioeconomic factors, and ethnic background. These values can also be subject to variability on the basis of diurnal or seasonal variation, endocrine changes, and the quality of the testing procedure and instruction. It is usually accepted that normal variations will be ±20% (ranging from 80% to 120%) of established norms. Lung volumes and capacities are usually expressed at body temperature and pressure, with the volume measured fully saturated with water vapor (BTPS). All lung volumes and capacities, except for residual volume, functional residual capacity, and total lung capacity, can be measured by simple spirometric measuring devices easily used at the bedside. Table 2-21 lists lung volumes and capacities under normal conditions and in obstructive and restrictive disorders.

Clinically, measurement of vital capacity (VC) assumes particular importance during assessment. The forced vital capacity (FVC) is usually equal to the VC. The FVC may be reduced in chronic obstructive lung diseases, whereas the VC may remain close to normal. Decreased FVC is common to restrictive diseases and ARDS. The FVC may also be reduced in obstructive processes such as emphysema and asthma because of the air trapping that results from airway compression during exhalation.

A normal VC ranges between 70 and 90 mL per kilogram of body weight. The vital capacity is used as an estimate of the patient's ventilatory reserve and lung compliance. The compliance of normal lungs changes directly with changes in functional residual capacity (FRC). Decreased FVC or compliance will contribute to decreased FRC, atelectasis, and increased respiratory rate accompanied by an increased work of breathing and an increase in pulmonary blood flow shunting, resulting in severe hypoxemia and possible respiratory failure. It is generally accepted that if the VC stays above 15 mL per kg body weight, the patient will be capable of responding to increased levels of cardiopulmonary stress. If the patient's VC is less than 10 mL per kg, ability to maintain prolonged spontaneous ventilation is in serious question, for this is considered the lowest level at which one maintains the capability to breathe.

Pulmonary Function Testing (PFT) Procedures

The vital capacity measurements discussed above can be subdivided into two further capacities: the inspiratory capacity and the expiratory capacity.

Table 2-21 Approximate Lung Volumes and Capacities

Measure	Normal	Obstructive Disorders	Restrictive Disorders
Tidal Volume	500 mL	500–700 mL	300–500 mL
Inspiratory Reserve	3500 mL	2500–3500 mL	2500 mL
Expiratory Reserve	1000 mL	700–1000 mL	700–1000 mL
Residual Volume	1000 mL	1200 mL	700–1000 mL
Inspiratory Capacity	3500 mL	3000–3500 mL	3000–3500 mL
Vital Capacity	4500 mL	3000–4500 mL	3000 mL
Forced Vital Capacity	4500 mL	3000 mL	3000 mL
Functional Residual Capacity	2000 mL	3000 mL	1500–2000 mL
Total Lung Capacity	6000 mL	7000 mL	4000 mL

Inspiratory capacity (IC) measurements record the largest gas volume that can be spontaneously inhaled from the resting and expiratory position. Approximately 70–75% of the vital capacity volume can be measured through an inspiratory capacity study. Changes in this volume parallel changes in VC as well as changes in lung compliance. Inspiratory capacity can be measured at the bedside.

Expiratory capacity (EC) measurements record the largest lung volumes that can be exhaled from the end resting expiratory position. The ERV (expiratory reserve volume) is approximately 20–25% of the VC. It is most sensitive to changes in position. The ERV may be calculated by subtracting the IC from the VC.

Functional residual capacity (FRC) measurements record the maximum amount of gas remaining in the lungs at the end expiratory level. The FRC cannot be directly measured as a lung capacity. Closely associated to the FRC value is the residual volume (RV), which is the amount of gas remaining in the lungs after a maximal expiratory effort. Like the FRC, it cannot be measured directly.

Three indirect techniques are commonly used to measure FRC:

1. Nitrogen washout: A patient breathes a sample of 100% gas for no more than 7 minutes, exhaling into a spirometric collecting system. The volume (%) of the nitrogen gas in the collected exhaled gas is measured. The FRC is determined by the formula

$$FRC = \frac{\% \ N_2 \ final}{\% \ N_2 \ atmospheric}$$

The residual volume is determined by subtracting the expiratory reserve volume from the calculated FRC.

2. Helium dilution: A patient breathes a known mixture of helium and air until equilibration occurs. The volume of gas collected in the spirometer is determined by the formula

$$Initial \ volume = \frac{He \ (added) \ (ml)}{\% \ He \ initial}$$

After the initial volume is known, the FRC can be determined by the following formula:

$$FRC = \frac{\% \ He \ initial - \% \ He \ final}{\% \ He \ final}$$

RV is then calculated by subtracting the ERV determined from spirometry from the FRC obtained indirectly.

In both of these methods accuracy is difficult to achieve, since smaller volumes result from air trapping. These tests can only measure airways that are in connection with the atmosphere and each other.

3. Body plethysmography (body box): This procedure is possible only if the patient is capable of going to the PFT lab. The patient must be able to sit in an enclosed box (either a pressure, volume, or flow box). Thoracic gas volume, residual volume, and total lung capacity can be measured. This technique has the advantage of being able to measure all the respiratory gases, whether directly exhaled or trapped in the alveoli.

These tests are performed to differentiate between obstructive diseases (increasing FRC) and restrictive ones (decreasing FRC). Modern pulmonary function technology has made it possible to perform two of these tests at the bedside somewhat easily. However, specialized equipment and a well-trained technologist are essential for the third test.

Total lung capacity (TLC) can be determined by combining the residual volume with VC measured spirometrically. Increases in TLC are indicative of obstructive disease; decreases suggest restrictive processes. The RV/TLC ratio indicates the percentage of TLC that is defined by the RV. Usually values greater than 35% are seen in the patient with hyperinflation, alveolar air trapping, and emphysema. These measurements have no strong predictive validity as to disability but are more diagnostic.

Radiologic estimates of TLC may be made; these are comparable in accuracy to measurements by other methods, particularly in the presence of severe air trapping. These radiologic techniques involve either surface field measurement of the lungs (planimetry) or a sectional division of the lungs into cylinders (ellipsoid method).

Flow volume loops are a very interesting graphical analytic method for measuring pulmonary function. This technique is used to measure the flow resistive properties of the lungs. Since airway resistance is inversely related to lung volume, the expiratory flow rate will change with decreasing lung volume. This method requires that the patient be able to make a forced exhalation and immediately follow it by a maximum inspiration back to TLC. The result of the test is a graphic representational drawing in which expiratory flow rates rise rapidly and then decrease to zero at residual volume. The information obtained from a flow volume loop includes vital capacity, flow rate (peak inspiratory and expiratory), and 25%, 50%, and 75% of vital capacity.

Closing volume studies measure the volume of gas remaining in the lung when the small airways begin to close during an expiratory effort. The test is usually performed by using a single-breath nitrogen test. As small airway obstruction progresses, the closing volume will become an increasingly larger percentage of the vital capacity.

Deadspace ventilation (V_D/V_T) testing has excellent clinical usefulness in assessing deadspace ventilation, that part of ventilation that does not participate in the gas exchange. The normal value for V_D/V_T is 0.3. In disease states there will be an increase in this value due to increases in alveolar deadspace (which is usually considered zero). The method for determining deadspace ventilation is quite simple and uses values for tidal volume, $PaCO_2$, and $PECO_2$ (partial pressure of carbon dioxide gas in the expired gas). Once this information is obtained, the V_D/V_T can be determined by applying the Bohr equation:

$$\frac{V_D}{V_T} = \frac{PECO_2 - PaCO_2}{PaCO_2}$$

The maximum expiratory flow rate (MEFR) is also known as the forced expiratory flow (FEF) rate 200–1200. This measurement represents the average flow rate for a liter of gas exhaled after the first 200 cc during an FVC maneuver. This measurement is a *good* assessment of the integrity of the larger airways. Normal range for this value is 6 L/sec, or 360 L/min. When this value is decreased, a restrictive or mechanical defect is present. Flow rates less than 1 L/sec are not uncommon in the patient with obstructive disease. This flow rate generally decreases with age and is lower in women than in men. The MEFR test is effort-dependent, so an alert and cooperative patient is necessary for optimal results. Current microprocessor technology allows this test to be performed at the bedside easily without extensive graphing and mathematical calculations.

Forced expiratory flow 25%–75% is a measurement of the average flow rate over the middle 50% of the FVC. It is well suited as an index of assessment for the small and medium-sized airways. Unlike the FEF 200–1200, this test is not effort-dependent. Reductions in the values obtained with this test, indicating obstructive disease, can be obtained earlier than results of other tests of pulmonary flow. Flows as low as 0.3 L/sec (20 L/min) can be found with severe obstruction and emphysema. This value also decreases with age. This measurement is easily attainable at the bedside using electronically controlled microprocessor devices.

Peak expiratory flow rate (PEFR) is a measurement of the maximal attainable flow rate during an expiration. Current technologies for the performance of this test require the full cooperation and maximal effort of the patient. The patient must blast out the gas in the lung, but not continue to expire to below normal expiratory levels. The Wright's peak flow meter uses a design that has become standard in all peak flow meters. The technology of peak flow devices has been so developed that the patient with airway obstructive lung processes may actually monitor his or her own pulmonary condition at home and direct self-care accordingly. Peak flows may be predicted by the following regression formula:

Males: [(0.144 × height in inches)
− (0.024 × age)] + 2.225
Females: [(0.090 × height in inches)
− (0.018 × age)] + 1.130

The peak flow is a rather *nonspecific* measurement of airway obstruction. Generally it is considered a measurement of flow in the upper airways. The average PEFR for the adult male is 10 L/sec (600 L/min), and the value is less for women.

Maximum voluntary ventilation (MVV) is the measurement of the largest volume of gas that can be breathed per minute by voluntary, conscious, and forced effort on the part of the patient. The MVV is measured by having the patient breathe as deeply and rapidly as possible. The effort required for this test is so substantial that a patient is asked to perform this maneuver for only 10, 12, or 15 seconds. The average value for this test is 160–170 L/min. The test exaggerates air trapping within the lungs in the obstructed patient. It is interesting that the test results may be within normal limits in the patient with restrictive disease because such a patient does not necessarily suffer impediments in muscular function.

Lung scans measure the regional distribution of ventilation. The patient inhales and exhales a gas mixture containing xenon-133, which is a radioactive substance. A scintillation camera monitors the gas flow within the lungs by tracking the distribution of the radioactive substance within the lungs. This procedure is a normal test for pulmonary embolism.

Perfusion lung scans require the injection of a radiolabeled particle, usually a gamma-emitting type of isotope such as iodine or technetium. The radioactive isotope is injected into the venous blood and is tracked by scintillation cameras as it flows through the pulmonary system. The use of the lung scan with the perfusion test can provide information on perfusion defects.

Pulmonary angiograms are used to confirm the presence of pulmonary embolism. A catheter is advanced into the pulmonary artery and radioopaque dye is rapidly injected into the artery. The diagnosis of pulmonary embolism is confirmed by abnormal filling within the artery or by an immediate cutoff of dye flow within the pulmonary vasculature. Usually this procedure is fairly minimal in risk, except in the presence of severe pulmonary hypertension or shock.

Diffusion (DLco) studies involve the inhalation of gas mixtures containing very low amounts (0.3%) of carbon monoxide. Through measurement of the volume of expired gas, the fractional concentration of carbon monoxide gas in expired gases, and the end-tidal and partial pressure of carbon monoxide, diffusion of this gas can be determined. Analysis of the diffusion rate of this gas determines the block or impairment gradient of oxygen within the alveolar system. Decreases from the expected diffusion rate can be due to decreased hematocrit, decreased pulmonary blood flow, decreased alveolar ventilation, pulmonary fibrosis, emphysema, pulmonary emboli, and pulmonary hypertension. Increases in diffusion rate can result from increased hematocrit, increased pulmonary blood flow, exercise, increased alveolar ventilation, and supine position.

Radiology

Various radiologic diagnostic procedures are available to facilitate assessment, diagnosis, and treatment of pulmonary disorders. These procedures include chest x-rays, bronchograms, and angiograms.

When assessing the patient using chest radiography, the practitioner must keep in mind some basic principles. The more dense a structure is, the more x-rays will be absorbed by the structure and the fewer x-rays will penetrate to the film. When almost all the x-rays are absorbed by a structure, the film will appear light or white. In the presence of air (and consequently less density), fewer x-rays are absorbed, allowing more of the film to be developed. Normally, only four types of densities are encountered in x-ray procedures.

1. Bone: The most dense of all naturally occurring substances within the body
2. Air: The least dense of all substances within the body. Because the major constituent of the normal lung is air, few x-rays are absorbed by normal lungs—thus the characteristic darkness of the chest x-ray
3. Fat: Adipose tissue is somewhat more dense than air and thus absorbs some x-rays.
4. Water: In radiographic analysis water makes a lighter image than fat, because water is more dense than fat.

Chest x-rays provide information regarding the following conditions:

Changes in the lung:
   a. areas of density
   b. bronchial thickening or dilution
   c. fibrotic markings
   d. thickening of diaphragmatic pleura
   e. consolidation; atelectasis
   f. pneumothorax; subcutaneous emphysema
   g. pleural fluid
   h. pulmonary edema
   i. pulmonary cancer
   j. hyperinflammation
   k. tracheal deviation

Positioning of invasive equipment or objects:
   a. chest tube
   b. endotracheal tube
   c. tracheostomy tube
   d. intravascular catheter
   e. nasogastric tube
Thoracic structures:
   a. pulmonary arteries
   b. mediastinum
   c. heart
   d. hemidiaphragm
   e. ribs[4]

Portable radiographs taken in the intensive care setting are usually taken in the anteroposterior (AP) projection. In this projection the heart is more distant from the film; therefore, the heart shadow is larger than the actual size of the heart. The left lateral view is sometimes preferred, because there is less cardiac magnification and a better view of the left lower lobe is afforded.

The right hemidiaphragm is dome-shaped and higher than the left because the liver is situated under it. The anterior portion of the liver should begin about the level of the fifth rib. The carina should be located about the point where the second rib joins the sternum (or at the level of the fourth thoracic vertebra). An endotracheal tube should be placed 2–5 cm above the carina. On a normal AP film, the tenth or eleventh posterior rib should be visible during a full inspiratory effort of the patient when the film is taken.

Chest film inspection should be undertaken systematically. Using a systematic inspection technique minimizes the likelihood of missing an important pathologic feature.

Atelectasis will appear on a chest x-ray as a density. Sometimes a mediastinal shift may be seen on the side with the density. A thorough working knowledge of topical, segmental, and subsegmental anatomy can help in determining the actual areas of collapse using the chest film.

A chest radiograph is essential in the diagnosis of pulmonary infection. The existence of new or progressive pulmonary infiltrates is considered sufficient evidence to suggest pulmonary infection. Infiltrates increase lung density and hence make the lungs appear more opaque (whiter) in appearance. Caution must be exercised with the use of x-ray for diagnostic purposes, for chest x-ray findings may lag as much as 24 to 48 hours behind other clinical findings.

In adult respiratory distress syndrome, the chest film will be opaque and show a honeycomb texture, with a butterfly shape. Some describe the "ground-glass" look of the whitened chest film. Such a chest film could mimic the picture of cardiogenic pulmonary edema, an acute pneumonitis process, or lung contusion. Thus, a chest x-ray cannot be counted on as the sole diagnostic for ARDS.

A chart of general radiologic findings in various lung processes is given in Table 2-22.

Laboratory Data

An in-depth discussion of acid-base balance and the functions of electrolytes is presented in the chapter on renal function. What follows is an overview of electrolytes critical to the functioning of the respiratory system, indicating clinical signs and significant causes of certain imbalances.

Normal sodium (Na^+) level is 135–145 mEq/L. Sodium promotes irritability of muscle tissues. This extracellular cation plays a major role in the conduction of nerve impulses.

Normal potassium (K^+) level is 3.5–5.5 mEq/L. Potassium greatly affects muscle contractions and plays a role in the conduction of nerve impulses. Even minor changes in the extracellular volume of

Table 2-22 Radiologic Findings in Pulmonary Disease

Process	Finding
Pneumonia	Opacity
ARDS	Opacity, honeycomb pattern
Chest trauma	Opacity, rib fractures
Chronic bronchitis	Enlarged heart, translucence, deepened or flattened diaphragm, air bronchogram (spikelike projections), increased AP diameter
Asthma	Hyperinflation (intercostal spaces almost parallel), translucence, deepened or flattened diaphragm, increased AP diameter
Asbestosis	Opacity, honeycomb pattern, enlarged heart
Congestive failure	Prominent pulmonary vessels, knarly lines
Pulmonary edema	Opacity, enlarged heart, prominent pulmonary vessels, knarly lines
Emphysema	Enlarged heart, translucence, deepened or flattened diaphragm
Cystic fibrosis	Enlarged heart, translucence, deepened or flattened diaphragm
Pneumothorax	Localized hyperlucency

this major intracellular cation can produce severe and profound clinical effects.

Normal chloride (Cl^-) level is 95–105 mEq/L. Chloride is a major extracellular anion that is very important in maintaining acid-base balance. Hypochloremia may cause shallow respirations, which are the start of a vicious cycle in the case of pneumonia, for pneumonias are, in turn, direct and significant causes of hypochloremia.

Hyperchloremia also affects respiratory effort, in that increased Cl^- causes symptoms including dyspnea and rapid deep breathing.

Normal magnesium (Mg^{++}) level is 1.3–2.5 mEq/L. Magnesium is a major intracellular cation that is significant in ATP function and affects acetylcholine release from the neuromuscular junction.

Mechanical Ventilation

The bulk movement of gases between the atmosphere and the lung occurs in response to a pressure gradient. The movement of gas at a given rate past a point is termed flow. As the gas flows through the system (the machine-patient complex), it encounters impedance, or resistance, the net result of which is the production and dispersion of pressure forces within the mechanical ventilation system and the lungs and thorax. In essence, mechanical ventilation should be considered a cooperation of distinctive and at times dysynergistic forces at the machine-patient interface. The physical factors affecting ventilation are flow, pressure, and volume. Manipulation of these parameters over time has significant effects; the combination of the above three factors must be considered when utilizing mechanical ventilation.

There are several important general concepts to understand in regard to mechanical ventilation. Although patients are placed on mechanical ventilators for various reasons, ventilatory muscle fatigue has come to be viewed as the primary factor mediating ventilator commitment. The patient who is unable to adequately ventilate the lungs experiences a resultant hypercarbia leading to respiratory failure.

Once respiratory failure (ventilatory or oxygenation) is suspected, and after all reasonable efforts at more conservative therapy and the patient's own natural respiratory drive have failed, mechanical ventilatory support can reasonably be assumed to be indicated. Intubation and mechanical ventilation are initiated. Support and maintenance of the patient while on the mechanical ventilator constitute the next phase of the process. Physiological, infectious, and mechanico-vascular parameters as well as prob-

lems related to machine dependability all require monitoring, assessment, interpretation, and intervention. Problem solving during the management of a patient on mechanical ventilation never stops. Continuous monitoring and appropriate interpretation for intervention must be based on sound knowledge and technique, the type of machine being used, and clinical data and their indications.

The importance of the human element in the patient-machine interface can *never* be disregarded. Critical care nurses, because of their close relationship with the patient, more often than not are obligated to bear the burden of caring. The skills and techniques related to acute support and patient rehabilitative preparation are numerous and technical in nature, and the patient's response to them varies.

Generally, the patient with primary respiratory failure (particularly in the case of severe acute or chronic exacerbation) who has been mechanically ventilated for 15 to 30 days has about a 70–80% chance of being weaned. Longer periods of mechanical ventilation range between one and five months. The estimated prevalence of chronic ventilator-dependent patients is 2.8 per 100,000 patients.

The support and treatment of the patient by mechanical means is an essential component of critical care medicine and life support. Thorough and appropriate involvement of respiratory care personnel trained to care for the patient on mechanical ventilation is necessary for the appropriate use of mechanical life support technologies.

Artificial Airway Management

The machine-patient interface is established through the use of an artificial airway, first indicated when a loss of protective muscle tone in the upper airway has occurred (a loss of patency in muscular integrity between the base of the tongue and the posterior pharyngeal wall). If the loss of muscle tone is partial in nature, it is accompanied by snoring sounds. The airflow noise is low and becomes louder with the increase of the obstruction; complete airway obstruction occurs with marked inspiratory muscular effort without the accompanying movement of air. At this point the patient makes obvious use of inspiratory accessory muscles. In the alert and conscious patient, panic and anxiety as well as a subjective sense of massive air hunger and choking will surface.

The first intervention in the treatment of soft airway obstruction is to relieve the obstruction through the simplest and most immediate maneuvers. The mechanical maneuvers include extending the neck and elevating the chin. The unconscious patient can often be moved into a lateral position, in which gravity and neck extension will naturally cause the airway to open.

In the critical care setting, artificial airways of the following types are often used:

Oropharyngeal and nasopharyngeal airways

Oral, endotracheal, and nasoendotracheal tubes

Tracheostomy tubes (fenestrated and nonfenestrated)

Tracheal buttons

Complications related to the use of these airways are not uncommon. First, with the use of such airways, natural body defense mechanisms are bypassed and contamination, colonization, and infection of the lower airway and tracheobronchial tree can occur. An effective cough is also inhibited by an artificial airway because it completely bypasses the vocal cords, or at least prevents effective use of the vocal cords. The artificial airway also markedly limits communication by the patient, although there are means of communicating with such patients. More radical complications of mechanical airways are numerous and include:

Orificial trauma

Hemorrhage

Technical and mechanical failure

Apnea

Esophageal rupture/fistula

Hypotension

Bronchospasm

Increased ICP

Airway obstruction and spasm

Sore throat

Stenosis of the airway

Granuloma formation

Displaced tube

Epistaxis

Maxillary sinusitis

Laryngeal nerve injury

Hypoxemia, including acute hypoxic encephalopathy

Vomiting, regurgitation, and aspiration

Esophageal, laryngeal, or endobronchial intubation

Barotrauma, pneumothorax

Cardiovascular stress

Vocal cord injury

Nerve damage

Ulceration

Obstruction of the eustachian tube

Pressure necrosis

Subcutaneous emphysema

Most artificial airways are made of polyvinyl chloride plastics especially suited for single uses; they possess low tissue toxicity and are fairly flexible, although less so than silicone rubber materials and devices. Most airway devices that are used for a period of time are anchored in the airway by a balloon containing air usually pressurized to no greater than 30 mm Hg, since at that pressure arterial capillary blood flow is seriously impeded as a result of capillary compression. Obviously any cuff pressure will also compromise mucosal blood flow, so inflation pressure should not exceed 20 mm Hg (25 cm H_2O) so as to allow arterial and venous flow through the ventilatory cycle.

Consideration should also be given to the appropriate size of suction catheter to be used with a given artificial oraltracheal, nasotracheal, or tracheal airway. Since each is sized differently, an approximate formula is

$$4(mm) + 2 = F \text{ or } \frac{F - 2}{4} = mm$$

where F indicates a French size catheter.

Positive Pressure Airway Therapy

The types of airway pressure therapy are numerous. Table 2-23 presents definitions and descriptions of the types available.

The decision to institute mechanical or auxiliary life support technologies is based on the need to support ventilation or oxygenation or to assist the respiratory musculature. This decision is made in circumstances that include the presence of apnea, the presence of acute respiratory failure, or the suspicion of impending ventilatory failure. Indications of the need for ventilatory support include depressed ventilatory drive, overloaded muscles due to excessive loads from increases in compliance and airway resistance, and muscular weakness. Indications for oxygenation support include V/Q mismatch (or shunts) and low perfusion states.

In determining the presence and degree of ventilatory distress or failure, pH serves as a better indicator than $PaCO_2$. A high $PaCO_2$ value is not necessarily sufficient cause to institute mechanical ventilation if the pH remains within acceptable range and the mental status of the patient remains intact. Usually a $PaCO_2$ value greater than 50 mm Hg

Table 2-23 Types of Airway Pressure Therapy

Type	Description
Positive airway pressure therapy	Positive pressure applied to the airway during any phase of the breathing cycle for the purposes of supporting or improving respiratory function
Positive pressure ventilation (PPV)	Positive pressure applied to the airway for the purpose of providing or augmenting inspiratory tidal volume
Full ventilatory support (FVS)	Provision of PPV in a manner ensuring that the patient *is not obligated* to contribute to the work of breathing required for maintenance of carbon dioxide (CO_2) homeostasis
Partial ventilatory support (PVS)	Provision of PPV in a manner that *obligates* the patient to provide some of the work of breathing required for maintenance of CO_2 homeostasis
Ventilator mode	A combination of mechanisms that governs the ventilator's function and determines the potential interactions between the patient and the ventilator
Inverse ratio ventilation (IRV)	Positive pressure ventilation intended to result in an inspiratory time equal to or greater than the expiratory time

Volume Preset Modes[a]

Type	Description
Control mode ventilation (CMV)	A volume preset mode in which the patient is not allowed to participate in any phase of the breathing cycle—*time initiated, volume limited, volume/time cycled*
Assist mode ventilation (AMV)	A volume preset mode in which the ventilator frequency is determined by the patient's inspiratory efforts—*pressure initiated, volume limited, volume/time cycled*
Assist/control mode ventilation (A/CMV)	Assist mode in which the ventilator frequency is determined by the patient's inspiratory efforts only when the patient's respiratory rate exceeds a preset control mode rate—*pressure or time initiated, volume limited, volume/time cycled*
Intermittent mandatory ventilation (IMV)	A ventilator system that allows spontaneous breathing via a continuous flow device between machine breaths delivered at preset time intervals—*time initiated, volume limited, volume/time cycled + spontaneous breathing*
Synchronized IMV (SIMV)	A ventilator system that allows spontaneous breathing via a demand flow device between machine breaths delivered in synchrony with a spontaneous inspiratory effort occurring within a preset time interval—*time/pressure initiated, volume limited, volume/time cycled*

Volume Variable Modes[b]

Type	Description
Pressure support ventilation (PSV)	A volume variable mode in which the ventilator frequency is determined by the patient's inspiratory efforts; a preset system pressure is rapidly achieved and maintained throughout inspiration by adjustment of machine inspiratory flow; and inspiration ends when the inspiratory flow falls below a preset minimal value—*pressure initiated, pressure limited, flow cycled*
Pressure control ventilation (PCV)	A volume variable mode in which inspiration is time initiated; a preset system pressure is rapidly achieved and maintained throughout inspiration by adjustment of machine inspiratory flow; and inspiration ends at a predetermined time—*time initiated, pressure limited, time cycled*
Airway pressure release ventilation (APRV)	A volume variable mode in which inspiration is time initiated; a preset system pressure is maintained throughout inspiration by a continuous flow–threshold resistor device; and inspiration ends at a predetermined time—*time initiated, pressure limited, time cycled + spontaneous breathing*

Positive End-Expiratory Pressure (PEEP)[c]

Type	Description
Continuous positive pressure ventilation (CPPV)	PEEP in conjunction with positive pressure breaths; CMV + PEEP, A/CMV + PEEP
Continuous positive airway pressure (CPAP)	PEEP in conjunction with a spontaneous breath through an apparatus designed to maintain airway pressure fluctuations above and below the baseline to no greater extent than would be present with normal spontaneous breathing
Expiratory positive airway pressure (EPAP)	PEEP in conjunction with a spontaneous breath through an apparatus designed to allow inspiratory flow only when inspiratory airway pressures descend below atmospheric

[a]Positive pressure modes that deliver a specified tidal volume unless predetermined safety limits are exceeded—volume limited modes.
[b]Positive pressure modes that deliver varying tidal volumes determined both by preset ventilator limits and patient factors—pressure, flow, or time limited.
[c]The maintenance of a positive airway pressure at the end of exhalation.
Source: Shapiro, A. In Sills, J. (1990). *Respiratory Care Certification Guide.* St. Louis: Mosby Year Book, p. 279.

accompanied by a pH of less than 7.30 is a good indication of the necessity for ventilatory support.

Ventilatory Failure

Progressive declines in $PaCO_2$ and pH usually indicate impending acute ventilatory failure. Ventilatory failure is caused by primary pulmonary abnormalities or pathologies that limit the mechanical ability of the lung to move air. Regardless of antecedent, impending ventilatory failure is characterized by an increase in the patient's work of breathing (WOB). As WOB increases, the patient experiences:

1. changes in the ventilatory pattern (total volume decreases and respiration rate increases)
2. accessory muscle use:
   With inspiration:
   Scalene
   Sternocleidomastoid
   Pectoralis major
   Trapezius
   With expiration:
   Rectus abdominis
   External oblique
   Internal oblique
   Transversus abdominis
   When inspiratory muscles contract, they elevate the thorax and increase the anteroposterior diameter, and when expiratory muscles contract, they increase abdominal pressure, so the diaphragm moves higher into the thoracic cage.
3. paradoxical breathing patterns
4. muscular retractions of head, neck, and thorax
5. decreased ventilatory reserve
   Vital capacity $< 10–15$ mL/kg
   Negative inspiratory force > -20 cm H_2O
   V_T a greater proportion of VC
6. deteriorating pH, $PaCO_2$, and PaO_2
7. increasing heart rate, respiratory rate, and blood pressure

A patient may require ventilatory support despite apparently adequate alveolar ventilation, for example, with metabolic acidosis, airflow obstruction, or neuromuscular weakness. Clinical wisdom suggests that if pH values greater than 7.60 or less than 7.25 are sustained, mechanical life support is indicated.

The patient who requires intubation of the airway and supplemental airway pressures (such as in PEEP therapy) for oxygenation can be observed to require high ventilatory energy and resultant work loads. Intervention directed toward decreasing ex-

cessive work of breathing is particularly indicated in the cardiovascularly stressed patient. Because of increased work of breathing such a patient also frequently demonstrates hypercarbia, acidosis, hypoxemia, and increased physiological and psychological stress. Often the patient's psychological stress is so intense that upon ventilatory commitment, the relief is great enough to cause decreasing central nervous system sympathetic tone and hypotension. The use of fluid therapy and/or vasopressor (β-1 sympathomimetic) drugs may be essential at this time.

When the patient is being supported by mechanical ventilation, increased work of breathing is present whenever the following are observed:

1. Exhalation during the inspiratory phase of the mechanical ventilator
2. Efforts at spontaneous ventilation during the inspiratory phase of the mechanical ventilator
3. The ventilator's pressure manometer reading deflecting more than 1 or 2 cm H_2O in the negative direction during the initiation of the machine-assisted breath or during IMV/SIMV

Most patients require full ventilatory support for the first 24–48 hours after commitment. This support can be achieved through one of several mechanisms, including control mode ventilation, assist/control ventilation, IMV/SIMV, mandatory minute ventilation, airway pressure release ventilation, pressure control–inverse ratio ventilation, and inspiratory pressure support.

The majority of patients committed to mechanical ventilation need only partial ventilatory support. This approach allows the patient to do some portion of the ventilatory work. The advantages of this approach are three: (1) ventilation provided is more like normal physiological ventilation, (2) gas distribution is closer to normal, and (3) mean intrathoracic pressure is lower.

Establishing Parameters of Ventilation

Minute Ventilation

When adjusting mechanical ventilation, the most important component to identify is the expired minute ventilation (Ve) and its effect on $PaCO_2$. In an adequate lung an increase in expired minute ventilation will result in a decrease in $PaCO_2$; that is, these two variables vary inversely with each other. A normal minute ventilation range for the adult patient is 5–7 Lpm (liters per minute).

The goal of adequate continuous mechanical ventilation is to provide ventilatory support to normalize physiological parameters such as $PaCO_2$, pH, and PaO_2. To provide this necessary support, an appropriate minute ventilation based on body weight, surface area, and metabolic activity must be established for the patient. A minute ventilation rate for a male with normal lungs and normal metabolic rate can be closely estimated using the following equation:

$$Ve = 4 \times body\ surface\ area$$

For females the equation is:

$$Ve = 3.5 \times body\ surface\ area$$

Body surface area is obtained by calculating the Dubois nomogram. The estimated Ve should be increased by 9% for every degree of body temperature above 37°C and decreased by the same percentage for every degree below normal. In cases of metabolic acidosis, it may be appropriate to increase Ve by as much as 20%.

Proper monitoring of minute ventilation is essential during mechanical ventilation to ensure an adequate $PaCO_2$ and to maintain a proper acid-base balance. As in the case of mechanical ventilatory monitoring, this monitoring should be performed at least every two hours in the critical care setting to provide indications of patient status. Decreasing expired minute ventilation can indicate either pathological or mechanical problems, including endotracheal or tracheostomy leak, faulty monitoring equipment, open/closed pneumothorax, acute alveolar air trapping, tracheoesophageal fistula, incorrect ventilator settings, ventilator circuit leaks, humidifier leaks, and bronchopleural fistula.

Tidal Volume

It is possible to vary and control minute ventilation to achieve the desired $PaCO_2$ independent of the design of the mechanical ventilator. The appropriate minute ventilation level is obtained by determining an appropriate tidal volume (the amount of gas that is moved in and out of the lung in one breath) and frequency (the number of cycles per minute).

$$Ve = V_T \times f$$

It is normal for tidal volumes of adults to range from 10 to 15 mL/kg. The respiratory rate can then be determined by dividing the predicted minute ventilation by the estimated tidal volume.

$$f = Ve/V_T$$

Frequency

The respiratory frequency, whether spontaneous, mechanical, or a combination of both, is dependent on inspiratory and expiratory time. With a normal respiratory rate of 12 breaths per minute, normal inspiratory time is 2 seconds in the adult. Frequency is most often described by the following relationship:

$$f = \frac{60\ seconds}{Ti + Te}$$

where

$$f = frequency$$
$$Ti = inspiratory\ time$$
$$Te = expiratory\ time$$

If inspiratory time is constant, the frequency will vary inversely with the expiratory time. If the expiratory time is constant, frequency will vary inversely with inspiratory time. And finally, if the frequency is constant (as when a rate control device is being used and is preset in control and IMV modes), then inspiratory and expiratory time will vary inversely with one another.

A concept related to frequency is the I:E ratio, which is the relationship of inspiratory to expiratory ventilatory cycle. During mechanical ventilation, the ratio should be optimized for each patient rather than routinely set at 1:2 or 1:3.

In the clinical setting, the I:E ratio should be monitored to establish the most mechanically efficient frequency consistent with the goal of minimizing cardiac dysfunction. There is significant risk of adverse effects of continuous positive airway pressure and mechanical ventilation on the cardiovascular system. During ventilation the mean airway pressure increases throughout the tracheobronchial tree and the alveoli, resulting in a mechanical compression of pulmonary capillaries and an increase in intrathoracic pressures. A decrease in venous return results from compression of the great veins returning blood to the heart. This positive pressure also interferes with the normal thoracic pump, which essentially milks blood flow through the great vessels in the thoracic cavity. The net effect of the above increased impedance to flow during the inspiratory cycle (when positive airway pressure is applied) is a decrease in left ventricular output.

Cardiovascular embarrassment The heart and great vessels are influenced by pressures similar to those that are in effect in the pleural space. Increased intrathoracic pressures caused by pressure ventilation reduce venous return. This phenomenon complicates the interpretation of central venous pressure (CVP) and pulmonary artery wedge pressure readings. Increases in the pulmonary vascular resistance measurement may indicate vascular injury, pulmonary thromboemboli, pneumothorax, increased blood viscosity, hypoxemia, acidosis, and hypercarbia, histamine release, vasoconstrictor drug effects, and compliance changes due to emphysema, fibrosis, or edema. In contrast, decreases in pulmonary vascular resistance through vasodilation or accessing of the vast vascular bed may result from increased left atrial pressure, increased pulmonary volume, drug effects, and increased pulmonary artery pressure. Increased levels of continuous airway pressure can increase right ventricular afterload sufficiently to cause RV dilation and therefore a reduction of left ventricular compliance.

Evidence suggests that reduction in cardiac output is likely to occur in the patient whose intrathoracic pressure rises and in the patient suffering volume depletion or impaired venous constrictive ability.

Monitoring of respiratory rate or frequency is best achieved when the nurse physically counts the frequency (even in the presence of monitors and alarm systems). Minute ventilation and tidal volume are usually measured by mechanical spirometers such as the Wright or Draeger respirometer or by electronic spirometers that have flow transducers and convert flow rate into volume using the following formula:

$$\text{Volume} = \text{flow rate} \times \text{time}$$

Oxygen Concentration

Inspired oxygen concentration should be established judiciously. Oxygen concentrations that would elevate the patient's PaO_2 above a level needed to sustain adequate ventilatory drive are strongly contraindicated. This is a particularly troublesome problem in the care of the chronic bronchitic patient with chronic hypercarbia and chronic hypoxemia. Such a patient requires low levels of PaO_2 and, thus, FIO_2 to prevent bradypnea. Furthermore, prolonged exposure to FIO_2 levels greater than 50% (for over 8 hours) causes oxygen toxicity, which can quickly lead to hypoxemia and decreased lung compliance.

Another risk is that oxygen concentrations greater than FIO_2 of .7, or 70% oxygen, will cause sudden displacement of nitrogen gas from the alveoli and tissue compartments, resulting in gas absorption atelectasis in already hypoventilated lung units. This absorption will lead to an increase in intrapulmonary

shunt, refractory hypoxemia, and finally, alveolar collapse. (This problem frequently arises in situations of low tidal volume and when a pressure-based ventilator mode is being used.)

Oxygen itself is a potent cellular oxidizer. The uncontrolled use of high oxygen concentrations ($FIO_2 = 1.0$) has been found to cause serious pulmonary changes in as little as 6 hours. Pathological changes can include:

Reduction in ciliary activity
Decreased protective macrophage activity
Endothelial cellular wall damage
Changes in surfactant production and activity
Decreased compliance
Decreased vital capacity
Decreased FRC
Progressive absorption atelectasis
Increased lung water
Decreased pulmonary capillary lung volume
Decreased diffusing capacity
Platelet aggregation in the pulmonary capillary
Capillary injury
Leaky lung capillaries
Acute lung injury

There are situations, however, that necessitate an increase in FIO_2 in order to maintain the patient's PaO_2 between 60 and 100 mm Hg. There is a linear relationship between FIO_2 and PaO_2 as long as the cardiovascular and alveolar ventilation systems are stable. This relationship suggests the following formula by which to achieve the necessary FIO_2:

$$\frac{\text{Known } PaO_2}{\text{Known } FIO_2} = \frac{\text{desired } PaO_2}{\text{desired } FIO_2}$$

Hypoventilation causes increased $PaCO_2$ and decreased PaO_2, resulting in hypoxemia. Without adequate restoration of physiologic ventilation, the arterial oxygen deficiency will not be reversed. Rarely is the hypoxemia that is accompanied by normal or adequate ventilation improved by use of mechanical ventilation unless there is a substantial unloading of the ventilatory muscles' work load and a major decrease in the oxygen consumption of those muscles.

Most arterial oxygen deficits are supported by means of oxygen therapy, cardiac support, positive end expiratory pressure, use of bronchial pulmonary hygiene techniques (suctioning), and sympathomimetic bronchodilators. Thus, it is important to realize that mechanical ventilation may not be the treatment of choice for the reversal of hypoxemia.

Positive End Expiratory Pressure (PEEP) Therapy

If an adequate PaO_2 cannot be maintained by an FIO_2 value of less than .5, or 50% oxygen, the decision to use PEEP should be made. PEEP is a method of preventing total exhalation of intrapulmonary gas and increasing lung volume by maintaining an end pressure gradient at which flow can no longer continue. Complete exhalation is retarded, allowing airway pressure to rise above atmospheric. Continuous positive airway pressure (CPAP) is an approach to maintaining a preset or desired PEEP level. PEEP should be administered via CPAP to restore the patient to normal FRC, thereby improving pulmonary compliance, decreasing the work of breathing, and improving the matching of ventilation to perfusion (decreased shunting). The above should result in an improved PaO_2 without increasing FIO_2.

With few exceptions, the use of PEEP/CPAP therapy is indicated for the restrictive ventilatory defect that has been proven to decrease. PEEP/CPAP therapy can restore normal oxygenation at a lower or safer (less toxic) FIO_2 level and improve pulmonary function.

PEEP values of 5–10 cm H_2O can be established in the patient suffering a homogeneous lung disease to increase the PaO_2 level. Sometimes it may be necessary to increase PEEP values to 10–20 cm H_2O; in such situations hemodynamic monitoring may be indicated, for adequate fluid replacement is required to maintain cardiac flow.

PEEP can be used safely in a situation of severely decreased lung compliance; the stiffness of the lung acts as a barrier to the PEEP pressure and minimizes its transmission to the rest of the pleural space, causing less cardiac compression.

Finally, PEEP should never be used in the case of localized lung disorders, as unaffected lung areas will become overdistended, causing hypoxemia and the increased risk of barotrauma and cardiac output compromise.

When PEEP therapy is instituted and compliance improvement can be identified, the highest values obtained occur when alveoli are maximally recruited. This clinical state is associated with a minimal ventilatory deadspace and decreased shunting, and is closely related to maximum oxygen delivery. The effectiveness of PEEP therapy can be monitored using the following parameters.

1. Arterial oxygen tension (PaO_2) or saturation (SaO_2). It is important to realize, however, that these measurements alone often prove inadequate.

2. Arterial-venous oxygen content difference (C a-v O_2). This measurement represents the volume of oxygen extracted from 100 mL of blood. It does not reflect the rate of oxygen consumption, however. In acute stress with adequate cardiovascular reserve, cardiac output increases, offsetting the increase in oxygen demands.

3. Lung Compliance. Static compliance reflects changes in the total lung-thorax compliance. This measure is affected by many extraneous variables.

4. Deadspace ventilation (Vd). The relationship between arterial and end tidal CO_2 may offer a significant measurement cutoff point, as effective compliance ends in positive pressure therapy when deadspace begins to increase.

5. Cardiac output. Inferred from the heart rate and blood pressure. This value must be measured using a properly placed pulmonary artery catheter.

6. Oxygen delivery. Cardiac output multiplied by the arterial oxygen content, multiplied by 10. It represents the total oxygen made available to the tissues per minute.

7. Intrapulmonary shunting calculations. Both arterial and pulmonary arterial blood samples are needed to calculate this variable. Shunt reductions of 15–20% are considered good cut-off points.

Finally, selected signs can indicate patient tolerance to PEEP/CPAP therapy. If the patient is tolerating the therapy well, one will see increases in PaO_2 and static lung compliance, decreased pulmonary vascular resistance and intrapulmonary shunting, and stable heart rate, pressures, and cardiac output. The patient not tolerating PEEP/CPAP will exhibit an increased PaO_2 (still), but this will be accompanied by significant changes in intrapulmonary shunting.

Alveolar Ventilation

Any volume of gas that enters the lung enters one of two anatomical spaces: the effective area of ventilation (the alveoli), or the ineffective area of ventilation (the conducting airways). Alveolar ventilation is the primary means by which the function of continuous mechanical ventilation is performed. The adequacy of alveolar ventilation is determined by the pathophysiological process present and the operational parameters of the mechanical ventilator. It is for this reason that the majority of ventilators used are volume-oriented rather than pressure-oriented; volume-oriented ventilators are certain to maintain a delivered tidal volume and minute ventilation regardless of decreasing lung compliance or increasing airway resistance.

As minute ventilation is increased, so is alveolar ventilation. Clinically (and mathematically), it has been shown that minute ventilation can be increased more by increasing tidal volume than by increasing ventilatory frequency. Increasing tidal volume does not increase ineffective ventilation or deadspace. The $PaCO_2$ level is the most direct reflection of alveolar ventilation.

Deadspace

Deadspace is composed of anatomic and alveolar deadspace and, when a patient is ventilated, the space wasted due to the ventilation system circuit:

Physiologic deadspace = alveolar deadspace
+ anatomic deadspace

Approximately one-third of each tidal breath ventilates the anatomic deadspace in the normal individual. Anatomic deadspace is usually equal to 1 mL per pound of body weight (about 150 mL in the normal adult). When a patient is intubated, the artificial airway is believed to reduce the anatomic deadspace by about 50%.

Alveolar deadspace is usually nil; so in the normal adult, physiologic deadspace equals the anatomic deadspace. However, in many pathologies ventilation may reach unperfused alveoli, which are ineffective in gas exchange. Thus, the volume of alveolar deadspace in such instances can increase to such magnitudes that it represents the major portion of deadspace, necessitating increases in minute ventilation. In such cases $PaCO_2$ levels will be out of proportion to delivered minute ventilation. The clinician may then estimate new minute ventilatory demands by the following equation:

$$\text{New Ve} = \text{Current Ve} \times \frac{\text{current } PaCO_2}{\text{desired } PaCO_2}$$

If respiratory acidosis continues even after correcting for an increase in alveolar volume, the patient may be experiencing significant deadspace resulting from too high an inspiratory flow rate or an uneven distribution of ventilation throughout the lungs. Reducing the flow rate, increasing expiratory time, or using a high tidal volume and slow ventilatory rate may be beneficial. Also, if the patient can be placed in a lateral position with the least affected lung in the dependent position, oxygenation may be improved.

Furthermore, if a patient is breathing rapidly, but maintaining a good tidal volume, minute ventilatory needs are not being met. This situation increases the work of breathing; the ventilator rate should be increased to decrease the work of breathing until the cause of the problem is identified. Tidal volume changes, in these situations, are limited by increasing changes in airway pressures and lung distensibility.

As mentioned above, another source of deadspace is the space added by the breathing circuit and humidifying system, called the mechanical deadspace. Thus,

Total dead space = physiologic deadspace
+ mechanical deadspace

A significant source for mechanical deadspace is lost in the compressible volume of the circuit, determined by:

$$\text{Comp. Vol.} = \frac{\text{known test volume (cc)}}{\text{plateau pressure (cm } H_2O)}$$

Most ventilator tubing systems have a 3–5 cc/cm H_2O value. Keeping an adequate level of water in the humidifying system will also reduce deadspace loss or compressible machine loss. Although it may be inconvenient to do so in the ICU, reducing the length of the circuit can decrease the effect of mechanical deadspace on the patient. In clinical practice, many hospitals do not take into account volume compression loss and tubing distensibility when determining tidal volume delivered to the adult patient, because the type of device that is most often used is a volume ventilator with sufficient capability to adjust to changing airway pressure and flows.

Airway Pressures

Airway pressures must also be considered. Historically, health care workers believed that airway pressures no greater than 40 cm H_2O were prudent; higher pressures were thought to cause barotrauma and cardiac compromise. As ventilatory techniques improved for the more critically ill patient, the belief evolved that whatever pressure was necessary to oxygenate and ventilate a patient should be used. It was thought that most patients could be adequately ventilated at peak pressures less than 60 cm H_2O. However, current evidence is causing practitioners to lower airway pressures in some instances to below 30 cm H_2O.

High peak airway pressures, high mean airway pressures, and high end expiratory pressures have all been linked to the potential for overinflation of alveoli and tissue rupture. The rupture of lung tissue can lead to complications such as pneumothorax, pneumomediastinum, pneumoperitoneum, or subcutaneous emphysema.

Barotrauma

The incidence of barotrauma correlates to increases of both mean and peak airway pressures. (The incidence of barotrauma in the clinical setting is about 5–10% of all ventilated patients.) However, barotrauma usually occurs when the patient simulates coughs, fights the ventilator, or is involved in maneuvers to increase intrathoracic pressure. Pleural puncture, whether spontaneous, lacerating, or traumatic, and lung necrosis can be aggravated in the presence of increased airway pressure. Barotrauma can obviously also occur during pleural biopsy, thoracentesis, and transthoracic aspirations. Other causes include necrotizing lung processes, excessive airway secretions, duration of ventilation, alveolar pressure, cycling pressure, severe unilateral lung pathology, and PEEP levels > 15 cm H_2O.

Persistent bronchopleural fistula, or leak, can also occur; if it does the patient has a poor chance of survival. Persistent leakage indicates the presence of a severe underlying disease process. The most common processes responsible include rupture of emphysematous blebs, necrotizing pneumonias, bronchiolitis obliterans, mechanical ventilation support for ARDS, subtotal pulmonary resections, and pharmacologic insults in the lung tissue.

Barotrauma must be prevented, not treated. Interventions aimed at preventing barotrauma include reducing peak and mean airway pressures by limiting tidal volumes and continuous positive airway pressures, allowing spontaneous breaths rather than machine-governed ventilation, reducing minute ventilation, establishing significant bronchial hygiene to minimize airway obstruction, improving lung/thorax distensibility, and decreasing peak flow of the system to a minimum that meets the patient's inspiratory demands without increasing work of breathing. In the event that barotrauma occurs despite preventive measures, care should include nutritional support to promote wound healing and visceral and parietal pleural pressure manipulations to facilitate the healing of pleural tears. Surgical intervention by tissue resection can be used to treat persistent pleural gas leaks. Chemical pleurodesis using bleomycin or doxorubicin has proven successful, although it is extremely difficult to accomplish, which mitigates against its use.

Oxygen Delivery and Airway Pressure

Increasing airway pressure and maintaining continuous airway pressure by mechanical support can affect oxygenation. However, if the cardiac output decrease is proportionately greater than the possible rise in circulating arterial oxygen content, the oxygen delivery capacity of the system will be hindered. More oxygen will be removed from hemoglobin molecules at the tissue level when slower perfusion and increased metabolic activity occur, resulting in more desaturated blood being returned to the failing pulmonary system. If this desaturated blood is returned to the damaged lung, capillary shunting (usually from atelectasis) can increase. Other true intrapulmonary and extrapulmonary shunts, such as space-occupying lesions, total airway obstruction, alveolar fluid, random collapse of alveoli, or increased surface tension, can continue to increase shunting above clinical margins of safety. The following are the clinical implications of various shunt values.

3–5% shunt: Normal anatomic shunt

<10% shunt: Clinically normal lungs

15–19% shunt: Intrapulmonary abnormality present but usually not severe enough to compromise the respiratory system

20–29% shunt: Significant intrapulmonary disease; may be life-threatening

>30% shunt: Requires aggressive cardiopulmonary life support

>60% shunt: If developed suddenly, prognosis is poor

Reduced mixed venous blood returned to the pulmonary system has a negative impact on arterial content after admixture (ventilation/perfusion inequality). Ventilation/perfusion inequality occurs under conditions of poorly ventilated alveoli or excessive blood flow, but in either case such a situation usually proves responsive to increases in oxygen concentrations. However, flow or tidal volume should not be reduced in an attempt to decrease the pressure and improve bronchodilation until it is ascertained that the machine pressure observed represents actual intrapulmonary airway pressure rather than a resistance to flow caused by too small an endotracheal or tracheostomy tube.

Problems with Mechanical Ventilation

Any application of mechanical ventilatory equipment places the patient at risk for problems relating to mechanical breathing. These can be minor or life-threatening.

The effects of pressure/volume ventilation are many and include:

Increased mean airway pressure
Increased mean intrathoracic pressure
Decreased venous return
Decreased cardiac output
Decreased urinary output
Gastrointestinal stress
Increased intracranial pressure
Increased deadspace ventilation
Increased work of breathing
Increased intrapulmonary shunt
Hyper/hypo ventilation
Psychological and affective stress

Because of the presence of the above risks, close monitoring and evaluation of the patient-machine interface is necessary. System monitoring should be performed as often as necessary; the following parameters should be checked.

1. Delivered FIO_2 should routinely and regularly be monitored.
2. Ventilator rate and timing factors should be checked by counting breaths per minute to assure calibration or identify abnormal breathing patterns.
3. Exhaled tidal volume is more appropriately measured in the event that there is an unidentified system leak present.
4. System flows should be adequate to meet minimal patient demands; outputs of these flows should be quantified.
5. Water or fluid reservoirs for temperature and humidification should be checked for fluid level.
6. The endotracheal tube cuff or seal should be functioning appropriately.
7. System alarms should be checked routinely to ensure that they are turned on and set appropriately and that the following alarms function properly:
    Patient/system disconnects
    Patient/system leaks
    Patient/system pressure fluctuations (including low PEEP)
    Patient/system volumes
    Patient/system humidity/heat systems
    Patient/system apnea
    Patient/system gas concentrations ($PaCO_2$ and FIO_2)

Patient/system airflow (machine and patient)
Patient/system power sources

Monitoring the response of the patient to mechanical ventilation should include assessment of the following:

Patient/system airway pressure
Mental status
Vital signs
Hemodynamic status
Arterial blood gases
Breath sounds
Chest radiography for tube placement and lung inflation
Cuff pressures
Patient's mechanical capacity, including negative inspiratory force, VC, spontaneous V_T, Ve, cough, and secretions
Work of breathing
Phase of synchronicity with mechanical demands
Complications of machine ventilation
Patient/system compliance
Problems associated with immobility
Patient/system resistance

Monitoring of the mechanically ventilated patient may need to be conducted as often as every hour (in the unstable patient) or every 4 hours (in the chronically ventilated patient). Ventilator parameters (tidal volume, frequency or minute ventilation, FIO_2, mode of mechanical ventilation, and PEEP levels) must be checked to ensure that they are set as ordered. Peak airway pressure, compliance, resistance, spontaneous ventilatory efforts, patient synchrony and comfort while on mechanical ventilation, exhaled tidal volumes, and the function and integrity of the cuff on the artificial airway must be assessed.

Arterial blood gas analysis should be performed whenever a change in the patient's clinical status or ventilator setting has occurred. It is usually recommended that an arterial blood gas be obtained at least 15 to 20 minutes after a change in parameters affecting ventilation. Recent evidence suggests that in the cardiovascularly stable patient for whom FIO_2 has been altered, a period of at least 10 minutes may elapse before the arterial gas is obtained. The critically ill patient on mechanical life support should have an indwelling arterial line inserted, monitored, and used to facilitate analysis of blood gases. Daily chest radiographs are recommended. Daily radiographs provide an index by which to determine if endotracheal tubes are migrating and may help to identify new pulmonary infiltrates or any early indication of barotrauma.

Meticulous care in the monitoring and adjustment of fluids and electrolytes is essential. Imbalances in fluid and electrolytes may occur as complications of mechanical ventilation. During continuous positive pressure ventilation, the normal patient has been found to experience a reduction in urinary output by as much as 50%, in part because of reduced renal blood flow caused by an alteration in the antidiuretic hormone (ADH), but primarily because ADH directly affects the baroreceptors. ADH is secreted by the pituitary gland, and the higher the level, the less urinary output there is. This gland is regulated by baroreceptors located throughout the body and cardiac atria. During mechanical ventilation, baroreceptor reflex activity in the aortic arch and carotid sinus signals a state of hypovolemia due to changes in right heart blood flow and pressure. The resulting increase in production of renin-angiotensin causes selective accumulation of abnormal amounts of fluid in the lungs, leading to heart failure.

Fluid therapy of the patient on mechanical ventilation must be undertaken cautiously, as overhydration in the face of increased ADH may lead to pulmonary edema. This may be exacerbated by decreased urinary output. The direct renal effects of positive pressure ventilation can be minimized with cautious intravascular volume expansion and the administration of low-dose dopamine therapy. Current data suggests that increased water retention may parallel increases in positive airway pressure. Water retention appears greater in conditions necessitating full ventilatory support and PEEP and lesser in conditions necessitating only partial ventilatory support and PEEP.

Finally, the principal reason for monitoring respiratory mechanics in the ICU patient is to examine and control forces inhibiting good lung expansion. Mechanical monitoring is indicated throughout the course of the patient's treatment. Esophageal studies, gas-dilution or washout studies, mass spectrometry, cardiopulmonary exercise studies, maximal ventilatory studies, and body plethysmography are not easily performed in the ICU but may be essential if further diagnosis must be made.

Lung Compliance

A primary index or measure of the lung-thorax relationship is compliance. It is essential to determine compliance in order to ascertain the pressure needed to hold a given volume. Compliance is proportional to lung volume, and thus to functional residual capacity (FRC). At constant FRC, changes in compliance represent changes in the lung or chest wall. In the normal lung during passive exhalation, the elastic forces of the lung and thorax oppose each other with equal magnitude. Any process that diminishes lung volume or the ability to generate pressure to increase lung volume causes a reduction in compliance. It is important to monitor compliance, for decreases in compliance can have serious ramifications, including decreased FRC, increased respiratory rate (that is, increased work of breathing), atelectatic phenomena, ventilation/perfusion mismatch (shunting), hypoxemia, and respiratory failure. Decreased compliance may indicate the need for any of the following:

1. appropriate body mobilization, repositioning every 1–2 hr with active and passive exercises to maintain muscular tone
2. chest physical therapy if secretions are present or suspected in any of the following conditions
   a. atelectasis
   b. acute/chronic bronchitis
   c. cystic fibrosis
   d. pneumonia
   e. bronchiectasis
3. deep breathing and coughing regimens
4. airway suctioning using appropriate catheter size and aspiration pressure to hyperoxygenate and hyperinflate
5. incentive spirometry
6. intermittent positive pressure breathing therapy (with neuromuscular impairment support and possible muscular conditioning). Volume-based therapy control of pressure to produce exhaled tidal volume > 1200–1500 cc or three times predicted tidal volume.
7. continuous positive airway pressure therapy (PEEP therapy): most aggressive conservative therapeutic approach before commitment to mechanical ventilation
   a. proper flow for system: 40 L/min flow for patient with normal/intact respiratory drive; 60–90 L/min flow for patient with increased ventilatory drive and respirations either tachypneic or hyperpneic
   b. appropriate technology for CPAP systems
   c. appropriate and secure interface for patient and CPAP system: secure and functional airway or well-fitting mask

d. monitoring and precautions to avoid gastric distension, reflux, and aspiration
e. effective airway protective mechanisms along with reasonable neurological status

8. Prolonged/chronic mechanical ventilatory support

The measure of compliance requires a measurement of volume and related pressure changes. Depending on the time and location of the pressure measurement, it may yield data on static, dynamic, effective, specific, lung, and lung-thorax compliance levels. When lung compliance is increased, the lungs will accept a greater volume of gas for each unit of pressure change. With decreased compliance, the lungs accept a smaller volume of gas per unit of pressure change. This relationship can be illustrated by the volume-pressure curve in Figure 2-40.

In contrast to a person breathing normally, the mechanically ventilated patient experiences changes in airway pressure across the lung and thorax, the measure of which indicate the compliance of the lung-thorax system. Lung compliance in such cases is expressed by the formula

$$CL = \hat{V}/\hat{P}I$$

In the ventilator supported patient, either $\hat{V}$ must be measured at the connection site of the endotracheal tube or the expired volume must be adjusted for loss of volume due to compressibility (expansion) of the circuit. The normal value for lung compliance in the mechanically ventilated patient is about 50 mL/cm/H_2O. Table 2-24 presents a list of disorders that limit lung expansion.

Peak airway pressures measure overall airway resistance in addition to elastic resistance. The type of compliance reflected by peak airway pressures is known as dynamic compliance because it includes both compliance and resistance components in the measure of impedance. Dynamic compliance decreases when airway resistance or peak airway pressures increase. Changes in dynamic compliance can often be reversed through simple maneuvers such as checking for the position of the endotracheal tube or suctioning the airway or by the administration of bronchodilators.

In general, the use of plateau pressures rather than peak pressures is usually indicated because they reflect airway pressure under a static condition of no flow and are therefore more representative of the distensibility of the lung system (static compliance). Causes of decreasing static compliance in the mechanically ventilated patient include air trapping, atelectasis, pleural effusion, changes in the chest wall (bony thorax lesions or muscle tension), pneumonia with consolidation, pulmonary edema, conditions that lead to abdominal distension, and pneumomediastinum. Reduced static compliance is an indication that ventilation is becoming less effective.

Through the technique of ventilating the lung at different volumes and recording both peak and plateau pressures, the clinician may plot both dynamic and static volume-pressure relationships. This procedure, if followed on a regular and systematic basis, may aid in planning intervention before significant injury to the patient occurs. The steps of the procedure are as follows.

1. Explain the procedure to the patient and attempt to elicit cooperation.
2. Inflate the balloon cuff of the artificial airway to eliminate leaks.
3. Occlude exhalation flow for each volume measurement.
4. Select a series of at least three tidal volumes, for example, 8, 10, and 12 mL/kg or 800, 1000, and 1200 mL.
5. Record peak airway pressure, plateau airway pressure, delivered tidal volume, and PEEP for each volume setting.
6. Return cuff pressure and all ventilator settings to normal level.
7. Plot the data.

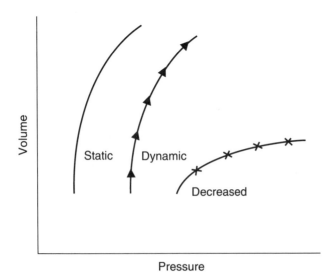

Figure 2-40 Volume-Pressure Curves Reflecting Lung Compliance

Table 2-25 describes pressure-volume changes in various pulmonary disorders.

Table 2-24 Disorders Limiting Lung Expansion

Type of Limitation	Etiology
Limitation of respiratory movements	Muscular dystrophy Neuromusclar junction problems Poliomyelitis Myasthenia gravis Depression of central respiratory centers
Limitation of thoracic cage expansion	Body deformities such as kyphoscoliosis Fractured ribs Massive obesity Fibrothorax (calcified pneumothorax or emphysema)
Limitations of lung expansibility	Lung cysts or tumors Pneumothorax Pleural effusion
Limitations of diaphragm movement	Ascites Pregnancy Phrenic nerve dysfunction
Limitation of quantity of lung tissue available	Surgical lobectomy Surgical pneumonectomy Bronchial obstruction with postoperative atelectasis
Pain	Pleurisy Recovering incision site from surgery Injured ribs Costochondritis

Source: Martin, D. (1988). *Respiratory Anatomy and Physiology*. St. Louis: The C.V. Mosby Company, p. 115.

Airway Resistance (R_{aw})

Pressures necessary to overcome the resistive forces offered by the lung are related to flow rate. Thus, the relationship between flow rate and resistance must always be quantified if comparisons are to be made. Resistance is usually described in cm H_2O/L/sec. Normal airway resistance (R_{aw}) is equal to 0.6–2.4 cm H_2O/L/sec; in the normal adult about 50% of the resistance to airflow occurs above the cricoid.

Resistance to airflow is determined by a number of factors, including viscosity of the gas, length of the delivery or transit tube, radius of the delivery or transit tube, rate of flow through the system, and change in the pressure gradient of the system. The most clinically significant of these factors is the radius of the airway, for a decrease in the radius effects a decrease in flow, according to Poiseuille's Law: flow is a function of the fourth power of the radius. That is, as the radius decreases by some factor or value, the resistance to flow will increase to the fourth power.

The importance of Poiseuille's r^4 factor of bronchial gas flow will become evident when the radius of the bronchi is severely reduced because of chronic inflammation, congestion, mucosal edema, or partial obstruction by mucous plugs. Airway resistance is also increased when the lumen of the airway is decreased due to bronchospasm, mucosal edema, or partial airway obstruction.

Physiologic effects of increased R_{aw} are remarkable, and include an uneven distribution of alveolar ventilation, increased ventilation/perfusion abnormalities, hypoxemia, increased work of breathing, increased oxygen consumption, fatigue, and hypoventilation. Treatment of increased airway resistance involves the administration of bronchodilators, sympathomimetic (β-2) agonists, mucolytic drugs, and methylxanthines, suctioning, and bronchial hygiene therapy.

Aerosol/Humidification Therapy

The goal of humidifying therapeutic gases is to increase the relative humidity of inspired gas to approximate a 50% relative humidity at room temperature. The practice is relatively safe, for humidification does not administer additional water vapor to the patient and rarely has been found to transmit nosocomial pneumonias (humidity is a vapor, not a particulate). In contrast, inadequate humidification has been proven to lead to decreased ciliary activity, drying and thickening of secretions,

Table 2-25   Pressure-Volume Changes in Pulmonary Disorders

Condition	Static Compliance	Dynamic Compliance	PaO$_2$	Pressure-Volume Curve	Treatment
Normal	Normal	Normal	Normal		None
Pulmonary edema	Decreased	Decreased	Decreased		Diuretics Digitalis Morphine Oxygen
ARDS	Decreased	Decreased	Decreased		PEEP therapy
Pneumothorax	Decreased	Decreased	Decreased		Chest tubes
Bronchospasm	Decreased	Decreased	Decreased		Bronchodilators

retention of thick secretions, airway obstruction, atelectasis, and pneumonia.

During continuous mechanical ventilation, heated humidifiers are most frequently used to supply fully saturated water vapor at body temperature to the patient with a bypassed airway. Gases introduced into the trachea at 32–34°C and saturated at that temperature mimic the conditions that prevail normally in the lung.

For short-term mechanical ventilation (1 to 2 days) and in the normovolemic patient, the use of hydroscopic condenser humidifiers (which capture all or most of the water vapor that crosses the membrane during exhalation and return it to the patient during the succeeding inspiration) is recommended. The principal value of this type of device is cost savings in the short term. These devices, however, are definitely contraindicated in the patient producing copious amounts of secretion, with bronchopleural fistulas, with substantial leaks in tracheal cuffs, or breathing with small tidal volumes on IMV.

Aerosol therapy is the application of water particles directly to the airway. Because secretions are hydrophilic (water absorbers), hydrating them can facilitate easy evacuation by suctioning or coughing. Furthermore, aerosol therapy is believed to help restore the effectiveness of the mucociliary escalator and thus has been found quite useful in the treatment of chronic bronchitis, bronchiectasis, pneumonia, cystic fibrosis, laryngeal edema, upper airway inflammation or burns, and laryngeotracheobronchitis.

It is important to realize that aerosol therapy is not without risk. The nurse must incorporate into care interventions to prevent the following complications:

1. Bronchospasm occurring following administration of bland aerosols and mucolytic agents. Bronchodilators should be given prior to bland aerosol therapy and with Mucomyst. There is support for the use of β$_2$ adrenergics

and Mucomyst therapy (aerosol nebulization with 3–5 cc of 10% strength Mucomyst). Bronkosol is recommended by some for its rapid onset and peak time compared to other sympathomimetic bronchodilators.

2. Cross contamination and nosocomial infection. Aerosols are considered good transport mechanisms for bacteria, as particulate water can carry mass. The nurse must monitor for pulmonary and upper respiratory infections and change the entire aerosol system daily.

3. Fluid overload. This problem has been identified particularly in the use of high-density aerosol generators such as ultrasonic nebulizers. Ultrasonic nebulizer output is between 3 and 6 mL/min, depending on the frequency assigned to the ultrasonic transducer by the Federal Communications Commission. Infants and patients with renal or congestive failure should be continuously monitored during the use of ultrasonic therapy.

Refractory upper airway obstruction or severe asthma may lead to hypoxemia and significant ventilation problems in the lung. When the patient inspires therapeutic gas mixtures with high concentrations of helium, the mixture possesses a lower viscosity than air and thus more readily moves through airways. Resistance to flow as well as the work of breathing are decreased.

Oxygenation Monitoring

Oxygenation can be monitored noninvasively. Continuous monitoring of saturation of oxygen (SpO_2) can be accomplished through pulse or ear oximetry, which transmits a red light beam through a perfused area such as an ear lobe, finger tip, or pinna of the ear.

Most oximeters compare the amount of light transmission at 640 and 810 nm (nanometers). The amount and type of absorption of light are determined, and the resulting saturation is presented. Oxyhemoglobin absorbs less light in the red region of the spectrum (640 nm) than does reduced hemoglobin. Many pulse oximeters provide some indication of the strength of the signal measured to allow the user to judge the quality of results. Since this signal reflects each arterial pulse, many pulse oximeters display heart rate as well as oxygen saturation. If the heart rate displayed on the oximeter is different from the actual heart rate of the patient, the SpO_2 should be held suspect. On the other hand, good agreement between the pulse rate and the oximeter rate is no guarantee that an accurate SpO_2 reading is being presented.

Factors that hamper the noninvasive measurement of SpO_2 include the presence of venous blood, intervening tissues, and skin pigmentation (oximeter readings are slightly less accurate on patients with dark skin color).

Most pulse oximeters are designed only to measure oxyhemoglobin. Dyshemoglobins such as carboxyhemoglobin (COHb) and methemoglobin (MetHb) are assumed not present in the standard range of findings in pulse oximetry. Because of this design feature, limited band wavelength pulse oximetry should not be used when carbon monoxide poisoning from smoke inhalation is suspected. Such pulse oximeters exhibit falsely low values at high concentrations of MetHb for oxygen saturations above 85%, and falsely high values for oxygen saturations below 85%. (This phenomenon may be due to the equal absorption of MetHb at both red and infrared wavelengths.) Other problems associated with pulse oximetry use are:

1. Vascular dyes depress SpO_2 measurements (methylene blue more so than indigo carmine or indocyanine green).
2. Ambient light from xenon lamps, fluorescent lights, and infrared lights interferes with readings. This can be controlled by isolating sensors and by wrapping the probe with light barriers.
3. The presence of black, blue, or green nail polish significantly lowers oximeter readings. Nail polish should be removed before a pulse oximeter is used.

The accuracy of pulse oximeters is also compromised by fluctuations in hemoglobin, in that higher levels of Hgb raise the saturation. The same is true in the case of acidosis or alkalosis: the former causes a rise in saturation, and the latter causes a decrease in saturation.

Certain normal saturation values resulting in PaO_2 changes are of practical interest to the clinician:

SpO_2	PaO_2
97%	90 mm Hg and higher
90%	60 mm Hg
80%	47 mm Hg
75%	40 mm Hg
50%	27 mm Hg

Oximetry may be valuable in monitoring the adult patient whose oxygenation status is unstable or who is being weaned from mechanical ventilation. Other areas where oximetry is particularly useful are in sleep studies and bronchoscopy studies, during suctioning on an unstable patient, and in the routine evaluation of a patient on oxygen therapy.

Patients should also be monitored by pulse oximetry whenever they are receiving sedatives or analgesics capable of interfering with airway protective reflexes. Significant decreases in intraoperative critical hypoxic episodes and recovery room events have been documented with the use of continuous pulse oximetry. The advantages of pulse oximetry include:

1. There is no membrane to replace.
2. It measures arterial pulse wave/heart rate.
3. It presents no risk of thermal injury.
4. It is effective in assessing chronic neonatal lung disease and lung problems in children and adults.

The disadvantages of pulse oximetry are related to the following:

1. increased cost of disposable sensor units
2. possible compression injuries caused by spring-loaded permanent sensor units
3. over-reliance on saturation values can lead to failure to monitor ventilation
4. unreliability for patients experiencing hypoperfusion states
5. not useful in determining eligibility for long-term oxygen; not a substitute for PaO_2 (arterial blood gas measurements)
6. false alarms caused by motion

Transcutaneous oxygen ($PtcO_2$) monitoring is dependent on the use of a heated (45°C) Clark or polarographic skin electrode. Heating the skin causes local vasodilation, and the gradient difference between the pO_2 of venous and arterial capillaries is almost eliminated. This process arterializes the skin blood vessels, and oxygen diffusion across the skin occurs; changes in skin oxygen tensions will reflect changes in PaO_2.

Skin metabolism and oxygen consumption vary with age and differences in skin thickness; thus, transcutaneous monitoring has not proven as successful a monitoring method in the adult patient.

Limitations of $PtcO_2$ monitoring include underestimation of PaO_2 during hyperoxemia or a compromised hemodynamic state, underestimation of PaO_2 in the adult patient, and the risk of skin blistering from the use of a heated electrode. The advantages of $PtcO_2$ include the fact that the $PtcO_2$ electrode is less subject to distortions such as those caused by movement, the fact that $PtcO_2$ can be assessed with $PaCO_2$, the ability to detect hyperoxemia, and the ability to more accurately estimate PaO_2 in cases of acute respiratory distress.

Oxygen pressure of mixed venous blood can be monitored by using a Swan-Ganz catheter and drawing blood samples or by taking fiber-optic real-time measurements. This measurement gives the nurse some indication of the level of oxygenation at the tissue level (since blood being measured is returning from that source). But it is important to realize that this measurement is only valid when circulatory function is intact and tissue oxygenation is unimpaired. If these conditions do not exist, normal (40 mm Hg) or supranormal levels for the PvO_2 measurement may be observed in the face of severe tissue hypoxia. Conditions that are associated with this discrepancy include hemorrhagic shock, septicemia, febrile states, congestive heart failure, and conditions of arterial admixture.

Carbon Dioxide Monitoring

Transcutaneous carbon dioxide ($TcPCO_2$) monitoring is similar to $PtcO_2$ monitoring, although different in that carbon dioxide is measured utilizing a modification of the Sveringhaus electrode. In order for the $TcPCO_2$ measurement to accurately reflect $PaCO_2$, cardiac output must be enough to prevent sluggish tissue perfusion accumulation of $PaCO_2$, which will falsely elevate the reading. When cardiac output is decreased and tissue perfusion is low, cell structures become hypoxic, and carbon dioxide and lactic acid accumulate. Buffering of the lactate with sodium bicarbonate further increases $PaCO_2$, causing $TcPCO_2$ to reflect tissue pCO_2 and not $PaCO_2$. $TcPCO_2$ monitoring has proven more valuable in neonates than in adults, as long as cardiac output and skin perfusion remain adequate.

Capnometry is the monitoring of exhaled carbon dioxide. Care should be taken when using this method, as the presence of secretions interferes with the readings. Increased respiratory rates also compromise the accuracy of capnometry measures, making the readings falsely low. The pressure of end-tidal carbon dioxide ($PetCO_2$) should represent alveolar $PaCO_2$. What it actually reflects is a mixture of exhaled gases from all of the millions of alveoli, thus a mixture of many different $PaCO_2$s. The measurement of end-tidal $PaCO_2$ is often used in conjunction with mechanical ventilation, particularly in the management of the unstable, acutely ill patient in need of multiple alterations in ventilatory and cardiovascular parameters. It is also used when weaning the long-term mechanically ventilated patient. The use of end-tidal measurements to detect esophageal intubation or tube slippage is now mandatory in the operative setting. Monitoring of this parameter is also valuable in situations of cardiac arrest. The prognosis is not good for the patient who demonstrates very low $PetCO_2$ levels (< 10 mm Hg) during resuscitation. ($PetCO_2$ serves as an indicator of pulmonary blood flow during resuscitative efforts.) The use of the difference between arterial and end-tidal carbon dioxide is believed by some to be the best way to monitor PEEP therapy; it is believed that the best ventilation/perfusion relationship can be established at the lowest difference level. However, this has not been consistently demonstrated. The best relationships between arterial and end-tidal carbon dioxide increases have been noted in pulmonary embolism, cardiac arrest, pulmonary hypoperfusion, high respiratory rate due to low tidal volume, and the use of positive pressure ventilation with PEEP.

Discontinuance and Weaning

The clinical goal of mechanical ventilation is to provide the pulmonary system with the extracorporal mechanical ventilatory support it needs. In addition, mechanical ventilation provides easy access to the lungs so as to maintain improved bronchial hygiene.

Effective and efficient application of the mechanical life support system can be found to decrease both myocardial and ventilatory work, allowing for rest and recuperation. Such a device, when used appropriately, can improve gas distribution throughout the complex system of the lung, thus improving ventilatory efficiency and oxygenation.

The decision to discontinue mechanical ventilation is made when there has been sufficient reversal of the pathophysiologic condition that necessitated ventilatory support. Before discontinuing such therapy it is important to document a number of parameters:

The absence of active pulmonary disease process
Stable hemodynamics
Adequacy of cardiovascular reserves
Adequacy of gas exchange capability
Adequacy of ventilatory capability
Adequate renal function
Adequate fluid and electrolyte balance
Adequacy of the CNS
Adequacy of nutritional status
Adequacy of psychological preparation
Minimal work of breathing imposed by the ventilator
Appropriate endotracheal tube size for patient
Adequacy of inspiratory flow demand and response
N.I.F. stronger than -20

Minimization of hidden or auto-PEEP
Appropriate selection of technique for discontinuance
Adequate staff and monitoring capability
Adequate control of infectious processes

Most patients require a very brief weaning period. Current experience suggests that only about 5% of all mechanically ventilated patients require a prolonged weaning phase. Factors determining the length of the weaning process are the weaning method used, the institutional protocol, the availability of adjunctive ventilatory modes, nutritional status, and the moderating influence of ventilatory muscle dysfunction or neuromuscular and neurological dysfunction. Procedures used to remove a patient from mechanical ventilation include:

1. T-piece trials: indicated when patient physiological status is acceptable and the ventilatory course brief. This method works best when there has been good postoperative anesthesia recovery and uncomplicated and relatively standard surgical or diagnostic procedures, and with younger patients without a history or evidence of cardiopulmonary disease.
2. Gradually decreasing IMV or SIMV rate: the use of IMV is believed to provide several important *potential* advantages for weaning, including:
   more uniform gas ventilation
   prevention of muscular weakness and atrophy
   prevention of respiratory alkalosis
   maintenance of adequate patient-machine synchrony
   reduction in cardiovascular side effects
   decreased risk of barotrauma due to lower mean airway pressures
3. Pressure support: many patients require simple pressure support when being weaned and after short periods of ventilator support.

Available research has not documented any significant hemodynamic difference between synchronized intermittent mandatory ventilation and intermittent mandatory ventilation. There is some evidence that work of breathing and oxygen consumption (VO_2) are increased with the use of demand-valve SIMV ventilation compared to other IMV systems. SIMV/IMV is the indicated mode when weaning must be gradual. This process may take as few as 6 hours or may last many months; it is begun when the individual is able to assume at least 20% of the work of breathing when using only *partial* ventilatory support. Mechanical set rates in the region of 8 to 12 breaths per minute are sufficient for most patients to start. Almost all current ventilators come equipped with IMV or SIMV modes. The majority of equipment failures associated with IMV or SIMV are due to disconnection of the patient from the system or circuit failure. When older IMV mechanical systems are used (requiring the addition of separate IMV/SIMV circuits), it is prudent to monitor the system with a low-pressure or apnea-disconnect audiovisual alarm system.

For the very long gradual wean, it is mandatory to continually assess the patient-machine interface as well as the patient's ventilatory and cardiovascular status. The most relevant bedside measurements include ABG's, compliance and resistance measurements, maximal inspiratory pressure measurements, vital capacity, daily chest radiography, flow measurements, and thoracic/abdominal wave form pattern analysis. Sufficient personnel and support to see this process through are essential.

Inspiratory pressure support is the most commonly used form of pressure-supported ventilation; it assists the intubated patient's spontaneous inspiratory effort with a clinician-selected amount of positive airway pressure. The patient initiates an inspiratory effort, and the mechanical ventilatory circuit is pressurized to the desired setting, holding constant at that setting until a certain minimum inspiratory flow rate is reached. In this approach to mechanical ventilation, the patient is able to control ventilatory timing and to interact with the set inspiratory pressure to establish inspiratory flow rate and tidal volume. This mode of ventilation makes spontaneous breathing more comfortable for the patient and allows the clinician to adjust the magnitude and characteristic of ventilatory work for the patient.

Pressure support ventilation should only be used in the patient with stable and dependable ventilatory drives. The patient in whom the work of breathing is high because of less than optimal endotracheal tube placement or fatigue can benefit greatly from the use of this adjuvant mode. The patient who is difficult to wean by other methods or who needs controlled reconditioning of ventilatory muscles may also benefit greatly. The advantages of this mode of weaning include increased patient comfort, decreased work of breathing, decreased oxygen consumption, and increased endurance conditioning.

Clinical parameters by which to assess a patient's readiness for weaning include:

1. an alert, awake, oriented individual (appropriate LOC)
2. an intact ventilatory drive (normal ventilatory pattern)
3. normal and stable vital signs
4. respiratory rate <30
5. intact airway protective reflexes (strong cough and ability to handle respiratory secretions)
6. Vital capacity >15 mL/kg, >1000–1200 cc, and 2–3 times tidal volume
7. Negative inspiratory force > −20 cm H_2O
8. Minute ventilation > 10 L/min
9. Adequate ABG's on less than 40% FIO_2
10. Deadspace value (V_D/V_T) less than .55
11. Shunt < 20% (optimally <15%)
12. P(A-a DO_2) (100%) <350 mm Hg
13. Tidal Volume >350 cc
14. <4–6 PVC/minute
15. Absence of dyspnea, neuromuscular fatigue, pain, diaphoresis, restlessness, use of accessory muscles, and cyanosis
16. Psychological preparedness
17. Clear or improving chest x-ray findings
18. Optimal nutritional status and caloric intake

Newer and Alternative Modes of Mechanical Ventilation

The search for alternative modes of mechanical ventilation was a response to various pathologies. There are several approaches to mechanical ventilation (as exemplified by basic volume, pressure ventilation, and negative pressure mechanical ventilators).

Pressure control inverse ratio ventilation (PC-IRV) was developed in response to problems of oxygenating the stiff lungs found in ARDS. Appropriate application of this mode necessitates well-trained and prepared clinicians, appropriate monitoring technology, and the correct mechanical ventilatory device. Patients should be chosen for this modality judiciously, as patient preparation and maintenance are crucial. The patient usually must be sedated and paralyzed during the use of this mode of ventilation because it is most uncomfortable.

In this type of ventilation a pressure-limited plateau of inspiration is used with a much longer inspiratory time phase; thus, shortening the expiratory time allows for passive ventilation. This is in marked contrast to conventional mechanical ventilation, in which the inspiratory phase of volume ventilation is shorter and the expiration time is lengthened. With this approach, gas is, in essence, stacked in the lungs, decreasing mean airway pressures and dynamically recruiting alveoli to improve oxygenation. Peak airway pressures are reduced. The result of this mode is the presence of the phenomenon of auto-PEEP, which, if not monitored and managed, can easily be overlooked. It is for this reason that some clinicians believe that standard modes of mechanical ventilation with high PEEP levels are more appropriate. The improved oxygenation that results from this mode is believed to be a result of applied PEEP and the effects of auto-PEEP. Significant problems with this mode are the increased possibility of cardiovascular embarrassment and barotrauma. This mode offers little benefit in the presence of severe airway obstruction. Currently there is little firm scientific evidence to support the use of this modality.

High-frequency jet ventilation is a technology that developed because of the high mortality rates associated with acute respiratory failure. High-frequency ventilation (HFV) is a generic term that describes all modes of mechanical ventilation in which supraphysiologic respiratory frequencies are used with small tidal volumes. At times, depending on the type of HFV used, tidal volumes are even less than the patient's deadspace. The application of HFV is beneficial to maintain oxygenation and carbon dioxide removal. It has been found to be especially successful in the presence of persistent bronchopleural fistula leaks; in such cases the application of HFV creates lower peak airway pressures for shorter time periods (resulting in the reduction of gas loss through the fistula, providing an enhanced opportunity to heal). Patients who have undergone laryngeal, tracheal, thoracic, or abdominal surgical procedures can benefit from this type of mechanical ventilation. But no data exist to suggest that this type of mechanical ventilation is an improvement over conventional ventilation. Current literature does not suggest that it is beneficial enough for widespread clinical use compared to conventional mechanical ventilation. The problem of bronchial mucous plugging with this type of mechanical ventilatory mode continues to be a significant one, for effective humidification systems for HFV are not yet perfected.

Extracorporal membrane oxygenation (ECMO) is a technological means of temporarily replacing (and at times augmenting) the functional gas exchange ability of the pulmonary system. There are essentially four modes utilized in the extracorporal circuit: arteriovenous, mixed, venoarterial, and venovenous. The venoarterial system is most commonly utilized. The purpose of ECMO is to give the pulmonary system time to heal after profound and serious insults by allowing the system to rest while providing for oxygenation and ventilation. However, it is important to understand that when resting the lungs by this method, pulmonary injury may still result through blood sludging and thrombosis in the pulmonary vasculature. It is a very specialized technique requiring special support and monitoring technologies, a large and extremely well-trained support

staff at all department levels, and readily available operating room and ICU space. ECMO can provide an acceptable means of life support for neonates with respiratory failure who have the potential to thrive. However, its use in the adult population is far less defined or understood.

Acute Lung Injury and Respiratory Failure

Acute lung injury (ALI) was described more than twenty years ago as adult respiratory failure. At that time one-half to two-thirds of all the patients with this respiratory disorder died. Recently, descriptions of acute lung injury disorders have been expanded to include a spectrum of pathologies similar in nature but with different degrees of severity. Despite advances in understanding of the underlying pathophysiology, improvements in critical care practice, and the availability of sophisticated mechanical ventilatory technology, the mortality rate associated with acute lung injury and respiratory failure and subsequent progression to ARDS has not changed significantly.

Clinical antecedents

Acute lung injury may be estimated to occur in the United States in approximately 175,000 patients per year. However, the majority of patients who develop acute lung injury and finally ARDS do *not* die from lung injury or other pulmonary problems, but from extrapulmonary causes. Only about 10% of the people who develop ALI actually die of pulmonary-related phenomena (that is, from refractory hypoxemia or respiratory acidosis).

A multitude of etiologic factors may produce respiratory failure leading to acute lung injury and subsequent ARDS. Among these are:

Infectious causes:
  Bacterial (gram-negative)
  Viral
  Fungal
  Parasitic
  Mycoplasma
Drug overdose:
  Heroin
  Barbiturates
  Methadone
  Morphine

Aspiration of liquid:
  Gastric fluids
  Fresh and salt water
  Hydrocarbon fluids
Trauma:
  Lung contusion
  Fat emboli
  Head injury
  Thoracic injury
  Nonthoracic injury (pelvis, long bones)
Inhaled toxins:
  Oxygen (in toxic amounts)
  Smoke
  Corrosive chemicals (chlorine, ammonia, phosgene, ozone, nitrogen dioxide)
Metabolic disorders:
  Pancreatitis
  Uremia
  Paraquat ingestion
Hematologic disorders:
  Massive blood transfusion (stored blood)
  Disseminated intravascular coagulation
  Hemorrhagic shock
  Cardiopulmonary bypass > 6 hours
Cardiac problems:
  Post-cardioversion
  Congestive heart failure
Pulmonary insults:
  Hypoperfusion
  Embolisms (fat, air, amniotic fluid)
  Salicylates
Abdominal processes
CNS disease with increased ICP
Immunologic reactions
Fluid overload
Goodpasture's syndrome
Eclampsia
Radiation-induced lung injury

Critical referents

ALI is a form of pulmonary edema of a noncardiogenic origin usually representing systemic intravascular inflammatory processes that escape the usual protective controls and lead to multi-organ system failure. The lungs initially sustain the most acute injury. As much as 60% of ALI can develop within 12–24 hours. Within 72 hours most individuals who are at risk of developing ALI will already have contracted it. Thus, ALI is not a slow and insidious process.

The pulmonary system may be the only organ system that manifests the development of system failure: the intravascular inflammation involves an increase (or activation) of a variety of mediators or potential markers for the inflammatory process that results in injury to the lung parenchyma. To date, the measurement of these blood-borne markers (or mediators) of ALI has not proven useful in predicting who will develop this form of injury. This diffuse inflammatory process (often initially observed in the pulmonary system) is probably multifaceted—several mechanisms and substances are necessary for triggering the pulmonary injury. The resultant injury, more than likely, differs from the original underlying pathology. Currently known mediators of ALI include neutrophils and platelets (formed blood elements); chemoattractants such as complement leukotrienes and platelet-activating factor (PAF); WBC products including O_2 radicals, proteases, and phospholipase products (PL); miscellaneous factors such as Factor VII, fibronectin, tumor necrosis factor, PLA2, and angiotensin-converting enzyme (ACE).

One underlying mechanism for the development of ALI is the role played by neutrophils. Neutrophils within the circulatory system become activated by inflammatory mediators and adhere to the endothelial surface of small blood vessels in the lung, releasing a series of inflammatory substances including toxic oxygen radicals, proteolytic enzymes, phospholipase products, and vasoactive substances. These substances lead to increased permeability of the capillary surface and a decrease in functional surfactant (which acts to maintain alveolar integrity) and initiate inflammatory cellular damage. Substances that attract neutrophils and platelets to endothelial surfaces include complement fragments, lipoxygenase products, platelet-activating factors, and bacterial peptides released by microorganisms. Figure 2-41 illustrates the process described above.

Fibronectin, a substance that occurs naturally in the bloodstream, combines with circulating bacteria and aids in the ingestion and destruction of bacteria by macrophages and neutrophils. Pathologies that reduce the amount of available fibronectin can reduce the opsonization process and increase the risk of sepsis. Bacterial peptides released by microorganisms may act as chemoattractants, causing neutrophilic adhesion and platelet aggregation on the endothelial surface.

Macrophage release of tumor necrosis factor is now implicated as an extremely important mediator of cellular injury in sepsis. Prostacyclin and coagulation Factor VII are products that result from cellular damage and that serve as mechanisms of this type of damage. Clinical measurement of Factor VII may

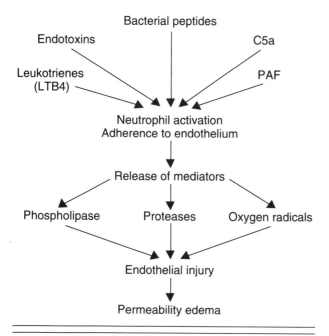

Figure 2-41 Activation of Neutrophils within the Circulatory System

provide a marker that can assist in the prediction of respiratory failure leading to ARDS. However, its activation may occur too late in the lung injury process to aid diagnosis of ALI. Furthermore, the assay procedure itself (which requires a 12- to 18-hour incubation period), is lengthy and tedious, although the process is being improved. The patient with septic endothelial injury who has significantly elevated Factor VII antigen levels is at greater risk of progressing to lung injury than patients whose antigen levels are normal.

The mechanism by which hyperoxia produces cellular damage is not fully established, but the general process can be described. Cellular metabolism involves a stepwise reduction of the ratio of oxygen to water. The byproducts of this complex chemical reaction, called free radicals, are highly reactive and destructive molecules associated with unregulated reactions of organic molecules. Such reactions are sufficient to damage cellular membranes and mitochondria as well as to inactivate cytoplasmic and nuclear enzyme systems, causing reduced mucociliary activity, interference with pulmonary surfactant, oxygen pneumonia, bronchopulmonary dysplasia, alveolar membrane formation, and retrolental fibroplasia.

Most mammalian cell lines contain intracellular mechanisms that protect against the untoward accumulation of free radicals. One such protective mechanism is superoxide dismutase (SOD), an enzyme

that inactivates oxygen radicals. Figure 2-42 maps the process of intracellular oxygen metabolism.

Several factors modify the development of oxygen toxicity. For example, the patient with COPD will be able to withstand prolonged oxygen exposure because of oxygen tolerance. Other factors can hasten or delay the onset of oxygen toxicity, including:

Hastened Onset or Severity:	*Delayed Onset or Severity:*
Adrenocortical hormones	Acclimatization to hypoxia
Adrenocorticotropic hormone	Adrenergic blocking agents
Carbon dioxide inhalation	Anesthesia
Convulsions	Antioxidants
Dexamethasone	Chlorpromazine
Dextroamphetamine	Gamma-aminobutyric acid
Epinephrine	Glutathione
Hyperthermia	Hypothermia
Insulin	Hypothyroidism
Norepinephrine	Immaturity
Paraquat	Intermittent O_2 exposure
Pulmonary toxic chemotherapy agents	Reserpine
Thyroid hormones	Vitamin E
Vitamin E deficiency	Tris-aminomethane
X-ray irradiation	

Arachidonic acid is a precursor substance for many substances that affect blood vessel patency, vascular permeability, and leukocyte or platelet aggregation at sites of vascular injury. Arachidonic acid is an unsaturated fatty acid, a precursor of certain prostaglandins (the cyclooxygenases D2, F2a, and G2). It becomes freely available to the circulatory

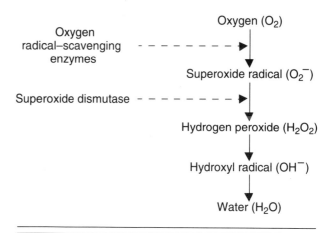

Figure 2-42 Intracellular Oxygen Metabolism

system and pulmonary capillaries when mast cells degranulate because of activation of phospholipase enzyme systems. The resulting prostaglandins stimulate platelet aggregation and cause fluid leak in inflamed tissues. The effects of prostaglandin formation include thrombosis of small arterioles, changes in vascular permeability, and pulmonary vasoconstriction.

Another significant mechanism for arachidonic acid is its conversion through the action of enzyme lipoxygenase to a series of 20-carbon fatty-acid derivatives known as leukotrienes. Leukotrienes play a significant role in mucus production, vascular permeability, and mucociliary clearance. The powerfully vasoconstrictive leukotrienes (such as C4, D4, and E4) are implicated in increasing pulmonary artery pressure and pulmonary vascular resistance.

The principle of activated complement fragments at one time was used to explain ALI. Complement participates as a cofactor in antigen-antibody reactions and other cellular defense mechanisms (cell lysis). Complement is believed capable of causing activation or attracting inflammatory cells; this process leads to cellular clumping and lysis, which causes the release of lysosomes and activates the neutrophils. The net result of complement activation (C5, C5a, and C3a) is increased vascular permeability and enhanced effect of free-oxygen radicals, causing further tissue damage. Current research suggests that complement activation is a nonspecific response and can occur both in ARDS patients who die and in those who survive. It does not predict respiratory failure leading to ARDS, nor is it sufficient to cause ALI.

Resulting signs and symptoms

About 60–70% of the patients who are considered at high risk for ALI will develop some degree of it. Of the patients who do experience an acute lung injury, most do so in conjunction with sepsis, major trauma, DIC, or aspiration of gastric contents. The combination of other physiologic insults (such as alveolar hyperoxia, hypotension, operative procedures lasting 8 hours or more, poor nutritional status, multiple transfusions, and interstitial pneumonic processes) increase the risk of respiratory failure leading to acute lung injury.

Acute lung injury is readily identified by the presence of an acute hypoxemia ($PaO_2 < 60$ mm Hg at a FIO_2 of 35–40%) with no apparent cause and in the absence of chronic lung disease and cardiogenic edema. Usually the patient's clinical history only suggests that the patient is "at risk." In examining the possible etiologic risk factors, the clinician should keep in mind that the presence of one risk factor creates a 20% chance of ALI, two risk factors create a 35% chance, and three risk factors indicate a 50% chance of ALI. Chest radiography at this point may reveal no pneumonic infiltrates or atelectasis but may show increased vascular markings in a relatively clear lung field. Respiratory work of breathing will be increased with a rapid respiratory rate (tachypnea) and an abnormal tidal volume (normal or slightly decreased). Often the earliest clinical indication that ALI may be present is the presence of respiratory alkalosis in the patient.

As ALI progresses to its most severe form (ARDS), increasing hypoxemia refractory to increases of inspired oxygen percentages will be manifested and confirmed by a severely decreased PaO_2/FIO_2 ratio (<150). There will be a markedly decreased pulmonary compliance (<50 cc/cm H_2O), and the work of breathing will be substantially increased. Chest radiographic findings will reveal a diffuse bilateral parenchymal infiltrate (of honeycombed or butterfly appearance). Wedge pressure tests will demonstrate a PWP of less than 18 mm Hg, confirming that the hypoxia and cardiopulmonary distress are not of cardiac origin. Diagnosticians may be unable to offer any other explanation as to what is wrong with the patient.

In response to the covert systemic biochemical phenomena occurring, pulmonary capillaries become engorged and the permeability of the alveolar/capillary membrane increases to create interstitial and intraalveolar edema and hemorrhage. Alveolar surfactant is destroyed or neutralized, and alveolar collapse and shunting ensue, with profound increases in a diffuse atelectasis. As the disease continues, an intraalveolar membrane of fibrin and cellular debris is deposited. Hyperplasia and swelling of Type 2 cells result and, in conjunction with other morphological changes, intraalveolar fibrosis develops. On autopsy, the lungs are heavy (as a result of the increase in lung water and blood-related products) and appear liverlike or "beefy."

It does not appear that the severity of ALI can be reduced even with rapid recognition and timely intervention. Presently the best that can be done is to identify the insult as early as possible and begin aggressive therapy, while aiming appropriate therapeutics toward the cause of the ALI process. Clinically, most supportive therapy is directed toward preventing any further complications of the process (toward sepsis and multi-organ failure).

In the presence of ALI one can expect to find an increase in respiratory rate, which is caused by several physiologic mechanisms:

1. Stimulation of the peripheral chemoreceptors due to the presence of hypoxemia
2. As lung compliance decreases, the patient must adjust to a smaller tidal volume, which increases respiratory rate. This change is the mechanico-physiologic system's attempt to minimize extreme levels of the work of breathing by preventing the sustained and immediate use of accessory muscles in ventilation.
3. During pulmonary congestion, capillary hypertension, alveolar wall edema, and (in the presence of serotonin and lung emboli) the juxtapulmonary-capillary receptors (J cells) are stimulated. This stimulation causes a reflex response characterized by rapid, shallow breathing patterns.

Cardiac output increases in the early phases of ALI and then later in the ARDS stage develops into a superimposed cardiovascular insufficiency. The performance of the ventricles decreases, causing further problems with tissue oxygenation. Increased pulmonary resistance, myocardial depression, preload decreases from PEEP, capillary leakage, myocardial stiffening, and contractility deficiencies can be identified.

Increased heart rate and blood pressure are characteristic of ALI and are indirect responses to increasing hypoxia and stimulation of the peripheral chemoreceptors in the carotid bodies. The pulmonary reflex to increase cardiac output serves as a compensatory mechanism to counteract the hypoxemia in ALI.

Fluid and electrolyte therapy is aimed at preventing excessive extravascular fluid, which may aggravate the noncardiogenic interstitial edema even further, thus promoting sluggish blood flow and cellular coagulation. If the patient is not suffering from hypoalbuminemia, crystalloid fluids should be administered. Diuretic therapy may be indicated to maintain the patient on the "dry" side without creating cardiovascular instability. Obviously, the patient's pulse, blood pressure, urinary output, and peripheral vasoconstriction must be monitored. Hemodynamic monitoring may also be indicated during ALI and in ARDS.

Nursing standards of care

Technological support of oxygenation through various technologies (PEEP and CPAP systems and mechanical ventilation) has historically been the front line therapy in the care of acute lung injury and respiratory failure. Providing the minimal FIO_2 necessary for adequate tissue oxygenation (PaO_2 of 60–70 mm Hg in a stable cardiovascular system with adequate hemoglobin) is of primary importance. It is also necessary to maintain the mixed venous oxygen level at 38–40 mm Hg to ensure adequate tissue oxygenation and prevent hypoxic shunting at the tissue level. Under most circumstances it is possible to adequately oxygenate the patient with FIO_2 levels below 50% if appropriate fluid therapy and cardiovascular support are provided.

The use of PEEP has been controversial to the extent that some believe that PEEP can serve more than a supportive role in the care of the patient with ALI. Current research findings, however, suggest that PEEP therapy can do nothing to stop ALI and its progression into ARDS. There is no evidence to suggest that mortality in the event of ARDS is decreased with the use of PEEP; it should be noted, however, that ARDS patients rarely die of refractory hypoxemia, but of other complications. PEEP is useful to treat hypoxemia and modify the manifestation of the lung injury (improve compliance), but it does nothing for the course of the pathology.

Improved ventilatory support, then, can be given little credit for affecting mortality rates in severe ALI. Its role might be considered more crucial if it could be proven to reduce infection and sepsis or even lessen lung injury due to the mechanical ventilatory response. But research reveals that as many patients suffering severe ALI who are mechanically ventilated die as do not die. However, the lungs are still considered the primary source for the development of sepsis, since normal protective mechanisms of the tracheobronchial tree are often assaulted and bypassed through the use of ventilatory support technologies. The absence of intubation and mechanical ventilation is no longer sufficient to preclude the development of sepsis syndrome and septic shock with worsening ARDS. Many clinicians believe that once ALI and its disseminated intravascular inflammatory response is triggered, the abdomen very often becomes the source of iatrogenic infection.

An aggressive search for the underlying causes of ALI, if they are not already known, must be of primary concern in the care of patients with the condition. Aggressive prevention and pharmacologic intervention to treat septic syndrome are also indicated. Criteria for septic syndrome are detailed in Chapter 9.

Finally, the diagnosis of pneumonia in the spectrum of ALI is always difficult because radiographic confirmation lags behind the clinical development and presentation of ALI. Later, in the presence of ARDS, evidence of pneumonia is hidden by overlying diffuse parenchymal infiltrates. Concomitantly, fever is already present and may offer little or no indication of new infection. Figure 2-43 summarizes the entire clinical course of acute lung injury and respiratory failure.

The specifics of nursing care are detailed in the following nursing care plan.

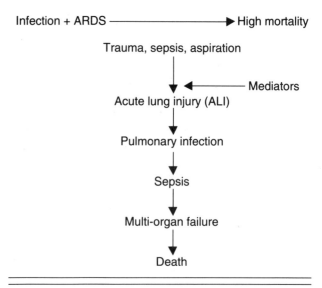

Figure 2-43   Clinical Course of Acute Lung Injury and Respiratory Failure

Nursing Care Plan for the Management of the Patient with Respiratory Failure

Diagnosis	Signs and symptoms	Intervention	Rationale
Alteration in respiratory function: hypoxemia	In the appropriate clinical context and with no other reason: $PaO_2 < 5(FIO_2)$; $PaO_2 <$ predicted for patient's age; $PaO_2 = 110 - \frac{1}{2}$ of patient's age; $PaO_2 < 75$ mm Hg on room air; $SaO_2 < 90\%$	Monitor ABGs frequently	To ascertain the presence of hypoxemia for appropriate choice of intervention
		Oxygen and ventilatory support as needed	To correct hypoxemia
	Increased work of breathing: increased respiratory rate; increased tidal volume	Monitor respiratory rate and tidal volume	To assess cardiopulmonary stress
		Place in semi- or high Fowler's position as indicated	To allow easiest breathing and full diaphragmatic descension
	Increased myocardial work: increased cardiac output; changes in BP; decreased level of consciousness; decreased capillary refill; cold and clammy skin; decreased urinary output	Assist with basic care regime	To conserve energy and prevent increases in cardiac oxygen demand
		Closely monitor VS and ECG and check for chest pain	Indications of ischemic damage and cardiac compromise
		Maintain patency of IV lines	To allow fast access in case of an emergency
		Avoid activity for half-hour after meal	To prevent further oxygen demand when blood is shunted to GI tract during digestion
	$PaCO_2$ 35–45 mm Hg or less	Assess closely for orthostatic hypotension	To prevent injury in the event of syncope associated with orthostatic hypotension
	Increased minute ventilation		
Impaired gas exchange due to alveolar hypoventilation and shunt effect	Increased work of breathing	Administer oxygen	PaO_2 should increase with increase in FIO_2
	Increased A-a gradient Normal or lower $PaCO_2$ Hypoxemia	Monitor chest x-ray	To assess lung volume and parenchymal status; to determine etiology of shunt; to monitor effectiveness of therapy

Nursing Care Plan for the Management of the Patient with Respiratory Failure

Diagnosis	Signs and symptoms	Intervention	Rationale
	Atelectasis: decreased lung compliance; decreased VC; decreased FRC; deceased V_T; increased respiratory rate	Monitor VC	To assess status of compliance and provide index of work of breathing and prognosis of patient's ability to maintain spontaneous ventilation
	Decreased breath sounds; dry crackles (rales); decreased fremitus; dull percussion note	Chest physical assessment	To fully monitor ventilatory ability of patient
	No improvement of PaO_2 with oxygen administration (refractory)	Institute mechanical ventilation	To assure adequate gas exchange in the event of ventilatory failure
	Radiographic findings of alveolar collapse and atelectasis; alveolar consolidation and pneumonia; excessive secretions	Increase FIO_2 then commit to PEEP to decrease shunt (at an FIO_2 of 1.0, every 10–15 mm Hg $p(A-a)O_2$ indicates 1% shunt); shunts > 25% are clinically significant and demand intervention	If PaO_2 does not increase by at least 10 mm Hg for every FIO_2 increase of 20%, shunt is considered refractory
		Monitor PaO_2	PaO_2 < 70 mm Hg will cause hypoxic pulmonary vasoconstriction, adding to shunting problem
		Appropriate bronchopulmonary hygiene techniques	To reinflate collapsed alveoli, mobilize retained secretions, remove thick, viscid secretions, decrease work of breathing, improve ventilation, decrease shunt

Diagnosis	Signs and symptoms	Intervention	Rationale
Potential for impaired gas exchange due to: fluid volume overload; ineffective airway clearance, atelectasis, or effusion; bronchospasm; inadequate supplemental O_2; inadequate tidal volume; secondary low cardiac output; excessive pulmonary vascular resistance; malpositioned ET tube, inadequate cuff volume; pneumothorax, hemothorax	Abnormal ABGs: $pO_2 < 80$ mm Hg; $pCO_2 < 35$ or $pCO_2 > 45$ mm Hg; $pH < 7.35$ or $pH > 7.45$; O_2 sat. $< 80\%$; $HCO_3 < 20$ or $HCO_3 > 26$ mEq/L; $BE < 0$ or $BE > 3$ Cyanosis ET tube cuff leak Lowered peak pressure Inadequate volume exchange Chest x-ray indicates atelectasis, effusion, pneumothorax, or hemothorax	Mechanically ventilate as ordered Closely monitor lung sounds for absent, unequal, diminished breath sounds, crackles (rales), wheezing, or asymmetric chest wall expansion; closely monitor ABGs PRN as indicated; obtain chest x-ray immediately and PRN for ET tube placement, lung expansion (pneumothorax), width of mediastinal shadow, presence of pleural fluid, or presence of foreign body	Ventilation support is needed until patient is stable Early indications of further respiratory compromise and/or complications
	Copious secretions Elevated respiratory rate, wheezing, air hunger, gasping, or asymmetrical chest wall expansion	Aggressive pulmonary toilet PRN with chest percussion therapy, incentive spirometry, and hyperinflation using 100% O_2 before and after suctioning; turn and reposition patient every 2 hours	To mobilize secretions, provide adequate oxygenation, and open closed alveoli
	Change in mental status	Monitor level of consciousness	Decreased level of consciousness may be first sign of anoxia
	Fluid overload	Assess for crackles (rales), S_3, and JVD (jugular vein distension) as indicated	Signs of respiratory failure leading to heart failure
		Monitor Na^+ and osmolarity	SIADH is common with pulmonary disease
		If patient is stable, promote extubation by holding sedation, elevating HOB (head of bed) 30 degrees, and decreasing IMV by increments of 2 to 4 breaths/min (if $pO_2 > 90$, pH between 7.35 and 7.45, and O_2 sat. 90–100%)	To assist patient to return to optimal breathing capacity as soon as possible (to prevent further atelectasis, secondary infection, etc.)

Nursing Care Plan for the Management of the Patient with Respiratory Failure

Diagnosis	Signs and symptoms	Intervention	Rationale
		Assist patient to position of comfort; semi- or high Fowler's position is best	To improve breathing patterns and lower diaphragm
		Administer oxygen as ordered	To counter problems with oxygenation
		Monitor heart rhythm	Tachycardia is commonly seen
		Review chest x-ray for signs of pulmonary edema	Pulmonary congestion can be clinically delayed up to 24 hours
	Dyspnea or decreased O_2 levels on ABGs	Monitor ABGs closely	Problems with oxygenation are commonly seen
Ineffective breathing pattern due to decreased compliance secondary to interstitial edema leading to: decreased surfactant; decreased alveolar stability; increased alveolar closure	Radiographic atelectasis Increased work of breathing	Monitor respirations and V_T; measure VC, Ve, and ABGs	To assess adequacy of breathing pattern and lung compliance; to follow improvement/ deterioration of patient
	Tachypnea Decreased V_T Increased Ve Decreased VC Use of accessory muscles	Incentive spirometry every hour: IC should be 3–4 times predicted V_T with 10–15 second inspiratory hold (sustained maximal inhalation)	To promote improved lung compliance; to treat atelectasis; to increase FRC; to decrease work of breathing; to improve inspiratory muscle tone
	Exertional dyspnea Decreased activity levels	Attempt to keep FIO_2 < 50% for an oxygen saturation ⩾ 90 mm Hg	Increased FIO_2 > 50% may lead to oxygen toxicity with fibrotic lung changes
	Hypoxemia Hypoxia Atelectic crackles (rales) Decreased bibasilar breath sounds Decreased chest movement	Administer IPPB therapy every 2–4 hours as ordered: exhaled V_T 1200–1500 per breath; sympathomimetic bronchodilator without normal saline to decrease CO_2 and work of breathing	To support ventilatory musculature if fatigue appears to be developing

Diagnosis	Signs and symptoms	Intervention	Rationale
		Monitor x-rays	To assess lung volumes and presence of atelectasis or pneumonia; diffuse bilateral or localized interstitial patterns with increased vascular shadows; decreased $PaCO_2$ and PaO_2; alveolar edema with a normal heart size; worsening hypoxia, $PaCO_2 <$ normal, decreasing lung compliance and FRC; alveolar edema and/or progression to fibrosis; severe hypoxemia with 100% O_2
		Administer PEEP by MASK/CPAP or intubation/mechanical ventilation with PEEP	To support ventilation, reverse hypercarbia, improve oxygenation, decrease work of breathing, prevent cardiopulmonary collapse, and support patient during crisis; to improve compliance by increasing intra-alveolar distending pressures; to increase FRC by recruiting unstable or closed alveoli; to promote oxygenation, which decreases myocardial and ventilatory work; to redistribute extravascular lung water; to decrease deadspace; to improve cardiac output and $C(a-v) O_2$; and to reduce shunt
		Aerosol/humidity therapy; suctioning; postural drainage and percussion; administer mucolytics and expectorants as ordered	To rehydrate airway; to improve mucociliary activity; to clear secretions; to maintain airway patency

Nursing Care Plan for the Management of the Patient with Respiratory Failure

Diagnosis	Signs and symptoms	Intervention	Rationale
		Mechanical ventilation	To decrease work of breathing and support oxygenation
Tissue hypoxia	Tachycardia Tachypnea Hyperventilation Dyspnea Cyanosis Hypertension Restlessness Confusion/disorientation	Monitor ABGs closely	To assess alveolar ventilation
		Monitor Ve	To assess total ventilation to provide an index of work of breathing affecting cardiopulmonary stress
	Early alkalosis leading to late respiratory acidosis Early alveolar hyperventilation leading to late severe alveolar hypoventilation Hypoxemia	Monitor for signs of cardiovascular and cardiopulmonary work	To determine acid-base balance and need for O_2 since there is no direct test for tissue hypoxia (can only evaluate hypoxemia)
		Emergent administration of increased FIO_2	To normalize PaO_2; to improve alveolar oxygen tension; to decrease work of breathing and myocardial work
		Use appropriate O_2 device	To maintain PaO_2 to prevent complications of hyperoxia; oxygen system should deliver flow (4 × Ve) to maintain desired FIO_2, prevent room air leakage into system, maintain adequate PaO_2 to at least level of inspired FIO_2, and reduce work of breathing
		Monitor oxygenation	Pulse oximetry should show O_2 sat. > 90%
Decreased tolerance of activity related to dyspnea	Dyspnea on exertion Fatigue Exaggerated increase in heart rate and BP on exertion	Assess level of activity tolerance (should be related to the New York Heart Association's classification for consistency)	Provides a baseline

Diagnosis	Signs and symptoms	Intervention	Rationale
		Assist patient to change position every 2 hours while on bedrest	To decrease risk of complications and promote venous return
		Check BP with patient in horizontal, sitting, and standing positions	To monitor for orthostatic hypotension
		Avoid activity for a half-hour to an hour after meals	May decrease chance of hypoxia due to increased blood flow to GI tract
		Monitor heart rate and BP with activity increases	To maintain heart rate within 10 bpm of resting heart rate and maintain systolic BP within 20 mm Hg of resting BP; if a drop occurs, it may indicate a drop in cardiac output
		Anticipate institution of progressive rehab	To provide controlled mechanism for increasing activity
		Encourage frequent rest periods	To prevent excessive fatigue
Potential for alteration in cardiopulmonary cerebral, renal, and peripheral tissue perfusion	Signs of altered cerebral perfusion: mental confusion, dizziness, syncope, convulsions and/or seizures, TIA, yawning	Rule out noncardiac causes of altered cerebral perfusion	To ascertain causative factor in order to choose appropriate intervention
	Signs of altered cardiopulmonary perfusion: angina and ischemic changes	Monitor for chest pain	To assist in prevention of and early intervention for ischemic cardiac damage
	Signs of altered renal perfusion: oliguria and anuria	Check urine output every 8 hours or every hour if oliguria occurs	To ascertain renal function
	Signs of altered peripheral perfusion: hypotension	Monitor BUN, creatinine, and K^+	Respiratory failure may eventually cause decrease in cardiac output to periphery from hypoxemia and related dysrhythmias

Nursing Care Plan for the Management of the Patient with Respiratory Failure

Diagnosis	Signs and symptoms	Intervention	Rationale
Potential for alteration in thought processes	Confusion Inability to concentrate	Provide protective environment: bed in low position with side rails up	Patient may become restless and be unsteady when getting up alone
		Reorient patient to environment	Frequent reminders of place and time help to improve patient's orientation
		Explain all procedures	Familiarity with surroundings, realistic expectations, and various sensory experiences help to decrease confused mental states
Potential for complications from pulmonary artery catheter	Infection Balloon rupture Kinking and/or dislodgement of catheter Dysrhythmia Pulmonary artery perforation	Assess patient's temperature and check catheter insertion site every 4 hours	Temperature elevation is sign that infection may be at IV site
		Discontinue use of IV as soon as possible and change site after 3–5 days	Per Centers for Disease Control standards; decreases chance of infection at site
		Inflate balloon with 1.5 cc of air or less	Overinflation may cause balloon rupture
		Observe balloon lumen for presence of blood	Indicates balloon rupture
		Monitor for PVCs, especially right-sided (appear as same deflection as normal beats)	May indicate irritation from catheter
		Continuously monitor PA waveform for continued wedge shape	Catheter expands after insertion because of body temperature, so is likely to extend into occluded position
		Monitor RV waveform	May indicate kinking or knotting of catheter, which requires repositioning

Diagnosis	Signs and symptoms	Intervention	Rationale
		Monitor for dampening of waveform	May indicate that a blood clot has formed, that the tip is against the arterial wall, or that the pressure bag is not inflated to 300 mm Hg
		Monitor for sudden onset of dyspnea, cough, or bloody expectorant	May indicate perforation of pulmonary artery
Potential for infection related to pulmonary congestion, indwelling lines, and Foley catheter	Elevated temperature	Encourage coughing and deep breathing; turn patient in bed every 2 hours while on bedrest	Help to prevent atelectasis, blood clots in legs, and pressure sores
		Change respiratory tubing every 24 hours	Per CDC specifications
		Increase activity as soon as indicated	To promote healing
		Monitor temperature every 4 hours	Sign of infection
	Increased WBCs	Assess WBC count	Sign of infection
		Maintain strict aseptic technique with invasive lines and indwelling catheters; change lines unless contraindicated: PAP every 72 hours, arterial lines every 7 days, tubing every 48 hours, IV bags every 24 hours; provide Foley care every 8 hours	Per CDC recommendation
		Assist in identifying source of infection: collect cultures; note atelectasis on chest x-ray; note sputum and urine characteristics; check insertion site for redness every 8 hours	Sites at risk of infection must be kept clean with aseptic technique; appropriate antibiotic therapy must be chosen
		Administer antibiotics as ordered	To combat infectious process

Nursing Care Plan for the Management of the Patient with Respiratory Failure

Diagnosis	Signs and symptoms	Intervention	Rationale
Altered nutritional status due to: anorexia and malaise; increased nutritional requirements resulting from stress of illness; less appealing taste of food related to low sodium content and changes in oral mucosa; changes in bowel routine; increased work of breathing	Too fatigued to eat	Auscultate bowel sounds	To evaluate GI peristalsis
	Too short of breath to eat	Help patient to eat slowly; use supplemental O_2 as needed	To facilitate nutritional intake
	Inadequate intake of food and fluids	Monitor I&O	To assess fluid balance
		Calculate calorie requirements	Calorie requirements may increase 200% in ARF
	Decreased albumin and lymphocytes	Monitor albumin and lymphocytes	To assess visceral proteins
	Decreasing body weight	Monitor weight	To monitor effect of diuretic therapy
	Complaints of lack of appetite	With patient, family, and dietary staff, assess appetite and food preferences and review what is allowed and what is best for optimal nutrition; provide preferred food as much as possible	To facilitate nutritional intake and status in any way possible
Potential for impaired skin integrity	Redness on pressure points	Assess skin integrity every 2–4 hours	To prevent skin breakdown
		Note redness on pressure points	Early signs of skin breakdown
		Use egg crate or air mattress	To relieve pressure on bony prominences
		Assist patient to turn every 2 hours	To improve circulation
		Institute skin care regimen	Dryness predisposes skin to break down

Diagnosis	Signs and symptoms	Intervention	Rationale
Patient lacks knowledge of disease process and prescribed regimen	Patient does not adhere to care plan	Assess patient's present understanding	Provides baseline
	Patient verbalizes lack of knowledge and understanding or exhibits anxiety and apprehension, especially during procedures and treatments	Institute teaching program for patient and family: normal lung function; pathology; risk factors; control of precipitating and aggravating factors; activity; diet; medications; weight monitoring; signs and symptoms of recurring respiratory failure; follow-up care	Increasing knowledge, understanding, and thus potential ability to adhere to regimen may decrease unnecessary rehospitalization
		Allow patient and family to ask questions and verify understanding of information	Patient may need reinforcement and several repetitions of information before it is fully understood and integrated

Medications Commonly Used in the Care of the Patient with Respiratory Failure

Medication	Effect	Major side effects
Furosemide or Bumex (Butedemide)	Inhibits reabsorption of sodium and chloride in the loop of Henle Diuresis Decreases pulmonary congestion	Hypokalemia Hypocalcemia Orthostatic hypotension Volume depletion and dehydration
Mucomyst (Acetylcysteine)	Increases production of respiratory tract fluids to thin secretions	Bronchospasm Nausea Hemoptysis
Expectorants	Increase production of respiratory tract fluids to thin secretion	Nausea Drowsiness
Crystalloid IV fluids	Fluid and electrolyte replacement	Aggravation of CHF Pulmonary edema Edema
Methylxanthines (Theophylline)	Bronchodilators Enhance ciliary movement to mobilize secretions Block histamine release from mast cells	Tachycardia Nervousness
Beta-adrenergic sympathomimetics (Isoproterenol, Albuterol)	Bronchodilate by enhancing sympathetic tone	Cardiac dysrhythmias Tremors Irritability

Adult Respiratory Distress Syndrome

Much like acute respiratory failure (but much more severe), adult respiratory distress syndrome (ARDS) is a rapidly progressive, diffuse pulmonary condition characterized by a noncardiogenic, high-permeability pulmonary edema resulting in hypoxemia, decreased lung compliance, and acute respiratory failure. ARDS is not considered a specific disease, but rather a syndrome of manifestations of deteriorating pulmonary status associated with a variety of clinical conditions.

The annual incidence of ARDS in the United States is over 150,000 cases. Despite over twenty years of research addressing the ARDS phenomenon, mortality rates remain as high as 60–70% for cases of ARDS in general[6] and 80–90% for cases of ARDS in conjunction with septic syndrome.[7] In the clinical setting ARDS may also be referred to as "stiff lung," "white lung," "wet lung," "adult hyaline membrane disease," "shock lung," or "Da Nang lung" (because the syndrome occurred and was discovered in the Vietnam war).

Clinical antecedents

One of the criteria frequently cited in the diagnosis of ARDS is a clinical risk factor. Clinical risk factors for ARDS can result either from direct pulmonary insult or from indirect systemic insult, as illustrated in Table 2-26. Most patients at risk for development of ARDS manifest signs and symptoms of the syndrome within 72 hours of exposure to the clinical risk factor.[8] Over 50% of ARDS cases are associated with trauma, sepsis, gastric aspiration, or nosocomial pneumonia.[9]

Critical referents

Pulmonary injury in ARDS is a result of the accumulation of protein-rich fluid in the alveoli secondary to increased microvascular permeability of the plasma proteins. Following the initial insult to the lungs, the complement cascade (including inflammatory mediators—histamine, serotonin, prostacycline, kinins, thrombaxanes, and metabolites of arachidonic acid) and the coagulation cascade are

Table 2-26 Conditions Associated with Adult Respiratory Distress Syndrome

Direct Pulmonary Insult	Indirect Pulmonary Insult
Aspiration*	Biological modifying agents
Embolism (air, fat, amniotic fluid)	Burns
Infectious pneumonia (viral, fungal, PCP, tuberculosis)*	Diabetic ketoacidosis
Inhaled toxins (smoke, toxic gases)	DIC
Ionizing radiation/radiation pneumonitis	Drug overdose (opiates, paraquat, salicylates, barbiturates)
Near-drowning	Heat stroke
Oxygen toxicity	Leukemia
Pulmonary contusion	Massive blood transfusions
	Multisystem trauma*
	Pancreatitis
	Post-cardioversion
	Sepsis*
	Shock (hypovolemic)
	Toxemia of pregnancy
	Uremia

*Conditions associated with over 50% of all ARDS cases.
Note: Cardiopulmonary bypass can result in both direct and indirect pulmonary insult.
Adapted from Bradley, R. B. (1987). Adult respiratory distress syndrome. *Focus on Critical Care 14* (5): 48–59; and Dal Nogare, A. R. (1989). Southwestern Internal Medicine Conference: Adult respiratory distress syndrome. *The American Journal of the Medical Sciences 298* (6): 413–429.

activated. Cascade activation results in the formation of platelets and protein microaggregates in the circulation, creating increased consumption of plasma proteins and lodging of platelets and protein aggregates in the pulmonary capillaries. Further protein consumption ensues.

In addition to protein consumption resulting from the lodging of platelets and protein microaggregates, chemotactic factors are released, which recruit and activate eosinophils and polymorphonuclear neutrophils (PMNs) into the pulmonary circulation. Adhesions of these granulocytes cause a release of noxious products (superoxide ions, hydrogen peroxide, hypochlorous acid, and hydroxyl ions). Along with degranulation and release of lysosomal enzymes by granulocytes, these noxious products create endothelial and Type I alveolar epithelial cell injury resulting in increased protein permeability at the capillary-alveolar barrier. High-permeability pulmonary edema ensues. Thick hyaline membranes from fibrin and cellular debris impede gas exchange. The physiological consequences of the process include decreased lung compliance and large intrapulmonary shunts.

As ARDS continues, hyperplasia of Type II alveolar epithelial cells occurs. Decreased surfactant production results in an increase in alveolar actelectasis.

There is proliferation of fibroblasts in the interstitial and alveolar spaces. An increase in collagen content in the lung is also hypothesized. Lung compliance is further compromised, and ventilation-perfusion abnormalities are exacerbated. A general overview of the pathophysiology of ARDS is presented in Figure 2-44.

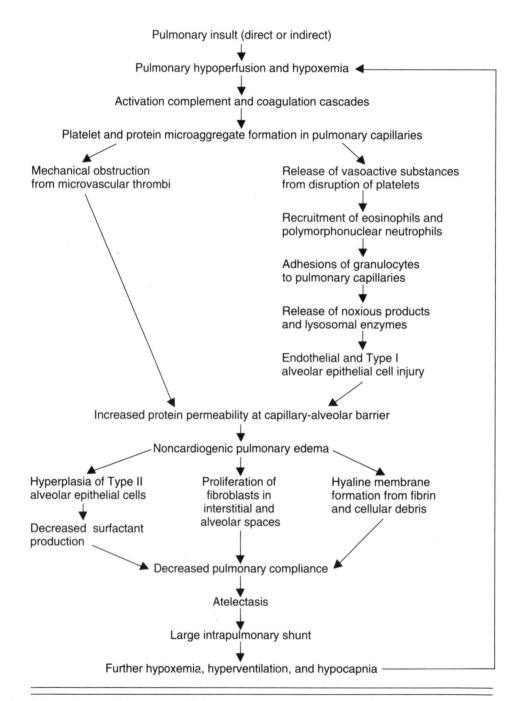

Figure 2-44 Pathophysiology Associated with ARDS
Source: Adapted from Cline, B. A., & Fisher, M. L. (1982). ARDS means emergency. Nursing 82, February: 62–67.

Resulting signs and symptoms

The diagnosis of ARDS continues to be based, for the most part, on three distinguishing characteristics: refractory hypoxemia associated with previously normal lungs; the presence of pulmonary edema (as evident by diffuse infiltrates on the chest x-ray); and decreased lung compliance.[10] A cardiogenic origin of pulmonary edema must be ruled out through assessment of ejection fractions or use of pulmonary capillary wedge pressure (PCWP) tests (see the section on cardiogenic shock in chapter 4). A comprehensive list of criteria used in the diagnosis of ARDS is provided in Table 2-27.

A recent development in the diagnosis of the presence and extent of ARDS is the Lung Injury Score, a tool developed by Murray in an attempt to quantify the extent of ARDS using clinical parameters.[11] The Lung Injury Score is determined by assessment of chest roentgenogram, degree of hypoxemia, positive end expiratory pressure requirements, and respiratory compliance.[12] The assessment is presented in Table 2-28.

Research studies have also identified two additional criteria that may be used in the diagnosis of ARDS in the future. The presence of terminal C56-9 complement complex, which indicates complement activation and inflammation, is one of these criteria. C56-9 complement complex can be detected by immunoassay up to 2 days prior to the onset of overt clinical symptomatology of ARDS (Stage III and Stage IV ARDS).[13] Further research is needed before

Table 2-27   Diagnostic Criteria for Adult Respiratory Distress Syndrome

Basis for Diagnosis	Indications
History	Previously normal lungs
Clinical condition	Acute onset of respiratory distress Presence of risk factor
Radiographic evidence	Diffuse infiltrates on chest x-ray

Physiologic parameters	Refractory hypoxemia
	  $PaO_2 < 50$ mm Hg with an $FIO_2 > 60\%$
	Total respiratory compliance
	  < 50 mL/cm H_2O
	Noncardiogenic origin (PCWP
	  < 12 mm Hg)

	Increased pulmonary shunt fraction

Adapted from Shale, D. J. (1987). The adult respiratory distress syndrome—20 years on. *Thorax* 42: 641–645.

Table 2-28   The Lung Injury Score

Score	Value
Chest roentgenogram score	
No alveolar consolidation	0
Alveolar consolidation confined to 1 quadrant	1
Alveolar consolidation confined to 2 quadrants	2
Alveolar consolidation confined to 3 quadrants	3
Alveolar consolidation in all 4 quadrants	4
Hypoxemia score	
PaO_2/FIO_2 > 300	0
PaO_2/FIO_2 225–299	1
PaO_2/FIO_2 175–224	2
PaO_2/FIO_2 100–174	3
PaO_2/FIO_2 < 100	4
PEEP score (when ventilated)	
PEEP > 5 cm H_2O	0
PEEP 6–8 cm H_2O	1
PEEP 9–11 cm H_2O	2
PEEP 12–14 cm H_2O	3
PEEP > 15 cm H_2O	4
Respiratory system compliance score (when available)	
Compliance > 80 mL/cm H_2O	0
Compliance 60–79 mL/cm H_2O	1
Compliance 40–59 mL/cm H_2O	2
Compliance 20–39 mL/cm H_2O	3
Compliance < 19 mL/cm H_2O	4

The final value is obtained by dividing the aggregate sum by the number of components that were used:

	Score
No lung injury	0
Mild to moderate lung injury	0.1–2.5
Severe lung injury (ARDS)	>2.5

Abbreviations: PaO_2/FIO_2 = ratio of arterial oxygen tension to inspired oxygen concentration ratio; PEEP = positive end-expiratory pressure.
Source: Murray, J., Matthay, M., Luce, J., and Flick, M. (1988). An expanded definition of adult respiratory distress syndrome. *American Review of Respiratory Disease 138:* 721.

this diagnostic method can be widely used. Edema fluid protein analysis has also been implicated in distinguishing cardiogenic pulmonary edema from increased permeability pulmonary edema. At this time techniques for measurement of edema fluid protein are not widely available.

Clinical manifestations of ARDS are divided into four stages: Stage I (injury), Stage II (latent period), Stage III (acute respiratory failure), and Stage IV (severe respiratory failure). The clinical manifestations of each stage are presented in Table 2-29. The hemodynamic profile of each stage is presented in Table 2-30.

In Stage I (injury), metabolic and perfusion abnormalities may develop as the body attempts to

Table 2-29   Clinical Manifestation of Adult Respiratory Distress Syndrome

Manifestation	Stage I	Stage II	Stage III	Stage IV
Clinical presentation	Hyperventilation with little or no respiratory distress; lungs typically clear to auscultation	Hyperventilation with subclinical respiratory distress; lungs clear or with diminished sounds on auscultation	Hyperventilation with shortness of breath; hypoxia; restlessness; disorientation; headache; tachycardia; peripheral vasoconstriction; crackles and wheezes on auscultation; occasional cough	Overt respiratory distress with profound shortness of breath and tachypnea; use of accessory muscles; intercostal, suprasternal, substernal, and supraclavicular retraction; diaphoresis; nasal flaring; cyanosis; somnolence; confusion; changes in vision; loss of coordination; impaired judgment; obtundation; coma; heart rate and blood pressure changes; progressive increase in positive airway pressure
Pathophysiology	Injury: ultrastructural changes in pulmonary capillary endothelial cells; underlying clinical process dominates clinical picture	Latent: microvascular permeability increasing; compression of peripheral airways; increased airway resistance	Acute respiratory failure: widespread damage to pulmonary capillary membrane resulting in widespread high protein edema; decreased lung compliance; intrapulmonary shunting	Severe respiratory distress: intra-alveolar hyaline membranes seen; proliferation of Type II pneumocytes; widespread interstitial fibrosis; severe intrapulmonary shunting; markedly decreased lung compliance
Arterial blood gases	Respiratory alkalosis: $PaCO_2$ level 30–40 mm Hg; PaO_2 level normal or slightly low	Respiratory alkalosis with slight hypoxemia: $PaCO_2$ level 25–30 mm Hg; PaO_2 level (RA) 60 mm Hg	Respiratory alkalosis with hypoxemia: $PaCO_2$ level 20–30 mm Hg; PaO_2 level 50–60 mm Hg; $P(A-a)O_2$ gradient increased	Severe hypoxemia: PaO_2 level < 40 mm Hg; CO_2 level > 45 mm Hg (a grave sign); $P(A-a)O_2$ gradient markedly increased
Chest x-ray	Normal	No infiltrates; congestion apparent in lung fields	Scattered infiltrates	Diffuse infiltrates and whited-out lung fields

Source: Darovic, G. O. (1987). *Hemodynamic Monitoring. Invasive and Noninvasive Clinical Application.* Philadelphia: W. B. Saunders Company, pp. 287–320.

adapt to the insult. Ultrastructural changes in the endothelial capillary membranes begin during this stage. Abnormalities in the hemodynamic profile as well as the clinical symptomatology reflect the underlying insult or injury.

Stage II (latent period) is characterized as a period of apparent stability. In actuality, microvascular permeability is increased, resulting in compression of peripheral airways. Clinical symptomatology remains subacute.

Stage III (acute respiratory failure) is characterized by the emergence of the first clinical signs and symptoms of pulmonary edema, reflecting the flooding of the alveoli with protein-rich fluid. By this stage

Table 2-30 Hemodynamic Changes with Adult Respiratory Distress Syndrome

Parameter	Stage I	Stage II	Stage III	Stage IV
Arterial pressure	Specific to type of insult	No change	No change	No change
Pulse pressure	Specific to type of insult	No change	No change	No change
CVP	Specific to type of insult	No change	No change	No change or slightly raised
SVR	Specific to type of insult	No change	No change or slightly low	No change or slightly raised
PVR	Specific to type of insult	No change	No change or slightly raised	Increased
PAP	Specific to type of insult	No change	No change or slightly raised	Increased
PCWP	Specific to type of insult	No change	No change	No change
Cardiac output	Specific to type of insult	No change	No change	No change or slightly decreased
SvO$_2$	Specific to type of insult	No change or slightly decreased	No change	Decreased

Source: Darovic, G. O. (1987). *Hemodynamic Monitoring. Invasive and Noninvasive Clinical Application.* Philadelphia: W. B. Saunders Company, pp. 287–320.

widespread damage to the pulmonary capillary membranes has occurred. Lymph flow to the area has increased, lung compliance has decreased, and intrapulmonary shunting is apparent. Mortality rates at this stage can reach 50% or more.

Stage IV (severe respiratory failure) is characterized by gross distortion of lung tissue related to decreased functioning of pulmonary capillaries secondary to microthrombolytic obstruction and the formation of fibrotic tissue. Lung compliance is markedly decreased, and extensive pulmonary shunting occurs secondary to massive pulmonary edema, actelectasis, and fibrosis. In the mechanically ventilated patient, peak airway pressures continue to rise, reflecting the loss of elasticity of the lungs.

Nursing standards of care

Treatment of ARDS remains supportive in nature, as no proven treatment modalities are available to reverse the underlying processes producing lung injury. Treatment strategies for ARDS often fail because of their supportive rather than curative nature and the extent of lung tissue damage evident when treatment is initiated.[14] Goals in the treatment of ARDS include:

1. Reversing the initiating insult

2. Providing adequate oxygenation while minimizing the risk of oxygen toxicity and barotrauma
3. Ensuring adequate pulmonary and systemic perfusion while minimizing the hydrostatic pressure of pulmonary vascular beds
4. Limiting further pulmonary damage and promoting lung recovery
5. Preventing further systemic insult (infection, stress ulcers)

The initial medical priority in the treatment of ARDS is correcting severe hypoxemia. Endotracheal intubation and mechanical ventilation are required to eliminate the high work of breathing seen in ARDS. Morphine sulfate in 3–5 mg increments is frequently administered to patients because of its ability to bronchodilate as well as to decrease sympathetically induced arteriolar and venous constriction resulting in preload, afterload, and cardiac work reduction and stroke volume increase.[15] Morphine sulfate also promotes a sense of well-being in the patient. Aminophylline, because of its bronchodilator effect, mild positive inotropic effect, and mild diuretic effect, may also be used, especially when bronchospasm complicates pulmonary edema.[16]

In addition to medications to promote adequate oxygenation, ventilator manipulation is used to reverse severe hypoxemia. Positive end expiratory pressure (PEEP) can be used in patients (and in nonintubated patients in the form of continuous positive airway pressure, CPAP) to improve oxygenation. The goal of PEEP is to maintain open alveoli at end expiration, which increases surface area for gas exchange, resulting in decreases in fractional inspired oxygen (FIO_2) requirements. Although in some cases adequate oxygenation can be achieved solely via administration of high FIO_2 (>80%), the risk of oxygen toxicity is dramatically increased with this approach. Oxygen toxicity is manifested by progressive hypoxemia and deterioration of lung compliance accompanied by increased intrapulmonary shunting; it can occur with prolonged exposure to higher FIO_2 (>50% FIO_2 for over 6–8 hours).[17] The goal of providing adequate oxygenation is to maintain PaO_2 levels higher than 55 mm Hg with an FIO_2 below 50% through the use of PEEP if necessary.[18] PEEP is contraindicated in the patient with chronic obstructive pulmonary disease (COPD), unilateral pulmonary disease, preexistent hypovolemia, pneumothorax, or increased intracranial pressure. PEEP may also create adverse cardiovascular side effects as well as barotrauma.

In addition to PEEP, several alternative modes of mechanical ventilation have been used in an attempt to maintain adequate oxygenation with ARDS. Pressure control inverse ratio ventilation (PC-IRV) involves altering the normal inspiration-to-expiration ratio (from 1:2 to > 1:1) in order to improve distribution of inspired gas, recruit and stabilize closed alveoli, decrease peak airway pressures (PAP), and potentially decrease oxygen consumption as a result of a decrease in the work of breathing.[19] In this mode of ventilation the patient frequently experiences the sensation of inability to breathe, and neuromuscular blocking agents in conjunction with sedation are indicated. PC-IRV is contraindicated in the patient with increased intracranial pressure or COPD. Potential adverse effects include hypotension related to compromised venous return, tachycardia, and arrhythmias. The longer the patient requires PC-IRV, the greater the risk of barotrauma.

Airway pressure release ventilation (APRV) is another ventilation mode that attempts to augment ventilation using periodic airway pressure release.[20] APRV employs a CPAP system, which allows the patient to breathe spontaneously without airway pressure fluctuations.[21] One major advantage of this mode of ventilation is that it lacks the adverse cardiovascular side effects seen with the other interventions. It should be noted, though, that this mode of treatment is still experimental.

High-frequency ventilation (HFV) involves the use of small volumes of gas delivered at rapid rates, resulting in small inspiratory and expiratory times.[22]

HFV results in adequate oxygenation as well as normocarbia, through a process called augmented dispersion. Augmented dispersion is described as a combination of the clearance of deadspace, or a fraction of it, in conjunction with the production of patterns of airflow that promote gas mixing throughout the lung.[23] The result is interregional mixing of gases, resulting in a more homogeneous distribution of gases, which ultimately enhances gas transport.[24] The benefits of HFV include improved alveolar ventilation, decreased barotrauma, and lack of adverse cardiovascular effects. Peak airway pressures and intrapulmonary shunting are reversed.

Finally, extracorporeal membrane oxygenation (ECMO) has also been used to support the patient while ARDS resolves. ECMO involves a partial cardiopulmonary bypass to potentiate oxygenation and carbon dioxide removal. To date ECMO has not been shown to improve overall survival rates in cases of ARDS.

A second major goal of medical intervention is the maintenance of adequate pulmonary and systemic perfusion. A Swan-Ganz catheter is used for optimal hemodynamic monitoring and to gain additional data regarding oxygenation status. Careful fluid management is crucial, to maintain adequate circulation and perfusion while avoiding fluid overload and further fluid leakage into the pulmonary tissue. Diuretics, fluid restrictions, and vasodilating agents may be used to reduce pulmonary capillary wedge pressures while maintaining cardiac output. Inotropic agents may be used in low cardiac output states. Opinions on the use of crystalloid versus colloid fluid replacement vary. The literature shows that many researchers now believe that because of the increased permeability of the pulmonary vasculature to protein, albumin easily crosses into the pulmonary interstitium, negating the beneficial effects of colloid administration. Based on this information, most clinicians currently advocate the use of crystalloids.[25]

Promoting lung recovery is another goal of medical intervention in ARDS. Many recent research studies have addressed the issue of promoting lung recovery in the patient with ARDS. The use of corticosteroids, in particular methylprednisolone, remains controversial. There is little support in the literature for the use of corticosteroids in ARDS, as they have no proven effect on lung recovery or improved prognosis.

Use of prostaglandin infusions in the treatment of ARDS in an attempt to decrease pulmonary hypertension has also been examined. Again, research does not support this treatment regimen, as findings indicate that prostaglandin infusions exacerbate deterioration of pulmonary gas exchange, worsening hypoxemia.[27]

Combination therapy including ibuprofen, methylprednisolone, cimetidine, benadryl, and ketanserin, as well as the use of ibuprofen alone, has shown promising results in altering cellular mediators, thereby reducing pulmonary hypertension and hypoxemia.[28] Further research is needed to support these findings. Surfactant replacement has also been examined as a potential mechanism for promotion of lung recovery.[29] Again, further research is needed to verify the effect and its applicability to the patient suffering ARDS.

Prevention and early detection of further systemic insult is another priority of medical management of ARDS. Protein-rich edema in the alveoli provide an excellent medium for bacterial growth and subsequent infection. Monitoring of WBC count and vital signs as well as the collection of routine cultures aid in early detection of infection. Selective gastric decontamination may be initiated to minimize gastrointestinal bacterial growth and the risk of aspiration gram-negative infection. Meticulous attention to aseptic technique is also necessary.

Use of antacids, cimetidine, and sucralfate to prevent stress ulcers and potential gastrointestinal hemorrhage is supported. Nutritional support is also advocated. Little information is available as to the recommended type of supplemental nutrition. Further research addressing the use of parenteral versus enteral feedings as well as the type of substrates to be used in hyperalimentation (high-protein versus high-glucose versus high-lipid content) is needed. Low-dose heparin therapy may also be indicated to prevent thrombosis, if coagulation studies are within normal limits.

Nursing management issues for cases of ARDS are related to the underlying clinical condition and the precipitating insult. The following care plan details specific nursing interventions applicable to the ARDS patient.

Nursing Care Plan for the Management of the Patient with Adult Respiratory Distress Syndrome

Diagnosis	Signs and symptoms	Intervention	Rationale
Potential for alteration in fluid status: overload	Edema Weight gain I > O Increased CVP Increased PCWP Changes in specific gravity of urine Decreased Hb/Hct Electrolyte abnormalities Signs of pulmonary edema	Monitor weight, fluid I&O, urine specific gravity, PAP, PCWP, cardiac output, and MAP	Loss of fluid to the pulmonary interstitium and alveoli may result in intravascular depletion, further exacerbating intrapulmonary shunting
		Monitor Hb/Hct and electrolytes	Intravascular overload will decrease Hb/Hct and alter electrolytes
		Administer diuretics as ordered	To minimize potential fluid in an attempt to prevent further pulmonary capillary leaks
		Monitor serum osmolarity	Can serve as reflection of hydration status
		Adhere strictly to fluid and sodium restrictions as ordered	To avoid fluid overload and retention leading to edema
		Monitor for crackles (rales) and S_3 heart sounds	Warn of pulmonary edema and impending heart failure
		Low-dose (2–5 mcg/kg/min) dopamine infusion	To provide increased renal perfusion to increase output
		Place patient in high or semi-Fowler's position for breathing	To promote full lung expansion and diphragmatic descension
Potential for alteration in fluid status: deficit	Decreased urine output Increased specific gravity of urine Weight loss Hypotension Tachycardia Thirst Change in mental status	Monitor patient's fluid status	To ascertain extent of deficit and provide appropriate rehydration
		Monitor patient's Hb/Hct and electrolytes	Fluid volume deficits result in hemo-concentration and electrolyte abnormalities

Diagnosis	Signs and symptoms	Intervention	Rationale
	Decreased CVP, cardiac output, MAP, PCWP, and PAP Hemoconcentration Electrolyte abnormalities	Administer vasoconstricting agents and/or fluids as ordered	Because of pulmonary capillary leaking, patient is kept mildly dehydrated but adequate perfusion (MAP > 60 mm Hg) is maintained to support ventilation-perfusion status and oxygenation of tissues
Ineffective airway clearance due to increased secretions and impaired respiratory function	Tenacious secretions	Monitor patient's respiratory status closely	To determine progression of syndrome and status of patient
	Cough	Provide frequent mouth care	To prevent drying of mucous membranes
	Atelectasis	Vigorous pulmonary toilet	Bronchial hygiene maximizes patient's existing ventilation
	Shunting		
	Hypoxemia		
		Suction every 2–4 hours and as needed using aseptic technique	Patient is unable to clear secretions because of decreased elasticity and compliance as well as compression of peripheral airways
		Administer humidified oxygen	To prevent upper airway drying and loosen secretions
		Administer bronchodilators based on patient tolerance (as ordered)	To enhance clearing of secretions
		Monitor for signs and symptoms of pulmonary infection: fever, atelectasis, hypoxia, shortness of breath	High-protein edema is an excellent medium for bacterial growth
		Use sedatives sparingly	To protect patient from further respiratory depression and to allow full cough effort
		Maintain adequate fluid balance	To keep secretions as wet and thin as possible

Nursing Care Plan for the Management of the Patient with Adult Respiratory Distress Syndrome

Diagnosis	Signs and symptoms	Intervention	Rationale
Ineffective airway clearance due to excessive secretions and impaired ability to cough	Weak and ineffective cough effort	If medically indicated, place patient in high Fowler's position to deep breathe and cough	Position allows diaphragm to descend and lungs to inflate as much as possible
		Instruct patient on good coughing technique (with deep breathing deep cough effort)	To increase effectiveness of cough effort
	Distant sounds, crackles (rales), gurgles (rhonchi), and wheezes on auscultation	Closely monitor for absent or diminished breath sounds	Early indications of respiratory compromise and/or complications
	Thick, tenacious sputum	Turn patient every 2 hours as medically indicated	To prevent pooling of secretions in dependent lung and improve circulation
	Chest x-ray indicates atelectasis		
		If medically indicated, encourage fluids	To thin secretions and allow easier movement of mucus by cilia
		Suction intubated patient as needed, using hyperventilation with 100% oxygen before and after suctioning; if indicated, lavage 1–3 cc sterile normal saline in ET tube before mechanically hyperventilating for suctioning	To mechanically promote loosening of secretions and ensure adequate oxygenation before and after suctioning
		Chest physical therapy as indicated	To promote breaking up mucus plugs and thick secretions and to clear specific lung fields
		Frequent and meticulous mouth care	To prevent further secretions from being aspirated and maintain good oral mucosa

Diagnosis	Signs and symptoms	Intervention	Rationale
		Position of safety and extreme caution during oral and tube feeding	To prevent aspiration of liquids or solids
Ineffective breathing pattern	In nonventilated patient: hyperventilation; hypoxemia; shortness of breath; cyanosis; changes in mental status In ventilated patient: hyperventilation (depending on mode); increasing PAP; hypoxemia; dyspnea; "bucking the ventilator"; changes in mental status Radiographic atelectasis Use of accessory muscles Decreased bibasilar breath sounds Decreased chest movement	Monitor patient's respiratory status: respiratory pattern; absent, unequal, or diminished breath sounds; wheezes or crackles (rales) with breath sounds; asymmetric chest wall expansion	Increasing edema and fibrosis cause lungs to lose elasticity and compliance, resulting in increased work with respirations
		Monitor V_T, VC, Ve, and ABGs	To assess adequacy of breathing pattern and lung compliance; to follow improvement/deterioration of patient
		Assist with intubation and initiation of mechanical support as needed	Mechanical ventilation is needed to provide adequate oxygenation and decrease work of breathing
		Administer neuromuscular blocking agents in conjunction with sedation	Especially when using alternative modes of ventilation, patient may experience the sensation of being unable to breathe and may then "buck the ventilator"; neuromuscular blockers allow for complete mechanical control of ventilation; sedation allows patient more comfort and less panic
		Monitor for adverse effects of mechanical ventilation	Decreased venous return and barotrauma are common adverse effects of modes of mechanical ventilation
		Incentive spirometry every hour; administer IPPB therapy as ordered in support of ventilatory musculature	To promote improved lung compliance; to treat atelectasis; to increase FRC; to decrease work of breathing; to improve inspiratory muscle tone

Nursing Care Plan for the Management of the Patient with Adult Respiratory Distress Syndrome

Diagnosis	Signs and symptoms	Intervention	Rationale
		HOB at 30 degrees	To allow for better respiratory effort
		Aggressive pulmonary toilet	To mobilize secretions, provide adequate oxygenation, and open closed alveoli
		Turn and reposition patient every 2 hours and as needed and tolerated	
		Allow for periods of rest; provide care in short sessions	To allow patient to rest to regain maximal strength for breathing
Impaired gas exchange due to pulmonary edema and respiratory failure	Hyperventilation Respiratory distress Agitation Hypoxia Headache Tachycardia Peripheral vasoconstriction Cough Cyanosis	Closely monitor patient's respiratory status	ARDS severely compromises pulmonary status; frequent assessment is crucial in determining progression of syndrome so as to plan, implement, and evaluate care
		Closely monitor patient's cardiovascular status	Loss of fluid to the pulmonary interstitium and alveoli can cause intravascular depletion, resulting in further intrapulmonary shunting
	Respiratory alkalosis: $PaCO_2 > 45$; $PaO_2 < 40$	Serial ABGs and pulse oximetry after ventilator changes	Refractory hypoxemia is a hallmark of ARDS; respiratory alkalosis is seen in early stages
	Altered lung sounds Inadequate volume exchange	Administer bronchodilators, FIO_2, mechanical ventilation as ordered: tidal volume that reduces $PaCO_2$; increase deadspace if necessary; PEEP	To ensure adequate oxygenation and correct hypoxemia To reduce shunting and improve gas exchange

Diagnosis	Signs and symptoms	Intervention	Rationale
		Turn patient every 2–4 hours as tolerated: vigorous pulmonary toilet (suction every 2–4 hrs and as needed)	To maximize functioning of existing alveoli in order to prevent further intrapulmonary shunting by preventing atelectasis
		When patient is stable, promote extubation as soon as possible by holding sedation, elevating HOB 30 degrees, incremental weaning	To assist patient to return to optimal breathing capacity as soon as possible and to prevent atelectasis and secondary infection
Potential for infection related to pulmonary congestion, indwelling lines, and Foley catheter	Elevated temperature	Encourage coughing and deep breathing; turn patient in bed every 2 hours while on bedrest, increase activity as soon as indicated	Helps to prevent atelectasis, blood clots in legs, and pressure sores
		Monitor temperature every 4 hours	Sign of infection
	Increased WBCs	Assess WBC count	Sign of infection
		Maintain strict aseptic technique with invasive lines and indwelling catheters; change lines unless contraindicated: PAP every 72 hours, arterial lines every 7 days, tubing every 48 hours, IV bags every 24 hours; provide Foley care every 8 hours	Per Centers for Disease Control recommendation
		Assist in indentifying source of infection: collect cultures; note atelectasis on chest x-ray; note sputum and urine characteristics; check insertion site for redness every 8 hours	Sites at risk of infection must be kept clean with aseptic technique; appropriate antibiotic therapy must be chosen

Nursing Care Plan for the Management of the Patient with Adult Respiratory Distress Syndrome

Diagnosis	Signs and symptoms	Intervention	Rationale
		Administer antibiotics as ordered	
Decreased tolerance of activity related to dyspnea	Dyspnea on exertion Fatigue Exaggerated increase in heart rate and BP on exertion	Assess level of activity tolerance (should be related to the New York Heart Association's classification for consistency)	Provides a baseline
		Assist patient to change position every 2 hours while on bedrest	To decrease risk of complications and promote venous return
		Check BP with patient in horizontal, sitting, and standing positions	To monitor for orthostatic hypotension
		Avoid activity for a half-hour to an hour after meals	May decrease chance of hypoxia due to increased blood flow to GI tract
		Monitor heart rate and BP with activity increases	To maintain heart rate within 10 bpm of resting heart rate and maintain systolic BP within 20 mm Hg of resting BP; if a drop occurs, it may indicate a drop in cardiac output
		Anticipate institution of progressive rehab	To provide controlled mechanism for increasing activity
		Encourage frequent rest periods	To prevent excessive fatigue

Diagnosis	Signs and symptoms	Intervention	Rationale
Anxiety due to respiratory distress	Agitation Restlessness Confusion Impaired concentration Hyperventilation Diaphoresis Tachycardia Sleeplessness Shakiness Facial tension Distracted behavior Withdrawal Nonadherence to treatment plan	Monitor patient's oxygenation status closely	ARDS is characterized by severe refractory hypoxemia
		Position patient to maximize respiratory status and minimize respiratory effort, based on patient tolerance	Dyspnea, shortness of breath, and hyperventilation are early signs of impending respiratory failure and cause high anxiety in patient, which only worsens respiratory status; positioning can decrease compression of diaphragm by abdomen and maximize ventilation-perfusion, decreasing sensations of inability to breathe
		Prepare patient for procedures and expected sensations	To minimize anxiety and maximize cooperation
		Ascertain patient's fears and anxieties	Baseline will allow nurse to know exactly what to address
		Ascertain patient's previous hospital experiences	Will help nurse to know how to best alleviate anxieties and support encouraging actions
		Provide emotional support as needed	To help patient and family deal with the situation in the best way possible
		Teach patient about what will happen in ICU: care routine, tubes, lines, ICU environment and visiting hours, how to improve breathing efforts, etc.	To help patient be prepared for what is to be experienced

Nursing Care Plan for the Management of the Patient with Adult Respiratory Distress Syndrome

Diagnosis	Signs and symptoms	Intervention	Rationale
		Administer analgesics and antianxiety agents as ordered (use of neuromuscular blocking agents requires sedation of patient)	To decrease anxiety and increase rest
Potential for impaired skin integrity	Redness on pressure points	Assess skin integrity every 2–4 hours	To prevent skin breakdown
		Note redness on pressure points	Early signs of skin breakdown
		Use egg crate or air mattress	To relieve pressure on bony prominences
		Assist patient to turn every 2 hours	To improve circulation
		Institute skin care regimen	Dryness predisposes skin to break down
Patient lacks knowledge of disease process and prescribed regimen	Patient does not adhere to care plan	Assess patient's present understanding	Provides baseline
	Patient verbalizes lack of knowledge and understanding or exhibits anxiety and apprehension, especially during procedures and treatments	Institute teaching program for patient and family: normal lung function; pathology; risk factors; control of precipitating and aggravating factors; activity; diet; medications; weight monitoring; signs and symptoms of recurring respiratory failure; follow-up care	Increasing knowledge, understanding, and thus potential ability to adhere to regimen may decrease unnecessary rehospitalization
		Allow patient and family to ask questions and verify understanding of information	Patient may need reinforcement and several repetitions of information before it is fully understood and integrated

Medications Commonly Used in the Care of the Patient with Adult Respiratory Distress Syndrome

Medication	Effect	Major side effects
Morphine sulfate	Analgesia/sedation Peripheral vasodilation Decreased systemic venous return Bronchodilation Relief of cardiac dyspnea	Hypotension Respiratory depression Nausea and vomiting Constipation Urinary retention
Aminophylline	Relaxation of smooth muscles of bronchial airways and pulmonary blood vessels	Restlessness Dizziness Palpitations Sinus tachycardia
Alupent	Beta-adrenergic stimulation Bronchodilation	Hypertension Palpitations Tachycardia
Ventolin (albuterol)	Beta-2-adrenergic stimulation of bronchial smooth muscles Prevention and relief of bronchospasm	Tremor, nervousness Tachycardia Palpitations

Diuretics:
  Furosemide
  Bumex
	Diuresis
	Decreased pulmonary congestion
		Hypokalemia
		Hypocalcemia
		Hypotension
		Volume depletion and dehydration

Acute Respiratory Infection

Although there are other forms of respiratory infection (infectious pleural effusion, bronchitis, empyema, and lung abscess), the primary focus of this section will be on bacterial and viral pneumonias, for the nursing care of all types of respiratory infection is similar, and the case of pneumonia provides a good model by which to plan care in the critical care setting. Pneumonia is also the respiratory infection most frequently seen.

Clinical antecedents

At greatest risk for respiratory infection are those whose physiological defenses are compromised, especially when the natural defenses are lowered by severe underlying illness. Colds and upper respiratory tract infections (e.g., sinusitis or strep throat) can lead to more serious illnesses by allowing bacterial invasion of the lower respiratory tract. The primary population at risk are the elderly and the chronically ill, especially those whose airway defenses and clearance mechanisms are compromised because of intubation or other clinical circumstances. Also at risk are those who are immunosuppressed, receiving corticosteroids, suffering cancer, being treated with chemotherapy or radiation therapy, undergoing treatment for organ transplantation, or suffering AIDS. Furthermore, any condition that interferes with normal lymphatic drainage of the lung (such as cancer of the lung, abdominal or thoracic surgery, or COPD) will predispose the patient to respiratory infection. The postoperative patient is especially at risk for bronchopneumonia, as anesthesia depresses the natural respiratory defenses and decreases the movement of the diaphragm. Depression of the central nervous system causing hypoventilation, whether from alcohol, drugs, or head injury, also predisposes the body to infectious processes. The patient over 50 years of age who contracts pneumonia has a higher risk of mortality than the younger patient, even when receiving prompt and appropriate antibiotic and pulmonary therapy.[30] Additional risk factors predisposing an individual to respiratory infection include a history of smoking, severe periodontal disease, chronic diseases such as diabetes, heart disease, or renal disease, poor living conditions, malnutrition and/or dehydration, exposure to air pollution, and inhalation of noxious substances.[31] Furthermore, almost all patients in critical care units today can be considered to be at risk, and it is the nurse who must take a primary role in preventing nosocomial infections.

Organisms that produce infection may be carried in the nasopharynx of a healthy or ill person at any time, and care must be exercised to prevent cross-contamination. Prevention is the best therapy, and the nurse must be alert to the possibility of infection, especially when caring for those at risk. Strict adherence to good aseptic technique is necessary to protect the severely immunologically compromised patient from cross-contamination from other patients, visitors, and staff. Finally, the patient who presents with recurring pneumonias should be examined for underlying diseases such as cancer of the lung, multiple myelomas, or others that predispose one to acute respiratory infections.[32]

Critical referents

In order for bacteria to invade the lung successfully, the ability of the lung to clear bacteria must be impaired as a result of compromises in the bactericidal ability of alveolar macrophages or increased susceptibility of the host to infection.[33] Once the lung is infected, an initial, acute, inflammatory response brings excess water and plasma proteins to the dependent areas of the lower lobes. Then red blood cells, fibrin, and polymorphonuclear leukocytes infiltrate neighboring alveoli, and the infectious bacteria are contained within segments of pulmonary lobes, in turn causing leukocytes and fibrin to consolidate within the involved area.[34]

The inflammatory exudate progresses through stages, including hyperemia and red and gray hepatization, and terminates in resolution. Hyperemia, also called the stage of congestion, is characterized by engorgement of the alveolar spaces with fluid and blood. The accumulation of edema fluid provides a rich medium for proliferation and spread of the original infecting organism through the lobes. Next, inflammation and injury occur in the stage known as the red hepatization stage, referring to the red appearance of affected cells, which have the consistency of liver tissue. Finally, the stage of gray hepatization occurs when increasing amounts of leukocytes infiltrate the alveoli, causing the tissue to become solid and grayish in color. During resolution, polymorphonuclear leukocytes are replaced by macrophages that are highly phagocytic and destroy the organisms.

When alveoli are filled with exudate or consolidation, they are unable to accept air, oxygen, and other gases. Sustained perfusion with poor ventilation occurs in the consolidated area, but is rarely severe enough to cause true hypoxemia. The infection resolves as exudate is lysed and reabsorbed by the neutrophils and macrophages. The lymphatics then carry exudate away from the site of infection, resulting in the restoration of the structure and function of the lung tissue. In some cases the resolution process does not occur; exudate converts to fibrous tissue, and the affected alveoli cease to function.[35] In the case of lung abscess, the area of pulmonary infection worsens to the point of parenchymal necrosis in multiple discrete lesions.

Different types of pneumonias also affect the pathophysiological processes experienced by the patient. Bacterial pneumonia is a consolidative inflammation that is caused by pathogenic microorganisms; it is a major culprit in compounding morbidity and mortality in the critically ill patient.[36] Lobar bacterial pneumonias are usually primary processes, not complications of other diseases.[37] Pneumococcal pneumonia is the most common bacterial pneumonia, and Streptococcus pneumoniae is the organism responsible for 80% or more of all community-acquired pneumonias. Some bacterial pneumonias present as bronchopneumonia with multiple, poorly defined areas of alveolar consolidation in one or both lungs. Organisms that can affect the lung in this way include streptococcus, hemophilus influenzae (which usually follows severe viral respiratory infections), pseudomonas (which causes a severe necrotizing pneumonitis and empyema), serratia, proteus, Escherichia coli, and the anaerobes. Staphylococcus may also surface in a pattern of bronchopneumonia, especially if the route of the infection is via the blood. It should be noted that these bronchopneumonias are often secondary to other predisposing conditions, including nosocomial pulmonary infections, which commonly result in bronchopneumonias.[38] These organisms may be opportunistic and lead to other infections or diseases in the patient who is already critically ill. The infection may then be complicated by abscess formation, empyema, and/or pleural effusion (all of which require draining by thoracentesis or chest tube).[39]

The incidence of gram-negative bacterial pulmonary infections is increasing at a rapid rate because of the widespread use of antibiotic therapy in today's clinical practice. This places the patient at risk for colonization of resistant gram-negative bacilli in the oropharynx. It is thought that up to 50% of nosocomial bacterial processes are due to gram-negative organisms. Other than antibiotic treatment, factors that predispose a patient to nosocomial infection include aspiration of oropharyngeal or gastric secretion, bypassing of normal mechanisms for clearance

of the respiratory tract, and the spread of infection to the lungs from other areas via the blood. (Such infections are opportunistic because they rarely occur in the immunocompetent or nondebilitated patient.[40])

Mycoplasmal pneumonia occurs most commonly in children and young adults with fibrinous pleurisy and interstitial pneumonia and in older adults in community hospital settings. The responsible organisms are smaller than bacteria, but are not classified as viruses. The disease tends to be self-limiting and is rare in persons between the ages of 45 and 70. A retrospective serologic diagnosis may be made, based on the fact that there is a rise in the serum complement, which fixes antibodies to the organism. Radiography proves it to be an interstitial pneumonia, often bilateral in nature. Rashes, upper respiratory infections, and bronchitis often precede a mycoplasma infection, which is transmitted by droplet infection. This pneumonia often occurs where people live and work together closely, such as in military units, schools, and dormitories, and incidences increase during the winter months.[41]

The infection that is viral in nature is frequently mild and self-limiting in the adult population, but can develop quickly and may be fatal if unattended. Viral pneumonias account for 50% of all pneumonias. Viral pneumonia may be suspected clinically, but a confirmed diagnosis is usually made retrospectively by serological studies. In adults, viral pneumonias are characterized by compromises in alveolar epithelial cells or the bronchioles.[42]

Precipitators of viral lung infection include common causative viruses such as influenza and chicken pox viruses, adenovirus, and parainfluenza viruses—organisms common in adults and transmitted by droplet infection. Additional causative agents include measles and cytomegalovirus; these viruses deplete the respiratory defense system and frequently predispose a patient to bacterial infection.[43]

In cases of fulminating viral infection, the alveoli are filled with fibrin, fluid, red blood cells, and macrophages. The patient affected in this manner also suffers severe hypoxemia, which does not respond to oxygen administration alone. Treatment for such a patient must be similar to that given the adult patient with respiratory distress syndrome. Fortunately such infections are rare, as the prognosis in this clinical situation is extremely grave. More commonly, patients present with patchy areas of viral pneumonitis not extensive enough to cause a severe loss of oxygen from the arterial blood.[44]

Pneumonia that complicates viral influenza is often bacterial, and the mortality rate from this type of pneumonia can be as high as 20%. Pneumonia due to varicella virus may complicate chicken pox in adults. Predisposing factors for viral pneumonia as a complication to chicken pox include chronic illness, steroid therapy, and chemotherapy.

Resulting signs and symptoms

The general signs and symptoms of pneumonia take many different forms and include fever and increased WBCs, bronchial inflammation manifested by cough and purulent sputum, shortness of breath, and decreased or absent breath sounds in the lobes affected.

Clinical manifestations of pneumococcal lung infection include fever, cough, leukocytosis, pleuritic chest pain, and production of a rusty colored or blood-streaked sputum. Hyperventilation will be apparent, with increased work of breathing. Breath sounds will be diminished or absent over affected lung fields. The elderly rarely exhibit these common symptoms of pneumonia initially; rather, the person may be lethargic, confused, and show signs of deterioration and exacerbation of other preexisting ailments. Complications, especially in the chronically ill and the elderly, include pleural involvement with empyema and pleuritis, lung abscess, bacteremia, and eventually respiratory failure.[45]

X-ray findings of bacterial pneumonia show an alveolar filling pattern that is soft, fluffy, and poorly demarcated, affecting one or both lungs. If an entire lobe is involved, an air bronchogram may serve as the most outstanding marker. In contrast, nosocomial bacterial lung infection is usually distributed throughout the lung in a lobar or segmental pattern.

Signs and symptoms of viral lung infection differ. The course of the disease may be very rapid, with an acute clinical episode of respiratory distress with or without fever, and it is possible for the terminal bronchioles to become damaged and then susceptible to bacterial infection, which can then spread to surrounding alveoli. Viral pneumonias are characterized by compromises in epithelial cells or the bronchioles. Pulmonary symptoms begin 2–5 days after the first symptoms of chicken pox, and typically include severe respiratory distress, cough, chest pain, hypoxemia, and hemoptysis. A pleural friction rub is present, and effusions may be found on auscultation, producing scattered crackles (rales) and gurgles (rhonchi).

Nursing standards of care

Therapy is aimed at treating the underlying infection and relieving symptoms. Initial antibiotic therapy is determined by gram stain and culture and sensitivity screens. Doses are prescribed according to what is recommended for serious infection, and are adjusted according to the individual patient's peak and trough serum levels. Basic life support is critical, and respiratory support and vigorous pulmonary toileting should be maintained.

Prevention, not treatment, of nosocomial bacterial infection in the critical care unit should be the goal. Nurses and other health care personnel must use the most scrupulous sterile technique when using respiratory therapy equipment and during suctioning. Finally, a meticulous program of infection control surveillance is absolutely essential in the critical care unit.

Specific nursing interventions include increasing the patient's natural resistance by encouraging good nutrition, rest, and positioning and monitoring contact with visitors and staff who may be suffering upper respiratory infections. Those patients who are highly susceptible (the elderly and the chronically ill) should be innoculated against influenza (if such protection is not contraindicated). In addition, the pneumococcal vaccine can be given to the healthy and to those at greatest risk (those suffering chronic diseases, COPD, or sickle cell anemia and those who are immunosuppressed). The nurse should be aware of the preoperative pulmonary function status of the surgical patient in order to assess possible postoperative complications. Immobilized patients should be repositioned every 2 hours and encouraged to maintain pulmonary toilet. Chest assessments should be conducted frequently, and pain relief should be afforded so that the nonintubated patient can breathe deeply and cough so as to prevent hypoventilation and atelectasis. Finally, adequate fluid intake without overhydration is indicated. The following nursing plan gives a detailed description of the care required by those suffering acute respiratory infections.

Nursing Care Plan for the Management of the Patient with Acute Respiratory Infection

Diagnosis	Signs and symptoms	Intervention	Rationale
Ineffective breathing pattern and cough related to infection of lung	Altered respiratory rate Unequal respiratory effort and rhythm Use of accessory muscles Ineffective cough	Monitor respiratory rhythm and rate and ABGs	To ascertain degree of respiratory compromise
		Determine causative organism (sputum sample for gram stain and culture)	To choose antibiotic (antifungal or antiviral) appropriate to infecting organism
		Pulmonary toilet: encourage coughing and deep breathing; change patient's position frequently; chest percussion with or without IPPB treatment	To loosen clogged sputum and mucus from airways to promote gas exchange and rid lung of medium in which infectious agents can multiply
		Auscultate for crackles (rales) and gurgles (rhonchi)	Warning signs of accumulation and pulmonary congestion leading to cardiac compromise
		Monitor chest x-ray	To ascertain extent of infectious involvement
		Administer antibiotic as ordered: monitor for side effects of antibiotics; dose according to peak and trough levels	To overcome the infection without further complications and with dose appropriate to patient
		Administer humidified oxygen via mask or intubation as ordered	To hydrate the lungs in order to thin mucus, promote ciliary movement of mucus, and prevent crusting of mucus in lung periphery
Potential for infection related to pulmonary congestion, indwelling lines, and Foley catheter	Elevated temperature	Encourage coughing and deep breathing; and turn patient in bed every 2 hours while on bedrest; increase activity as soon as indicated	Helps move secretions pooling in dependent lung regions to prevent atelectasis, blood clots in legs, and pressure sores

Nursing Care Plan for the Management of the Patient with Acute Respiratory Infection

Diagnosis	Signs and symptoms	Intervention	Rationale
		Change respiratory tubing every 24 hours	Per CDC specifications
		Monitor temperature every 4 hours	Sign of infection
	Increased WBCs	Assess WBC count	Sign of infection
		Maintain strict aseptic technique with invasive lines and indwelling catheters; change lines unless contraindicated: PAP every 72 hours, arterial lines every 7 days, tubing every 48 hours, IV bags every 24 hours; provide Foley care every 8 hours	Per Centers for Disease Control recommendation
		Assist in identifying source of infection: collect cultures; note atelectasis on chest x-ray; note sputum and urine characteristics; check insertion site for redness every 8 hours	Sites at risk of infection must be kept clean with aseptic technique; appropriate antibiotic therapy must be chosen
		Administer antibiotics as ordered	To combat infectious process
Decreased tolerance of activity related to dyspnea	Dyspnea on exertion Fatigue Exaggerated increase in heart rate and BP on exertion	Assess level of activity tolerance (should be related to the New York Heart Association's classification for consistency)	Provides a baseline
		Assist patient to change position every 2 hours while on bedrest	To decrease risk of complications and promote venous return

Diagnosis	Signs and symptoms	Intervention	Rationale
		Check BP with patient in horizontal, sitting, and standing positions	To monitor for orthostatic hypotension
		Avoid activity for a half-hour to an hour after meals	May decrease chance of hypoxia due to increased blood flow to GI tract
		Monitor heart rate and BP with activity increases	To maintain heart rate within 10 bpm of resting heart rate and maintain systolic BP within 20 mm Hg of resting BP; if a drop occurs, it may indicate a drop in cardiac output
		Anticipate institution of progressive rehab	To provide controlled mechanism for increasing activity
		Encourage frequent rest periods	To prevent excessive fatigue
Potential for alteration in gas exchange	Dyspnea or decreased O_2 levels on ABGs	Monitor ABGs closely	Problems with oxygenation are commonly seen
	Fluid overload	Assist patient to position of comfort; semi- or high Fowler's position is best	To improve breathing patterns and lower diaphragm
		Assess for rales, S_3, and JVD every 4 hours and as needed	Signs of respiratory failure with resultant heart failure
		Administer oxygen as ordered	To counter problems with oxygenation
		Monitor heart rhythm	Tachycardia is commonly seen
		Review chest x-ray for signs of pulmonary edema	Pulmonary congestion can be clinically delayed up to 24 hours
	Change in mental status	Monitor level of consciousness	Decreased level of consciousness may be first sign of anoxia

Nursing Care Plan for the Management of the Patient with Acute Respiratory Infection

Diagnosis	Signs and symptoms	Intervention	Rationale
Alteration in respiratory function: hypoxemia	In the appropriate clinical context and with no other reason: $PaO_2 < 5(FIO_2)$; $PaO_2 <$ predicted for patient's age; $PaO_2 = 110 - \frac{1}{2}$ of patient's age; $PaO_2 < 75$ mm Hg on room air; $SaO_2 < 90\%$	Monitor ABGs frequently	To ascertain the presence of hypoxemia for appropriate choice of intervention
		Oxygen and ventilatory support as needed	To correct hypoxemia
	Increased work of breathing: increased respiratory rate; increased tidal volume	Monitor respiratory rate and tidal volume	To assess cardiopulmonary stress
		Place in semi- or high Fowler's position as indicated	To allow easiest breathing and full diaphragmatic descension
	Increased myocardial work: increased cardiac output; changes in BP; decreased level of consciousness; decreased capillary refill; cold and clammy skin; decreased urinary output	Assist with basic care regime	To conserve energy and prevent increases in cardiac oxygen demand
		Closely monitor VS and ECG and check for chest pain	Indications of ischemic damage and cardiac compromise
		Maintain patency of IV lines	To allow fast access in case of an emergency
		Avoid activity for half-hour after meal	To prevent further oxygen demand when blood is shunted to GI tract during digestion
	$PaCO_2$ 35–45 mm Hg or less	Assess closely for orthostatic hypotension	To prevent injury in the event of syncope associated with orthostatic hypotension
	Increased minute ventilation		

Diagnosis	Signs and symptoms	Intervention	Rationale
Potential for impaired gas exchange due to: fluid volume overload; ineffective airway clearance, atelectasis, or effusion; bronchospasm; inadequate supplemental O_2; inadequate tidal volume; secondary low cardiac output; excessive pulmonary vascular resistance; malpositioned ET tube, inadequate cuff volume; pneumothorax, hemothorax	Abnormal ABGs: $pO_2 < 80$ mm Hg; $pCO_2 < 35$ or $pCO_2 > 45$ mm Hg; $pH < 7.35$ or $pH > 7.45$; O_2 sat. $< 80\%$; $HCO_3 < 20$ or $HCO_3 > 26$ mEq/L; BE < 0 or BE > 3	Mechanically ventilate as ordered	Ventilation support is needed until patient is stable
	Cyanosis	Closely monitor lung sounds for absent, unequal, diminished breath sounds, crackles (rales), wheezing, or asymmetric chest wall expansion; closely monitor ABGs PRN as indicated; obtain chest x-ray immediately and PRN for ET tube placement, lung expansion (pneumothorax), width of mediastinal shadow, presence of pleural fluid, or presence of foreign body	Early indications of further respiratory compromise and/or complications
	ET tube cuff leak		
	Lowered peak pressure		
	Inadequate volume exchange		
	Chest x-ray indicates atelectasis, effusion, pneumothorax, or hemothorax		
	Copious secretions	Aggressive pulmonary toilet PRN with chest percussion therapy, incentive spirometry, and hyperinflation using 100% O_2 before and after suctioning; turn and reposition patient every 2 hours	To mobilize secretions, provide adequate oxygenation, and open closed alveoli
	Elevated respiratory rate, wheezing, air hunger, gasping, or asymmetrical chest wall expansion		
	Change in mental status	Monitor level of consciousness	Decreased level of consciousness may be first sign of anoxia
	Fluid overload	Assess for crackles (rales), S_3, and JVD (jugular vein distension) as indicated	Signs of respiratory failure leading to heart failure
		Monitor Na^+ and osmolarity	SIADH is common with pulmonary disease
		If patient is stable, promote extubation by holding sedation, elevating HOB (head of bed) 30 degrees, and decreasing IMV by increments of 2 to 4 breaths/min (if $pO_2 > 90$, pH between 7.35 and 7.45, and O_2 sat. 90–100%)	To assist patient to return to optimal breathing capacity as soon as possible (to prevent further atelectasis, secondary infection, etc.)

Nursing Care Plan for the Management of the Patient with Acute Respiratory Infection

Diagnosis	Signs and symptoms	Intervention	Rationale
Anxiety due to respiratory distress	Agitation Restlessness Confusion Impaired concentration Hyperventilation Diaphoresis Tachycardia Sleeplessness Shakiness Facial tension Distracted behavior Withdrawal Nonadherence to treatment plan	Monitor patient's oxygenation status closely	ARDS is characterized by severe refractory hypoxemia
		Position patient to maximize respiratory status and minimize respiratory effort, based on patient tolerance	Dyspnea, shortness of breath, and hyperventilation are early signs of impending respiratory failure and cause high anxiety in patient, which only worsens respiratory status; positioning can decrease compression of diaphragm by abdomen and maximize ventilation-perfusion, decreasing sensations of inability to breathe
		Prepare patient for procedures and expected sensations	To minimize anxiety and maximize cooperation
		Ascertain patient's fears and anxieties	Baseline will allow nurse to know exactly what to address
		Ascertain patient's previous hospital experiences	Will help nurse to know how to best alleviate anxieties and support encouraging actions
		Provide emotional support as needed	To help patient and family deal with the situation in the best way possible
		Teach patient about what will happen in ICU: care routine, tubes, lines, ICU environment and visiting hours, how to improve breathing efforts, etc.	To help patient be prepared for what is to be experienced

Diagnosis	Signs and symptoms	Intervention	Rationale
		Administer analgesics and antianxiety agents as ordered (use of neuromuscular blocking agents requires sedation of patient)	To decrease anxiety and increase rest
Altered nutritional status due to: anorexia and malaise; increased nutritional requirements resulting from stress of illness; less appealing taste of food related to low sodium content and changes in oral mucosa; changes in bowel routine; increased work of breathing	Too fatigued to eat	Auscultate bowel sounds	To evaluate GI peristalsis
	Too short of breath to eat	Help patient to eat slowly; use supplemental O_2 as needed	To facilitate nutritional intake
	Inadequate intake of food and fluids	Monitor I&O	To assess fluid balance
		Calculate calorie requirements	Calorie requirements may increase 200% in ARF
	Decreased albumin and lymphocytes	Monitor albumin and lymphocytes	To assess visceral proteins
	Decreasing body weight	Monitor weight	To monitor effect of diuretic therapy
	Complaints of lack of appetite	With patient, family, and dietary staff, assess appetite and food preferences and review what is allowed and what is best for optimal nutrition; provide preferred food as much as possible	To facilitate nutritional intake and status in any way possible

Medications Commonly Used in the Care of the Patient with Acute Respiratory Infection

Medication	Effect	Major side effects
Penicillins: Ampicillin Nafcillin Mezlin	Bactericidal (inhibit cell-wall synthesis) Broad-spectrum activity	Hypersensitivity (rash, urticaria, anaphylaxis)
Cephalosporins: Ancef Mefoxin Cefotan	Inhibit cell-wall synthesis, promoting osmotic instability Broad-spectrum activity	Pseudomembranous colitis Anaphylaxis GI disturbance
Valium	Depresses the limbic and subcortical level of the brain Antianxiety agent Sedative	Drowsiness, lethargy Cardiovascular collapse
Morphine sulfate	Analgesia/sedation Peripheral vasodilation Bronchodilation Relief of cardiac dyspnea	Hypotension Respiratory depression Constipation Urinary retention

Status Asthmaticus

Respiratory diseases associated with decreased expiratory flow rates (as indicated by FEV_1) include bronchitis, emphysema, and asthma. Those who suffer from these conditions live with a small respiratory reserve and easily develop acute respiratory failure. Asthma and bronchitis have reversible components, and asthmatic patients may be symptom-free between episodes, in contrast to patients who suffer from emphysema, which is irreversible. If asthma is not controlled, patients may end up in the intensive care unit for treatment for acute respiratory compromises caused by spasmodic contractions of smooth muscle in the walls of the smaller bronchi and bronchioles, sometimes leading to failure.

Clinical antecedents

There are several classifications of asthma, which are based on precipitating events and clinical antecedents. Extrinsic asthma is caused by a hypersensitivity reaction to inhaled allergens and is mediated by immunoglobulin E (IgE-mediated). It is diagnosed through positive skin tests and documented correlation with exposure to possible allergens. The major offenders include house dust, mold spores, pollens, feathers, and animal dander. Prognosis is good for those who suffer from this type of asthma, especially if they are able to avoid the irritants.

Intrinsic asthma does not appear to have a definite cause, but infection is often present. Skin tests of the common allergens are usually negative (non-IgE-mediated). Precipitating factors can include strong odors or fumes such as those associated with paints, chemicals, heavily scented flowers, tobacco smoke and other air pollutants, and perfumes. Cold air, sudden barometric changes, and even emotionally charged events can lead to attacks of intrinsic asthma.[46]

Finally, there are two other types of asthma: mixed asthma, which occurs as a combination of an allergic reaction and an infection, and aspirin-induced asthma, which is a type of intrinsic asthma induced by aspirin and other related medications.

Critical referents

The active stage of an asthma attack (the spasm of the bronchial smooth muscle) is thought to be due to a markedly hyperactive response of the smooth muscle to an irritant. This endogenous hyperresponsivity is thought to be caused by physiological imbalance occurring in neurologic innervation and chemical mediation as well as a breakdown of airway defenses due to inflammation. Vasoactive chemical substances (leukotrienes) are responsible for the ensuing acute airway constriction and bronchospasm, mucus production, and airway inflammatory response. Leukotrienes may serve to potentiate the effects of other substances on the airways as well.[47] Allergens reacting with mast cells coated with immunoglobulin E cause a release of histamine, prostaglandins, serotonin, and bradykinin, which are normally inhibited by cyclic adenosine monophosphate (CAMP).[48]

Furthermore, a neurological imbalance (beta blockade) exists between the sympathetic and parasympathetic innervation of the bronchi. Beta-adrenergic receptors (specifically, beta-2) in the airways are responsible for relaxation of bronchial smooth muscles when stimulated by CAMP. When beta-2 stimulation is low or blocked, CAMP is lower, and bronchoconstriction and hyperactivity occur.

Cardiopulmonary vessels are supplied with beta-1 receptors. When these receptors are stimulated, vasoconstriction and other side effects such as tachycardia, arrhythmias, and blood pressure changes occur. Without beta stimulation, bronchoconstriction can be caused by a variety of stimulations including hyperventilation, extreme temperature and humidity changes, emotional disturbances, infection, and the typical response to allergens. Another effect of beta-2 stimulation is bronchial relaxation, since stimulation increases CAMP. Figure 2-45 provides a flow chart of the effects experienced in response to alterations in sympathetic and parasympathetic influences in the development of bronchospasm.

In some individuals, irritation of the upper airway may cause bronchoconstriction via stimulation of the vagus nerve, and this is exacerbated by the parasympathetic stimulation, which encourages mucus secretion and is responsible for the cough, bronchonstriction, and hyperventilation that accompany bronchospasm. Edema of the bronchial wall and mucus hypersecretion also occur in the asthma response, and because of this increased production of secretions, local areas of atelectasis occur in spite of the resulting coughing, which frequently stimulates more bronchospasm. Capillary blood flow through and around these areas of alveolar collapse results in increased shunting, which, in turn, produces severe hypoxemia. In addition, marked pulmonary hyperinflation and higher residual volumes are evidenced, with increases of total lung inflation of up to 30%.

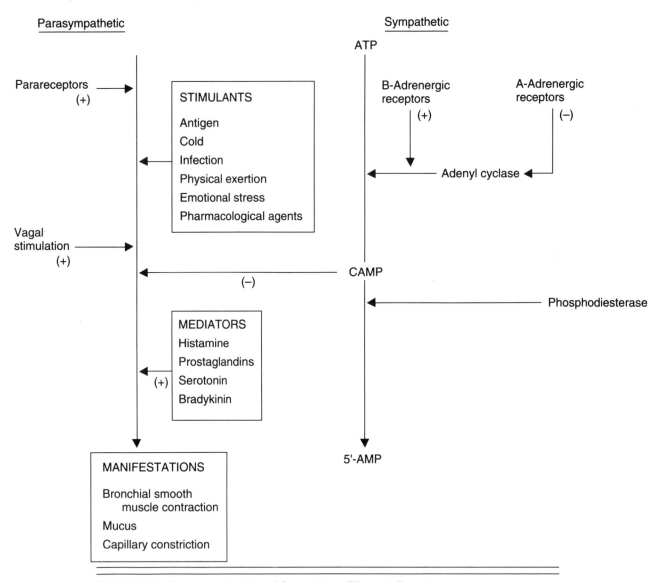

Figure 2-45 Parasympathetic and Sympathetic Effects in Bronchospasm
Source: Adapted from Kinney, M., Packa, D., Dunbar, S. (1988). *AACN's Clinical Reference for Critical Care Nursing* (2nd Edition). New York: McGraw-Hill, p. 802.

When the lung is overinflated, it becomes stiff and lung compliance lessens, which increases the work of breathing. It is at this point that the patient begins to perceive dyspnea, the hallmark of an asthma attack. In the beginning stages, the patient's $PaCO_2$ is low (because of the hyperventilation), but as the bronchospasm continues and the patient tires, $PaCO_2$ elevates, sometimes to very high levels. The vicious cycle is now initiated: dyspnea is exacerbated by anxiety, leading (again) to hyperventilation and weakened ventilatory effort with resultant hypercapnia. At this point the ventilation-perfusion mismatch that caused the hypercapnia may worsen enough for the patient to require mechanical ventilatory support. Figure 2-46 depicts the process diagrammati-

cally. Finally, cardiac effects are evidenced: (1) cyanosis due to inadequate oxygenation occurs, (2) elevated intrathoracic pressures interfere with venous return to the right ventricle, (3) dehydration secondary to hyperventilation decreases circulating volume, so cardiac output falls and vascular collapse results, and (4) tachycardia results as the heart makes a compensatory effort to overcome the above stressors placed on the cardiovascular system.

Resulting signs and symptoms

The clinical presentation of a patient in status asthmaticus is unmistakable. The critical care nurse

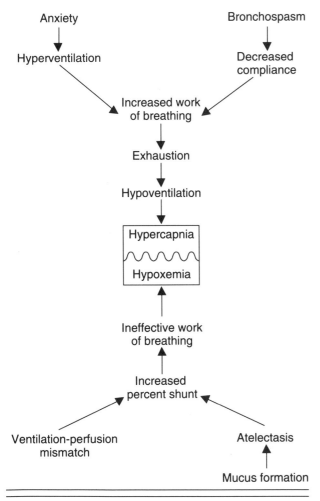

Figure 2-46 Effects of Bronchospasm

poxemic, diaphoretic, cyanotic, and, if these are severe enough, may be unresponsive from lack of oxygen to the brain.

The length of an acute asthma attack varies from 20 or 30 minutes to 1 hour, if conducive to medication, or as long as days or weeks. The frequency of attacks is even more variable, with some patients experiencing acute episodes only once or twice a year and others suffering chronic respiratory distress with frequent exacerbations and acute inflammatory responses.

Pulmonary diagnostics reveal airway obstruction; pulmonary function studies show decreased expiratory gas flow, forced expiratory volume, and forced vital capacity. Because air is trapped distal to spasmodic bronchioles during expiration, functional residual capacity is increased. Pulmonary function studies during attacks usually reflect marked improvement after treatment with bronchodilators; results can be compared to those of studies conducted during symptom-free periods to ascertain the patient's degree of responsiveness to drug therapy.

Laboratory data also reflect the degree of airway obstruction being experienced by the patient. Serial ABGs provide important information about the degree of hypoxemia present and how well the patient responds to medical interventions. Initially, PaO_2 levels will be as low as 40 mm Hg, pH will be normal, and $PaCO_2$ levels may be within normal range or slightly lower, due to the compensatory hyperventilatory effort. Increasing levels of $PaCO_2$ and falling pH levels indicate decompensation as the patient tires from the effort to breathe. Blood counts indicate elevations of eosinophils stemming from infections or inflammation.

Chest x-rays should also be taken when a patient is in asthmatic crisis. Often the initial picture will be normal, or the film may show air trapping. Hyperinflation is evidenced by a lower than usual placement of the diaphragm. Because x-rays do not provide more productive diagnostic information, they are primarily a mechanism by which to ascertain the presence of other pulmonary complications such as pneumothorax, mediastinal emphysema, or infectious processes (including mucous plugs), which are indicated in an x-ray by collapsed segments of lung.

ECG monitoring is maintained (especially during the acute stages of an asthma attack) in order to detect rhythm changes indicative of strain of the right heart.

Increased neutrophil and eosinophil counts document the infectious process associated with extrinsic asthma. Sputum samples should be collected and tested for identification of possible infectious organisms. In the case of mild asthma, the sputum will

sees this type of patient at the point in the attack at which the bronchospasm can no longer be relieved by bronchodilators and gas exchange is interrupted by obstruction of distal airways. Symptoms include nasal inflammation, flushing of the upper body, nausea and vomiting, wheezing, and cyanosis. The primary symptom, though, is extreme dyspnea accompanied by difficulty in forcing air out of the lungs (wheezing). Harsh coughing comes as the result of bronchospasm, and as the attack progresses, the dyspnea and wheezing worsen and coughing becomes productive. The patient is so dyspneic that only short verbal responses can be made (if talking is even possible). The chest is hyperresonant, and breath sounds are diminished. Pulse is rapid and thready, and heart sounds are distant. In severe attacks, paradoxical pulsus is present with diminished volume on inspiration as a result of decreased filling of the right atrium caused by decreased lung compliance from pulmonary overdistention and increased pressures in the alveoli. The patient is hy-

appear foamy, clear, or white. In more serious cases of asthma, it will be thicker and more tenacious. Asthma, with infection, produces sputum that is purulent green or yellow.

Nursing standards of care

The cause of an asthma attack is usually identifiable from a carefully compiled patient history. Once the implicated bronchial irritants are identified, every effort should be made to avoid them. Respiratory infection must be treated immediately, and drugs that may cause bronchospasm (propranolol, etc.) should be avoided.

Careful attention to bronchial hygiene is most important for the asthmatic patient in order to maintain an open airway and prevent any ventilation-perfusion mismatch and problems that result from it. Adequate hydration, either by mouth or intravenously, is essential to prevent dehydration caused by hyperventilation. Adequate fluid intake is also essential to prevent the thickening and drying (crusting) of mucus in the irritated airways.

Medications are usually administered in a stepwise manner; one drug is added to the treatment regimen at a time, and dosage is adjusted to achieve the maximum benefit. The use of medications is coordinated with other factors such as control of the environment and possibly immunotherapy.

Cromolyn sodium has proven to be effective in preventing attacks in approximately 50% of asthmatic patients, when delivered as a powder propelled from a hand-held dispenser. The drug is not a bronchodilator, but appears to block the release of the chemical mediators of bronchospasm from the bronchial mucosa. It should be noted that this drug should not be given once bronchospasm has begun.[49]

Isoetharine with phenylephrine (Bronkosol) is available as a metered aerosol and can also be administered via nebulization. It is a selective β-2 agent that is especially useful in patients in bronchospasm who are hypoxic and present with an underlying tachycardia and/or coronary artery disease. Metaproterenol (Alupent, Metaprel) is reported to have fewer cardiac stimulatory side effects than drugs such as isoproterenol, and the β-1 side effects are thought to be similar. Terbutaline (Brethine) has a higher β-2:β-1 ratio than either isoproterenol or metaproterenol, and has very little alpha activity. Oral administration of this drug has a tendency to produce muscular tremor and nervousness. Subcutaneous injections (0.125–0.25 mg, repeated in 30 minutes

with no more than 0.5 mg every 4 hours) have been demonstrated to be especially useful in the critical care setting.

Beclomethasone (Vanceril) is a metered inhaled steroid delivered at 50 μg per puff. It is thought that up to 2 mg per day is safe and without significant steroid effects. Most asthmatic patients require smaller doses, and many who are steroid-dependent have been switched from oral preparations, which may cause Cushing's syndrome, to the safer aerosol preparation.

Steroids are frequently used to diminish the nonspecific inflammatory response and inhibit release of chemical mediators that promote bronchoconstriction. The reason for the beneficial effect of steroids in cases of asthma is not fully understood. It is thought that steroids:

> prevent antibody-antigen reactions by inhibiting the antibody formation,
>
> prevent the formation or storage of mediators such as histamines, and
>
> prevent nonspecific inflammatory processes.

Steroids potentiate sympathomimetic drugs, probably via the β-2 receptors, with the result that smooth muscles relax and circulating levels of CAMP increase. Anti-inflammatory steroids (glucocorticoids) are helpful in status asthmaticus of any origin.[50]

Once the patient is stabilized, prednisone is the oral steroid prescribed for maintenance therapy. It is similar to hydrocortisone in action, although more potent. During an attack it may be given in large doses of 40–70 mg per day for 5 to 7 days, and then it is titrated to a maintenance dose of 5–20 mg per day. However, there is a risk that Cushing's syndrome will develop with long-term use. Many patients do well on alternate-day dose schedules, which tend to decrease side effects. In status asthmaticus in the critical care unit, intravenous hydrocortisone (Solu-Cortef) is given in doses of 250–500 mg, followed by 100–250 mg every 3 hours.

Bronchodilators are used on a short-term basis to reverse the effects of the asthma attack, and on a long-term basis to maintain ventilatory capacity as close to normal as possible. (Most asthmatics can be well maintained on oral bronchodilators.) Sympathomimetics are available in aerosol form and include epinephrine (the least active), isoproterenol, and metaproterenol. Sympathomimetic aerosols are primarily used to prevent or block an attack or to provide relief until oral medication takes effect (usually 30 to 120 minutes). Subcutaneous (epinephrine and terbutaline) or intravenous (aminophylline) bronchodilators may be necessary for severe asthma attacks. The major problem with these medications, however, is the potential for overuse, which causes complications of dehydration of the bronchial tree and/or serious cardiac arrhythmias. Sedatives should not be given unless the patient is intubated because of the accompanying depressant effect on the respiratory drive.

Bronchodilators are also important drugs for the patient with bronchospasm. Intravenous epinephrine was used extensively in the past, but has been replaced by aminophylline and inhaled drugs. Epinephrine, because of its A, β-1, and β-2 effects, is a potent bronchodilator, but has major cardiovascular and nervous system side effects. Isoproterenol is one of the most potent β-2 stimulators and also has strong β-1 effects; it therefore potentiates a risk of inotropic and chronotropic cardiac stimulation. The methylxanthines are currently the most popular drugs for treating bronchospasms, since they inhibit phosphodiesterase activity, thus preventing the breakdown of CAMP and promoting bronchial relaxation. Additional benefits of theophylline include an increase in cardiac output, decrease in venous pressure, dilation of pulmonary vascular bed, improved renal circulation, and cerebral stimulation. There are side effects with theophylline, but in contrast to other drugs, the most serious side effect of this pharmacological agent is increasing gastric secretions and possible gastric bleeding. This side effect is more common with the oral preparation of the drug, but also remains a factor as long as blood levels of the drug are high; the best clinical results are obtained when blood levels of theophylline are close to toxic. Hepatic metabolism and renal excretion of the drug are also often impaired, thus the serum drug levels should be monitored daily in the critical care unit. Gastric pH should also be monitored, and antacids should be used to control possible gastric complications.

Nursing diagnoses are individualized for each patient. Nursing care and interventions for the patient suffering status asthmaticus are outlined in the following care plan.

Nursing Care Plan for the Management of the Patient with Status Asthmaticus

Diagnosis	Signs and symptoms	Intervention	Rationale
Ineffective airway clearance related to bronchial constriction and retained secretions	Tenacious secretions Ineffective cough effort Distant sounds, crackles (rales), gurgles (rhonchi), and wheezes on auscultation Chest x-ray indicates atelectasis Shunting Hypoxemia	Monitor patient's respiratory status closely	To determine progression of syndrome and status of patient
		If indicated, place patient in high Fowler's position to deep breathe and cough	To allow diaphragm to descend and lungs to inflate as much as possible
		Turn patient every 2 hours as medically indicated	To prevent pooling of secretions and improve systemic and pulmonary circulation
		Instruct patient on coughing technique, including deep breathing and deep cough effort (using diaphragm, not throat)	To increase efficacy of cough effort
		Vigorous pulmonary toilet	To improve existing ventilation and rid patient of infection source and media
		Suction every 2–4 hrs and as needed, using aseptic technique	To clear secretions patient is unable to clear because of decreased elasticity and compliance and compression of airway
		If medically indicated, encourage fluids to maintain fluid balance	To thin secretions and allow easier movement of mucus by cilia
		Suction intubated patient as needed, hyperventilating with 100% O_2 before and after suctioning; if indicated, lavage 1–3 cc sterile NS in ET tube before mechanically hyperventilating	To mechanically promote loosening of secretions and to assure adequate oxygenation before and after suctioning

Diagnosis	Signs and symptoms	Intervention	Rationale
		Chest physical therapy as indicated	To promote breaking up of mucus plugs and thick secretions and to clear specific lung fields
		Frequent and meticulous mouth care	To prevent further secretions from being aspirated and to maintain condition of oral mucosa
		Place patient in position of safety and use extreme caution during oral and tube feeding	To prevent aspiration of liquids or solids
		Administer humidified oxygen	To prevent drying of upper airway and to loosen secretions
		Administer bronchodilators based on patient tolerance, as ordered	Enhances clearing of secretions and opening up of airways
		Monitor for signs and symptoms of pulmonary infection: fever, atelectasis, hypoxia, shortness of breath	Clogged airways are fertile areas for growth of bacteria
		Use sedatives sparingly	To protect patient from further respiratory depression and to allow full cough effort
Alteration in respiratory function: hypoxemia	In the appropriate clinical context and with no other reason: $PaO_2 < 5(FIO_2)$; $PaO_2 <$ predicted for patient's age; $PaO_2 = 110 - \frac{1}{2}$ of patient's age; $PaO_2 < 75$ mm Hg on room air; $SaO_2 < 90\%$	Monitor ABGs frequently	To ascertain the presence of hypoxemia for appropriate choice of intervention
		Oxygen and ventilatory support as needed	To correct hypoxemia
	Increased work of breathing: increased respiratory rate; increased tidal volume	Monitor respiratory rate and tidal volume	To assess cardiopulmonary stress
		Place in semi- or high Fowler's position as indicated	To allow easiest breathing and full diaphragmatic descension

Nursing Care Plan for the Management of the Patient with Status Asthmaticus

Diagnosis	Signs and symptoms	Intervention	Rationale
	Increased myocardial work: increased cardiac output; changes in BP; decreased level of consciousness; decreased capillary refill; cold and clammy skin; decreased urinary output	Assist with basic care regime	To conserve energy and prevent increases in cardiac oxygen demand
		Closely monitor VS and ECG and check for chest pain	Indications of ischemic damage and cardiac compromise
		Maintain patency of IV lines	To allow fast access in case of an emergency
		Avoid activity for half-hour after meal	To prevent further oxygen demand when blood is shunted to GI tract during digestion
	$PaCO_2$ 35–45 mm Hg or less	Assess closely for orthostatic hypotension	To prevent injury in the event of syncope associated with orthostatic hypotension
	Increased minute ventilation		
Decreased tolerance of activity related to dyspnea	Dyspnea on exertion	Assess level of activity tolerance (should be related to the New York Heart Association's classification for consistency)	Provides a baseline
	Fatigue		
	Exaggerated increase in heart rate and BP on exertion		
		Assist patient to change position every 2 hours while on bedrest	To decrease risk of complications and promote venous return
		Check BP with patient in horizontal, sitting, and standing positions	To monitor for orthostatic hypotension
		Avoid activity for a half-hour to an hour after meals	May decrease chance of hypoxia due to increased blood flow to GI tract
		Monitor heart rate and BP with activity increases	To maintain heart rate within 10 bpm of resting heart rate and maintain systolic BP within 20 mm Hg of resting BP; if a drop occurs, it may indicate a drop in cardiac output

Diagnosis	Signs and symptoms	Intervention	Rationale
		Anticipate institution of progressive rehab	To provide controlled mechanism for increasing activity
		Encourage frequent rest periods	To prevent excessive fatigue
Impaired gas exchange due to increased shunting	Hyperventilation Respiratory distress Agitation Hypoxia Headache Tachycardia Peripheral vasoconstriction Cough Cyanosis Changes in acid-base balance Altered lung sounds Inadequate volume exchange	Closely monitor respiratory status	Asthma crisis severely compromises respiratory status; frequent assessment is crucial in determining clinical progression of the condition so as to plan, implement, and evaluate care
		Closely monitor cardiovascular status	Loss of fluid to the pulmonary interstitium and alveoli causes intravascular depletion, resulting in further intrapulmonary shunt
		Serial ABGs and pulse oximetry after ventilator changes; assist with insertion of arterial line	Respiratory acidosis must be treated with sodium bicarb and appropriate O_2 therapy; arterial line gives easy access for frequent arterial blood draws
		Administer bronchodilators, FIO_2, mechanical ventilation as ordered: tidal volume that reduces $PaCO_2$; deadspace as necessary; PEEP as necessary; minimal FIO_2	To ensure adequate oxygenation and correct hypoxemia without depressing respiratory drive from too much oxygen To reduce shunting and improve gas exchange
		Turn patient every 2–4 hours as tolerated; vigorous pulmonary toilet; suction every 2–4 hours and as needed	To maximize functioning of existing alveoli in order to prevent further intrapulmonary shunting by preventing atelectasis

Nursing Care Plan for the Management of the Patient with Status Asthmaticus

Diagnosis	Signs and symptoms	Intervention	Rationale
		When patient is stable, promote extubation as soon as possible by holding sedation, elevating HOB 30 degrees, using incremental weaning	To assist patient to return to optimal breathing capacity as soon as possible and to prevent atelectasis and secondary infection
Potential for alteration in cardiac output related to congestive failure	Decreased cardiac output as measured directly with pulmonary artery catheter: CO < 3 L/min CI < 2 L/min/m²	Monitor CO and CI closely	To facilitate early intervention
	Decreased BP	Administer vasoactive medications as ordered (Dobutamine, Inocor)	Maintain adequate perfusion in vital organs and periphery
	Reduced peripheral tissue perfusion (evidenced by decreased distal pulses, cool extremities, and sluggish capillary refill)	Promote rest and avoid isometric activities; use bedside commode as indicated; avoid Valsalva maneuver; monitor capillary refill and pulses	Isometrics increase peripheral vascular resistance, thereby increasing the workload of the heart and thus the work of breathing
	Lethargy	Monitor ECG; administer drugs to maintain normal sinus rhythm as ordered	Dysrhythmias can decrease filling time, thus decreasing cardiac output
	Dyspnea		
	Arrhythmias such as PVCs, heart blocks, SVT, PAT, AF, and AFL	Correct fluid imbalances	To maintain cardiac function and output within appropriate parameters
	Ischemia: CPK > 180 IU/L, MBs > 15 IU/L, new ECG ischemic changes	Provide appropriate oxygen therapy	To increase oxygenation of cardiac tissue to prevent ischemic damage leading to infarction
	Increased preload		
	(Crackles) rales	Vigorous pulmonary toilet, IPPB, and breathing treatments	To promote clearing of secretions and clogged airways

Diagnosis	Signs and symptoms	Intervention	Rationale
Inadequate tissue perfusion related to reduction in oxygen intake	Agitation Confusion Anxiety Headache Tachycardia Tachypnea Dyspnea Cyanosis Restlessness Hypoxemia Early alkalosis Late acidosis	Closely monitor patient's mental status	Subtle changes in mental status and headache may serve as first indicators that hypoxia is present
		Maintain HOB at 30 degrees or more; control external environment; allow rest periods	To allow for full respiratory effort, prevent agitation, and allow patient to maintain comfortable position
		Administer pain medication as ordered, but avoid depressing respiratory effort	To alleviate headache
		Monitor ABGs closely	To assess alveolar ventilation
		Monitor Ve	To assess total ventilation to provide an index of work of breathing affecting cardiopulmonary stress
		Emergent administration of increased FIO_2	To normalize PaO_2, improve alveolar oxygen tension, decrease work of breathing, and decrease myocardial work
		Use appropriate O_2 device	To maintain pO_2 to best prevent complications of hyperoxia; oxygen system should deliver flow ($4 \times Ve$) to maintain desired FIO_2, prevent room air leaking into system, maintain adequate PaO_2 (at least level of inspired FIO_2), and reduce work of breathing
		Monitor oxygenation	Pulse oximetry should show O_2 sat. $> 90\%$

Nursing Care Plan for the Management of the Patient with Status Asthmaticus

Diagnosis	Signs and symptoms	Intervention	Rationale
Potential for alteration in fluid status: deficit related to hyperventilation accompanied by lung water loss, diaphoresis, and diuresis from aminophylline administration	Decreased urine output Increased specific gravity of urine Weight loss Hypotension Tachycardia Thirst Change in mental status Decreased CVP, cardiac output, MAP, PCWP, and PAP Hemoconcentration Electrolyte abnormalities	Monitor patient's fluid status, CVP, and pressure readings Monitor patient's Hb/Hct and electrolytes Administer vasoconstricting agents and/or fluids as ordered	To ascertain extent of deficit and provide appropriate rehydration Fluid volume deficits result in hemoconcentration and electrolyte abnormalities Because of pulmonary capillary leaking, patient is kept mildly dehydrated but adequate perfusion (MAP > 60 mm Hg) is maintained to support ventilation-perfusion status and oxygenation of tissues
Potential for infection related to pulmonary congestion, bronchial irritation, altered nutrition, indwelling lines, and Foley catheter	Elevated temperature Increased WBCs Increased pulse Chest x-ray changes indicative of infectious process in lungs	Encourage coughing and deep breathing; turn patient in bed every 2 hours while on bedrest; increase activity as soon as indicated Monitor temperature every 4 hours Assess WBC count Maintain strict aseptic technique with invasive lines and indwelling catheters; change lines unless contraindicated: PAP every 72 hours, arterial lines every 7 days, tubing every 48 hours, IV bags every 24 hours; provide Foley care every 8 hours	Helps to prevent atelectasis (which supplies fertile ground for infection), blood clots in legs, pressure sores Sign of infection Sign of infection Per Centers for Disease Control recommendation

Diagnosis	Signs and symptoms	Intervention	Rationale
		Assist in identifying source of infection: collect cultures; note atelectasis on chest x-ray; note sputum and urine characteristics; check insertion site for redness every 8 hours	Sites at risk of infection must be kept clean with aseptic technique; appropriate antibody therapy must be chosen
		Administer antibiotics as ordered	To overcome infectious agent
		Encourage adequate oral intake of food and fluids	To promote healing and good nutritional status to fight infection; to thin mucus and promote ciliary movement of secretions
Altered nutritional status due to: anorexia and malaise; increased nutritional requirements resulting from stress of illness; less appealing taste of food related to low sodium content and changes in oral mucosa; changes in bowel routine; increased work of breathing	Too fatigued to eat	Auscultate bowel sounds	To evaluate GI peristalsis
	Too short of breath to eat	Help patient to eat slowly; use supplemental O_2 as needed	To facilitate nutritional intake
	Inadequate intake of food and fluids	Monitor I&O	To assess fluid balance
		Calculate calorie requirements	Calorie requirements may increase 200% in ARF
	Decreased albumin and lymphocytes	Monitor albumin and lymphocytes	To assess visceral proteins
	Decreasing body weight	Monitor weight	To monitor effect of diuretic therapy
	Complaints of lack of appetite	With patient, family, and dietary staff, assess appetite and food preferences and review what is allowed and what is best for optimal nutrition; provide preferred food as much as possible	To facilitate nutritional intake and status in any way possible

Nursing Care Plan for the Management of the Patient with Status Asthmaticus

Diagnosis	Signs and symptoms	Intervention	Rationale
Anxiety due to respiratory distress related to severe dyspnea	Agitation Restlessness Confusion Impaired concentration Hyperventilation Diaphoresis Tachycardia Sleeplessness Shakiness Facial tension Distracted behavior Withdrawal Nonadherence to treatment plan	Monitor patient's oxygenation status closely	Asthmatic crisis can decrease lung ability for gas exchange
		Position patient to maximize respiratory status and minimize respiratory effort, based on patient tolerance	Dyspnea, shortness of breath, and hyperventilation are early signs of impending respiratory failure and cause high anxiety in patient, which exacerbates condition; positioning decreases compression of diaphragm by abdomen and maximizes ventilation-perfusion, decreasing sensations of inability to breathe
		Prepare patient for procedures and expected sensations	To minimize anxiety and maximize cooperation
		Ascertain patient's fears and anxieties	Baseline will allow nurse to know exactly what to address
		Ascertain patient's previous hospital experiences	Will help nurse to know how to best alleviate anxieties and support encouraging actions
		Provide emotional support as needed	To help patient and family deal with the situation in the best way possible
		Teach patient about what will happen in ICU: care routine, tubes, lines, ICU environment and visiting hours, how to improve breathing efforts, etc.	To help patient be prepared for what is to be experienced

Diagnosis	Signs and symptoms	Intervention	Rationale
		Administer analgesics and antianxiety agents as ordered (use of neuromuscular blocking agents requires sedation of patient)	To decrease anxiety and increase rest
Lack of knowledge of disease process and prescribed regimen	Patient does not adhere to care plan	Assess present understanding and teach patient and family from that point	Provides baseline and direction for teaching
	Patient verbalizes lack of knowledge and understanding of asthma and what precipitates asthmatic crises	Institute teaching program about: normal lung function; pathology of asthma risk factors; control of precipitating and aggravating factors; activity; diet; medications; signs and symptoms of recurring respiratory crisis	Lifestyle changes will be required, but are difficult to accomplish without much teaching and assistance; increasing patient's knowledge and understanding and thus potential to adhere to regimen may decrease unnecessary complications or exacerbations of asthma, and make rehospitalization unnecessary
	Patient expresses anxiety and apprehension, especially during procedures and treatments		
	Patient does not distinguish between permitted and prohibited activities		
	Patient is unable to describe diagnosis, prognosis, and care regimen	Allow patient and family to ask questions and verify information	Patient and family may need personal reinforcement and several repetitions of information before it is fully understood and integrated
	Patient is unable to identify professional services available for support	Instruct patient on services and resources available	Patient and family will receive more compre-hensive and effective service if all available resources are tapped
	Patient does not know when to call nurse or MD for assistance	Review signs and symptoms that can be used as warning signals of approaching asthmatic crisis	To allow for early diagnosis and treatment of respiratory crisis and its complications
	Patient and family make inappropriate requests and display hypervigilance	Delegate one resource and support person to the family to assist them through crisis periods; suggest ways family can assist in care	Consistency in problem solving and care improves quality of decisions; participating in patient care decreases family anxiety

Medications Commonly Used in the Care of the Patient with Status Asthmaticus

Medication	Effect	Major side effects
Epinephrine	Stimulates alpha and beta receptors of autonomic nervous system Potent bronchodilator with rapid onset of action Vasoconstriction	Tachycardia Arrhythmias Nausea and vomiting Palpitations Hypertension Nervousness and tremor Bad taste
Metaproterenol (Metaprel, Alupent)	Beta-adrenergic stimulator Bronchodilator	Tachycardia Hypertension
Terbutaline sulfate (Brethine)	Promotes relaxation of bronchial smooth muscles lasting 4–6 hours	Tachycardia Tremors Nervousness
Cromolyn sodium (Intal)	Inhibits degranulation of sensitized mast cells after exposure to antigen Contraindicated for acute asthma attacks and status asthmaticus	Irritation of throat and trachea Cough Hypersensitivity
Bronkosol	Relaxes bronchial smooth muscles by acting on beta-2-adrenergic receptors	Palpitations Tremors Headache
Bechomethasone (Vanceril)	Synthetic corticosteriod with anti-inflammatory action (used prophylactically; has no immediate benefit in acute asthma crisis)	Hoarseness Oral dryness Weight gain
Methylxanthines: Theophylline Aminophylline	Relaxes bronchial smooth muscles Increases cardiac output Decreases venous pressure Dilates pulmonary vascular bed Improves renal circulation and cerebral stimulation	Epigastric pain and gastric bleeding Nausea and vomiting Headache Palpitations Agitation Seizures Increased alertness

Medication	Effect	Major side effects

Steroids:
  Prednisone
  Prednisolone
  Solu-Cortef
  Hydrocortisone
	Inhibit allergic reactions	Fluid retention
		Weight gain
		Hypertension
		Cushing syndrome
		Gastritis; gastric ulcers
		Adrenal suppression
		Hypokalemia
		Psychosis
		Glucose imbalances

Anticholinergics: Atropine	Reduces bronchial smooth muscle contractions and bronchial mucous secretions	Oral dryness Thirst Loss of taste Nausea and vomiting Arrhythmias Headache

Acute Pulmonary Embolus

An embolus is an undissolved mass that travels in the bloodstream and results in an occlusion of a blood vessel. Pulmonary emboli (PE) can be venous thromboemboli or air, fat, or catheter emboli. A pulmonary embolus is an obstruction of one or more pulmonary arteries by a dislodged thrombus that originated somewhere in the venous system or in the right side of the heart.

It is important to keep in mind two facts in regard to pulmonary embolus: (1) the risk of PE can be reduced if prophylactic measures are initiated; (2) misdiagnosis of PE occurs frequently because of the inherently nonspecific signs and symptoms. It can be mistaken for pulmonary infarction (similar to myocardial infarction), which involves necrosis of lung tissue resulting from disruption of the blood supply. Careful assessment is necessary to discover clear and substantiated evidence of pulmonary embolus.

Thromboembolus

Pulmonary thromboembolism is a common condition that complicates the hospitalization course of many patients. Pulmonary emboli occur 500,000 to 650,000 times annually and cause 50,000 deaths.[51]

Clinical antecedents

The health care team must anticipate and prevent emboli whenever possible and be alert for conditions that increase the likelihood of different types of emboli. Thromboemboli may result from blood stasis, venous wall abnormalities, clotting abnormalities, or irrigation of clotted catheter tips. (Virchow described these contributing factors that predispose the patient to thrombus formation in 1846.) Venostasis remains the leading cause of deep vein thrombosis (DVT). Contributing factors include prolonged bed rest, immobility due to old age or muscular weakness, and obesity. Long intraoperative procedures in which cardiac output is reduced lead to a decrease in limb perfusion. Myocardial infarctions, atrial fibrillation or standstill, severely decreased myocardial contractility, and congestive heart failure also decrease cardiac output. Other patients at risk include those suffering trauma to the pelvis (especially surgical trauma) or lower extremities (especially hip fractures), those with varicose veins, and those who are pregnant, postoperative, or septic from drug abuse complications.

Venous wall abnormalities can result from venous punctures or incisions, trauma, sepsis, major body burns, or atherosclerosis or can occur in those whose professions or work situations require long periods of standing or sitting. Persons suffering injury to the endothelial lining of the blood vessels, which can lead to intravascular clotting, are also at risk.

Factors that change coagulation factors have been under investigation as possible causes of thrombus formation. An increase in PE has been documented during pregnancy and in women who take oral contraceptives. Abrupt discontinuation of anticoagulation therapy has also been documented as increasing the risk of PE. Formation of thrombus is enhanced by hypercoaguability and the release of serotonin. Disorders that cause abnormal blood clotting include thrombocytosis, cancer, and dehydration.

Factors that create risk of air emboli include surgery in the peritoneal cavity, air in intravenous lines, or breakage of a pulmonary artery catheter balloon. Fat emboli can result from long-bone fractures (especially of the tibia or femur), sternal splitting incisions (as in open-heart surgery), the use of pump oxygenation during cardiopulmonary bypass, or trauma to subcutaneous fat. Catheter emboli can occur if a small piece of catheter breaks off and moves through a blood vessel and eventually becomes lodged.

Critical referents

Once a thrombus has formed, it can dislodge and travel via the circulation and become lodged in the pulmonary artery. The thrombus may dislodge spontaneously, although it is more common for a PE to occur as a result of the jarring of a clot from the vessel wall by mechanical forces such as standing suddenly (usually during the first ambulation) or changing the rate of blood flow with a Valsalva maneuver.[52] These situations can usually be prevented by an alert health care team.

The size and location of the embolus determine the physiologic effect. Symptoms will therefore range from none to cardiovascular collapse. Smaller emboli tend to settle in the distal branches of the pulmonary artery at the periphery of the lung. The severity of the event is greater when a large number of small emboli travel to the lungs at the same time or when one large embolus blocks a larger vessel. Small emboli tend to be multiple and recurrent and may continue undiagnosed until they eventually lead to pulmonary embarrassment. The resulting blockage or increased resistance of blood flow has both respiratory and hemodynamic implications.

In the early stages the number of perfused alveoli decreases, thus increasing deadspace and causing "wasted ventilation." Ventilatory deadspace is the result of lack of perfusion of ventilated alveoli. This results in a ventilation-perfusion (V/Q) mismatch. Since no gas exchange can occur, bronchoalveolar hypocarbia (decreased alveolar CO_2) results, causing the bronchial smooth muscle to contract, which leads to bronchoconstriction and shrinking of the alveoli. This constriction leads to an unequal distribution of ventilation, increased airway resistance, and increased work of breathing. Constriction, though, might be considered a protective mechanism, because the amount of wasted ventilation is reduced. The air that is inspired is forced into alveoli that are functioning, rather than into those where diffusion of gases cannot occur. However, the constriction is not enough to correct or normalize the V/Q ratio.[53] As the condition worsens, hypercapnea results. Atelectasis is the end result of bronchoalveolar constriction.

An additional mechanism that leads to alveolar collapse is the reduction of surfactant. The reduction in surfactant levels is possibly due to the effect of decreased blood flow to alveolar cells producing surfactant. Surfactant levels begin to decrease 24 to 48 hours after obstruction of blood flow.

Hemodynamic changes that may result from pulmonary emboli appear to be a function of the extent of impedance to pulmonary blood flow and of the patient's cardiopulmonary status before the event. The primary result of obstruction is an increase in pulmonary vascular resistance, and the right ventricle must maintain enough pressure to force blood through that increased resistance. An increase in pulmonary artery pressure (PAP) will be noted. If the pulmonary hypertension is severe enough, the right ventricle will not be able to override it and will fail. Tachycardia and decreased cardiac output will often be observed clinically. Other signs of right ventricular failure include jugular vein distention (JVD), hepatomegaly, and peripheral edema. A large embolus that obstructs the main pulmonary artery at its bifurcation to the right and left main branches leads to acute cor pulmonale, severe shock, and often sudden death; the progression is illustrated in Figure 2-47. Often the PE is not completely obstructing the pulmonary artery, and the cardiopulmonary changes are not as severe.

Research reports have indicated that the release of serotonin from platelets that surround the embolus may be involved in the constrictive response of the bronchioles and terminal lung units. Other factors that may lead to bronchoconstriction include the release of various chemical mediators such as thromboxanes, prostaglandins, and histamine. These may produce asthma-like symptoms that contribute to an

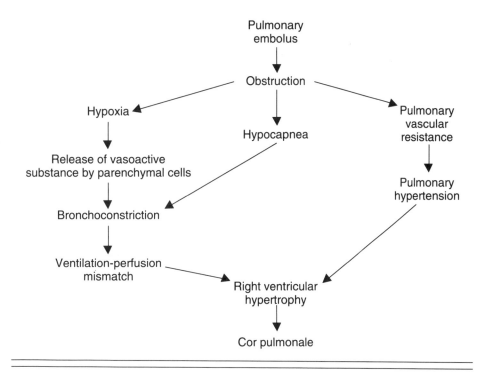

Figure 2-47 Pathophysiology of Pulmonary Embolus Leading to Cor Pulmonale

initial misdiagnosis. Bronchoconstriction necessarily involves the areas that are affected by the embolus and often involves functioning alveoli as well. Perfusion exists with little or no ventilation because of the constriction of alveoli, leading to areas of atelectasis and shunting (which may explain the arterial hypoxemia that is often manifested with PE). Pulmonary hypertension is a second factor that contributes to an increase in shunting. The result is a decrease in diffusion of gases in the lung.

In summary, three main factors lead to ventilation-perfusion mismatching in PE: the deadspace effect on alveoli that are ventilated but not perfused, secondary to the obstruction of the blood flow from the thrombus; shunting of blood past nonventilated alveoli that have collapsed secondary to atelectasis; and the absence of both ventilation and perfusion evidenced in silent units (alveoli that have shut down completely).

A pulmonary embolus is resolved by absorption and fibrosis, and activation of the intrinsic fibrinolytic system may restore pulmonary circulation within hours or days. This process may begin within a few hours after a small episode. Clots may be partly or totally dissolved by the fibrinolytic system.

Pulmonary infarction is another possible end result of PE, but it is uncommon. Usually when an infarct develops, there is an underlying pulmonary disease that has already impaired the pulmonary circulation or increased pulmonary congestion, causing cardiac compromises. Pulmonary infarction is characterized by marked consolidation, usually from hemorrhage, and is often associated with pleuritic pain from pleurisy or effusion. The infarct may undergo necrosis and become infected, resulting in a lung abscess. Healing of the involved lung results in some degree of fibrosis and scar tissue.

Resulting signs and symptoms

The signs and symptoms of PE vary greatly. The embolus may be clinically silent, with no symptoms at all. Because of the vagueness of presenting clinical signs and symptoms, PE may be misdiagnosed. Usually a sudden onset of dyspnea is the most common complaint. This dyspnea may be mild, moderate, severe, or transient in nature and, unless the embolus is severe, may be the only symptom. A severe embolus may produce chest pain. Tachypnea that continues is also suggestive of PE. An increased intensity of the pulmonary S_2 heart sound is found with pulmonary hypertension. Other findings include nonspecific crackles (rales), a slight tempera-

ture elevation, a gallop rhythm, and sometimes signs of phlebitis. A cough, often with hemoptysis, frequently occurs. Pain may be absent, mild, or severe; it may present as pleural pain or a deep, crushing substernal pain that may be confused with that associated with a myocardial infarction. Clinical signs of PE may include splinting of the affected side, cyanosis, distended neck veins, tachycardia with an increased pulmonic sound, and an S_3 or S_4 gallop. Atrial dysrhythmias may also occur. Crackles (rales), wheezing, and decreased breath sounds in the affected areas are frequent clinical findings. Anxiety, apprehension, and restlessness are common responses to hypoxemia. Palpitations and weakness, profuse perspiration, nausea, and vomiting often are seen. If the embolus is massive, cardiovascular collapse may occur, leading to sudden shock, seizures, or cardiopulmonary arrest. Hypotension with peripheral vasoconstriction and cyanosis may be seen.

When a pulmonary infarct has occurred, the symptoms are more specific. Cough, hemoptysis, and pleuritic pain are common. There may be signs of consolidation, pleural effusion, and infection of the infarct. Bronchial breathing, pleural friction rub, and high fever are hallmarks of pulmonary infarct. Infarction is not a usual complication of PE, so these symptoms are rare.

As stated above, the clinical signs and symptoms of PE are frequently subtle, and definitive diagnosis is often difficult. Laboratory tests are usually not specific but are useful to rule out other pulmonary diseases. Leukocytosis is rare (except in infarctions) but may differentiate a diagnosis of pneumonia. Arterial blood gas analysis is useful, especially in cases of massive PE, when hypoxemia, hypocarbia, and respiratory alkalosis occur. In such cases the alveolar-arterial pCO_2 difference is greater than normal because of increased deadspace and compensatory hyperventilation. The presence of an underlying pulmonary disease may complicate the assessment of blood gas reports. Arterial blood gas changes may help to confirm the diagnosis of PE; however, normal ABGs do not rule it out.

Chest x-rays and ECG results are also vague. As with the ABGs, a normal chest x-ray (which is seen frequently) does not exclude the diagnosis of PE. Any abnormalities seen on x-ray, such as elevated diaphragm, atelectasis, or pleural effusion, may be seen in the unaffected patient at any given moment. Subtle changes that may indicate PE include differences in the diameter of vessels that are normally equal in size (one may be blocked and the other may have to accommodate the increase in blood flow); abrupt cessation of a vessel due to obstruction; shadow from an embolus with no distal perfusion;

and diaphragmatic elevation. ECG changes are usually confirmed by the presence of a filling defect or an abrupt cutoff of an artery. Classic ECG changes include a new right axis deviation or right bundle branch block, prominent P waves, and ST elevations that occur diffusely across precordial leads. Finally, small peripheral emboli may not be seen on angiography, but these small emboli, if present, rarely cause symptoms or consequences of embolism worthy of investigation. Venous doppler studies or venograms can confirm the presence of distal thromboses in patients with existing deep vein thromboses; however, such distal thromboses are often not easily noted.

The most commonly used diagnostic study is a ventilation-perfusion (VQ) scan, which can indicate severe VQ mismatch. A positive result on a VQ scan is important and indicates a high probability of PE; however, a negative or a nonspecific result does not always rule out the possibility of PE. In addition, false positive results may arise from ventilation-perfusion mismatches resulting from obstructive lung disease. The most definitive diagnostic exam for pulmonary embolism is the pulmonary angiogram, in which a dye injected into the vena cava is traced as it circulates throughout the lung. Isolated areas of malperfusion related to PE can be detected and embolism can thereby be confirmed. This diagnostic test may also be used to administer thrombolytic agents to treat pulmonary embolism.

Nursing standards of care

Preventive measures must be taken to reduce the likelihood of embolization. First, a careful history must be elicited from each patient, to identify those who may be at risk. Many interventions are suggested by Virchow's observations of contributing factors, including: (1) decreasing venous stasis through the use of antiembolic stockings or sequential compression stockings, which maintain venous flow; (2) assisting the patient with active or passive exercises; (3) elevating the supine patient's legs about 15 degrees to encourage venous flow unless contraindicated and avoiding constant Fowler's position; (4) reducing venous wall trauma by avoiding venous punctures in the legs whenever possible; (5) observing catheter insertion sites for inflammation and phlebitis; (6) protecting I.V. lines from clotting and not irrigating them forcefully if they are clotted; (7) preventing dehydration to maintain normal coaguability; (8) routinely administering low-dose heparin as ordered. (A preventive dose of heparin has proven effective in the prevention of PE, especially in the patient undergoing major surgical procedures who is over 40 years of age.[54])

Supportive therapy is necessary for adequate cardiopulmonary functioning. Oxygen administered by cannula, face mask, or endotracheal tube may be necessary for adequate oxygenation. The use of inotropic and pressor drugs may be necessary to maintain cardiac output. However, the patient is often severely vasoconstricted and may be unresponsive to catecholamines. Sympathomimetics may also exacerbate the tachycardia; hence, alpha-adrenergic agonists such as phenylephrine may be preferred. Volume-loading agents such as Dextran 40 or 70 may be used to increase pulmonary blood flow to unperfused segments. (If flow is increased and more evenly distributed, arterial saturation will improve.) A secondary benefit of Dextran is its anticoagulant properties.

Should an embolus be confirmed, treatment will have three main objectives: anticoagulation to prevent further thrombosis, direct clot lysis when indicated, and cardiopulmonary supportive therapy. Continuous intravenous heparin remains the drug of choice for anticoagulant therapy. A baseline coagulation profile must be done before therapy is initiated. Usually an initial loading dose of 2000–5000 U of heparin is administered, followed by 800–1200 U per hour in order to maintain adequate anticoagulation. Anticoagulant levels should be determined on a periodic basis (usually twice a day initially and then once a day). The Lee-White clotting time should remain about 2 to 2½ times normal. The partial thromboplastin time (PTT) should also be elevated to 2 to 2½ times normal.

Heparin therapy should continue for 7 to 10 days. There are other factors to consider, however. When the patient is ready to ambulate, the extent of the venostasis and the preexisting condition should be considered before heparin therapy is discontinued. As long as the patient is on extended bedrest (a major risk factor), therapy should be continued. The transition to oral anticoagulants can be made as soon as the patient is moving about. Prothrombin time (PT) is used to determine the amount of warfarin required to maintain anticoagulation. Heparin should be maintained until a therapeutic PT is achieved. The length and course of anticoagulant therapy are dependent on the number of risk factors that originally predisposed the patient to thrombosis.

Streptokinase and urokinase are used as thrombolytic agents in cases of massive PE with hemodynamic consequences. These substances are especially indicated for use in the case of massive PE in a patient for whom surgical intervention is contraindicated. Studies of these drugs have shown that they reduce the size of the obstruction earlier and provide a more rapid restoration of hemodynamic properties than heparin alone. But no formal evidence regarding morbidity or mortality improvements with the use of either of these thrombolytics exists. Streptokinase, a protein of hemolytic streptococci, is thought to activate plasminogen, a fibrinolytic enzyme precursor. The effect of this drug can be seen 24 hours after administration. The patient must be observed for adverse reactions, including allergic reactions, bleeding, and a low-grade fever. Urokinase, also an activator of plasminogen, is an enzyme found in human urine. The maximum effect of urokinase can be observed within 12 to 24 hours of administration of the enzyme. Streptokinase and urokinase therapy should be followed by heparin and/or warfarin therapy in order to prevent further thrombosis.

Even though great advances have been made in pharmacological treatment modes, surgery may be indicated for the patient suffering massive PE (50% obstruction) or repeated pulmonary emboli. The patient who does not respond to the more conservative pharmacological therapy or who has life-threatening complications (or in whom anticoagulation therapy is contraindicated) may require surgery. Primary surgery, a pulmonary embolectomy, is rather risky, for it requires location of the embolus by pulmonary angiography and the use of cardiopulmonary bypass with all of its potential complications. The other surgical procedure, the use of the intracaval "umbrella" or "filter," also involves risk, for the devices cause progressive obstruction of the vena cava as they trap dislodged clots, and endothelial irritation can be produced at the insertion site. This procedure is less involved than pulmonary embolectomy, however, and may be performed under local anesthesia. A reduced mortality rate in patients treated by this procedure has been documented. Recently the use of the Greenfield filter (very similar to the intracaval "umbrella") has become the surgical intervention of choice because of a low incidence of vena cava obstruction.[55] After insertion of an umbrella or filter the patient requires long-term anticoagulation therapy, and constant monitoring for filter occlusion in the form of superior or inferior vena cava syndrome is necessary.

The main emphasis in the treatment of PE should be on prevention, however, especially of deep vein thrombosis. The literature suggests that low-dose heparin therapy is the best prophylactic measure for the patient at risk. Studies have also been conducted to evaluate the use of aspirin, dyparimadole, warfarin, and Dextran 40 or 70; but the heparin regimen has resulted in fewer bleeding problems and no problems relating to clotting time or PTT.

Nonpharmacologic treatments such as early ambulation, elastic stockings, and elevation of the legs have not been proven to significantly reduce the risk of deep vein thrombosis, especially in the patient most at risk. The nurse is clearly the member of the health team who will be in the best position to ascertain the presence of risk and to implement preventive measures specific to the needs of the patient. The care plan at the end of this section outlines what must be done for patients with pulmonary embolism.

Fat Embolus

Fat emboli occur more often than they are actually seen clinically. The embolization is often not accompanied by clinical symptoms, and the disorder is not ascertained until it is found on autopsy, when the patient is found to have had multiple fat deposits throughout the body, especially in the cerebral and pulmonary circulation.

Clinical antecedents

A fat embolism arises from the microembolization of fat, which creates obstruction of blood flow and an inflammatory reaction around the vessels affected. Fat embolism manifests itself 12 to 24 hours after such injuries as long-bone fractures or major soft-tissue trauma, which are the leading causes of this problem. Sometimes embolization occurs after osteomyelitis, cardiopulmonary bypass, burns, poisonings, pancreatitis, and renal transplant. Up to 5% of all those who suffer major orthopedic trauma develop a fat embolism.[56] Usually the large emboli become lodged in the pulmonary vasculature, but smaller emboli circulate to other parts of the body.

Two precipitating events lead to the formation of fat emboli: (1) intramedullary adipose tissue, disrupted by the pathological process that occurs when long bones fracture, enters the venous circulation, and (2) circulating cyclomicrons clump together into fat droplets as a response to intravascular biochemical changes occurring with trauma. The adipose tissue or the fat droplets then circulate until they become lodged in organ vasculature.[57]

Critical referents

Fat emboli are drawn from the originating tissue into the venous circulation because of a pressure gradient. The fat globules are made up of neutral (saturated) fat and fatty acids (unsaturated). Fat emboli circulate in the pulmonary vasculature and can travel as far as the brain, heart, kidney, skin, posterior pituitary, or eye. Systemic fat emboli can be broken down into liquid form and often cause partial or temporary obstruction of vessels. It is thought that as emboli enter the capillaries they break into smaller particles. The smaller emboli continue to circulate through the system and lungs until they eventually become small enough to be removed by phagocytosis. As the fat is broken down by lipases in the plasma and macrophages, fatty acids, which cause an inflammatory reaction, are released.

Fat emboli lodging in the smaller arteries of the gray matter of the brain may cause infarcts, which may or may not be hemorrhagic. In contrast, fat emboli in the heart may be a product of fatty degeneration, and resulting symptoms, if present, are mild and reversible. If fat emboli travel to the kidneys, petechiae can result but have not been linked to tubular necrosis or renal failure. Fat emboli have been known to occur in the retinal vessels and can cause blind spots in the eyes, but these resolve with few lasting effects. In these cases petechiae also appear in the conjunctiva of the eyelids. Skin rash, especially on the anterior chest, neck, and axillary folds, is a strong indication of fat emboli, especially if it appears in conjunction with increased deadspace, right ventricular failure, or decreased cardiac output.

Fat deposits in the lungs can lodge in the smaller arteries and arterioles until pulmonary arterial pressures escalate enough to cause cor pulmonale. At the same time, free fatty acids formed by lipases breaking down the fat droplets cause a capillary leak in the pulmonary bed. Thrombocytopenia (causing petechiae) occurs as a complication of platelet aggregation. Finally, arterial hypoxemia is almost always present.

Resulting signs and symptoms

Most cases of fat emboli are asymptomatic and remain undiagnosed. However, severe fat emboli may develop quickly and cause death if left unchecked. Emboli reach the lung within minutes, and early signs of hypoxemia may be seen. Classic symptoms can develop within hours or up to 4 days after the injury, although the latter is rare. Most symptoms develop before the third day after a traumatic insult. In addition to mild hypoxemia, there may be subtle mental changes (confusion) within the first 24 hours. Respiratory distress, changes in behavior, a slight disorientation, and increases in pulse and temperature serve as early warning signs of fat em-

boli. In partial embolization the cerebral and pulmonary symptoms and skin rash may be absent. Once manifested, these symptoms usually disappear in a week with adequate treatment.

The more severely affected patient will show signs of severe respiratory compromise similar to ARDS. A petechial rash usually appears within 24 hours. Cerebral effects can lead to coma and death, probably as a result of brainstem infarction. Other less severe clinical findings include fat in the sputum (due to leakage in the alveoli), lipuria, decreased hematocrit readings (because of trapping of red blood cells), thrombocytopenia, and possibly ECG changes such as right-axis deviation and ventricular strain. An elevated serum lipase level may appear about the third day after the injury, and may be a guide to prognosis. Chext x-ray is usually normal initially, but when the syndrome is full-blown, noncardiac pulmonary edema is present. Before pulmonary edema develops, the x-ray may show an elevated diaphragm due to pneumoconstriction, decreased or absent vascular markings, or dilation of the main pulmonary artery and right ventricle. Pulmonary angiography may show a filling defect due to an embolus or a cutoff due to a complete occlusion. Ventilation-perfusion scans will define an area of normal ventilation with decreased or absent perfusion if a fat embolus is present.[58] ABG results show low pO_2 and pCO_2 levels.

Nursing standards of care

The prevention of fat emboli should be of primary concern upon admission of a patient suffering a long-bone fracture or trauma or undergoing surgery. The fracture should be splinted as soon as possible with particular care to avoid over-manipulation. The use of pneumatic tourniquets during surgery on long bones has been shown to decrease the possibility of fat reaching the lungs. (The tourniquets should not be removed until the bone has been stabilized in a splint.) The use of oxygen to correct any hypoxemia is clearly indicated, and it is thought that the use of oxygen therapy may inhibit the passage of the emboli through the lungs. In cases of severe respiratory compromise, the use of mechanical ventilation with PEEP may be indicated.

The prophylactic use of heparin, dextran, and steroids has been advocated, but conflicting reports on all of these drugs exist, and further study is indicated. Corticosteroids, however, have proven effective in reducing incidence of fat embolism if administered to the high-risk patient within 12 hours of trauma.[59] Lipolytic drugs are contraindicated because their use may dissolve larger fat globules into smaller ones and increase circulation of the particles through the lungs. (They may also be harmful because of the local inflammatory reaction they cause; it has been suggested that glucose and insulin be used to counteract this reaction.[60])

If shock occurs and embolectomy is necessary, the patient is placed on cardiopulmonary bypass while the pulmonary artery is incised and the embolus removed. The workload of the right ventricle must be reduced as much as possible; thus the patient should rest. Emotional stress should be prevented by placing the patient in a quiet and calm atmosphere; analgesics should be administered to control pain and relieve anxiety.

Nursing care of any patient who has suffered trauma or fracture of any long bone includes recognition of any subtle changes relating to respiratory or neurological status. The baseline admission should include a good neurological and respiratory assessment, including arterial blood gases. The nurse should be aware of any slight change in these measurements and suspect a fat embolism in the patient who has experienced significant trauma.

Chest pain should be relieved by administering analgesics as necessary, providing supplemental oxygen, and encouraging relaxation. In the event of a ventilation-perfusion mismatch and resulting poor gas exchange, the nurse should watch for signs of progressive hypoxemia and hypocapnia or hypercapnia. Bedrest is mandatory for the patient, and the head of the bed should be elevated. The patient should be given assistance with activities that may increase dyspnea. The care plan at the end of this section delineates what must be done for the patient with fat embolism.

Air Embolus

Under certain conditions entrance of air into the circulatory system can result in the same pathological changes found when the embolus is solid. A 100 cc dose of air is lethal. Even though this is a large amount, smaller amounts can occlude small vessels if introduced into the system rapidly. Lesser amounts of air can also lead to frothing in the circulatory system.

Clinical antecedents

Air that enters the bloodstream does so primarily through the venous system because venous pressure can reach levels below atmospheric pressure. Other conditions or practices that can lead to air emboli include air bubbles in intravenous infusion, tubal insufflation, pneumoperitoneum, uterine douches, hemodialysis, surgeries of the neck, neurosurgical procedures, open-heart surgery, retroperitoneal air injection, irrigation of nasal sinuses, chest trauma, and rapid decompression.

Critical referents

The role of subatmospheric pressure in the development of air embolus was mentioned above. If the venous system is open to the atmosphere, air enters the circulation; thus there is a risk of air embolus during neurosurgical procedures performed with the patient in the sitting position, surgery of the neck, and venous catheterization. Any portion of the venous system that is above the level of the heart is under subatmospheric pressure, and risk of air embolus is present if the venous circulation is interrupted. Additionally, if the surgery involves the major venous sinuses of the brain, risk is increased, because sinus walls are rigid and do not collapse when opened, thus allowing large amounts of air to rush in. Use of ultrasonic doppler neurosurgical procedures assists in the detection of an air embolus. With the transducer at the level of the right atrium, minute bubbles of air can be identified.

An air embolus may develop after cardiac surgery if air has been trapped in the right or left side of the heart during the surgical procedure. Air in the left side of the heart can cause the serious problem of myocardial ischemia as well as presenting the possibility of the passage of air through the aorta and into the cerebral circulation. Air must be withdrawn from the heart before a cardiopulmonary bypass is terminated.

Air embolism following the insertion of a central venous pressure (CVP) line occurs most often because of an opening in the catheter system, usually through a disconnected or open line. The tip of the catheter is placed in the superior vena cava or right atrium, which is subatmospheric during inspiration. When part of the system is open to the atmosphere, air rushes in during inspiration. Catheters placed in the veins of the neck may also cause development of air embolus because of the negative venous pressure when the head is in the upright position.

An increase in air pressure can also cause an air embolism. Chest trauma, tubal insufflation, and pneumoperitoneum can allow air to enter the venous system as a result of an increase in air pressure relative to venous pressure. In the case of chest trauma, lung damage may result when communication is established between the venous system and the bronchi. Forced expiration or mechanical ventilation can also force air into the open venous system, which will result in air embolus. Tension pneumothorax may produce a similar situation.

Gas embolus is similar to air embolus but is mainly experienced by underwater divers and people exposed to increased atmospheric pressure. With high atmospheric pressure, increased hydrogen, oxygen, and nitrogen become dissolved in the blood. If the person is placed in a lower atmospheric pressure too rapidly, these gases come out of solution. The hydrogen and oxygen are reabsorbed, but the nitrogen remains out of solution. Atoms of nitrogen join together, forming large nitrogen bubbles, which may obstruct the vascular tree. There may be activation of the clotting mechanism downstream of the bubbles and a loss of plasma volume, which results in hemoconcentration because of transcapillary leakage of plasma fluid. Placing the patient in a hyperbaric chamber for treatments forces the nitrogen back into solution.

Resulting signs and symptoms

As mentioned, the most common method for air to enter the venous system is via an intravenous infusion line. Air may enter either slowly or rapidly. Signs and symptoms will vary with the amount of air and the speed at which it is pulled into the venous system. A slow infusion of air will result in decreased peripheral resistance, and any physiological changes that are seen are the result of pulmonary vasculature compromises. Rapid infusions cause total pulmonary artery obstruction and circulatory collapse.

ECG changes in a patient with an air embolus include a peaked P wave and, later, ST depression. Once cardiovascular problems have developed, a churning sound will be heard on auscultation of the right ventricle; the sound is strong confirmation of an air embolism in the ventricle. Central venous pressure rises gradually during a slow infusion of air, and pulmonary artery pressure increases as well. The blood pressure decreases, and the pulse rate increases. Signs of shock are seen as peripheral resistance decreases. With a large bolus of air, cardiovascular collapse occurs because of an air lock in the right ventricle. The rise in pulmonary artery pressure is not usually evident in such cases because severe circulatory collapse can occur in sections, and thus the air embolus is not pumped into the pulmonary artery.

Nursing standards of care

Effects of an air embolus can be fatal in minutes. Complete resuscitation should be started immediately. The patient with an air embolus should be placed with the head down and on the left side; otherwise any embolus in the right heart remains there. (Air bubbles will float to the right atrium and away from the pulmonary artery.) In the case of a large bolus of air, inflow to the right heart may also be obstructed, so such positioning of the patient may not prove effective. Intracardiac aspiration of the air may be accomplished by way of a subclavian or central line advanced to the right atrium. The success of this maneuver depends on early detection of the air embolus and prompt aspiration and intervention.

The following care plan details nursing care and interventions for acute pulmonary embolus.

Nursing Care Plan for the Management of the Patient with Acute Pulmonary Embolus

Diagnosis	Signs and symptoms	Intervention	Rationale
Alteration in respiratory function: hypoxemia	In the appropriate clinical context and with no other reason: $PaO_2 < 5(FIO_2)$; $PaO_2 <$ predicted for patient's age; $PaO_2 = 110 - \frac{1}{2}$ of patient's age; $PaO_2 < 75$ mm Hg on room air; $SaO_2 < 90\%$	Monitor ABGs frequently	To ascertain the presence of hypoxemia for appropriate choice of intervention
		Oxygen and ventilatory support as needed	To correct hypoxemia
	Increased work of breathing: increased respiratory rate; increased tidal volume	Monitor respiratory rate and tidal volume	To assess cardiopulmonary stress
		Place in semi- or high Fowler's position as indicated	To allow easiest breathing and full diaphragmatic descension
	Increased myocardial work: increased cardiac output; changes in BP; decreased level of consciousness; decreased capillary refill; cold and clammy skin; decreased urinary output	Assist with basic care regime	To conserve energy and prevent increases in cardiac oxygen demand
		Closely monitor VS and ECG and check for chest pain	Indications of ischemic damage and cardiac compromise
		Maintain patency of IV lines	To allow fast access in case of an emergency
		Avoid activity for half-hour after meal	To prevent further oxygen demand when blood is shunted to GI tract during digestion
	$PaCO_2$ 35–45 mm Hg or less	Assess closely for orthostatic hypotension	To prevent injury in the event of syncope associated with orthostatic hypotension
	Increased minute ventilation		
Potential for alteration in gas exchange related to ventilation-perfusion mismatch and shunting from pulmonary emboli	Dyspnea	Monitor ABGs closely	Problems with oxygenation are commonly seen
	Decreased O_2 levels on ABGs		
	Fluid overload	Assist patient to position of comfort: semi- or high Fowler's position is best	To improve breathing patterns and lower diaphragm

Diagnosis	Signs and symptoms	Intervention	Rationale
		Assess for crackles (rales), S_3, and JVD every 4 hours and as needed	Signs of respiratory failure with resultant heart failure
		Administer oxygen as ordered	To counter problems with oxygenation leading to hypoxemia
		Monitor rhythm	Tachycardia is commonly seen
		Review chest x-ray for signs of increasing pulmonary thromboembolism and cor pulmonale	Note that signs of pulmonary congestion can be clinically delayed up to 24 hours
	Changes in mental status	Monitor level of consciousness	Decreased level of consciousness may be first sign of anoxia
		Administer IV fluids and/or vasopressor as ordered	To increase BP when patient is hypotensive and to preserve right ventricular filling pressure
		Treat for heart failure if present	To maintain perfusion to lungs
		Provide rest between treatments	To decrease oxygen demand
		Turn patient every 2 hours as tolerated	To minimize ventilation-perfusion shunting effects
Potential for alteration in cardiopulmonary, cerebral, renal, and peripheral tissue perfusion related to emboli	Signs of altered cerebral perfusion: mental confusion; dizziness; syncope; convulsions and/or seizures; TIA; yawning	Rule out nonpulmonary causes of altered cerebral perfusion	To ascertain the need for interventions not relating to the pulmonary system and choose appropriate intervention according to underlying disorder
	Signs of altered cardiopulmonary perfusion: angina and ischemic changes	Monitor for chest pain	
	Signs of altered renal perfusion: oliguria and anuria	Check urine output every 8 hours or every hour if oliguria occurs	To assess kidney function

Nursing Care Plan for the Management of the Patient with Acute Pulmonary Embolus

Diagnosis	Signs and symptoms	Intervention	Rationale
	Signs of altered peripheral perfusion: hypotension; cyanosis; distant or absent peripheral pulses	Monitor BUN, creatinine, and K^+	Respiratory failure may eventually cause decrease in cardiac output to periphery from hypoxemia and related dysrhythmias
Tissue hypoxia	Tachycardia Tachypnea Hyperventilation Dyspnea Cyanosis Hypertension Restlessness Confusion/disorientation Early alkalosis leading to late respiratory acidosis Early alveolar hyperventilation leading to late severe alveolar hypoventilation Hypoxemia	Monitor ABGs closely	To assess alveolar ventilation
		Monitor Ve	To assess total ventilation to provide an index of work of breathing affecting cardiopulmonary stress
		Monitor for signs of cardiovascular and cardiopulmonary work	To determine acid-base balance and need for O_2 since there is no direct test for tissue hypoxia (can only evaluate hypoxemia)
		Emergent administration of increased FIO_2	To normalize PaO_2; to improve alveolar oxygen tension; to decrease work of breathing and myocardial work
		Use appropriate O_2 device	To maintain PaO_2 to prevent complications of hyperoxia; oxygen system should deliver flow ($4 \times$ Ve) to maintain desired FIO_2, prevent room air leakage into system, maintain adequate PaO_2 to at least level of inspired FIO_2, and reduce work of breathing
		Monitor oxygenation	Pulse oximetry should show O_2 sat. $> 90\%$

Diagnosis	Signs and symptoms	Intervention	Rationale
Ineffective breathing pattern due to shunting effect of pulmonary embolus and thoracic pain	Radiographic atelectasis Increased work of breathing: 　tachypnea and 　　decreased V_T Increased Ve Decreased VC Exertional dyspnea Decreased activity levels Hypoxemia Hypoxia Atelectic crackles (rales) Decreased bibasilar breath sounds Decreased chest movement	Monitor respirations and V_T; measure VC, Ve, and ABGs	Reflect adequacy of breathing pattern; prognostic if $V_T < 1000$ cc or if patient is unable to sustain spontaneous ventilation; to follow improvement/deterioration of patient
		Incentive spirometry every hour IC should be 3–4 times predicted V_T with 10–15 second inspiratory hold (sustained maximal inhalation)	To promote improved lung function; to prevent atelectasis; to increase FRC; to decrease work of breathing; to improve inspiratory muscle tone
		Monitor x-rays	To assess lung volumes; diffuse bilateral or localized interstitial patterns with increased vascular shadows leading to decreased $PaCO_2$ and PaO_2; changing left ventricle size; worsening hypoxia, pulmonary hypertension; alveolar edema and/or progression to fibrosis; severe hypoxemia with 100% O_2
		Supplemental oxygenation as indicated	To provide adequate oxygenation in the face of inefficient breathing effort and shunting
		Administer diuretics as ordered	To overcome fluid overload in event of congestive failure and pulmonary hypertension
		Administer thrombolytics as ordered	To dissolve emboli in lungs, decreasing deadspace and shunting to allow effective gas exchange

Nursing Care Plan for the Management of the Patient with Acute Pulmonary Embolus

Diagnosis	Signs and symptoms	Intervention	Rationale
Ineffective cough effort related to thoracic pain from pulmonary embolus	Weak cough effort Complaints of pain on inspiration and coughing Ineffective, nonproductive cough effort Pulmonary congestion	Medicate for pain a half-hour prior to respiratory treatments and coughing and deep breathing exercises; monitor for possible side effects such as lethargy or decreased respiratory status	To allow for maximal benefit from treatment and full chest expansion (medications for pain are counterproductive if found to further depress respiratory effort)
		Place patient in position of comfort to allow for adequate lung expansion and aeration	Patient will "guard" affected area and not fully expand chest on breathing or coughing if in pain
		Encourage use of pillow, blanket, or roll to splint chest when coughing	To support chest wall when coughing to decrease discomfort (even more important if patient has incisions or tubes near the affected area)
Potential for infection related to pulmonary embolus, indwelling lines, and Foley catheter	Elevated temperature	Encourage coughing and deep breathing; turn patient in bed every 2 hours while on bedrest	Help to prevent atelectasis, blood clots in legs, and pressure sores
		Change respiratory tubing every 24 hours	Per CDC specifications
		Increase activity as soon as indicated	To promote healing
		Monitor temperature every 4 hours	Sign of infection
	Increased WBCs	Assess WBC count	Sign of infection
		Maintain strict aseptic technique with invasive lines and indwelling catheters; change lines unless contraindicated: PAP every 72 hours, arterial	Per CDC recommendation

Diagnosis	Signs and symptoms	Intervention	Rationale
		lines every 7 days, tubing every 48 hours, IV bags every 24 hours; provide Foley care every 8 hours	
		Assist in identifying source of infection: collect cultures; note atelectasis on chest x-ray; note sputum and urine characteristics; check insertion site for redness every 8 hours	Sites at risk of infection must be kept clean with aseptic technique; appropriate antibiotic therapy must be chosen
		Administer antibiotics as ordered	To combat infectious process
Potential for bleeding related to anticoagulant therapy	Bleeding from venipuncture insertion sites	Minimize intramuscular injections	To avoid possible bleeding into muscle or hematoma formation
	Black stools	If venipuncture is necessary, place pressure over site for 10 minutes	To prevent bruising and sloughing of tissue
	GI distress and bleeding		
	Bleeding gums	Screen stools, emesis, and NG drainage for occult blood every 4 hours and PRN	To monitor for internal bleeding and presence of ulcer
		Screen urine for RBC every 4 hours and PRN	To monitor for internal bleeding and kidney damage
		Administer antacid as prescribed	To protect from possible stress ulcer
		If patient is at high risk for ulcer, measure abdominal girth every shift	To assess for internal bleeding
		Teach patient not to brush teeth and gums vigorously	To prevent gum damage and bleeding
		Prohibit prolonged sitting or crossing of legs and use antiembolic stockings as indicated	To prevent further risk of thrombus formation

Nursing Care Plan for the Management of the Patient with Acute Pulmonary Embolus

Diagnosis	Signs and symptoms	Intervention	Rationale
		Monitor signs of overanticoagulation: bleeding gums, nosebleeds, bruising, hematuria, black stools	To identify early signs of overanticoagulation to prevent possible complications of bleeding/hemorrhage
Decreased tolerance of activity related to dyspnea	Dyspnea on exertion Fatigue Exaggerated increase in heart rate and BP on exertion	Assess level of activity tolerance (should be related to the New York Heart Association's classification for consistency)	Provides a baseline
		Assist patient to change position every 2 hours while on bedrest	To decrease risk of complications and promote venous return
		Check BP with patient in horizontal, sitting, and standing positions	To monitor for orthostatic hypotension
		Avoid activity for a half-hour to an hour after meals	May decrease chance of hypoxia due to increased blood flow to GI tract
		Monitor heart rate and BP with activity increases	To maintain heart rate within 10 bpm of resting heart rate and maintain systolic BP within 20 mm Hg of resting BP; if a drop occurs, it may indicate a drop in cardiac output
		Anticipate institution of progressive rehab	To provide controlled mechanism for increasing activity
		Encourage frequent rest periods	To prevent excessive fatigue

178

Diagnosis	Signs and symptoms	Intervention	Rationale
Altered nutritional status due to: anorexia and malaise; increased nutritional requirements resulting from stress of illness; less appealing taste of food related to low sodium content and changes in oral mucosa; changes in bowel routine; increased work of breathing	Too fatigued to eat	Auscultate bowel sounds	To evaluate GI peristalsis
	Too short of breath to eat	Help patient to eat slowly; use supplemental O_2 as needed	To facilitate nutritional intake
	Inadequate intake of food and fluids	Monitor I&O	To assess fluid balance
		Calculate calorie requirements	Calorie requirements may increase 200% in ARF
	Decreased albumin and lymphocytes	Monitor albumin and lymphocytes	To assess visceral proteins
	Decreasing body weight	Monitor weight	To monitor effect of diuretic therapy
	Complaints of lack of appetite	With patient, family, and dietary staff, assess appetite and food preferences and review what is allowed and what is best for optimal nutrition; provide preferred food as much as possible	To facilitate nutritional intake and status in any way possible

Medications Commonly Used in the Care of the Patient with Acute Pulmonary Embolus

Medication	Effect	Major side effects
Heparin	Anticoagulant; binds with antithrombin III and lipoproteins; a naturally occurring component of plasma (which maintains the intravascular fluidity of blood)	Hemorrhage Hematuria Epitaxis Ecchymosis Bleeding gums Tarry stools
Oral anticoagulants: Warfarin Dicumarol	Prothrombin depression and depression of hepatic synthesis of factors II, VII, IX, and X, which compete with vitamin K function of clotting	Bleeding complications (as above) Diarrhea Congenital malformations in fetus
Plasma substitutes: Dextran 70 Dextran 40	Glucose polymer used to expand plasma volume and maintain blood pressure in the event of shock; interferes with normal clotting by coating platelets; restores flow to microcirculation; improves tissue perfusion by reducing blood viscosity	Increased clotting time Fluid volume overload Renal complications
Thrombolytics (fibrinolytics): Streptokinase Urokinase	Dissolves clots by way of the endogenous fibrinolytic system, which converts plasminogen to plasmin, which digests fibrin threads and fibrinogen; all of the above lyse the clot; fibrinolytic enzymes dissolve thrombi (urokinase is nonantigenic, streptokinase is not)	Bleeding complications (as above) Tachycardia Joint pain Anaphylactic reaction (streptokinase) Fever and chills
Morphine sulfate	Analgesia/sedation Peripheral vasodilation Decreased systemic venous return Bronchodilation Relief of congestive dyspnea	Hypotension Respiratory depression Nausea and vomiting Constipation Urine retention

Medication	Effect	Major side effects
Digitalis	Increased contractility Lengthened refractory period of AV node; decreased left ventricular end diastolic pressure; increased ventricular automaticity	Tachycardia AV blocks, bradycardia GI upset Headache Drowsiness Confusion Double vision
Diuretics	Diuresis Decreased pulmonary congestion	Hypokalemia Hypocalcemia Hypomagnesemia Altered glucose metabolism

Thoracic Trauma

Thoracic trauma includes injuries to the chest wall, lung parenchyma and airways, and aorta and heart. Injuries to the chest wall can include simple rib fractures, multiple rib fractures (flail chest), hemothorax, penetrating wounds, pulmonary hemorrhage, and pneumothorax (to be discussed later in the chapter). Trauma to the lung parenchyma and airways include pulmonary hematoma and contusion, compression injury, shock lung, and tracheobronchial injury. Finally, direct injury to the heart or aorta can occur, and information regarding this type of injury is presented in the chapter on the cardiovascular system. Blunt trauma comprise 90% of all thoracic injuries and generally take the form of pneumothorax, hemothorax, or chest wall injuries.

Clinical antecedents

Most chest trauma (about 60%) occurs as a result of motor vehicle accidents, and the driver is usually injured more seriously than passengers because of the steering wheel. (The dashboard rarely causes injury to the chest area.) Other causes of chest trauma include work-related accidents, home falls and other accidents, sports accidents, assault, and suicide attempts. Men are injured more often than women, and most of the injured males are in their twenties.

Simple Rib Fractures

Simple rib fracture is diagnosed when the rib is fractured and all possibility of intrathoracic injury has been ruled out. Most simple rib fractures occur from some type of blow—usually in younger adults in catastrophe, but the elderly become more at risk for simple rib fracture when the rib cage loses compressibility due to bone brittleness.

Critical referents

There are two types of simple rib fractures: those that result from a direct injury, which causes a fracture directly adjacent and interior to the point of impact (known as "en dedans") from overflexion; and those that result from an indirect injury, which occurs from an anteroposterior compressive blow that causes rib fracture on the outer rib curve away

from the site of injury ("en dehors"). The two types are illustrated in Figure 2-48.

Resulting signs and symptoms

Whether the fracture is en dedans or en dehors serves as indication of what type of injury to expect, if any: with the former, lung parenchyma injury can be anticipated, and with the latter, the mediastinum may be damaged. Even in the absence of internal injury or flail chest, simple rib fractures almost always affect ventilation, for they are extremely painful. Because of the pain, the patient restricts chest movement when breathing and suppresses any cough, thus increasing the risk of accumulation of bronchial secretions leading to atelectasis and even bronchopneumonia.

Nursing standards of care

Intervention is aimed at eliminating the pain in order to preserve respiratory function. Mild to strong analgesia may be needed, and if this does not provide pain relief, Lidocaine or other anesthetic agents may be injected. Immobilization of the ribs by taping or binders assists the patient in deep breathing and coughing. The most drastic measure taken is to perform an intercostal nerve block for relief of pain; this approach has proven to be more effective and longer acting than anesthetic injection.

Multiple Fractured Ribs (Flail Chest)

Flail chest consists of multiple rib fractures that cause the chest wall to become unstable during inspiration and expiration. The sternum may also be fractured.

Critical referents

External blows to different areas of the chest wall can cause flail chest. The syndrome can manifest itself differently and different tissues and regions of the lung can be affected in different ways, depending on the direction of the blow relative to the body.

Anterior flail chest can involve ribs 2 through 6. The false ribs are usually not affected, for they are supple and pliable enough not to break unless they

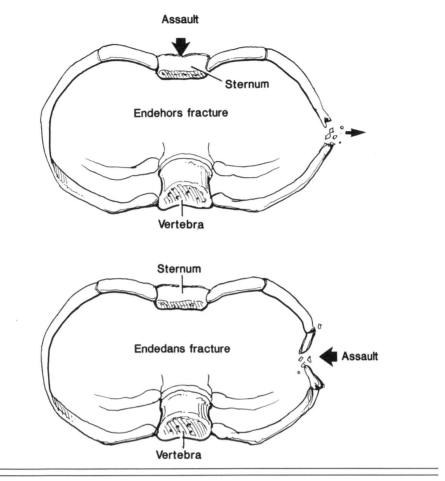

Figure 2-48 Simple Rib Fractures

receive a significant assault. Because ribs 2 through 6 are involved, injury to the pleural cavities accompanies anterior flail chest. Significant paradoxical movement of the chest on breathing is noted: during inspiration the affected region is sucked inward, and during expiration it bulges outward. Prognosis can be poor in such instances because of the serious injury to the pleural cavities.

Lateral flail chest occurs only in the region of external impact. Multifocal fractures usually are found on each rib, thus respiratory chest movement and gas exchange are severely impaired. There is an even more significant risk of mortality if the chest is involved bilaterally, causing the "soft thorax" syndrome.

Posterior flail chest, seen very rarely, involves the dorsal side of the chest. Paradoxical breathing motion may not be evident with this type of flail chest, for the fractured ribs are held in place by the dorsal muscles. Also, when the patient is positioned supinely, little extra movement of posterior regions of the lung are allowed.

Resulting signs and symptoms

In addition to the paradoxical breathing movements involved in the three types of flail chest, other signs and symptoms directly reflect the other tissues that are injured (for example, the myocardium or lung parenchyma). Because flail chest prevents the appropriate chest wall movement for the bellows motion of breathing, inadequate ventilation and all its complications result. Air will cease to move in and out of the trachea and will only move back and forth within the chest. In the severely injured patient, flail chest is fatal. In less severe cases, bronchial secretions are not coughed up, atelectasis develops, hemoptysis can occur, and hypoxia and hypercapnia are almost always present. The patient will try to compensate by breathing more rapidly and shallowly, will appear cyanotic, and will be tachycardic.

The interruption of the normal chest wall allows a considerable reversal of intrathoracic negative pressure. Pneumothorax and cardiopulmonary collapse may develop in a very short time if the patient is not supported immediately. Later, if the patient survives, the risk of hemothorax and tension pneumothorax is great. If the myocardium is damaged (contusions or lacerations) as well, ECG readings will reflect mild to severe ischemic changes in the areas affected. ABG results will reflect hypercapnia and hypoxia.

Nursing standards of care

Basic life support must be provided. Rigid or semirigid supports should be placed around the chest as a temporary measure until internal stabilization of the chest wall by intubation and mechanical ventilation with PEEP is accomplished. The patient should also be paralyzed and sedated as needed to prevent extra movements accompanying the work of breathing and to allow for maximal effectiveness of the mechanical ventilator. Chest tubes may be indicated. The patient will require long-term critical care, for mechanical ventilation will be necessary for at least two or three weeks in order to allow time for the fractured ribs and lung parenchyma to begin to heal. Surgical thoracotomy may also be indicated to repair damage to operable sites in the lung. More detail regarding nursing interventions is provided in the accompanying nursing care plan.

Hemothorax

Simply defined, a hemothorax is the collapse of a lung from an accumulation of blood in the pleural space. It commonly occurs as a result of either blunt or penetrating trauma and may occur alone or in combination with pneumothorax. The severity of this condition ranges from negligible to life-threatening. The most common precipitating factor for hemothorax is blunt or penetrating trauma to the chest or upper abdomen. Rib fractures and injury to the pulmonary parenchyma or thoracic aorta account for over 50% of the incidence of symptomatic hemothoraxes.[61] The great vessels may also be torn from the aortic arch, particularly in acceleration/deceleration injuries. Common sources of bleeding are summarized in Table 2-31. There is also risk of iatrogenic hemothorax, which occurs in association with subclavian vein cannulation as a result of laceration of the vessel during insertion of the catheter or as a result of a gradual erosion of the vessel by the catheter rubbing against the wall of the vessel. Risk factors also include hemothorax, which has been

Table 2-31 Common Sources of Bleeding Associated with Hemothorax

Ribs

Pulmonary

Heart

Aorta or pulmonary vasculature

Thoracic vessels (internal mammary artery, intercostal artery, or supraaortic vessels)

Diaphragm

Spleen

Liver

reported, although rarely, in association with mediastinal tumors, anticoagulant therapy, and sudden acute changes in intrathoracic pressure.[62]

Critical referents

The low pressure of the pulmonary vasculature allows most sources of bleeding to tamponade if not treated with surgical intervention. Most adults can remain asymptomatic with up to 400 mL of blood pooling; however, if bleeding continues and accumulation is greater than 400 mL, pulmonary function will be compromised.[63] The resulting hemothorax displaces the affected lung, which eventually results in the collapse of the alveoli. As the size of the lesion increases, so will the degree of ventilatory impairment. If the bleeding continues, the space occupied by the accumulating blood will cause the mediastinum to shift away from the lesion, leading to compression of the heart and aortic arch. The resulting mechanical restriction of cardiac motion (contractility), compounded by the falling blood volume (preload), will quickly lead to hypovolemic shock and hemodynamic failure. Finally, the bleeding will eventually slow or stop, either when the pressures on both side of the pleural space equalize or when death occurs.

Resulting signs and symptoms

During the early phases of an isolated hemothorax, the patient may exhibit no obvious symptoms. Thus, any patient suffering injuries or a pathology involving the chest or upper abdomen should be considered at risk for developing this complication.

Signs of respiratory difficulty are typically the first to be exhibited. The patient may appear dyspneic and complain of feeling short of breath. Frequently, the breath sounds become muffled or absent over the affected lung, and the area will sound dull when manually percussed. If the hemothorax is large enough to cause a mediastinal shift, the patient will exhibit the typical signs of a shifting of the point of maximum intensity (PMI), jugular vein distention (JVD), and tracheal deviation away from the affected side.

The patient requiring mechanical ventilation presents a special challenge, since the endotracheal tube itself may cause pain and anxiety and makes communication difficult. Such a patient may demonstrate the symptoms described above and will, in addition, exhibit acute changes in airway pressure readings. If the patient is placed on volume control settings such as assist control (CMV or SIMV), peak inspiratory pressures may increase precipitously as the affected lung collapses. Depending on the patient's level of consciousness, the ventilator's pressure limit alarm may actually serve as the primary indicator of hemothorax, well before any apparent physical symptoms develop.

Initially, arterial blood gas results may also appear normal. The patient who is experiencing shock or pain may hyperventilate to compensate and maintain normal minute volume (Ve). Thus, ABGs should always be viewed in light of the clinical exam. As the size of the hemothorax increases, signs of impaired ventilation (such as an increase in $PaCO_2$ and a decrease in pH, PaO_2, and SaO_2) become evident.

A massive hemothorax, defined as a 1.5–4.0 L blood loss into the pleural space, is life-threatening. A patient suffering such a large hemothorax will exhibit symptoms of hypovolemic shock, including tachycardia, hypotension, and low central venous or pulmonary artery pressures. If left untreated, these symptoms will progress to full cardiac arrest. If a pulmonary artery catheter is in place, the cardiac output will remain stable initially, because of a compensatory increase in the patient's systemic vascular resistance. However, cardiac output will eventually fall if blood volume continues to decline and blood is not replaced. Laboratory data will reveal a progressive lowering of hematocrit levels.

A chest x-ray is the most effective means of confirming the diagnosis of hemothorax. The affected area will range from gray to totally opaque, and any mediastinal shift will be evident. The chest x-ray is especially useful, for it often reveals the hemothorax before the patient becomes clinically symptomatic.

Nursing standards of care

Medical intervention is targeted to sustaining life and treating symptoms. A needle thoracentesis may be performed to drain a small hemothorax. This procedure involves the insertion of a large-gauge needle, usually under fluoroscopy, at the level of the lesion.

In the event of a more extensive hemothorax, insertion of a large-bore, 30–40 French chest tube is the most common therapy. The procedure allows the blood and clot formations to drain and the lung to re-expand. The usual insertion site is at the fourth, fifth, or sixth intercostal space on the midaxillary line. After insertion, the chest tube is connected to an underwater seal system with 20–30 cm of suction pressure. Soon after the evacuation of the hemothorax, the ABGs and chest x-ray should be reevaluated. Serial chest x-rays are necessary to confirm re-expansion of the lung. The nurse must assess the patient's clinical status frequently. Close monitoring of the amount and type of drainage from the chest tube is essential in order to evaluate the efficacy of the therapy. Frank bloody drainage of over 200 mL per hour for 2 consecutive hours may be indicative of additional injuries, and in such cases exploratory thoracotomy may be indicated.

In the case of massive hemothorax, the nurse will assist in resuscitation efforts and other life support measures, after which the primary responsibilities will be blood replacement and the use of volume expanders. Autotransfusion is frequently used in such cases to restore volume.

In addition to monitoring the patient's clinical status and chest tube drainage, the critical care nurse must remain cognizant of the patient's and family's emotional status. Frequent, clear explanations of procedures and why they are performed, in addition to measures to relieve pain, will lessen the patient's anxiety.

Once the patient is stabilized and the chest tube has been inserted or the thoracotomy has been completed, the nurse should continue to assess the patient for symptoms of pulmonary contusion, which frequently occurs as a complication of a collapsed lung. Rigorous pulmonary toilet as indicated, including incentive spirometry, coughing and deep breathing, or postural drainage and cupping, may prevent further complications. The accompanying nursing care plan indicates more specific care to be provided to patients suffering hemothorax.

Penetrating Wounds

A penetrating wound through the chest wall into the pleural cavity constitutes a sucking wound that is considered a dire emergency. With an open pneumothorax, depending on the extent of the wound, bellows breathing is rendered ineffectual, and air is moved in and out of the lungs through the wound. Adequate ventilation and gas exchange are impossible. Death results quickly from hypoxia and carbon dioxide retention.

Gunshot wounds present a particular clinical challenge, for the nurse must understand principles of ballistics in order to care for the patient. Care does not involve just treating what is apparent; different types of bullets behave differently upon impact. A small, low-caliber, low-velocity bullet creates a clean wound. Risk of mortality is present only in the event that the bullet penetrates a vital organ. In contrast, a large-caliber bullet that enters the body sideways as a result of yawing or tumbling often explodes intrathoracic viscera. This results in life-threatening complications. Finally, a high-velocity, large-caliber bullet enters the body at a point and creates an apparently clean wound. But some bullets are made to explode internally, and even if not, such a bullet produces shock waves that create further cavernous damage.

Critical referents

Penetrating wounds can be divided into three classes according to location: median wounds, which usually also involve the myocardium; cervicothoracic wounds, which involve the trachea and/or large vessels; and lateral wounds, which involve the lower thorax and diaphragm and can extend further down into the spleen, colon, or liver. Regardless of location, negative chest pressure is compromised by a penetrating wound, and effusion, hemothorax, hypoxia, and hypercarbia occur; shock can develop within minutes. Concomitant risk of tamponade is high in this type of injury. Air embolus and diaphragmatic perforation are also frequently seen.

Resulting signs and symptoms

Signs and symptoms of injuries associated with penetrating wounds are similar to those already described for other types of lung injuries. Hypoxia, cyanosis, and hypercapnia are present. Hemorrhagic shock may also be evident. Tamponade or hemorrhage due to cardiac perforation, bleeding from a lacerated internal mammary artery or other systemic vessel, and tension pneumothorax may be manifested. Respiratory and cardiac arrest may follow quickly.

Nursing standards of care

Basic life support must be provided. All other care depends on the type of presenting wound and the complications that surface. If the patient is in severe respiratory and cardiac distress, assessment for tamponade, internal hemorrhage, air embolism (especially if the patient is ventilated on PEEP), and pneumothorax should be performed. In such cases, the treatment of choice is usually surgical correction of the injury. Postoperative care is similar to that provided in the case of other thoracic and cardiac surgeries.

If the patient is unstable but is not "crashing," the situation is most often due to hemorrhage or air leak causing asphyxia. Resuscitation measures are indicated, and chest tubes should be inserted to remove air and fluid and to restore normal intrapleural pressure for lung expansion. Otherwise the patient is mechanically ventilated to provide for adequate ventilation, gas exchange, and tissue perfusion. The accompanying nursing care plan provides further specifics regarding responsibilities of the critical care nurse in the treatment of such injuries.

Pulmonary Hemorrhage

Pulmonary hemorrhage results from pulmonary and cardiac lacerations, intercostal vessel rupture, or rupture of the aorta. In rare cases it can be due to bleeding from the abdominal region flooding transdiaphragmatically into the pulmonary region. Patients suffering cavitating infectious processes such as necrotizing pseudomonas or invasive aspergillosis are at risk for pulmonary hemorrhage. Patients with coagulation disorders such as hemophilia, thrombocytopenia, uremia, hepatic failure, or DIC are also at risk for pulmonary hemorrhage. It can be minute or massive, progressive or full-blown. More often than not, if a frank wound is not apparent, pulmonary hemorrhage can be traced to pharmacologically induced injury. The use of anticoagulants such as heparin and warfarin (Coumadin) increases the risk of intrapulmonary hemorrhage.

Critical referents

In effect, intrapulmonary hemorrhage causes a pleural effusion/pleural edema type of syndrome. Bleeding occurs interstitially, causing the pulmonary interstitial fluid pressure to rise from normally negative values to within a positive range. Damage to the pulmonary capillary membrane occurs, and plasma colloid osmotic pressure is decreased, causing even more fluids to be drawn into the pulmonary interstitial space. Interstitial fluid volume can only rise about 50% (about 100 cc) before alveolar epithelial membranes rupture, causing what was in the interstitial spaces to flood the alveoli. If this process continues unchecked, death can occur by drowning, in effect.

Resulting signs and symptoms

Signs and symptoms of intrapulmonary hemorrhage mimic those of pulmonary edema. Gas exchange in the lungs is impeded by the accumulation of blood and serosanguineous fluid. The patient is short of breath, agitated, pale, and cyanotic. Severe tachypnea results as the patient tries to breathe enough oxygen. The skin becomes cold and clammy. Work of breathing becomes very labored. Interestingly enough, hemoptysis is rarely manifested, for all the blood remains in the interstitial and alveolar regions. Lung sounds include gurgles (rhonchi) and wheezes throughout the areas affected or diminished breath sounds in areas of severe hemorrhage. ABG results show a considerable lowering of PaO_2 and increases in $PaCO_2$, as well as high peak airway pressures and poor compliance; in addition the patient exhibits severe hypoxia leading to extreme acidotic states. Obviously, hematocrit and hemoglobin levels fall.

The chest x-ray shows diffuse interstitial infiltrates, which often cannot be differentiated from fluids seen in other syndromes, such as ARDS, for example. Reabsorption and improvement of x-ray findings are slow and lag behind the clinical findings by several days. Differentiation of blood from fluid or atelectasis is possible with a chest CT.

Nursing standards of care

Care supplied to the patient suffering pulmonary hemorrhage is targeted at supporting respiratory efforts to assure adequate ventilation, gas exchange, and tissue perfusion. If the hemorrhage is believed to be a complication of pharmacological agents, discontinuing the offending drug is indicated; if the hemorrhage is due to clinical disorders, these must be corrected. Respiratory support must be provided during the sometimes slow resolution of drug-induced lung damage. The following nursing care plan gives details of the care of the patient suffering thoracic trauma.

Nursing Care Plan for the Management of the Patient with Thoracic Trauma

Diagnosis	Signs and symptoms	Intervention	Rationale
Ineffective breathing pattern related to inadequate ventilation secondary to thoracic trauma	Dyspnea	Maintain patent airway	To ensure adequate ventilation
	Tachypnea	Closely monitor breathing patterns and VT	To ascertain type and extent of injury and effects on breathing adequacy
	Muffled or absent breath sounds		
	Use of accessory muscles	Monitor chest x-rays	To follow development of injury and efficacy of treatment; to assess tamponade; to ascertain placement of chest tubes and ET tube
	Chest dull to percussion		
	Asymmetrical chest expansion		
	Abnormal ABGs: $PaO_2 < 80$; $PaCO_2 > 45$; pH < 7.35; $SaO_2 < 90\%$; $HCO_3 > 26$	Aerosol/humidity therapy; supplemental O_2 or mechanical ventilation as needed	To maintain optimal oxygenation and lung hydration; to obtain internal stabilization in the case of flail chest
	Exertional dyspnea	Splint thoracic cage as indicated	To immobilize chest wall for breathing and prevention of pain
	Decreased activity levels		
	Hypoxemia	Assist with chest tube management and/or thoracentesis as indicated; dress CT insertion site with vaseline gauze dressing	To drain hematoma and air and reinflate lung lobes by normalizing negative lung pressure; dressing protects against air leak
	Radiographic lobular collapse, atelectasis, and flail chest		
		PEEP administration by MASK/CPAP or intubation	To ventilate lung; to reverse hypercarbia; to improve oxygenation; to decrease work of breathing; to prevent cardiopulmonary collapse; to decrease deadspace and shunt; to improve CO and AV content difference
		Vigorous pulmonary toilet including incentive spirometry, coughing and deep breathing, postural drainage and cupping, and IPPB treatments	To prevent further pulmonary congestion and complications; to promote improved breathing; to better ventilate and oxygenate the lungs

Diagnosis	Signs and symptoms	Intervention	Rationale
Alteration in respiratory function: hypoxemia	In the appropriate clinical context and with no other reason: $PaO_2 < 5(FIO_2)$; $PaO_2 <$ predicted for patient's age; $PaO_2 = 110 - \frac{1}{2}$ of patient's age; $PaO_2 < 75$ mm Hg on room air; $SaO_2 < 90\%$	Monitor ABGs frequently	To ascertain the presence of hypoxemia for appropriate choice of intervention
		Oxygen and ventilatory support as needed	To correct hypoxemia
	Increased work of breathing: increased respiratory rate; increased tidal volume	Monitor respiratory rate and tidal volume	To assess cardiopulmonary stress
		Place in semi- or high Fowler's position as indicated	To allow easiest breathing and full diaphragmatic descension
	Increased myocardial work: increased cardiac output; changes in BP; decreased level of consciousness; decreased capillary refill; cold and clammy skin; decreased urinary output	Assist with basic care regime	To conserve energy and prevent increases in cardiac oxygen demand
		Closely monitor VS and ECG and check for chest pain	Indications of ischemic damage and cardiac compromise
	$PaCO_2$ 35–45 mm Hg or less	Maintain patency of IV lines	To allow fast access in case of an emergency
	Increased minute ventilation		
Potential for alteration in gas exchange related to ventilation-perfusion mismatch and shunting from injury	Dyspnea	Monitor ABGs closely	Problems with oxygenation are commonly seen
	Decreased O_2 levels on ABGs		
	Fluid overload	Assist patient to position of comfort; semi- or high Fowler's position is best	To improve breathing patterns and lower diaphragm
		Assess for crackles (rales), S_3, and JVD every 4 hours and as needed	Signs of respiratory failure with resultant heart failure
		Administer oxygen as ordered	To counter problems with oxygenation leading to hypoxemia
		Monitor rhythm	Tachycardia is commonly seen

Nursing Care Plan for the Management of the Patient with Thoracic Trauma

Diagnosis	Signs and symptoms	Intervention	Rationale
		Review chest x-ray for signs of fractures, hemorrhage, lung collapse, and diaphragmatic injury	To ascertain type and degree of injury
	Changes in mental status	Monitor level of consciousness	Decreased level of consciousness may be first sign of anoxia
		Administer IV fluids and/or vasopressors as ordered	To increase BP when patient is hypotensive and to preserve right ventricular filling pressure
		Treat for heart failure if present	To maintain perfusion to lungs
		Provide rest between treatments	To decrease oxygen demand
		Turn patient every 2 hours as tolerated	To minimize ventilation-perfusion shunting effects and risk of atelectasis
		Increase FIO_2; commit to PEEP if indicated	To decrease shunt and ensure adequate oxygenation
Potential for impaired gas exchange due to: ineffective airway clearance, atelectasis, effusion; inadequate ventilation and/or supplemental O_2; low hematocrit and hemoglobin; hypervolemia treatment	Abnormal ABGs: $pO_2 < 80$ mm Hg; $pCO_2 < 35$ or > 45 mm Hg; $pH < 7.35$ or > 7.45; $sO_2 < 80\%$; $HCO_3 < 20$ or > 26 mEq/L; $BE < 0$ or > 3 Cyanosis ET tube cuff leak Lowered peak pressure Inadequate volume exchange	Mechanically ventilate as required Closely monitor lungs for absent, unequal, diminished breath sounds, crackles, (rales), wheezing, or asymmetric chest wall expansion; closely monitor ABGs PRN and after ventilator changes; obtain chest x-ray immediately upon intubation and PRN for ET tube	Ventilation support is needed until patient is stable Early indications of further respiratory compromise and/or complications

Diagnosis	Signs and symptoms	Intervention	Rationale
	Chest x-ray indicates atelectasis, effusion, pneumothorax, or hemothorax	placement, lung expansion (pneumothorax), presence of pleural fluid	
	Elevated respiratory rate, wheezing, air hunger, gasping, copious secretions, or asymmetrical chest wall expansion	Pulmonary toilet PRN with chest percussion therapy, incentive spirometry, and hyperinflation using 100% O_2 before and after suctioning; turn and reposition patient every 2 hours	To mobilize secretions, provide adequate oxygenation, and open closed alveoli
		Elevate HOB 30 degrees	To assist patient to return to optimal breathing capacity (to prevent atelectasis, infection, etc.)
	Fluid imbalances; decreased serum osmolality; increased specific gravity of urine; increased sodium levels	Maintain fluid balance	To mobilize secretions and facilitate maximal gas exchange
	Fluid volume deficits lead to hypotension, anemia	Monitor CT drainage for color/consistency	To ascertain amount of bleeding from CT
		Perform Hct on drainage after removing sample through sampling port	To ascertain need for blood replacement
		Use of autotransfusion as indicated; contraindicated in elderly and very young, those infected with blood-borne diseases, or the hematologically compromised; administer per regular transfusion protocol	Per CDC specifications

Nursing Care Plan for the Management of the Patient with Thoracic Trauma

Diagnosis	Signs and symptoms	Intervention	Rationale
Potential for skin breakdown due to: restriction in movement; pain/discomfort; impaired thoracic movement; depression; diaphoresis or drainage into patient's bed; additional conditions such as diabetes, peripheral vascular disease, obesity, etc.; low cardiac output; poor tissue perfusion; altered nutritional status; weakness/fatigue	Imposed restriction of movement, including body mechanics, medical protocol, etc.	Apply air mattress to bed	To prevent pressure spots on skin
	Impaired coordination or decreased muscle strength preventing independent movement	Assist patient with required movements; turn patient a quarter turn every 1–2 hours	To prevent injury and facilitate movement
	Reluctance to attempt movement	Encourage movement as medically indicated	To promote lung expansion and ventilation
	Redness over pressure points	Inspect skin pressure points including occiput, sacrum, coccyx, heels, and elbows every 2 hours	To prevent skin breakdown
		Passive range of motion for all extremities	To prevent irritation of pressure points
		Keep patient dry	To prevent skin breakdown
		Maintain and supplement nutrition as needed	To maintain supply of vital nutrients to skin
		Consult enterostomal therapist for actual breakdown	For optimal care planning and intervention
Potential for infection related to penetrating and open wounds, chest tubes, accumulated blood, indwelling lines, and Foley catheter	Elevated temperature Congestion	Encourage coughing and deep breathing; turn patient in bed every 2 hours while on bedrest	Help to prevent atelectasis, blood clots in legs, and pressure sores
		Change respiratory tubing every 24 hours	Per CDC specifications
		Increase activity as soon as indicated	To promote healing
		Monitor temperature every 4 hours	Sign of infection

Diagnosis	Signs and symptoms	Intervention	Rationale
	Increased WBCs	Assess WBC count	Sign of infection
		Maintain strict aseptic technique with invasive lines and indwelling catheters; change lines unless contraindicated: PAP every 72 hours, arterial lines every 7 days, tubing every 48 hours, IV bags every 24 hours; provide Foley care every 8 hours	Per Centers for Disease Control recommendation
		Assist in identifying source of infection: collect cultures; note atelectasis on chest x-ray; note sputum and urine characteristics; check insertion site for redness every 8 hours	Sites at risk of infection must be kept clean with aseptic technique; appropriate antibiotic therapy must be chosen
		Administer antibiotics as ordered	To combat infectious process
Decreased tolerance of activity related to dyspnea	Dyspnea on exertion Fatigue Exaggerated increase in heart rate and BP on exertion	Assess level of activity tolerance	Provides a baseline
		Assist patient to change position every 2 hours while on bedrest; assist patient with range of motion exercises	To decrease pooling of secretions in lung fields and risk of complications and to promote venous return
		Monitor heart rate and BP with activity increases	To maintain heart rate within 10 bpm of resting heart rate and maintain systolic BP within 20 mm Hg of resting BP; if a drop occurs, it may indicate a drop in cardiac output
		Anticipate institution of progressive rehab	To provide controlled mechanism for increasing activity
		Encourage frequent rest periods	To prevent excessive fatigue
		Group nursing activities together	To ensure rest periods and to prevent overexertion

Nursing Care Plan for the Management of the Patient with Thoracic Trauma

Diagnosis	Signs and symptoms	Intervention	Rationale
Potential for alteration in cardiopulmonary, cerebral, renal, and peripheral tissue perfusion related to hemorrhage or injury	Signs of altered cerebral perfusion: mental confusion; dizziness; syncope; convulsions and/or seizures; TIA; yawning	Rule out nonpulmonary causes of altered cerebral perfusion	To ascertain the need for interventions not relating to the pulmonary system and choose appropriate intervention according to underlying disorder
	Signs of altered cardiopulmonary perfusion: angina and ischemic changes	Monitor for chest pain	
	Signs of altered renal perfusion: oliguria and anuria	Check urine output every 8 hours or every hour if oliguria occurs	To assess kidney function
	Signs of altered peripheral perfusion: hypotension, cyanosis, distant or absent peripheral pulses	Monitor BUN, creatinine, & K^+	Respiratory failure may eventually cause decrease in cardiac output to periphery from hypoxemia and related dysrhythmias
		Assist patient with range of motion exercises, deep breathing and coughing, leg exercises; provide antiembolic stockings as indicated	To promote peripheral circulation; to prevent venous pooling, thrombi, and ischemic skin tissue breakdown
Tissue hypoxia	Tachycardia Tachypnea Hyperventilation Dyspnea Cyanosis Hypertension Restlessness Confusion/disorientation	Monitor ABGs closely	To assess alveolar ventilation
		Monitor Ve	To assess total ventilation to provide an index of work of breathing affecting cardiopulmonary stress
	Early alkalosis leading to late respiratory acidosis	Monitor for signs of cardiovascular and cardiopulmonary work	To determine acid-base balance and need for O_2 since there is no direct test for tissue hypoxia (can only evaluate hypoxemia)

Diagnosis	Signs and symptoms	Intervention	Rationale
	Early alveolar hyperventilation leading to late severe alveolar hypoventilation Hypoxemia	Emergent administration of increased FIO$_2$	To normalize PaO$_2$; to improve alveolar oxygen tension; to decrease work of breathing and myocardial work
		Use appropriate O$_2$ device	To maintain PaO$_2$ to prevent complications of hyperoxia; oxygen system should deliver flow (4 × Ve) to maintain desired FIO$_2$, prevent room air leakage into system, maintain adequate PaO$_2$ to at least level of inspired FIO$_2$, and reduce work of breathing
		Monitor oxygenation	Pulse oximetry should show O$_2$ sat. > 90%
Discomfort related to: injury; headache from hypoxia; myocardial ischemia; imposed physical restrictions accompanying the use of IV, Foley catheter, invasive monitoring	Headache Complaints of chest pain on breathing and coughing Increased heart rate and blood pressure	Have patient report and describe the pain: location, onset, and precipitator; duration; characteristics	To assess pain, specifically from the patient's perspective
		Assess physical signs and indicators of pain	To provide further indicators of pain
		Explore the use of measures to improve physical comfort: repositioning, back rubs, increased O$_2$, relaxation techniques	To promote comfort and alleviate fatigue
		Administer prescribed analgesics PRN especially before pulmonary toilet	To alleviate discomfort; to promote progressive pulmonary toilet (care must be taken not to depress respiratory effort and efficacy)
		Determine effectiveness of interventions and therapies	To choose best measures

Nursing Care Plan for the Management of the Patient with Thoracic Trauma

Diagnosis	Signs and symptoms	Intervention	Rationale
Anxiety due to respiratory distress related to injury, thoracic pain on breathing, and severe dyspnea	Agitation Restlessness Confusion Impaired concentration Hyperventilation Diaphoresis Tachycardia Sleeplessness Shakiness Facial tension Distracted behavior Withdrawal Nonadherence to treatment plan	Monitor patient's oxygenation status closely	Lung injuries greatly decrease ability for gas exchange
		Position patient to maximize respiratory status and minimize respiratory effort, based on patient tolerance	Dyspnea, shortness of breath, and hyperventilation are early signs of impending respiratory failure and cause high anxiety in patient, which only worsens respiratory status; positioning can decrease compression of diaphragm by abdomen and maximize ventilation-perfusion, decreasing sensations of inability to breathe
		Prepare patient for procedures and expected sensations	To minimize anxiety and maximize cooperation
		Ascertain patient's fears and anxieties	Baseline will allow nurse to know exactly what to address
		Ascertain patient's previous hospital experiences	Will help nurse to know how to best alleviate anxieties and support encouraging actions
		Provide emotional support as needed	To help patient and family deal with the situation in the best way possible

Diagnosis	Signs and symptoms	Intervention	Rationale
		Teach patient about what will happen in ICU: care routine, tubes, lines, ICU environment and visiting hours, how to improve breathing efforts, etc.	To help patient be prepared for what is to be experienced
		Administer analgesics and antianxiety agents as ordered (use of neuromuscular blocking agents required sedation of patient)	To decrease anxiety and increase rest

Medications Commonly Used in the Care of the Patient with Thoracic Trauma

Medication	Effect	Major side effects
Epinephrine	Stimulates alpha and beta receptors of autonomic nervous system Potent bronchodilation with rapid onset of action Vasoconstriction	Tachycardia Arrhythmias Nausea and vomiting
Steroids: Prednisone Prednisolone Solu-Cortef Hydrocortisone	Intermediate-acting synthetic form of hydrocortisone but 3–5 times more potent Inhibits allergic reactions	Fluid retention Weight gain Hypertension Cushing syndrome Gastritis; gastric ulcers Adrenal suppression Hypokalemia Psychosis Glucose imbalances
Antibiotics according to gram stain, culture, and sensitivity	Depends on specific antibiotic	Depends on specific antibiotic
Plasma substitutes: Dextran 70 Dextron 40	Glucose polymer used to expand plasma volume and maintain blood pressure in the event of shock Interferes with normal clotting by coating platelets Restores flow to microcirculation Improves tissue perfusion by reducing blood viscosity	Increased clotting time Fluid volume overload Renal complications
Morphine sulfate	Analgesia/sedation Peripheral vasodilation Decreased systemic venous return Bronchodilation Relief of congestive dyspnea	Hypotension Respiratory depression Nausea and vomiting Constipation Urine retention

Pulmonary Aspiration

Pulmonary aspiration is the introduction of foreign, nongaseous substances into the lower respiratory tract as a result of depression of inherent reflex protective mechanisms, structural changes such as fistulas, which allow spillage of swallowed material, and invasive factors such as the introduction of a nasogastric tube or the like. Aspirated materials may be solids, which create situations requiring immediate action, or gastric contents and other fluids.

Aspirations in the lung lead to an inflammatory response involving the airways and alveoli, which eventually results in infection of the parenchyma and/or pneumonia. There are many organisms that will cause such infectious processes if introduced into the lung, and these include aerobic and anaerobic bacteria, viruses, mycoplasmas, fungal agents, protozoa, and helminths. Noninfectious precipitators include solids, gastric contents, vegetable or mineral oils, liquid petroleum, water (in the case of drowning), toxic or caustic chemicals, dusts, gases, or smoke from fires. Once the patient is stabilized, immobility and chronic illness may complicate the clinical status, resulting in pneumonia or flu-like symptoms.

Clinical antecedents

Aspiration results when material is propelled into the alveolar system and most frequently occurs when eating, after vomiting, or with drowning. The only effective therapy for choking when eating is to remove the obstruction. Aspiration of food particles and/or gastric contents is relatively common and is associated mostly with impaired consciousness resulting from such conditions as cardiac arrest, seizures, strokes, uremia, hepatic failure, and general anesthesia. Conditions that affect the ability of the patient to swallow (such as esophageal motility problems stemming from hiatal hernia, stroke, or cancer) are also prime antecedents of aspiration. Most frequent, though, is the situation in which food or fluid is passively or actively vomited and then aspirated into the trachea and lungs. This type of aspiration, known as Mendelson's syndrome, can occur during the induction of anesthesia, during surgery, or postoperatively, as the patient recovers from anesthesia.

Aspiration pneumonia may take one of three different forms: acute aspiration pneumonia (septic pneumonitis or Mendelson's syndrome), chronic aspiration pneumonia, and lipoid pneumonia.[64] Acute aspiration pneumonia results from the aspiration of hydrochloric acid (gastric content), food, and other foreign substances. (In such cases the vomitus can be evaluated for content or appearance to ascertain risk of irritation and inflammation. At the same time any mechanical obstruction must be eliminated so as to lower the risk of respiratory distress for the patient.)

In drowning or near-drowning, aspiration of water usually causes laryngospasm, which, although intense, is not severe enough to protect the alveoli from introduction of the fluid. Pulmonary surfactant is washed out, and the alveoli collapse, resulting in negative interalveolar hydrostatic pressure and fluid accumulation. The end result in such cases is severe hypoxemia and acidosis. The close similarity between near-drowning and ARDS may be due in part to the washing out of the surfactant from the alveolar linings. If drowning occurs in salt water, hyperosmolar fluid is aspirated into the lungs and then fluid is pulled from the vascular tree into the alveoli to achieve equilibrium. Regardless of the type of fluid, in the case of drowning, fluid and electrolyte abnormalities will occur; their degree depends on the volume and type of aspirant. The victim of freshwater aspiration will be hypervolemic and will experience hemodilution and red cell lysis within minutes of the time the water is absorbed into the circulation. Additional problems associated with drowning can include the occurrence of pneumonia and lung abscess from aspiration of infectious foreign matter. It should be noted that if the catastrophe occurs in hypothermic conditions, prognosis is improved, for in such circumstances oxygen demand is greatly reduced.

Other predisposing conditions for acute aspiration pneumonia include trauma, burns, use of general anesthesia, unconsciousness, and the placement of nasogastric or endotracheal tubes. With acute aspiration pneumonia there is usually a latent period after the aspiration and before the onset of respiratory distress. In some cases pneumonia may develop as long as 2 weeks after the initial traumatic event.

Chronic aspiration pneumonia is a localized consolidation of dependent portions or bilateral midzones of the lungs occurring as a result of repeated aspirations of small amounts of infected pharyngeal secretions. This type of aspiration pneumonia is especially common in the chronic alcoholic, the drug abuser, and the patient who is obtunded. Common predisposing factors to chronic aspiration pneumonia are conditions such as hiatal hernia, disorders affecting the mechanics of swallowing, and the presence of nasogastric and endotracheal tubes.

Lipoid pneumonia results from aspiration of milk, mineral oil, or oily nose drops. The presence of lipid macrophages in the inflammatory exudate indicates that fats have been aspirated and have caused an acute or chronic pneumonia.

Critical referents

The specific pathophysiology involved in the event of choking is quite straightforward: air exchange is prohibited and asphyxia results. Initially, the presence of hypoxia vigorously drives the work of breathing, but without success. Death occurs within minutes if the victim is left unaided. In contrast, if a smaller solid becomes lodged in the pulmonary system, it swells from hydration in the bronchial tree, impeding the flow of gases in and out of the lumen. Foreign solids also interfere with the lungs' ability to rid themselves of foreign and irritating material. When aspiration of gastric contents occurs (either acutely or chronically), it causes a chemical irritation and destruction of the mucosa of the tracheobronchial tree (because of the high acidic value of gastric juices, pH < 3). Once in the lungs gastric juices damage the alveolar-capillary barrier, especially in dependent portions of the affected lobes. The damage causes a significant compromise in the permeability of pulmonary blood vessels, the precursor to significant plasma shifts. Pulmonary arterial pressure rises to very high levels; simultaneously, histamine released by mast cells in the area further lowers the efficacy of the alveolar-capillary barrier, allowing alveolar overhydration. Shunting of blood to unventilated areas of the lung occurs at this point, causing arterial hypoxemia. The severity of the patient's reaction depends on the physiologic status and the amount and acidity of the aspirant.

Resulting signs and symptoms

The event of choking is a traumatic one, and the patient will experience acute asphyxia. Respiratory distress—bronchospasm, dyspnea, tachycardia, chest pain, and cyanosis—may or may not begin immediately upon aspiration. Severe hypoxia frequently occurs and, if not treated, may result in adult respiratory distress syndrome. Severe hypoxemia frequently occurs, along with pulmonary edema. Coughing is the predominant symptom, but it may be absent in the critically ill if mechanisms suppressing the cough reflex are present. In the event of sputum production, sputum will be purulent, and

identification of infectious organisms by gram stain may prove difficult. Glucose testing of sputum is also helpful; it may provide valuable clues to the diagnosis of silent aspiration in the event of enteral feedings.

Aspiration pneumonias are usually found to involve gram-negative bacilli such as Klebsiella pneumoniae (which may be multilobar), Pseudomonas aeruginosa (also multilobar and predominating in the lower lobes), Escherichia coli, and enterobacteria (appear throughout the pulmonary tract, including the lower lobes). Atelectasis and small pleural effusions are common. Such pneumonias are especially severe in the critical care patient because of the complication of early necrosis of lung tissue and rapid abscess formation.[65]

Bacterial aspiration pneumonias produce a localized infiltrate resulting in bronchial breath sounds. In contrast, viral pneumonias manifest in a more diffuse manner and produce chest sounds of scattered crackles (rales) and gurgles (rhonchi).

Nursing standards of care

Prevention of pulmonary aspiration is the best course, and the nurse must constantly monitor patients who are at high risk. Common practices that decrease the incidence of such aspirations include (1) elevating the head of the bed of the debilitated patient receiving tube feedings or experiencing mechanical disorders of the swallowing reflexes; (2) positioning the patient suffering impaired reflexes in a lateral position; (3) assuring the seal of the cuff of tracheostomy or endotracheal tubes; and (4) withholding food and liquid for at least 8 hours prior to anesthesia. Enteral feedings can be monitored through the use of food coloring or methylene blue dye added to the feeding. Small or silent aspiration will be evidenced by endotracheal suctioning of the dye.

If a solid is aspirated, the Heimlich maneuver should be executed. If, in spite of close monitoring, solids or fluids are introduced into the lungs, the patient should be turned on his or her side and suctioned immediately. The maintenance of oxygenation and circulation is of paramount importance. Bronchoscopy can be performed to remove consolidated foreign material lodged in regions that are reachable. Bronchial washings are definitely contraindicated, for the risk of washing the foreign body further into the system is high. If the patient is not intubated and has no need to be, 100% humidified oxygen should be supplied by facial mask. If severe respiratory distress results, endotracheal intubation and mechanical ventilation with PEEP will be required. Whether there is a need for intubation or not, the primary goal is to provide enough oxygen to overcome the arterial hypoxemia caused by the aspirant.

When extensive damage to the alveolar-capillary membrane occurs, a shift of fluid to the alveoli and interstitium from the intravascular space occurs. Hypotension and dehydration result, and immediate volume replacement is indicated. Whether to administer crystalloids or colloids in such a case remains controversial; what is certain is that volume replacement must be accomplished judiciously to protect damaged lung tissue from high fluid pressures.

Protection of the patient from infection is also critical in the case of aspiration. Aspiration can cause a large invasion of bacteria into a sterile field. Obstruction by the foreign body or fluid impedes mucociliary action that usually propels contaminants out of the lung; furthermore, because of the fluid shift, the ability of leukocytes to reach the area of contamination is greatly compromised. Postural drainage positioning may facilitate removal of aspirant and enhance blood and lymph flow to injured areas. Cultures of suctioned material should be made to ascertain whether organisms have been introduced into the lung. Broad-spectrum antibiotics should be administered until the infectious organism is identified.

Chest x-rays should be obtained daily to chart the progress and effects of aspiration pneumonia, in order to plan and implement appropriate interventions. Chemical aspiration injury usually begins to resolve within 5 to 7 days if properly treated. Vigorous respiratory toileting is extremely important for the respiratory health of the patient. Positioning of the patient so that the affected lung is not dependent for extended periods of time will serve to improve the ventilation-perfusion ratio and prevent settling of congestant and aspirant. Serial arterial blood gas analyses will suggest appropriate oxygen therapy.

Bronchodilators and mucolytics to mobilize secretions may be indicated. Clinical experience has proven steroid therapy of little value. If steroids are chosen (despite current practice not to include them in the treatment regimen), they may be administered intravenously or via an endotracheal tube, and the nurse must closely monitor the patient's response to such medications.

Nursing responsibilities in the care of a patient who has suffered pulmonary aspiration are to prevent further respiratory distress and infection and provide support for healing. Appropriate interventions are outlined in the following nursing care plan.

Nursing Care Plan for the Management of the Patient with Pulmonary Aspiration

Diagnosis	Signs and symptoms	Intervention	Rationale
Potential for impaired gas exchange due to: aspiration; retention of secretions; ineffective airway clearance; atelectasis; inadequate tidal volume; excessive pulmonary vascular resistance	Dyspnea Cyanosis Increased work of breathing Hypoxemia Decreased breath sounds Dull percussion note Abnormal ABGs: $pO_2 < 80$ mm Hg; $pCO_2 < 35$ or > 45 mm Hg; $pH < 7.35$ or > 7.45; O_2 sat. $< 80\%$; $HCO_3 < 20$ or > 26 mEq/L; BE < 0 or > 3	Closely monitor ABGs; monitor lungs for absent, unequal, diminished breath sounds, crackles (rales), wheezing, or asymmetric chest wall expansion	Early indications of further respiratory compromise and/or complications .
		Closely monitor chest x-ray for presence of foreign substance or body, ET tube placement, lung expansion, presence of pleural fluid	To assess lung and parenchymal status; to determine presence of foreign substance; to monitor effectiveness of therapy
		Monitor level of consciousness	Decreased level of consciousness may be first sign of anoxia
	Inadequate volume exchange	Assess for S_3 and JVD	Signs of respiratory failure leading to heart failure
	Elevated respiratory rate, wheezing, air hunger, gasping, and/or asymmetrical chest wall expansion	Monitor VC	To assess status of lung and serve as an index of work of breathing and prognosis of ability to maintain spontaneous ventilation
	Atelectasis Decreased lung compliance, VC, FRC, and V_T Increased respiratory rate No improvement of PaO_2 with oxygen administration (refractory) Increased A-a gradient Radiographic findings of alveolar collapse and atelectasis, alveolar consolidation, and secretions Copious secretions	Administer oxygen as ordered; institute mechanical ventilation; increase FIO_2, then commit to PEEP to decrease shunt (at FIO_2 of 1.0, every 10–15 mm Hg P(A-a) O_2 indicates 1% shunt; (shunt greater than 25% requires PEEP); monitor PAO_2	If PaO_2 does not increase by at least 10 mm Hg for every FIO_2 increase of 20%, it is considered refractory; $PAO_2 < 70$ mm Hg will cause hypoxic pulmonary vasoconstriction, adding to shunting problem
		Assist patient to position of comfort; semi- or high Fowler's position is best	To improve breathing patterns and allow full descension of diaphragm

Diagnosis	Signs and symptoms	Intervention	Rationale
	Changes in mental status	Aggressive pulmonary toilet PRN with chest percussion therapy, incentive spirometry, and hyperinflation using 100% O_2 before and after suctioning	To mobilize secretions; to reinflate collapsed alveoli; to remove thick, viscid secretions; to promote oxygenation; to decrease work of breathing; to improve ventilation; and to decrease shunt
		Turn and reposition patient every 2 hours	To prevent pooling of secretions in dependent lung fields; to promote circulation
		If patient is stable, promote extubation by: holding sedation; elevating HOB 30 degrees; decreasing IMV by increments of 2–4 breaths/min if $PO_2 > 90$, pH between 7.35 and 7.45, and O_2 sat. 90–100%	To assist patient to return to optimal breathing capacity as soon as possible (to prevent further atelectasis, secondary infection, etc.)
		Culture secretions and administer appropriate antibiotics	To overcome infectious agent causing further secretions and consolidation
Ineffective breathing pattern due to shunting effect of aspiration	Radiographic atelectasis Increased work of breathing Tachypnea and decreased V_T Increased Ve Decreased VC Exertional dyspnea Decreased activity levels Hypoxemia Hypoxia Atelectic crackles (rales)	Monitor respirations and V_T; measure VC, Ve, and ABGs	Reflect adequacy of breathing pattern; prognostic if $V_T < 1000$ cc or if patient is unable to sustain spontaneous ventilation; to follow improvement/deterioration of patient
		Incentive spirometry every hour; IPPB every 2–4 hours; bronchodilators as ordered	To promote improved lung function; to prevent atelectasis; to increase FRC; to decrease work of breathing; to improve inspiratory muscle tone

Nursing Care Plan for the Management of the Patient with Pulmonary Aspiration

Diagnosis	Signs and symptoms	Intervention	Rationale
	Decreased bibasilar breath sounds Decreased chest movement	Monitor x-rays	To assess lung volumes; diffuse bilateral or localized interstitial patterns with increased vascular shadows indicate decreased $PaCO_2$ and PaO_2; changing left ventricle size indicates worsening hypoxia, pulmonary hypertension; alveolar edema and/or progression to fibrosis indicate severe hypoxemia with 100% O_2
		Supplemental oxygenation as indicated; PEEP; mechanical ventilation	To support ventilation, to reverse hypercarbia, to improve oxygenation, to decrease work of breathing; to prevent cardiopulmonary collapse
		Aerosol/humidity therapy; vigorous pulmonary toilet with postural percussion and drainage	To rehydrate airway; to improve mucociliary activity; to clear secretions; to maintain airway
Ineffective airway clearance due to aspiration, increased secretions, and impaired ability to cough	Weak and ineffective cough effort	Place patient in high Fowler's position to deep breathe and cough	To allow maximal diaphragm descension and lung inflation
		Instruct patient on good coughing technique: deep breathing and deep cough effort (not from throat)	To increase effectiveness of cough effort

Diagnosis	Signs and symptoms	Intervention	Rationale
	Distant sounds, crackles (rales), gurgles (rhonchi), and wheezes on auscultation	Closely monitor for absent or diminished breath sounds	Early indications of further respiratory compromise and/or complications
	Thick, tenacious sputum	Turn patient every 2 hours as medically indicated	To prevent pooling of secretions in dependent lung and to improve circulation
	Chest x-ray indicates obstruction, atelectasis	If medically indicated, encourage fluids	To thin secretions and to allow easier movement of mucus by cilia
		If patient is intubated, suction as needed, using hyperventilation with 100% oxygen before and after suctioning; if indicated, lavage 1–3 cc sterile NS in ET tube before mechanically hyperventilating for suctioning	To mechanically promote loosening of secretions and to ensure adequate oxygenation before and after suctioning
		Chest physical therapy as indicated	To promote breaking up aspirant, mucus plugs, and thick secretions and to clear specific lung fields
		Frequent and meticulous mouth care	To prevent further secretions from being aspirated and to maintain good oral mucosa
		Position patient safely and use extreme caution during oral and tube feeding	To prevent further aspiration of liquids or solids
Tissue hypoxia due to obstruction by aspirant	Tachycardia Tachypnea Hyperventilation Dyspnea Cyanosis Hypertension Restlessness Confusion/disorientation	Monitor ABGs closely	To assess alveolar ventilation
		Monitor Ve	To assess total ventilation to provide an index of work of breathing affecting cardiopulmonary stress

Nursing Care Plan for the Management of the Patient with Pulmonary Aspiration

Diagnosis	Signs and symptoms	Intervention	Rationale
	Early alkalosis leading to late respiratory acidosis	Monitor for signs of cardiovascular and cardiopulmonary work	To determine acid-base balance and need for O_2 since there is no direct test for tissue hypoxia (can only evaluate hypoxemia)
	Early alveolar hyperventilation leading to late severe alveolar hypoventilation	Emergent administration of increased FIO_2	To normalize PaO_2; to improve alveolar oxygen tension; to decrease work of breathing and myocardial work
	Hypoxemia	Use appropriate O_2 device	To maintain PaO_2 to prevent complications of hyperoxia; oxygen system should deliver flow ($4 \times Ve$) to maintain desired FIO_2, prevent room air leakage into system, maintain adequate PaO_2 to at least level of inspired FIO_2, and reduce work of breathing
		Monitor oxygenation	Pulse oximetry should show O_2 sat. $> 90\%$
		Turn and reposition patient every 2 hours; provide range of motion exercises as indicated	To promote circulation; to prevent venous pooling
		Provide good skin care	To prevent skin breakdown from tissue ischemia
Potential for infection related to aspirant, indwelling lines, and Foley catheter	Elevated temperature Increased WBCs Congestion	Encourage coughing and deep breathing; turn patient in bed every 2 hours while on bedrest	Helps to prevent atelectasis (a source of infection); moves secretions
		Increase activity as soon as indicated	To promote circulation and healing

Diagnosis	Signs and symptoms	Intervention	Rationale
		Monitor temperature every 4 hours	Sign of infection
		Assess WBC count	Sign of infection
		Maintain strict aseptic technique with invasive tubes and indwelling catheters; change lines unless contraindicated: PAP every 72 hours, arterial lines every 7 days, tubing every 48 hours, IV bags every 24 hours; provide Foley care every 8 hours	Per Centers for Disease Control recommendation
		Assist in identifying source of infection: collect cultures; note atelectasis on chest x-ray; note sputum and urine characteristics; check insertion site for redness every 8 hours	Sites at risk of infection must be kept clean with aseptic technique; appropriate antibiotic therapy must be chosen
		Administer antibiotics as ordered; observe for complications	To combat infectious process without causing renal failure and superinfections
Decreased tolerance of activity related to dyspnea from obstructed airways	Dyspnea on exertion	Assess level of activity tolerance	Provides a baseline
	Fatigue		
	Exaggerated increase in heart rate and BP on exertion	Assist patient to change position every 2 hours while on bedrest; assist patient with range of motion exercises	To decrease pooling of secretions in lung fields and risk of complications and to promote venous return
		Monitor heart rate and BP with activity increases	To maintain heart rate within 10 bpm of resting heart rate and maintain systolic BP within 20 mm Hg of resting BP; if a drop occurs, it may indicate a drop in cardiac output

Nursing Care Plan for the Management of the Patient with Pulmonary Aspiration

Diagnosis	Signs and symptoms	Intervention	Rationale
		Anticipate institution of progressive rehab	To provide controlled mechanism for increasing activity
		Encourage frequent rest periods	To prevent excessive fatigue
		Group nursing activities together	To ensure rest periods and to prevent overexertion
Altered nutritional status due to: anorexia and malaise; increased nutritional requirements resulting from stress of illness	Too fatigued to eat	Auscultate bowel sounds	To evaluate GI peristalsis
	Too short of breath to eat	Help patient to eat slowly; use supplemental O_2 as needed	To facilitate nutritional intake
	Inadequate intake of food and fluids	Monitor I&O	To assess fluid balance
		Calculate calorie requirements	Calorie requirements may increase 200% in ARF
	Decreased albumin and lymphocytes	Monitor albumin and lymphocytes	To assess visceral proteins
	Decreasing body weight	Monitor weight	To monitor effect of diuretic therapy
	Complaints of lack of appetite	With patient, family, and dietary staff, assess appetite and food preferences and review what is allowed and what is best for optimal nutrition; provide preferred food as much as possible	To facilitate nutritional intake and status in any way possible

Medications Commonly Used in the Care of the Patient with Pulmonary Aspiration

Medication	Effect	Major side effects
Bronchodilators: Epinephrine	Stimulate alpha and beta receptors of autonomic nervous system; potent bronchodilation with rapid onset of action Vasoconstriction	Tachycardia Arrhythmias Nausea and vomiting

Metaproterenol:
  Metaprel
  Alupent
	Beta-adrenergic stimulator
	Bronchodilator
		Tachycardia
		Hypertension

Terbutaline: Brethine	Bronchial smooth muscle relaxation lasting 4–6 hours	Tachycardia Tremors Nervousness

Methylxanthines:
  Theophylline
  Aminophylline
	Relaxes bronchial smooth muscles; increases cardiac output; decreases venous pressure; dilates pulmonary vascular bed; improves renal circulation and cerebral stimulation	Epigastric pain and gastric bleeding
		Nausea and vomiting
		Headache
		Palpitation
		Agitation
		Seizures
		Increased alertness

Steroids:
  Prednisone
  Prednisolone
  Solu-Cortef
  Hydrocortisone
	Inhibit allergic reactions	Fluid retention
		Weight gain
		Hypertension
		Cushing syndrome
		Gastritis; gastric ulcers
		Adrenal suppression
		Hypokalemia
		Psychosis
		Glucose imbalances

Antibiotics according to gram stain, culture, and sensitivity	Depends on specific antibiotic	Depends on specific antibiotic

Air Leak Syndrome

Air leak syndrome occurs any time air is allowed in the pleural space. Under normal conditions the pleural cavity is completely free of any gaseous substance, and the two pleural surfaces are in constant contact, gliding smoothly against one another. The lungs inflate upon inspiration and deflate on expiration because of their elasticity and because the pressure in the pleural cavity is less than that in the lungs. On inspiration, the size of the thoracic cavity increases, and the lungs become filled with air at atmospheric pressure, expanding until they fill the enlarged thoracic space. As they expand, the lungs are stretched so much that they have a tendency to pull away from the chest wall, creating a slight negative pressure (less than atmospheric). When an air leak occurs, air is sucked into the pleural space, the negative pressure that maintains the lung in its expanded position is lost, and the lung collapses. What results is a pneumothorax. It is interesting to note that in the past, induced pneumothorax was used as a form of treatment for pulmonary tuberculosis—a practice deemed not best for the patient once its consequences were fully understood!

Clinical antecedents

Air leak syndrome can arise in one of three different ways:

1. entry of gas into the pleural space from the lung via a perforation in the visceral pleura,
2. entry of gas from outside the body through a perforation in the chest wall, or
3. formation of gas by a gas-forming microorganism, causing an empyema in the pleural space.[66]

Spontaneous pneumothorax usually occurs without apparent cause, although it may be related to mass-occupying lesions of the lung such as cancer or empyema; in any case the pathophysiological process is similar to that of other pneumothorax conditions. In contrast, tension pneumothorax occurs when pressures in the pleural cavity rise to positive levels (higher than atmospheric), causing the lung to collapse and the mediastinum to shift to the unaffected side, thus compressing that lung. Antecedents of tension pneumothorax include clinical situations in which pressure is allowed to build up in the pleural cavity, for example: the clamping or occlusion of already placed chest tubes; groaning, shouting, or coughing by the patient; use of positive pressure ventilation; and bronchial spasms. The most serious antecedent of a spontaneous pneumothorax is a wound in the chest wall, which serves as a one-way valve. Air enters through the perforation upon inspiration but cannot escape on expiration because the edges of the wound are forced together and closed. Thus, with each breath more air is allowed in, and as it does not find a way out, pressures continue to build to very high levels, and tension pneumothorax eventually results.

A simple closed pneumothorax (illustrated in Figure 2-49) is one that occurs in the absence of an external wound, is usually partial in nature (although complete pneumothorax may occur), and is without complication once treated. About 86% of all pneumothoraxes are closed.[67] Most commonly, a simple closed pneumothorax occurs spontaneously. It is seen most frequently in male cigarette smokers between the ages of 20 and 40.[68] In the intensive care unit, spontaneous simple closed pneumothorax often occurs as a complication of mechanical volume ventilation. It can also occur accidentally during insertion of a subclavian catheter if the physician inadvertently punctures the space. Likewise, the breaking of the sternum or a rib during cardiopulmonary resuscitation can cause injury to the lung. Finally, a simple closed pneumothorax can occur as a respiratory complication of COPD or cancer. Although they are simple, care must be taken in the treatment of such pneumothoraxes, for they can be aggravated into more serious life-threatening degrees of injury.

A closed pneumothorax is considered to be moderate when about 30% lung expansion is involved. This type of pneumothorax is also rather uncomplicated but can become serious. A complete closed pneumothorax is just what the name suggests: the lung collapses completely. Risk is high that this type of pneumothorax will evolve into a very serious clinical episode.

Open pneumothoraxes (illustrated in Figures 2-50 and 2-51), often referred to as "sucking wounds," occur when injury opens the lung and/or pleural space directly. Knife wounds, gunshot wounds, and catastrophes such as vehicle accidents are usually the cause of such injuries, which result in direct communication between the pleural cavity and the external atmosphere.

An open pneumothorax presents more risk than simply collapse of the lung. With an open pneumothorax (sucking wound), a mediastinal flutter (portrayed in Figure 2-52) is set in motion: the mediastinum swings back and forth in concert with inspiratory and expiratory movements. On inspira-

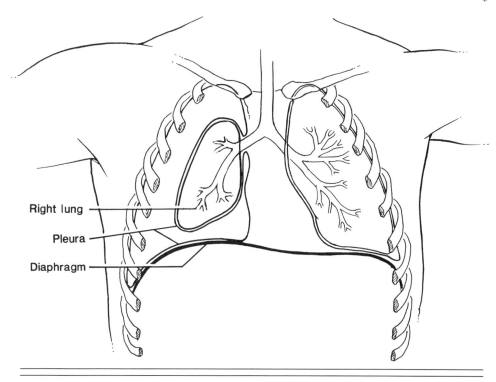

Figure 2-49   Simple Closed Pneumothorax

tion, because of the difference in pressures, air is more easily sucked through the wound than through the bronchus and the mediastinum swings toward the partially inflated unaffected lung, thus increasing the size of the pleural cavity on the affected side. Then, during expiration, air once again passes through the wound to the outside, causing the mediastinum to swing to the affected side. The resultant

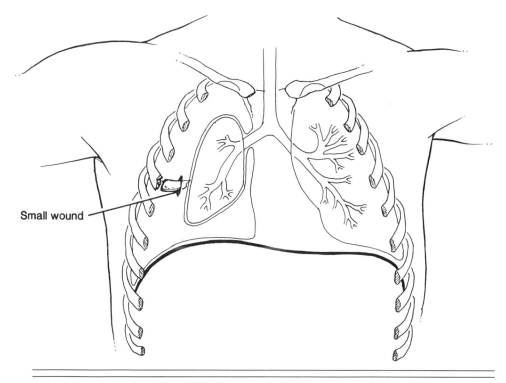

Figure 2-50   Open Pneumothorax

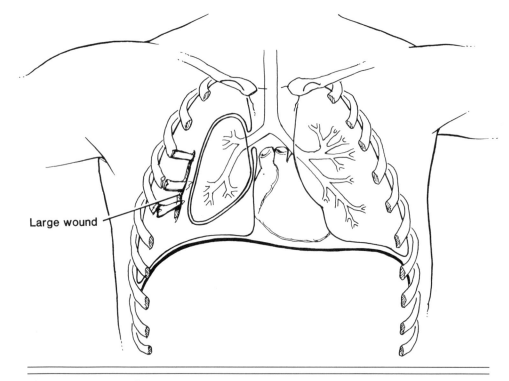

Figure 2-51   Large Open Pneumothorax

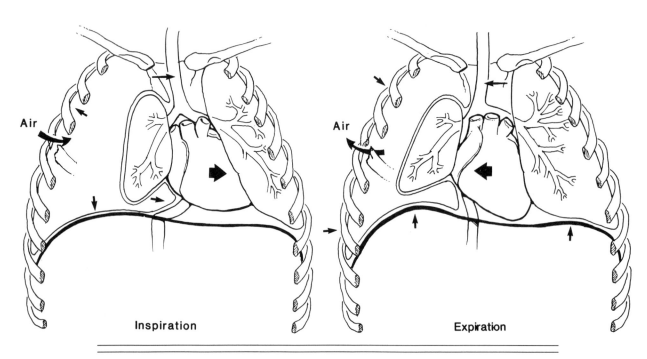

Figure 2-52   Mediastinal Flutter

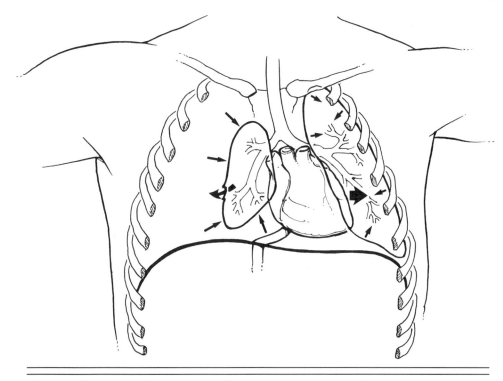

Figure 2-53 Tension Pneumothorax Causing Compression and Circulatory Collapse

rebreathing that occurs effectively increases dead-space and, if left untreated, causes extensive pulmonary collapse, cardiovascular collapse, shock, and death.

Critical referents

Spontaneous pneumothorax usually occurs in the patient already suffering some sort of diffuse pulmonary disorder, as a result of a spontaneous rupture of a small (usually previously undetected) subpleural alveolar cyst or emphysemic bleb. This type of pneumothorax is known to be recurring; about 30% recur, and in up to 10% of cases, the previously unaffected lung collapses sometime in the future.[69] Pre-existing adhesions between the pleural layers may further complicate the spontaneous pneumothorax to the extent that intrapleural hemorrhage occurs.

Tension pneumothorax occurs when air is drawn into the pleural cavity in any of the situations described above. If a lung collapses completely, a shift of the mediastinum to the unaffected side causes two things to occur: (1) the unaffected lung is compressed, thus impeding ventilatory processes even further; and (2) circulatory collapse results, due to a fall in cardiac output caused by increasing intratho-

racic pressures that inhibit venous return (see Figure 2-53). The reduced cardiac output is exacerbated by rotation of the heart caused by the shift of the mediastinum, which causes occlusion of the vena cava. Shock ensues very rapidly if the condition is not treated.

Resulting signs and symptoms

Signs of pneumothorax are straightforward and reflect the degree of severity of the injury. Typically, the clinical presentation of a spontaneous pneumothorax is the occurrence of a sudden, unilateral chest pain (corresponding to the affected side and more common on the left than on the right), closely followed by shortness of breath and increased work of breathing. The patient experiences much difficulty in breathing, even without exercise, activity, coughing, or shouting. Not all patients experience pain, however; it seems to occur more often in those with histories of some underlying pulmonary affliction. Chest wall movement on inspiration and expiration will be uneven; the affected side will not expand as much as the other. Fremitus may be decreased or absent, and chest percussion will produce hyperresonant or tympanic sounds; breath sounds will be distant or even absent. The degree of pulmonary collapse seen on roentgenographic diagnostic examination is moderate and may not show clearly on films taken during inspiration. But on films taken during expiration, air around the partially collapsed lung can be seen more easily and clearly. Furthermore, upon close examination of the films, a small accumulation of fluid can be seen in the dependent portions of the pleural space.

Tension pneumothorax is manifested by asphyxia, hyperresonance of the chest accompanied by distant or absent breath sounds, severe respiratory distress, shallow breathing, severe chest pain, tachycardia, and a drop in blood pressure and cardiac output. A significant enlargement of the affected pleural cavity can be seen on radiographic film, accompanied by a shift of the mediastinum and flattening of the diaphragm. Crepitus (subcutaneous emphysema) may or may not be present, depending on the nature of the originating assault.

A patient with an open pneumothorax exhibits the above characteristics in conjunction with an open chest wound, which may be very small but connecting or very large and cavernous. The extent of the wound depends on the type and severity of the original assault.

Nursing standards of care

Treatment of those suffering air leak disorders almost always involves the insertion of one or more chest tubes. Treatment of a spontaneous pneumothorax depends on the degree of lung involvement and level of intrapleural pressure. If minimal, the patient is supplied supplemental oxygen and is closely observed for signs of worsening or further complication. Restriction of strenuous exercise is recommended until re-expansion of the lung occurs naturally. Once the offending leak seals, the lung usually re-expands spontaneously.

In the case of a moderate, closed, uncomplicated pneumothorax, a simple needle puncture (Figure 2-54) to rid the pleural space of gas or fluid may suffice. In those suffering more extensive air leaks, the insertion of a single chest tube intercostally through the chest wall into the pleural cavity prevents additional accumulation of air and promotes re-expansion of the lung (see Figure 2-55). The patient is mechanically ventilated when lung collapse and compromise are extensive enough to inhibit adequate ventilatory effort, but the risk of tension

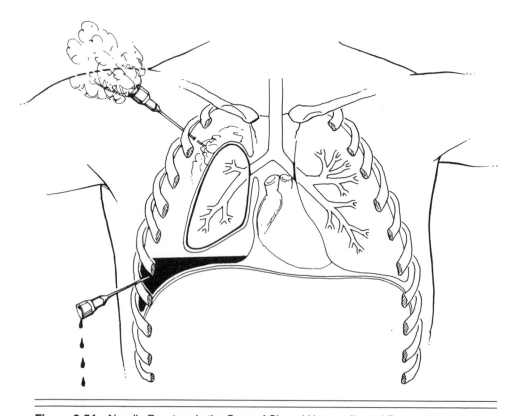

Figure 2-54   Needle Puncture in the Case of Closed Uncomplicated Pneumothorax

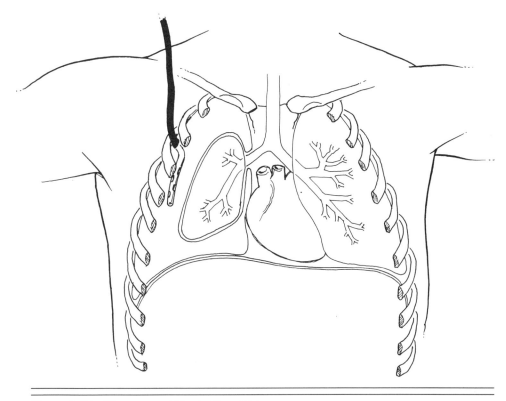

Figure 2-55 Placement of Single Chest Tube

pneumothorax increases significantly with the initiation of mechanical ventilation, so drainage of the cavity *must* be accomplished before the patient is placed on mechanical ventilation, especially positive pressure ventilation.

With an open pneumothorax the chest should be closed first and then drained; if drainage is attempted before closure, the effort will be useless and tension pneumothorax will result. Likewise, drainage must be complete, or the risk of tension pneumothorax will remain very high after the wound is closed (see Figure 2-56). Chest tubes are inserted; one into the second or third intercostal space to accomplish pressure changes in order to reinflate the lung, and the other in the eighth or ninth intercostal space to drain the cavity of fluid. Underwater seal (see Figure 2-57) or chest tube suction should be initiated; once tubes are in place and operating, the risk of tension pneumothorax is greatly lessened. It is only then that the patient should be placed on positive pressure ventilation.

In all cases of tension pneumothorax, immediate drainage of the pleural cavity is indicated. Once the chest is drained, the injury can be assessed to ascer-

tain the causative factor. Chest tubes must be connected to some form of pressure drainage system (Figure 2-58). Ventilation should be accomplished mechanically, for the risk of bilateral chest collapse is high, and if it occurs it will prove life-threatening in a very short period of time.

In some cases, in spite of all attempts to reinflate the lung through insertion of chest tubes, pressure suction intervention, or mechanical ventilation, the affected lung remains deflated. An open thoracotomy is then indicated to remedy the source of the persistent pneumothorax and to debride the wound. Thoracotomy is also indicated when the pneumothorax has recurred three or more times on the affected side and, obviously, in the event of bilateral lung collapse. During the surgery, after the injury has been mended, the surgeon will make abrasions on both surfaces of the pleura so as to cause adhesions to form between the chest wall and lung. Such adhesions have proved to significantly decrease the incidence of recurrent pneumothorax.

Following is a detailed plan for the care of the patient suffering from air leak syndrome.

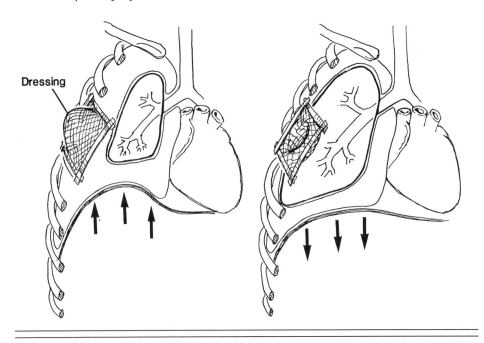

Figure 2-56   How Tension Pneumothorax Arises with Occlusive Dressing and Undrained Pneumothorax

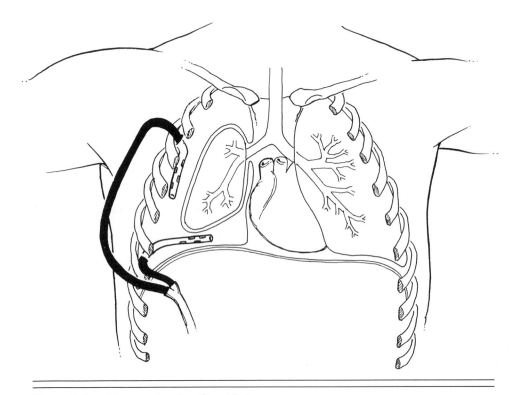

Figure 2-57   Placement of Two Chest Tubes

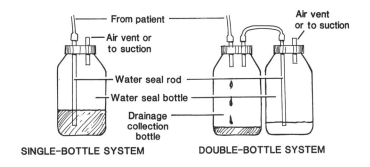

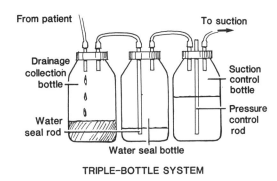

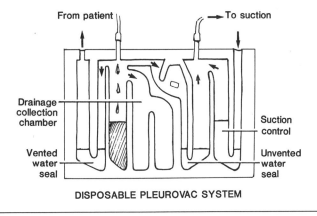

Figure 2-58 Various Forms of Pressure Drainage Systems

Nursing Care Plan for the Management of the Patient with Air Leak Syndrome

Diagnosis	Signs and symptoms	Intervention	Rationale
Ineffective breathing pattern related to inadequate ventilation	Dyspnea Tachypnea Muffled or absent breath sounds Use of accessory muscles Chest dull to percussion Asymmetrical chest expansion Abnormal ABGs: $PaO_2 < 80$; $PaCO_2 > 45$; pH < 7.35; $SaO_2 < 90\%$; $HCO_3 > 26$ Exertional dyspnea Decreased activity levels Hypoxemia Radiographic lobular collapse, atelectasis, and flail chest	Maintain patent airway	To ensure adequate ventilation
		Closely monitor breathing patterns and V_T	To ascertain type and extent of injury and effects on adequacy of breathing
		Monitor chest x-rays	To follow development of injury and assess efficacy of treatment; to assess tamponade; to ascertain placement of chest tubes and ET tube
		Aerosol/humidity therapy; supplemental O_2 or mechanical ventilation as needed	To maintain optimal oxygenation and lung hydration; to obtain internal stabilization in case of flail chest
		Splint thoracic cage as indicated	To immobilize chest wall for breathing and prevention of pain
		Assist with chest tube management and/or thoracentesis as indicated	To drain hematoma and air and reinflate lung lobes by normalizing negative lung pressure
		PEEP administration by MASK/CPAP or intubation	To ventilate lung; to reverse hypercarbia; to improve oxygenation; to decrease work of breathing; to prevent cardiopulmonary collapse; to decrease deadspace and shunt; to improve CO and AV content difference
		Vigorous pulmonary toilet including incentive spirometry, coughing and deep breathing, postural drainage and cupping, and IPPB treatments	To prevent further pulmonary congestion and complications; to promote improved breathing; to better ventilate and oxygenate the lungs

Diagnosis	Signs and symptoms	Intervention	Rationale
Alteration in respiratory function: hypoxemia	In the appropriate clinical context and with no other reason: $PaO_2 < 5(FIO_2)$; $PaO_2 <$ predicted for patient's age; $PaO_2 = 110 - \frac{1}{2}$ patient's age; $PaO_2 < 75$ mm Hg on room air; $SaO_2 < 90\%$	Monitor ABGs frequently Oxygen and ventilatory support as needed; PEEP	To ascertain the presence of hypoxemia for appropriate choice of intervention To correct hypoxemia
	Increased work of breathing: increased respiratory rate, increased tidal volume	Monitor respiratory rate and tidal volume Place in semi- or high Fowler's position as indicated	To assess cardiopulmonary stress To allow easiest breathing and full diaphragmatic descension
	Increased myocardial work: increased cardiac output; changes in BP; decreased level of consciousness; decreased capillary refill; cold and clammy skin; decreased urinary output	Assist with basic care regime Closely monitor VS and ECG and check for chest pain Maintain patency of IV lines	To conserve energy and prevent increases in cardiac oxygen demand Indications of ischemic damage and cardiac compromise To allow fast access in case of an emergency
	$PaCO_2$ 35–45 mm Hg or less Increased minute ventilation		
Potential for alteration in gas exchange related to ventilation-perfusion mismatch, lung collapse, and shunting from injury	Dyspnea Decreased O_2 levels on ABGs Fluid overload	Monitor ABGs closely Assist patient to position of comfort: semi- or high Fowler's position is best Assess for crackles (rales), S_3, and JVD every 4 hours and as needed	Problems with oxygenation are commonly seen To improve breathing patterns and lower diaphragm Signs of respiratory failure leading to heart failure

Nursing Care Plan for the Management of the Patient with Air Leak Syndrome

Diagnosis	Signs and symptoms	Intervention	Rationale
		Administer oxygen as ordered	To counter problems with oxygenation leading to hypoxemia
		Monitor rhythm	Tachycardia is commonly seen
		Review chest x-ray for signs of fractures, hemorrhage, lung collapse, and diaphragmatic injury	To ascertain type and degree of injury
	Changes in mental status	Monitor level of consciousness	Decreased level of consciousness may be first sign of anoxia
		Administer IV fluids and/or vasopressors as ordered	To increase BP when patient is hypotensive and to preserve right ventricular filling pressure
		Treat for heart failure if present	To maintain perfusion to lungs
		Provide rest between treatments	To decrease oxygen demand
		Turn patient every 2 hours as tolerated	To minimize ventilation-perfusion shunting effects and risk of atelectasis
		Increase FIO_2; commit to PEEP if indicated	To decrease shunt and ensure adequate oxygenation
Potential for impaired gas exchange due to: ineffective airway clearance, atelectasis, effusion, lung collapse; inadequate ventilation and/or supplemental O_2; low hematocrit and hemoglobin; hypervolemia treatment	Abnormal ABGs: $pO_2 < 80$ mm Hg; $pCO_2 < 35$ or > 45 mm Hg; pH < 7.35 or > 7.45; O_2 sat. $< 80\%$; $HCO_3 < 20$ or > 26 mEq/L; BE < 0 or > 3

Cyanosis

ET tube cuff leak

Lowered peak pressure | Mechanically ventilate as required

Closely monitor for absent, unequal, or diminished breath sounds, crackles (rales), wheezing, or asymmetric chest wall expansion; closely monitor ABGs PRN and after ventilator changes; obtain chest | Ventilation support is needed until patient is stable

Early indications of further respiratory compromise and/or complications |

Diagnosis	Signs and symptoms	Intervention	Rationale
	Inadequate volume exchange	x-ray immediately upon intubation and PRN for ET tube placement, lung expansion (pneumothorax), presence of pleural fluid	
	Chest x-ray indicates atelectasis, effusion, pneumothorax, or hemothorax		
	Elevated respiratory rate, wheezing, air hunger, gasping, copious secretions, or asymmetrical chest wall expansion	Pulmonary toilet PRN with chest percussion therapy, incentive spirometry, and hyperinflation using 100% O_2 before and after suctioning; turn and reposition patient every 2 hr	To mobilize secretions, provide adequate oxygenation, and open closed alveoli
		Elevate HOB 30 degrees	To assist patient to return to optimal breathing capacity (to prevent atelectasis, infection, etc.)
	Fluid imbalances; decreased serum osmolality; increased specific gravity of urine; increased sodium levels	Maintain fluid balance	To mobilize secretions and facilitate maximal gas exchange
Risk of injury related to complications from chest tube insertion and maintenance	Absence of fluid fluctuation corresponding to breathing movements in chest tube drainage system	Monitor fluid fluctuation in system; notify MD of change	Fluid fluctuation indicates patency of system
	Chest tubes clamped unnecessarily	Do not clamp chest tubes except in event of a leak	Clamping chest tubes for prolonged periods increases risk of tension pneumothorax
	Bubbling in water seal	Monitor water seal; notify MD of bubbling	Bubbling may indicate air leak
	Chest tube drainage > 100 cc/hr; change in amount of drainage	Monitor type and amount of chest tube drainage; notify MD if > 100 cc/hr or if tube entry site becomes reddened	May indicate hemorrhage or new bleeding

Nursing Care Plan for the Management of the Patient with Air Leak Syndrome

Diagnosis	Signs and symptoms	Intervention	Rationale
	Kinked tubing	Protect chest tubes from kinking at all times	Kinked tubing increases risk of tension pneumothorax and clotted tubing
	Respiratory difficulty or cyanosis and chest pressure	Closely monitor respiratory rate and pattern; closely monitor for cyanosis and chest pressure	May be early indicator of chest tube malfunction leading to recurrence of lung deflation
	Crepitation	Monitor for crepitation	May indicate chest tube dislodgement
	Hemorrhage	Monitor for signs of bleeding and Hgb and Hct	To ascertain bleeding complication
	Water seal unit not intact	While assessing for respiratory distress: 1. Clamp chest tube unless there has been a large air leak 2. Reestablish a closed system 3. Unclamp tubes 4. Notify MD	To prevent deflation of lung and, in the event of a large leak, tension pneumothorax
	Tubing disconnected	While assessing for respiratory distress: 1. Clamp chest tube 2. Cleanse tubing connection sites with antiseptic solution 3. Reconnect tubing 4. Unclamp tubes 5. Notify MD	To prevent deflation of lung and occurrence of tension pneumothorax
	Chest tube dislocated	While assessing for respiratory distress: 1. Cover site with sterile dressing (vaseline, if possible) and tape occlusively 2. Notify MD	To prevent air being sucked into pleural cavity and deflation of affected lung

Diagnosis	Signs and symptoms	Intervention	Rationale
	Patient shows signs or complains directly of pain in association with chest tubes	Administer analgesics as ordered and before pulmonary toilet	To promote patient's effort to breathe fully; to facilitate vigorous pulmonary toilet
	Patient lacks knowledge about care activities regarding chest tubes; expresses anxiety related to chest tube placement	Teach patient and family about: purpose and function of chest tubes; coughing and deep breathing and pulmonary toilet techniques; appropriate use of analgesics; need for assistance with moving and turning; notifying nurse in the event of shortness of breath, dislocation of chest tube, increased bleeding in tube or on dressing, etc.; ventilatory and oxygen support; positioning of chest tube and drainage system	To allay fears of patient and family and facilitate full cooperation with care regimen; to prevent injury
Potential for infection related to penetrating and open wounds, chest tubes, accumulated blood, indwelling lines, and Foley catheter	Elevated temperature Congestion	Encourage coughing and deep breathing; turn patient in bed every 2 hours while on bedrest	Help to prevent atelectasis, blood clots in legs, and pressure sores
		Change respiratory tubing every 24 hours	Per CDC specifications
		Increase activity as soon as indicated	To promote healing
		Monitor temperature every 4 hours	Sign of infection
	Increased WBCs	Assess WBC count	Sign of infection

Nursing Care Plan for the Management of the Patient with Air Leak Syndrome

Diagnosis	Signs and symptoms	Intervention	Rationale
		Maintain strict aseptic technique with invasive lines and indwelling catheters; change lines unless contraindicated: PAP every 72 hours, arterial lines every 7 days, tubing every 48 hours, IV bags every 24 hours; provide Foley care every 8 hours	Per Centers for Disease Control recommendation
		Assist in identifying source of infection: collect cultures; note atelectasis on chest x-ray; note sputum and urine characteristics; check insertion site for redness every 8 hours	Sites at risk of infection must be kept clean with aseptic technique; appropriate antibiotic therapy must be chosen
		Administer antibiotics as ordered	To combat infectious process
		Maintain closed system for chest tube drainage	To protect system from introduction of bacteria and to maintain patency
Decreased tolerance of activity related to dyspnea	Dyspnea on exertion Fatigue	Assess level of activity tolerance	Provides a baseline
	Exaggerated increase in heart rate and BP on exertion	Assist patient to change position every 2 hours while on bedrest	To decrease pooling of secretions in lung fields and risk of complications and to promote venous return
		Monitor heart rate and BP with activity increases	To maintain heart rate within 10 bpm of resting heart rate and maintain systolic BP within 20 mm Hg of resting BP; if a drop occurs, it may indicate a drop in cardiac output

Diagnosis	Signs and symptoms	Intervention	Rationale
		Anticipate institution of progressive rehab	To provide controlled mechanism for increasing activity
		Encourage frequent rest periods	To prevent excessive fatigue
		Group nursing activities together	To ensure rest periods and to prevent overexertion
Potential for alteration in cardiopulmonary, cerebral, renal, and peripheral tissue perfusion	Signs of altered cerebral perfusion: mental confusion; dizziness; syncope; convulsions and/or seizures; TIA; yawning	Rule out nonpulmonary causes of altered cerebral perfusion	To ascertain the need for interventions not relating to the pulmonary system and choose appropriate intervention based on underlying disorder
	Signs of altered cardiopulmonary perfusion: angina and ischemic changes	Monitor for chest pain	
	Signs of altered renal perfusion: oliguria and anuria	Check urine output every 8 hours or every hour if oliguria occurs	To assess kidney function
	Signs of altered peripheral perfusion: hypotension; cyanosis; distant or absent peripheral pulses	Monitor BUN, creatinine, and K^+	Respiratory failure may eventually cause decrease in cardiac output to periphery from hypoxemia and related dysrhythmias
		Assist patient with range of motion exercises, deep breathing and coughing, leg exercises; provide antiembolic stockings as indicated	To promote peripheral circulation; to prevent venous pooling and thrombi; to prevent ischemic skin tissue breakdown

Nursing Care Plan for the Management of the Patient with Air Leak Syndrome

Diagnosis	Signs and symptoms	Intervention	Rationale
Discomfort related to: injury; headache from hypoxia; insertion of chest tubes; myocardial ischemia; imposed physical restrictions accompanying the use of IVs, Foley catheter, invasive monitoring	Headache Complaints of chest pain on breathing and coughing Increased heart rate and blood pressure	Have patient report and describe the pain: location; onset and precipitator; duration; characteristics	To assess pain specifically from the patient's perspective
		Assess physical signs and indicators of pain	To provide further indicators of pain
		Explore the use of measures to improve physical comfort: repositioning; back rubs; increased O$_2$; relaxation techniques	To promote comfort and alleviate fatigue
		Administer prescribed analgesics PRN especially before pulmonary toilet	To alleviate discomfort; to promote progressive pulmonary toilet (care must be taken not to depress respiratory effort and efficacy)
		Determine effectiveness of interventions and therapies	To choose best measures
		Monitor chest tubes for placement, drainage, and patency; milk chest tubes as ordered	To maintain patency of chest tubes to facilitate inflation of affected lung and adequate drainage of pleural cavity
Tissue hypoxia	Tachycardia Tachypnea Hyperventilation Dyspnea Cyanosis Hypertension Restlessness Confusion/disorientation	Monitor ABGs closely Monitor Ve	To assess alveolar ventilation To assess total ventilation to provide an index of work of breathing affecting cardiopulmonary stress

Diagnosis	Signs and symptoms	Intervention	Rationale
	Early alkalosis leading to late respiratory acidosis Early alveolar hyperventilation leading to late severe alveolar hypoventilation Hypoxemia	Monitor for signs of cardiovascular and cardiopulmonary work	To determine acid-base balance and need for O_2 since there is no direct test for tissue hypoxia (can only evaluate hypoxemia)
		Emergent administration of increased FIO_2	To normalize PaO_2; to improve alveolar oxygen tension; to decrease work of breathing and myocardial work
		Use appropriate O_2 device	To maintain PaO_2 to prevent complications of hyperoxia; oxygen system should deliver flow ($4 \times Ve$) to maintain desired FIO_2, prevent room air leakage into system, maintain adequate PaO_2 to at least level of inspired FIO_2, and reduce work of breathing
		Monitor oxygenation	Pulse oximetry should show O_2 sat. $> 90\%$
Anxiety due to respiratory distress related to injury, thoracic pain on breathing, presence of chest tubes, and severe dyspnea	Agitation Restlessness Confusion Impaired concentration Hyperventilation Diaphoresis Tachycardia Sleeplessness Shakiness Facial tension Distracted behavior Withdrawal Nonadherence to treatment plan	Monitor patient's oxygenation status closely	Lung injuries greatly decrease ability for gas exchange
		Position patient to maximize respiratory status and minimize respiratory effort, based on patient tolerance	Dyspnea, shortness of breath, and hyperventilation are early signs of impending respiratory failure and cause high anxiety in patient, which only worsens respiratory status; positioning can decrease compression of diaphragm by abdomen and maximize ventilation-perfusion, decreasing sensations of inability to breathe

Diagnosis	Signs and symptoms	Intervention	Rationale
		Prepare patient for procedures and expected sensations	To minimize anxiety and maximize cooperation
		Ascertain patient's fears and anxieties	Baseline will allow nurse to know exactly what to address
		Ascertain patient's previous hospital experiences	Will help nurse to know how to best alleviate anxieties and support encouraging actions
		Provide emotional support as needed	To help patient and family deal with the situation in the best way possible
		Teach patient about what will happen in ICU: care routine, tubes, lines, ICU environment and visiting hours, how to improve breathing efforts, etc.	To help patient be prepared for what is to be experienced
		Administer analgesics and antianxiety agents as ordered (use of neuromuscular blocking agents requires sedation of patient)	To decrease anxiety and increase rest

Medications Commonly Used in the Care of the Patient with Air Leak Syndrome

Medication	Effect	Major side effects
Morphine sulfate	Analgesia/sedation Peripheral vasodilation Decreased systemic venous return Bronchodilation Relief of congestive dyspnea	Hypotension Respiratory depression Nausea and vomiting Constipation Urinary retention

Steroids:
  Prednisone
  Prednisolone
  Solu-Cortef
  Hydrocortisone
	Intermediate-acting synthetics of hydrocortisone but 3–5 times more potent; inhibit allergic reactions	Fluid retention; weight gain
		Hypertension
		Cushing syndrome
		Gastritis; gastric ulcers
		Adrenal suppression
		Hypokalemia
		Psychosis
		Glucose imbalances

Antibiotics according to gram stain, culture, and sensitivity	Per specific antibiotic	Per specific antibiotic

Plasma substitutes:
  Dextran 70
  Dextran 40
	Glucose polymers used to expand plasma volume and maintain blood pressure in the event of shock; interfere with normal clotting by coating platelets; restore flow to microcirculation; improve tissue perfusion by reducing blood viscosity	Increased clotting time
		Fluid volume overload
		Renal complications

Methylxanthines:
  Theophylline
  Aminophylline
	Relax bronchial smooth muscles; increase cardiac output; decrease venous pressure; dilate pulmonary vascular bed; improve renal circulation and cerebral stimulation	Epigastric pain and gastric bleeding; nausea and vomiting
		Headache
		Palpitation
		Agitation
		Seizures
		Increased alertness

Metaproterenol:
  Metaprel
  Alupent
	Beta-adrenergic stimulator
	Bronchodilator
		Tachycardia
		Hypertension

Terbutaline (Brethine)	Bronchial smooth muscle relaxation lasting 4–6 hours	Tachycardia Tremors Nervousness

CHAPTER 2 POST-TEST

1. When a mucus plug blocks a bronchiole:
   a. perfusion of blood distal to the plug creates a right-to-left shunt.
   b. gas exchange will continue in alveoli distal to the plug if perfusion to the same alveoli continues.
   c. "regional atelectasis" occurs, thus decreasing PaO_2.
   d. all of the above occur.

2. If a patient presents with a pAO_2 of 72 mm Hg, a PaO_2 of 68 mm Hg, and a $PaCO_2$ of 70 mm Hg while breathing room air, the patient is probably suffering:
   a. venous-to-arterial shunting due to severe atelectasis.
   b. diffusion impairment due to ARDS.
   c. hypoventilation due to respiratory depression.
   d. hyperventilation due to anxiety.

3. An increase in respiratory rate would normally result from:
   a. hyperthermia.
   b. a decrease in blood pH.
   c. exercise.
   d. all of the above.

4. Normal respiratory rate and effort result from:
   a. impulses sent from neurons in the medulla.
   b. impulses sent from the pons.
   c. impulses sent in response to stretch receptors in the lungs.
   d. all of the above.

5. Needlessly administering oxygen at 100% results in depressed breathing because:
   a. central chemoreceptors are depressed and peripheral centers then respond to decreased oxygen tension.
   b. peripheral chemoreceptors are depressed while central centers respond.
   c. chemoreceptors respond normally, but the integrative center is depressed.
   d. both central and peripheral centers are depressed.

6. A vagus nerve response would cause breathing to:
   a. increase in rate and depth.
   b. increase in rate and decrease in depth.
   c. decrease in rate and depth.
   d. remain unchanged.

7. Maximal minute volume is attained by which of the following actions?
   a. voluntary hyperventilation
   b. exercise

   c. inhalation of 6% oxygen
   d. inhalation of 10% oxygen

8. An increase in alveolar pCO_2 results in:
   a. an increase in blood pH.
   b. an increase in plasma HCO_3 concentration.
   c. a decrease in respiratory minute volume.
   d. an increase in resistance to blood flow through the brain.

9. Clinical criteria for intubation include all *except*:
   a. PaO_2 less than 50.
   b. central neurologic injury.
   c. blood pH less than 7.30.
   d. $PaCO_2$ greater than 50.

10. A patient experiences the following ABG values while being mechanically ventilated with $V_T = 1000$, $FIO_2 = 35\%$, PEEP = 5, and SIMV = 8:
    $PaO_2 = 60$
    $PaCO_2 = 53$
    pH = 7.30
    $HCO_3 = 24$

    What ventilatory changes should be made to improve the ABG results?
    a. increase the SIMV rate
    b. decrease the SIMV rate
    c. increase the SIMV and increase the FIO_2
    d. decrease the SIMV and increase the FIO_2

11. To ensure that accurate ABG values are attained after ventilatory changes, the nurse should wait to draw the blood at least:
    a. 5 minutes
    b. 10 minutes
    c. 30 minutes
    d. 60 minutes

12. Nursing assistance with intubation may include all of the following *except*:
    a. placing the patient in Trendelenburg position.
    b. having sedatives and paralytic agents on hand.
    c. setting up suction devices and ambu bag.
    d. having a syringe available to inflate the cuff.

13. The assist-control mode on a ventilator differs from SIMV in that:
    a. the minute ventilation on the SIMV is constant.
    b. when on the assist-control mechanism, the patient triggers the ventilator and automatically receives the preset tidal volume.

c. when on the assist-control mechanism, the preset respiratory rate is the maximum rate the patient will receive regardless of effort.

d. when on the SIMV mechanism, the patient will receive machine-delivered preset tidal volumes each time a breath is generated.

14. Pressure support ventilation:
a. delivers a fixed tidal volume with every ventilator-delivered breath.
b. augments the patient's respiratory effort with a preset amount of inspiratory pressure.
c. potentiates the resistance to gas flow caused by the endotracheal tube.
d. is best used with the unconscious patient.

15. A patient may be considered to be at risk for oxygen toxicity if oxygen concentrations are equal to or greater than:
a. 40%.
b. 50%.
c. 60%
d. 70%.

16. Signs and symptoms of oxygen toxicity include all of the following *except*:
a. reduced peak airway pressures.
b. subscapular and pleuritic pain.
c. cough.
d. increased secretions.

Refer to the following clinical vignette in answering questions 17 through 22.

A 58-year-old female weighing 50 kilograms returns from surgery still intubated and being mechanically ventilated on a Bear ventilator with the following settings:

$V_T = 750$
$SIMV = 20$
$FIO_2 = 40\%$

The patient indicates that she is in pain and appears anxious. You observe her respiratory rate to be 35 breaths per minute, her ABG values are as follows:

$pH = 7.50$
$PaCO_2 = 33$
$PaO_2 = 65$
$HCO_3 = 21$

17. The patient's ABG values indicate:
a. respiratory acidosis.
b. metabolic acidosis.
c. respiratory alkalosis.
d. metabolic alkalosis.

18. The probable cause for these blood gas values is:
a. inadequate tidal volume resulting in inadequate gas exchange.
b. too much deadspace created from the tubing connecting the patient to the ventilator.
c. anxiety secondary to pain from surgical procedure.
d. ventilation rate set too low.

19. A normal tidal volume for this patient would be:
a. 800 cc.
b. 900 cc.
c. 5–10 cc/kg normal body weight.
d. 10–15 cc/kg normal body weight.

20. If a cuff leak were to occur on this patient, it would probably be due to all of the following *except*:
a. an insufficient amount of air instilled in cuff.
b. a lower airway pressure, creating the need for a higher cuff pressure.
c. a leak in the inflation port.
d. displacement of the endotracheal tube.

21. Which of the following statements is *not* true?
a. If the cuff is observed to have a hole in it, the patient must be reintubated.
b. If the patient experiences high airway pressures, a higher cuff pressure is required.
c. The patient had a normal airway pressure, so she should have had a cuff pressure of approximately 30 mm Hg.
d. High pressure alarms may indicate that the patient is not receiving the prescribed tidal volume.

22. When auscultating the patient's breath sounds, the proper way to use the stethoscope is:
a. with the bell held firmly against the chest.
b. with the bell held lightly against the chest.
c. with the diaphragm held firmly against the chest.
d. with the bell held loosely against the chest to avoid friction.

ENDNOTES

1. Rau, J. (1988). *Respiratory Therapy Pharmacology*, 3rd edition. Chicago: Year Book Medical Publishers, p. 151.

2. Grimes, J., Burns, E. (1992). *Health Assessment in Nursing Practice*. 3d edition. Boston: Jones and Bartlett Publishers, Inc., pp. 269–274.

3. Barnes, T., Lisbon, A., Fulks, J. (1988). *Respiratory Practice*. Chicago: Year Book Medical Publishers, Inc., p. 159.

4. Ibid, p. 118.

5. Dal Nogare, A. (1989). Southwestern Internal Medicine Conference: Adult respiratory distress syndrome. *The American Journal of Medical Sciences* 298(6): 413–429.

6. Bernard, G., Luce, J., Serung, C., Rinaldo, J., Tate, R., Sibbold, W., Karimen, K., Higgins, S., Bradley, R., Metz, C., Harris, T., Brigham, K. (1987). High dose corticosteroids in patients with the adult respiratory distress syndrome. *The New England Journal of Medicine* 316(25): 1565–1570.

7. Shale, D. (1987). The adult respiratory distress syndrome—20 years on. *Thorax* 42: 641–645.

8. Ibid.

9. Dal Nogare, A., op. cit.

10. Petty, T. (1988). ARDS: Refinement of concept and redefinition. *American Review of Respiratory Disease* 138: 724.

11. Murray, J., Matthay, M., Luce, J., Flick, M. (1988). An expanded definition of adult respiratory distress syndrome. *American Review of Respiratory Disease* 138: 720–723.

12. Ibid.

13. Langlois, P., Gawryl, M. (1988). Accentuated formation of the terminal C56-9 complement complex in patient's plasma precedes development of the adult respiratory distress syndrome. *American Review of Respiratory Diseases* 138: 720–723.

14. Dal Nogare, A., op. cit.

15. Darovic, G. (1987). *Hemodynamic Monitoring. Invasive and Noninvasive Clinical Application*. Philadelphia: W. B. Saunders Company, pp. 287–320.

16. Ibid.

17. Holloway, N. (1984). *Nursing the Acutely Ill Adult*. 2nd edition. Menlo Park, California: Addison-Wesley Publishing Company, Inc., pp. 374–464.

18. Dal Nogare, A., op. cit.

19. Weilitz, P. (1989). New modes of mechanical ventilation. *Critical Care Nursing Clinics of North America* 1(4): 689–695.

20. Ibid.

21. Downs, J., Stock, M. (1987). Airway pressure release ventilation: A new concept in ventilatory support. *Critical Care Medicine* 15: 459.

22. Burns, S. (1990). Advances in ventilator therapy. *Focus on Critical Care* 17(3): 227–237.

23. Rossing, R., Slutsky, A., Lehr, J., Drinker, P., Kamm, R., Drazen, J. (1981). Tidal volume and frequency dependence of carbon dioxide elimination by high frequency ventilation. *New England Journal of Medicine* 301: 1375–1379.

24. Burns, S., op. cit.

25. Bradley, R. (1987). Adult respiratory distress syndrome. *Focus on Critical Care* 14(5): 48–59; Holloway, N., op. cit.; Rodman, G., Kirby, R. (1983). Post-traumatic respiratory failure: Role of fluid therapy. *Contemporary Anesthesia Practice* 6: 119–135; Petty, R., Fowler, A. (1982). Another look at ARDS. *Chest* 82: 98–104.

26. Bernard, G., et al., op. cit; Bone, R., Fisher, Jr., C., Clemmer, R., Slotman, G., Metz, C. (Methylprednisolone Severe Sepsis Study Group) (1987). Early methylprednisolone treatment for septic syndrome and the adult respiratory distress syndrome. *Chest* 92(6): 1032–1036; Luce, J., Montgomery, A., Marks, J., Turner, J., Metz, C., Murray, J. (1988). Ineffectiveness of high-dose methylprednisolone in preventing parenchymal lung injury and improving mortality in patients with septic shock. *American Review of Respiratory Disease* 138: 62–68; Dal Nogare, A., op. cit.

27. Cline, B., Fisher, M. (1982). ARDS means emergency. *Nursing 82*. 62–67. February.

28. Sielaff, J., Sugarman, H., Tatum, J., Kellum, J., Blocher, C. (1987). Treatment of porcine pseudomonas ARDS with combination drug therapy. *The Journal of Trauma* 27(12): 1313–1321.

29. Enhorning, G. (1989). Surfactant replacement in adult respiratory distress syndrome. *American Review of Respiratory Distress* 140: 281–283.

30. Brunner, L., Suddarth, D. (1986). *Lippincott Manual of Nursing Practice*. 4th edition. Philadelphia: J. P. Lippincott; Holloway, N. (1988). *Nursing the Critically Ill Adult*. 4th edition. Menlo Park, California: Addison-Wesley, pp. 154–278.

31. Luckman, J., Sorenson, K. (1987). *Medical-Surgical Nursing: A Psychophysiological Approach*. 3rd edition. Philadelphia: W. B. Saunders Company, pp. 1159–1384.

32. Brunner, L., Suddarth, D., op. cit.

33. Bullock, B., Rosendahl, P. (1988). *Pathophysiology: Adaptations and Alterations in Function*. 2nd edition. Glenview, Illinois: Scott-Foresman.

34. Ibid.

35. Ibid.

36. Kinney, M., Packa, D., Dunbar, S. (1988). *AACN's Clinical Reference for Critical Care Nursing*. 2nd edition. New York: McGraw-Hill, pp. 485–542.

37. Ibid.; Bullock, B., Rosendahl, P., op. cit.

38. Kinney, M., Packa, D., Dunbar, S., op. cit.

39. Bullock, B., Rosendahl, P., op. cit.; Kinney, M., Packa, D., Dunbar, S., op. cit.

40. Ibid.

41. Bullock, B., Rosendahl, P., op. cit.

42. Ibid.

43. Luchman, J., Sorensen, K., op. cit.

44. Kinney, M., Packa, D., Dunbar, S., op. cit.

45. Bullock, B., Rosendahl, P., op. cit.

46. Brunner, L., Suddarth, D., op. cit.

47. Holloway, N. (1988), op. cit.

48. Kinney, M., Packa, D., Dunbar, S., op. cit.

49. Govoni, L., Hayes, J. (1985). *Drugs and Nursing Implications*. Connecticut: Appleton-Century-Crofts.

50. Ibid.; Kinney, M., Packa, D., Dunbar, S., op. cit.

51. Brunner, L., Suddarth, D., op. cit.; Holloway, N., op. cit.; Kinney, M., Packa, D., Dunbar, S., op. cit.

52. Kinney, M., Packa, D., Dunbar, S., op. cit.

53. Kinney, M., Packa, D., Dunbar, S., op. cit.

54. Holloway, N. (1988), op. cit.

55. Kinney, M., Packa, D., Dunbar, S., op. cit.

56. Fishman, A. (1988). *Pulmonary Diseases and Disorders*. 2nd edition, volume 2. New York: McGraw-Hill Book Company, p. 1081.

57. Ibid.

58. Holloway, N. (1988), op. cit.

59. Fishman, A., op. cit., p. 1082.

60. Kinney, M., Packa, D., Dunbar, S., op. cit.

61. Besson, A., Saegesser, F. (1983). Chest trauma and associated injuries. In Oradell, N. (ed.). *Medical Economics* 1: 276–287.

62. McMahon, M. (1973). Hazards of central venous catheterization. *British Medical Journal* 3: 353; Bardosi, L., Mostafa, S., Wilkes, R., Wenstone, R. (1988). Contralateral haemothorax: A late complication of subclavian vein cannulation. *British Medical Journal* 60: 461–463; Templeton, P., Vainright, J., Rodriquez, A., Diaconis, J. (1988). Mediastinal tumors presenting as spontaneous hemothorax, simulating aortic dissection. *Chest* 93: 828–830; MacDonald, R., Kelly, J. (1975). Cervico-mediastinal hematoma following sneezing. *Anesthesia* 30: 50–53.

63. Hurn, P. (1988). Thoracic injuries. In Cardona, V., Hurn, P., Mason, P., Scanlon-Schlipp, A., Veise-Berry, S. (eds.). *Trauma Nursing From Resuscitation Through Rehabilitation.* Philadelphia: W. B. Saunders.

64. Kinney, M., Packa, D., Dunbar, S., op. cit., pp. 449–490.

65. Brunner, L., Suddarth, D., op. cit.

66. Hinshaw, H., Murray, J. (1980). *Diseases of the Chest.* Philadelphia: W. B. Saunders Company, p. 904.

67. Besson, A., Saegesser, F. (1983). *Color Atlas of Chest Trauma and Associated Injuries.* Oradell, New Jersey: Medical Economics Books, p. 249.

68. Lewis, S., Collier, I. (1983). *Medical-Surgical Nursing: Assessment and Management of Clinical Problems.* New York: McGraw-Hill Book Company, p. 489.

69. Hinshaw, H., Murray, J., op. cit., p. 905.

3 The Nervous System

CHAPTER 3 PRE-TEST

1. Impending or slow bleeding from a rupturing aneurysm or an arteriovenous malformation may be treated with:
   a. blood products and sedation.
   b. pentobarbital and steroids.
   c. Verapamil and Amicar.
   d. phenobarbital and mechanical ventilator–induced hypocarbia.

2. When eliciting a central pain response, which of the following choices is *not* considered acceptable nursing practice?
   a. supraorbital pressure
   b. pinching of nailbeds
   c. pinching of muscle tissue of extremities
   d. compression of achilles tendon

3. Drainage from the nose that is positive for glucose and accompanies a head injury indicates that the patient:
   a. had eaten just prior to the accident.
   b. has sustained a CSF leak.
   c. has diabetes mellitus.
   d. is suffering bacterial infection.

4. The blood-brain barrier is least permeable to:
   a. glucose.
   b. H_2O.
   c. electrolytes.
   d. gas molecules.

5. Which of the following would be contraindicated in a patient suffering increased intracranial pressure?
   a. osmotic diuretics
   b. steroids
   c. fluid limitation
   d. flat positioning

6. Which of the following is most likely to result in an increase in intracranial pressure?
   a. increased intrathoracic pressure
   b. hyperventilation
   c. mild hypovolemia
   d. increased intracranial compliance

7. Cerebral blood flow (CBF):
   a. normally varies greatly with changes in the blood pressure.
   b. increases when intracranial pressure is close to the mean arterial pressure.
   c. increases in response to a high pCO_2 due to vasodilation.
   d. decreases in response to a low pCO_2 due to vasoconstriction.

8. An intraventricular drain is preferable to a subarachnoid screw when:
   a. CSF needs to be drained off.
   b. it is placed in the epidural space.
   c. it has an internal transducer and therefore need not be calibrated.
   d. cerebral pressure is less than 50 mm Hg.

Overview of the Nervous System

The nervous system is the coordinating system of the body and is composed of the central nervous system (CNS, consisting of the brain and spinal cord) and the peripheral nervous system (the cranial nerves, the spinal nerves, and the autonomic nervous system, which includes the sympathetic and parasympathetic systems). The basic physiologic functions of this system are the transmission of nerve impulses and the initiation of reflex actions.

Anatomy and Physiology of the Nervous System

The nervous system is highly organized and developed to regulate and integrate activities affecting all systems of the body.

Cellular Structure of the Nervous System

The nervous system is composed of two basic types of cells: neurons and neuroglia. The neuron is the structural and basic functional unit of the nervous system. The average adult human brain contains more than 10 billion neurons and, after the age of 35, loses 100,000 neurons daily. The functions of neurons include the conduction of nerve impulses, the reception of impulses from other neurons, and the transference of information across the synaptic cleft to other neurons or muscle or organ cells.

Figure 3-1 presents structural details of neurons. Each neuron consists of a cell body, dendrites, and axons. The cell body performs the metabolic functions of the cell and includes fibers of various lengths. The dendrites are short branching fibers extending from the cell body, which receive and conduct impulses toward the cell body. As illustrated in Figure 3-1, the axons, which are single fibers, conduct impulses away from the cell body to a muscle or gland.

The second type of nervous system cell is the neuroglial cell. Neuroglial cells provide nourishment and structural support to the central nervous system. There are four main types of neuroglial cells: oligodendrocytes, astrocytes, ependymal cells, and microglial cells. Oligodendrocytes are support cells whose main function is the production of lipoprotein, which protects the axons and forms the myelin

sheath. The myelin sheath is a protein-lipid covering formed by Schwann cells, which encircle the axon except at periodic interruptions known as nodes of Ranvier (see Figure 3-1). The primary function of astrocytes (astroglia) is to provide nourishment and support for the neurons. Astrocytes contribute to the formation of the blood-brain barrier. Ependymal cells line the ventricular system and spinal cord and aid in the production of cerebrospinal fluid. Finally, the microglial cells are phagocytic cells that remove and digest waste products of the neurons.

A functional classification of neurons is based on the direction of the nerve impulses. Sensory neurons, called afferent neurons, carry impulses from receptors in the skin and sensory organs to the brain and spinal cord. Motor neurons, called efferent neurons, convey impulses from the brain and spinal cord to effector organs, muscles, or glands.

Physiology of Nerve Impulses

Membrane depolarization begins when a stimulus of sufficient magnitude, or threshold intensity, is applied to a neuron. A stimulus that excites a neuron and creates an impulse is called the action potential. As illustrated in Figure 3-2, depolarization causes an increased permeability of the cell membrane, resulting in an exchange of ions. Sodium ions flow into the cell while potassium ions move out. In myelinated nerves, impulses travel quickly, moving from one node of Ranvier to the next in saltatory conduction; nerve impulses conducted along unmyelinated axons travel continuously along the entire fiber and move more slowly. The time during which a nerve membrane is unable to be excited by another stimulus during depolarization is called the absolute refractory period. The period following the absolute refractory period, when an action potential can be produced with a stronger than normal stimulus, is called the relative refractory period. Following depolarization, the cell repolarizes and returns to its resting membrane potential.

Communication between adjacent neurons occurs at the synapse, where the axon of one neuron meets the dendrite, cell body, or axon of another neuron. The action potential of the presynaptic neuron causes the release of a neurotransmitter from the synaptic vesicles. Either an excitatory or inhibitory transmitter is secreted into the postsynaptic cleft. Acetylcholine, norepinephrine, dopamine, and serotonin are excitatory neurotransmitters, and gamma-aminobutyric acid (GABA) is an inhibitory neurotransmitter. Graded responses, in contrast to the all-or-nothing phenomenon associated with nerve impulse transmission, are produced in the postsyn-

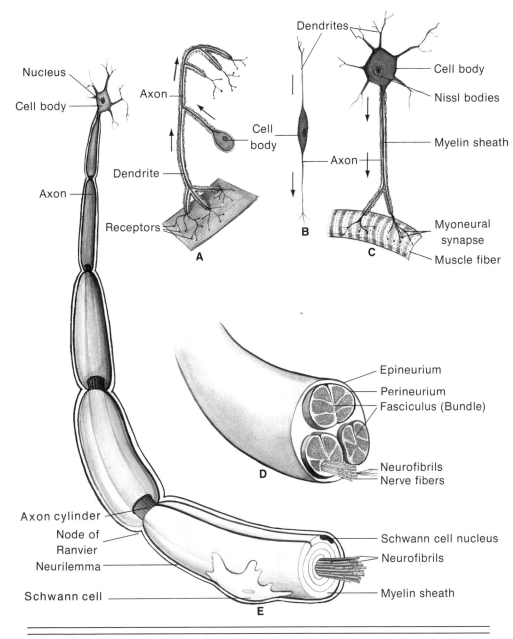

Figure 3-1 The Neuron. (A) monopolar sensory neuron, (B) bipolar retinal neuron, (C) multipolar motor neuron, showing a muscle-nerve synapse, (D) typical nerve structure, (E) enlarged extension of an axon.

aptic membrane, depending on the synaptic input received from the neurotransmitter. An excitatory neurotransmitter causes the membrane of the postsynaptic neuron to depolarize. An inhibitory neurotransmitter causes hyperpolarization, in which only the permeability to potassium and chloride is changed and the transmission of impulses is delayed. Excitatory postsynaptic potential (EPSP) refers to depolarizing responses, and inhibitory postsynaptic potential (IPSP) refers to hyperpolarizing responses.

Coverings of the Central Nervous System

Scalp

The scalp is composed of skin and hair, subcutaneous tissue, the galea aponeurotica (a thick band of fibrous tissue), and the pericranium. The subcutaneous tissue is vascular but has a poor vasoconstrictive capacity. The subgleal space is between the subcutaneous tissue and the pericranium and permits mobil-

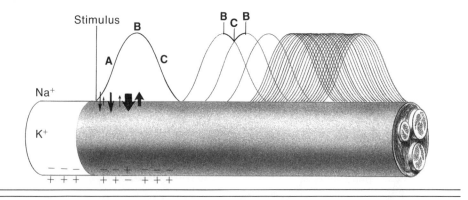

Figure 3-2   Conduction of a Nerve Impulse

ity of the scalp. The scalp protects the brain by helping to absorb some of the force of any external blow.

Skull

The skull is a bony framework composed of eight bones fused to form a solid, rigid unit (see Figures 3-3 and 3-4). The primary function of the cranium, the portion of the skull that encloses the brain, is protection. The bones that comprise the cranium are the frontal, parietal, temporal, occipital, ethmoid, and sphenoid bones. Behind the frontal bone is the eth-

moid, which houses the cribriform plate, where the olfactory nerve fibers exit the nasal cavity. The sphenoid bone, a wedge-shaped bone, resembles a bat's wings and separates the anterior and middle fossa of the brain. The sella turcica is a depression in the sphenoid bone that houses the pituitary gland.

Meninges

The meninges are membranes that encase and protect the brain and spinal cord. These membranes, illustrated in Figure 3-5, are the dura mater, arachnoid, and pia mater.

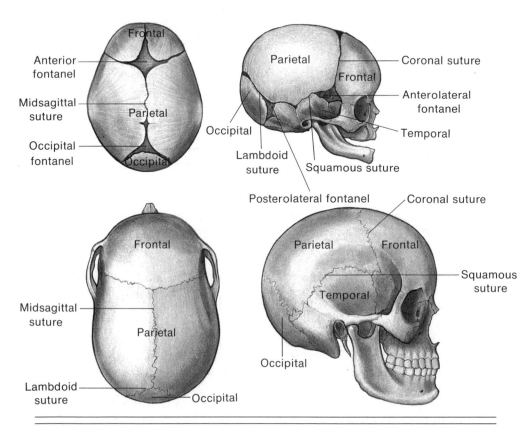

Figure 3-3   Superior and Lateral Views of Fetal and Adult Skulls

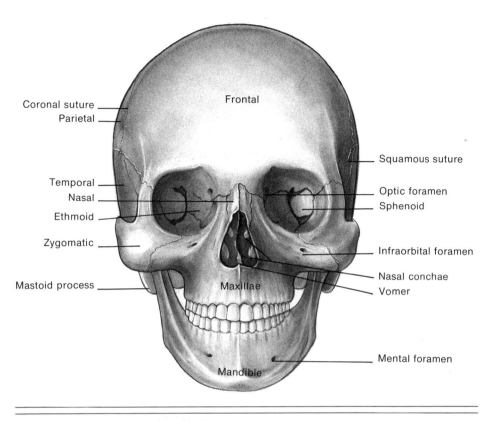

Figure 3-4   Frontal View of the Skull

The dense outermost layer is the dura mater, and it consists of two layers: the periosteal and the meningeal layers. The dura mater is a tough, semi-translucent, and inelastic membrane. Its outer layer forms the periosteum of the inner skull, and its meningeal layer is folded to create several compartments. Figure 3-5 also depicts how the venous channels that form the dural sinuses are situated between these two layers of the dura mater. Folds in the dura form the following anatomical landmarks of the brain:

Falx cerebri: descends vertically, separating the right and left cerebral hemispheres

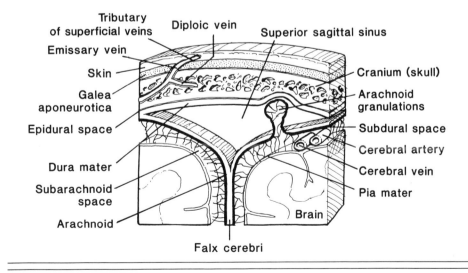

Figure 3-5   Membranes and Venous Channels of the Brain

Tentorium cerebelli: a double fold, tentlike in shape, separating the cerebral hemispheres from the cerebellum

Falx cerebelli: separates the two lateral lobes of the cerebellum

The middle meningeal layer is called the arachnoid. It is a delicate, fibrous, and elastic membrane between the dura mater and the pia mater. The subarachnoid space (SAS) between the arachnoid and the pia mater is a spongy, weblike structure filled with CSF.

The most delicate, vascular, and inner meningeal layer is the pia mater. The pia mater adheres closely to the entire surface of the brain.

The epidural (or extradural) space is a potential space between the outer layer of the dura and the skull. This potential space may become a real space as a result of epidural hematoma from laceration of the middle meningeal artery and/or skull fracture. A second potential space is the subdural, which lies between the dura mater and the arachnoid. Subdural hematomas, usually venous in origin, result from tearing of the dural veins and are also associated with head trauma.

Ventricular System

The ventricular system (illustrated in Figure 3-6) includes four large fluid chambers called ventricles: two lateral ventricles, the third ventricle, and the fourth ventricle. The lateral ventricles are the largest and extend into all the lobes of the brain. The fora-men of Monro is a small opening that connects the lateral ventricles and the third ventricle. The cerebral aqueduct of Sylvius, which is the narrowest passage for cerebrospinal fluid, connects the third and fourth ventricles. The fourth ventricle, the smallest, lies between the brainstem and the cerebellum. Cerebrospinal fluid exits the fourth ventricle through three openings. It flows through the two lateral foramina of Luschka and over the cerebral hemispheres. The foramen of Magendie routes the cerebrospinal fluid into the cisterna magna and around the spinal cord.

Cerebrospinal Fluid

Cerebrospinal fluid (CSF) is a clear, colorless, odorless fluid produced mainly in the choroid plexus (network of capillaries) of the ventricles. The normal ranges for characteristics of CSF are presented in Table 3-1. This fluid is constantly being produced at a rate of 20 cc per hour, or 500 cc per day, and circulates throughout the brain and spinal cord (see Figure 3-7). At any time, there will be 130–150 cc of CSF in the ventricular system. The entire volume will usually be replaced several times daily. The rate of production of CSF is influenced by cerebral metabolism, blood osmotic pressure, and hydrodynamic forces of blood flow. Arachnoid villi are projections into the dural venous sinuses that reabsorb the CSF into the superior sagittal sinus. The movement of CSF is affected by hydrostatic pressure and active transport mechanisms.

The functions of CSF are to support and protect

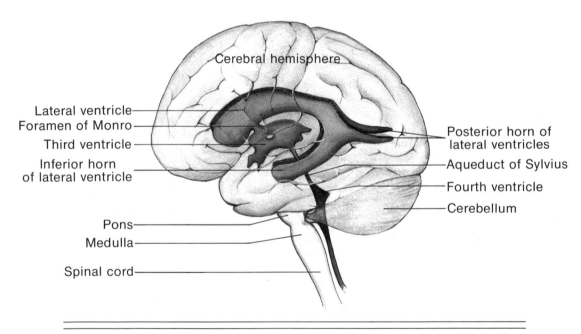

Figure 3-6   The Ventricular System

Table 3-1 Normal Ranges of Characteristics of Cerebrospinal Fluid

Characteristic	Normal Range
Appearance	Clear, colorless, odorless
Protein composition	15–45 mg/100 mL
Glucose	50–70 mg/100 mL
WBC count	0–5 cells/mm
pH	7.35–7.40
Specific gravity	1.005–1.009
Pressure	70–200 mm H$_2$O
Culture	Negative

the brain and spinal cord, maintain homeostasis of the CNS, and compensate for changes in intracranial volume and pressure. The blood–cerebrospinal fluid barrier is a special mechanism between the CSF and the blood to promote the entry of needed substances and prevent the entry of harmful substances.

Cerebral Circulation

Cerebral blood flow is vital for normal brain function. Brain tissue undergoes irreversible changes very quickly when deprived of adequate blood supply. The brain normally receives 750 mL (or 15% of the cardiac output) of blood every minute. Cerebral blood flow is maintained by several protective responses. Autoregulation helps to maintain a constant flow by altering the diameter of resistance of arterioles over a range of perfusion pressures. Cere-

bral blood flow is increased when the carbon dioxide concentration of the blood becomes elevated, causing a vasodilation of the cerebral vessels, thereby increasing blood flow and removing carbon dioxide. Brain ischemia is a strong stimulus that also triggers a vasodilation mechanism to increase cerebral blood flow in order to maintain adequate perfusion.

Cerebral circulation is portrayed in Figure 3-8. The brain receives arterial blood from two pairs of arteries: internal carotids and vertebral arteries. Both of these anastomose at the base of the brain in the circle of Willis, providing a mechanism for collateral circulation.

The anterior cerebral circulation comprises the internal carotid arteries. The common carotid branches at the level of the thyroid to form the external and internal carotid arteries. The internal carotid enters the cranial cavity of the petrous portion of the temporal bone and passes through the cavernous sinus and sphenoid bone before merging into the circle of Willis. Larger cerebral vessels arising from the internal carotid include the anterior communicating, the anterior cerebral, the middle cerebral, and the posterior communicating arteries (see Figure 3-9). The middle cerebral artery is the largest branch of the internal carotid artery and provides two-thirds of the blood supply to the cerebral hemispheres. The posterior communicating artery branches from the internal carotid artery and connects with the posterior cerebral artery.

The posterior cerebral circulation comprises the vertebral arteries. The vertebral arteries arise from the subclavian arteries and enter the skull through the foramen magnum. Vessels arising from the ver-

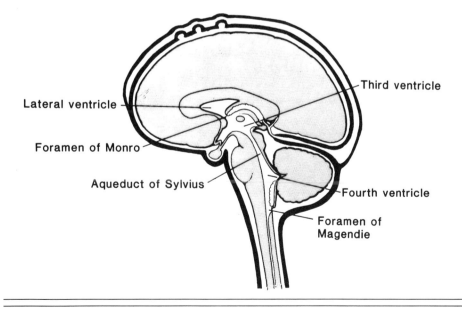

Figure 3-7 Circulation of Cerebrospinal Fluid

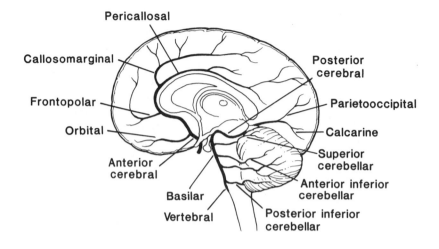

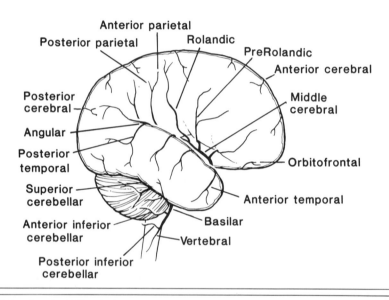

Figure 3-8 Cerebral Circulation

tebral arteries include the anterior and posterior spinal arteries as well as the posterior inferior artery. At the lower border of the pons, the vertebral arteries merge to form the basilar artery. The basilar artery gives off the anterior and posterior inferior cerebellar arteries, the pontine branches, the superior cerebellar artery, and the posterior cerebral artery.

Venous Drainage

Venous drainage is provided by the venous sinuses and the superficial and deep cerebral veins (see Figure 3-10). In cerebral venous drainage no valves are involved, and drainage occurs mainly through the dural sinuses and the vascular channels created by the two dural layers. Venous blood is emptied into the internal jugular vein and returned to the systemic circulation.

The superior sagittal sinus originates in the frontal lobe and lies along the border of the falx cerebri. The inferior sagittal sinus travels along the border of the falx cerebri and joins the straight sinus. The straight sinus is a continuation of the great cerebral vein that joins the superior sagittal sinus. Transverse sinuses are continuations of the superior sagittal sinus and travel laterally along the skull to the internal jugular. Other sinuses include cavernous, circular, superior petrosal, inferior petrosal, basilar, sphenoparietal, and occipital.

Superficial cerebral veins cover the surface of the cerebral hemispheres and include the superior cerebral, superficial middle cerebral, and inferior cerebral veins. The deep cerebral veins lie beneath the corpus callosum and include the basal, internal cerebral, and great cerebral veins.

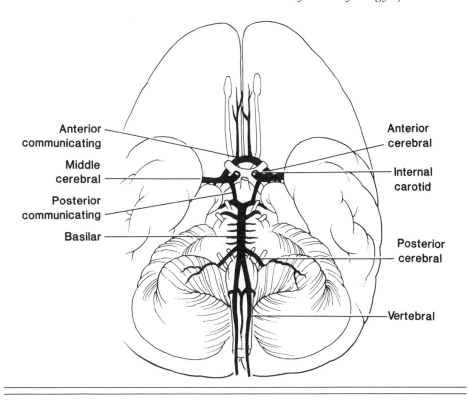

Figure 3-9 Basilar and Internal Carotid Arteries

Blood-Brain Barrier

The blood-brain barrier functions as a protective mechanism and maintains a homeostatic environment for the neurons. It consists of a network of capillary endothelial cells and astroglial cells. Movement of substances to the brain depend on particle size, lipid solubility, chemical dissociation, and protein-binding potential. Substances such as water, carbon dioxide, oxygen, and glucose easily cross the blood-brain barrier; the uptake of ions is much slower. Alterations in the blood-brain barrier caused by brain injury, certain drugs, tumors, or toxic substances may result in an increased permeability.

Cerebral Cortex

The cerebral cortex is the largest and most highly developed part of the brain. It is composed of two cerebral hemispheres (left and right) and four pairs of lobes (frontal, parietal, temporal, and occipital). The outer layer is composed of gray matter (neurons), and the inner layer of white matter (nerve fibers).

Cerebral Hemispheres

The surface of the cerebral hemispheres is increased by folds and convolutions called gyri. Sulci are the shallow grooves on the surface of the brain.

Fissures (deep sulci) are the large separations in the cerebral hemispheres (see Figure 3-11). The following are important anatomical landmarks in neuroanatomy:

> Longitudinal fissure: separates left and right hemispheres
> Lateral fissure of Sylvius: separates temporal lobe from frontal and parietal lobes
> Central fissure of Rolando: separates frontal lobe from parietal lobe
> Parieto-occipital fissure: separates occipital lobe from parietal and temporal lobes

It is generally accepted that in most people one side of the brain (the dominant hemisphere) is more highly developed. The left hemisphere is more involved in verbal, linguistic, arithmetic, and analytic functions. The right hemisphere is more involved with nonverbal skills, spatial-visual association, musical abilities, and holistic functioning. A large percentage of the population has a highly developed left hemisphere and is right-handed. In most cases, but not always, left-handed people have a right dominant hemisphere. Severe damage to the dominant hemisphere in an adult results in severe neurological deficits.

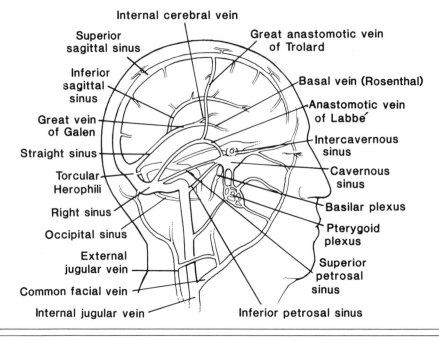

Figure 3-10 Venous Drainage of the Brain

The corpus callosum is the bundle of thick nerve fibers that connects the cerebral hemispheres.

Frontal Lobes

The frontal lobes are divided into the motor cortex, the premotor area, the prefrontal area, and Broca's area. The motor cortex lies anterior to the central fissure and transmits impulses that control fine voluntary motor activity (corticospinal tract). The spatial arrangement of the motor cortex is illustrated in Figure 3-12, where the positioning of body parts indicates the specific areas of the motor cortex that innervate them. The premotor area lies immediately anterior to the motor cortex and is involved in extrapyramidal motor control. The prefrontal area lies in the anterior portion of the frontal lobe and influences higher intellectual functions such as attention, abstract thinking, judgment, ethics, memory, and emotional responses as well as autonomic functions associated with emotional responses. The prefrontal areas are important to maintaining the individual's focus of attention and help to establish long-term memory.[1] Broca's area is located at the base of the motor cortex in the inferior frontal gyrus. This area is involved with the motor activities in the formulation of speech. Damage to Broca's area in the dominant hemisphere results in expressive aphasia.

Parietal Lobes

The parietal lobes are located posterior to the central fissure of Rolando (see Figure 3-11). The parietal lobes are responsible for processing sensory information in the primary sensory cortex. The arrangement of the primary sensory cortex resembles that of the motor cortex (see Figure 3-12). Sensory association areas analyze specific sensory information from the thalamus. The parietal lobes interpret size, shape (stereognosis), weight, texture, consistency, and two-point discrimination. They also play an important role in the awareness of body parts and spatial orientation. Touch, awareness of position (proprioception), pressure, and vibration are identified in the parietal lobes. Damage to the parietal lobes causes perceptual deficits such as agnosia (inability to interpret sensory input) and body neglect (common in stroke patients).

Temporal Lobes

Also illustrated in Figure 3-11 are the temporal lobes, which are located inferior to the lateral fissure of Sylvius. They are mainly involved in the interpretation of hearing, taste, smell, and balance. Wernicke's area is located in the parietal and temporal lobes and is a primary auditory receptive area. This area controls the comprehension and meaning of the spoken and written language. Damage to

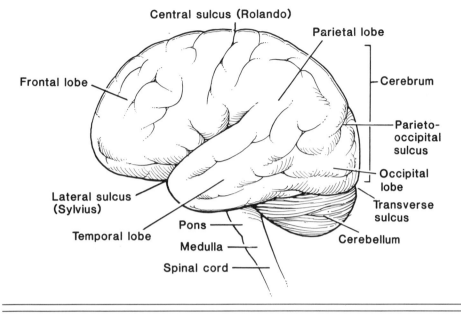

Figure 3-11   Cerebral Sulci and Lobes

Wernicke's area may cause receptive aphasia. In the primary auditory areas, sounds are received and interpreted. There is an integration of auditory, visual, and somatic impulses in the association areas.

Occipital Lobes

The occipital lobes are superior to the cerebellum and contain primary visual association areas and primary receptive areas for vision. Visual association

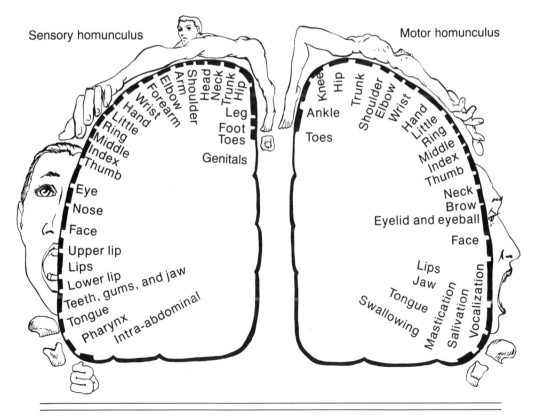

Figure 3-12   Sensory and Motor Areas of the Cortex

allows identification and recognition of objects. Damage to the visual association areas results in the inability to recognize and identify objects (visual agnosia).

Limbic System

The limbic system (rhinencephalum) is located at the border of the lateral ventricle on the medial surface of each cerebral hemisphere. Its major functions are primitive behaviors, personality, expression of emotions, instincts, sexual desire, and recent memory.

Diencephalon

The diencephalon includes the thalamus, the hypothalamus, the subthalamus, and the epithalamus.

The thalamus consists of two large oval masses of gray matter that form the lateral wall of the third ventricle. It acts as a final relay station and processing center for all ascending and descending sensory impulses (except for olfactory pathways). Therefore, the thalamus is responsible for coordinating and regulating the activities of the cerebral cortex. Additional activities include involvement of the limbic system and the reticular activating system and perception of sensations, such as pain, touch, pressure, and temperature.

The hypothalamus forms the base of the diencephalon and is located near the pituitary gland and above the midbrain. The hypothalamus is connected to the pituitary gland by the pituitary stalk. The optic chiasm, located at the floor of the hypothalamus, is where the optic tracts cross. Functions of the hypothalamus include regulation of activity of the autonomic nervous system, temperature regulation, maintenance of water balance through regulation of the antidiuretic hormone (ADH), control of appetite, release of hormones of the pituitary gland, emotional response, sexual activity, and influences on the reticular activating system. In summary, the hypothalamus can be described as being involved with homeostasis of the internal environment of the body and behavior patterns.

The subthalamus is located below the thalamus and internal capsule. The subthalamus is involved in the voluntary motor activities.

The epithalamus forms a thin roof over the third ventricle. The pineal body (epiphysis) is a part of the epithalamus. The pineal body is diagnostically useful because it is a midline structure and its calcification is usually radiopaque.

Basal Ganglia

The basal ganglia are several masses of gray matter located deep in the cerebral hemispheres (see Figure 3-13). Each basal ganglion includes the caudate nucleus, claustrum (both components of basal ganglia development), amygdaloid body, and lentiform nucleus (globus pallidus and putamen). Corpus striatum refers to the lenticular nucleus and caudate nuclei.

The structures that comprise the basal ganglia are associated with the extrapyramidal system. The exact function is unknown; however, the basal ganglia are believed to act as a relay station between the cerebral motor cortex and the thalamus. Dysfunction in the basal ganglia is associated with neurotransmitter disorders such as Parkinson's disease and Huntington's disease and movement disorders such as chorea and athetosis.

Internal Capsule

The internal capsule is a band of white fibers located between the thalamus and the basal ganglia (see Figure 3-14). The internal capsule consists of fiber tracts ascending and descending from the cerebral cortex. Demyelinating diseases and hemorrhagic cerebrovascular accidents are pathological conditions commonly involving the internal capsule.

Cerebellum

The cerebellum is located in the posterior fossa, posterior to the pons and the medulla. The cerebellum is attached to the brainstem by three paired bundles of nerve fibers, which transmit and receive nerve impulses: the inferior peduncles, the middle peduncles, and the superior peduncles. The cerebellum is composed of the cortex, a gray outer covering; the connecting pathways, which consist of white matter; and four pairs of deep cerebellar nuclei (dentate, globose, emboliform, and fastigia). The cerebellum is primarily involved with the coordination of muscular activity. It influences the reflexes for regulation of muscle tone, maintenance of equilibrium and posture, and voluntary movement. Cerebellar control is ipsilateral; that is, the right side of the cerebellum controls the right side of the body, and the left side of the cerebellum controls the left side of the body. Injury to the cerebellum may cause cerebellar ataxia, hypotonia, abnormal postural reflexes, tremors, past pointing, inability to perform rapid alternating movements, speech disturbances, and nystagmus.

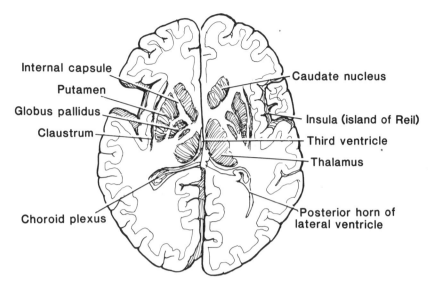

Horizontal sections through cerebrum at two levels to show basal ganglia

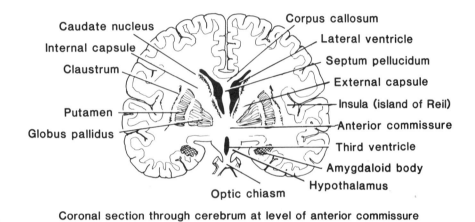

Coronal section through cerebrum at level of anterior commissure

Figure 3-13 Basal Ganglia

Brainstem

The brainstem is divided into three major areas: midbrain (mesencephalon), pons (metencephalon), and medulla oblongata (myelencephalon).

The reticular activating system (RAS) extends from the lower brainstem to the cerebral cortex. The RAS is involved in the regulation of cycles of sleep and wakefulness. It plays an important role in maintaining wakefulness and directing attention to specific areas of mental activity.

Midbrain

The midbrain is a short segment of the brainstem between the diencephalon and the pons. The nuclei of cranial nerves III and IV, the red nucleus, and the substantia nigra are located in the midbrain. The roof of the midbrain holds the tectum, which is composed of the superior colliculi (involved with the optic system) and the inferior colliculi (involved with the auditory system). Large bundles of fibers called cerebral peduncles pass through the midbrain.

Pons

The pons is located between the midbrain and the medulla. The nuclei of cranial nerves V through VIII are situated in the pons, and various ascending and descending fiber tracts pass through the pons. The pattern of respiration is influenced by the pons.

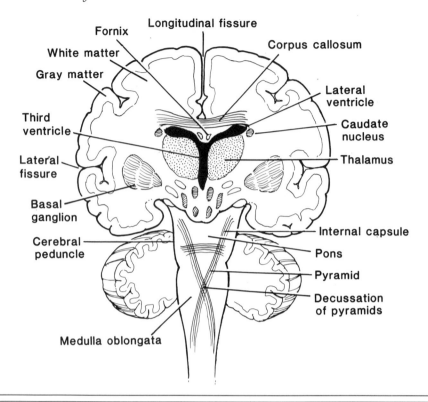

Figure 3-14   Coronal Section of the Brain

Medulla Oblongata

The medulla oblongata is the last division of the brain, extending from the pons and becoming continuous with the spinal cord. The nuclei of cranial nerves IX through XII, along with ascending and descending fiber tracts, are located in the medulla. Centers involved in the control of swallowing, vomiting, respiration, and vasomotor activity are also located in the medulla. It is in the medulla that the majority of the tracts decussate, or cross to the opposite side, and descend the spinal cord.

Table 3-2 gives the structure and function of the primary divisions of the brain.

Peripheral Nervous System

The peripheral nervous system includes the spinal nerves, the cranial nerves, and the autonomic nervous system.

Spinal Nerves

There are 31 pairs of spinal nerves, all of which originate in dorsal and ventral root fibers of the spinal cord: 8 pairs arise in the cervical region, 12 in the thoracic, 5 in the lumbar, 5 in the sacral, and 1 in the coccygeal. The dorsal root fibers are sensory, and the ventral root fibers are motor. All spinal nerves leave the vertebral canal by passing between adja-

cent vertebrae and then immediately branch into two rami: the dorsal (posterior) ramus that supplies segments of the skin, bones, joints, and muscles of the back, and the ventral (anterior) ramus that supplies segments of the trunk and limbs.

At the cervical, lumbar, and sacral levels, elaborate networks of nerves carrying fibers of neurons from several spinal cord segments at once are formed. These networks are called plexuses (see Figure 3-15). They are described below.

Cervical plexus: The cervical plexus is formed by the ventral rami of the top four cervical nerves. The phrenic nerve (which controls the diaphragm) originates from the cervical plexus, and injuries to this region may result in respiratory paralysis. Frequently, the phrenic nerve is "nicked" in an effort to arrest reflex disorders such as hiccups.

Brachial plexus: The axillary, median, radial, and ulnar nerves originate in the brachial plexus, which stems from the ventral rami of the fifth through eighth cervical nerves and the first thoracic nerve. Damage to this region results in various disorders of the upper extremities.

Lumbar plexus: The lumber plexus originates in the ventral rami of the second through fourth lumbar nerves. The femoral nerve arises from

Table 3-2 Structure and Function of Major Divisions of the Brain

Brain Part	Subdivisions	Structure or Location	Function
Cerebrum	Telencephalon	Largest part of brain; made up of two hemispheres, each divided into four lobes	Provides for sensations, emotions, voluntary actions, mental processes and consciousness
	Basal ganglia	Masses of gray matter located deep in cerebral hemispheres	Extrapyramidal motor activity
Cerebellum	Cortex Connecting pathways Nuclei	Second largest part of brain; composed of both gray and white matter	Coordination, equilibrium, synchronized muscle movement
Diencephalon	Thalamus	There is a right and a left thalamus; made up of many cell bodies of neurons	Acts as relay station for sensory input; association of sensations and emotions
	Hypothalamus	Lies under the thalamus; one of smallest structures of the brain	Helps control many of the internal organs and vital functions; helps control endocrine performance; controls the waking state
Brainstem	Mesencephalon (midbrain)	Lies between pons and diencephalon, is connected to the cerebellum by the superior cerebellar peduncle	Some motor and sensory functions, as well as visual and auditory pathways
	Pons	Lies between the midbrain and medulla	Houses some motor and sensory pathways
	Medulla	Located at terminal portions of brainstem	Contains all the vital centers and is responsible for respiration, heartbeat, and blood pressure; contains sensory and motor pathways
	Reticular formation (reticular activating system)	Diffuse network of fibers that project from brainstem to cortex	Ascending formation controls wakefulness and sleep; descending formation inhibits or enhances neurons controlling skeletal muscle activity

this plexus. Injury to this area results in hip and leg disorders.

Sacral plexus: The ventral rami of the fourth and fifth lumbar nerves and the first through fourth sacral nerves form the sacral plexus. The sciatic, peroneal, tibial, and pudendal nerves originate in this region. Injury to this area results in various disorders below the waist. An overview of these plexuses is provided in Table 3-3.

Cranial Nerves

There are 12 pairs of cranial nerves, which exit through the foramen of the skull (see Figure 3-16). Cranial nerves I (olfactory) and II (optic) are nerve fiber tracts and not true nerves. Each cranial nerve is classified as sensory, motor, autonomic, or some combination of these. Table 3-4 gives the classification and function of each cranial nerve.

Olfactory nerve (I) Sensory fibers innervating nasal mucous membranes pass through the cribriform plate to the olfactory bulb in the frontal lobe. Receptors in the nasal mucosa are responsible for smell. Injury to the olfactory nerve results in loss of the sense of smell (anosmia).

Optic nerve (II) The optic nerve contains fibers arising from the retina, which pass through the optic foramen to the brainstem. The two optic nerves meet at the optic chiasm, where some fibers decussate. These fibers continue as optic tracts to the occipital cortex. The optic nerve is a sensory nerve concerned with vision, specifically relating to retinal rods and cones. Injury to the optic nerve causes visual deficits and blindness.

Oculomotor nerve (III) The oculomotor nerve arises from the midbrain and travels close to the internal carotid artery in the cavernous sinus. The

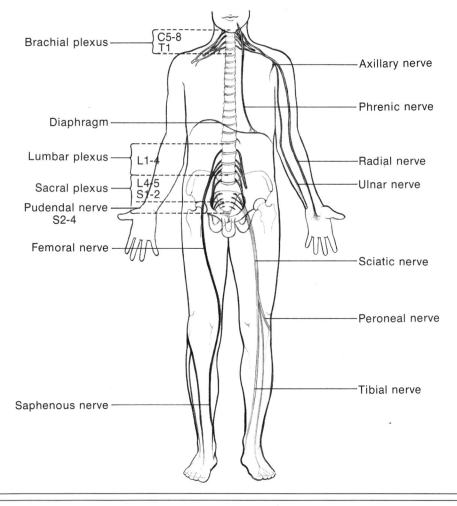

Brachial plexus — [C5-8 / T1]

Axillary nerve

Phrenic nerve

Diaphragm

Lumbar plexus — [L1-4]

Radial nerve

Ulnar nerve

Sacral plexus — [L4/5 / S1-2]

Pudendal nerve S2-4

Femoral nerve

Sciatic nerve

Peroneal nerve

Tibial nerve

Saphenous nerve

Figure 3-15 The Spinal Plexuses

oculomotor nerve innervates the muscle (levator palpebrae superioris) that elevates the upper eyelid and constricts the pupil (sphincter pupillae of the iris) in response to light and accommodation (ciliaries of the lens). The oculomotor nerve also innervates four of the six muscles responsible for movement of the eyeball. Such movement is controlled in the following manner: medial recti control medial and inward movements; superior recti, upward movements; inferior recti, downward movements; and inferior oblique recti, upward and outward movements. Injury to the oculomotor nerve may cause ptosis (drooping of the upper eyelid), loss of ability to adduct the eye, and loss of pupillary constriction. Abnormal pupillary dilation may occur with interruption of the parasympathetic nerves as a result of brainstem compression or an intracranial lesion.

Trochlear nerve (IV) The trochlear nerve arises from the midbrain posterior to the oculomotor nuclei. The trochlear nerve innervates the superior oblique muscle of the eyeball, which allows downward and inward eye movements. Injury to the trochlear nerve causes an impairment of the downward gaze.

Trigeminal nerve (V) Sensory and motor fibers from the trigeminal nerve arise in the pons and are the largest cranial nerves. The motor component supplies the muscles of mastication (temporalis and masseter), corneal reflex, and jaw reflex. The three sensory divisions are the ophthalmic, maxillary, and mandibular branches. The ophthalmic branch conveys sensation to the eyes, lacrimal gland, paranasal sinuses, nasal mucosa, nose, and forehead. The maxillary branch conveys sensation to the skin of the nose, the upper jaw, the teeth, the upper lip, the cheeks, the hard palate, the maxillary sinuses, and the nasal mucosa. The mandibular branch conveys sensation to the meninges, the lower lip, the chin, the ear, the mucous membranes, the lower jaw, and the tongue. Injury to the trigeminal nerve may cause

Table 3-3 The Cervical, Brachial, Lumbar, and Sacral Plexuses

Plexus	Origin	Principal Nerve(s)	Result of Damage
Cervical	C1–4	Phrenic	Respiratory paralysis; death
Brachial	C5–8; T1	Axillary	Weakened abduction and rotation of arm
		Median	Impaired flexion and abduction of hand; loss of flexion and abduction of thumb and index finger; loss of thumb apposition
		Radial	Wristdrop
		Ulnar	Clawhand
Lumbar	L2–4	Femoral	Loss of extension of leg and flexion at hip
			Lumbago—inflammation
Sacral	L4–5; S1–4	Sciatic	Loss of extension at hip and flexion at knee
			Sciatica—inflammation
		Peroneal	Footdrop

difficulty in chewing, deviation of the jaw, loss of facial sensations, and loss of the corneal reflex. Trigeminal neuralgia (tic douloureux) is an extremely painful condition that occurs along the maxillary and mandibular branches from pressure on the nerve.

Abducens nerve (VI) The abducens nerve arises from the lower border of the pons and enters the orbit with cranial nerves III and IV. The abducens nerve innervates the lateral rectus muscle and rotates the eyeball outward (laterally). Injury to the abducens nerve results in a loss of ability to turn the eye laterally.

Facial nerve (VII) The facial nerve arises from the lower border of the pons and exits the cranium

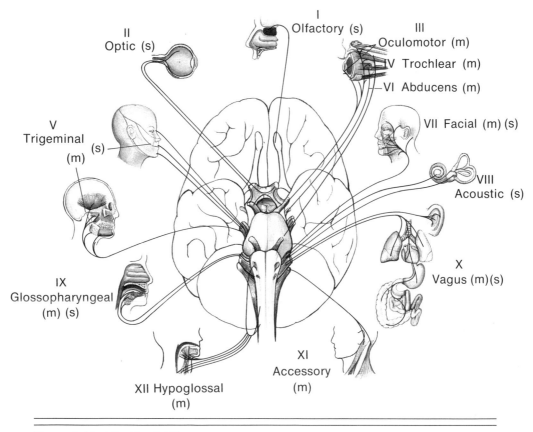

Figure 3-16 The Cranial Nerves

Table 3-4 Classification and Function of Cranial Nerves

Number	Name	Classification	Function
I	Olfactory	Sensory	Carries impulses of smell to the brain
II	Optic	Sensory	Special nerve of the sense of sight
III	Oculomotor	Motor and autonomic	Concerned with contraction of most of the eye muscles (the extrinsics)
IV	Trochlear	Motor	Supplies motor fibers for movement of the superior oblique muscle of the eye
V	Trigeminal	Motor and sensory	Largest cranial nerve and chief sensory nerve of the face and head; motor fibers extend to the muscles of mastication
VI	Abducens	Motor	Supplies motor fibers to the lateral rectus muscle of the eye
VII	Facial	Sensory and motor	Sensory fibers supply the anterior two-thirds of the tongue (taste) and the lacrimal and salivary glands; motor fibers supply the muscles of facial expression
VIII	Acoustic (Vestibulocochlear)	Sensory	Contains sense fibers for hearing and balance (semicircular canals of the internal ear)
IX	Glossopharyngeal	Sensory, motor, and autonomic	Sensory fibers supply the posterior third of the tongue (taste), tonsils, and pharynx; motor fibers control the swallowing muscles in the pharynx
X	Vagus	Sensory, motor, and autonomic	Longest cranial nerve and only one to leave the cranial region; motor and sensory fibers innervate most of the organs of the thoracic and abdominal cavities; the nerve acts as a cardiac inhibitor and bronchial constrictor
XI	Accessory	Motor	Controls the major trapezius and sternocleidomastoid muscles of the neck
XII	Hypoglossal	Motor	Controls movements of the tongue

through the internal acoustic meatus. The sensory component of the facial nerve innervates the taste buds of the anterior two-thirds of the tongue, as well as certain salivary and lacrimal glands. The motor fibers of the facial nerve innervate all muscles of the face involved in facial expressions and eyelid closure. Injury to the facial nerve causes a paralysis of the facial muscles (Bell's palsy) associated with a loss of ability to close the eyelid, a loss of taste in the anterior portion of the tongue, and decreased tearing and salivation.

Acoustic nerve (VIII) The acoustic nerve enters the cranial cavity through the internal acoustic meatus and arises from the brainstem behind the middle cerebellar peduncle. The acoustic nerve has two branches: cochlear and vestibular. The cochlear division is involved in hearing, and the vestibular division is associated with maintaining equilibrium and coordinating head and eye movements. Injury to the cochlear branch causes deafness, and injury to the

vestibular branch causes vertigo, tinnitus, nausea, and nystagmus.

Glossopharyngeal nerve (IX) The glossopharyngeal nerve arises from the medulla and includes sensory, motor, and autonomic components. The sensory component innervates taste on the posterior third of the tongue, the pharynx, and the soft palate. Special receptors in the carotid body and carotid sinus influence control of respiration, blood pressure, and the heart. There is also parasympathetic innervation of the parotid glands. The motor component participates with the vagus nerve in the swallowing mechanism. Injury to the glossopharyngeal nerve causes an impairment of sensation in the palate and the pharynx, which results in difficulty in swallowing. Such injury is also associated with a loss of sense of taste in the posterior part of the tongue and a disturbance of the carotid body and carotid sinus.

Vagus nerve (X) The vagus nerve arises in the medulla and is the only cranial nerve that travels beyond the neck through the thorax to the abdomen. The vagus receives sensory fibers from the external ear, the auditory canal, and the tympanic membrane. Sensory and motor fibers innervate abdominal and thoracic organs, pharynx, larynx, and trachea. Many of the parasympathetic fibers are innervated by the vagus, which controls swallowing, speech, and movement of the pharynx and soft palate. Injury to the vagus results in difficulty in swallowing, impairment of voice, and autonomic disturbances.

Spinal accessory nerve (XI) The spinal accessory nerve arises from the lower medulla and upper cervical spinal cord. Motor fibers supply the upper trapezius and sternocleidomastoid muscles and allow shoulder shrugging and head movement. Some fibers in association with the vagus supply motor nerves for swallowing and speech. Injury causes an impairment in the ability to rotate the head and raise the shoulder of the affected side.

Hypoglossal nerve (XII) The motor fibers of the hypoglossal nerve originate in the medulla. The hypoglossal nerve innervates the muscles of the tongue and is important in speech, mastication, and swallowing. Therefore, injury causes difficulty with speaking, chewing, and swallowing.

Autonomic Nervous System

The autonomic nervous system (ANS) is also referred to as the involuntary nervous system. As the name implies, it is responsible for maintaining homeostasis of the internal environment at an unconscious level. A developing body of science pertinent to this area is biofeedback, enabling humans to learn to control emotional responses that trigger physiological responses.

The two major divisions of the ANS are the sympathetic and the parasympathetic (see Figure 3-17). The sympathetic and parasympathetic divisions are activated by the higher cortical centers and the spinal cord. The body's internal environment is regulated by dual innervation except for the sweat glands, certain blood vessels to skeletal muscles, and the adrenals. The two neuron chains of the ANS are as follows:

> Preganglionic neuron: the presynaptic neuron that is located in the brainstem or spinal cord
>
> Postganglionic neuron: the postsynaptic neuron that is located in an outlying ganglion or sympathetic chain and innervates a designated organ

Sympathetic division The sympathetic division arises from the lateral horns of the gray matter of the spinal cord between T1 and L2. Figure 3-18 shows the general organization of the sympathetic nervous system. Short preganglionic fibers leave the spinal nerve and pass through the white ramus into one of the ganglia of the sympathetic chain. At the sympathetic chain, the preganglionic fibers synapse with postganglionic fibers, travel upward and downward in the chain to synapse at higher or lower levels, pass through the chain and synapse in an outlying sympathetic ganglion, or pass through the chain and travel to the adrenal medulla without synapsing.

Many long postganglionic fibers originating from the sympathetic trunk or outlying ganglia travel through the gray rami before reaching the designated organ. As a general guideline, sympathetic outflow is distributed as follows: the sympathetic fibers from T1 generally pass up the sympathetic chain into the head; those from T2 into the neck; those from T3, T4, T5, and T6 into the thorax; those from T7, T8, T9, T10, and T11 into the abdomen; and those from T12, L1, and L2 into the legs.[2]

Parasympathetic division The parasympathetic system is commonly referred to as the craniosacral system. Preganglionic neurons exit the gray matter of the brainstem via the cranial nerves (III, VII, IX, and X) and the sacral segments of the spinal cord (S2, S3, and S4). Most preganglionic neurons have long axons that run without interruption until they synapse with postganglionic neurons peripherally or on visceral structures. In contrast to the sympathetic system, the parasympathetic system has long preganglionic neurons and (usually) short postganglionic neurons.

Preganglionic neurons of the parasympathetic system include the vagus nerve (75% of the activity), which innervates the thoracic (heart and lungs) and abdominal viscera. The pelvic nerve innervates the descending colon, rectum, bladder, lower ureters, and external genitalia affecting sexual activity. Parasympathetic fibers of the third cranial nerve (oculomotor) supply constrictor, sphincter, and ciliary muscles of the eye. Fibers of the seventh cranial nerve (facial) innervate the lacrimal, submandibular, sublingual, nasal, oral, and pharyngeal muscles. Fibers of the ninth cranial nerve (glossopharyngeal) innervate the parotid gland.

Physiology of the autonomic nervous system The ANS is the locus of the fight or flight phenomenon. The sympathetic system is more active during stressful situations, corresponding to the fight response. Release of norepinephrine from the postganglionic neurons mobilizes body responses. Heart rate and blood pressure are increased, the coronary arteries dilate, the bronchioles of the lung dilate and secre-

254

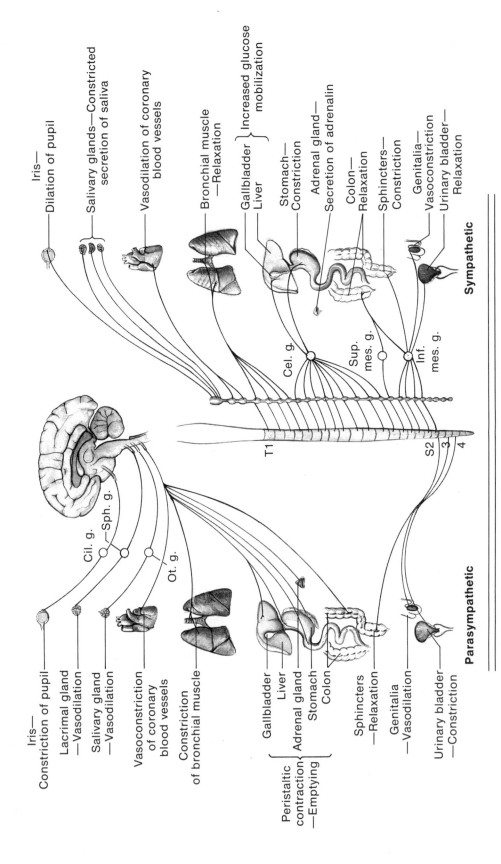

Iris—
Dilation of pupil

Salivary glands—Constricted
secretion of saliva

Vasodilation of coronary
blood vessels

Bronchial muscle
—Relaxation

Gallbladder
Liver } Increased glucose
mobilization

Stomach—
Constriction

Adrenal gland—
Secretion of adrenalin

Colon—
Relaxation

Sphincters—
Constriction

Genitalia—
Vasoconstriction

Urinary bladder—
Relaxation

Sympathetic

Cel. g.

Sup.
mes. g.

Inf.
mes. g.

T1

S2
3
4

Sph. g.

Cil. g.

Ot. g.

Parasympathetic

Iris—
Constriction of pupil

Lacrimal gland
—Vasodilation

Salivary gland
—Vasodilation

Vasoconstriction
of coronary
blood vessels

Constriction
of bronchial muscle

Gallbladder
Liver
Adrenal gland
Stomach
Colon } Peristaltic
contraction
—Emptying

Sphincters
—Relaxation

Genitalia
—Vasodilation

Urinary bladder
—Constriction

Figure 3-17 The Parasympathetic and Sympathetic Divisions

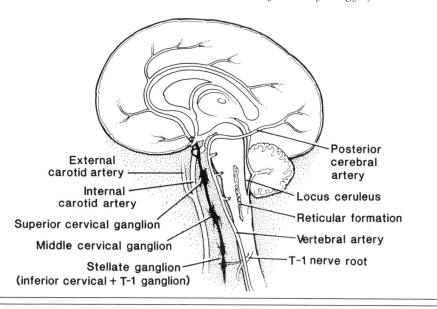

Figure 3-18 The Sympathetic Nervous System

tions decrease, the pupils dilate, and there is a vasoconstriction of peripheral blood vessels. The parasympathetic system is associated with the conservation and restoration of energy, corresponding to the flight response. In this response, the heart rate and blood pressure are decreased, the bronchioles of the lung constrict and secretion increases, the pupils constrict, and there is an increase of gastrointestinal activity.

It is important to note that both sympathetic and parasympathetic activity may cause excitatory and inhibitory effects in certain organs. Further information on the parasympathetic and sympathetic systems is supplied in Table 3-5.

The sympathetic and parasympathetic nerve fibers secrete either acetylcholine or norepinephrine. Fibers that secrete acetylcholine are referred to as cholinergic. Fibers that secrete norepinephrine are said to be adrenergic. All preganglionic neurons secrete acetylcholine and are cholinergic. The postganglionic neurons of the parasympathetic system are also cholinergic. Most of the postganglionic sympathetic neurons are adrenergic and secrete norepinephrine (with the exception of neurons to the sweat glands, a few blood vessels in skeletal muscles, and the adrenals). The effects of cholinergic fibers are short-acting and localized because acetylcholine is quickly deactivated by the enzyme cholinesterase. In

Table 3-5 Characteristics of the Parasympathetic and Sympathetic Divisions of the Autonomic Nervous System

Parasympathetic	Sympathetic
Craniosacral	Thoracolumbar
Cholinergic	Adrenergic
Long preganglionic fibers secrete acetylcholine	Short preganglionic fibers secrete acetylcholine
Short postganglionic fibers secrete acetylcholine	Long postganglionic fibers secrete norepinephrine
Site of origin is found in cranial nerves III, VII, IX, and X and in sacral segments S2 to S4	Site of origin is found in the lateral horn of the gray matter of the spinal cord from T1 to L2
Has a specifically localized and fast response	Has a widespread, slow, and relatively long-lasting response
Enzymes broken down by cholinesterase	Enzymes broken down by monoamine oxidase and catechol-o-methyl transferase

Table 3-6 Parasympathetic and Sympathetic Effects

Structure or Function	Parasympathetic Cholinergic Effects	Sympathetic Adrenergic Effects
Pupil of eye	Constricted	Dilated
Lacrimal, salivary glands	Vasodilated	Vasoconstricted
Circulation		
Heart rate and force of beat	Decreased	Increased
Blood pressure	Decreased	Increased
Blood vessels of skin and abdominal viscera		Constricted
Blood vessels in heart and skeletal muscles	Constricted	Dilated
Respiration		
Bronchioles of lung	Constricted	Dilated
Breathing rate	Decreased	Increased
Digestion		
Peristalsis	Increased	Decreased
Stomach	Increased	Inhibited
Intestine	Increased	Inhibited
Adrenal medulla		Increased
Integument		
Sweat gland secretion		Increased
Blood vessels of skin	Dilated	Constricted
Genitourinary		
Bladder	Constricted	Dilated
Genital organs	Vasodilated	Vasoconstricted

contrast, the effects of adrenergic fibers are slower and are more widely spread because norepinephrine is more slowly inactivated.

A summary of the twofold functioning of the ANS is provided in Table 3-6.

Assessment of the Nervous System

Neurological assessment is conducted to evaluate nervous system function. Such an evaluation is important to the nurse in determining specific therapeutic interventions and assisting the health care team in establishing an appropriate and timely medical treatment plan. Achieving the optimal level of care for the critically ill neurological patient largely depends on the nurse's ability to perform neurological assessment and interpret the clinical findings so as to intervene appropriately. The critical care nurse is responsible for establishing a baseline neurological assessment and then performing frequent neurological assessments to monitor the patient's responses and detect any early signs of nervous system dysfunction. A neurological flow sheet standardizes the documentation of such assessments and facilitates

recording. Changes in neurological status as well as trends can then be easily identified.

Neurological assessment is a combined responsibility of nurses and doctors. The medical domain includes identifying the location and etiology of the pathological process, determining appropriate medical and surgical treatments, and directing members of the health care team toward delivery of the medical treatment plan. The nursing domain complements the medical domain and consists of determining the influence of illnesses or disabilities on the patient's and family's life-style and providing direction for care with a focus on the goal of maximizing potential.

A comprehensive neurological examination includes the following components:

1. Health history:
    present illness, chief complaint
    personal history
    family history
2. Cerebral function:
    level of consciousness, mental status
    orientation
    memory
    thought process, content
    mood
3. Cranial nerve functions

Table 3-7 CNS Functions and Corresponding Findings for a Neurological Assessment

System Function	Assessment Findings
Level of consciousness	Alertness Orientation to person, place, and time Episodes of fainting or loss of consciousness Distortions of reality, orientation, or sense of self Presence of seizures Changes in patterns of sleep or circadian rhythms Use of consciousness-altering drugs Mood swings and emotionality
Cognition	Presence of short- or long-term memory loss Changes in ability to concentrate, read, speak, or understand words Inability to use problem-solving techniques or judgment skills Spatial disorientation or distortion
Speech	Intelligible and clear patterns of speech Presence of hoarseness Ability to articulate
Movement/coordination	Presence of weakness, discoordination, tremors, or paralysis Presence of uncoordinated gait/movements Difficulty in swallowing Difficulty in performing activities of daily living
Sensory	Alterations in sense of smell, vision, hearing, taste, or sensation Tactile tingling or numbness
Ingestion and digestion	Changes in appetite Presence of indigestion, cramps, nausea, or vomiting
Elimination	Urinary incontinence, retention, frequency, urgency, or burning Presence of diarrhea, incontinence, cramping, or constipation
Oxygenation	Hypoxia, or shortness of breath
Circulation	Claudication or thrombophlebitis Presence of transient ischemic attacks or stroke Postural hypotension, dizziness, or fainting Peripheral edema, skin blanching, and capillary refill Exercise intolerance
Sexual response	Alterations in sexual interests, activities, responses, or ability

4. Motor function
5. Cerebellar function
6. Reflexes
7. Sensory status
8. Vital signs
9. Diagnostic evaluation

The following tools may be used to perform a neurological assessment: stethoscope, otoscope, safety pin, wisp of cotton, flashlight, tongue blade, Snellen chart, reading materials, lemon, peppermint, vinegar, sugar, salt, ophthalmoscope, tuning fork, reflex hammer, millimeter ruler, some coins, and some keys.

Health History

The health history can provide invaluable information relating to the patient's neurological condition.

Table 3-7 presents a list of CNS functions for the nurse to investigate with patients, family members, or any other individual able to provide information. Additional factors to consider in a health history for a neurological exam are the individual's age, developmental level, language skills, cognitive deficits, occupation, working history, education, health care practices, medications, and medical history. The use of prescribed and over-the-counter medications, whether in compliance with instructions or not, is an important factor. It is also important to explore with patients their usual practices with respect to alcohol consumption and use of illegal drugs. Excessive use of alcohol or drug abuse should be confirmed with a family member and communicated to the entire health care team. Any information about exposure to toxic substances or travel abroad (especially to third world countries) may assist the team in diagnostic evaluation. Information pertaining to the family health history (heredity/familial diseases) is important in diagnosing neurological conditions and establishing the appropriate medical treatment plan.

Cerebral Function

Consciousness and Mental Status

The level of consciousness (LOC) is evaluated first in a neurological assessment. It is the earliest and most sensitive indicator of neurological change. A change in LOC is one of the first signs of neurological deterioration. Changes in neurological status may occur gradually over a period of days or weeks or very rapidly in a few minutes or hours. Table 3-8 lists the categories used to describe various levels of consciousness.

The Glasgow Coma Scale (GCS) is a standardized tool used to assess the neurological status of the trauma patient in order to predict prognostic outcomes. The GCS has gained wide acceptance internationally in the evaluation of the level of consciousness of the acutely ill head-injured patient. It is a valuable assessment tool for easily and quickly detecting neurological changes. However, a more detailed neurological assessment tool is necessary once the patient's condition stabilizes. As Table 3-9

Table 3-8 Clinical Presentation of Consciousness Levels

Level of Consciousness	Clinical Presentation
Alert and oriented	Responds immediately and appropriately to external stimuli
	Oriented to person, place, and time
Lethargic	Drowsy
	Short attention span
	Frequently drops off to sleep
	May be difficult to arouse, but responses are appropriate once aroused
Stuporous	Inappropriate responses to verbal commands
	Extremely difficult to arouse
Semicomatose	Little movement seen
	Inability to respond to verbal commands
	Nonpurposeful reflex action when stimulated with noxious stimuli
Comatose	No movements of extremities seen
	No response to verbal or noxious stimuli

Table 3-9 Glasgow Coma Scale Ratings

Function	Clinical Presentation	Score
Eye opening	Spontaneously	4
	To voice	3
	To noxious stimuli	2
	None	1
Verbal responses	Oriented	5
	Confused	4
	Inappropriate words	3
	Incomprehensible sounds	2
	Makes no noise	1
Motor responses	Obeys commands	6
	Localized responses	5
	Flexion withdrawal	4
	Abnormal flexion	3
	Abnormal extension	2
	None	1

shows, the GCS is divided into three sections: eye opening, verbal responses, and motor responses. The patient receives a total numerical value for each section. A maximum score of 15 indicates an alert and oriented patient; a minimum score of 3 reflects the status of one in a deep coma.

Orientation

Orientation to time, place, and person are determined to assess a level of cognitive function. The patient is asked to state the current month, date and day of the week, and year. If the patient has difficulty in accomplishing this task, it may be helpful to ask the patient to identify past or upcoming holidays. Questions attempting to assess orientation to time are the questions most frequently answered incorrectly with a change in LOC. Testing orientation to place is done by asking the patient to communicate his or her present location. The patient is asked to state his or her name to determine orientation to person. For the patient unable to communicate verbally (for example, a patient who is ventilated, tracheostomied, or aphasic), an alternate method of communication must be established. A communication board, hand signals, or writing materials are assistive devices that may be used in such circumstances.

Memory

Both recent and distant memory should be tested in a neurological assessment. Asking the patient to recall events surrounding the hospitalization is the means used to evaluate recent memory. Distant memory can be tested by asking the patient to recall the dates of significant life events such as births and marriages of family members. The patient with neurological dysfunction may experience difficulty re-calling such information, especially the most recent events.

Thought Process and Content

The patient's capacity for concentration and at-tention span are important to assess. A patient's general knowledge can be assessed by asking ques-tions regarding current news events. Thought pro-cesses will reflect a patient's insight and personal interpretation of daily experiences. The patient with impaired thought processes will most likely exhibit poor judgment and problem-solving ability, lack of insight concerning personal limitations, and inability to perform abstract thinking.

Mood

The patient's mood is another component of cognitive function that can be observed during a neurological assessment. When possible, the patient should be encouraged to describe his or her present mood. The nurse can best assess the appropriateness of the response by matching exhibited body lan-guage to the situational circumstance to ascertain whether the patient's verbalization is reflected non-verbally. Behaviors that may reflect mood deficits include depression, irritability, and severe anxiety.

Cranial Nerve Functions

A thorough neurological examination includes as-sessment of the cranial nerves. A description of the assessment of cranial nerves I through XII is detailed in Table 3-10. It must be realized, though, that routine neurological assessment will not include all 12 cranial nerves. In a life-threatening situation, the stability of the patient will dictate what components of a neurological assessment should be performed.

Cranial Nerve I (Olfactory)

An assessment of this nerve is accomplished by having the patient identify familiar and nonirritating odors (coffee, peppermint, and lemon) separately and with each nostril. The patient should close his or her eyes during the testing to avoid visual cues.

Cranial Nerve II (Optic)

To assess visual acuity, the patient should be instructed to cover one eye and read a newspaper positioned 15 to 18 inches from the face. This proce-dure should be repeated for each eye. The same test can be accomplished using a Snellen chart from a distance of 20 feet.

To evaluate visual fields, the patient is asked to cover one eye and look directly at the examiner's

nose, distanced 2 feet away. The examiner holds two fingers out to the side and slowly brings them in from the periphery of four quadrants. The patient is re-quested to identify when the examiner's fingers first enter the visual field. Fields of vision are similar in quadrants for the patient and the examiner, so the examiner can anticipate when the patient should see the finger movement. Further specialized testing is necessary to confirm the presence of any visual dysfunctions. Visual field defects caused by inter-ruption of visual pathways at various locations are depicted in Figure 3-19.

Cranial Nerves III, IV, and VI (Oculomotor, Trochlear, and Abducens)

The third, fourth, and sixth cranial nerves are always tested together. The examiner can assess extraocular movement by asking the patient to follow an object through all fields of gaze on both the right and left sides. The third cranial nerve controls me-dial, upward, and downward eye movement. The fourth cranial nerve controls downward and inward eye movement. The sixth cranial nerve controls lat-eral eye movement. The sixth cranial nerve is tested by requesting the patient to attempt to look in the lateral direction. A check of whether the eyes are symmetrical when at rest is also made. Clinical find-ings such as limited eye movements, gaze distur-bances, diplopia, and nystagmus should be noted at this time.

The third cranial nerve also controls the muscles that constrict the pupil and elevate the upper eyelid.

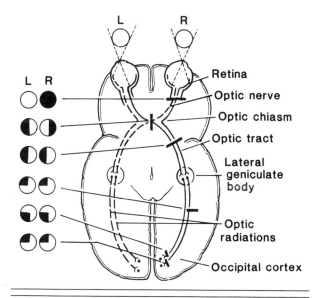

Figure 3-19 Visual Field Changes Corresponding to Se-lected Visual Pathway Injuries

Table 3-10 Assessment of Cranial Nerves

Cranial Nerve	Technique	Common Problems
I. Olfactory	1. Have client close eyes. 2. Close off client's naris by placing pressure against the side with an index finger. 3. Hold substance (soap, lemon, coffee) near naris. 4. Ask client to identify substance. 5. Repeat procedure for the remaining naris.	Anosmia.
II. Optic	Use techniques for evaluating visual acuity, visual fields, eye grounds.	Decreased or loss of visual acuity, visual field defects, changes in optic nerve disk.
III. Oculomotor	1. Inspect eyelids. 2. Inspect pupil sizes and reaction to light, accommodation, and convergence. 3. Check EOMS. 4. Note whether eyes are symmetrical at rest.	Ptosis of eyelid. Dilated pupil.
IV. Trochlear	1. Check EOMS. 2. Note whether eyes are symmetrical at rest.	Unable to gaze in nasally downward direction.
V. Trigeminal	1. Check corneal reflex and three sensory divisions (ophthalmic, maxillary, and mandibular) with a cotton wisp, pinprick, and temperature (hot and cold water–filled test tubes). 2. Observe for jaw deviation. 3. Palpate masseter muscle while teeth are clenched and unclenched. 4. Have client open lower jaw against resistance (place your hand under lower jaw to provide resistance).	Brain stem lesion, herpes zoster, tic douloureux. Masseter and temporalis muscle weakness with myasthenia gravis and amyotrophic lateral sclerosis (ALS).
VI. Abducens	1. Check EOMS. 2. Note whether eyes are symmetrical at rest.	Unable to gaze in lateral direction.
VII. Facial	1. Observe for symmetry at rest and while client smiles, frowns, clenches teeth, blows out cheeks, purses lips. 2. Test for sweet and salty taste sensation on anterior two-thirds of tongue. 3. Dip applicator in salt-water solution. 4. Ask client to extend tongue and identify taste before retracting tongue into mouth. 5. Place applicator on anterior portion of tongue. 6. Rinse mouth with water. 7. Repeat procedure with sugar-water solution.	Bell's palsy. Change in taste sensation. Decrease in salivation and tearing.

VIII. Auditory or acoustic	1. Weber test
	2. Rinne test
	3. Special tests
	   a. Audiometry examination
	   b. Caloric test
		Decreased or loss of hearing.
		Acoustic neuroma.

IX. Glosso-pharyngeal	1. Observe for difficulty swallowing. 2. Check gag reflex. 3. Test for bitter and sour taste sensation on posterior one-third of tongue using quinine water and vinegar respectively.	Dysphasia, decreased gag reflex, glossopharyngeal neuralgia, and change in taste sensation.
X. Vagus	1. Observe for difficulty swallowing as client drinks water. 2. Check uvular reflex.	Hoarseness or aphonia, regurgitation of water through the nose.
XI. Spinal accessory	1. Have client shrug shoulders against resistance (place your hands on client's shoulders). 2. Observe scapula. 3. Place hand on side of client's forehead. 4. Ask client to flex his head against your hand. 5. Repeat on opposite side of face.	Drooping of shoulder, unable to raise arm above head. Scapula displaced downard and maybe slight winging.
XII. Hypoglossal	1. Have client stick out tongue. 2. Have client move tongue against resistance (tongue blades or examiner's finger on outside of cheek). 3. Observe for scalloping or indentation along edge of tongue.	Tongue deviation, weakness, atrophy.

(Ptosis is the drooping of the upper eyelid.) To obtain the maximal response, pupillary reaction should be assessed in a room with subdued lighting. The pupil size is observed before and after a bright light is shone directly into each pupil. The patient should look straight ahead while the light source is introduced from a side angle. The pupil size is recorded before the light stimulus is introduced. The size, shape, equality, and reaction of each pupil to the light stimulus is examined. A direct light reflex is the constriction of the pupil when stimulated by light. A consensual light response occurs when there is pupillary constriction in the eye not receiving the direct light stimulus. Anisocoria (unequal pupils) may be normal for some individuals or may indicate significant neurological dysfunction. Table 3-11 presents some abnormal pupillary responses related to specific cerebral injuries.

Testing eye movement in the unconscious or comatose patient is accomplished by evaluating the oculocephalic reflex (doll's eyes) and the oculovestibular reflex (calorics). The oculocephalic reflex is tested by holding open the upper eyelids while turning the patient's head rapidly from side to side. In patients with an intact brainstem, the eyes will move slightly in the direction opposite to that of the head (doll's eyes); lack of such movement indicates absence of the oculocephalic reflex, signifying deep coma and severe brainsteam damage.

To ascertain oculovestibular reflex, the patient's tympanic membrane must be intact. With the patient in the supine position with the head elevated 30 degrees, the ear is slowly irrigated with ice water by the physician. For the patient with an intact brainstem, this stimulation will cause horizontal nystagmus with slow movement toward the irrigated ear and rapid movement to the opposite side. In the comatose patient, there may be no rapid eye movement, dysconjugate eye movement, or no discernible eye movement. This reflex is tested on the opposite side after 5 minutes. Irrigations can also be performed with warm water; in that case the fast component occurs on the same side as the irrigation. The mnemonic "cows" is helpful to recall the direction of the fast component: *c*old, *o*pposite; *w*arm, *s*ame.

Cranial Nerve V (Trigeminal)

The fifth cranial nerve has a sensory and motor component. The sensory component controls facial sensation and can be tested by lightly touching different areas of the patient's face with a wisp of cotton and sterile pin while the patient's eyes are

Table 3-11 Clinical Presentation of Pupils with Selected Neurological Injuries

Clinical Presentation	Clinical Antecedents	Injury
	Bilaterally equal, small, reactive pupils caused by: Metabolic coma Supratentorial lesion	Diencephalic bilateral damage
	Bilaterally equal, small, nonreactive pupils resulting from the loss of sympathetic innervation caused by: Opiate drug effects Pontine hemorrhage	Pontine damage
	Bilaterally midpositioned, nonreactive pupils resulting from a nuclear midbrain lesion (pupils are unequal and irregular) or a lesion in the dorsal aspect of the midbrain (pupils remain bilaterally round and regular) caused by: Hemorrhage Infarct Transtentorial herniation Tumor	Midbrain damage
	Fixed and dilated ipsilateral pupil caused by compression of the oculomotor nerve on the posterior cerebral artery or tentorium	Oculomotor nerve compression
	A unilaterally small pupil, ptosis of the eyelid, and the absence of sweating on the affected side caused by: Descending sympathetic fiber compromise in the upper cord or ipsilateral brainstem Ascending sympathetic fiber compromise in the head or neck Transtentorial herniation	Hypothalamic damage
	Bilaterally fixed and dilated pupils caused by: Atropine Terminal brain damage	Severe anoxia Death

closed. The patient is requested to identify when and where touch is applied to each side of the face. The motor function of this nerve is tested by asking the patient to tightly clamp the jaw. The nurse palpates the masseter muscles bilaterally, assessing for motor strength and symmetry.

Cranial Nerve VII (Facial)

The seventh cranial nerve has both motor and sensory components. The motor function of this nerve is not routinely assessed, but can be by requesting the patient to raise both eyebrows, wrinkle the forehead, wink, puff out the cheeks, frown, and smile in a way as to show teeth. Asymmetrical movement, decreased facial grimace, and any abnormal movements are noted. The sensory function of the seventh cranial nerve is associated with the taste fibers of the anterior two-thirds of the tongue. The patient is asked to identify the taste of sweet, salty, sour, and bitter substances on each side of the tongue.

Cranial Nerve VIII (Acoustic)

The eighth cranial nerve is responsible for hearing and control of balance. The nurse assesses hearing capability by placing a ticking watch several inches from the patient's ears in various positions. The patient's ability to hear these sounds is estimated, and obvious defects are noted.

Cranial Nerves IX and X (Glossopharyngeal and Vagus)

The ninth and tenth cranial nerves control swallowing, gag reflex, and vocalizing. The nurse first asks the patient to open the mouth and say "ah." The soft palate moves upward while the uvula remains midline. To test the gag reflex, the nurse strokes the back of the patient's throat on each side of the posterior pharynx with a tongue blade. This reflex may be diminished or absent in some normal people. If the gag reflex is present, the ability to swallow is assessed by observing the patient drinking fluid. Finally, the quality of the voice is evaluated for hoarseness, nasal sounds, and dysarthria.

The sensory component of the ninth cranial nerve controls taste in the posterior one-third of the tongue. The testing technique is the same as that used for testing of the sensory component of the seventh cranial nerve.

Cranial Nerve XI (Spinal Accessory)

The eleventh cranial nerve controls shoulder shrugging and neck movement and innervates the trapezius and sternocleidomastoid muscles. Evaluation of the trapezius is accomplished by having the patient shrug both shoulders upward against the resistance of the examiner's hand. To evaluate the sternocleidomastoid, the patient is asked to turn the head to each side and forward against the resistance of the examiner's hand. Motor strength, atrophy, and spasm are noted.

Cranial Nerve XII (Hypoglossal)

The twelfth cranial nerve controls tongue movement. The patient is instructed to stick out the tongue. The examiner assesses the tongue in both a midline position and laterally against a tongue blade. The tongue is further evaluated for asymmetry, atrophy, deviations from the midline, fasciculation (slight muscle flickerings), and spasms.

Examination of the following is considered adequate for routine ICU screening for cranial nerve function:

Cranial nerve III assessing pupil response and movement of the upper eyelids

Cranial nerve IV assessing eye and extraocular movements

Cranial nerve VI assessing eye and extraocular movements

Cranial nerves V and VII assessing corneal reflex and facial symmetry

Cranial nerves IX and X assessing gag reflex

Motor Function

An assessment of motor function includes muscle size, muscle tone, muscle strength, coordination, and abnormal responses. It is most important that the nurse assess motor responses on each side of the body and note differences.

The nurse assesses muscle size for bilateral symmetry by inspection and palpation. Hypertrophy, atrophy, or flattening of the muscle masses is noted. To confirm differences, a tape measure can be used to measure muscle mass precisely.

Muscle tone is assessed by palpating major muscles for firmness and performing passive range of motion exercises. Disturbances of muscle tone include spasticity, rigidity, and flaccidity. To test motor strength of the upper extremities, the patient is asked to grasp and squeeze the examiner's index and middle finger. Hand grips should be compared for strength and equality, allowing for slight increases in strength on the dominant side. The patient is next asked to raise the arms above the head and then to flex each arm against increasing resistance applied by the examiner. The strength of motor responses is graded using the standard numerical scale provided in Table 3-12.

Concurrently, it is important for the nurse to assess arm drifts. The patient is instructed to extend the arms straight forward with palms up and eyes closed for 10–20 seconds. The weaker arm will noticeably drift downward and pronate.

To test the lower extremities, the patient is instructed to lift each leg off the bed with and without resistance. Plantar flexion and dorsiflexion of the foot are evaluated by asking the patient to push downward and pull upward against resistance of the examiner's hand.

To test motor function of an unconscious patient obviously requires a different approach. If the patient does not respond to verbal or tactile stimuli (shake and shout), a painful stimulus is applied to elicit a motor response. The least amount of stimulus that will elicit a response is used. Noxious stimuli include a squeeze of the sternocleidomastoid muscle, pressure to the nailbeds, and a sternum rub. Responses to such stimuli are judged purposeful when the patient attempts to push the stimulator away or withdraws the affected extremity from the pain generation. A nonpurposeful response occurs when the patient attempts but is unable to remove the source of painful stimulus or move away from the painful stimulus.

To assess arm weakness in the unconscious patient, the examiner lifts the patient's arm as it is in a neutral position and then releases the arm. The weaker arm will fall quickly, and the stronger, or normal, arm will fall more slowly to its previous position. To assess leg weakness, the legs are tested from a neutral position; the knees are bent with the feet placed flat on the bed. Leg movement is noted when the feet are released. The weaker leg will fall quickly, leaving the hip outwardly rotated. The stronger, or normal, leg may remain in the position momentarily before slowly returning to its previous position.

Two abnormal motor responses that indicate serious cerebral damage are decortication and decerebration. Decortication is characterized by flexion of the arms, wrist, and fingers with adduction in the upper extremities and extension, internal rotation, and plantar flexion of the lower extremities.[3] Decortication is hyperflexion of the upper extremities and hyperextension of the lower extremities. In contrast, decerebration is characterized by rigid extension, adduction, and hyperextension of the extremities. Of these two abnormal motor responses, decerebration indicates greater cerebral dysfunction. Figure 3-20 illustrates the two abnormal postures as exhibited by the comatose patient.

Finally, the patient suffering from inflammation of the meninges should be tested for nuchal rigidity and presence of Kernig's sign. While the patient is in a supine position, the examiner should place a hand behind the patient's head and attempt to flex the neck forward so as to allow the chin to touch the chest. Expressions of pain and resistance to movement are noted. Flexion of the patient's hips and knees in response to this forward neck flexion is called Brudzinski's sign. Kernig's sign is tested for by slowly extending the patient's knee when the hip is in a flexed position of 90 degrees. Expressions of pain and resistance imply a positive Kernig's sign.

Cerebellar Function

Cerebellar function is evaluated by assessing coordination and balance. Two characteristics of the upper extremities should be examined:

1. Rapid alternating movements: While in a sitting position, the patient is asked to pat both knees simultaneously with the palms and

Table 3-12 Grading Scale for Strength of Motor Response

Letter Scale	Percent Scale	Number Scale	Interpretation
Normal (N)	100%	5	Normal power
Good (G)	75%	4	Muscle can make full normal movement but not against resistance
Fair (F)	50%	3	Muscle cannot move against resistance or make full normal movement but can make normal movement against gravity
Poor (P)	25%	2	Full muscle movement possible with force of gravity eliminated
Trace (T)	10%	1	No movement of limb or joint, but contraction is visible or palpable
Zero (0)	0%	0	Total paralysis

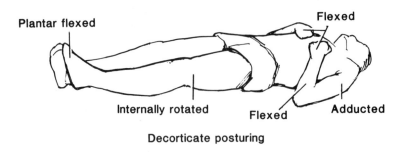

Decorticate posturing

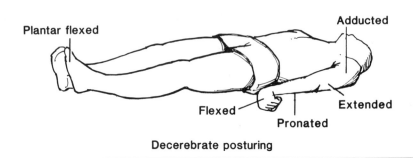

Decerebrate posturing

Figure 3-20 Abnormal Postures in the Comatose Patient

then the backsides of the hands as rapidly as possible.

2. Point-to-point testing: The patient is instructed to touch the examiner's finger with the index finger and then to touch his or her own nose. This is repeated as the examiner changes the position of his or her finger. The accuracy and smoothness of the movement are observed. Past pointing and incoordination are abnormal findings.

Three characteristics of the lower extremities are assessed:

1. Postural stability: The patient is observed standing feet together with the eyes opened and closed. A positive Romberg occurs if the patient sways or loses balance.
2. Tandem walking: The patient is observed walking a straight line placing one foot directly in front of the other.
3. Heel-to-shin movement: If the patient is not able to stand, he or she should be instructed to close the eyes and to then move each foot down the shin of the opposite leg. The accuracy of the movement or any uncoordinated movements are noted.

Reflexes

Evaluation of reflexes during the neurological examination provides important information about both the conscious and unconscious patient. Reflexes are classified in three categories: deep tendon reflexes, superficial reflexes, and pathological reflexes.

Deep tendon reflexes (DTR), also referred to as muscle stretch reflexes, are examined when the patient's muscles are midline in a relaxed position. As illustrated in Table 3-13, the tendon is briskly tapped with a reflex hammer at the muscle insertion over the bony prominence, and the contraction of the muscle is observed. Tendon reflexes are graded using the standard numerical scale presented in Table 3-14.

Superficial reflexes are elicited by stroking the skin with a light touch or by using a firm object. The important superficial reflexes include the abdominal, cremasteric, bulbocavernosus, corneal, pharyngeal, uvular, perineal, and plantar reflexes. Table 3-15 provides an overview of the assessment of the superficial reflexes.

To test the corneal reflex, the examiner should approach the patient from the side and then touch the cornea lightly with a fine wisp of cotton. The patient should be assessed for a normal, strong, decreased, or absent blink response.

To test the plantar reflex, the examiner firmly strokes the lateral aspect of the sole of the patient's foot, using one continuous stroke from the heel to the ball. The Babinski reflex, an abnormal response in the adult, is dorsiflexion of the great toe, which may or may not be accompanied by fanning of the other toes. A positive Babinski in adults is clinically significant and implies damage to the corticospinal tract.

Pathological reflexes are associated with frontal lobe involvement, cerebral atrophic diseases, cortex and brain injury, and encephalitis. Table 3-16 presents an overview of common pathological reflexes.

Sensory Status

Basic assessment of sensory status consists of evaluating the patient's responses to touch, superficial pain, and temperature, and his or her awareness of position. Assessment of the sensory function will depend on the acuity level of the patient. Each side of the patient's body should be evaluated and compared to the other side. The following terms are frequently used in reporting sensation responses:

Graphesthesia: the ability to recognize numbers and letters written on the palm of the hand

Stereognosis: the ability to recognize, by touch, objects placed in the hand

Anesthesia: absence of sensation

Hypesthesia: decreased sensation

Hyperesthesia: excessive sensitivity

To assess the patient's response to touch, the examiner lightly touches different areas of the patient's skin with a wisp of cotton. The patient notifies the examiner when the sensation is felt.

The examiner uses both the sharp and dull surfaces of an open safety pin to test the sensation of superficial pain. Starting distally and moving proximally, the examiner asks the patient to identify the sensation of sharp or dull. When examining spinal cord injured patients, it is especially important that the test be performed in conjunction with a dermatome chart in order to identify the sensation loss and to assist in determining the level of the injury.

Temperature response can be assessed by applying test tubes filled with warm and cold water to various parts of each side of the patient's body. The patient is asked to identify the different sensations in the various locations.

Awareness of position, or proprioception, is tested by determining if a patient can identify the position of his or her finger or toe when it is moved either up or down while the patient's eyes are closed. The test should be performed with each extremity.

Table 3-13 Assessment of Deep Tendon Reflexes

Reflex	Percussion Site	Response	CNS Dermatomes
Biceps	Biceps tendon Place your thumb on tendon cord in midantecubital space with client's elbow flexed. Strike your thumbnail with percussion hammer. 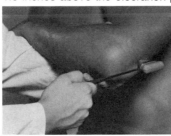	Biceps contraction	Cervical 5 and 6
Triceps	Triceps tendon Strike tendon with percussion hammer about 1.5 inches above the olecranon process.	Elbow extension; triceps contraction	Cervical 6–8

(continued)

Table 3-13 Assessment of Deep Tendon Reflexes (*continued*)

Reflex	Percussion Site	Response	CNS Dermatomes
Brachioradialis	Styloid process of radius Strike tendon about 2 inches above the wrist on the radial [thumb] side of the arm. 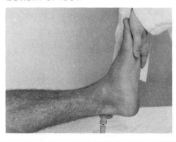	Pronation of forearm and hand	Cervical 5 and 6
Patellar	Patellar tendon Strike tendon immediately below the patella (knee cap)	Knee extension	Lumbar 2–4
Achilles	Achilles tendon Strike heelcord as you gently apply pressure to bottom of foot.	Plantar flexion of foot	Sacral 1 and 2

Table 3-14 Grading Scale for Tendon Reflexes

Grade	Symbols	Interpretation
0	0	Absent (indicate whether reinforcement used)
1	+	Diminished but present
2	++	Normal; average
3	+++	Normal: brisker than average—may or may not indicate pathology
4	++++	Hyperactive: very brisk—most often pathologic
5	+++++	Hyperactive with clonus

Vital Signs

Vital signs are included in a neurological assessment because changes in them may serve as late signs of changes in neurological status.

Alterations in Cardiovascular Function

Increases in intracranial pressure cause a decrease in cerebral blood flow, and cerebral ischemia stimulates the sympathetic response. This powerful compensatory mechanism maintains adequate blood flow to the brain by raising the systolic pressure and creating a widening of the pulse pressure. Hypotension may be due to cerebral decompensation or other

Table 3-15   Assessment of Superficial Reflexes

Reflex	Stimulus Site	Response	CNS Dermatomes
Abdominal		Umbilicus moves toward area stroked	Upper thoracic 7–9
Cremasteric		Scrotum elevates	Thoracic 12 and lumbar 1
Plantar		Toes flex	Sacral 1 and 2
Anal	Rectal stimulation by gloved finger	Contraction of anal sphincter	Sacral

medical conditions, and other neurological signs should be considered in conjunction with the presenting hypotension.

Baroreceptors in the aorta and carotid bodies are sensitive to increases in blood pressure and stimulate the vagus to slow the heart rate. Pressure on the medullary centers of the brain due to highly increased intracranial pressure results in bradycardia.

Cardiac dysrhythmias are common in the patient experiencing specific neurological conditions. The following are possible dysrhythmias exhibited in acute neurological situations:

Large, upright T waves with long Q-T intervals
Q waves with ST depression

Supraventricular tachycardia
Atrial flutter/fibrillation
Sinus bradycardia and/or arrest
Junctional rhythms
AV blocks or dissociation
Premature ventricular contractions
Ventricular flutter/fibrillation

Alterations in Respiration

Respiratory status is indicative of brainstem dysfunction. Abnormal respiratory patterns reflect neurological dysfunction at different levels of the brain

Table 3-16 Overview of Pathological Reflexes

Reflex	How Elicited	Response If Present
Babinski (upper motor neuron damage)	Stroke lateral aspect of sole of foot	Extension of great toe and fanning of the toes
Chaddock (upper motor neuron damage)	Stroke lateral aspect of foot beneath the lateral malleolus	Same as above
Oppenheim (upper motor neuron damage)	Stroke anteromedial tibial surface	Same as above
Gordon (upper motor neuron damage)	Squeeze calf muscles firmly	Same as above
Hoffmann (upper motor neuron damage)	Flick terminal phalanx of middle finger downward	Flexion of thumb and/or fingers (clawing)
Ankle clonus (upper motor neuron damage)	Sudden, brisk dorsiflexion of foot with knee flexed and applying sustained and moderate pressure	Exaggerated rhythmic up-and-down movements of foot (a rapidly exhaustible clonus may be normal)
Kernig's sign (meningeal irritation)	Straight leg raising or below knee extension with thigh flexed on abdomen	Limitation with pain down posterior thigh
Brudzinski's sign (meningeal irritation)	Flexing chin on chest	Limitation with pain

(see Table 3-17). Metabolic dysfunction also influences respirations and must be carefully interpreted through arterial blood gas analysis.

Alteration in Temperature

The patient's temperature should be closely monitored to prevent extreme fluctuations and neurological deterioration. Hypothermia can occur with spinal shock, destructive lesions of the hypothalamus or brainstem, and coma. Hyperthermia can be caused by infection, subarachnoid hemorrhage, and destructive lesions of the hypothalamus. Regardless of cause, hyperthermia requires immediate and aggressive management to prevent further increases in metabolic demands.

Diagnostic Evaluation

Neurodiagnostic testing provides valuable clinical information with minimal risk to the patient. Advances in diagnostic imaging have greatly assisted the medical team in making fast and accurate diagnoses. The nurse's role in facilitating diagnostic testing includes education of the patient to prepare him or her for the procedure, patient preps, monitoring the patient during and following the test, and documenting the patient's response to the tests.

Electroencephalography (EEG) is the graphic recording and analysis of electrical activity occurring in the cerebral hemispheres. Although an EEG cannot be used to diagnose different intracranial pathophysiologies, abnormalities in EEG recordings indicate the presence of abnormal conditions. The EEG can be used to differentiate epilepsy from other disorders and to confirm metabolic disturbances and sleep disorders. It is used as the primary diagnostic tool in the event of brain death. The EEG may also be used during neurovascular surgery to monitor cerebral activity. Electrodes are placed over the surface of the brain cortex, and changes in the electrical activity of the brain cells are recorded.

A complete neurological examination includes x-rays of the skull and spine. These are helpful in detecting the presence of fractures, abnormalities of the base of the skull and cranial vault, increased intracranial pressure, tumors, calcifications, subluxations, and degenerative changes.

The computerized tomography (CT) scan is extremely valuable in quickly and accurately diagnosing various intracranial pathologies, such as head and spinal cord trauma, tumors and abscesses, hydrocephalus, and cerebral edema. The CT scan provides a three-dimensional computerized composite of x-ray images along axial planes. Detailed outlines

Table 3-17 Respiratory Patterns Reflecting Neurological Dysfunctions

Type	Respiratory Pattern	Neuroanatomical Location
Cheyne-Stokes respiration		Usually bilateral in cerebral hemispheres Sometimes cerebellar Midbrain Upper pons
Central neurogenic hyperventilation		Low midbrain Upper pons
Apneustic breathing		Mid pons Low pons
Cluster breathing		Low pons High medulla
Ataxic breathing		Medulla
	├── 1 minute ──┤	

Source: Gifford, R. & Plant, M., Abnormal respiratory patterns in the comatose patient caused by intracranial dysfunction. *Journal of Neurosurgical Nursing* 7(1):58, July, 1975.

of bone, tissue, and fluid demarcations are created. These images may be enhanced with a contrast medium.

Cerebral angiography is extremely useful in diagnosing vessel patency, vasospasm, aneurysms, arteriovenous malformations, and the presence of intracranial lesions causing displacement or narrowing of the vessels. Angiography is the radiographic visualization of intracranial or extracranial circulation made visible by the injection of radio-opaque contrast medium into the brachial or femoral artery. Possible complications include allergic reactions to the dye, pulmonary emboli, thrombosis, stroke, and vasospasm.

Digital subtraction angiography (DSA) may be used as a diagnostic tool for patients with suspected vascular pathologies. It is a computerized radiographic technique for visualization and examination of the extracranial circulation. A series of the target area (mask image) is taken after the injection of a contrast medium. The computer subtracts anything common between the images and produces an enhanced radiographic image of the contrast medium in the vessels. A DSA is less expensive and less invasive and therefore poses fewer potential complications than cerebral angiography.

Magnetic resonance imaging (MRI) signifies a

new era in diagnostic imaging. It is useful in accurately diagnosing cerebral edema, tumor size and extent, brain infarct, hemorrhage, seizures, degenerative diseases, and congenital anomalies. Detailed and sharp images of internal structures are created from radiofrequency signals as atomic nuclei are caused to oscillate by forces of a magnetic field. This is accomplished without the use of radiation or dyes using magnetic fields and radiowaves. The distinct advantage of MRI is that it can differentiate blood vessels from soft tissue and provide better visualization of the brainstem and posterior fossa structures. Scans are not recommended for patients with metallic equipment such as aneurysm clips, pacemakers, bullet fragments, gold fillings, and prosthetic devices, since these devices may be affected by magnetic fields. Use of MRIs with critically ill patients on ventilators or on IVs with pumps is also contraindicated for the same reason.

Myelography is helpful in the diagnosis of herniated intravertebral disc, spinal cord tumor, and trauma to the spinal cord. A myelogram is a radiographic examination of the spinal cord and the vertebral column after injection of a radio-opaque substance into the subarachnoid space via lumbar puncture. Postprocedure care depends on the type of contrast medium used. Oil-based medium requires strict bedrest (flat) for 24 hours, forced fluids, and frequent vital and neurological assessment. Water based medium requires the head of the bed to be elevated at 30 degrees for 8 hours, forced fluids, and no phenothiazines.

A lumbar puncture (LP) is performed to obtain cerebrospinal fluid (CSF) for laboratory analysis, to determine CSF pressure, to inject radio-opaque substance for x-ray visualization, and to induce spinal anesthesia. Analyses of CSF serve as primary indicators of several neurological disorders. Table 3-18 presents an overview of the various normal and abnormal characteristics of CSF.

To perform a lumbar puncture, a spinal needle is inserted into the lumbar subarachnoid space, usually between the fourth and fifth lumbar vertebrae. Brainstem herniation, infection, and headache are possible complications of the procedure, and care should be taken to prevent these from occurring. A lumbar puncture is contraindicated in the patient suffering from increased intracranial pressure, because a sudden reduction in pressure may cause brain herniation.

Evoked potentials (EP) measure electrical activity in the brain in response to various sensory stimuli. Auditory (AEP), visual (VEP), brainstem auditory evoked response (BAER), and somatosensory (SSEP) are the various types of EP. Evoked potentials provide useful diagnostic information for detecting lesions and evaluating CNS injury of comatose patients and those experiencing neuromuscular disorders.

Electromyography (EMG) records the electrical activity of skeletal muscles in response to stimuli of various intensities and duration. EMG is helpful to diagnose and monitor peripheral nerve and neuromuscular diseases.

Positron emission tomography (PET) measures cerebral blood flow and metabolism. It is the only diagnostic test to measure physiological and biochemical processes in the nervous system. The patient either inhales or is injected with a radioactive isotope, which acts as a tracer. A gamma scanner measures the radioactive uptake, and a computer produces a video image. This image corresponds to the location in the brain where the radioactive material is absorbed and cellular metabolism is occurring. The PET scan is used in research related to neurotransmitter function, brain metabolism of certain agents, and behavioral disturbances that have a physiological basis.

Table 3-18 Normal and Abnormal Characteristics of Cerebrospinal Fluid

Characteristic	Normal	Abnormal
Appearance	Clear, colorless	Pink or red that clears after 5–10 mL is withdrawn indicates traumatic tap; nonclearing pink or red indicates subarachnoid hemorrhage; xanthrochromic (yellow) fluid is caused by presence of pigments: 1. Bilirubin appears 2 to 3 days after subarachnoid hemorrhage; remains 2 to 3 weeks 2. Oxyhemoglobin appears after intracranial hemorrhage 3. Methemoglobin found when blood is encapsulated (chronic subdural hematoma)
Pressure	70–180 mm H_2O	Less than 50 mm H_2O indicative of spinal block; more than 200 mm H_2O can occur in expanding mass lesions, cerebral edema, cerebral hemorrhage, or thrombosis
Specific gravity	1.007	
Glucose	50–80 mg/100 mL (80 percent of plasma glucose)	Decrease seen in acute bacterial meningitis, tubercular meningitis, meningeal carcinomatosis, but not significant of itself
Protein	15–45 mg/100 mL	Elevations seen in tumor, infection, demyelinating disease, polyneuropathy
Gamma globulin	12–20 percent of total protein	Gamma globulin increased in tertiary syphilis, subacute encephalitis, and multiple sclerosis
Cellular content Erythrocytes Leukocytes	0 0–6 lymphocytes/mm^3	1,000/mm^3 or more seen in central nervous system infection; also occurs with brain or spinal tumor and multiple sclerosis

Source: Snyder, Mariah (1983). *A Guide to Neurological and Neurosurgical Nursing.* New York: John Wiley & Sons, Inc., p. 56.

Increased Intracranial Pressure

Intracranial pressure (ICP) is generally referred to as a pressure exerted by brain tissue, intracranial blood, and cerebrospinal fluid (CSF) within the cranial vault. Normal ICP is a dynamic phenomenon dependent on the pressure of the total volume of these intracranial contents within an intact skull. Increased ICP is caused by imbalances between the rates of secretion and absorbtion of CSF or uncompensated changes in the volume of intracranial blood or brain tissue.

Increased intracranial pressure is an actual or potential problem for many neurological patients. Significantly increased ICP that is prolonged presents a threat to cerebral circulation and may result in life-threatening situations unless tended to as soon as possible.

Clinical antecedents

Table 3-19 outlines antecedents to increased ICP in various types of neurological disorders.

Table 3-19 Antecedents to Increased ICP

Disorder	Precipitating Factors
Hydrocephalus	Obstruction of CSF pathways as found with aqueductal stenosis Deficient CSF absorption as found with subarachnoid hemorrhage Oversecretion of CSF as found with choroid plexus tumor
Craniocerebral trauma	Intracranial hematoma (epidural or subdural) Intracerebral hemorrhage Subarachnoid hemorrhage Cerebral edema (cytotoxic or vasogenic) Cerebrovascular accident (CVA)
Infectious processes	Meningitis Encephalitis Ventriculitis Intracranial abscess
Neoplasms	Primary CNS tumors Metastatic tumors
Metabolic disorders	Inappropriate ADH syndrome Metabolic encephalopathy (hypoxia or anoxia)

Source: Adapted from the American Association of Neuroscience Nurses, (1984). *Core Curriculum for Neuroscience Nursing.* Chicago: American Association of Neuroscience Nurses, p. 180.

Critical referents

The intracranial volume of the normal adult brain varies, but generally is composed of 80% brain mass, 10% blood, and 10% CSF. The Monro-Kellis hypothesis proposes that these intracranial volumes enclosed within the rigid container of the skull are fixed. An increase in the volume of one intracranial component requires a decrease in another in order for the composite volume and pressure to remain constant. Increases in ICP occur as a result of an imbalance in this volume-pressure relationship. Lundberg's classification of ICP is presented in Table 3-20.

Compensation within the rigid fixed container of the adult skull is minimal because of the restricted movement of the intracranial contents. Accommodation and autoregulation are the primary compensatory mechanisms triggered to maintain adequate cerebral blood flow (CBF). Intracranial components can accommodate volume increases by (1) shunting of CSF into the spinal subarachnoid space, (2) increasing CSF absorption by the venous sinuses, (3) decreasing cerebral blood volume by displacement into the venous sinuses, or (4) displacement of brain tissue.

The autoregulatory mechanism of the brain regulates the diameter of the cerebral blood vessels to maintain a constant rate of CBF in response to a wide range of systemic arterial pressures. In the presence of autoregulation, CBF is not altered with mean systemic arterial pressures (MSAP) between 60 and 160 mm Hg.[4] When cerebral autoregulation is impaired, blood flow to the brain becomes dependent on the systemic arterial pressure (SAP). As blood pressure rises, the CBF increases, as does the ICP. As blood pressure decreases, the CBF also falls, causing cerebral ischemia.

The intracranial compliance, the rate of expansion of the volume (the faster the rate, the greater the rise in ICP), the volume of the mass and intracranial compartment, and impairment of CSF reabsorption

Table 3-20 Lundberg's Classification of ICP

Classification	Pressure Range
Normal	<10 mm Hg
Slightly elevated	11–20 mm Hg
Moderately elevated	21–40 mm Hg
Severely elevated	>40 mm Hg

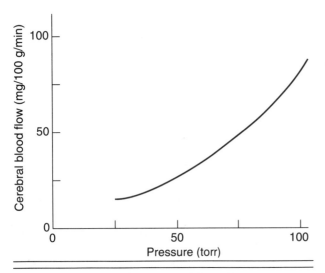

Figure 3-21   Cerebral Pressure-Volume Curve

are all factors affecting compensation. The pressure-volume curve shown in Figure 3-21 graphically illustrates the relationship between intracranial pressure and volume blood flow. Initially, increases in volume cause no increases in ICP, followed by only slight increases in ICP. As compensation begins to fail, small increases in volume result in significant increases in ICP. A critical point is reached when compensation is lost and brain compliance is decreased. At this point slight increases in volume cause severe increases in ICP. Decompensation occurs when compensation capacities fail to maintain ICP equilibrium. If compensation is exhausted, severe increases in ICP compromise CBF and cerebral perfusion pressure (CPP). It is generally considered that when CPP, the blood pressure gradient at which brain cells are being perfused, drops below 60 mm Hg, cerebral ischemia results. Brain death results when CBF ceases and ICP equals SAP. The following formula is used to calculate CPP:

$$MSAP - ICP = CPP$$

where

> MSAP = mean systemic arterial pressure
> ICP = intracranial pressure
> CPP = cerebral perfusion pressure

Resulting signs and symptoms

Neurological assessment in conjunction with diagnostic evaluation is the most accurate and reliable method of determining increases in ICP when a continuous intracranial pressure-monitoring device is not available. Establishing a baseline assessment and performing frequent ongoing assessments will help to detect early signs of increased ICP. The signs and symptoms of increased ICP in the early and later stages are presented in Table 3-21.

Decreased level of consciousness (LOC)   Alterations in LOC are the most sensitive and reliable indicators of neurological changes. Subtle early changes include lethargy, confusion, disorientation, restlessness, and apathy. As ICP continues to increase and deterioration in the LOC progresses, the patient will become comatose.

Headache and vomiting   Patients with increased ICP may complain of an intermittent, mild headache, which may worsen upon awakening. Various activities such as coughing and sneezing may also increase the discomfort. Vomiting may be caused by direct compression of the vomiting center located in the medulla. This vomiting may be associated with nausea and be projectile in nature.

Visual disturbances and pupillary dysfunction   Visual impairments may occur early in the development of increased ICP as the result of increased pressure on the visual pathways causing blurred vision, visual field deficits, and diplopia. Papilledema (optic nerve compression) is usually considered a late finding of increased ICP.

Pupillary changes reflect the degree of the brain compression. Increased ICP in the midbrain causes the pupil to dilate, become slightly oval in appearance, and respond sluggishly to light. Further increases in ICP can result in a dilated, nonreactive pupil, ipsilateral to the area of brain compression. Bilateral dilated and fixed pupils occur in later stages of increased ICP and indicate brainstem herniation.

Motor dysfunction   In the early stages of increased ICP, extremity drifts and contralateral hemiparesis occur as motor fibers in the brainstem are compressed. During the later stages, abnormal posturing such as decortication and decerebration result from brainstem compression. In decompensation, bilateral flaccidity occurs following brainstem herniation.

Alterations in vital signs   Blood pressure and pulse remain relatively stable during the early stages of rising ICP. Changes in blood pressure and pulse occur in the later stages of increased ICP as the brainstem becomes compressed. As ICP rises, CPP becomes threatened, and cerebral ischemia results. This powerful stimulus triggers the systemic arterial pressure to increase while the diastolic pressure decreases or remains unchanged, creating a widened pulse pressure. The vagal response of bradycardia

Table 3-21 Clinical Manifestation of Increased ICP in Early and Late Stages

Early Clinical Presentation of Increased ICP	Late Clinical Presentation of Increased ICP
Level of Consciousness 　Disorientation 　Lethargic 　Restless	Level of Consciousness 　Deterioration 　Decreasing Glasgow Coma Scale rating 　Coma
Visual Responses 　Blurred vision 　Diplopia 　Visual field deficits	Visual Responses 　Signs of pupillary dysfunction; dilated, oval pupils are sluggish to nonreactive to light 　Papilledema
Motor Function 　Extremity drift 　Contralateral hemiparesis 　Seizure	Motor Function 　Decortication 　Decerebration 　Bilateral flaccidity
Sensory Function 　Impaired	Sensory Function 　Loss of brainstem reflexes 　—corneal 　—gag
Vital Signs 　Stable	Vital Signs 　Cushing response: rising systolic BP, widening pulse pressure, bradycardia
Discomfort 　Vague complaints of headache 　Projectile vomiting	Respiratory Function 　Hyperventilation 　Cheyne-Stokes (diffuse hemisphere involvement) 　Apneustic breathing (brainstem involvement) 　Ataxic breathing 　Pulmonary edema
	Reflexes 　Positive Babinski 　Chewing 　Sucking
	Acid-Base Balance 　Hypercarbia 　Hypoxemia

(full and bounding heart rate) is stimulated by increases in pressure. This late clinical finding of ICP is called the Cushing response.

Alterations in respiration with increasing ICP vary, depending on the area of the brain involved. Alterations in temperature are usually associated with hypothalamic dysfunction. In the early stages of increased ICP, temperature elevations may or may not be present. Temperature elevations are frequently observed during the later stages of increased ICP.

Nursing standards of care

The medical management of patients with increased ICP includes identifying the patient at risk and treating the underlying cause to restore the ICP to within a normal range. The following medical protocols are most commonly used in the overall management of increased ICP (see Table 3-22).

Hyperventilation by controlled mechanical ventilation is a well-established form of treatment for reducing increased ICP. Hypoxia is known to markedly alter cerebral blood flow, thus increasing pressure. Hyperventilation therapy to reduce $PaCO_2$ to between 25 and 30 mm Hg will maintain adequate oxygenation and vasoconstrict the cerebral arteries. This action reduces intracranial volume and facilitates the compensatory cerebral blood flow mechanism to decrease ICP.

Controlling cerebral perfusion pressure is accomplished by the use of routine blood pressure management techniques, relaxation, and treatment of temperature increases. Concurrently, promoting

Table 3-22   Medical Management of Increased ICP

Treatment Modality	Methods	Management Goals/Parameters

Ventilation	Adequate airway
	  Positioning
	  Intubation
	Mechanical ventilation
	  Hyperventilation
	  Use of PEEP
	Suctioning
		Desired blood gas values
		P_aO_2 80–100 mm Hg
		P_aCO_2 25–35 mm Hg

Cerebral perfusion pressure control	Blood pressure control
	  Reduce noxious stimuli
	  Muscle relaxants
	  Antihypertensive drugs
	  Volume replacement
	  Drugs to manage hypotension
		Low–normal CPP
		CPP = MSAP − ICP
		(normal range 45–160 mm Hg)

	Promoting cerebral venous return
	  Elevation of head of bed 30 degrees
	  Head positioning to reduce venous pressure
	Temperature control
	  Antipyretic drugs
	  Cooling blanket
		Low–normal CPP
		CPP = MSAP − ICP
		(normal range 45–160 mm Hg)
		Normothermia

Drugs
  Hyperosmolar agents
	Mannitol (20% solution)
	  Initial dosing: 1.0–2.0 g/kg intravenously, over 10–60 minutes
	  Multiple dosing: 0.25–0.50 g/kg intravenously every 4–6 hours
		Decrease brain volume

	Glycerol (50% or 75% solution)
	  Initial dosing: 1.0–1.5 g/kg by nasogastric tube
	  Multiple dosing: 0.5–1.0 g/kg by nasogastric tube every 3–4 hours
		Decrease brain volume

Steroids	Dexamethasone
	  Initial dosing: 10 mg IV or per NG
	  Multiple dosing: 4 mg IV or per NG every 6 hr
	Methylprednisolone
		Decrease brain volume

Diuretics	Furosemide Acetazolamide	{ Decrease CSF production { Decrease brain volume
Barbiturates	Sodium thiopental Pentobarbital	Decrease cerebral blood flow

Intracranial surgery	Mass removal
	  Burr holes
	  Craniotomy
		Decrease brain compression and brain shifts

	CSF shunting
	  Ventricular drain
	  Ventriculoperitoneal shunt
	  Ventriculoatrial shunt
		Decrease CSF volume

	Brain removal Bone removal	Decrease brain volume Decrease brain compression

Source: Snyder, Mariah. (1983). *A Guide to Neurological and Neurosurgical Nursing.* New York: John Wiley & Sons, Inc, p. 114–115.

cerebral venous return by elevating the head of the bed and positioning the patient's head so that compression of the jugular is prevented can help to decrease perfusion pressure.

Drug therapy for increased ICP is widespread. Hyperosmolar agents, steroids, and diuretics are all prescribed to treat intracranial hypertension. Barbiturate therapy in the treatment of uncontrolled ICP is attempted when conventional treatments have not been effective. A state of uncontrolled hypertension exists when the ICP exceeds 20 mm Hg for more than 30 minutes and fails to respond to less aggressive treatment. The goal of barbiturate therapy is to decrease cerebral metabolism in an attempt to lower ICP to a safe range. Loading and maintenance doses of pentobarbital (nembutal) or thiopental (pentothal) are administered to induce a state of coma. A vasopressor is usually necessary to maintain adequate MSP and CPP during this time. Continuous monitoring of ICP, ECG, arterial pressure, pulmonary artery pressure, and arterial blood gases are indicated in the management of barbiturate therapy to achieve hemodynamic stability.

Surgical management is chosen when ICP increases occur too rapidly for other mechanisms to be effective or when other interventions do not help the progress of the patient. Shunting of CSF fluid may help to reduce normal brain volume, and drilling burr holes and removal of bone can be performed in the event of severe ICP problems. Evacuation of neurohematomas, abscesses, tumors, and localized necrotic brain tissue can also be accomplished surgically.

Intracranial monitoring ICP monitoring is widely used in the therapeutic management of patients with cerebral insults. Direct ICP monitoring provides continuous information about ICP status and brain compliance in response to various therapeutic measures. Contraindications for ICP monitoring include abnormalities of blood clotting, collapsed or displaced ventricles (intraventricular monitoring), and a cerebral aneurysm in close proximity to the monitoring catheter.[5] As Figure 3-22 shows, three methods are used for ICP monitoring: intraventricular catheter (IVC), subarachnoid screw (bolt), and epidural transducer. These methods are described below.

Intraventricular catheter (IVC) A small catheter is inserted via a twist drill hole into the frontal horn of the lateral ventricle (preferably on the nondominant side). The IVC is connected to a stopcock, pressure tubing, collection drainage bag, and transducer for continuous monitoring. Advantages to the use of an IVC are accurate and reliable pressure recordings and access for CSF drainage and sampling. The disadvantages include the risk of intracranial hemorrhage, infection, rapid CSF drainage, and/or ventricular collapse.

Subarachnoid screw The subarachnoid screw is

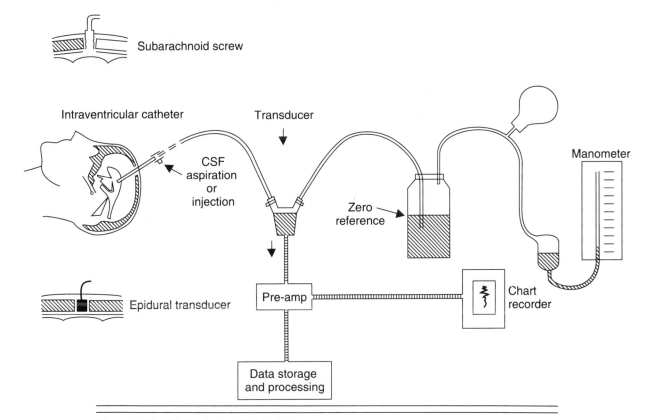

Figure 3-22 Methods for ICP Monitoring
Source: Adapted from Snyder, Mariah. (1983). *A Guide to Neurological & Neurosurgical Nursing.* New York: John Wiley & Sons, Inc., p. 111.

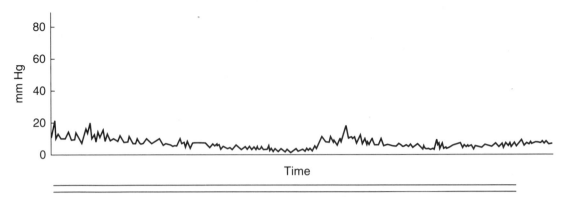

Figure 3-23   Normal ICP Waveform

firmly inserted through a twist drill hole in the skull with the base resting in the subarachnoid space. It is attached to a stopcock, pressure tubing, and transducer for continuous monitoring. Intracranial pressure measurements with the screw are less accurate than those with the IVC because the pressure is transmitted through the brain tissue. Advantages realized with the use of a subarachnoid screw include the ease of placement, reduced risk of brain penetration, and lower risk of infection compared to the IVC. Disadvantages of this method include the requirement of a closed skull, the inability to withdraw CSF, and the risk of hemorrhage during insertion.

Epidural Transducer   A small fiber-optic sensor is implanted in the epidural space through a burr hole in the skull. The epidural technique is the least invasive of the types of ICP monitoring. Thus, the risks of insertion and infection are low. The greatest disadvantages of the use of the epidural transducer are the low degree of accuracy and the inability to access CSF.

Interpreting ICP waveforms   Waveforms are produced by pulsations from the choroid plexus and transmitted through CSF. A normal ICP waveform is displayed in Figure 3-23. There are three types of abnormal waveforms: A, B, and C waves. The nurse should understand the clinical significance of these, which are illustrated in Figure 3-24. ICP waveforms that appear abnormal (dampened, heightened, or absent) may be related to problems in the pressure monitoring system. Potential causes of abnormal waveforms include a change in the patient's position in relation to the transducer, a need for calibration, a loose connection in the monitoring system, an air bubble in the tubing, or an occlusion somewhere in the system. Mastering troubleshooting techniques is important in the management of continuous ICP monitoring.

Nursing interventions have a direct impact on the management of increased ICP. The goal of nursing care is to prevent and control ICP. The following nursing care plan describes standard interventions used with individuals suffering from increased ICP.

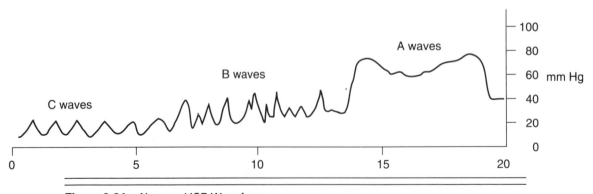

Figure 3-24   Abnormal ICP Waveforms

Nursing Care Plan for the Management of the Patient with Increased Intracranial Pressure

Diagnosis	Signs and symptoms	Intervention	Rationale
Potential alteration in comfort related to increased ICP	Headache Nausea Projectile vomiting	Maintain HOB at 30 degrees	Elevation of the head promotes venous drainage and decreases ICP
		Administer pain medication as ordered and initiate comfort measures	Alleviating or decreasing pain or discomfort helps to decrease ICP by decreasing MAP; comfort measures decrease agitation, thus decreasing ICP
Potential for alteration in cerebral perfusion related to increased ICP due to nursing activities, emotional upset, and agitation	Higher ICP readings Anxiety Agitation	Control external stimulation from the environment (noise, temperature, light, and odors)	Reducing external stimulation may help to decrease patient's activity and startle responses, thus decreasing ICP
		Prevent unnecessary disturbances	Nursing activities can lead to anxiety and agitation
		Approach patient in a calm and reassuring manner; provide soft stimuli (light touch, soft music, pleasant and familiar sounds)	Calm and quiet environment helps prevent drastic increases in ICP
		Plan activities to allow adequate rest times	Fatigue exacerbates agitation responses
		Monitor increases in ICP to learn what causes them and organize activities to minimize time and intensity of stimulation	To limit time and intensity of activities that challenge (stress) the patient and raise ICP
		Assist family to communicate with patient in a calm and quiet manner; counsel family to avoid emotionally stimulating the patient	Teaching of family may help to prevent unnecessary startles, excessive stimulation, and agitation that can lead to rises in ICP

Nursing Care Plan for the Management of the Patient with Increased Intracranial Pressure

Diagnosis	Signs and symptoms	Intervention	Rationale
Potential for impaired gas exchange related to inadequate ventilation, hypercapnia, hypoxemia, and increased secretions	Hypercapnia Hypoxemia Increased secretions	Maintain airway; ensure adequate ventilation	To promote adequate oxygen exchange
		Assess color of skin and mucous membranes; monitor trends in ABGs	Assessment of signs of oxygenation and blood gas analysis evaluate adequacy of respiratory function
		Hyperventilation therapy to maintain $PaCO_2$ between 25 and 30 mm Hg (or as prescribed); notify MD if $PaCO_2 < 25$ mm Hg	Hyperventilation blows off carbon dioxide, thus reducing $PaCO_2$ levels, which causes vasoconstriction, thereby decreasing ICP; $PaCO_2 < 25$ mm Hg may impair autoregulation
		Closely monitor patient's response to PEEP	PEEP may increase intrathoracic pressure
	Respiratory crackles, gurgles, and wheezes	Hyperoxygenate and hyperventilate with 100% O_2 before and after suctioning	To help reduce the risk of hypoxemia and hypercapnia, which cause cerebral vasodilation
		Avoid suctioning for more than 15 seconds per each insertion of catheter	Prolonged suctioning causes hypoxemia and agitation
		Assess neck veins for jugular venous distention	To determine increased CVP
Potential for impaired venous drainage of the brain from incorrect positioning and agitation	Impaired venous drainage and increased ICP	Maintain head and neck in a neutral position with HOB elevated 15–30 degrees	To reduce the risk of impaired venous drainage and increased ICP
		Assist patient in turning and moving in bed	Avoiding excessive activities, strain, and incorrect positioning decreases the risk of increasing intra-abdominal and intra-thoracic pressures, which may increase ICP
		Instruct patient to exhale while moving	
		Perform passive ROM exercises	

Diagnosis	Signs and symptoms	Intervention	Rationale
		Avoid isometric exercises	
		Avoid extreme flexion of the hip	
		Avoid flexion, extension, and rotation of the head	
		Prevent the Valsalva maneuver	The Valsalva maneuver increases intrathoracic pressure, which increases MAP and ICP
		Implement a bowel program	To help prevent constipation and the need to strain
Potential for injury and increases in ICP due to seizure activity	Seizure activity	Administer anticonvulsants as prescribed (Dilantin, Valium, and phenobarbital)	Prophylactic anticonvulsants in therapeutic doses (to achieve optimal effectiveness) help to prevent seizure activity
		Monitor therapeutic drug levels	
		Institute seizure precautions as needed (padded bed rails, oral airway, suction equipment, and supplemental oxygen)	To protect the patient from injury
Potential for alteration (decrease) in cerebral perfusion pressure (CPP) due to rising ICP	CPP < 60 mm Hg Rising ICP trends	Notify the MD	To initiate immediate medical intervention to prevent cerebral ischemia
		Conduct frequent neurological assessments	To detect early changes in neurological status
		Initiate nursing measures to decrease ICP	Decreased agitation and increased quiet and comfort help to decrease ICP
		Organize patient's activities to prevent further increases in ICP	To avoid rises in ICP from activity stressors

Nursing Care Plan for the Management of the Patient with Increased Intracranial Pressure

Diagnosis	Signs and symptoms	Intervention	Rationale
		Provide hyperventilation therapy and hyperoxygenate prior to suctioning	To decrease ICP and prevent further increases in ICP related to nursing activities
		Administer volume expanders, vasopressors, and antihypertensives as prescribed; monitor hemodynamic parameters (CVP, wedge pressures, and cardiac output)	To maintain adequate CPP and hemodynamic stability
Potential for increased cerebral metabolism related to temperature elevations	Shivering Temperature elevation	Monitor temperature every 4 hours	Elevated temperatures increase cerebral oxygen demand and cerebral blood flow
		Assess and treat the cause of increased temperature (such as superimposed infection or hypothalamic dysfunction); apply hypothermia blanket	To maintain normothermia and help control shivering (shivering increases oxygen consumption and metabolic rates, which exhaust glycogen stores and produce acidosis)
Potential for fluid and electrolyte imbalance related to antidiuretic hormone imbalance, fluid restrictions, gastrointestinal suctioning, and hyperthermia	Volume excess	Accurately monitor I&O and urine specific gravity	To ascertain fluid balance status
	Volume depletion	Assess for signs of volume depletion or excess	To ascertain fluid balance status
	Electrolyte imbalances	Closely monitor electrolyte status, hematocrit, BUN, creatinine, and serum osmolality	To detect imbalances and determine renal function
		Adhere strictly to fluid restrictions	To avoid overhydration and cerebral edema
		Maintain temperature within normal limits	To prevent rises in ICP

Diagnosis	Signs and symptoms	Intervention	Rationale
		Assess for presence of bowel sounds and abdominal distention; measure gastric output and test pH every 8 hours; if pH < 5, administer antacids as ordered	Gastric retention and aspiration of gastric contents increase intra-abdominal and intrathoracic pressures
		Consult with dietician and initiate nutritional support as soon as appropriate; initiate tube feeding if needed	Early nutritional support promotes strength leading to recovery
Potential for anxiety due to: fear of unknown, fear of death, fear of pain, fear of disability, lack of knowledge regarding hospital procedures and routines	Facial tension Distracting behavior Low attention span Withdrawal Twitching and shaking of extremities Inappropriate laughter or behavior Diaphoresis Tachycardia Nonadherence to treatment plan	Ascertain patient's fears and anxieties	Will allow the nurse to know just what to address
		Ascertain patient's previous hospital experiences (own as well as others')	Will help the nurse to know how to best alleviate anxieties and support positive attitudes
		Ascertain readiness to learn	Need to begin patient and family education when ready
		Teach patient about routines of hospital and care regimen: tubes, lines, ICU routines, visiting hours, pain medication, moving, and deep breathing and coughing; provide patient with educational booklets	To help patient and family be prepared for what is to be experienced
		Sedate as ordered PRN	To help patient relax
		Provide emotional support as needed	To help patient and family deal with the situation in the best way possible
		Consult with social worker, chaplain, etc., as needed	Multidisciplinary team effort provides broader, more comprehensive care

Nursing Care Plan for the Management of the Patient with Increased Intracranial Pressure

Diagnosis	Signs and symptoms	Intervention	Rationale
Potential for skin breakdown due to: restriction of movement; pain/discomfort; drug-induced neuromuscular or musculoskeletal impairment; depression; body stiffness; diaphoresis or drainage into patient's bed; independent variables such as diabetes, peripheral vascular disease, obesity, etc.	Imposed restriction of movement, including body mechanics, medical protocol, etc.	Place air mattress on bed	To prevent pressure spots on skin
	Impaired coordination or decreased muscle strength preventing independent movement	Assist with required movements; quarter turn every 1–2 hours	To prevent overexertion and to facilitate movement
	Reluctance to attempt movement	Encourage movement within safety parameters	To prevent injury and facililate movement
	Redness over pressure points	Inspect pressure points, including occiput, sacrum, coccyx, heels, and elbows, every 2 hours	To prevent skin breakdown
		Passive range of motion for all extremities	To prevent pressure spots
		Keep patient dry	To prevent skin breakdown
		Maintain and supplement nutrition as needed	To maintain vital nutrients to skin
		Consult enterostomal therapist	To provide for optimal care planning and intervention and to prevent skin breakdown
	Elevated temperature	Keep patient dry when diaphoretic	To prevent skin breakdown
Potential for ineffective coping by the patient or family related to: situational crisis, maturational crisis, personal vulnerability	Verbalization of inability to cope	Assess family's usual coping mechanisms	Questions and concerns of patient and family must be answered even if not voiced
	Inability to ask for emotional help	Assist family to identify alternative coping mechanisms; identify and acknowledge family's needs	Optimal coping must be accomplished for maximal healing

Diagnosis	Signs and symptoms	Intervention	Rationale
	Inability to meet role expectations	Provide information to patient and family regarding diagnosis and supportive services	Patient and family must be helped through role redefinition
	Prolonged progression of disease or disability	Support patient and family through role transition time	To help patient and family make transition
		Encourage open communication among patient, family, and health care team	To facilitate problem solving and care planning
		Reinforce simple explanations to patient and family	During times of crisis, care must be taken not to cause information overload
	Exhaustion	Provide rest periods and offer nutrition; plan visiting schedule to accommodate interventions as well as family's schedule and rest periods; restrict visitors as appropriate	To maximize strength; to improve quality of family time as well as provide for needed rest
	Fear and anxiety	Delegate one resource and support person to assist family communication	Consistency in problem solving and care improves quality of decisions
	Inappropriate requests or hypervigilance by patient and/or family	Suggest approaches for family to assist in patient's care	Participatory care decreases family's anxiety
	Inability to solve problems	Assist patient and family to identify problems and work together to solve them	Sometimes patients and families are unable to anticipate possible problems
	Unreasonable and/or excessively frequent requests (excessive use of call light)	Assist family in caring for patient and problem solve about how to continue such care after discharge	Personal involvement in care decreases anxiety while increasing self-confidence and skills
		Encourage progressively independent activities	To avoid rushing patient and family into too much responsibility for care

Nursing Care Plan for the Management of the Patient with Increased Intracranial Pressure

Diagnosis	Signs and symptoms	Intervention	Rationale
Potential for self-care deficit due to: muscle deconditioning; disturbance of sleep pattern; fear of overexertion; anxiety; decreased tolerance of activity	Weak muscles resulting from bedrest	Encourage activities safe to patient: minor self-care, passive ROM	To allow time for patient to regain strength
	Reports of headaches	Assess discomfort and encourage patient to request medication as appropriate	To allow for maximal rest and decreased ICP
	Fatigue	Assess patient's need for rest and sleep and incorporate rest periods during the day	To allow for needed rest and to promote relaxation and healing
	Increased heart rate and respiratory rate upon minimal activity	Facilitate calm environment (lighting, noise, interruptions, etc.)	To prevent agitation and discomfort, leading to increased ICP
	Repetitive fast speech, indicating anxiety	Encourage patient's participation in scheduling and carrying out daily care to decrease anxiety through familiarity	To prevent anxiety leading to overexhaustion and to facilitate adequate rest
Potential for infection due to: immunosuppressive therapy, IV lines, indwelling Foley, endotracheal intubation, stress	Increased temperature	Tylenol 600 mg every 4 hours PRN as ordered	To alleviate fevers
	WBC > 10,000 mm³	Implement thorough hand washing between patient contacts; implement universal isolation precautions if indicated	To prevent spread of infections
	Redness, exudate, or increased tenderness at IV or ICP insertion site	Routine IV care with povidone-iodine solution, telfa dressing, and foam tape	To prevent infections
		Change peripheral IV sites at least every 3 days or with any signs of infection or infiltration; change IV tubing every 48 hours	IV fluid is especially fertile medium for bacterial growth

Diagnosis	Signs and symptoms	Intervention	Rationale
		Culture suspected origins of infection	To administer antibiotics that bacteria are sensitive to
	Changes in characteristics of sputum: tan, brown, yellow, or green color and/or foul odor	Nonvigorous pulmonary toilet	To prevent and/or treat pulmonary congestion that can lead to infections (without increasing neurological stressors)
	Chest x-ray indicative of atelectasis		
	Decreased or absent breath sounds locally		
	Sediment in urine or foul-smelling urine; WBCs in urine; hesitancy, frequency, urgency, burning, difficulty starting stream, incontinence, and/or inability to void	Routine Foley care every 8 hrs; push fluids if taking fluids and not neurologically contraindicated	To prevent urinary tract infections
Potential for alteration in bowel function or constipation due to: decreased mobility, change in eating patterns, side effects of medications, decreased fluid volume	Reports of feeling constipated, "full" feeling in abdomen, inability to move bowels	Assess abdomen for bowel sounds, softness, and appearance and ask patient about discomfort at least every 12 hours	For early diagnosis of constipation in order to prevent Valsalva maneuver and to intervene before serious problems occur
	Decreased or absent bowel sounds	Encourage progressive activity as tolerated	To stimulate peristalsis
	Inadequate oral fluid/food intake as evidenced on I&O records and calorie counts	Reassure patient that constipation is frequently a problem during bedrest	So patient will not become overly concerned
	Symptoms of dehydration: poor skin turgor, sunken eyes, intake less than output, weight loss	Assess for signs of dehydration and encourage oral intake within fluid restriction limits	Hydration impedes constipation
		Closely monitor electrolytes	Dehydration leads to electrolyte imbalance

Nursing Care Plan for the Management of the Patient with Increased Intracranial Pressure

Diagnosis	Signs and symptoms	Intervention	Rationale
	Absence of bowel movement for more than 2 days	Implement bowel regimen as ordered: milk of magnesia 30 mL p.o. every HS; consult with dietician about increased fiber in diet as indicated; rehydrate patient as ordered via IV or oral fluids (as neurologically indicated)	Patient may need extra help to have regular bowel movements
		Reduce narcotic consumption when feasible	Narcotics inhibit bowel activity
Knowledge deficit concerning increased ICP, complications, diagnostic tests, and treatments	Communicates lack of knowledge Exhibits behavior indicating knowledge deficit	Educate patient and family about the significance of increased ICP, complications, diagnostic tests, and treatments	A higher level of understanding may improve compliance with established regime
		Assess level of understanding and reinforce content	Reinforcement promotes learning

Medications Commonly Used in the Care of the Patient with Increased Intracranial Pressure

Medication	Effect	Major side effects

Hyperosmotic agents:
  Mannitol
  Glycerol
	Reduction in brain water by creating an osmotic gradient between tissue and plasma
	Reduction of intracranial pressure within 1–3 hours by rapid diuresis
		Diuresis
		Electrolyte imbalances
		Rebound of increased intracranial pressure

Corticosteroids:
  Dexamethasone
  Prednisone
  Hydrocortisone
  Methylprednisolone
	Reduction of cerebral edema by stabilizing the capillary endothelial junction and reducing cerebrovascular permeability
	Promotes integrity of cells to inhibit flow of intracellular fluid to extracellular space
		Opportunistic infection
		Cushing's syndrome
		Nervousness
		Hyperglycemia
		Electrolyte imbalances
		Menstrual irregularities
		Skin rash
		Gastric irritation

Diuretics:
  Furosemide
  Ethacrynic acid
	Loop diuretic
	Decrease in intracranial pressure within 2–4 hours
		Hypokalemia
		Hypocalcemia
		Hypomagnesemia
		Altered glucose metabolism

Barbiturates:
  Phenobarbital
  Primidone
	Control of seizure activity by raising the seizure threshold of cells
	CNS depressant
	Lowered cerebral metabolism
		Drowsiness leading to coma
		Confusion
		Respiratory depression
		Hypotension
		Renal failure
		Blood dyscrasias
		Hypocalcemia

Vasopressors:
  Dobutamine
  Dopamine
  Phenylephrine
	Inotropic with alpha-adrenergic stimulant
	Vasoconstrictor
	Decreased tissue perfusion
		Headache
		Hypotension
		Vasoconstriction
		Dyspnea
		Ectopic arrhythmias

Anticonvulsant:
  Phenytoin (Dilantin)
  Valproic acid
	Prevention of seizures by stabilizing the cell threshold of excitation and inhibiting the spread of impulses to adjacent tissue	CNS depression
		Cardiovascular collapse
		Nausea and vomiting
		Vertigo
		Ataxia
		Hypotension
		Coagulation defects

Valium	Decreases force of seizures by relaxing the skeletal muscles and depressing the reticular activating and limbic systems	Respiratory depression Increased frequency of generalized tonic-clonic seizures

Medications Commonly Used in the Care of the Patient with Increased Intracranial Pressure

Medication	Effect	Major side effects
Carbamazepine	Analgesic Decreases complex partial, simple partial, and generalized tonic-clonic seizures	Nausea and vomiting Vertigo Drowsiness Aplastic anemia Hepatotoxicity Inappropriate secretion of ADH
Antipyretic (Aspirin)	Analgesic Anti-inflammatory Alters the temperature regulation center of the hypothalamus	Interference with synthesis of prothrombin Inhibition of platelet adhesiveness leading to hemorrhage Tinnitus Hypothrombinemia
Analgesic (Codeine)	Inhibits transmission of pain impulses at the subcortical level	Respiratory depression Decreased peristalsis Drowsiness

Head Trauma

Head trauma encompasses injuries that cause damage to the skull, brain, and/or intracranial vessels. The clinical course of head trauma depends primarily on the type of injury sustained. However, several commonalities are found among the various injuries in physiological progression and clinical care. The following discussion will present the precursors, pathophysiological processes, signs and symptoms, and accepted practices used in the care of individuals suffering from different categories of injury to the skull, brain, and intracranial vessels.

Trauma to the Skull

Injury to the skull occurs in the form of skull fractures, and these are classified by type as linear, depressed, or compound (open) and also by location. Linear skull fractures, the most commonly seen, occur as clean breaks in the skull bone without any inward depression of the bone toward the brain. In contrast, depressed skull fractures involve inward movement of the bone toward the brain tissue. Compound fractures are breaks in the bone that are accompanied by open cuts or lacerations in the scalp. Locations of skull fractures include the frontal, orbital, temporal, parietal, posterior fossa, and basilar areas.

Clinical antecedents

Events leading up to all types of skull fractures include falls, accidents, gunshot wounds, and blows to the head. Risk factors range from personal lifestyles and habits of the victims to unpredictable accidents. Many skull fractures can be prevented through the safe use of weapons and sports apparatus and the enforcement of seat belt and helmet safety standards. Low-velocity assaults cause linear skull fractures. Depressed skull fractures occur as a result of very hard blows to the head area. Compound skull fractures are a direct result of severe and penetrating injuries.

Critical referents

Linear skull fractures Individuals suffering from linear fractures very rarely (if ever) sustain associated brain tissue damage. Some type of blow to the head results in a clean and uncomplicated disruption of the skull.

Depressed skull fractures When a blow to the head results in a depression of skull bone into the brain tissue, a more complicated injury occurs. Direct damage to the brain tissue may occur in the form of concussion, contusion, hematoma, or hemorrhage and may develop into a full-blown case of increased ICP. Dural tears may be involved, as well as direct perforation of venous sinuses. Brain tissue damage usually remains localized directly beneath the point of impact; however, depending upon the acceleration, force, and impact of the blow and the resulting jostling of brain tissue, the risk of unforeseen complications is present.

Compound skull fractures Compound skull fractures occur with scalp cuts and lacerations directly above or in proximity to the fracture line. Foreign objects and bone fragments frequently penetrate the brain tissue and can cause dural tears leading to hematoma or hemorrhage. Introduction of bacteria through the lacerations into the brain tissue place these patients at very high risk for infection.

Resulting signs and symptoms

Linear skull fractures Linear skull fractures can be diagnosed from x-rays of the skull. Usually no accompanying neurological deficits are experienced, since the break is clean and without brain tissue involvement. There may be a complete absence of neurological symptoms.

Depressed and compound skull fractures Signs and symptoms of depressed and compound skull fractures depend on the area in which the fracture occurs and the extent of injury to the adjacent brain tissue. Frequently a very apparent indentation and/or open wound in the patient's head is noticeable upon visual check. More specific symptoms manifested with injuries to selected locations are detailed in Table 3-23.

Nursing standards of care

Linear skull fractures Close observation leading to early recognition and expedient intervention is what is required in the care of the linear skull fracture patient. A hematoma may develop at the time of injury or several hours later, so frequent neurological checks are required. After a brief observation period

Table 3-23 Symptoms Manifested with Skull Fractures in Selected Neurological Regions

Location of Fracture	Symptoms
Frontal	Pneumocranium CSF drainage from the nose Cortex rhinorrhea
Orbital	Periorbital ecchymosis (raccoon eyes)
Temporal	Ecchymosis behind the ear (Battle's sign) CSF drainage from the ear (otorrhea) Cortex otorrhea
Parietal	Loss of hearing Loss of taste Facial paralysis Ecchymosis behind the ear (Battle's sign) CSF drainage from the ear (otorrhea) Cortex otorrhea Tympanic bulging from blood and/or CSF pooling
Posterior fossa	Visual field deficits Cortical blindness Occipital ecchymosis Loss of coordination

Basilar	CSF or blood drainage in external auditory canal
	CSF drainage from the nose (rhinorrhea)
	Ecchymosis behind the mastoid (Battle's sign)
	Periorbital ecchymosis (raccoon eyes)
	Tympanic membrane bulging from pooling of blood or CSF
	Cranial nerve disturbances:
	   Facial paralysis or paresis
	   Hearing impairment
	   Tinnitus
	   Nystagmus
	   Conjugate deviation of gaze
	   Vertigo

that results in negative findings, the patient can usually be discharged to the care of a significant other. In the event of unforeseen complications (which almost always result in increased ICP), patients are managed according to guidelines specified in the preceding section on increased intracranial pressure.

Depressed and compound skull fractures Surgical elevation and/or removal of bony fragments and other objects is usually medically indicated. Surgical repair of dural tears, hematomas, and/or hemorrhage may also be attempted. Once surgery has been accomplished, medical and nursing care follows the postoperative care regimen detailed in the section on craniotomies. One additional point to emphasize is

the need for appropriate antibiotic treatment to overcome the high risk of infection caused by the introduction of foreign objects and bacteria at the injury site.

Brain Tissue Injury

Injury to the brain tissue falls into three basic categories, which are, in order of severity, concussion, cerebral contusion, and hematoma.

Clinical antecedents

As in the case of injury to the skull, events leading to brain tissue injury range from falls and accidents to gunshot wounds and blows to the head. Risk factors are similar to those in regard to skull injuries, and prevention is also the same. A concussion is usually caused by a stunning blow to the head, somewhat similar to a precordial thump. Cerebral contusions occur as a result of brain movement within the skull that is caused by blows to the head. Sometimes the blow is of such consistency that opposing forces are strong enough to drive the brain back against the opposite skull surface with such force that a more severe injury directly opposite the original point of impact results. Finally, hematomas are usually associated with a fracture (again caused by an external blow) along the distribution of the middle meningeal artery in the temporal region.

Critical referents

Concussions are traumatic injuries causing transient neuronal dysfunction of an immediate but short-term nature. A concussion is basically an electrical event, causing momentary depolarization, in which the brain tissue experiences no lasting changes.

Cerebral contusions result in petechial damage (bruising) to the brain tissue as a result of brain movement within the skull. Bruising occurs either at the site of impact of the blow or far from the initial injured area in a contrecoup manner, where the brain is bounced away from the point of impact with force enough to cause bruising at the opposing reverberated point within the skull. Areas of the brain most frequently experiencing contusions are the frontal and temporal lobes and the brainstem.

Finally, hematomas may occur epidurally, subdurally, or intracerebrally. Epidural hematomas are arterial bleeds, generally originating from the middle meningeal artery, which occur in the epidural space between the skull and the dura. In contrast, subdural hematomas are collections of venous blood in the subdural space between the dura and the arachnoid. Intracerebral hematomas occur when bleeding into the parenchyma develops. Depending on the size and location of the bleed, brain shifting can result.

Resulting signs and symptoms

A history and physical examination are important to the diagnosis. The history should pay particular attention to details of the accident or causal event and should be taken from an eyewitness, if possible. Special attention should be given to any period of unconsciousness, no matter how short. Radiographs, CT scans, and other radiologic tests may be indicated by the history and physical presentation. It is wisest to assume the worst-case scenario and err on the side of caution and conservatism than to miss a clinical sign indicating progressing neurological involvement.

The signs of a concussion are immediate and transient. Short episodes of neurological deficits such as loss of consciousness, loss of balance or coordination, or short-term and temporary amnesia or disorientation occur. Prompt recovery occurs, and any neurological deficit assessed during neurological checks soon disappears (usually within 24 hours).

Manifestations of a cerebral contusion depend on the extent and location of the injury. The patient suffering contusions frequently loses consciousness and, because of the very high risk of immediate or delayed edema either in the defined areas of bruising or diffusely throughout the brain tissue, is known to develop signs of increased ICP (refer to Table 3-21).

The patient who experiences epidural hematomas also usually loses consciousness. These hematomas may surface rapidly or may be manifested after a period of apparent neurological intactness. Regardless of time of clinical manifestation, because the bleeding is arterial and under high pressure, extensive morbidity and mortality can occur within very short periods of time. Frequently, this individual regains consciousness for a short period of time and then deteriorates rather rapidly. Complaints of headache are almost always voiced upon regaining consciousness, and then the patient experiences progressive compromises in responsiveness. Signs and symptoms of increased ICP occur, along with further manifestations of specific brain region involvement. If the hematoma is left unchecked, the extradural collection of blood can become great enough to cause

the uncus of the temporal lobe to begin to herniate down through the tentorium, resulting in a true neurosurgical emergency.

Signs and symptoms of subdural hematomas may occur acutely or in a delayed and chronic manner (occurring weeks after the assult). These bleeds are less of an immediate emergent nature than epidural hematomas because they are venous rather than arterial bleeds, but still carry high risk for morbidity and mortality. General signs include those of increased ICP and may occur immediately or progressively. As with epidural hematomas, local areas of involvement elicit specific clinical presentations.

Manifestations of intracerebral hematomas depend on the location and extent of injury and how much exacerbation from edema occurs to the tissue. Usually, decreased reactivity and responsiveness occurs early on, and if left untreated, the condition progresses in severity, producing symptoms of uncal herniation.

Nursing standards of care

Care of the patient suffering from concussion involves close neurological observation for a short period of time. If the patient remains unremarkable upon neurological assessment, discharge with instructions about reporting any indications of developing complications is indicated.

Management of cerebral contusions is targeted at basic life support and controlling cerebral edema. This is accomplished by closely observing the patient and initiating early interventions as indicated by assessment and diagnosis.

Medical management of epidural, subdural, and intracerebral hematomas depends on the type and rate of progression of the signs and symptoms of neurological deterioration. Basic life support is of primary importance. Seizure precautions are frequently instituted. Burr holes are often indicated, and hyperosmolar fluids and steroids are administered to help reduce increased ICP. Surgical intervention is frequently indicated (depending on whether the location is in an operable area) to ligate the bleeder and evacuate the hematoma. In concert with the medical management, nurses must closely monitor the patient. Delays in diagnosis and treatment can result in life-threatening situations. In addition, care reflects practices developed for the individual suffering from increased ICP. Postoperative care is administered as detailed in the section on care of neurosurgical patients.

Nursing Care Plan for the Management of the Patient with Head Trauma

Diagnosis	Signs and symptoms	Intervention	Rationale
Potential alteration in comfort related to increased ICP	Headache Nausea Projectile vomiting	Maintain HOB at 30 degrees	Elevation of the head promotes venous drainage and decreases ICP
		Administer pain medication as ordered and initiate comfort measures	Alleviating or decreasing pain or discomfort helps to decrease ICP by decreasing MAP; comfort measures decrease agitation, thus decreasing ICP
Potential for alteration in cerebral perfusion related to increased ICP due to nursing activities, emotional upset, and agitation	Higher ICP readings Anxiety Agitation	Control external stimulation from the environment (noise, temperature, light, and odors)	Reducing external stimulation may help to decrease patient's activity and startle responses, thus decreasing ICP
		Prevent unnecessary disturbances	Nursing activities can lead to anxiety and agitation
		Approach patient in a calm and reassuring manner; provide soft stimuli (light touch, soft music, pleasant and familiar sounds)	Calm and quiet environment helps prevent drastic increases in ICP
		Plan activities to allow adequate rest times	Fatigue exacerbates agitation responses
		Monitor increases in ICP to learn what causes them and organize activities to minimize time and intensity of stimulation	To limit time and intensity of activities that challenge (stress) the patient and raise ICP
		Assist family to communicate with patient in a calm and quiet manner; counsel family to avoid emotionally stimulating the patient	Teaching of family may help to prevent unnecessary startles, excessive stimulation, and agitation that can lead to rises in ICP

Diagnosis	Signs and symptoms	Intervention	Rationale
Alteration in cerebral perfusion related to increased ICP related to pathophysiology	Increased ICP Altered level of consciousness	Establish baseline for neurological functions; assess for changes by comparing ongoing assessments to baseline	To compare clinical findings to detect early changes in neurological functions
		Maintain fluid restriction and accurate I&O records	To help control ICP
		Monitor ABGs for hypocapnia	$PaCO_2 < 25$ mm Hg may impair autoregulation
		Maintain in a semi-Fowler's position with head in a neutral position except when contraindicated (with subdural hematoma and infratentorial approach)	To facilitate venous drainage
		Instruct patient to exhale with movement	To prevent Valsalva maneuver, which increases intrathoracic pressure, which increases ICP
	Anxiety	Control external stimulation (noise, light, temperature)	To prevent agitation and startle response, which cause increased ICP
	Agitation	Approach patient calmly and reassuringly	Nursing activities can lead to agitation
	Decreased pupillary response	Plan activities to allow for adequate rest	Fatigue exacerbates agitation responses
	Motor dysfunction	Monitor ICP increases to learn what causes them and organize activities to minimize stimulation	To limit time and intensity of activities that stress the patient and raise ICP
		Assist family to communicate calmly and quietly and to avoid emotionally stimulating the patient	To prevent excessive stimulation, agitation, and unnecessary startles, which cause rises in ICP

Nursing Care Plan for the Management of the Patient with Head Trauma

Diagnosis	Signs and symptoms	Intervention	Rationale
Alteration in respiratory function related to ineffective breathing patterns and airway clearance, impaired gas exchange, and immobility	Abnormal ABGs: $pO_2 < 80$ mm Hg; $pCO_2 < 35$ or > 45 mm Hg; pH < 7.35 or > 7.45; O_2 sat. $< 80\%$; $HCO_3 < 20$ or > 26 mEq/L; BE < 0 or > 3

Dyspnea

Hypoxemia

Hypercapnia

Copious secretions

Atelectasis

Elevated respiratory rate, wheezing, air hunger, gasping, or asymmetrical expansion of chest wall | Assess breathing pattern frequently

Maintain airway and mechanically ventilate postoperatively as required

Closely monitor ABGs PRN and after ventilator changes; closely monitor for absent, unequal, or diminished breath sounds, crackles, wheezing, or asymmetrical chest wall expansion

Aggressive pulmonary toilet (as neurologically indicated) PRN with chest percussion therapy, incentive spirometry, and hyperinflation using 100% oxygen before and after suctioning; turn and reposition patient every 2 hours (within neurological indications)

If stable, promote extubation as soon as possible by: holding sedation, elevating HOB 30 degrees, incremental weaning (as indicated neurologically) | To evaluate respiratory function

To ensure adequate ventilation

To discover early indications of respiratory compromise and/or complications

To mobilize secretions, provide adequate oxygenation, and open closed alveoli

To assist patient to return to optimal breathing capacity as soon as possible and to prevent atelectasis and secondary infection |

Diagnosis	Signs and symptoms	Intervention	Rationale
Potential for impaired gas exchange related to inadequate ventilation, hypercapnia, hypoxemia, and increased secretions	Hypercapnia Hypoxemia Increased secretions	Maintain airway; ensure adequate ventilation	To promote adequate oxygen exchange
		Assess color of skin and mucous membranes; monitor trends in ABGs	Assessment of signs of oxygenation and blood gas analysis evaluates adequacy of respiratory function
		Hyperventilation therapy to maintain $PaCO_2$ between 25 and 30 mm Hg (or as prescribed); notify MD if $PaCO_2 < 25$ mm Hg	Hyperventilation blows off carbon dioxide, thus reducing $PaCO_2$ levels, which causes vasoconstriction, thereby decreasing ICP; $PaCO_2 < 25$ mm Hg may impair autoregulation
		Closely monitor patient's response to PEEP	PEEP may increase intrathoracic pressure
	Respiratory crackles, gurgles, and wheezes	Hyperoxygenate and hyperventilate with 100% oxygen before and after sucitoning	To help reduce the risk of hypoxemia and hypercapnia, which cause cerebral vasodilation
		Avoid suctioning for more than 15 seconds per each insertion of catheter	Prolonged suctioning causes hypoxemia and agitation
		Assess neck veins for jugular venous distention	To determine increased CVP
Potential for impaired venous drainage of the brain from incorrect positioning and agitation	Impaired venous drainage and increased ICP	Maintain head and neck in a neutral position with HOB elevated 15–30 degrees	To reduce the risk of impaired venous drainage and increased ICP
		Assist patient in turning and moving in bed	Avoiding excessive activities, strain, and incorrect positioning decreases the risk of increasing intra-abdominal and intrathoracic pressures, which may increase ICP
		Instruct patient to exhale while moving	
		Perform passive ROM exercises	
		Avoid isometric exercises	
		Avoid extreme flexion of the hip	
		Avoid flexion, extension, and rotation of the head	

Nursing Care Plan for the Management of the Patient with Head Trauma

Diagnosis	Signs and symptoms	Intervention	Rationale
		Prevent the Valsalva maneuver	The Valsalva maneuver increases intrathoracic pressure, which increases MAP and ICP
		Implement a bowel program	To help prevent constipation and the need to strain
Potential for physical injury related to sensorimotor deficits, cognitive impairment, altered level of consciousness, or seizure activity	Motor deficits Agitation	Maintain a safe environment by: placing bed in low position with wheel brakes in locked position, side rails up, call light within easy reach, assistive devices within reach; arranging furniture and equipment for safe use by patient; providing adequate lighting at HS; providing nonskid foot wear	To promote safety and decrease risk of physical injury
		Identify patient's safety needs and establish safety guidelines with patient and family; reinforce guidelines frequently	To promote learning of safety practices by patient and family
	Seizures	Administer anticonvulsants as prescribed and monitor therapeutic levels	To help prevent seizures through attaining of optimal drug effectiveness
		Institute seizure precautions (padded bed rails, oral airway, suction equipment, and supplemental oxygen)	To decrease the risk of physical injury in the event of seizures
	Confusion	Reorient patient frequently	To increase patient's awareness of surroundings

Diagnosis	Signs and symptoms	Intervention	Rationale
	Anxiety	Explain patient care activities	To help alleviate anxiety
	Restlessness	Assess causes of restlessness (hypoxemia, pain, bladder distention) and plan care appropriate to need	To decrease risk of restlessness and agitation leading to possible accidental injury
		Use physical restraints only when necessary	To promote safety and reduce agitation
Potential for fluid and electrolyte imbalance related to antidiuretic hormone imbalance, fluid restrictions, gastrointestinal suctioning, and hyperthermia	Volume excess	Accurately monitor I&O and urine specific gravity	To ascertain fluid balance status
	Volume depletion	Assess for signs of volume depletion or excess	To ascertain fluid balance status
	Electrolyte imbalances	Closely monitor electrolyte status, hematocrit, BUN, creatinine, and serum osmolality	To detect imbalances and determine renal function
		Adhere strictly to fluid restrictions	To avoid overhydration and cerebral edema
		Maintain temperature within normal limits	To prevent rises in ICP
		Assess for presence of bowel sounds and abdominal distention; measure gastric output and test pH every 8 hours; if pH < 5, administer antacids as ordered	Gastric retention and aspiration of gastric contents increase intra-abdominal and intrathoracic pressures
		Consult with dietician and initiate nutritional support as soon as appropriate; initiate tube feeding if needed	Early nutritional support promotes strength leading to recovery
Potential for infection due to: surgical procedure, IV lines, indwelling Foley, endotracheal intubation, stress, CSF leak	Increased temperature	Tylenol 600 mg every 4 hours PRN as ordered	To alleviate fevers
	WBC > 10,000 mm^3	Implement thorough hand washing between patient contacts; implement universal isolation precautions if indicated	To prevent spread of infections

Nursing Care Plan for the Management of the Patient with Head Trauma

Diagnosis	Signs and symptoms	Intervention	Rationale
	Redness, exudate, or increased tenderness at IV or ICP insertion site	Routine care with povidone-iodine solution, telfa dressing, and foam tape	To prevent infections
		Change peripheral IV sites at least every 3 days or with any signs of infection or infiltration; change IV tubing every 48 hours	IV fluid is especially fertile medium for bacterial growth
		Culture suspected origins of infection	To administer appropriate antibiotics
	Changes in characteristics of sputum: tan, brown, yellow, or green color and/or foul odor	Nonvigorous pulmonary toilet	To prevent and/or treat pulmonary congestion leading to infections (without increasing neurological stressors)
	Decreased or absent breath sounds locally		
	Sediment in urine or foul-smelling urine; WBCs in urine; hesitancy, frequency, urgency, burning, difficulty starting urination, incontinence, and/or inability to void	Routine Foley care every 8 hours; push fluids if taking fluids and not neurologically contraindicated	To prevent urinary tract infections
	Altered LOC, headache, meningeal signs	If CSF leak suspected, test drainage with dextrostix (CSF will test positive for glucose)	To assess for early signs of wound infection, CSF leak, or meningitis, requiring prompt treatment
Alteration in tissue integrity of oral/nasal membrane due to trauma of transsphenoidal and oral surgical procedures	Red, swollen mucous membranes	Assess oral mucous membranes and gingival incisional line	To detect signs of infection
	Nasal bleeding	Provide mouth care every 4 hours and PRN with toothettes, using 1 part NS/1 part hydrogen peroxide/1 part Cepacol	To remove dried blood and clean mouth
	Complaints of pain	Lightly cleanse upper gingiva	To cleanse while protecting incision line

Diagnosis	Signs and symptoms	Intervention	Rationale
	Dry lips	Apply lip balm PRN	To promote comfort
		Administer high-humidity oxygen via face tent or mask	To provide moisture to mucous membranes
		Instruct patient to use toothbrush only on lower teeth until after 10 days	To prevent tearing of gingival incision
		Instruct patient to avoid sneezing and blowing the nose	To prevent stress on nasal membranes and graft site
		Keep accurate record of I&O	To monitor fluid balance
Alteration in patterns of urinary elimination due to decreased LOC, decreased mobility, and presence of urinary catheter	Urinary retention or incontinence	Report abnormal amount, color, or odor of urine and unusual frequency and pain of urination	To determine and treat early signs of urinary tract infection
		Monitor serum creatinine, BUN, urine specific gravity, UA, and urine C&S	To evaluate renal function
		Determine regular pattern of urination and structure bladder training accordingly	To establish optimal urine elimination
		Assess for urinary retention and plan catheterization regime accordingly	To assist patient to adequately empty bladder
Potential for alteration in bowel function or constipation due to: decreased mobility, change in eating patterns, side effects of medications, decreased fluid volume, postoperative paralytic ileus	Reports of feeling constipated, "full" feeling in abdomen, inability to move bowels	Assess abdomen for bowel sounds, softness, and appearance, and ask patient about discomfort at least every 12 hours	For early diagnosis of constipation in order to intervene before serious problems occur
	Decreased or absent bowel sounds	Encourage progressive ambulation and activity as indicated	To stimulate peristalsis
	Inadequate oral fluid/food intake as evidenced on I&O records and calorie counts	Reassure patient that constipation is frequently a postoperative problem	So patient will not become overly concerned

Nursing Care Plan for the Management of the Patient with Head Trauma

Diagnosis	Signs and symptoms	Intervention	Rationale
	Symptoms of dehydration: poor skin turgor, sunken eyes, intake less than output, weight loss	Assess for signs of dehydration and encourage oral intake unless on fluid restriction	Hydration impedes constipation
		Closely monitor electrolytes	Dehydration leads to electrolyte imbalance
	Absence of bowel movement for more than 2 days	Implement bowel regimen as ordered: milk of magnesia 30 mL p.o. every HS; consult with dietician about increased fiber in diet as indicated; rehydrate patient as ordered via IV or oral fluids	Patient may need extra help to start peristalsis postoperatively
		Reduce narcotic consumption when feasible	Narcotics inhibit bowel activity
Potential for skin breakdown due to: restriction of movement; pain/discomfort; drug-induced neuromuscular or musculoskeletal impairment; depression; body stiffness; diaphoresis or drainage into patient's bed; independent variables, such as diabetes, peripheral vascular disease, obesity, etc.	Imposed restriction of movement, including body mechanics, medical protocol, etc.	Place air mattress on bed	To prevent pressure spots on skin
	Impaired coordination or decreased muscle strength preventing independent movement	Assist with required movements; quarter turn every 1–2 hours	To prevent overexertion and to facilitate movement
	Reluctance to attempt movement	Encourage movement within safety parameters	To prevent injury and facilitate movement
	Redness over pressure points	Inspect pressure points, including occiput, sacrum, coccyx, heels, and elbows, every 2 hours	To prevent skin breakdown
		Passive range of motion for all extremities	To prevent pressure spots

Diagnosis	Signs and symptoms	Intervention	Rationale
		Keep patient dry	To prevent skin breakdown
		Maintain and supplement nutrition as needed	To maintain vital nutrients to skin
		Consult enterostomal therapist	To provide for optimal care planning and intervention and to prevent skin breakdown
	Elevated temperature	Keep patient dry when diaphoretic	To prevent skin breakdown
Alteration in rest/sleep pattern related to continuous environmental stimuli, ICU routine, and interrupted sleep	Disturbances in rest/sleep pattern	Determine the patient's established rest/sleep pattern and organize nursing activities to accommodate it as much as possible	To accommodate to patient's normal pattern
	Exhaustion	Structure nursing activities to provide for fewer interruptions at normal time of sleep; design schedule to balance daytime activities with periods of uninterrupted sleep	To maximize patient's ability to relax, rest, and sleep
	Inability to fall asleep	Provide comfort measures and assistive devices individualized to patient's need; explore the possibility of relaxation therapy	To promote comfort and sleep
	Interrupted rest periods	Plan visiting schedule to accommodate interventions as well as family's schedule and rest periods; restrict visitors as appropriate	To maximize quality of family time as well as provide for needed rest
Alteration in comfort related to: surgery, headache, dehydration, imposed physical restrictions	Headache Discomfort related to the use of IVs, Foley catheter, or invasive monitoring	Request patient to report and describe the presence of pain: location, onset and precipitator, duration, characteristics	To facilitate assessment of pain, specifically from the patient's perspective
		Assess physical signs and indicators of pain	To provide further indicators of pain

Nursing Care Plan for the Management of the Patient with Head Trauma

Diagnosis	Signs and symptoms	Intervention	Rationale
		Explore the use of comfort measures: repositioning, backrubs, massage, relaxation techniques	To promote comfort and alleviate fatigue
		Administer prescribed analgesics PRN or as ordered	To alleviate discomfort
		Determine the effectiveness of interventions and therapies	To facilitate maximal comfort measures
Potential for impaired verbal communication related to: decreased LOC, cerebral edema, dysphasia, endotracheal tube, tracheostomy	Receptive, global, or expressive aphasia	Assess patient's ability to hear, understand, and speak	To determine patient's ability to communicate
	Frustration during communication attempts	Teach appropriate strategies to promote communication: using assistive materials such as writing implements and communication board, reducing environmental distractions, decreasing anxiety, decreasing speed of communication, using simple commands with gestures	To help patient identify and use appropriate strategies to facilitate communication
		Face the patient and establish eye contact to provide support and reassurance during communication attempts	To encourage patient's efforts
		Consult with speech therapist	To allow for early rehabilitation
	Uneasiness and impatience of family during communication attempts	Teach family successful strategies for communication with patient	To promote family communication and cohesion

Diagnosis	Signs and symptoms	Intervention	Rationale
Disturbance in body concept related to: neurological deficits, cranial nerve dysfunction (facial palsy, decreased corneal reflex), hair loss from surgical procedure	Alterations in body concept	Assess patient's and family's interpretation of change in body concept	To establish baseline
	Anxiety during visiting hours	Encourage patient and family to express feelings	To help alleviate feelings of anxiety and promote adjustment
	Inability of family to comfortably and calmly look at and interact with patient	Assist family in adapting to patient's body changes and appearance	To achieve maximal level of self-esteem for patient and acceptance and support from family
	Lack of knowledge of available support services	Consult with hospital and community support services	To help patient and family make use of appropriate resources
Potential for ineffective coping by the patient or family related to: situational crisis, maturational crisis, personal vulnerability	Verbalization of inability to cope	Assess family's usual coping mechanisms	Questions and concerns of patient and family must be answered even if not voiced
	Inability to ask for emotional help	Assist family to identify alternative coping mechanisms; identify and acknowledge family's needs	Optimal coping must be accomplished for maximal healing
	Inability to meet role expectations	Provide information to patient and family regarding diagnosis and supportive services	Patient and family must be helped through role redefinition
	Prolonged progression of disease or disability	Support patient and family through role transition time	To help patient and family make transition
		Encourage open communication among patient, family, and health care team	To facilitate problem solving and care planning
		Reinforce simple explanations to patient and family	During times of crisis, care must be taken not to cause information overload
	Exhaustion	Provide rest periods and offer nutrition; plan visiting schedule to accommodate interventions as well as family's schedule and rest periods; restrict visitors as appropriate	To maximize strength; to improve quality of family time as well as provide for needed rest

Nursing Care Plan for the Management of the Patient with Head Trauma

Diagnosis	Signs and symptoms	Intervention	Rationale
	Fear and anxiety	Delegate one resource and support person to assist family communication	Consistency in problem solving and care improves quality of decisions
	Inappropriate requests or hypervigilance by patient and/or family	Suggest approaches for family to assist in patient's care	Participatory care decreases family's anxiety
	Inability to solve problems	Assist patient and family to identify problems and work together to solve them	Sometimes patients and families are unable to anticipate possible problems
	Unreasonable and/or excessively frequent requests (excessive use of call light)	Assist family in caring for patient and problem solve about how to continue such care after discharge	Personal involvement in care decreases anxiety while increasing self-confidence and skills
		Encourage progressively independent activities	To avoid rushing patient and family into too much responsibility for care
Potential for self-care deficit due to: muscle deconditioning, disturbance of sleep pattern, fear of overexertion, anxiety, decreased tolerance of activity	Weak muscles resulting from bedrest	Encourage activities safe to patient: minor self-care, passive ROM	To allow time for patient to regain strength
	Reports of headaches	Assess discomfort and encourage patient to request medication as appropriate	To allow for maximal rest and decreased ICP
	Fatigue	Assess patient's need for rest and sleep and incorporate rest periods during the day	To allow for needed rest and to promote relaxation and healing
	Increased heart rate and respiratory rate upon minimal activity	Facilitate calm environment (lighting, noise, interruptions, etc.)	To prevent agitation and discomfort, leading to increased ICP
	Repetitive fast speech, indicating anxiety	Encourage patient's participation in scheduling and carrying out daily care to decrease anxiety through familiarity	To prevent anxiety leading to overexhaustion and to facilitate adequate rest

Diagnosis	Signs and symptoms	Intervention	Rationale
Potential for anxiety due to: fear of unknown; fear of death; fear of pain; fear of disability; lack of knowledge regarding hospital procedures and routines	Facial tension Distracting behavior Low attention span Withdrawal Twitching and shaking of extremities Inappropriate laughter or behavior Diaphoresis Tachycardia Nonadherence to treatment plan	Ascertain patient's fears and anxieties	Will allow the nurse to know just what to address
		Ascertain patient's previous hospital experiences (own as well as others')	Will help the nurse to know how to best alleviate anxieties and support positive attitudes
		Ascertain readiness to learn	Need to begin patient and family education when ready
		Teach patient about routines of hospital and care regimen: tubes, lines, ICU routines, visiting hours, pain medication, moving, and deep breathing and coughing; provide patient with educational booklets	To help patient and family be prepared for what is to be experienced
		Sedate as ordered PRN	To help patient relax
		Provide emotional support as needed	To help patient and family deal with the situation in the best way possible
		Consult with social worker, chaplain, etc., as needed	Multidisciplinary team effort provides broader, more comprehensive care
Potential for alteration in health maintenance due to lack of knowledge of: diagnosis, surgical procedure, medication regimen, activity, medical follow-up, referrals, home management	Inability to describe personal diagnosis and how it relates to type of surgery and prognosis	Instruct patient and family about diagnosis, surgery, and prognosis with as many repetitions as needed	Patient and family must understand in order to adhere to prescribed regimen, which will promote healing and optimal level of functioning
		Encourage questions and open discussion of problems and concerns	To allow for clear understanding and acceptance

Nursing Care Plan for the Management of the Patient with Head Trauma

Diagnosis	Signs and symptoms	Intervention	Rationale
	Inability to describe prescribed regimen and reasons for it	Instruct about medications, diet, and followup arrangements: what, why, care options, plan of daily schedule	To promote understanding and thus adherence to prescribed regimen
	Does not distinguish between permitted and prohibited progression of activities	Include discussion of: activities in routine, balancing rest and activity, progression of activities, resumption of sexual roles and activities	To facilitate progressive resumption of activities without overdoing it and increasing risk of untoward event
	Does not know about followup appointments	Help patient and family to arrange followup plans before discharge	To promote continuity of care
	Lacks information pertaining to home management and followup arrangements	Explore discharge plans and home management with patient and family	To facilitate expeditious discharge
	Inability to identify professional and community services available for support	Review patient and family needs and available services and resources; refer to appropriate rehabilitation facilities	To enable patient and family to utilize available resources and services to attain most comprehensive care possible

Medications Commonly Used in the Care of the Patient with Head Trauma

Medication	Effect	Major side effects
Hyperosmotic agents: Mannitol Glycerol	Reduction in brain water by creating an osmotic gradient between tissue and plasma Reduction of intracranial pressure within 1–3 hours by rapid diuresis	Diuresis Electrolyte imbalances Rebound of increased intracranial pressure
Corticosteroids: Dexamethasone Prednisone Hydrocortisone Methylprednisolone	Reduction of cerebral edema by stabilizing the capillary endothelial junction and reducing cerebrovascular permeability Promotes integrity of cells to inhibit flow of intracellular fluid to extracellular space	Opportunistic infection Cushing's syndrome Nervousness Hyperglycemia Electrolyte imbalances Menstrual irregularities Skin rash Gastric irritation
Diuretics: Furosemide Ethacrynic acid	Loop diuretic Decrease in intracranial pressure within 2–4 hours	Hypokalemia Hypocalcemia Hypomagnesemia Altered glucose metabolism
Barbiturates: Phenobarbital Primidone	CNS depressant Lowered cerebral metabolism Control of seizure activity by raising the seizure threshold of cells	Drowsiness leading to coma Confusion Respiratory depression Hypotension Renal failure Blood dyscrasias Hypocalcemia
Vasopressors: Dobutamine Dopamine Phenylephrine	Inotropic with alpha-adrenergic stimulant Vasoconstrictor Decreased tissue perfusion	Headache Hypotension Vasoconstriction Dyspnea Ectopic arhythmias
Anticonvulsants: Phenytoin Valproic Acid	Prevention of seizures by stabilizing the cell threshold of excitation and inhibiting the spread of impulses to adjacent tissue	CNS depression Cardiovascular collapse Nausea and vomiting Vertigo Ataxia Hypotension Coagulation defects
Antibiotics (chosen according to infectious agent)	Overcoming of infectious agent	Specific to antibiotic agent chosen
Valium	Decreases force of seizures by relaxing the skeletal muscles and depressing the reticular activating and limbic systems	Respiratory depression Increased frequency of generalized tonic-clonic seizures

Medications Commonly Used in the Care of the Patient with Head Trauma

Medication	Effect	Major side effects
Carbamazepine	Analgesic Decreases complex partial, simple partial, and generalized tonic-clonic seizures	Nausea and vomiting Vertigo Drowsiness Aplastic anemia Hepatotoxicity Inappropriate secretion of ADH
Antipyretic (Aspirin)	Analgesic Anti-inflammatory Alters the temperature regulation center of the hypothalamus	Interference with synthesis of prothrombin Inhibition of platelet adhesiveness leading to hemorrhage Tinnitus Hypothrombinemia
Analgesic (codeine)	Inhibits transmission of pain impulses at the subcortical level	Respiratory depression Decreased peristalsis Drowsiness

Cerebral Aneurysm and Subarachnoid Hemorrhage

A cerebral aneurysm is a localized dilatation of the artery wall from a weakness in the vessel. Sudden bleeding into the subarachnoid space (SAS) as a result of trauma, hypertension, ruptured arteriovenous malformation, or aneurysm is called subarachnoid hemorrhage (SAH). Subarachnoid hemorrhage from a ruptured cerebral aneurysm and the associated complications of rebleeding, vasospasm, hypothalamic dysfunction, and hydrocephalus present one of the greatest challenges of critical care. A thorough knowledge of the causative factors, clinical presentation, complications, and treatment is vitally important in the care of the patient with this problem.

In spite of great progress in the prompt diagnosis and surgical management of the patient suffering from SAH, the morbidity and mortality rates remain unacceptably high.[6] The poor prognosis of SAH is overwhelming; approximately 28,000 new cases of ruptured aneurysm (12 per 100,000) occur in North America every year.[7] As a result of the primary insult, 10,000 people will die or suffer severe disability. Another 8,000 will die or be disabled as a result of secondary complications such as rebleeding (3,000), vasospasm (3,000), and medical and surgical complications (2,000). Fewer than one in three survivors ever return to their premorbid state.

Clinical antecedents

The causes of cerebral aneurysm are unknown, but the following conditions are associated with the more clinically advanced event of subarachnoid hemorrhage:[8]

Severe hypertension and arteriosclerosis

Arteriovenous malformation

Congenital defects

Blood dyscrasias such as leukemia, sickle cell anemia, thrombocytopenic purpura, and anticoagulation

Intracranial neoplasms

Infectious conditions and inflammation such as with syphilis

Direct traumatic damage to cerebral arteries

Cocaine abuse

Critical referents

Most aneurysms occur where there is a junction created by the bifurcation of arterial vessels along the circle of Willis. Eighty-five percent of these aneurysms involve the anterior portion of the circle of Willis, the internal carotid artery at the junction of the middle cerebral artery, the posterior communicating artery, and the anterior cerebral arteries at the junction of the anterior cerebral artery and the anterior communicating artery. The remaining 15% involve the vertebral-basilar system. Common sites include the junctions of the posterior cerebral, posterior communicating, and basilar arteries. The bifurcations of the vertebral arteries are also possible sites (Refer to Figure 3-9.)

Aneurysms are localized dilatations of the inner lining of the cerebral vessels, which may be caused by a weakness from a degenerative change or a congenital defect. Although the precise etiology of aneurysms is unclear, these conditions, in association with the contributing factors listed above, may be involved in the development of SAH. Aneurysms can also have multiple sites with bilateral locations and never rupture.

Intracranial aneurysms are often classified according to form (e.g., microscopic, dissecting, fusiform, giant, or saccular) and according to causal factor (e.g., atherosclerotic, traumatic, inflammatory, or congenital). Of all aneurysms, 90% are berry (saccular); these have a ball shape with a neck or stem. Fusiform aneurysms develop from atherosclerosis and are wide with an irregular dilatation. These aneurysms rarely rupture. Dissecting aneurysms are associated with trauma and are caused by blood being forced between layers of the arterial wall. Mycotic aneurysms are rare; they develop from a septic embolus lodged in the arterial lumen and are often associated with bacterial endocarditis. Traumatic aneurysms are usually associated with intracranial damage and injury to the middle meningeal artery.

When an aneurysm ruptures, blood under high pressure is forced into the SAS, resulting in SAH. Under severe pressure, blood may be forced to enter surrounding brain tissue, causing intracranial hemorrhage and infarction; the ventricles, causing hydrocephalus; or the subdural space, causing a subdural hematoma. Death can occur as a result of a massive bleed from increased ICP and brainstem compression leading to brain herniation. A clot is formed over the ruptured aneurysm. Blood in the subarachnoid space irritates the meninges (causing meningeal signs) and may obstruct the flow of CSF (causing hydrocephalus). The serious complications of SAH are rebleeding, vasospasm, hypothalamic dysfunction, and hydrocephalus.

Rebleeding   Rebleeding following the rupture of an aneurysm is associated with a high mortality rate. Rebleeding occurs most frequently during the first 24 hours, and the rate of incidence decreases gradually over a 2-week period.[9] Rebleeding is frequently caused by dissolution of the clot in conjunction with hypertension. The symptoms of rebleeding include severe headache, nausea, vomiting, hypertension, further neurological deterioration, respiratory arrest, coma, and death.

Medical management of rebleeding is aimed at decreasing the amount of bleeding until surgery can be performed. Cautious use of antihypertensives to control blood pressure may be beneficial when cerebral perfusion pressure is adequate and vasospasm is not present. The use of antifibrinolytic agents such as Amicar (epsilon-aminocaproic acid) to prevent rebleeding from occurring (by stabilizing the clot and preventing lysis) remains controversial. Complications associated with the use of antifibrinolytic agents are hydrocephalus, vasospasm, pulmonary embolus, and deep venous thrombosis; and the risks of this therapy may exceed any benefit realized.

Vasospasm   It is commonly estimated that vasospasm occurs in 30–60% of all patients surviving SAH. Vasospasm is the leading cause of morbidity and mortality with ruptured aneurysms. Narrowing of the cerebral arteries comprising the circle of Willis and its branches results in ischemia. There are two classifications of vasospasm: angiographic and clinical. Angiographic vasospasm is the focal and occasionally diffuse narrowing of the dye column in the major cerebral arteries, and clinical vasospasm is the syndrome of ischemic consequences of the narrowing of cerebral arteries. Although the time course of each type of vasospasm is similar, up to 70% of patients experiencing SAH may develop arterial narrowing, but only 20–35% exhibit neurological deficits.[10] Vasospasm can be linked to the contact of the extravasated blood clots in the SAS with cerebral arteries. The patient who undergoes surgery prior to the rupturing of the aneurysm rarely develops vasospasm. The frequency and development of vasospasm may be related to the amount of blood in the SAS. The occurrence of vasospasm is usually associated with higher clinical grades, which reflect an impaired neurological status or deteriorating condition (refer to the grading scale in Table 3-24).

The pathogenesis of cerebral vasospasm remains unknown and poorly understood. The following are hypothesized as clinical antecedents to the arterial

Table 3-24   Hunt and Hess Grading Scale

Grade	System
0	Unruptured
I	Asymptomatic Minimal headache Slight nuchal rigidity
Ia	No acute meningeal reactions Fixed neurological deficit
II	Moderate to severe headache Nuchal rigidity No neurological deficit other than cranial nerve deficit
III	Drowsiness Confusion Mild focal deficit
IV	Stupor Moderate to severe hemiparesis Possible early decerebrate rigidity Possible vegetative disturbances
V	Deep coma Decerebrate rigidity Moribund appearance

narrowing evidenced: (1) contraction of the cerebral arterial smooth muscle secondary to vasoactive substances in the CSF, (2) impairment of vasodilatory activity, (3) proliferative vasculopathy, (4) immunoreactive processes, (5) inflammatory processes, and (6) mechanical phenomena.[11]

The clinical presentation of vasospasm depends largely on the location of the brain that is affected, the degree of spasm, the cerebral perfusion pressure, and autoregulation mechanisms. The onset of vasospasm is insidious; it rarely occurs before the 4th day after the SAH and peaks around the 7th day.[12] Vasospasm may persist for a few days or last up to 2 weeks. Symptoms may be transient or progressive, ranging from minor manifestations such as confusion and focal neurological deficits to major ones such as coma and death.

In the absence of a clear understanding of the pathogenesis of vasospasm, effective therapies for medical management have not yet been established. Specific pharmacological agents for vasospasm have had only limited success. Recently, investigations into the use of calcium-blocking agents such as Nifedipine and Nimodipine for the prevention and reversal of cerebral narrowing have been initiated. Advantages to the use of these agents include decreased platelet aggregation, lysis of erythrocytes, and decreased endothelial damage.

The goals of management of vasospasm center on increasing cerebral perfusion pressure, resolving the ischemic events, and decreasing the risk of recurrence. Intravascular volume expansion and pharmacologically induced arterial hypertension are recognized as effective treatment regimens if instituted before cerebellar infarction develops. Adequate perfusion pressure can be maintained by using hypervolemic/hypertensive therapies and decreasing ICP. However, the risks of rebleeding, increased ICP, and pulmonary edema must be considered and carefully managed before surgery.

Hypothalamic dysfunction Hypothalamic dysfunction occurs frequently after the rupture of an aneurysm. Direct pressure on the hypothalamus as a consequence of hematoma or hydrocephalus interferes with regular function. Hyponatremia several days after the rupture is the most common fluid and electrolyte disturbance experienced. The exact cause of hyponatremia remains unknown, but it is thought to be related more to a loss of sodium in the urine than to the syndrome of inappropriate antidiuretic hormone secretion.[13] Decreased serum osmolarity and increased urine osmolarity and sodium are associated with hyponatremia. Possible clinical presentations of hyponatremia include changes in the level of consciousness, confusion, fatigue, seizures, headache, vomiting, and coma. Finally, medical management of hyponatremia includes free water restriction and volume expansion with colloids and blood to replace intravascular volume and maintain adequate cerebral perfusion pressure.

Another complication of hypothalamic dysfunction is increased stimulation of the sympathetic nervous system. Increased circulating catecholamines cause symptoms of increased sympathetic activity including flushing, diaphoresis, dilated pupils, decreased gastric motility, increased serum glucose, elevated temperature, hypertension, and tachycardia.[14] The severity of the hypothalamic disturbance corresponds to the severity of vasospasm. Electrocardiogram abnormalities accompanying hypothalamic dysfunction may include peaked P waves, short P-R intervals, elongated Q-T segments, large U waves, and peaked T waves.[15] Sinus and nodal bradycardia, wandering atrial pacemaker, paroxysmal atrial tachycardia, atrial fibrillation, arterioventricular block, atrioventricular dissociation, and premature ventricular contractions may occur in the first 48 hours after SAH and may be transient in nature.[16]

Hydrocephalus Hydrocephalus is a frequent complication of a ruptured aneurysm. Obstructive hydrocephalus can result from a hematoma obstructing the flow of CSF; communicating hydrocephalus is caused by the decreased reabsorption of bloody CSF.

Treatment of either includes placement of an intraventricular catheter or ventriculoperitoneal shunt. In an emergency situation, an intraventricular catheter is usually inserted in order to control ICP, or osmotic diuretics (Mannitol) and corticosteroids (Decadron) may be administered.

Resulting signs and symptoms

The Hunt and Hess grading scale (Table 3-24) is frequently referred to for the classification of SAH. Clinical grades are used to describe the patient's neurological status and prognosis.

The individual who experiences aneurysm rupture is usually 45 to 65 years of age, and is more likely to be female than male (3:2). Aneurysm rupture can occur at any time and is often associated with periods of activity. An estimated 40–60% of patients may experience warning signs (referred to as prodromal signs) prior to the rupture of the aneurysm. Prodromal signs include a slight to severe headache, neck and back pain, fever, malaise, vertigo, nausea, vomiting, cranial nerve palsies (especially the oculomotor nerve), diplopia, and blurred vision. These signs usually occur when minor leaks begin, and they serve as important warning signals indicating the imminent risk of a major bleed. Prompt diagnosis is critical. Timely surgical intervention before the aneurysm ruptures can reduce morbidity and mortality rates. Because the effects of SAH are so severe, common medical practice tends toward extensive screening of those considered most at risk: those with a familiy history of aneurysm, uncontrolled hypertension, onset of severe headache, polycystic kidney disease, fibromuscular dysplasia, coarctation or hypoplasia of the aorta, or diseases of vascular walls (such as Marfan's syndrome and Ehlers-Danlos syndrome).[17]

The abrupt onset of symptoms usually occurs rapidly. The classic sign of a ruptured aneurysm is a sudden, excruciating headache, often described as "the worst headache of my life." The patient may describe hearing a snap or a burst at the time of the rupture as well. Nausea, vomiting, headache, mild fever, photophobia, irritability, restlessness, hyperesthesia, nuchal rigidity, Kernig's sign, Brudzinski's sign, and seizures are also possible symptoms. Depending on the location and severity of the bleed, the patient may experience varying alterations in level of consciousness, ranging from confusion to coma. A transient loss of consciousness frequently occurs at the onset of rupture, as the ICP suddenly rises and the CPP is reduced. Additional signs exhibited at this moment include palsy of the third, fourth, and fifth cranial nerves, subhyaloid hemorrhage (irregular blots of blood on the retina), homonomous hemianopia, and focal neurological deficits. Finally, clinical manifestations of complications such as vasospasm, rebleeding, increased ICP, and hypothalamic dysfunction contribute to the clinical presentation of SAH.

Nursing standards of care

The most successful outcomes of care for the patient in this classification are achieved through prevention. Early recognition and prompt intervention constitute the ideal; unfortunately, most patients present only after the aneurysm has ruptured. Current medical practices offer limited hope of recovery in the face of the many devastating complications of SAH.

The definitive treatment for aneurysm rupture is surgical intervention to obliterate the sac and remove the clot. Surgical approaches include clipping the aneurysm neck, encasement with a self-hardening plastic coating, carotid ligation to obliterate or reduce the size of the aneurysm, induced thrombosis, and extracranial-intracranial bypass.[18]

The optimal time to perform the surgery remains controversial. Traditionally, the scheduling of surgery was delayed in an attempt to stabilize the patient and decrease the risk of life-threatening complications. In the face of the grim morbidity and mortality rates, the decision for early surgical intervention (within 1–3 days of the SAH) is gaining widespread acceptance. Considerations to be addressed in the deliberations about performing early surgery include the ability to prevent rebleeding, the ability to remove the clot (thus reducing the incidence of vasospasm), the extent to which ischemic complications are prevented and/or treated, the presence of psychological needs, and the need to be concerned about length of hospitalization.[19] Those favoring delayed surgery (after 3 days to 2 weeks) prefer to wait until the patient has had time to recover from the initial insult. By the time the initial recovery has been reached, the brain is usually less swollen, permitting easier dissection of the aneurysm. Other considerations during the planning of surgical intervention are the patient's clinical presentation in regard to scoring on the Hunt and Hess scale, age, medical history, location of the aneurysm, and occurrence of complications. At present, the decision as to when to perform surgery is made according to individual practices of neurosurgeons and protocols established by various medical centers. A clearer definition of the optimal time for surgery is needed to standardize the medical management of such cases.

The initial diagnosis and choice of intervention are often suggested by the clinical course and presentation. A CT scan can be performed immediately upon admission to identify the presence of subarachnoid blood and other underlying clinical conditions. When brain herniation and rebleeding are not considered to be risks, diagnostic lumbar punctures may be performed. Gross bloody CSF, elevated protein levels, and a high opening pressure are common indicators of aneurysm rupture. Angiography is also used diagnostically in cases of SAH, but because of its invasive properties, several risks accompany its use. Although not as accurate, transcranial doppler ultrasound, a noninvasive technique, is useful in the detection of the narrowing of the cerebral arteries that is suggestive of vasospasm and is a promising alternative to angiography.

Nursing care for the critically ill patient with SAH is extremely challenging. The nurse's goals are to maintain adequate cerebral perfusion pressure, prevent rebleeding, and minimize the effects of vasospasm. By performing continuous neurological assessment and alerting the medical staff to changes, the nurse can play a crucial role in promoting the optimal level of recovery for SAH patients. Neurological assessment includes ascertaining LOC, pupillary response, speech responses, motor status, and presence of pronator drift. The nursing assessment protocol presented in Table 3-25 will further assist the nurse with early detection of vasospasm. Knowledge of what artery may be affected by vasospasm helps to guide the nurse in performing and interpreting the neurological assessment. Early recognition of changes in a patient's neurological status facilitates prompt initiation of appropriate treatment.

In addition to conducting neurological assessment, the nurse should maintain precautions for the SAH patient whenever possible. These precautions include use of a private room, maintaining a quiet environment and restricting visitors, keeping the lighting subdued, adhering to strict bedrest without television or radio, and avoiding the Valsalva maneuver.

Further interventions include the use of mechanical ventilation in order to assure adequate oxygenation in the presence of neurological deterioration. Hyperventilation to reduce the level of carbon dioxide in the blood and vasoconstrict the arteries to help decrease cerebral edema is frequently indicated. During intubation, meticulous hygiene is important to help prevent pulmonary complications. Arterial blood gas monitoring is also crucial to ensure the

Table 3-25 Nursing Assessment Protocol for the Detection of Vasospasm

Data	Source	Frequency
Past medical and nursing history: present and past family illnesses; physiological, psychosocial, cultural and developmental effects of health status and functioning	Patient and family Medical records Health care personnel	Once
Chronology of events leading to admission: onset, description, and duration of symptoms; alleviating and aggravating factors	Patient and family	Once

Baseline Assessment:
  Review of general systems: vital signs, physical, sensory/perceptual/pain, oxygenation, nutrition, fluid and electrolyte/elimination, activity/sleep
  Neurological status: cerebral function, cerebellar function, motor function, cranial nerves, sensory function, reflexes
	Physical exam	Once

Diagnostics: CT, angiogram, ECG, lab	Diagnostic exams	Once

Trend analyses
  Review of general systems:
    vital signs
    physical
    sensory/perceptual/pain
    oxygenation
    nutrition
    fluid and electrolyte/elimination
    activity/sleep
  Neurological status: cerebral function, cerebellar function, motor function, cranial nerves, sensory function, reflexes
	Physical exam	Comparisons:
		5 minutes–4 hours
		4 hours–daily
		Hourly
		1 hour–8 hours
		Daily
		1 hour–8 hours
		Daily
		Hourly

Diagnostics:
  CT
  angiogram
  ECG
  lab
	Diagnostic exams	Comparisons:
		Daily–biweekly
		Weekly
		Continuous
		Hourly–daily

adequacy of efforts to maintain cerebral perfusion. Depending on the neurological status of the patient, hemodynamic monitoring may be indicated for evaluating cardiovascular responses to hypervolemic/hypertensive therapy. Peripheral edema, tachycardia, respiratory crackles (rales), and distended neck veins are all signs of pulmonary edema or congestive heart failure from excess fluid volume.[20] Electrocardiogram monitoring is also used to identify changes in cardiac rhythms and to detect dysrhythmias. Finally, close monitoring of electrolytes and fluid status is necessary for early detection of fluid and electrolyte imbalances.

In conclusion, subarachnoid hemorrhage can strike suddenly and have devastating effects. Anxiety associated with fear of life-threatening complications, poor prognosis, apparent neurological deficits, and fear of surgery can be extremely trying for the patient and family. Thus, patient and family teaching are essential to patient care. Offering emotional support, communicating realistic expectations, conducting educational sessions, and reinforcing the physician's explanations will be helpful to the patient and family. Consulting with appropriate resource and support groups should also be attempted in order to provide the most comprehensive care possible. The standard practice for the care of the SAH patient is outlined in the following nursing care plan.

Nursing Care Plan for the Management of the Patient with Cerebral Aneurysm and Subarachnoid Hemorrhage

Diagnosis	Signs and symptoms	Intervention	Rationale

Potential for anxiety due to:
  fear of unknown,
  fear of death,
  fear of disfigurement,
  fear of pain,
  fear of disability,
  lack of knowledge regarding hospital procedures and routines
	Facial tension
	Distracting behavior
	Low attention span
	Withdrawal
	Twitching and shaking of extremities
	Inappropriate laughter or behavior
	Diaphoresis
	Tachycardia
	Nonadherence to treatment plan
		Ascertain patient's fears and anxieties	Will allow the nurse to know just what to address

		Ascertain patient's previous hospital experiences (own as well as others')	Will help the nurse to know how to best alleviate anxieties and support positive attitudes
		Ascertain readiness to learn	Need to begin patient and family education when ready
		Teach patient about routines of lab, radiology, ECG, house staff, possible surgery, incisions, tubes, lines, operation length, ICU routine, visiting hours, pain medication, and deep breathing and coughing; provide patient education booklets; give ICU tour if desired	To help patient and family be prepared for what is to be experienced
		Sedate as ordered PRN	To help patient relax
		Provide emotional support as needed	To help patient and family deal with the situation in the best way possible
		Consult with social worker, chaplain, etc., as needed	Multidisciplinary team effort provides broader, more comprehensive care

Potential for ineffective coping by the patient or family related to:
  severity of illness,
  sudden hospitalization,
  personal vulnerability,
  imposed physical restrictions
	Verbalization of inability to cope	Assess family's usual coping mechanisms	Questions and concerns of patient and family must be answered even if not voiced

	Inability to ask for emotional help	Assist family to identify alternative coping mechanisms; identify and acknowledge family's needs	Optimal coping must be accomplished for maximal healing

314

Diagnosis	Signs and symptoms	Intervention	Rationale
	Inability to meet role expectations	Provide information to patient and family regarding diagnosis and supportive services	Patient and family must be helped through role redefinition
	Prolonged progression of disease or disability	Support patient and family through role transition time	To help patient and family make transition
		Encourage open communication among patient, family, and health care team	To facilitate problem solving and care planning
		Reinforce simple explanations to patient and family	During times of crisis, care must be taken not to cause information overload
	Exhaustion	Provide rest periods and offer nutrition; plan visiting schedule to accommodate interventions as well as family's schedule and rest periods; restrict visitors as appropriate	To maximize strength; to improve quality of family time as well as provide for needed rest
	Fear and anxiety	Delegate one resource and support person to assist family communication	Consistency in problem solving and care improves quality of decisions
	Inappropriate requests or hypervigilance by patient and/or family	Suggest approaches for family to assist in patient's care	Participatory care decreases family's anxiety
Potential for alteration in health maintenance due to lack of knowledge of: diagnostic tests; surgical procedure; medications; diet; activity; hospital routine	Inability to describe personal diagnosis and how it relates to type of surgery	Instruct patient and family about diagnostics, procedures, and routines	Patient and family must understand diagnosis and prognosis
		Encourage questions and discussion of problems and concerns	To allow for greatest learning

Nursing Care Plan for the Management of the Patient with Cerebral Aneurysm and Subarachnoid Hemorrhage

Diagnosis	Signs and symptoms	Intervention	Rationale
	Communicates lack of knowledge Does not distinguish between permitted and prohibited activities	Organize frequent teaching sessions to educate patient and family about: SAH pathology, diagnostics, ICU routines, appropriate precautions, medications, explanations by physician	To facilitate healing by promoting adherence to regimen and prevent complications resulting from inappropriate activities
	Inability to identify professional services available for support	Instruct about available services and resources	To provide comprehensive and effective service to patient and family

Potential for impaired gas exchange due to:
  ineffective airway clearance, atelectasis, effusion;
  inadequate ventilation and/or supplemental oxygen;
  low hematocrit and hemoglobin;
  treatment for hypervolemia
	Abnormal ABGs:
	  $pO_2 < 80$ mm Hg
	  $pCO_2 < 35 > 45$ mm Hg
	  pH < 7.35 or > 7.45
	  O_2 sat. $< 80\%$
	  $HCO_3 < 20$ or > 26 mEq/L
	  BE < 0 or > 3
	
	Cyanosis
	
	ETT cuff leak
	
	Lowered peak pressure
	
	Inadequate volume exchange
	
	Chest x ray indicates atelectasis, effusion, pneumothorax, or hemothorax
		Mechanically ventilate as required
		
		Closely monitor lung sounds for absent, unequal, diminished breath sounds, crackles, wheezing, or asymmetric chest wall expansion; closely monitor ABGs PRN and after ventilator changes; obtain chest x ray immediately upon intubation and PRN for ETT placement, lung expansion (pneumothorax), presence of pleural fluid
			Ventilation support is needed until stabilization
			
			Early indications for ensuing respiratory compromise and/or complications

	Elevated respiratory rate, wheezing, air hunger, gasping, copious secretions, or asymmetric chest wall expansion	Pulmonary toilet PRN with chest percussion therapy, incentive spirometry, and hyperinflation using 100% O_2 before and after suctioning (within neurological safety parameters); turn and reposition every 2 hours	To mobilize secretions, provide adequate oxygenation, and open closed alveoli in a neurologically safe manner

Diagnosis	Signs and symptoms	Intervention	Rationale
		Elevate HOB 30 degrees	To assist patient to optimal breathing capacity (to prevent atelectasis, infection, etc.)
	Fluid imbalances, decreased serum osmolality and increased urine specific gravity and sodium levels	Maintain fluid balance within neurological safety parameters	To mobilize secretions and to facilitate maximal gas exchange
Alteration in cerebral perfusion related to increased ICP, vasospasm, and rebleed	CPP < 60 mm Hg Altered level of consciousness	Notify the MD	To initiate immediate medical intervention to prevent cerebral ischemia
	Neurological deterioration Pronator drift	Conduct frequent checks of neurological and hemodynamic parameters (CVP, wedge pressures, and cardiac output)	To detect early changes in neurological status
	Anxiety and agitation	Organize activities to prevent unnecessary disturbances and allow adequate rest	Reducing external stimuli and activity and allowing adequate rest help to decrease ICP
		Approach patient in a calm and reassuring manner; provide soft stimuli (light touch, soft music, pleasant and familiar sounds)	Nursing activities can lead to anxiety and agitation, which cause increases in ICP
		Monitor increases in ICP to learn what causes them and organize activities to minimize time and intensity of stimulation	To limit time and intensity of activities that challenge (stress) the patient and raise the ICP
		Assist family to communicate with patient in a calm and quiet manner and to avoid emotionally stimulating the patient	Family teaching may help to prevent unnecessary startles, excessive stimulation, and agitation that can lead to rises in ICP

Nursing Care Plan for the Management of the Patient with Cerebral Aneurysm and Subarachnoid Hemorrhage

Diagnosis	Signs and symptoms	Intervention	Rationale
		Provide hyperventilation therapy and hyperoxygenate prior to suctioning	To decrease ICP and to prevent further increases in ICP related to nursing activities
		Administer volume expanders, vasopressors, and antihypertensives as prescribed	To maintain adequate CPP and hemodynamic stability
Alteration in fluid volume (excess or deficit) related to hypervolemia therapy and hypothalamic dysfunction	Fluid imbalance CO < 3 L/min CI < 2 L/min/m²	Assess cardiovascular status for signs of volume depletion or excess in: cardiac output, cardiac index, ECG	To evaluate cardiac function and ability to maintain adequate fluid volume perfusion
	Increased/decreased serum osmolality Increased/decreased urine specific gravity and sodium	Maintain hypervolemia therapy as prescribed to keep: CVP at 10–12 mm Hg; wedge pressure at 18–20 mm Hg; urine < 200 cc/hr	To provide for adequate volume and to maintain neural perfusion
		Limit oral intake; adhere to low sodium diet	To prevent/correct fluid retention and overload
	Electrolyte imbalance	Closely monitor electrolyte status, hematocrit, BUN, creatinine, and serum osmolality	To correct imbalances in order to maintain optimal system functioning
	Increased pulmonary congestion	Pulmonary toilet as per neurological safety parameters	To allow optimal respiratory gas exchange and oxygen perfusion

Diagnosis	Signs and symptoms	Intervention	Rationale
Impaired physical mobility related to imposed physical restrictions	Imposed restriction of movement, including body mechanics	Maintain alignment of head, neck, and body	To prevent complications of immobility
	Decreased muscle strength preventing independent movement	Perform skin massage and passive/active ROM exercises	To maintain joint and muscle mobility and increase circulation
	Signs of impeded circulation in extremities (redness over pressure points)	Apply antiembolism stockings; assess lower extremities for tenderness, redness, warmth, and pain	Helps to identify and decrease venous stasis and deep vein thrombosis
		Place air mattress on bed	To prevent pressure spots on skin
	Impaired coordination while in bed, which impedes independent movement	Assist with required movements; quarter turn every 1–2 hours	To prevent overexertion and to facilitate movement
Potential for alteration in bowel function or constipation due to: decreased mobility; change in eating patterns; side effects of medications; decreased fluid volume	Reports of feeling constipated, "full" feeling in abdomen, inability to move bowels	Assess abdomen for bowel sounds, softness, and appearance and ask patient about discomfort at least every 12 hours	For early diagnosis of constipation in order to intervene before serious problems occur
	Decreased or absent bowel sounds	Encourage progressive ambulation and activity as tolerated	To stimulate peristalsis
	Inadequate oral fluid/food intake as evidenced on I&O records and calorie counts	Reassure patient that constipation is frequently a problem when on fluid restrictions	So patient will not become overly concerned
	Symptoms of dehydration: poor skin turgor, sunken eyes, intake < output, weight loss	Assess for signs of dehydration and encourage oral intake within fluid restriction limits	Hydration impedes constipation
		Closely monitor electrolytes	Dehydration leads to electrolyte imbalance
	Absence of bowel movement for more than 2 days	Implement bowel regimen as ordered: Milk of magnesia 30 mL PO every HS; consult with dietician about increased fiber in diet as indicated	Patient may need extra help to facilitate peristalsis

Nursing Care Plan for the Management of the Patient with Cerebral Aneurysm and Subarachnoid Hemorrhage

Diagnosis	Signs and symptoms	Intervention	Rationale
Potential for alteration in nutritional status due to: hypothalamic dysfunction; altered LOC; anorexia and malaise; increased nutritional requirements resulting from physical stress; less appealing taste of food related to low sodium content; constipation, diarrhea, abdominal cramping, or flatus	Complaints of lack of appetite Eating only small portions Trend for weight loss Decreased fluid intake Pain or discomfort GI depression	Assess appetite with patient and family and determine what sounds appealing and is allowed Monitor tray after meals to assess amount eaten Calculate calories Weigh daily Dietary consult Provide preferred foods as much as possible	To facilitate patient's nutritional status in any acceptable way To monitor patient's intake accurately To help meet body's requirement for calories
Alteration in comfort related to meningeal irritation and imposed physical restrictions	Headache, neck pain Nausea Projectile vomiting Nuchal rigidity Photophobia Hyperthermia	Maintain HOB at 30 degrees Maintain aneurysm precautions Administer analgesic, sedation, and antipyretics as ordered; turn and position Group nursing activities together	Elevation of the head promotes venous drainage and decreases ICP To decrease stimulation, reduce risk of rebleed, and decrease ICP To promote comfort To ensure rest periods
Potential for skin breakdown due to: restriction of movement; pain/discomfort; drug-induced neuromuscular or musculoskeletal impairment; depression	Imposed restriction of movement, including body mechanics, medical protocol, etc. Impaired coordination or decreased muscle strength preventing independent movement	Place air mattress on bed Assist with required movements; quarter turn every 1–2 hours	To prevent pressure spots on skin To prevent overexertion and to facilitate movement

Diagnosis	Signs and symptoms	Intervention	Rationale
body stiffness; diaphoresis or drainage into patient's bed; independent variables such as diabetes, peripheral vascular disease, obesity, etc.; low cardiac output; poor tissue perfusion; altered nutritional status; weakness/fatigue	Reluctance to attempt movement	Encourage movement within safety parameters	To prevent injury and facilitate movement
	Redness over pressure points	Inspect pressure points, including occiput, sacrum, coccyx, heels, and elbows, every 2 hours	To prevent skin breakdown
		Passive range of motion for all extremities	To prevent pressure spots
		Keep patient dry	To prevent skin breakdown
		Maintain and supplement nutrition as needed	To maintain vital nutrients to skin
		Consult enterostomal therapist	To provide for optimal care planning and intervention and to prevent skin breakdown
	Elevated temperature	Keep patient dry when diaphoretic	To prevent skin breakdown
Potential for gastrointestinal irritation related to hypothalamic dysfunction and medication	Gastrointestinal hemorrhage	Assess GI status	To allow for timely intervention
	Guaiac-positive stools	Report guaiac-positive stools	To allow for timely intervention
	Nausea and vomiting	Administer antacids with steroids	To decrease gastric irritation
	Complaints of lack of appetite	Assess with patient and family what is appealing and within dietary restrictions; dietary consult to provide preferred foods as much as possible	To facilitate the meeting of body's requirements for calories for optimal healing
	Complaints of gastric pain or discomfort	Progress diet as tolerated Administer antacids	To prevent gastric distress caused by foods the stomach is not ready to tolerate while maintaining adequate calorie intake

Nursing Care Plan for the Management of the Patient with Cerebral Aneurysm and Subarachnoid Hemorrhage

Diagnosis	Signs and symptoms	Intervention	Rationale
Potential for physical injury related to seizure activity, altered LOC, and possible falls	Confusion Agitation Seizures	Maintain a safe environment by: administering anticonvulsants as prescribed and monitoring therapeutic levels; instituting seizure precautions (padded bed rails, oral airway suction equipment, and supplemental oxygen)	To decrease risk of physical injury, help prevent seizures, and obtain optimal effectiveness of drugs
		Reorient patient frequently	To increase patient's awareness of surroundings
		Explain care activities to patient	To help alleviate patient's anxiety
		Assess causes of restlessness (hypoxemia, pain, bladder distention) and plan care appropriately	To decrease risk of increased agitation leading to possible accidental injury
		Restraints PRN	To promote patient's safety

Medications Commonly Used in the Care of the Patient with Cerebral Aneurysm and Subarachnoid Hemorrhage

Medication	Effect	Major side effects
Nitroprusside	Vasodilator with a direct action on vascular smooth muscle	Nausea and vomiting Muscle twitching Hypotension
Nitroglycerin	Vasodilation leading to increased coronary blood supply and decreased myocardial oxygen demand	Hypotension Headache
Hydralazine Minoxidil Diazoxide	Vasodilator with a direct action on vascular smooth muscle, leading to relaxed arterioles, decreased vascular resistance, and increased cardiac output	Angina Nausea and vomiting Tachycardia Headache Flushing Hypotension
Furosemide Ethacrynic acid	Loop diuretic Decreased pulmonary congestion	Hypokalemia Hypocalcemia Hypomagnesemia Altered glucose metabolism
Trimethaphan Phentolamine	Ganglionic blocker inhibiting the peripheral sympathetic nervous system	Orthostatic hypotension Ileus Urinary retention Blurred vision Dry mouth
Reserpine Guanethidine	Peripheral adrenergic antagonist inhibiting peripheral sympathetic nervous system	Drowsiness Nausea and vomiting Tremors Bradycardia Dyspnea Fatigue
Methyldopa Clonidine	Centrally stimulates alpha-adrenergic receptors leading to decreased peripheral vascular resistance	Drowsiness Dry mouth Vertigo Depression Gastrointestinal upsets
Atenolol Propranolol Timolol	Beta-adrenoreceptor antagonist	Postural hypotension Dizziness and syncope Palpitations Dry mouth

Medications Commonly Used in the Care of the Patient with Cerebral Aneurysm and Subarachnoid Hemorrhage

Medication	Effect	Major side effects
Antifibrinolytic agent: Amicar	Enhances hemostasis Inhibition of plasminogen activation	Nausea and vomiting Dizziness Hypotension Tinnitus Diarrhea Headache

Calcium channel blockers:
  Nifedipine
  Nimodipine
	Arterial spasm inhibitor
	Reduces arterial pressure
	Reduces oxygen utilization
		Hypotension
		Congestive heart failure
		Dizziness or lightheadedness
		Headache
		Weakness
		Nausea and vomiting

Acute Spinal Cord Injury

Acute spinal cord injury (SCI) is a complex, multisystem injury, which is most often traumatic in nature. The effects of acute SCI are as diverse as the multitude of individual precipitating factors and characteristics of the injury. Acute SCI can affect virtually every body system, and the effects can range from slight to profound. The nursing care needs of the patient with acute SCI are as diverse as the effects of the injury. The patient requires close surveillance and often swift and aggressive intervention to preserve neurological function or even, at times, life. The care that the SCI patient receives from the moment of injury until the pathogenic mechanisms subside days and weeks later has a significant effect on the long-term functional outcome.

Clinical antecedents

The predominant cause of acute SCI is trauma, with a reported annual incidence of 32.1 per million in the United States. Most traumatic SCIs in the United States result from motor vehicle crashes (47.7%), followed by falls and falling objects (20.8%), acts of violence such as gunshot wounds and stabbings (14.6%), and sports activities, especially diving, football, and skiing (14.2%).[21] Traumatic SCI occurs most frequently in persons who are between 16 and 30 years of age (61.1%) and are males (82%).

There are also a variety of diseases or conditions that may result in nontraumatic acute spinal cord damage. These include intraspinal tumors (although damage is usually more chronic), various infectious and inflammatory diseases of the spinal cord and meninges, intraspinal abscesses, and iatrogenic complications of surgical and diagnostic procedures (for example, surgical ligation during abdominal surgery). Although the pathogenesis and treatments of these disorders are quite different, many similarities exist in the nursing care of patients with acute SCI of varying etiologies. Traumatic SCI will therefore be the main focus of this discussion.

Critical referents

Injury to the spinal cord most often occurs as a result of traumatic force that causes a disturbance in the structural integrity of the spine and its support-ing ligaments. Once the structural integrity of the spine has been interrupted, the spinal cord is highly susceptible to injury. Spinal integrity can be disrupted by a direct insult (blunt or penetrating trauma), compression of the spine from a downward or upward force (especially in falls or diving), or hyperflexion, hyperextension, or extreme rotation of the head or trunk (especially in motor vehicle accidents and sports injuries). Less commonly, a traumatic force can be transmitted through the spine to the spinal cord and cause injury without apparent damage to the spine or ligaments.

The injury that the spinal cord sustains is due, in part, to individual factors such as the size of the vertebral canal. A wider canal allows more movement of the spine or spinal cord without compression of the cord. The spinal canal narrows with age and may be more narrow in individuals with cervical spondylosis, osteoarthritis, or congenital anomalies of the spine.

The most common mechanisms of injury to the spinal cord are contusion, concussion, compression, laceration, and ischemia. These mechanisms produce the initial injury to the neurons and blood vessels of the spinal cord. A contusion, or bruising, of the cord can occur if a hard object (a vertebrae or disk) strikes the cord. This may result in small petechial hemorrhages within the cord tissue. A concussion may be caused if the cord is struck or stretched and electrochemical disruption occurs within the cord without any morphological changes. In such cases complete recovery usually occurs within hours. Compression occurs when fractured or dislocated bones, displaced ligaments, extruded disk materials, or hematomas produce pressure on the cord. Laceration, or penetration, of the cord can also occur, particularly with knife or gunshot injuries. Ischemia may also be a mechanism of SCI if blood flow to the spinal cord is interrupted by compression or laceration.

A variety of other traumatic injuries may be associated with a spinal cord injury, particularly one caused by a motor vehicle accident. Associated brain, head, neck, chest, and orthopedic trauma are commonly found.

The acute injury stage The acute injury stage begins immediately following the injury and lasts for hours or even days, depending on the injury, the treatment, and the patient's response. In more severe cases, the acute process may persist for several weeks. Following the initial injury, the spinal cord undergoes a chain of events that leads to further morphological destruction. This process is characterized by a vicious cycle of ischemia, edema, and

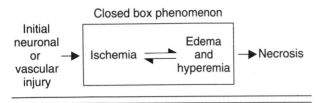

Figure 3-25   Acute Injury Stage of SCI

hyperemia, which occurs within the limited space of the vertebral canal and eventually leads to necrosis of the cord (see Figure 3-25). The initial injury leads to a focal ischemia of damaged neuronal and vascular tissue in the cord, which results in (1) disrupted electrical condition of damaged neurons and (2) increased permeability of damaged capillaries. Edema occurs as a result of increased capillary permeability. Hyperemia (increased blood volume) and vasoconstriction occur in response to ischemia and the release of prostaglandins and vasoactive amines (various neurotransmitters and histamine) at the injury site. Edema and hyperemia at the injury site compress surrounding neurons and blood vessels as pressure inside the vertebral canal rises. Once pressure on the surrounding tissue exceeds the perfusion pressure, ischemia occurs, resulting in more widespread edema and hyperemia. Eventually, if uninterrupted, this process will result in necrosis of spinal cord tissue.

Electrochemical conduction is disrupted by both initial traumatic mechanisms and spreading ischemia, if present. If conduction loss becomes widespread across the spinal cord and connections between the spinal cord and cortical and brainstem control centers are disrupted, then spinal shock occurs. Because normal facilitation or excitation by the brain and brainstem are inhibited, the spinal cord at and below the level of injury ceases to function during spinal shock.

The subacute stage   Following the retreat of the acute destructive process within the cord, a recovery and reparative phase begins. As swelling subsides, the electrical conduction of intact neurons returns, and spinal shock, if present, subsides. The return of neurological function may occur immediately, but more often occurs slowly, over months. Macrophage removal of necrotic debris occurs during this stage. Overgrowth of regenerating neuroglia during this stage (gliosis) may inhibit functional regeneration of neurons. The recovery of electrical conduction in damaged (nonintact) neurons within the spinal cord is limited, and functional regeneration does not occur.

Resulting signs and symptoms

Upon admission, gross physical presentations of SCI may include deformity, swelling, or limited movement of the spine, particularly in the neck. A tenderness or space between spinous processes may be present. Pain may or may not be present. There may be evidence of other trauma to the head, chest, abdomen, or extremities.

Motor and sensory symptoms   Motor and sensory functions are the most important indicators of the spinal cord's neurological integrity. The location and degree of motor or sensory dysfunction is indicative of the level and severity of SCI. Figure 3-26 illustrates the motor and sensory functions mediated by each level of the spinal cord.

The type of SCI is classified according to motor and sensory impairment. Table 3-26 presents the SCI terminology recommended by the American Spinal Injury Association (ASIA).

Injury to the spinal cord usually causes both upper motor neuron and lower motor neuron symptoms. A lower motor neuron injury is caused when the dorsal horn nuclei of the lower motor neurons are damaged. This results in a loss of motor function mediated by the spinal cord at that level. For example, an injury to the dorsal horn nuclei at C5 (a C4 SCI) damages the nerves that control the deltoids and the biceps. Therefore, these muscles would present as flaccid and areflexic. An upper motor neuron injury is caused when the axons of the corticospinal tract are damaged during injury. Because these neurons carry messages from the motor cortex to the spine to control conscious motor function, an injury to them affects conscious motor control below the level of injury. Reflex motor control within the spinal cord itself still takes place below the level of injury. Therefore, the muscles below the level of upper motor neuron injury will be spastic.

Spasticity with SCI is generally due to upper motor neuron injury but may be due to a disturbance of neurons from subcortical motor centers inhibiting or exciting the reflex centers. Spasticity may involve segmental reflexes and single muscle groups (for example, all leg and trunk muscles on one side).

Normal and abnormal reflexes may be seen below the level of injury. The return of deep tendon reflexes without conscious sensation or control is an indicator that spinal shock has subsided. Pathological reflexes (such as the Babinski reflex) may also be seen following spinal shock. These generally indicate a disturbance of neurons from inhibitory subcortical motor centers.

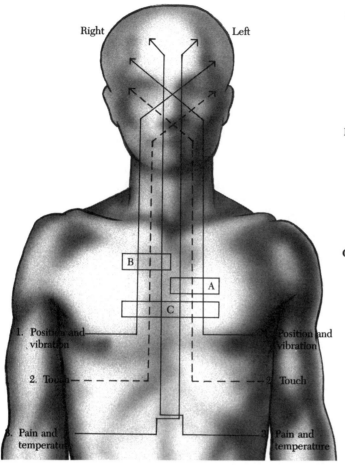

A. **Left lateral cord lesion**
1. Loss of pain and temperature of right side below level of lesion
2. Loss of touch of left side below level of lesion
3. Loss of position and vibration sense on left side of body below level of cord lesion

B. **Right lateral cord lesion**
1. Loss of pain and temperature of left side below level of lesion
2. Loss of touch on right side below level of lesion
3. Loss of position and vibration sense on right side of body below level of cord lesion

C. **Total cord lesion**
1. Loss of pain and temperature in all areas below level of lesion
2. Loss of touch in all areas below level of lesion
3. Loss of position and vibration sense in all areas below level of cord lesion

Figure 3-26   Spinal Cord Lesions and Associated Sensory Loss

Table 3-26   The American Spinal Injury Association's Classification of Spinal Cord Injuries

Term	Definition
Neurological level of injury	The lowest (most caudal) neurological segment with both normal motor and sensory function.
Complete injury	No preservation of any motor and/or sensory function.
Incomplete injury	Preservation of any motor and/or sensory function below the zone of injury (including sacral sensory sparing).
Quadriplegia-quadriparesis	Impairment or loss of motor and/or sensory function in the cervical neurological segments secondary to damage of neural elements within the spinal cord.
Paraplegia-paraparesis	Impairment or loss of motor and/or sensory function in the thoracic, lumbar, or sacral neurological segments secondary to damage of neural elements within the spinal canal. This includes cauda equina and conus medullaris injuries, but does not include root avulsion or peripheral nerve injury outside the neural canal.

Some degree of respiratory impairment may be caused by an SCI above the T12 level. However, respiratory distress is generally not seen in the patient with injuries below C5, unless there is associated head, neck, or chest trauma. Injury at the T9–T12 segments can affect abdominal muscle function, with a resulting impairment of coughing and forceful expiration. Injury at the T1–T7 segments may affect intercostal muscle function and thus impair forceful inspiration or expiration.

Injury at the C3–C5 level will cause some degree of diaphragmatic impairment and respiratory distress. With injury at the C5 level, phrenic nerve innervation is usually sufficient to maintain diaphragmatic respiration, unless spinal cord swelling causes compression at higher levels. Injury at the C4 level results in respiratory paralysis during the acute stage of SCI, with a later return of weak diaphragmatic breathing. Injury at the C3 level or above results in permanent impairment of diaphragmatic function and the need for permanent ventilatory assistance.

Finally, spinal shock (a widespread loss of electrical conduction across the spinal cord) can occur during any of the above. In spinal shock, essentially all spinal cord functions at and below the level of injury are depressed. Symptoms include flaccid paralysis, loss of autonomic reflexes resulting in hypotension (with injury above T6), and bowel and bladder dysfunction. Spinal shock corresponds to the period of acute spinal cord pathology and may resolve in just days or, perhaps, weeks.

Autonomic system symptoms Understanding autonomic nervous system (ANS) symptoms requires knowledge of the anatomy involved. Most of the parasympathetic control over the heart, the major blood vessels, and the digestive tract originates from the cranial vagus nerve above the spinal cord. A small number of parasympathetic spinal nerves that mediate the function of the bowel and genito-urinary systems originate from the spinal cord at the S2–S4 level. The sympathetic nervous innervation to the entire body originates from spinal cord levels T1 through L1. Sympathetic innervation to the major blood-storing vessels (liver, spleen, intestines, and legs) occurs below T6.

Life-threatening cardiovascular symptoms that may occur as a result of SCI include hypotension, slowed heart rate, a loss of temperature autoregulation, and autonomic hyperreflexia. These symptoms occur most frequently and severely with complete injuries but occur to a lesser degree with upper thoracic injuries (see Table 3-27). With complete cervical injuries, a functional sympathectomy occurs during spinal shock because the vagus nerve exerts its control over the cardiovascular and digestive systems without any sympathetic reflex response. Hypotension and bradycardia may result in a profound decrease in cardiac output with cervical SCI when the patient is in spinal shock. If untreated, cardiac output may be unable to support adequate cerebral perfusion. Following spinal shock, the quadriplegic patient's baseline blood pressure and heart rate are typically lower than normal. Ortho-

Table 3-27 Major Autonomic Symptoms with Spinal Cord Injury

Level of Spinal Cord Injury	Common Symptoms	Problems That May Occur In Less Severe Form
C1–C8	Hypotension Slowed heart rate Loss of temperature autoregulation Venous stasis and complications Autonomic hyperreflexia Gastric hypersecretion and paralytic ileus Reflex bowel, bladder, and erection	
T1–T4	Venous stasis and complications Reflex bowel, bladder, and erection	Hypotension Slowed heart rate Loss of temperature autoregulation Autonomic hyperreflexia
T4–T5	Venous stasis and complications Reflex bowel, bladder, and erection	Hypotension Autonomic hyperreflexia
T6–S1	Venous stasis and complications Reflex bowel, bladder, and erection	
S2–Coccygeal	Arreflexic bowel, bladder, and erection	

static hypotension may be a long-term problem in quadriplegic patients. Hypotension and bradycardia may occur during spinal shock with injuries between T1 and T5, but are usually not as severe.

A loss of temperature autoregulation is also problematic with complete cervical injuries and, to a lesser degree, upper thoracic injuries. The patient with disturbed temperature autoregulation tends to vary in body temperature toward extremes in environmental temperatures. This problem improves only slightly in the patient with complete injuries following spinal shock.

Autonomic dysreflexia is an abnormal response of the ANS to a noxious stimulus (usually an overdistended bladder or bowel) that occurs with SCI above the T6 level. Autonomic hyperreflexia is characterized by a hyperreflexic sympathetic response above the injury level and a hyperreflexic parasympathetic response below the level of injury. It results in (1) headaches that are pounding and severe in nature and have a sudden onset, (2) elevations in blood pressure (ranging from 140/90 to 300/60), (3) bradycardia, (4) profuse sweating above the level of injury, (5) nasal stuffiness, and (6) anxiety.

Dependent edema, deep venous thrombosis, and pulmonary embolus may occur as a result of venous stasis due to lost or diminished vasomotor control and flaccid paralysis. Blood hypercoagulation may also be a contributing factor. These complications most commonly develop during spinal shock and become clinically evident between 3 and 5 weeks after injury. One study documented the incidence of subclinical pulmonary embolus and deep venous thrombosis to be 42%.[22] As vasomotor reflexes return and activity increases, the risk of these complications decreases.

Gastrointestinal symptoms that occur after SCI may include paralytic ileus and gastric hypersecretion. These are more commonly experienced with complete cervical injuries but may be seen with upper thoracic injuries, as outlined in Table 3-27. Paralytic ileus, evidenced by a loss of bowel sounds, usually occurs immediately but may be delayed as long as 2 days.[23] Paralytic ileus may resolve within a day or may last a week or longer. Copious secretions of acidic gastric juices are particularly problematic in the cervically injured patient because they generally occur concurrently with paralytic ileus. The combined effects of gastric hypersecretion, NPO status, steroid therapy, and local irritation from NG tube insertion place the patient at high risk for gastric ulceration. Ensuing malnutrition may quickly become an exacerbation in the SCI patient because of paralytic ileus and metabolic demands resulting from traumatic stress. Weight loss, fatigue, and weakness

may result within days after SCI if appropriate measures are not instituted in a timely manner.

A disturbance in control and sensation of the bowel, bladder, and genitals is common with SCI at any level; the parasympathetic centers mediating these functions are located in the lowest area of the spinal cord (S2–S4). All of these organs require an intact reflex arc with the sacral centers in order to function properly. During spinal shock, complete SCI at any level results in areflexic bowel, bladder, and genital function (erection, engorgement). Following spinal shock, varying amounts of control and sensation may return. With complete injuries above the S2–S4 level, reflex functions of the bowel, bladder, and genitals remain intact, but conscious control and sensation are disturbed. With complete injury at the S2–S4 level, bowel, bladder, and genital reflexes are disrupted, and the affected organs are likely to remain dysfunctional.

Psychosocial symptoms Following an SCI, the patient experiences a multitude of stressors that may lead to problems in coping. Psychological stressors include memories of the traumatic incident, emergency care, intensive medical/nursing treatment, the ICU environment, and the person's perception of functional losses. Coping strategies typically include anger, denial, and/or depression, and these may become pathological in extended circumstances. In a small number of patients, confusion and psychotic episodes occur.

Diagnostics Radiological assessment provides the most definitive diagnostic information necessary to treat SCI. Such assessment must be accomplished as quickly as possible after the injury. It generally includes (1) multiple conventional radiographs for identification of fractures and dislocations, (2) computerized tomography (with or without contrast) for assessment of narrowing in the spinal canal from vertebral compression, bone fragments, or epidural hemorrhage, and (3) myelography (used less frequently) for assessment of spinal cord compression and intraspinal lesions. The use of MRI, though valuable, is usually not practical during acute SCI; therefore, its use is generally limited to assessment of post-traumatic complications such as syringomyelia.

Nursing standards of care

Medical and surgical interventions upon admission are aimed at (1) preserving vital cardiovascular and respiratory function, (2) relieving the SCI and preserving neurological function, and (3) treating associated traumatic injuries. Since the preservation of neurological function is directly related to swift and appropriate intervention, treatment of SCI optimally occurs in a fully equipped trauma center, where these interventions can be performed rapidly and simultaneously. Unfortunately, with some injuries (those caused by infarction or transection), preserving neurological function is not possible.

Emergency medical intervention aimed at maintaining cardiovascular and respiratory function is often essential to preserve life as well as maintain spinal cord perfusion and oxygenation. Cardiovascular monitoring, including ECG and arterial and/or pulmonary artery catheters, is usually necessary to monitor hemodynamic status. With cervical and upper thoracic injuries, intravenous access is obtained, and vasopressor therapy is usually needed to maintain blood pressure. Care must be taken to prevent system overload by the administration of crystalloids, which increases the risk of edema at the injury site. Endotracheal intubation and mechanical ventilation are usually needed to maintain ventilation with an injury above the C5 level and may also be needed for anesthesia. High-dose corticosteroid therapy is sometimes administered to prevent edema at the injury site, although its effectiveness has never been substantiated.

Surgical intervention is aimed at alleviating the mechanism of injury, when possible, and preventing further harm. Vertebral alignment is obtained by traction, manual manipulation, or surgical reduction, if necessary. Immediate laminectomy may be indicated to eliminate compression and/or relieve edema. However, surgery is optimally performed when neurological function and swelling have stabilized. Surgical stabilization procedures most often include fusion and wiring in the cervical spine and Harrington rod and Olerud plate stabilization in the thoracic and lumbar spine. External vertebral stabilization is attained by traction for certain cervical injuries; however, because of advances in surgical techniques and the use of the Halo Vest for immobilization, long-term traction is no longer indicated. A variety of spinal orthoses are available, and utilization is based on surgeon preference.

Additional medical interventions in the ICU include placement of an NG tube and NPO status for the patient with paralytic ileus and placement of a Foley catheter for all SCI patients. Measures such as subcutaneous heparin may be ordered to prevent complications of venous stasis.

Nursing management of SCI requires a comprehensive, holistic approach to the patient. Necessary nursing interventions are (1) careful surveillance for deterioration in neurological status or development of adverse symptoms indicating physiological deterioration or complication, (2) administration and evaluation of medical interventions to maintain physiological homeostasis and prevent complications, and (3) psychosocial support and ongoing communication with the patient and family regarding the injury and the treatment regimen. Because of the enormous number of individual variables and circumstances surrounding the injury, no two cases of SCI will be exactly the same. The following nursing care plan outlines standard practices used in the care of the SCI patient.

Diagnosis	Signs and symptoms	Intervention	Rationale
Potential risk of permanent injury due to acute spinal cord injury	Vertebral misalignment showing on x-ray Pain at injury site Motor and/or sensory impairment	Monitor sensory and motor levels and compare to baseline (frequency based on acuity of injury)	To identify expanding spinal cord lesions
		Administer corticosteroids as ordered	To minimize inflammation at the injury site
		Maintain spinal alignment at all times and per physician order: do not turn patient; do not raise the head of the bed until the fracture is reduced or stabilized	To prevent impingement of fractured, dislocated spinal fragments into the vertebral canal
		Maintain head, neck, trunk, and hips in a neutral position when turning (log roll technique) and positioning patient	To prevent hyperflexion or extension, twisting, or torquing of the spine
		Use of immobilization devices to follow protocol: apply device continuously unless otherwise ordered; assure complete spinal alignment when device is opened; keep HOB flat when device is opened	To assure safety of patient and prevent accidental hyperflexion or extension, twisting, or torquing of the spine
		Monitor cervical traction frequently to assure proper function: weights and pulleys, pins and bolts, clearance of knot from pulley When moving patient, always have one person monitoring traction	To prevent accidental injury from use of improperly functioning traction equipment

Nursing Care Plan for the Management of the Patient with Acute Spinal Cord Injury

Diagnosis	Signs and symptoms	Intervention	Rationale
		Use of Stryker frame to follow protocol: assure that all pads and straps are properly placed before turning (particularly head and chin straps); check all safety points before turning (two-person check is best);	To assure safety of patient during turning and to prevent accidental hyperflexion or extension, twisting, or torquing of the spine
		turn patient slowly	To avoid hypotensive and/or bradycardic episodes
Potential for alteration in bowel function due to paralytic ileus	Gastric distension Absent bowel sounds Vomiting or high gastric (NG) output	Maintain NPO 2–3 days following injury or until ileus resolves	Normal time range for onset of paralytic ileus is 2–3 days
		Monitor bowel sounds each shift and PRN	
		Use vented NG tube or intermittent suction (per orders)	Appropriate tube or suction minimizes GI irritation
		Measure abdominal girth every shift or PRN	To ascertain retention and bowel distention
		Monitor replacement therapy in comparison to NG and urine output	Fluid and electrolyte imbalances lead to multisystem problems
		Monitor blood chemistry (especially sodium and potassium)	
		Prevent rectal distention (use suppositories or rectal tube PRN)	
Potential for impaired integrity of gastric tissue related to gastric ulceration and/or bleeding	Frank blood or "coffee ground" gastric output or vomitus	Continue all measures outlined in care plan relating to paralytic ileus	To minimize GI irritation

Diagnosis	Signs and symptoms	Intervention	Rationale
	Loose, tarry stool with occult blood	Administer antacids as ordered for pH < 3	To decrease stomach acidity
	Abdominal pain or referred shoulder pain	Administer cimetidine as ordered	To decrease gastric secretions
	Hemorrhagic shock	Check stools and NG aspirate for occult blood	To monitor for further sign of GI bleed
		Monitor Hgb and Hct	These are further indications of bleeding
		Administer iced saline lavage as ordered	To vasoconstrict gastric circulatory bed and control gastric bleeding
		Administer blood/IV replacement therapy as ordered	To maintain adequate circulation and tissue perfusion
		Discontinue steroid therapy as ordered	To decrease gastric secretions
		Control pain with analgesics or muscle relaxants	To promote the patient's comfort
Potential for alteration in body temperature due to interruption of autonomic nervous control	Temperature above or below normal	Adjust environmental and bed temperature to patient, avoiding extremes	Impaired thermoregulation inhibits body compensation to room temperature
	Diaphoresis above the level of injury, particularly of the face	Tepid sponge bath or cooling blanket to cool patient slowly, not exceeding 1 °C every 15 minutes	To cool patient, but not so quickly as to cause ventricular irritability
	Absence of shivering below the level of injury	Adjust bed coverings according to patient's need	To mediate exposure to environmental temperature
		Administer IV fluids as ordered	Elevated temperatures can cause dehydration
Potential for altered bowel elimination due to disturbance in conscious control and/or spinal reflexes	Constipation Impaction Bowel incontinence Abdominal distention	Monitor bowel movements on a daily basis	To prevent complications of constipation
		Manually check bowel for presence of stool and remove any stool in lower rectum; administer bowel elimination procedure per protocol (usually digital stimulation or	Patient may be unable to move bowels independently

Diagnosis	Signs and symptoms	Intervention	Rationale
		suppository or manual removal) every other day or PRN if stool is present	
		Perform procedure at a consistent time (preferably after a meal) and while patient is lying on left side or is on commode chair	To use gastrocolic reflex To provide for proper bowel position
		Use anesthetic cream for patient with sensation or autonomic dysreflexia	To alleviate discomfort and promote ease of procedure without resistance
		Give stool softener and/or fiber laxative as indicated	To facilitate proper stool consistency and prevent constipation
		Give mild laxative if bowel elimination procedure is ineffective and intake is adequate	To facilitate bowel movements
		Assure adequate fluid intake (between 2 and 3 L/day)	To prevent constipation and promote softer stools
Decreased cardiac output due to hypotension and bradycardia	Hypotension	Closely monitor BP and ECG continuously during spinal shock	To allow early intervention and prevention of complications
		Administer vasopressors as ordered	To treat severe hypotension
	Bradycardic arrhythmias Oliguria	Use physiological methods to promote cardiac output (Ace wraps, antiembolic stockings, abdominal binders)	To promote cardiac output
		Observe heart rate closely during suctioning	To observe for and prevent vasovagal response

Diagnosis	Signs and symptoms	Intervention	Rationale
		Administer atropine or antiarrhythmic as ordered	To overcome bradycardic episodes
	Reduced peripheral tissue perfusion evidenced by decreased distal pulses and mottled and cool extremities	Monitor cardiac output and CVP closely, especially in neurogenic shock	Hemodynamic measurements guide in decision making during shock management
		Avoid fluid overload	To prevent edema (especially spinal cord and pulmonary)
		Administer vasoactive drugs as ordered	To increase cardiac index
	Dyspnea	Supply supplemental oxygen as ordered; raise head of bed	To promote adequate oxygenation
		Advance activity slowly (when spine is stabilized) based on BP and patient's reports of dizziness: 1. raise head of bed 2. out of bed to chair 3. ambulation	Activity intolerance is caused by loss of autoregulation of BP
Alteration in comfort due to central and peripheral nerve damage, denervated muscles, and spasticity	Subjective report of pain or paresthesia	Distinguish pain, spasm, and paresthesia	To select appropriate intervention
		Administer medications PRN as ordered (analgesics, antispasmodics)	To alleviate pain, decrease spasticity, and promote comfort
		Institute comfort measures	Comfort measures decrease agitation and promote rest
Impaired communication due to endotracheal or tracheal intubation and respiratory paralysis	Intubation Loss of breath control	Establish a means of comunication (eye blinks, tongue movements, talking tracheostomy tube, clicking, or communication board)	To promote interaction with patient and to better meet his or her needs
		Don't leave patient alone for extended periods of time	So patient will not become fearful

Nursing Care Plan for the Management of the Patient with Acute Spinal Cord Injury

Diagnosis	Signs and symptoms	Intervention	Rationale
Impaired physical mobility related to denervation of skeletal muscle, spasticity, and imposed physical restrictions	Decreased muscle strength and tone	Maintain splints (especially hand and foot) as ordered	To prevent contractures
	Imposed restriction of movement	Maintain head, neck, and body alignment	To prevent complications of immobility
	Decreased range of motion	Assist with ROM exercises at least twice daily, allowing patient to do as much as possible	To maintain joint and muscle mobility and to increase circulation while preventing fatigue
		Try to calm patient during activity	Anxiety increases spasticity
	Signs of impeded circulation in extremities (redness over pressure points)	Apply antiembolism stockings; assess for tenderness, redness, warmth, and pain	To identify and decrease venous stasis and deep vein thrombosis
	Impaired small motor coordination	Assist with required movements	To facilitate patient's movement
	Spasm	Avoid sudden moves; note changes in spasm; explain spasticity to patient	May be due to noxious stimuli (full bladder, impaction, decubitus ulcer, etc.)
Potential dysreflexia related to abnormal autonomic reflexes	Headache	Emergency procedure:	
	Nausea	1. call for assistance	
		2. take vital signs	May need to administer antihypertensive agent
	Hypertension (very high increases compared to baseline)		To decrease BP
	Bradycardia	3. elevate head of bed	
		4. monitor symptoms carefully	
	Sweating, goose bumps, and flushing above injury level	5. drain bladder (catheterize or check indwelling catheter) if no bladder distention: check rectum, administer anesthetic ointment and disimpact (once symptoms subside)	Most common cause of autonomic hyper-reflexia is bladder distention
	Nasal congestion		

Diagnosis	Signs and symptoms	Intervention	Rationale
		6. if above is ineffective, consult MD immediately 7. continue to look for other noxious stimuli (skin breakdown, etc.)	
		Ascertain causative factors and take measures to prevent recurrence	To prevent dysreflexic episodes in the future
Altered nutrition (less than body's requirements) related to prolonged NPO status and paralytic ileus	Complaints of lack of appetite	Consider TPN if NPO status is prolonged	To provide for adequate nutritional support
	Weakness and fatigue Decrease in body weight since admission	Begin PO or NG feedings as soon as paralytic ileus or risk of is over	To facilitate patient's nutritional progress
	Decreased Hgb and Hct	Assess swallowing ability carefully with first feedings	Swallowing may be impaired by injury or device

	Decreased serum albumin and protein	Work with dietician to assure adequate nutritional intake:
		    need for additional protein;
		    need for different food consistency;
		    need for supplement;
		    need for small, frequent meals
			Accelerated protein catabolism occurs in response to trauma; patient's swallowing reflex may be impaired; patient may need iron for Hgb, etc.; patient may tolerate small, frequent meals better

Potential for impaired skin integrity related to:
    decreased sensation,
    restriction in movement,
    pain and discomfort,
    neuromuscular impairment,
    depression,
    diaphoresis or drainage into patient's bed
	Imposed restriction of movement	Turn and position as tolerated by patient	To promote circulation and prevent pressure spots on skin

		Use mattress or overlay appropriate to patient's condition	Typical foam overlays are inadequate for SCI patients
	Impaired coordination of movement	Assist with required movements; avoid common causes of injury: bedpans, poor transfer techniques, heating appliances, ice packs, injections below injury line	To prevent injury and facilitate movement

Nursing Care Plan for the Management of the Patient with Acute Spinal Cord Injury

Diagnosis	Signs and symptoms	Intervention	Rationale
	Decreased muscle strength preventing independent movement	Assist with required movements; turn every 1–2 hours; passive ROM as indicated	To prevent injury and facilitate movement
		Maintain and supplement nutrition as needed	To maintain vital nutrients to skin
	Reluctance to attempt movement	Premedicate PRN as ordered to decrease discomfort accompanying movement	To prevent injury and facilitate movement
	Redness over pressure points or skin lesions	Check skin when changing position or increasing time in sitting/lying position, especially at bony prominences and around devices	To ascertain quality of skin and prevent skin breakdown
	Elevated temperature	Keep patient dry	To prevent skin breakdown
	Skin breakdown	Consult enterostomal therapist	To provide for optimal care planning and intervention
Potential for ineffective coping by the patient and/or family related to: stress of SCI, stress of ICU, personal vulnerability	Verbalization of inability to cope	Assess family's usual coping mechanisms	To ascertain how best to facilitate coping
	Inability to ask for emotional help	Assist family to identify alternative coping mechanisms; identify and acknowledge patient and family needs	Optimal coping must be accomplished for maximal healing
	Withdrawal		
	Prolonged course of disability	Support patient and family through role transition period	Family must be supported through role definition for family cohesiveness

Diagnosis	Signs and symptoms	Intervention	Rationale
		Encourage open communication between family and health care team; resolve conflicts with open discussion and negotiation; discuss implications of negative coping behaviors	Problem solving and planning will be facilitated
	Exhaustion	Monitor and structure environment as needed to decrease/increase stimuli as appropriate	To alleviate sensory deprivation or overstimulation
		Provide regular rest periods	To maximize rest
	Fear and anxiety	Continually inform patient of interventions and rationales	During times of crisis care must be taken not to cause information overload at any one time
		Allow and expect maximal patient independence; assist patient in maintaining control and privacy	To overcome patient anxiety and increase self-assurance
	Inappropriate requests or hypervigilance by patient and/or family	Suggest approaches for family to assist in patient's care	Participatory care decreases family's anxiety
Potential for altered respiratory function related to denervated respiratory muscles	Abnormal ABGs: $pO_2 < 80$ mm Hg; $pCO_2 < 35$ or > 45 mm Hg; pH < 7.35 or > 7.45; O_2 sat. $< 80\%$; $HCO_3 < 20$ or > 26 mEq/L; BE < 0 or > 3	Monitor respiratory parameters closely during the first 3 days following injury in patients with C5 or C6 involvement	Spinal cord edema may cause phrenic nerve impairment
	Cyanosis	Monitor for respiratory insufficiency and cardiac dysrhythmia carefully when patient is prone on a turning frame	Diaphragmatic breathing is inhibited in prone position
	Dyspnea, tachypnea		
	Diminished breath sounds	Use NG tube until patient is able to swallow and control breathing function	To prevent aspiration

Nursing Care Plan for the Management of the Patient with Acute Spinal Cord Injury

Diagnosis	Signs and symptoms	Intervention	Rationale
		Encourage coughing, deep breathing, and incentive spirometry in unintubated patients; use quad coughing technique	To prevent atelectasis
		Perform chest physiotherapy and postural drainage as indicated	To mobilize secretions and prevent atelectasis
		If patient requires artificial ventilation, use jaw thrust technique	To prevent further spinal cord damage
		Begin mobilization as soon as possible	To mobilize secretions and prevent atelectasis
Potential for altered peripheral and cardiopulmonary tissue perfusion related to disturbance in autonomic nervous control and venous stasis	Signs of altered peripheral perfusion: hypotension; peripheral edema; redness, heat, pain, or tenderness in calf or thigh; asymmetrical calves and thighs	Assess pulses, extremities, and BP every 1–2 hours and as needed; measure calf and thigh circumference on admission and daily until out of bed at least 6 hours daily	To monitor for deep venous thrombosis or compromised circulation in extremities
		Perform ROM to extremities at least four times daily; apply antiembolism stockings, Ace wraps, and/or abdominal binders; administer prophylactic therapy (usually heparin 5,000 U subcutaneously every 12 hours)	To prevent venous pooling
		Assure proper positioning for the legs	To prevent compression of veins in popliteal space
		Avoid venipuncture in legs	Trauma to veins increases the risk of deep venous thrombosis

Diagnosis	Signs and symptoms	Intervention	Rationale
	Signs of altered cardiopulmonary perfusion: angina, ischemic changes on ECG, pulmonary embolus, tachypnea or dyspnea, pleural friction rub	Monitor for chest pain	Early detection will help to prevent/allay cardiac complications
		Encourage deep breathing and coughing and turning on a routine schedule	To improve circulation
		Administer supplemental oxygen as needed	To allow for adequate oxygenation
Alteration in patterns of urinary elimination related to disturbance in conscious control and/or spinal elimination reflexes	Bladder distention Bladder incontinence Residual urine volume	Maintain in-dwelling catheter while patient requires frequent urinary monitoring or is hemodynamically unstable (at least 2–3 days following injury)	To prevent overdistention and damage to bladder and to avoid causing dysreflexia
		Restrict fluid to 2 L/day when medically indicated and initiate an intermittent catheterization program every 4 hours when intake has stabilized: return to an in-dwelling catheter if scheduled catheterizations are over 500 cc; reassess fluid restriction and catheterization schedule; advance intermittent catheterization to every 6 hours when catheterization volumes remain below 500 cc	To facilitate success of intermittent catheterization, which decreases the risk of urinary infection and helps patient regain functional control
		If patient voids, obtain residual urine volumes	To evaluate emptying of bladder
		Obtain urological evaluation before advancing program beyond 6 hours	Functional voiding may be subclinically inadequate

Nursing Care Plan for the Management of the Patient with Acute Spinal Cord Injury

Diagnosis	Signs and symptoms	Intervention	Rationale
Potential for alteration in health maintenance due to lack of knowledge of SCI	Verbalizes lack of knowledge Inability to describe diagnosis and care	Assess readiness to learn each topic and give only information appropriate to learning ability and readiness	To allow for greatest amount of learning
	Exhibits behaviors of nonadherence to care regimen Evidence of denial	Make sure patient understands the function of the spinal cord, effects of SCI, and rationale for current intervention	To facilitate healing and prevent complications resulting from deviations from prescribed regimens
	Anxiety	Reiterate information	To promote understanding

Medications Commonly Used in the Care of the Patient with Acute Spinal Cord Injury

Medication	Effect	Major side effects
Vasopressors: Dobutamine Dopamine Phenylephrine	Inotropic with alpha-adrenergic stimulation Vasoconstrictor Decreased tissue perfusion	Headache Vasoconstriction Hypotension Dyspnea Ectopic arrhythmias
Corticosteroids: Dexamethasone Prednisone Hydrocortisone Methylprednisolone	Reduction of cerebral edema by stabilizing the capillary endothelial junction and reducing cerebrovascular permeability; promotes integrity of cells to inhibit flow of intracellular fluid to extracellular space	Opportunistic infection Cushing's syndrome Nervousness Hyperglycemia Electrolyte imbalances Menstrual irregularities Skin rash Gastric irritation
Heparin	Anticoagulation	Bleeding

Space-Occupying Neurological Lesions

A lesion is simply any structural or functional alteration in tissue produced by injury or disease. Neurological lesions that are of a space-occupying nature are more serious than such lesions occurring in other parts of the body, for the neurological system is confined to a limited and uncompromising physical area: the skull. Harmful displacement of brain tissue or very high intracranial pressure occurs as a result of a space-occupying neurological lesion.

Clinical antecedents

Space-occupying lesions that occur neurologically are caused by hemorrhage, hematomas, abscesses, and tumors. Hemorrhages and hematomas are discussed in the section on intracranial hemorrhage, and abscesses are reviewed in the section on neurological infections; only tumors will be discussed here.

An intracranial neoplasm, or tumor, is a pathological overgrowth of tissue that involves regions within the skull, including brain tissue, cranial nerves, meninges, or the pituitary gland. An intracranial tumor is either benign or malignant and may be of a primary nature (originating within the brain) or a secondary nature (occurring as a consequence of the metastasis of a malignancy elsewhere in the body). Tumors are classified according to the neurological region from which the neoplasm arises as supratentorial or infratentorial. Supratentorial tumors present as cerebral (gliomas, including glioblastomas, astrocytomas, and oligodendrogliomas, or meningiomas) or midline (pituitary and pineal tumors and craniopharyngiomas). Infratentorial tumors present as hemangioblastomas, meningiomas, and acoustic schwannomas. Approximately half of all intracranial neoplasms are classified as gliomas, all of which are malignant.

Antecedents to primary intracranial tumors are relatively unknown. Such things as smoking and carcinogens are implicated, but precipitating events and risk factors cannot be clearly defined. Brain tumors are most commonly seen in males between the ages of 35 and 55, but do occur in women (at a lesser incidence) and at any age. Cerebellar tumors are the most common brain tumors found in children, followed by pituitary gland tumors. The antecedent to a secondary intracranial tumor is the primary tumor from which the metastasis originated.

Critical referents

The glioblastoma multiforme (astrocytoma grades 3 and 4 and malignant glioma) is the most common of the primary intracranial neoplasms and occurs in the frontal and temporal lobes or the cerebral hemispheres (rarely in the cerebellum or brainstem) and does not metastasize outside of the central nervous system. This type of tumor is irreversibly malignant and has a rapid growth rate, resulting consistently in fatality within 9–12 months (rarely as long as 2 years). This primary tumor is fibrillary in nature, affects the cell protoplasm, and is found to infiltrate extensively across cerebral commissures into adjacent lobes. Surgical removal of the primary tumor can be accomplished by gross resection, but because of its infiltration, recurrence occurs within months of excision.

Low-grade astrocytoma and oligodendroglioma occur less frequently than glioblastoma multiforme. They grow in the cerebral hemispheres at a slower rate and are less malignant, perhaps because they contain calcifications. Because they are slow-growing, diagnosis of these types of tumor sometimes cannot be made until they have been present for years. Over the years, the structure of the tumor tissue can become more complex or be broken down into simpler forms, so the degree of malignancy does not remain consistent throughout the tumor; in fact, it is highly variable. For this reason, it is difficult to assign a prognosis to such cases. Usually, the patient with these tumors survives 3 to 5 years after surgery and radiation treatment. Recurrence of the tumor can occur and, if in an operable location, can be treated in the same manner.

The meningioma is a rather common but benign tumor that arises from arachnoidal cells. It occurs mostly in women who are between the ages of 40 and 50 years. Surgical removal is usually an effective treatment for a meningioma because it is well circumscribed and usually unable to infiltrate areas outside of the dura, dural sinuses, or adjacent bone. If complete resection is accomplished, survival rates are high and extended.

The pituitary adenoma is classified on an endocrinological basis as nonfunctioning or hypersecreting and is generally slow-growing. This type of tumor is usually benign and is manifested through endocrinological changes such as hyperprolactinemia, amenorrhea, and hypopituitarism. It can progress into the sella turcica, leading to visual compromises.

The pineal tumor arises in the midbrain and frequently leads to hydrocephalus. It can also infiltrate anteriorly into the hypothalamus, causing diabetes insipidus, or into the optic pathways. This type of tumor is not fast-growing, but it can metastasize through the CSF. It does respond fairly well to treatment, being sensitive to radiation therapy. In the rare event that it does not respond to that therapy, complete surgical resection can be accomplished. Survival after therapy is usually long-term with the tumor nonrecurrent.

The craniopharyngioma is a benign tumor that arises from squamous cells in the pituitary stalk. It occurs congenitally and usually manifests in children and young adults. It can cause compromises in the optic nerve or hypothalamus and can also lead to hydrocephalus. Because of its location, surgical intervention is very risky, so radiation therapy is the treatment of choice.

The hemangioblastoma is an overgrowth of arterial or venous tissue that consumes blood provided by the blood vessel in order to grow. It is slow-growing and very rare. This type of tumor usually forms in the parietal cortex in proximity to middle cerebral vessels, which can act as feeders. Surgical clipping of the feeder vessels followed by removal of the growth is the treatment of choice. Minimal disability is frequently a consequence of the surgical manipulation.

The acoustic schwannoma is a slow-growing tumor of the Schwann cells of peripheral nerves. It is usually found in the intracranial cavity but frequently occurs bilaterally and in conjunction with other cranial and spinal tumors. The acoustic schwannoma is usually encapsulated and puts pressure on adjoining tissue rather than infiltrating it. If diagnosed early, the prognosis for the patient with this type of tumor is good, for surgical excision can be accomplished on a small neoplasm by the translabyrinthine approach rather than by craniectomy. Survival rates are high for patients following successful surgical removal of smaller lesions. Larger tumors eventually cause increased intracranial pressure and ultimately brainstem compression.

Resulting signs and symptoms

Clinical presentation of intracranial tumors is mostly due to effects of the destruction of surrounding tissue, the local accumulation of metabolites, and increased intracranial pressure. Generally, headache, nausea and vomiting, and seizure activity are seen in varying degrees. Motor and sensory dysfunction occurs in response to specific regional involvement. Primary signs and symptoms associated with each specific tumor are as follows:

Glioblastoma multiforme: according to location affected

Astrocytoma and oligodendroglioma: delayed and according to location affected

Meningioma: according to location affected

Pituitary adenoma: asymptomatic unless hypersecreting, in which case symptoms can include hyperprolactinemia, female amenorrhea and male impotence, hypopituitarism, visual field losses, Cushing's disease

Pineal tumor: Parinaud's syndrome, noncommunicating hydrocephalus, diabetes insipidus

Craniopharyngioma: increased intracranial pressure, optic compromises, depressed pituitary function

Hemangioblastoma: according to location affected

Acoustic schwannoma: deafness, tinnitus, unsteadiness and imbalance, loss of corneal reflex, facial numbness and weakness, ataxia

Nursing standards of care

Medical management of the patient with intracranial tumors includes surgery, radiation, chemotherapy, or a combination of the three. Surgery, the most often utilized of these treatments, is indicated when the tumor is located in a easily accessible region of the brain. Radiation and/or chemotherapy are chosen when the tumor is of an infiltrating, nonencapsulating nature and is responsive to such intervention or is considered to be in an inoperable region of the brain. Chemotherapy is indicated only when the tumor has destroyed the blood-brain barrier, for most drugs cannot cross this barrier when it is intact.

Nursing care in the intensive care unit is provided in concert with the medical regimen in order to provide protection from injury and further complications. Details are provided in the sections on increased intracranial pressure and craniotomy.

Craniotomy for Correction of Space-Occupying Lesions

A craniotomy is a common neurosurgical procedure usually performed for the removal of an intracranial tumor or for the purpose of obtaining a biopsy.

Clinical antecedents

A craniotomy may be performed in an emergency or as a routine procedure, depending on the underlying pathology. Possible indications include intracranial lesions and hematomas, cerebral abscesses and aneurysms, arteriovenous malformation, nerve decompression, hydrocephalus, and excision of seizure foci.

Advances in technology such as laser surgery, stereotaxic surgery, and microsurgery (neurosurgery using a microscope) continue to refine and shape neurosurgical practices. Laser surgery allows precise tumor resection by vaporization as well as entry into formerly nonaccessible areas. Adjacent brain tissue is not injured, and since brain manipulation is reduced, there is less postoperative cerebral edema. Stereotaxic surgery, based on a three-dimensional concept, permits precise localization to any area in the brain. The procedure is conducted under local anesthesia and guided by a CT scanner using the stereotaxic frame for external reference points. A burr hole is made, and the dura is opened for access to the intracranial contents. Clinical applications include tumor biopsy; aspiration of hematomas, colloid cysts, and abscesses; craniopharyngiomas; implantation of interstitial radiation; ablative procedures for extrapyramidal disorders; and localization of seizure focus. The following terms relate to various aspects of craniotomy:

Burr hole(s): a hole or series of holes in the cranium made in preparation for neurosurgery

Craniotomy: a surgical opening of the skull to gain access to the brain

Craniectomy: removal of a portion of the skull

Cranioplasty: replacement of portion of the removed skull with a synthetic material to provide protection for the brain

Supratentorial approach: surgical approach used to gain access to the lobes of the cerebral hemispheres above the tentorium

Infratentorial approach: surgical approach used to gain access to the brainstem and cerebellum below the tentorium

Transsphenoidal approach: a transnasal approach through the submucosa gum area and sphenoid sinus to the sella turcica for access to the pituitary gland

Critical referents

Specific pathophysiological characteristics of various neurological disorders that require craniotomy are detailed below.

Intracranial lesions, tumors, and hematomas Lesions, tumors, or hematomas in the brain may be primary or secondary, and lesions and tumors may be malignant or benign. Hematomas may occur from intracranial hemorrhage into the epidural, subdural, or subarachnoid space. Subdural hematomas usually result from a laceration or damage of the subdural veins. Epidural hematomas are usually found in the temporal fossa and are formed by bleeding from the middle meningeal artery. Subarachnoid hemorrhage is discussed in the section on subarachnoid aneurysms.

Lesions and tumors are classified according to the tissue within which they originate, and unless treated successfully, result in eventual death from increasing size and resulting increased ICP, if not from metastasis and secondary complications. Table 3-28 summarizes the various types of lesions and tumors according to tissue of origin and location of occurrence.

Intracranial lesions, tumors, and hematomas are surgically treated according to the type and location

Table 3-28 Originating Tissue and Location of Intracranial Lesions and Tumors

Type	Originating Tissue	Location
Metastatic	Lungs Thyroid Kidney Breast Prostate	Cerebral cortex Diencephalon
Arteriovenous malformation	Arteries Veins	Parietal cortex
Pituitary	Pituitary gland	Pituitary gland
Meningioma	Endothelial cells Angioblasts Fibrous tissue	Arachnoid villi Dura mater Base of hemisphere
Glioma		
Astrocytoma	Astrocytes Glial cells	White matter of temporal and frontal lobes
Medulloblastoma	Supportive tissue	Brainstem Fourth ventricle Posterior fossa
Glioblastoma	Glioblast	Cerebral hemispheres
Oligodendroglioma	Glial cells Dendrites	Cerebral hemispheres Cerebellum Frontal lobe Basal ganglia
Ependymoma	Ependymal epithelium	Fourth ventricle Lateral ventricles

of the disorder. Sometimes complete removal can be accomplished, but at other times only a reduction in size can be attempted with the goal being to relieve the symptoms and extend limited survival time.

Intracranial abscesses Intracranial abscesses may occur epidurally, subdurally, within the subarachnoid space, or in the actual brain and ventricle tissue. They are caused by chemical irritants (contrast media used in diagnostic tests); bacteria such as Staphylococcus aureus, Streptococcus pneumoniae, Hemophilus influenzae, and Neisseria meningitidis; viruses such as herpes simplex; and fungi. They are inflammatory conditions within the cranium that may have originated from infections via penetrating wounds, the bloodstream, the CSF, the spinal nerves, or the nasopharyngeal and oral cavities. Inflammation results, production of CSF increases, and intracranial pressure rises. Any resultant purulent drainage accumulates within the brain tissue or can be spread to other areas of the brain and spinal cord by the CSF. CSF characteristics indicative of the inflammatory process include the presence of bacteria or viruses, increased CSF pressures, increased WBCs, and increased protein. Primary abscesses, if not treated in a timely manner, can easily and quickly result in systemic infections. Depending on the characteristics of an abscess, surgical drainage or removal (if encapsulated in benign regions of the brain) is attempted.

Hydrocephalus Cerebrospinal fluid circulates around the spinal cord and over the convexities of the brain and is resorbed into large venous sinuses in the dura. Even if the flow of CSF is obstructed (by congenital abnormalities, tissue inflammation, or tumors), secretion continues, resulting in a damming effect in the ventricles proximal to the obstruction. The ventricles become distended and dilated and compression and damage of brain tissue occurs (see Figure 3-27).

Surgical intervention entails a shunting procedure, in which a one-way-valved tube is inserted into the dilated ventricle and rerouting of the CSF fluid (frequently into the peritoneal cavity or into the jugular vein extending into the right atrium) is accomplished.

Epileptic foci If an epileptic has a clearly indentifiable seizure focus in a benign area of the nondominant portion of the brain, surgical excision of that focus may be indicated. These surgical resections are

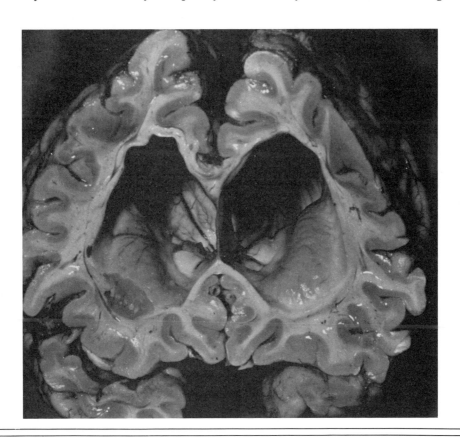

Figure 3-27 Cross Section of Brain Revealing Marked Dilation of Ventricles Associated with Hydrocephalus

usually performed in the corpus callosum or cortical regions of the brain.

Resulting signs and symptoms

The above neurological disorders result in the following signs and symptoms.

Intracranial lesions, tumors, and hematomas Clinical manifestations of intracranial lesions, tumors and hematomas include increased ICP, changes in level of consciousness, headache, nausea and vomiting, papilledema, seizure activity, focal and functional neurological deficits (depending on the area affected), and personality changes. The section on neurological assessment provides information regarding indicators of involvement of specific areas of the brain.

Intracranial abscesses Severe headache accompanied by photophobia and high fever are the landmarks of the patient suffering from intracranial abscesses. Signs of increased ICP may also be manifest; these include drowsiness, confusion, and seizures. As with intracranial lesions, tumors, and hematomas, focal and functional neurological deficits (depending on the area affected) also occur.

Hydrocephalus Signs and symptoms of hydrocephalus mirror the manifestations of increased ICP. These include headache, decreased level of consciousness, blurred vision, vomiting, and restlessness.

Epileptic foci Epileptic seizures of various types may have a clearly defined seizure focus. Manifestations include tonic-clonic seizure activity resulting in loss of consciousness, stiffening of the body, and subsequent jerking of extremities. Another manifestation may be a staring episode preceded by a moment of confusion. Sometimes partial seizures occur, involving shaking of one area of the body or lip smacking, hypersalivation, and facial automatism. A variety of psychosensory symptoms may also occur during partial seizures, including visual or auditory distortions, vertigo, and alterations in memory and other thought processes such as directing of attention and forced thinking. Finally, autonomic symptoms that occur during such seizures may include gastrointestinal involvement as well as respiratory and cardiovascular complications.

Nursing standards of care

To promote optimal recovery of the patient undergoing a craniotomy, the critical care nurse must be knowledgeable about the specific nursing and medical practices used to care for such a patient.

Preoperative considerations A crucial role of the nurse in the management of the craniotomy patient is to provide emotional support and preoperative teaching to the patient and family. Preparing the patient and family for the ICU experience is important in helping to decrease postoperative anxiety. An assessment of the patient's and family's level of understanding, anxiety, fears, cultural practices, religious beliefs, and use of support systems will help the nurse to structure appropriate educational sessions. Information should be presented according to the individual's ability and readiness to learn.

Beyond the usual physical, mental, and emotional workup done on all critical care patients, a detailed assessment to establish the baseline of neurological function is most important for early detection of neurological changes following surgery. Specific areas of neurological assessment include level of consciousness, pupillary reaction and eye movement, motor and reflex status, and vital signs.

Postoperative considerations One of the most frequently presented complications of craniotomy is increased intracranial pressure. Increased ICP resulting from hemorrhage, cerebral edema, and hydrocephalus is potentially life-threatening and easily becomes so without early recognition and prompt management. Please refer to the care plan for the management of the patient with increased ICP for details of care to be provided should this complication arise.

Respiratory complications are also frequently seen in the craniotomy patient. Common complications are atelectasis, pneumonia, and pulmonary emboli. Nursing interventions to promote optimal respiratory function are of primary importance in the prevention of these complications. Humidified air, suctioning during pulmonary toilet (unless neurologically contraindicated), frequent turning, breathing exercises with assistive devices such as the incentive spirometer, and chest physiotherapy are helpful in the prevention and management of respiratory complications.

Since respiratory complications may occur in spite of nurses' efforts to prevent them, it is important that the critical care nurse be able to recognize them early for prompt intervention. The clinical presentation of pulmonary embolism varies and is often nonspecific. Symptoms may include chest pain, fever, hypoxia, hypotension, tachycardia, and dyspnea. In the event of pulmonary embolism, nursing management is directed toward supporting cardiovascular and respiratory function, preventing recurrent emboli, and alleviating discomfort. Surgical management includes (1) transvenous placement of a Greenfield filter to trap emboli and allow blood flow, (2) vein ligation, and (3) embolectomy. Anticoagulants, frequently administered as an intervention for pulmonary emboli, may be contraindicated in the neurosurgical patient at risk for hemorrhage.

The craniotomy patient is usually placed on prophylactic anticonvulsant therapy to prevent seizure activity. Dilantin is generally the drug of choice. Seizure activity may be focal or generalized and may be caused by alcohol withdrawal, an expanding intracranial lesion, inflammatory trauma from surgery, or metabolic or fluid and electrolyte imbalances.

Meningitis is another possible complication of craniotomy. The patient who has an associated infection or traumatic injuries or who has undergone a transsphenoidal hypophysectomy, placement of a subarachnoid bolt, or insertion of a ventricular drain is more at risk for developing meningitis. Astute assessment by the nurse can detect early signs of meningitis and allow the initiation of prompt treatment. Strict measures to prevent the development of meningitis should be instituted. Prophylactic antibiotic therapy is frequently initiated to help prevent the development of infection.

Thrombophlebitis is a common complication of the neurosurgical patient. Clinical presentation includes edema surrounding the thrombus, pain in the calf with dorsiflexion of the ankle (positive Homan's sign), redness, and warmth. Prophylactic measures to help reduce the incidence of thrombophlebitis include the administration of low-dose heparin, application of elastic stockings, intermittent pneumatic leg compression, range of motion exercises, and early ambulation as soon as it is neurologically indicated. Treatment for thrombophlebitis includes bed rest, use of elastic stockings, elevation of the involved extremity, and anticoagulation therapy if not neurologically contraindicated.

Other complications can occur secondarily to the postoperative treatment for craniotomy. Steroid therapy, commonly part of the postoperative treatment of the craniotomy patient, may contribute to gastric irritation, ulceration, and hemorrhage. Clinical presentation includes guaiac-positive stools, a gradual drop in hemoglobin, and coffee-ground emesis. Active bleeding warrants discontinuing the steroid therapy or at least reducing the dosage. An antacid regime in combination with medication such as Zantac or Tagamet is used to help decrease gastric hemorrhage.

A slight elevation in temperature is common during the early postoperative period and is caused by atelectasis and/or cerebral irritation. Hyperthermia increases cerebral metabolism, thereby increasing ICP. Nursing interventions to control the detrimental effects of hyperthermia include the administration of antipyretic medications such as Tylenol, controlling the climate of the patient's immediate environment, removing excess clothing from the patient, applying tepid baths, and placing the patient on a hypothermia blanket. Temperature elevations not responding to these interventions require further investigation in order to identify the source, whether infectious or neurological in nature.

Loss of corneal reflex (cranial nerve V) results in an inability to blink the eye. Nursing interventions to protect the cornea from abrasion and ulceration include frequent administrations of eye drops or ointment, placement of an eye shield, and taping the eyelids closed.

Paralysis of the facial nerve (cranial nerve VII) causes severe weakness on one side of the face and the inability to completely close the affected eye. Nursing interventions are directed at protecting the cornea from injury. Food and fluids should be introduced on the unaffected side to facilitate chewing and swallowing. A loss of the gag reflex (cranial nerve IX and X) and of function of the hypoglossal nerve (cranial nerve XII) implies varying degrees of dysphagia. A detailed assessment of the patient's swallowing mechanism should be performed prior to the initiation of feedings. Consultation with a speech pathologist can assist in this evaluation.

The development of diabetes insipidus is a common transient problem following surgery near the pituitary gland (transsphenoidal hypophysectomy). The cranial presentation includes thirst, copious and rapid urinary output, low urine specific gravity, and hypernatremia. Accurate hourly measurements of intake and output and frequent measurements of urine specific gravity are important for determining the management of such cases. Fluid and electrolyte replacement are usually indicated; therefore, the patient is not placed on strict fluid restriction as is usual with craniotomy patients. Vasopressin (Pitressin) is the medication of choice for diabetes insipidus during the acute stages. Desmopressin acetate (DDAVP), administered intranasally, is used in the long-term management of diabetes insipidus.

The syndrome of inappropriate antidiuretic hormone (SIADH) may be caused by operative manipulation, the presence of cerebral irritation, meningitis, or overadministration of vasopressin. The clinical presentation of SIADH includes headache, nausea and vomiting, anorexia, irritability, altered level of consciousness, hyponatremia, hypocalcemia, low serum osmolarity, low urinary output with high urine sodium and osmolality, muscle weakness, and seizures. In less acute cases, a fluid restriction may be adequate to prevent complications, but if the patient is at risk for seizures from severe hyponatremia, more aggressive measures are warranted. Administration of 3% hypertonic saline (to replace the depleted sodium chloride) and drug therapy such as Lasix and Declomycin (to induce diuresis) may be indicated.

Periorbital edema may be a result of the manipulation that occurs during surgical procedures such as a frontal craniotomy or transsphenoidal hypophysectomy. Application of cool compresses may help to alleviate swelling and discomfort. Commonly, headache caused by postoperative swelling exacerbated by a constricting dressing can usually be relieved by mild analgesics or codeine.

Fever, dehydration, periorbital edema, headache, skin irritation along the suture lines, and trauma to the nasal and oral mucous membranes also contribute to the patient's pain. Imposed physical restrictions such as those accompanying a patient's stay in the ICU as well as the placement of a foley catheter, IV, arterial line, and central venous pressure and intracranial monitoring devices can further discomfort the patient during the critical postoperative period. Individualized nursing interventions to maximize comfort during the time following surgery can prove to be invaluable in promoting the early recovery of the craniotomy patient.

The patient undergoing transsphenoidal surgery may have a graft of muscle or fascia from the anterior thigh or abdomen packed into the sella turcica to prevent leakage of CSF. Vaseline packing is inserted into each nare to help control bleeding. With bilateral nasal packing, the postoperative transsphenoidal patient will need to breathe through the mouth. A moustache dressing is taped to cover the nasal packing and collect serosanguinous drainage.

Positioning   Positioning is an important consideration in the care of the craniotomy patient and the type of positioning required depends on the surgical procedure and underlying pathology. Following a supratentorial craniotomy, the head of the patient's bed is elevated 30–45 degrees to promote venous and cerebrospinal fluid drainage to help decrease intracranial pressure. If there are no complications, progressive mobilization is instituted on the second postoperative day. When the infratentorial approach has been used, the patient is kept flat for 48 hours, followed by gradual head elevations. Supporting the head and maintaining body alignment while turning the patient are important. The patient who has a bone flap is turned and repositioned in ways to avoid the operative side. The patient recovering from a subdural hematoma may be kept flat in bed for some initial period, followed by gradual elevations of the head. This position promotes subdural drainage, increases intracranial pressure (thereby reducing the possibility of reaccumulation of fluid), and decreases the risk of hemorrhage from the tearing of dural veins.

Further considerations concerning the management of the craniotomy patient are detailed in the following nursing care plan.

Nursing Care Plan for the Management of the Patient with Space-Occupying Lesions

Diagnosis	Signs and symptoms	Intervention	Rationale
Alteration in respiratory function related to ineffective breathing patterns and airway clearance, impaired gas exchange, and immobility	Abnormal ABGs: $pO_2 < 80$ mm Hg; $pCO_2 < 35$ or > 45 mmHg; pH < 7.35 or > 7.45; O_2 sat. $< 80\%$; $HCO_3 < 20$ or > 26 mEq/L; BE < 0 or > 3 Dyspnea Hypoxemia Hypercapnia Copious secretions Atelectasis Elevated respiratory rate, wheezing, air hunger, gasping, or asymmetrical expansion of chest wall	Assess breathing pattern frequently Maintain airway Mechanically ventilate postoperatively as required Closely monitor ABGs PRN postoperatively and after ventilator changes; closely monitor lungs for absent, unequal, diminished breath sounds, crackles, wheezing, or asymmetrical chest wall expansion Aggressive pulmonary toilet (as neurologically indicated) PRN with chest percussion therapy, incentive spirometry, and hyperinflation using 100% oxygen before and after suctioning Turn and reposition patient every 2 hours (within neurological indications) Promote extubation of stable patient as soon as possible by: holding sedation, elevating HOB 30 degrees, incremental weaning (as neurologically indicated)	To evaluate respiratory function To ensure adequate ventilation To ascertain early indications of ensuing respiratory compromise and/or complications To mobilize secretions, provide adequate oxygenation, and open closed alveoli To assist patient to return to optimal breathing capacity as soon as possible and to prevent atelectasis and secondary infection

Nursing Care Plan for the Management of the Patient with Space-Occupying Lesions

Diagnosis	Signs and symptoms	Intervention	Rationale
Alteration in cerebral perfusion related to increased ICP	Increased ICP Altered level of consciousness	Establish baseline for neurological function and assess for changes by comparing ongoing assessment to baseline	To compare clinical findings to detect early changes in neurological function
		Maintain fluid restriction and accurate I&O	To help control ICP
		Monitor ABGs for hypo- or hypercapnia	$PaCO_2 < 25$ mm Hg or > 55 mm Hg may impair autoregulation
	Decreased pupillary response	Maintain in a semi-Fowler's position with head in a neutral position except when contraindicated (with subdural hematoma and infratentorial approach)	To facilitate venous drainage
		Instruct patient to exhale with movement	To prevent Valsalva maneuver, which increases intrathoracic pressure, which increases ICP
	Anxiety	Control external stimulation (noise, light, temperature)	To prevent agitation and startle response, which cause increased ICP
	Agitation	Approach patient calmly and reassuringly	Nursing activities can lead to agitation
		Plan activities to allow adequate rest	Fatigue exacerbates agitation
	Motor dysfunction	Monitor ICP increases to learn what causes them and organize activities to minimize stimulation	To limit time and intensity of activities that stress the patient and raise ICP
		Assist family to communicate calmly and quietly and to avoid emotionally stimulating the patient	To prevent excessive stimulation, agitation, and unnecessary startles, which cause rises in ICP

Diagnosis	Signs and symptoms	Intervention	Rationale
Alteration in tissue integrity of oral/nasal membrane due to trauma of transsphenoidal and oral surgical procedures	Red, swollen mucous membranes Nasal bleeding Complaints of pain	Assess oral mucous membranes and gingival incisional line	To detect signs of infection
		Provide mouth care every 4 hours and PRN with Toothettes, using 1 part NS/1 part hydrogen peroxide/1 part Cepacol	To remove dried blood and clean mouth
		Lightly cleanse upper gingiva	To cleanse while protecting incision line
		Apply lip balm PRN	To promote comfort
	Dry lips	Administer high humidity oxygen via face tent or mask	To provide moisture to mucous membranes
		Instruct patient to use toothbrush only on lower teeth until after 10 days	To prevent tearing of gingival incision
		Insruct patient to avoid sneezing and blowing the nose	To prevent stress on nasal membranes and graft site
		Keep accurate I&O records	To monitor fluid balances
Alteration in patterns of urinary elimination due to decreased level of consciousness, decreased mobility, and presence of urinary catheter	Urinary retention or incontinence	Report abnormal amount, color, or odor of urine and unusual frequency or pain of urination	To determine and treat early signs of urinary tract infections
		Monitor serum creatinine, BUN, urine specific gravity, UA, and urine C&S	To evaluate renal function
		Determine regular pattern of urination and structure bladder training accordingly	To establish optimal urinary elimination
		Assess for urinary retention and plan catheterization regime accordingly	To assist patient to adequately empty bladder

Nursing Care Plan for the Management of the Patient with Space-Occupying Lesions

Diagnosis	Signs and symptoms	Intervention	Rationale
Potential for alteration in bowel function or constipation due to: decreased mobility, change in eating patterns, side effects of medications, postoperative paralytic ileus, decreased fluid volume	Reports of feeling constipated, "full" feeling in abdomen, inability to move bowels	Assess abdomen for bowel sounds, softness, and appearance and ask patient about discomfort at least every 12 hours	For early diagnosis of constipation in order to intervene before serious problems occur
	Decreased or absent bowel sounds	Encourage progressive activity as tolerated	To stimulate peristalsis
	Inadequate oral fluid/food intake as evidenced on I&O records and calorie counts	Reassure patient that constipation is frequently a problem postoperatively	So patient will not become overly concerned
	Symptoms of dehydration: poor skin turgor, sunken eyes, intake less than output, weight loss	Assess for signs of dehydration and encourage oral intake within fluid restriction limits	Hydration impedes constipation
		Closely monitor electrolytes	Dehydration leads to electrolyte imbalance
	Absence of bowel movement for more than 2 days	Implement bowel regimen as ordered: milk of magnesia 30 mL p.o. every HS; consult with dietician about increased fiber in diet as indicated; rehydrate patient as ordered via IV or oral fluids (as neurologically indicated)	Patient may need extra help to have regular bowel movements
		Reduce narcotic consumption when feasible	Narcotics inhibit bowel activity

Diagnosis	Signs and symptoms	Intervention	Rationale
Potential for fluid and electrolyte imbalance due to fluid loss, antidiuretic hormone imbalance, gastrointestinal suctioning, and hyperthermia	Volume excess	Accurately monitor I&O and urine specific gravity	To ascertain fluid balance status
	Electrolyte imbalances, such as hypernatremia or hyponatremia	Closely monitor electrolyte status: hematocrit, BUN, creatinine, and serum osmolality	To detect imbalances and determine renal function (hyponatremia can precipitate seizures)
	Large and rapid urine output		
	Abnormal serum osmolality	Administer ADH replacement therapy as prescribed	To help concentrate urine and prevent fluid losses
		Adhere strictly to fluid restrictions	To avoid overhydration, leading to cerebral edema
		Maintain temperature within normal limits	To prevent rises in ICP
		Measure gastric output and test pH every 8 hours; if pH < 5, administer antacids as ordered	To prevent gastric acidity
		Consult dietician and initiate nutritional support as soon as appropriate; initiate tube feeding if needed	Early nutritional support promotes fluid and electrolyte balances and provides strength, leading to recovery
Potential for physical injury related to sensorimotor deficits, cognitive impairment, altered level of consciousness, or seizure activity	Motor deficits Agitation	Maintain a safe environment by: placing bed in low position with wheel brakes in locked position, side rails up, call light within easy reach, assistive devices within reach; arranging furniture and equipment for safe use by patient; providing adequate lighting at HS; providing nonskid foot wear	To promote safety and decrease risk of physical injury
		Identify patient's safety needs and establish safety guidelines with patient and family; reinforce guidelines frequently	To promote learning of safety practices by patient and family

Nursing Care Plan for the Management of the Patient with Space-Occupying Lesions

Diagnosis	Signs and symptoms	Intervention	Rationale
	Seizures	Administer anticonvulsants as prescribed and monitor therapeutic levels	To help prevent seizures through attaining of optimal drug effectiveness
		Institute seizure precautions (padded bed rails, oral airway, suction equipment, and supplemental oxygen)	To decrease the risk of physical injury in the event of seizures
	Confusion	Reorient patient frequently	To increase patient's awareness of surroundings
	Anxiety	Explain patient care activities	To help alleviate anxiety
	Restlessness	Assess causes of restlessness (hypoxemia, pain, bladder distention) and plan care appropriate to need	To decrease risk of restlessness and agitation leading to possible accidental injury
		Use physical restraints only when necessary	To promote safety and reduce agitation
Potential for infection due to: surgical procedure, IV lines, indwelling Foley, endotracheal intubation, stress, CSF leak	Increased temperature	Tylenol 600 mg every 4 hours PRN as ordered	To alleviate fevers
	WBC > 10,000 mm^3	Implement thorough hand washing between patient contacts; implement universal isolation precautions if indicated	To prevent spread of infections
	Redness, exudate, or increased tenderness at IV or ICP insertion site	Routine care with povidone-iodine solution, telfa dressing, and foam tape	To prevent infections
		Change peripheral IV sites at least every 3 days or with any signs of infection or infiltration; change IV tubing every 48 hours	IV fluid is especially fertile medium for bacterial growth
		Culture suspected origins of infection	To administer appropriate antibiotics

Diagnosis	Signs and symptoms	Intervention	Rationale
	Changes in characteristics of sputum: tan, brown, yellow, or green color and/or foul odor	Nonvigorous pulmonary toilet	To prevent and/or treat pulmonary congestion leading to infections (without increasing neurological stressors)
	Decreased or absent breath sounds locally		
	Sediment in urine or foul-smelling urine; WBCs in urine; hesitancy, frequency, urgency, burning, difficulty starting urination, incontinence, and/or inability to void	Routine Foley care every 8 hours; push fluids if taking fluids and not neurologically contraindicated	To prevent urinary tract infections
	Altered LOC, headache, meningeal signs	If CSF leak suspected, test drainage with dextrostix (CSF will test positive for glucose)	To assess for early signs of wound infection, CSF leak, or meningitis, requiring prompt treatment
Alteration in rest/sleep pattern related to continuous environmental stimuli, ICU routine, and interrupted sleep	Disturbances in rest/sleep pattern	Determine the patient's established rest/sleep pattern and organize nursing activities to accommodate it as much as possible	To accommodate to patient's normal pattern
	Exhaustion	Structure nursing activities to provide for fewer interruptions at normal time of sleep; design schedule to balance daytime activities with periods of uninterrupted sleep	To maximize patient's ability to relax, rest, and sleep
	Inability to fall asleep	Provide comfort measures and assistive devices individualized to patient's need; explore the possibility of relaxation therapy	To promote comfort and sleep
	Interrupted rest periods	Plan visiting schedule to accommodate interventions as well as family's schedule and rest periods; restrict visitors as appropriate	To maximize quality of family time as well as provide for needed rest

Nursing Care Plan for the Management of the Patient with Space-Occupying Lesions

Diagnosis	Signs and symptoms	Intervention	Rationale
Potential for self-care deficit in areas of hygiene, toileting, feeding, and mobility related to postoperative restrictions, decreased LOC, and impaired ability to recognize self-care needs	Inability to perform self-care activities independently	Assess neurological deficits	To identify and meet self-care needs
		Encourage patient to function as independently as possible; assist with minor self-care, passive ROM; provide equipment and assistance as appropriate	To promote highest level of independence
		Encourage patient to participate in scheduling and carrying out daily care	To prevent overexhaustion and to facilitate adequate rest while encouraging independence
		Consult with occupational therapist and physical therapist to plan strategies to promote self-care activities incorporating safety measures	To reduce the risk of physical injury while promoting self-care abilities and activities
		Teach family about ways to encourage the patient's independence	To promote autonomy and initiate planning for early discharge
Potential for impaired verbal communication related to decreased LOC, cerebral edema, dysphasia, endotracheal tube, and tracheostomy	Receptive, global, or expressive aphasia	Assess patient's ability to hear, understand, and speak	To determine patient's ability to communicate
	Frustration during communication attempts	Teach appropriate strategies to promote communication: using assistive materials such as writing implements and communication board, reducing environmental distractions, decreasing anxiety, decreasing speed of communication, using simple commands with gestures	To help patient identify and use appropriate strategies to facilitate communication

Diagnosis	Signs and symptoms	Intervention	Rationale
		Face the patient and establish eye contact to provide support and reassurance during communication attempts	To encourage patient's efforts
		Consult with speech therapist	To allow for early rehabilitation
	Uneasiness and impatience of family during communication attempts	Teach family successful strategies for communication with patient	To promote family communication and cohesion
Disturbance in body concept related to neurological deficits, cranial nerve dysfunction (facial palsy, decreased corneal reflex), and hair loss from surgical procedure	Alterations in body concept	Assess patient's and family's interpretation of change in body concept	To establish baseline
	Anxiety during visiting hours	Encourage patient and family to express feelings	To help alleviate feelings of anxiety and promote adjustment
	Inability of family to comfortably and calmly look at and interact with patient	Assist family in adapting to patient's body changes and appearance	To achieve maximal level of self-esteem for patient and acceptance and support from family
	Lack of knowledge of available support services	Consult with hospital and community support services	To help patient and family make use of appropriate resources

Potential for alteration in health maintenance due to lack of knowledge of:
    diagnosis;
    surgical procedure;
    medication regimen;
    activity;
    medical follow-up;
    referrals;
    home management
	Inability to describe personal diagnosis and how it relates to type of surgery and prognosis	Instruct patient and family about diagnosis, surgery, and prognosis with as many repetitions as needed	Patient and family must understand in order to adhere to prescribed regimen, which will promote healing and optimal level of functioning

		Encourage questions and open discussion of problems and concerns	To allow for clear understanding and acceptance

	Inability to describe prescribed regimen and reasons for it	Instruct about medications, diet, and followup arrangements:
		    what,
		    why,
		    care options,
		    plan of daily schedule
			To promote understanding and thus adherence to prescribed regimen

Nursing Care Plan for the Management of the Patient with Space-Occupying Lesions

Diagnosis	Signs and symptoms	Intervention	Rationale
	Does not distinguish between permitted and prohibited progression of activities	Include discussion of: activities in routine, balancing rest and activity, progression of activities, resumption of sexual roles and activities	To facilitate progressive resumption of activities without overdoing it and increasing risk of untoward event
	Does not know about followup appointments	Help patient and family to arrange follow-up plans before discharge	To promote continuity of care
	Lacks information pertaining to home management and followup arrangements	Explore discharge plans and home management with patient and family	To facilitate expeditious discharge
	Inability to identify professional and community services available for support	Review patient and family needs and available services and resources; refer to appropriate rehabilitation facilities	To enable patient and family to utilize available resources and services to attain most comprehensive care possible
Potential for skin breakdown due to: restriction of movement; pain/discomfort; drug-induced neuromuscular or musculoskeletal impairment; depression; body stiffness; diaphoresis or drainage into patient's bed; independent variables such as diabetes, peripheral vascular disease, obesity, etc.	Imposed restriction of movement, including body mechanics, medical protocol, etc.	Place air mattress on bed	To prevent pressure spots on skin
	Impaired coordinated or decreased muscle strength preventing independent movement	Assist with required movements; quarter turn every 1–2 hours	To prevent overexertion and to facilitate movement
	Reluctance to attempt movement	Encourage movement within safety parameters	To prevent injury and facilitate movement
	Redness over pressure points	Inspect pressure points, including occiput, sacrum, coccyx, heels, and elbows, every 2 hours	To prevent skin breakdown
		Passive range of motion for all extremities	To prevent pressure spots

Diagnosis	Signs and symptoms	Intervention	Rationale
		Keep patient dry	To prevent skin breakdown
		Maintain and supplement nutrition as needed	To maintain vital nutrients to skin
		Consult enterostomal therapist	To provide for optimal care planning and intervention and to prevent skin breakdown
	Elevated temperature	Keep patient dry when diaphoretic	To prevent skin breakdown
Potential for anxiety due to: fear of unknown, fear of death, fear of pain, fear of disability, lack of knowledge regarding hospital procedures and routines, risk of surgery, loss of body function, loss of hair	Facial tension Distracting behavior Low attention span Withdrawal Twitching and shaking of extremities Inappropriate laughter or behavior Diaphoresis Tachycardia Nonadherence to treatment plan	Ascertain patient's fears and anxieties	Will allow the nurse to know just what to address
		Ascertain patient's previous hospital experiences (own as well as others')	Will help the nurse to know how to best alleviate anxieties and support positive attitudes
		Ascertain readiness to learn	Need to begin patient and family education when ready
		Teach patient about diagnostics, routines of hospital and care regimen: surgery, tubes, lines, ICU routines, visiting hours, pain medication, moving, and deep breathing and coughing; provide patient with educational booklets	To help patient and family be prepared for what is to be experienced
		Sedate as ordered PRN	To help patient relax
		Provide emotional support as needed	To help patient and family deal with the situation in the best way possible
		Consult with social worker, chaplain, etc., as needed	Multidisciplinary team effort provides broader, more comprehensive care

Nursing Care Plan for the Management of the Patient with Space-Occupying Lesions

Diagnosis	Signs and symptoms	Intervention	Rationale
Potential for ineffective coping by the patient or family related to: surgery, situational crisis, maturational crisis, personal vulnerability	Verbalization of inability to cope	Assess family's usual coping mechanisms	Questions and concerns of patient and family must be answered even if not voiced
	Inability to ask for emotional help	Assist family to identify alternative coping mechanisms; identify and acknowledge family's needs	Optimal coping must be accomplished for maximal healing
	Inability to meet role expectations	Provide information to patient and family regarding diagnosis and supportive services	Patient and family must be helped through role redefinition
	Prolonged progression of disease or disability	Support patient and family through role transition time	To help patient and family make transition
		Encourage open communication among patient, family, and health care team	To facilitate problem solving and care planning
		Reinforce simple explanations to patient and family	During times of crisis, care must be taken not to cause information overload
	Exhaustion	Provide rest periods and offer nutrition; plan visiting schedule to accommodate interventions as well as family's schedule and rest periods; restrict visitors as appropriate	To maximize strength; to improve quality of family time as well as provide for needed rest
	Fear and anxiety	Delegate one resource and support person to assist family communication	Consistency in problem solving and care improves quality of decisions
	Inappropriate requests or hypervigilance by patient and/or family	Suggest approaches for family to assist in patient's care	Participatory care decreases family's anxiety

Diagnosis	Signs and symptoms	Intervention	Rationale
Alteration in comfort related to: surgery, headache, dehydration, imposed physical restrictions	Headache Discomfort related to the use of IVs, Foley catheter, or invasive monitoring	Request patient to report and describe the presence of pain: location, onset and precipitator, duration, characteristics	To facilitate assessment of pain, specifically from the patient's perspective
		Assess physical signs and indicators of pain	To provide further indicators of pain
		Explore the use of comfort measures: repositioning, backrubs, massage, relaxation techniques	To promote comfort and alleviate fatigue
		Administer prescribed analgesics PRN or as ordered	To alleviate discomfort
		Determine the effectiveness of interventions and therapies	To facilitate maximal comfort measures

Medications Commonly Used in the Care of the Patient with Space-Occupying Lesions

Medication	Effect	Major side effects
Corticosteroids: Dexamethasone Prednisone Hydrocortisone Methylprednisolone	Reduces cerebral edema by stabilizing the capillary endothelial junction and reducing cerebrovascular permeability Promotes integrity of cells to inhibit flow of intracellular fluid to extracellular space	Opportunistic infection Cushing's syndrome Nervousness Hyperglycemia Electrolyte imbalances Menstrual irregularities Skin rash Gastric irritation
Hyperosmotic agents: Mannitol Glycerol	Reduces brain water by creating an osmotic gradient between tissue and plasma Reduces intracranial pressure within 1–3 hours by rapid diuresis	Diuresis Electrolyte imbalances Rebound of increased intracranial pressure
Carbamazepine	Analgesic Decreases complex partial, simple partial, and generalized tonic-clonic seizures	Nausea and vomiting Vertigo Drowsiness Aplastic anemia Hepatotoxicity Inappropriate secretion of ADH
Valium	Decreases force of seizures by relaxing the skeletal muscles and depressing the reticular activating and limbic systems	Respiratory depression Increased frequency of generalized tonic-clonic seizures
Anticonvulsants: Phenytoin (Dilantin) Valproic acid	Prevents seizures by stabilizing the cell threshold of excitation and inhibiting the spread of impulses to adjacent tissue	CNS depression Cardiovascular collapse Nausea and vomiting Vertigo Ataxia Hypotension Coagulation defects
Barbiturates: Phenobarbital Primidone	Control of seizure activity by raising the seizure threshold of cells CNS depressant Lower cerebral metabolism	Drowsiness leading to coma Confusion Respiratory depression Hypotension Renal failure Blood dyscrasias Hypocalcemia
Nitrosoureas: Carmustine Lomustine Semustine	Antineoplastic agency with ability to cross the blood-brain barrier	Leukopenia Thrombocytopenia

Intracranial Hemorrhage

Intracranial hemorrhages result primarily from cerebral hemorrhage, subarachnoid hemorrhage, or arteriovenous malformation. Hemorrhagic cerebrovascular incidents are generally associated with longstanding hypertension and arteriosclerosis of the cerebral arteries, and occur most frequently in patients between 50 and 75 years of age. Other possible causes of hemorrhage include inflammatory changes accompanying acute infections, systemic disease, and metastatic tumors; angiographic diagnostics; sickle cell anemia; cancer; trauma; use of anticoagulants; and blood dyscrasias.

Intracranial hemorrhage is classified into four types: epidural, subdural, subarachnoid, and intracerebral. This section will address all but subarachnoid hemorrhage, which was thoroughly investigated in the section on cerebral aneurysms.

Epidural, Subdural, and Intracerebral Hematoma

A hematoma is simply a mass of coagulated blood collected in an area of tissue. It can occur epidurally, subdurally, or intracerebrally.

Clinical antecedents

Hematomas are usually associated with a skull fracture caused by an external blow along the distribution of the middle meningeal artery in the temporal region. Events leading to this type of injury include falls and blows to the head. Risk factors range from personal life-styles and habits to unpredictable accidents.

Critical referents

Epidural hematomas are arterial bleeds that generally originate from the middle meningeal artery and occur in the epidural space between the skull and the dura. In contrast, subdural hematomas are collections of venous blood in the subdural space between the dura and the arachnoid. Intracerebral hematomas occur when bleeding into the parenchyma develops.

Resulting signs and symptoms

Patients experiencing epidural hematomas usually lose consciousness. Symptoms may surface rapidly or may be manifested in a delayed manner. Because the bleeding is of an arterial nature and under high pressure, extensive morbidity and mortality can occur within very short periods of time. Complaints of headache, almost always voiced by the conscious patient, are followed by progressive signs of compromised responsiveness. Signs and symptoms of increased intracranial pressure occur, and further manifestations of involvement of one or more specific brain regions coincide (as detailed in the section on head trauma). If the hematoma remains unchecked, extradural accumulation of blood can become great enough to cause the uncus of the temporal lobe to begin to herniate down through the tentorium, resulting in a true neurosurgical emergency.

Signs and symptoms of subdural hematomas occur acutely or in a delayed manner (sometimes weeks after the assault). Since these bleeds are venous rather than arterial, they are less emergent than epidural hematomas, but still carry a high risk of morbidity and mortality. General signs include those of increased intracranial pressure, and local areas of involvement define specific clinical manifestations.

The clinical manifestations of intracerebral hematomas depend on the location and extent of the bleed and the amount of general tissue edema present. Early in the clinical course, the patient exhibits decreased reactivity and responsiveness. In later stages, the patient can worsen to the point of producing signs of uncal herniation.

Nursing standards of care

Medical management of a hematoma depends on the type and the rate of progression of symptoms indicating neurological deterioration. Basic life support and seizure precautions are of primary importance. Burr holes, hyperosmolar fluids, and steroids are used to help reduce increased intracranial pressure. Surgical intervention is indicated to ligate the bleeder and evacuate the lesion if it is in an operable area of the brain.

Intracranial Hemorrhage

Intracranial hemorrhage may be due to a rupture of an arteriole, capillary, or vein in the cerebral hemispheres, or more rarely, in the cerebellum or brainstem.

Clinical antecedents

Those who have longstanding hypertension are especially at risk for intracranial hemorrhage because hypertension and atherosclerosis weaken the very small penetrating blood vessels deep in the brain. Men suffer from this disease more than women and mostly during the fifth through seventh decades. Hemorrhage caused by vascular damage due to long-term hypertension is usually evidenced in the putamen, thalamus, pons, and cerebellum. Other diseases such as cancer, blood dyscrasias, and sickle cell anemia can also weaken blood vessels. Finally, infiltrating tumors can erode away the outside of a vessel until hemorrhage results.

Critical referents

Before hemorrhagic changes transpire, several pathophysiological changes have already taken place. First, lipohyalinosis and fibrinoid necrosis result from constant strain on the vessels from hypertension. These processes, in turn, drastically weaken the arteriolar muscularis of the vessel. If the hypertension is left untreated, the weakened arteriolar muscularis allows ruptures in the intimal portion of the vessel. Microdissections of the affected tissue result, and these are the direct precursors to hemorrhage. Most hemorrhages first develop as small liquid hematomas, which eventually progress along fiber tracts within the brain tissue, tearing neighboring venules and capillaries. These add to the original hematoma, amplifying the lesion. Edema then occurs, causing compression and damage in the surrounding tissue, placing it at risk for hemorrhage, which left untreated, occurs in short amounts of time. This, in turn, starts the whole process over, causing a reiterative, or snow-balling, effect. In con-

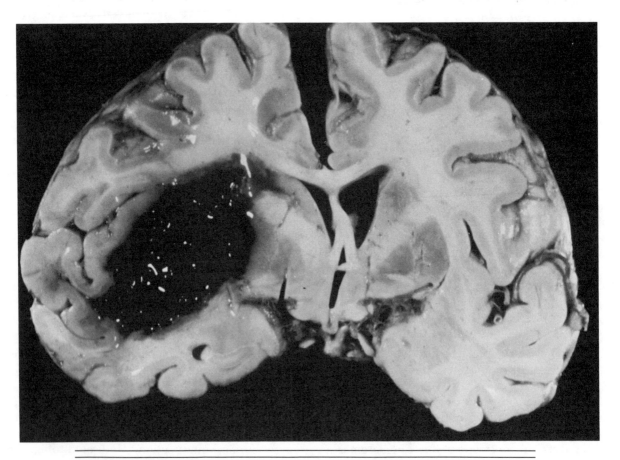

Figure 3-28   Cross Section of Brain Illustrating Intracerebral Hemorrhage with Associated Compression and Displacement of Ventricles

trast, when many small cerebral hemorrhages are noted, it is usually secondary to blood dyscrasias, vasculitis, and neoplasms, where tissue damage occurs as a result of infiltrating lesions or pathological breakdown of cellular structure.

Regardless of precipitating factor, when intracranial hemorrhage occurs, a cerebral vessel ruptures, and bleeding into the brain tissue and meninges results. As mentioned above, common sites of hemorrhage include the putamen, internal capsule, white matter, thalamus, pons, and cerebellar hemispheres. Bleeding into these areas causes widespread destruction of adjacent brain tissue, which in turn, results in infarction of the compressed tissue. The extravasated blood acts as a space-occupying lesion, compressing and displacing brain tissue. A large mass resulting from a massive hemorrhage may cause brain shifting (as illustrated in Figure 3-28) and brainstem compression, which eventually lead to coma and death.

A high mortality rate is generally associated with extensive intracranial hemorrhages, but in the event of a bleed not so extensive, an improvement in the patient's neurological status may be observed as the extravasated blood is gradually reabsorbed and cerebral edema is resolved. Prognosis for recovery from a small hemorrhage is usually good.

Resulting signs and symptoms

Varying degrees of neurological deficits ranging from transient, mild, severe, to rapid cerebral deterioration and death can occur as a result of intracranial hemorrhage. Clinical manifestations reflect the size of the infarct and the area of the brain involved.

With respect to initial clinical presentation, an intracranial hemorrhage is similar to ischemic stroke and infarction. Thus a CT scan is the most important diagnostic test to perform as soon as possible, for it enables easy differentiation between hemorrhage and infarction. Although the onset of hemorrhage is abrupt and without warning, symptoms progress rapidly. Differentiation between hemorrhagic and embolic strokes and thrombotic strokes is also fairly straightforward: the first two types frequently occur during periods of activity; the latter occurs during periods of inactivity, rest, and even during sleep. Regardless of the type of hemorrhage, the classic clinical presentation includes sudden onset of severe headache, confusion, vomiting, nuchal rigidity, seizure activity, hemiplegia on the contralateral side,

ipsilateral dilated pupil, papilledema, increased ICP, and a rapid progression of neurological deterioration. Further signs and symptoms directly reflect the location of the hemorrhage and are detailed in Table 3-29.

Nursing standards of care

Medical management of an intracranial hemorrhage is directed at prevention of further hemorrhage, resolution of the hematoma, and/or surgical intervention to evacuate or aspirate the clot. Prompt diagnosis is essential, particularly when the cerebellum is involved, because when immediate surgery to relieve tissue compression is indicated, it must be undertaken as soon as possible so as to prevent rapidly ensuing increases in intracranial pressure and brain tissue death. Supportive care consists of providing basic life-sustaining measures and managing systemic and intracranial hypertension to within what is considered normal range. Steroids or other antiedema medications are administered if the patient exhibits signs of cerebral edema (such as extreme drowsiness) or impending herniation. Anticonvulsants are usually withheld until actual signs of

Table 3-29 Signs and Symptoms of Intracranial Hemorrhage According to Location

Location	Signs and Symptoms
Putaminal	Visual field deficits Dysphasia Progressive hemiparesis Hemiplegia Sensory deficits
Thalamic	Impaired vertical gaze Small ipsilateral pupil Sensory deficits Hemiparesis
Cortical and subcortical	Sensory deficits Lateralizing headache Hemianopsia
Pontine	Stupor Coma Small but reactive pupils Total paralysis leading to cessation of breathing
Cerebellar	Occipital headache Dysarthria Severe ataxia Nausea and vomiting

seizure activity surface. If the hemorrhage is due to some clotting abnormality, one of the following is administered, depending on the precipitator: platelets (for thrombocytopenia), fresh frozen plasma or vitamin K (for coumadin), or protamine (for heparin). Finally, the size and location of the clot, along with the patient's prognosis, are carefully evaluated when surgery is considered.

Priorities for nursing the acute intracranial hemorrhage patient are to support vital function, to prevent further complications, and to begin rehabilitation. The following nursing care plan outlines the standard critical care practices used in the management of this patient.

Nursing Care Plan for the Management of the Patient with Intracranial Hemorrhage

Diagnosis	Signs and symptoms	Intervention	Rationale
Potential for alteration in respiratory function related to: altered level of consciousness, ineffective airway clearance, injury to respiratory center, pulmonary embolus	Abnormal ABGs: $pO_2 < 80$ mm Hg $pCO_2 < 35$ and > 45 mm Hg pH < 7.35 and > 7.45 O_2 sat $< 80\%$ $HCO_3 < 20$ and > 26 mEq/L BE < 0 or > 3	Assess breathing pattern frequently	To evaluate respiratory function
		Position to facilitate drainage of oral secretions (HOB at 30–60 degrees)	To ensure adequate ventilation
	Dyspnea	Maintain airway and mechanically ventilate as required	To assess for ensuing respiratory compromise and/or complications
	Hypoxemia	Closely monitor ABGs; closely monitor for absent, unequal, or diminished breath sounds, crackles, wheezing, or asymmetrical chest wall expansion	
	Hypercapnia		
	Copious secretions		
	Atelectasis		
	Elevated respiratory rate, wheezing, air hunger, gasping, or asymmetrical expansion of chest wall	Aggressive pulmonary toilet (as neurologically indicated) PRN with chest percussion therapy, incentive spirometry, and hyperinflation using 100% oxygen before and after suctioning; turn and reposition patient every 2 hours (within neurological indications)	To mobilize secretions, provide adequate oxygenation, and open closed alveoli
		If intubated, promote extubation as soon as possible by: holding sedation; elevating HOB 30 degrees; incremental weaning (as indicated neurologically)	To assist patient to return to optimal breathing capacity as soon as possible and to prevent atelectasis and secondary infection

Nursing Care Plan for the Management of the Patient with Intracranial Hemorrhage

Diagnosis	Signs and symptoms	Intervention	Rationale
Potential for impaired gas exchange related to inadequate ventilation, hypercapnia, hypoxemia, and increased secretions	Hypercapnia Hypoxemia Increased secretions	Maintain airway; ensure adequate ventilation	To promote adequate oxygen exchange
		Assess color of skin and mucous membranes; monitor trends in ABGs	Assessment of signs of oxygenation and blood gas analysis evaluates adequacy of respiratory function
		Hyperventilation therapy to maintain $PaCO_2$ between 25 and 30 mm Hg (or as prescribed); notify MD if $PaCO_2 < 25$ mm Hg	Hyperventilation blows off carbon dioxide, thus reducing $PaCO_2$ levels, which causes vasoconstriction, thereby decreasing ICP; $PaCO_2 < 25$ mm Hg may impair autoregulation
		Closely monitor patient's response to PEEP	PEEP may increase intrathoracic pressure
	Respiratory crackles, gurgles, and wheezes	Hyperoxygenate and hyperventilate with 100% oxygen before and after sucitoning	To help reduce the risk of hypoxemia and hypercapnia, which cause cerebral vasodilation
		Avoid suctioning for more than 15 seconds per each insertion of catheter	Prolonged suctioning causes hypoxemia and agitation
		Assess neck veins for jugular venous distention	To determine increased CVP
Potential for alteration in cerebral perfusion related to: ischemic injury, cerebral edema, increased ICP	Agitation	Control hyperstimulation from the external environment (noise, temperature, light, and odors) and prevent unnecessary disturbances	Reducing external environmental stimulation may help to decrease patient's activity and startle responses, thus decreasing ICP
	Anxiety	Approach patient in a calm and reassuring manner	Nursing activities can lead to anxiety and agitation

Diagnosis	Signs and symptoms	Intervention	Rationale
	Altered level of consciousness	Provide soft stimuli (light touch, soft music, pleasant and familiar sounds)	Calm and quiet environment helps prevent drastic increases in ICP
	Sensory and motor disturbances		
		Plan activities to allow adequate rest times	Fatigue exacerbates agitation responses
	Higher ICP readings	Monitor increases in ICP to learn what causes them and organize activities to minimize time and intensity of stimulation	To limit activities that challenge (stress) the patient and raise ICP
	Aphasia	Assist family to communicate with patient in a calm and quiet manner and to maintain patience	Teaching of family may help to prevent unnecessary startles, excessive stimulation, agitation, and frustration when attempting to speak, which can lead to rises in ICP
		Counsel family to avoid emotionally stimulating the patient	
	Headache	Maintain HOB at 30 degrees	Elevation of the head promotes venous drainage and decreases ICP
		Administer pain medication as ordered and provide comfort measures	Alleviating or decreasing pain or discomfort helps to decrease ICP by decreasing MAP; comfort measures decrease agitation and thus ICP
Potential for impaired venous drainage of the brain from incorrect positioning and agitation	Impaired venous drainage and increased ICP	Maintain head and neck in a neutral position with HOB elevated 15–30 degrees	To reduce the risk of impaired venous drainage and increased ICP
		Assist patient in turning and moving in bed	Avoiding excessive activities, strain, and incorrect positioning decreases the risk of increasing intra-abdominal and intrathoracic pressures, which may increase ICP
		Instruct patient to exhale while moving	
		Perform passive ROM exercises	
		Avoid isometric exercises	

Nursing Care Plan for the Management of the Patient with Intracranial Hemorrhage

Diagnosis	Signs and symptoms	Intervention	Rationale
		Avoid extreme flexion of the hip	
		Avoid flexion, extension, and rotation of the head	
		Prevent the Valsalva maneuver	The Valsalva maneuver increases intrathoracic pressure, which increases MAP and ICP
		Implement a bowel program	To help prevent constipation and the need to strain
Potential for injury and increases in ICP due to seizure activity	Seizure activity	Administer anticonvulsants as prescribed (Dilantin, Valium, and phenobarbital)	Prophylactic anticonvulsants in therapeutic doses (to achieve optimal effectiveness) help to prevent seizure activity
		Monitor therapeutic drug levels	
		Institute seizure precautions as needed (padded bed rails, oral airway, suction equipment, and supplemental oxygen)	To protect the patient from injury
Potential for alteration (decrease) in cerebral perfusion pressure (CPP) due to rising ICP	CPP < 60 mm Hg Rising ICP trends	Notify the MD	To initiate immediate medical intervention to prevent cerebral ischemia
		Conduct frequent neurological assessments	To detect early changes in neurological status
		Initiate nursing measures to decrease ICP	Decreased agitation and increased quiet and comfort help to decrease ICP
		Organize patient's activities to prevent further increases in ICP	To avoid rises in ICP from activity stressors

Diagnosis	Signs and symptoms	Intervention	Rationale
		Provide hyperventilation therapy and hyperoxygenate prior to suctioning	To decrease ICP and prevent further increases in ICP related to nursing activities
		Administer volume expanders, vasopressors, and antihypertensives as prescribed; monitor hemodynamic parameters (CVP, wedge pressures, and cardiac output)	To maintain adequate CPP and hemodynamic stability
Potential for increased cerebral metabolism related to temperature elevations	Shivering Temperature elevation	Monitor temperature every 4 hours	Elevated temperatures increase cerebral oxygen demand and cerebral blood flow
		Assess and treat the cause of increased temperature (such as superimposed infection or hypothalamic dysfunction); apply hypothermia blanket	To maintain normothermia and help control shivering (shivering increases oxygen consumption and metabolic rates, which exhaust glycogen stores and produce acidosis)
Alteration in cerebral perfusion related to increased ICP related to pathophysiology	Increased ICP Altered level of consciousness	Establish baseline for neurological functions; assess for changes by comparing ongoing assessments to baseline	To compare clinical findings to detect early changes in neurological functions
		Maintain fluid restriction and accurate I&O records	To help control ICP
		Monitor ABGs for hypocapnia	$PaCO_2 < 25$ mm Hg may impair autoregulation
		Maintain in a semi-Fowler's position with head in a neutral position except when contraindicated (with subdural hematoma and infratentorial approach)	To facilitate venous drainage

Nursing Care Plan for the Management of the Patient with Intracranial Hemorrhage

Diagnosis	Signs and symptoms	Intervention	Rationale
		Instruct patient to exhale with movement	To prevent Valsalva maneuver, which increases intrathoracic pressure, which increases ICP
	Anxiety	Control external stimulation (noise, light, temperature)	To prevent agitation and startle response, which cause increased ICP
	Agitation	Approach patient calmly and reassuringly	Nursing activities can lead to agitation
	Decreased pupillary response	Plan activities to allow for adequate rest	Fatigue exacerbates agitation responses
	Motor dysfunction	Monitor ICP increases to learn what causes them and organize activities to minimize stimulation	To limit time and intensity of activities that stress the patient and raise ICP
		Assist family to communicate calmly and quietly and to avoid emotionally stimulating the patient	To prevent excessive stimulation, agitation, and unnecessary startles, which cause rises in ICP
Potential for fluid and electrolyte imbalance due to fluid loss, antidiuretic hormone imbalance, gastrointestinal suctioning, and hyperthermia	Volume excess	Accurately monitor I&O and urine specific gravity	To ascertain fluid balance status
	Electrolyte imbalances, such as hypernatremia or hyponatremia	Closely monitor electrolyte status: hemocrit, BUN, creatinine, and serum osmolality	To detect imbalances and determine renal function (hyponatremia can precipitate seizures)
	Large and rapid urine output		
	Abnormal serum osmolality	Initiate ADH replacement therapy as prescribed	To help concentrate urine and prevent fluid losses
		Adhere strictly to fluid restrictions	To avoid overhydration leading to cerebral edema
		Maintain temperature within normal limits	To prevent rises in ICP

Diagnosis	Signs and symptoms	Intervention	Rationale
		Measure gastric output and test pH every 8 hours; if pH < 5, administer antacids as ordered	To prevent gastric acidity
		Consult with dietician and initiate nutritional support as soon as appropriate; initiate tube feeding if needed	Early nutritional support promotes fluid and electrolyte balances and provides strength, leading to recovery
Potential for infection due to: surgical procedure, IV lines, indwelling Foley, endotracheal intubation, stress, CSF leak	Increased temperature	Tylenol 600 mg every 4 hours PRN as ordered	To alleviate fevers
	WBC > 10,000 mm^3	Implement thorough hand washing between patient contacts; implement universal isolation precautions if indicated	To prevent spread of infections
	Redness, exudate, or increased tenderness at IV or ICP insertion site	Routine care with povidone-iodine solution, telfa dressing, and foam tape	To prevent infections
		Change peripheral IV sites at least every 3 days or with any signs of infection or infiltration; change IV tubing every 48 hours	IV fluid is an especially fertile medium for bacterial growth
		Culture suspected origins of infection	To administer appropriate antibiotics
	Changes in characteristics of sputum: tan, brown, yellow, or green color and/or foul odor	Nonvigorous pulmonary toilet	To prevent and/or treat pulmonary congestion leading to infections (without increasing neurological stressors)
	Decreased or absent breath sounds locally		
	Sediment in urine or foul-smelling urine; WBCs in urine; hesitancy, frequency, urgency, burning, difficulty starting stream, incontinence, and/or inability to void	Routine Foley care every 8 hours; push fluids if taking fluids and not neurologically contraindicated	To prevent urinary tract infections

Nursing Care Plan for the Management of the Patient with Intracranial Hemorrhage

Diagnosis	Signs and symptoms	Intervention	Rationale
	Altered LOC, headache, meningeal signs	If CSF leak suspected, test drainage with dextrostix (CSF will test positive for glucose)	Assess for early signs of wound infection, CSF leak, or meningitis, requiring prompt treatment
Potential for physical injury related to: confusion, sensory-perceptual deficits, seizure activity, altered level of consciousness, emotional lability, possible falls	Confusion	Reorient patient frequently as to surroundings, time, and routine activities	To increase patient's awareness of surroundings
	Seizure activity	Maintain a safe environment by: administering anticonvulsants as prescribed and monitoring therapeutic levels; instituting seizure precautions (padded bed rails, oral airway, suction equipment, and supplemental oxygen)	To help prevent seizures and decrease risk of physical injury
	Agitation and impulsive behavior	Assess causes of restlessness (hypoxemia, pain, bladder distention) and plan care appropriately	To decrease risk of increased agitation leading to possible accidental injury
	Visual field deficits	Place objects within areas of vision and reorient patient to other areas frequently	To increase patient's awareness of surroundings and ability to function within them
	Poor judgment and denial of deficit	Increase patient's awareness of deficit and limitations; teach ways to adapt	To help decrease risk of physical injury and increase independent functioning

Diagnosis	Signs and symptoms	Intervention	Rationale
	Neglect of affected side	Help patient to do passive ROM with extremities of affected side	To prevent complications of immobility and to increase self-care efforts
	Disorientation	Restraints PRN	To remind patient not to get up without assistance and to promote safety
Impaired physical mobility due to motor disturbances	Hemiplegia	Maintain body alignment with assistive devices (pillows, footboard)	To prevent complications of immobility
	Decreased muscle strength and tone	Maintain splints (especially hand and foot) as ordered	To prevent contractures
	Paresis	Consult with physiotherapist and initiate rehab program when condition is stable	To promote early recovery
	Decreased range of motion	Assist with ROM exercises at least every 2–4 hours, allowing patient to do as much as possible	To maintain joint and muscle mobility and to increase circulation while preventing patient fatigue
		Try to calm patient during activity	Anxiety increases spasticity
	Signs of impeded circulation in extremities (redness over pressure points)	Apply antiembolism stockings; assess for tenderness, redness, warmth, and pain	Helps to identify and decrease venous stasis and deep vein thrombosis
	Impaired small motor coordination	Assist with required movements	To facilitate patient's movement
Potential for skin breakdown due to: restriction of movement; pain/discomfort; neuromuscular impairment; depression; body stiffness, diaphoresis or drainage into patient's bed independent	Restriction of movement, including body mechanics	Place air mattress on bed	To prevent pressure spots on skin
	Impaired coordination or decreased muscle strength preventing independent movement	Assist with required movements; quarter turn every 1–2 hours	To prevent overexertion and to facilitate movement
	Reluctance to attempt movement	Encourage movement within safety parameters	To prevent injury and facilitate movement

Nursing Care Plan for the Management of the Patient with Intracranial Hemorrhage

Diagnosis	Signs and symptoms	Intervention	Rationale
variables such as diabetes, peripheral vascular disease, obesity, etc.; low cardiac output; poor tissue perfusion; altered nutritional status; weakness/fatigue	Redness over pressure points	Inspect pressure points, including occiput, sacrum, coccyx, heels, and elbows, every 2 hours	To prevent skin breakdown
		Passive range of motion for all extremities	To prevent pressure spots
		Keep patient dry	To prevent skin breakdown
		Maintain and supplement nutrition as needed	To maintain vital nutrients to skin
		Consult enterostomal therapist	To provide for optimal care planning and intervention and to prevent skin breakdown
	Elevated temperature	Keep patient dry when diaphoretic	To prevent skin breakdown
Potential for alteration in bowel function or constipation due to: decreased sensation and muscle tone, altered level of consciousness, decreased mobility, change in eating patterns, side effects of medications, decreased fluid volume	Reports of feeling constipated, "full" feeling in abdomen, inability to move bowels	Assess abdomen for bowel sounds, softness, and appearance and ask patient about discomfort at least every 12 hours	For early diagnosis of constipation in order to intervene before serious problems occur
	Decreased or absent bowel sounds	Encourage progressive activity as tolerated	To stimulate peristalsis
	Inadequate oral fluid/food intake as evidenced on I&O records and calorie counts	Reassure patient that constipation is frequently a problem during bedrest	So patient will not become overly concerned

378

Diagnosis	Signs and symptoms	Intervention	Rationale
	Symptoms of dehydration: poor skin turgor, sunken eyes, intake less than output, weight loss	Assess for signs of dehydration and encourage oral intake within fluid restriction limits	Hydration impedes constipation
		Closely monitor electrolytes	Dehydration leads to electrolyte imbalance
	Absence of bowel movement for more than 2 days	Implement bowel regimen as ordered: milk of magnesia 30 mL p.o. every HS; consult with dietician about increased fiber in diet as indicated	Patient may need extra help to have regular bowel movements
Alteration in urinary elimination due to: decreased sensation, impaired muscle tone, altered level of consciousness, urinary tract infection	Urinary retention or incontinence	Assess voiding patterns (I&O, frequency, incontinence, retention)	Evaluation of urinary elimination pattern helps patient to attain optimal urinary functioning
		Foley catheter to be removed as soon as possible	The risk of UTI is greater with indwelling catheter
		Institute a bladder training program as soon as possible	To establish regular bladder function
	Urinary infection: sediment in urine; WBCs in urine; hesitancy, frequency, urgency, burning, difficulty starting stream, or inability to void	Administer antibiotics as ordered	To prevent or fight any infection
		Urine C&S (routine/fungal/gram stain) when indicated or as ordered	For early detection and treatment of urinary tract infections
		Routine catheter care every 8 hours	To prevent infection
Potential for alteration (decrease) in nutritional status related to: altered level of consciousness, absent gag reflex, dysphagia	Weight loss	Weigh daily	To determine weight losses or gains
	Decreased fluid intake	Assess skin turgor	To assess for dehydration
	Caloric intake less than body requirements	Consult with dietitian	To determine nutritional needs and plan nutritional support
	Depressed swallowing mechanism	Consult with speech pathologist to assist in evaluation of swallowing mechanism	To evaluate ability of patient to swallow (to prevent injury from choking, etc.)

Diagnosis	Signs and symptoms	Intervention	Rationale
	Inability to feed self	Assist with feeding as appropriate	To facilitate improvement in patient's nutritional status
	Complaints of lack of appetite	Assess patient's appetite with patient and family and what is preferred within accepted diet	To facilitate improvement in patient's nutritional status
Alteration in rest/sleep pattern related to continuous environmental stimuli, ICU routine, and interrupted sleep	Disturbances in rest/sleep pattern	Determine the patient's established rest/sleep pattern and organize nursing activities to accommodate it as much as possible	To accommodate to patient's normal pattern
	Exhaustion	Structure nursing activities to provide for fewer interruptions at normal time of sleep; design schedule to balance daytime activities with periods of uninterrupted sleep	To maximize patient's ability to relax, rest, and sleep
	Inability to fall asleep	Provide comfort measures and assistive devices individualized to patient's need; explore the possibility of relaxation therapy	To promote comfort and sleep
	Interrupted rest periods	Plan visiting schedule to accommodate interventions as well as family's schedule and rest periods; restrict visitors as appropriate	To maximize strength; to improve quality of family time as well as provide for needed rest
Alteration in comfort related to: surgery, headache, dehydration, imposed physical restrictions	Headache Discomfort related to the use of IVs, Foley catheter, or invasive monitoring	Request patient to report and describe the presence of pain: location, onset and precipitator, duration, characteristics	To facilitate assessment of pain, specifically from the patient's perspective

Diagnosis	Signs and symptoms	Intervention	Rationale
		Assess physical signs and indicators of pain	To provide further indicators of pain
		Explore the use of comfort measures: repositioning, backrubs, massage, relaxation techniques	To provide further indicators of pain
		Administer prescribed analgesics PRN or as ordered	To alleviate discomfort
		Determine the effectiveness of interventions and therapies	To facilitate maximal comfort measures
Potential for impaired verbal communication related to decreased LOC, cerebral edema, dysphasia, endotracheal tube, tracheostomy and cerebral injury	Aphasia	Assess patient's ability to hear, understand, and speak	To determine patient's ability to communicate
	Frustration during communication attempts	Teach appropriate strategies to promote communication: using assistive materials such as writing implements and communication board, reducing environmental distractions, decreasing anxiety, decreasing speed of communication, using simple commands with gestures	To help patient identify and use appropriate strategies to facilitate communication
		Face the patient and establish eye contact to provide support and reassurance during communication attempts	To encourage patient's efforts
		Consult with speech therapist	To allow for early rehabilitation
	Uneasiness and impatience of family during communication attempts	Teach family successful strategies for communication with patient	To promote family communication and cohesion

Nursing Care Plan for the Management of the Patient with Intracranial Hemorrhage

Diagnosis	Signs and symptoms	Intervention	Rationale
Disturbance in body concept related to neurological deficits	Alterations in body concept	Assess patient's and family's interpretation of change in body concept	To establish baseline
	Anxiety during visiting hours	Encourage patient and family to express feelings	To help alleviate feelings of anxiety and promote adjustment
	Inability of family to comfortably and calmly look at and interact with patient	Assist family in adapting to patient's body changes and appearance	To achieve maximal level of self-esteem for patient and acceptance and support from family
	Lack of knowledge of available support services	Consult with hospital and community support services	To help patient and family make use of appropriate resources

Potential for anxiety due to:
  fear of unknown,
  fear of death,
  fear of pain,
  fear of disability,
  lack of knowledge regarding hospital procedures and routines
	Facial tension
	Distracting behavior
	Low attention span
	Withdrawal
	Twitching and shaking of extremities
	Inappropriate laughter or behavior
	Diaphoresis
	Tachycardia
	Nonadherence to treatment plan
		Ascertain patient's fears and anxieties	Will allow the nurse to know just what to address

		Ascertain patient's previous hospital experiences (own as well as others')	Will help the nurse to know how to best alleviate anxieties or support positive attitudes
		Ascertain readiness to learn	Need to begin patient and family education when ready
		Teach patient about routines of hospital and care regimen: tubes, lines, ICU routines, visiting hours, pain medication, moving, and deep breathing and coughing; provide patient with educational booklets	To help patient and family be prepared for what is to be experienced
		Sedate as ordered PRN	To help patient relax

Diagnosis	Signs and symptoms	Intervention	Rationale
		Provide emotional support as needed	To help patient and family deal with the situation in the best way possible
		Consult with social worker, chaplain, etc., as needed	Multidisciplinary team effort provides broader, more comprehensive care
Potential for ineffective coping by the patient or family related to: situational crisis, maturational crisis, personal vulnerability, severity and chronicity of impairment	Verbalization of inability to cope	Assess family's usual coping mechanisms	Questions and concerns of patient and family must be answered even if not voiced
	Inability to ask for emotional help	Assist family to identify alternative coping mechanisms; identify and acknowledge family's needs	Optimal coping must be accomplished for maximal healing
	Inability to meet role expectations	Provide information to patient and family regarding diagnosis and supportive services	Patient and family must be helped through role redefinition
	Prolonged progression of disease or disability	Support patient and family through role transition time	To help patient and family make transition
		Encourage open communication among patient, family, and health care team	To facilitate problem solving and care planning
		Reinforce simple explanations to patient and family	During times of crisis, care must be taken not to cause information overload
	Exhaustion	Provide rest periods and offer nutrition; plan visiting schedule to accommodate interventions as well as family's schedule and rest periods; restrict visitors as appropriate	To maximize strength; to improve quality of family time as well as provide for needed rest
	Fear and anxiety	Delegate one resource and support person to assist family communication	Consistency in problem solving and care improves quality of decisions

Nursing Care Plan for the Management of the Patient with Intracranial Hemorrhage

Diagnosis	Signs and symptoms	Intervention	Rationale
	Inappropriate requests or hypervigilance by patient and/or family	Suggest approaches for family to assist in patient's care	Participatory care decreases family's anxiety
	Inability to solve problems	Assist patient and family to identify problems and work together to solve them	Sometimes patients and families are unable to anticipate possible problems
	Unreasonable and/or excessively frequent requests (excessive use of call light)	Assist family in caring for patient and problem solve about how to continue such care after discharge	Personal involvement in care decreases anxiety while increasing self-confidence and skills
		Encourage progressively independent activities	To avoid rushing patient and family into too much responsibility for care

Potential for self-care deficit due to:
  sensory and cognitive impairment,
  muscle deconditioning,
  disturbance of sleep pattern,
  fear of overexertion,
  anxiety,
  decreased ability and tolerance for activity
	Inability to perform activities of daily living independently	Place assistive equipment in visual field	To allow as much independence as possible

	Body neglect	Assist with physical hygiene as needed	To facilitate personal hygiene
	Visual field deficit	Instruct patient to turn head to compensate for visual field deficit	To increase awareness of what is in blind spots

	Weak muscles resulting from physical deficits and bedrest	Encourage activities safe to patient:
		  minor self-care,
		  passive ROM
			To allow time for patient to regain strength and ability to function

	Fatigue	Assess patient's need for rest and sleep and incorporate rest periods during the day	To allow for maximal rest and decreased ICP
	Increased heart rate and respiratory rate upon minimal activity	Progressive activities as tolerated; encourage patient's participation in scheduling and carrying out daily care	To prevent fatigue, agitation, and discomfort, leading to increased ICP
	Unsupervised attempts to get out of bed, etc.	Protect patient from injury	Patient's poor judgment can lead to risky behavior, possibly resulting in injury

Diagnosis	Signs and symptoms	Intervention	Rationale
Potential for alteration in health maintenance due to lack of knowledge of: diagnosis, surgical procedure, medication regimen, activity, medical follow-up, referrals, home management	Inability to describe personal diagnosis and how it relates to type of surgery and prognosis	Instruct patient and family about diagnosis, surgery, and prognosis with as many repetitions as needed	Patient and family must understand in order to adhere to prescribed regimen, which will promote healing and optimal level of functioning
		Encourage questions and open discussion of problems and concerns	To allow for clear understanding and acceptance
	Inability to describe prescribed regimen and reasons for it	Instruct about medications, diet, and followup arrangements: what, why, care options, plan of daily schedule	To promote understanding and thus adherence to prescribed regimen
	Does not distinguish between permitted and prohibited progression of activities	Include discussion of: activities in routine, balancing rest and activity, progression of activities, resumption of sexual roles and activities	To facilitate progressive resumption of activities without overdoing it and increasing risk of untoward event
	Does not know about followup appointments	Help patient and family to arrange followup plans before discharge	To promote continuity of care
	Lacks information pertaining to home management and followup arrangements	Explore discharge plans and home management with patient and family	To facilitate expeditious discharge
	Inability to identify professional and community services available for support	Review patient and family needs and available services and resources; refer to appropriate rehabilitation facilities	To enable patient and family to utilize available resources and services to attain most comprehensive care possible

Medications Commonly Used in the Care of the Patient with Intracranial Hemorrhage

Medication	Effect	Major side effects

Anticonvulsants:
  Phenytoin (Dilantin)
  Valproic acid
	Prevent seizures by stabilizing the cell threshold of excitation and inhibiting the spread of impulses to adjacent tissue	CNS depression
		Cardiovascular collapse
		Nausea and vomiting
		Vertigo
		Ataxia
		Hypotension
		Coagulation defects

Barbiturates:
  Phenobarbital
  Primidone
	Control seizure activity by raising the seizure threshold of cells
	CNS depressant
	Lower cerebral metabolism
		Drowsiness leading to coma
		Confusion
		Respiratory depression
		Hypotension
		Renal failure
		Blood dyscrasias
		Hypocalcemia

Hyperosmotic agents:
  Mannitol
  Glycerol
	Reduce brain water by creating an osmotic gradient between tissue and plasma
	Reduce intracranial pressure within 1–3 hours by rapid diuresis
		Diuresis
		Electrolyte imbalances
		Rebound increased intracranial pressure

Carbamazepine	Analgesic Decreases complex partial, simple partial, and generalized tonic-clonic seizures	Nausea and vomiting Vertigo Drowsiness Aplastic anemia Hepatotoxicity Inappropriate secretion of ADH
Valium	Decreases force of seizures by relaxing the skeletal muscles and depressing the reticular activating and limbic systems	Respiratory depression Increased frequency of generalized tonic-clonic seizures

Corticosteroids:
  Dexamethasone
  Prednisone
  Hydrocortisone
  Methylprednisolone
	Reduce cerebral edema by stabilizing the capillary endothelial junction and reducing cerebrovascular permeability
	Promotes integrity of cells to inhibit flow of intracellular fluid to extracellular space
		Opportunistic infection
		Cushing's syndrome
		Nervousness
		Hyperglycemia
		Electrolyte irregularities
		Menstrual irregularities
		Skin rash
		Gastric irritation

Neurological Infections

Brain abscesses and empyema, encephalitis, and meningitis are the three primary infectious conditions found in the brain, and all are related to bacterial, viral, or fungal infections.

Brain Abscess and Empyema

An intracranial abscess is a localized collection of purulent exudate resulting from a streptococcal, Escherichia coli, pneumococcal, Klebsiella, Proteus, or staphylococcal infection in the brain. An abscess is usually secondary to some infectious process occurring elsewhere in the body.

An empyema is also an accumulation of purulent exudate, but it occurs subdurally and is most commonly associated with sinus or ear infection. It can also be found with a skull trauma or intracranial surgery. Most rarely, empyema can be clinically present in meningitis cases, but this most often happens in the pediatric population.

Clinical antecedents

Brain abscess occurs as a direct extension of bacterial infection somewhere in the cranial cavity or, less frequently, hematogenously from endocarditis, congenital heart disease, lung abscess, or systemic infections. Ear, sinus, and teeth abscesses are causative antecedents to brain abscess. Finally, head trauma or intracranial surgery may precipitate the incidence of a brain abscess. Extradural abscess occurs between the dura and the skull, and subdural abscess (or empyema) occurs between the dura and the arachnoid. If the abscess is secondary to infectious complications of the ear, it usually forms in the temporal lobe or cerebellum; nasal and sinus infections lead to brain abscess in the frontal lobe. An empyema usually stays localized subdurally.

Critical referents

The formation of a brain abscess occurs in two stages. The first stage involves an acute encephalitis without a defined area of pus formation. The infection is diffuse, and peripheral edema and brain tissue damage occur. Brain abscess, during this stage, is seen on radiography as diffuse and of a low density and mimics other growing lesions of the brain. If untreated, within 2–4 weeks the core of this diffuse purulent formation becomes semiliquid and brain tissue begins to necrose. As time progresses, this semiliquid granulates into layers that localize the abscess: the inner layer consisting of pus cells; the second, granulating tissue; and the third, inflamed neuroglia. Tomography can show a donut effect (a shadow around the low-density abscess).

In contrast, an empyema forms in response to infectious complications of sinus and ear infections. Infecting agents infiltrate into the subdural space and fester until a full-blown empyema is formed.

Resulting signs and symptoms

Manifestations of brain abscess and empyema are usually insidious and subacute. Diagnosticians must be particularly alert to the possibility of an abscess or empyema, because symptoms can be very similar to other indicators of brain lesion, hemorrhage, hematoma, etc. It may be extremely difficult to differentiate brain tumor, viral encephalitis, chronic meningitis, and brain abscess. A definitive diagnosis is often established only after surgical exploration, for attempting lumbar puncture on individuals suspected of brain abscess is contraindicated (and culture of CSF does not disclose the organism of infection). Arteriography is the most reliable diagnostic test for determining the presence and location of subdural empyema (interpretation of a CT scan can miss the shadow so close to the skull, especially if it is small). On arteriography, an empyema appears as a collection of fluid. Further tests confirm the infectious nature of the fluid. If left untreated for long periods because of inaccurate diagnosis, a brain abscess can rupture into the ventricular system, causing bacterial ventriculitis and acute meningitis. In contrast, an empyema remains localized but can grow unchecked, frequently mimicking symptoms of subdural hematomas, including papilledema, increased intracranial pressure, seizure, and fever.

Headache usually occurs with an abscess, and it may be persistent and severe or intermittently mild on changes of posture. If the abscess is in the cerebellar region, the headache usually originates in the suboccipital region and can radiate down into the neck and cervical areas. If the abscess is in the frontal lobe, the headache may be diffuse, and inattention and apathy progress to impaired memory and drowsiness. As the abscess grows, symptoms are the same as for any expanding lesion in the brain. These include mental deterioration and neurological compromise progressing to coma and death. About half of all patients suffering brain abscesses experience focal symptoms, which coincide with the neurological region affected. Seizures may or may not occur. Fever may be present as a result of the infectious state, but once the abscess has become encapsulated, the core body temperature returns to normal.

Nursing standards of care

Medical management of a brain abscess depends on the stage and location of involvement. If discovered during the first stage of diffuse infection, an abscess is usually responsive to appropriately selected antibiotic therapy. Many brain abscesses contain multiple organisms, so results of cultures and gram stains guide in the prescription, and medications are administered in doses equal to that given for full-blown meningitis.

For a brain abscess that is discovered after encapsulation (as is usually the case), treatment entails antibiotic therapy before and after surgery, surgical drainage of the purulent cavity by craniotomy or needle aspiration, and the administration of anticonvulsants and medications to discourage the formation of edema and inflammation. What constitutes the best method of surgical treatment remains controversial. Needle aspiration may require multiple aspirations, which increase the risk of further contaminating surrounding tissue, and surgical excision may be considered radical or overkill. The rule of thumb has become that, if the lesion is superficial and readily accessible, surgical removal should be attempted. Needle aspiration should be performed on these abscesses located deep within the recesses of the brain. Furthermore, the patient at eminent risk for increased intracranial pressure should be treated surgically.

In the case of empyema, surgical drainage is almost always indicated. Antibiotic therapy is instituted before surgery and continues in high doses for at least three weeks postoperatively. If the empyema has caused increased intracranial pressure, mannitol is indicated, followed by steroids if pressures remain high for more than a couple hours after mannitol administration.

Nursing interventions coincide with medical practice. Efforts are directed toward maintaining basic life functions, preventing further complications, overcoming infection, and alleviating symptoms.

Encephalitis

Encephalitis is a serious, frequently fatal, inflammation of the brain tissue, which is usually viral in nature. Mortality rates in those infected can reach as high as 20%. Virus particles enter the brain via the bloodstream or along nerves from other virally infected locations in the body.

There are three classes of viruses: neurotropic, pantropic, and viscerotropic. Neurotropic viruses, those which primarily infect the nervous system, cause the St. Louis type of encephalitis, rabid encephalitis, herpes simplex and herpes zoster, and poliomyelitis. Pantropic viruses infect the meninges and include mumps, mononucleosis, and lymphocytic choriomeningitis. Viscerotropic viruses include the various influenza-type infections and very rarely, if ever, affect the nervous system.

Clinical antecedents

Encephalitis is epidemically caused by virus-laden transmissions from rabid animals, mosquitoes, or ticks, or can be contracted in association with mumps, herpes simplex, and arboviruses such as in St. Louis and western and eastern equine encephalitis.

Critical referents

Incubation periods of viruses depend on the inherent immunity of specific cells to the infectious agent, on the degree of protection provided by the blood-brain barrier, and on the susceptibility of specific brain cells to the infecting agent. Incubation periods, thus, can range from as little as 2 weeks to as long as 6 months.

Pathophysiological processes occurring in encephalitis begin with degenerative changes in nerve cells. Cellular infiltration progresses to inflammation of grey matter, but damage can also be evidenced in white matter and the meninges. Other specific changes reflect the route of infection and the type of infectious agent.

Herpes simplex produces destructive lesions in the frontal and anterior temporal lobes. Acute cases of rabies cause severe inflammation in the brainstem and are associated with high mortality rates. In measles and mumps, damage to the nerve cells and glia occur, and demyelination is the primary differentiating process specific to this type of encephalitis.

Resulting signs and symptoms

Different types of encephalitis exhibit different clinical manifestations. Most forms, though, usually start out as innocuous bouts of mild fever accompanied by headache and malaise and drowsiness. As the infection intensifies, fever persists and worsens, confusion can develop into stupor and coma, and signs of CNS involvement progress to respiratory arrest, paralysis, and absence of reflexes. Intracranial edema to the point of herniation can occur, and seizures are frequently very difficult to control. CSF pressures can raise to very high levels with most types of encephalitis. Pupils become unequal and react poorly to light, and nystagmus is frequently apparent. It is very important to note that even if a patient exhibits severely advanced signs of neurological involvement and compromise, aggressive therapy should still be supplied, for even patients at this very critical stage can fully recover.

Nursing standards of care

Management of encephalitis depends directly on the accurate and timely diagnosis of the viral infection. Antiviral medications are indicated, but extreme care must be followed when administering such drugs, for several side effects are known to occur. Seizure control must be attempted, and antiedema medications are initiated. As above, nursing care is provided in concert with the medical regimen and is targeted at protection from injury and further complication.

Meningitis

Meningitis is an inflammatory reaction within the pia and arachnoid meninges caused by bacteria, viruses, parasites, or fungi. Bacterial meningitis is a serious life-threatening condition requiring early recognition, prompt initiation of antibiotic therapy, and effective nursing management. The focus of this section will be bacterial meningitis, because it is the most frequently found.

Clinical antecedents

Specific organisms enter the central nervous system by various routes. Organisms may enter the CNS via the blood, cerebrospinal fluid (CSF), a traumatic injury, the uterus, and the oral or nasopharyngeal passages. Infectious microorganisms most commonly enter the central nervous system through the systemic circulation. Dural tearing, which creates a cerebrospinal fluid leak progressing to otorrhea and rhinorrhea, may quickly lead to a central nervous system infection if left untreated. Sepsis, septic emboli, endocarditis, pneumonia, neurosurgical infection, osteomyelitis, and occasionally insect bites and otitis media are possible causes of meningitis.

The most common infectious agents of bacterial meningitis are hemophilus influenzae, Neisseria meningitidis, and Streptococcus pneumoniae. The causative organisms of bacterial meningitis are identified in Table 3-30. Predisposing pathogens or diseases leading to subacute meningitis can vary widely, as is illustrated in Table 3-31. Regardless of precipitating factors, one primary risk factor is age. The very young and very old tend to be more commonly affected by meningitis. Susceptibility to meningitis can be increased by certain factors that are directly involved with immune compromise:

Immunoglobulin deficiency
Malignancy
Radiation therapy
Immunosuppressive therapy
Debilitation
Malnutrition
Exposure to precipitating microorganisms
Various underlying infectious processes
HIV infection
Congenital defects

Critical referents

Microorganisms enter the subarachnoid space and spread quickly through the CSF to the brain and spinal cord. A purulent exudate, formed in the acute inflammatory response, covers the entire cerebral cortex. An accumulation of this exudate may interfere with the circulation of CSF, causing obstructive or communicating hydrocephalus. Associated with this inflammatory reaction is hyperemia of the meningeal vessels. Severe meningeal infections and irritation may result in cerebral edema. Cerebral edema in the presence of hydrocephalus further increases intracranial pressure. Thrombosis and bleeding may occur as cerebral circulation becomes impaired. Neuronal damage and brain infarction occur when the blood supply to the neurons is severely compromised. As the exudate accumulates over the base of the brain, it may extend into the sheaths of the cranial and spinal nerves and into the perivascular spaces of the cerebral cortex, resulting in an associated encephalitis.[24] After several weeks

Table 3-30   Selected Risk and Precipitating Factors and Causative Organisms
for Bacterial Meningitis

Risk and Precipitating Factors	Organism	Disease
Risk Factors 　Infancy 　Adulthood 　Alcoholism Precipitating Factors 　Infection of the sinuses 　Otitis media 　Pneumonia 　Head trauma or surgery 　Skull fractures 　Sickle cell anemia crises 　Splenectomy	Streptococcus pneumoniae	Pneumococcal Meningitis
Risk Factor 　<20 years of age Precipitating Factors 　Systemic infection 　Septicemia	Neisseria meningitidis	Meningococcal Meningitis
Risk Factor 　Childhood Precipitating Factors 　Upper respiratory infection 　Ear infection 　Flu	Hemophilus influenzae	Hemophilus Influenzae Meningitis
Risk Factor 　Adulthood Precipitating Factors 　Bacteremia 　Parameningeal abscess 　Neurosurgery 　Skull trauma	Staphylococcus aureus	Staphylococcal Meningitis
Risk Factors 　Leukemia 　Lymphoma Precipitating Factor 　Invasion of vessel wall by blasts	Malignant cells	Malignant Meningitis

without effective therapy, fibrotic changes of the arachnoid layer may cause fibrosis and scar tissue formation. Complications that occur with the progression of symptoms include hydrocephalus, mental retardation, paralyses, coma, seizures, cranial nerve dysfunction, and herniation syndrome.

Resulting signs and symptoms

Although there are many causative organisms of meningitis, the signs and symptoms are evidenced similarly. The onset of symptoms in viral meningitis is less severe than in bacterial meningitis and is nonspecific. In infants and children, the typical symptoms of meningitis may not even be present. Clinical manifestations include fever, refusal of feedings, vomiting, diarrhea, irritability, listlessness, shrill crying, bulging fontanels, and seizures. Initial signs and symptoms of meningitis in the adult include fever, headache, malaise, vomiting, changing levels of consciousness, confusion, restlessness, agitation, hyperirritability, hypersensitivity, hyperalgesia, muscle hypotonia, and seizures. Signs of meningeal irritation include nuchal rigidity, photophobia (intense sensitivity to light), Kernig's sign (pain and resistance upon leg extension), and Brudzinski's sign (neck flexion produces reactive flexion of thigh and knee). Cranial nerve dysfunction

Table 3-31 Selected Risk and Precipitating Factors and Pathologies of Subacute Meningitis

Risk and Precipitating Factors	Pathology	Disease
Tuberculosis	Myobacterium tuberculosis	Bacterial meningitis
Unpasteurized dairy products Close and frequent contact with farm animals	Brucella	Bacterial meningitis
Age (neonates, elderly) Diabetes Alcoholism Immunosuppression	Listeria monocytogenes	Bacterial meningitis
Homosexuality AIDS Syphilis	Mycoplasma pneumonae	Bacterial meningitis
Contaminated water Contact with farm animals	Leptospira	Bacterial meningitis
Drug addiction Homosexuality Hemophilia Blood transfusions	HIV	Viral meningitis
Contact with mice and hamsters Contact with farm animals	Lymphocytic choriomeningitis	Viral meningitis
Genital herpes (virus transmitted to neonates during delivery)	Herpes simplex 2	Viral meningitis
AIDS Diabetes Immunosuppression	Cryptococcus	Fungal meningitis
Neonates: AIDS Immunosuppression Organ transplantation	Toxoplasmosis	Parasitic meningitis
Swimming in natural water supplies	Amoebae	Parasitic meningitis

may occur from the inflammation and vascular changes. Oculomotor involvement results in ptosis, strabismus, and pupil abnormalities. An involvement of the acoustic cranial nerve (VIII) causes deafness, nystagmus, and vertigo. Facial paresis results when the facial cranial nerve (VII) is involved. Hyponatremia from inappropriate secretion of antidiuretic hormone and disseminated intravascular coagulation are possible complications. Finally, a characteristic petechial rash may assist in the identification of meningococcal meningitis.

When left untreated, later clinical findings may include increased intracranial pressure due to hydrocephalus and cerebral edema. Clinical presentation at this stage includes further deterioration in the level of consciousness progressing to coma, weak and rapid pulse, and respiratory difficulties.

A differential diagnosis is based on the results of a lumbar puncture and analysis of cerebrospinal fluid. A summary of common findings of CSF analysis is presented in Table 3-32.

Nursing standards of care

Early diagnosis of meningitis relies primarily on patient history, clinical presentation, and laboratory cultures. The most effective therapy for meningitis is early recognition and prompt initiation of appropriate antibiotic therapy. The medical management of aseptic viral meningitis focuses on treatment of symptoms and supporting homeostasis once the diagnosis is confirmed. A lumbar puncture and examination of CSF are crucial in determining the presence and differential diagnosis of meningitis. When herniation is identified as a risk, a CT scan is warranted prior to the lumbar puncture to help

Table 3-32 Results of CSF Analysis with Different Types of Meningitis

	Cells	Protein	Glucose	Culture
Normal Values	0–10 Lymphs	15–45 mg/100 mL	60–80 mg/100 mL	Negative
Infectious Bacterial Meningitis	10–10,000 Polys	70–600 mg/100 mL	<60 mg/100 mL	Positive for aerobes and/or anaerobes
Viral Meningitis	10–2,000 Polys 10–1,000 Lymphs	20–100 mg/100 mL	60–80 mg/100 mL	Positive for viruses
Fungal Meningitis	10–1,000 Lymphs	100–500 mg/100 mL	40–60 mg/100 mL	Positive for fungi
Tubercular Meningitis	10–1,000 Lymphs	100–500 mg/100 mL	40–60 mg/100 mL	Positive for AFB

identify the etiology of increased intracranial pressure. (Performing a lumbar puncture in the presence of increased intracranial pressure presents the risk of cerebral herniation in and of itself.) Skull, chest, and sinus x-rays, along with blood cultures and cultures of infected sites, the nose, and the throat, may be helpful in identifying the presence of any infectious process exacerbating the case. Table 3-33 summarizes what should be ascertained in the clinical and laboratory evaluation of a patient presenting with signs indicating the possibility of acute meningitis.

In concert with the physician, the critical care nurse has an important role in the prevention and early intervention of bacterial meningitis for the patient at risk. Clinical assessment may assist in the identification of meningitis and facilitate prompt treatment. The patient with acute meningitis is critically ill and requires specialized nursing interventions for optimal recovery. Priorities for nursing management of the patient suffering from meningitis are as follows:

Assessment of neurological status for early recognition of complications

Administration of antibiotic therapy according to the physician's established medication schedule to maintain therapeutic serum drug levels

Table 3-33 Elements of Clinical Evaluation for Suspected Cases of Meningitis

Type of Assessment	Factors to Consider
History	Risk factors including alcoholism, diabetes, drug addiction, HIV, AIDS, leukemia, immunosuppression, chemotherapy, head trauma, or neuroprocedures Incidence and duration of past infections such as sinusitis, pneumonia, and otitis Incidence and duration of past diseases such as syphilis, genital herpes, and tuberculosis Complaints of headache, photophobia, lethargy Nausea and vomiting Fever and chills Incidence and duration of irritability, restlessness, and periods of confusion Presence of generalized seizures
Physical Examination	Orientation Level of consciousness and response Motor weakness Cranial nerve palsies Sensory deficits Kernig's sign Positive Brudzinski's sign Signs of ear, nose, and throat infections Signs of pneumonia Presence of rashes
Laboratory Findings	Cultures of CSF, nasal swabs, and aspirates of skin lesions Serum electrolytes and glucose Prothrombin times

Maintenance of vital functions including controlling intracranial pressure, supporting respiratory and circulatory function, and monitoring fluid and electrolyte balances

Prevention of complications and maintenance of patient safety

Provision of comfort measures and supportive care aimed at relieving symptoms of fever, headache, photophobia, and irritability.

More specifically, the following nursing care plan outlines the standard critical care practices for managing the patient suffering from meningitis.

Nursing Care Plan for the Management of the Patient with Neurological Infection

Diagnosis	Signs and symptoms	Intervention	Rationale
Alteration in comfort related to meningeal irritation	Headache Photophobia Meningeal signs Subjective report of pain	Elevate HOB to 30 degrees	To facilitate venous drainage
		Maintain a quiet and darkened room	To decrease external stimulation and promote rest
		Administer analgesic, sedation, and antipyretic as ordered and evaluate patient's response; turn and position patient to promote comfort	To alleviate pain and promote comfort and relaxation and to monitor effectiveness of intervention
		Group nursing activities together	To decrease number of occasions requiring painful manipulations and to ensure rest periods
Alterations in sensory perceptions related to increased sensitivity to visual, auditory, and tactile stimulation	Hyperirritability Hyperalgesia Photophobia	Provide a nonstimulating environment by controlling noise and reducing lighting	To help decrease sensory overload (a darkened room is recommended in the event of photophobia)
		Group nursing activities together	To avoid unnecessary stimulation
		Approach patient in a calm and gentle manner	To help decrease effects of hyperirritability and hyperalgesia
		Assess mental status and select appropriate stimulus	To avoid confusion and overstimulation while simultaneously decreasing the risk of sensory deprivation (which frequently occurs during ICU stays)
Alteration in respiratory function related to ineffective breathing patterns and airway clearance, increased secretions, immobility, and inadequate ventilation	Abnormal ABGs: $pO_2 < 80$ mm Hg; $pCO_2 < 35$ or > 45 mm Hg; pH < 7.35 or > 7.45; O_2 sat. $< 80\%$; $HCO_3 < 20$ or > 26 mEq/L; BE < 0 or > 3	Assess breathing pattern frequently	To evaluate respiratory function
		Maintain airway and mechanically ventilate postoperatively as required	To ensure adequate ventilation

Diagnosis	Signs and symptoms	Intervention	Rationale
	Dyspnea Hypoxemia Hypercapnia Copious secretions Atelectasis Elevated respiratory rate, wheezing, air hunger, gasping, or asymmetrical expansion of chest wall	Closely monitor ABGs PRN and after ventilator changes; closely monitor for absent, unequal, or diminished breath sounds, crackles, wheezing, or asymmetrical chest wall expansion	To discover early indications of respiratory compromise and/or complications
		Aggressive pulmonary toilet (as neurologically indicated) PRN with chest percussion therapy, incentive spirometry, and hyperinflation using 100% oxygen before and after suctioning; turn and reposition patient every 2 hours (within neurological indications)	To mobilize secretions, provide adequate oxygenation, and open closed alveoli
		If stable, promote extubation as soon as possible by: holding sedation, elevating HOB 30 degrees, incremental weaning (as indicated neurologically)	To assist patient to return to optimal breathing capacity as soon as possible and to prevent atelectasis and secondary infection
Potential for alteration in cerebral tissue perfusion related to: ischemic injury, cerebral edema, increased ICP, inflammation of meninges	Agitation	Control external hyperstimulation from the environment (noise, temperature, light, and odors) and prevent unnecessary disturbances	Reducing external environmental stimulation may help to decrease patient's activity, irritation, and startle responses, thus decreasing ICP
	Anxiety	Approach patient in a calm and reassuring manner	Nursing activities can lead to anxiety and agitation
	Altered level of consciousness	Provide soft stimuli (light touch, soft music, pleasant and familiar sounds)	Calm and quiet environment helps prevent drastic increases in BP and thus ICP

Nursing Care Plan for the Management of the Patient with Neurological Infection

Diagnosis	Signs and symptoms	Intervention	Rationale
	Sensory and motor disturbances	Plan activities to allow adequate rest times	Fatigue exacerbates agitation responses
	Higher ICP readings	Monitor increases in ICP to learn what causes them and organize activities to minimize time and intensity of stimulation	To limit time and intensity of activities that challenge (stress) the patient, causing greater oxygen demand and raising ICP
		Assist family to communicate with patient in a calm and quiet manner; counsel family to avoid emotionally stimulating the patient	Teaching of family may help to prevent unnecessary startles, excessive stimulation, agitation, and frustration, leading to rises in ICP
	Headache	Maintain HOB at 30 degrees	Elevation of the head promotes venous drainage and decreases ICP
		Administer pain medication as ordered and initiate comfort measures	Alleviating or decreasing pain or discomfort helps to decrease ICP by decreasing MAP; comfort measures decrease agitation and thus ICP
Potential alteration in comfort related to increased ICP	Headache Nausea Projectile vomiting	Maintain HOB at 30 degrees	Elevation of the head promotes venous drainage and decreases ICP
		Administer pain medication as ordered and initiate comfort measures	Alleviating or decreasing pain or discomfort helps to decrease ICP by decreasing MAP; comfort measures decrease agitation, thus decreasing ICP

Diagnosis	Signs and symptoms	Intervention	Rationale
Potential for alteration in cerebral perfusion related to increased ICP due to nursing activities, emotional upset, and agitation	Higher ICP readings Anxiety Agitation	Control external stimulation from the environment (noise, temperature, light, and odors)	Reducing external stimulation may help to decrease patient's activity and startle responses, thus decreasing ICP
		Prevent unnecessary disturbances	Nursing activities can lead to anxiety and agitation
		Approach patient in a calm and reassuring manner; provide soft stimuli (light touch, soft music, pleasant and familiar sounds)	Calm and quiet environment helps prevent drastic increases in ICP
		Plan activities to allow adequate rest times	Fatigue exacerbates agitation responses
		Monitor increases in ICP to learn what causes them and organize activities to minimize time and intensity of stimulation	To limit time and intensity of activities that challenge (stress) the patient and raise ICP
		Assist family to communicate with patient in a calm and quiet manner; counsel family to avoid emotionally stimulating the patient	Teaching of family may help to prevent unnecessary startles, excessive stimulation, and agitation that can lead to rises in ICP
Potential for fluid and electrolyte imbalance due to fluid loss, antidiuretic hormone imbalance, inadequate intake, gastrointestinal suctioning, and hyperthermia	Volume excess	Accurately monitor intake and output, weight, and urine specific gravity	To ascertain fluid balance status
	Hyponatremia Hypertonic urine with increased specific gravity	Closely monitor electrolyte status: hematocrit, BUN, creatinine, and serum osmolality	To detect imbalances and determine renal function (hyponatremia can precipitate seizures)
	Abnormal serum osmolality	Adhere strictly to fluid restrictions	To help prevent overhydration and hyponatremia and to control ICP and avoid cerebral edema
	Hyperthermia	Maintain temperature within normal limits	To prevent rises in ICP

Nursing Care Plan for the Management of the Patient with Neurological Infection

Diagnosis	Signs and symptoms	Intervention	Rationale
		Measure gastric output and test pH every 8 hours; if pH < 5, administer antacids as ordered	To prevent gastric acidity
		Consult with dietician and initiate nutritional support as soon as appropriate; initiate tube feeding if needed	Early nutritional support promotes fluid and electrolyte balances and provides strength leading to recovery
Potential for physical injury related to altered sensory perception, sensorimotor deficits, cognitive impairment, altered level of consciousness, or seizure activity	Motor deficits Agitation Hyperirritability	Maintain a safe environment by: placing bed in low position with wheel brakes in locked position, side rails up, call light within easy reach, assistive devices within reach; arranging furniture and equipment for safe use by patient; providing adequate lighting at HS; providing nonskid foot wear	To promote safety and decrease risk of physical injury
		Identify patient's safety needs and establish safety guidelines with patient and family; reinforce guidelines frequently	To promote learning of safety practices by patient and family
	Seizures	Administer anticonvulsants as prescribed and monitor therapeutic levels	To help prevent seizures through attaining of optimal drug effectiveness
		Institute seizure precautions (padded bed rails, oral airway, suction equipment, and supplemental oxygen)	To decrease the risk of physical injury in the event of seizures

Diagnosis	Signs and symptoms	Intervention	Rationale
	Confusion	Reorient patient frequently	To increase patient's awareness of surroundings
	Anxiety	Explain patient care activities	To help alleviate anxiety
	Restlessness	Assess causes of restlessness (hypoxemia, pain, bladder distention) and plan care appropriate to need	To decrease risk of restlessness and agitation leading to possible accidental injury
		Use physical restraints only when necessary	To promote safety and reduce agitation
Hyperthermia related to inflammatory response to CNS infection	Elevated temperature	Monitor temperature closely	To accurately determine temperature
	Shivering	Observe for signs of shivering and institute measures to decrease them	Shivering increases metabolic rate
		Obtain specimens for cultures as indicated	Cultures can contribute to the diagnosis of meningitis
		Consult with infectious disease control department	To assist in the planning of care of infected patient
		Institute isolation precautions according to hospital procedure (strict respiratory and universal precautions are recommended for meningitis)	To prevent spread of infection to other patients
	Diaphoresis	Provide a cool environment	To help control drastic increases in temperature leading to increased ICP and oxygen demand
		Remove excess clothing and linen	To mediate exposure to environmental temperature

Nursing Care Plan for the Management of the Patient with Neurological Infection

Diagnosis	Signs and symptoms	Intervention	Rationale
		Implement cooling measures as needed (tepid sponge bath or hypothermia blanket to cool patient slowly, not exceeding 1°F every 15 minutes); administer antipyretics as prescribed	To help control drastic increases in temperature leading to increased ICP and oxygen demand
		Administer antibiotics as prescribed	To help alleviate cause of hyperthermia
		Administer IV fluids as prescribed	Elevated temperatures can cause dehydration
Potential for impaired verbal communication related to decreased LOC, cerebral edema, dysphasia, endotracheal tube, and tracheostomy	Receptive, global, or expressive aphasia	Assess patient's ability to hear, understand, and speak	To determine patient's ability to communicate
	Frustration during communication attempts	Teach appropriate strategies to promote communication: using assistive materials such as writing implements and communication board, reducing environmental distractions, decreasing anxiety, decreasing speed of communication, using simple commands with gestures	To help patient identify and use appropriate strategies to facilitate communication
		Face the patient and establish eye contact to provide support and reassurance during communication attempts	To encourage patient's efforts
		Consult with speech therapist	To allow for early rehabilitation
	Uneasiness and impatience of family during communication attempts	Teach family successful strategies for communication with patient	To promote family communication and cohesion

Diagnosis	Signs and symptoms	Intervention	Rationale
Disturbance in body concept related to neurological deficits, cranial nerve dysfunction (facial palsy, decreased corneal reflex), and hair loss from surgical procedure	Alterations in body concept	Assess patient's and family's interpretation of change in body concept	To establish baseline
	Anxiety during visiting hours	Encourage patient and family to express feelings	To help alleviate feelings of anxiety and promote adjustment
	Inability of family to comfortably and calmly look at and interact with patient	Assist family in adapting to patient's body changes and appearance	To achieve maximal level of self-esteem for patient and acceptance and support from family
	Lack of knowledge of available support services	Consult with hospital and community support services	To help patient and family make use of appropriate resources
Potential for skin breakdown due to: restriction of movement; pain/discomfort; drug-induced neuromuscular or musculoskeletal impairment; depression; body stiffness; diaphoresis or drainage into patient's bed; independent variables such as diabetes, peripheral vascular disease, obesity, etc.	Imposed restriction of movement, including body mechanics, medical protocol, etc.	Place air mattress on bed	To prevent pressure spots on skin
	Impaired coordination or decreased muscle strength preventing independent movement	Assist with required movements; quarter turn every 1–2 hours	To prevent overexertion and to facilitate movement
	Reluctance to attempt movement	Encourage movement within safety parameters	To prevent injury and facilitate movement
	Redness over pressure points	Inspect pressure points, including occiput, sacrum, coccyx, heels, and elbows, every 2 hours	To prevent skin breakdown
		Passive range of motion for all extremities	To prevent pressure spots
		Keep patient dry	To prevent skin breakdown
		Maintain and supplement nutrition as needed	To maintain vital nutrients to skin
		Consult enterostomal therapist	To provide for optimal care planning and intervention and to prevent skin breakdown

Nursing Care Plan for the Management of the Patient with Neurological Infection

Diagnosis	Signs and symptoms	Intervention	Rationale
	Elevated temperature	Keep patient dry when diaphoretic	To prevent skin breakdown
Alteration in rest/sleep pattern related to continuous environmental stimuli, ICU routine, and interrupted sleep	Disturbances in rest/sleep pattern	Determine the patient's established rest/sleep pattern and organize nursing activities to accommodate it as much as possible	To accommodate to patient's normal pattern
	Exhaustion	Structure nursing activities to provide for fewer interruptions at normal time of sleep; design schedule to balance daytime activities with periods of uninterrupted sleep	To maximize patient's ability to relax, rest, and sleep
	Inability to fall asleep	Provide comfort measures and assistive devices individualized to patient's need; explore the possibility of relaxation therapy	To promote comfort and sleep
	Interrupted rest periods	Plan visiting schedule to accommodate interventions as well as family's schedule and rest periods; restrict visitors as appropriate	To maximize strength; to improve quality of family time as well as provide for needed rest
Potential for alteration in bowel function or constipation due to: decreased mobility, change in eating patterns, side effects of medications, postoperative paralytic ileus, decreased fluid volume	Reports of feeling constipated, "full" feeling in abdomen, inability to move bowels	Assess abdomen for bowel sounds, softness, and appearance and ask patient about discomfort at least every 12 hours	For early diagnosis of constipation in order to intervene before serious problems occur
	Decreased or absent bowel sounds	Encourage progressive activity as tolerated	To stimulate peristalsis
	Inadequate oral fluid/food intake as evidenced on I&O records and calorie counts	Reassure patient that constipation is frequently a problem postoperatively	So patient will not become overly concerned

Diagnosis	Signs and symptoms	Intervention	Rationale
	Symptoms of dehydration: poor skin turgor, sunken eyes, intake less than output, weight loss	Assess for signs of dehydration and encourage oral intake within fluid restriction limits	Hydration impedes constipation
		Closely monitor electrolytes	Dehydration leads to electrolyte imbalance
	Absence of bowel movement for more than 2 days	Implement bowel regimen as ordered: milk of magnesia 30 mL p.o. every HS; consult with dietician about increased fiber in diet as indicated; rehydrate patient as ordered via IV or oral fluids (as neurologically indicated)	Patient may need extra help to start peristalsis postoperatively
		Reduce narcotic consumption when feasible	Narcotics inhibit bowel activity
Potential for anxiety due to: fear of unknown, fear of death, fear of pain, fear of disability, lack of knowledge regarding hospital procedures and routines, risk of surgery, loss of body function, loss of hair	Facial tension Distracting behavior Low attention span Withdrawal Twitching and shaking of extremities Inappropriate laughter or behavior Diaphoresis Tachycardia Nonadherence to treatment plan	Ascertain patient's fears and anxieties	Will allow the nurse to know just what to address
		Ascertain patient's previous hospital experiences (own as well as others')	Will help the nurse to know how to best alleviate anxieties and support positive attitudes
		Ascertain readiness to learn	Need to begin patient and family education when ready
		Teach patient about diagnostics, routines of hospital and care regimen: surgery, tubes, lines, ICU routines, visiting hours, pain medication, moving, and deep breathing and coughing; provide patient with educational booklets	To help patient and family be prepared for what is to be experienced

Nursing Care Plan for the Management of the Patient with Neurological Infection

Diagnosis	Signs and symptoms	Intervention	Rationale
		Sedate as ordered PRN	To help patient relax
		Provide emotional support as needed	To help patient and family deal with the situation in the best way possible
		Consult with social worker, chaplain, etc., as needed	Multidisciplinary team effort provides broader, more comprehensive care
		Assist patient and family in identifying effective coping skills	To help patient and family effectively manage situation
Potential for ineffective coping by the patient or family related to: surgery, situational crisis, maturational crisis, personal vulnerability	Verbalization of inability to cope	Assess family's usual coping mechanisms	Questions and concerns of patient and family must be answered even if not voiced
	Inability to ask for emotional help	Assist family to identify alternative coping mechanisms; identify and acknowledge family's needs	Optimal coping must be accomplished for maximal healing
	Inability to meet role expectations	Provide information to patient and family regarding diagnosis and supportive services	Patient and family must be helped through role redefinition
	Prolonged progression of disease or disability	Support patient and family through role transition time	To help patient and family make transition
		Encourage open communication among patient, family, and health care team	To facilitate problem solving and care planning
		Reinforce simple explanations to patient and family	During times of crisis, care must be taken not to cause information overload

Diagnosis	Signs and symptoms	Intervention	Rationale
	Exhaustion	Provide rest periods and offer nutrition; plan visiting schedule to accommodate interventions as well as family's schedule and rest periods; restrict visitors as appropriate	To maximize strength; to improve quality of family time as well as provide for needed rest
	Fear and anxiety	Delegate one resource and support person to assist family communication	Consistency in problem solving and care improves quality of decisions
	Inappropriate requests or hypervigilance by patient and/or family	Suggest approaches for family to assist in patient's care	Participatory care decreases family's anxiety
	Inability to solve problems	Assist patient and family to identify problems and work together to solve them	Sometimes patients and families are unable to anticipate possible problems
	Unreasonable and/or excessively frequent requests (excessive use of call light)	Assist family in caring for patient and problem solve about how to continue such care after discharge	Personal involvement in care decreases anxiety while increasing self-confidence and skills
		Encourage progressively independent activities	To avoid rushing patient and family into too much responsibility for care
Potential for self-care deficit due to: muscle deconditioning; disturbance of sleep pattern; fear of overexertion; anxiety; decreased tolerance of activity	Weak muscles resulting from bedrest	Encourage activities safe to patient: minor self-care, passive ROM	To allow time for patient to regain strength
	Reports of headaches	Assess discomfort and encourage patient to request medication as appropriate	To allow for maximal rest and decreased ICP
	Fatigue	Assess patient's need for rest and sleep and incorporate rest periods during the day	To allow for needed rest and to promote relaxation and healing
	Increased heart rate and respiratory rate upon minimal activity	Facilitate calm environment (lighting, noise, interruptions, etc.)	To prevent agitation and discomfort, leading to increased ICP

Diagnosis	Signs and symptoms	Intervention	Rationale
	Repetitive fast speech, indicating anxiety	Encourage patient's participation in scheduling and carrying out daily care to decrease anxiety through familiarity	To prevent anxiety leading to overexhaustion and to facilitate adequate rest
Potential for alteration in health maintenance due to lack of knowledge of : diagnosis, medication regimen, activity, medical followup, referrals, home management	Anxiety	Explain hospital routines and restrictions and reasons for them	To decrease anxiety and improve adherence
	Communicates lack of knowledge or is unable to describe diagnosis and how it relates to prognosis	Instruct patient and family about diagnosis and prognosis with as many repetitions as needed; encourage questions and open discussion of problems and concerns	Patient and family must understand in order to adhere to prescribed regimen, which will promote healing and optimal level of functioning
	Inability to describe prescribed regimen and reasons for it	Instruct about medications, diet, and followup care: what, why, care options, plan of daily schedule	To allow for clear understanding and acceptance
	Does not distinguish between permitted and prohibited activities	Discuss activities in routine, balancing rest and care, and progression of care	To facilitate adherence to regimen and progressive resumption of activities without overdoing it and increasing risk of complications

Medications Commonly Used in the Care of the Patient with Neurological Infection

Medication	Effect	Major side effects
Ampicillin	Antibiotic therapy for Escherichia coli and Hemophilus influenzae	Allergic reactions Nephritis Anaphylaxis Hemolytic anemias Bone marrow depression
Penicillin G	Antibiotic therapy for Neisseria meningitidis, Streptococcus and Diplococcus	As for Ampicillin
Nafcillin	Antibiotic therapy for Staphylococcus	As for Ampicillin
Gentamycin	Antibiotic therapy for Pseudomonas	Nephrotoxicity Anaphylaxis Ototoxicity
Carbenicillin	Antibiotic therapy for Pseudomonas and Escherichia coli	Allergic reactions Nephritis Anaphylaxis Hemolytic anemias Bone marrow depression
Chloramphenicol	Antibiotic therapy for Neisseria, Streptococcus, Staphylococcus, Escherichia coli, and Pseudomonas	Erythropoietic depression Thrombocytopenia Nausea Diarrhea
Corticosteroids: Dexamethasone Prednisone Hydrocortisone Methylprednisolone	Reduce cerebral edema by stabilizing the capillary endothelial junction and reducing cerebrovascular permeability Promote integrity of cells to inhibit flow of intracellular fluid to extracellular space	Opportunistic infection Cushing's syndrome Nervousness Hyperglycemia Electrolyte imbalances Menstrual irregularities Skin rash Gastric irritation
Hyperosmotic agents: Mannitol Glycerol	Reduce brain water by creating an osmotic gradient between tissue and plasma Reduce intracranial pressure within 1–3 hours by rapid diuresis	Diuresis Electrolyte imbalances Rebound increased intracranial pressure

Medications Commonly Used in the Care of the Patient with Neurological Infection

Medication	Effect	Major side effects
Anticonvulsants: Phenytoin (Dilantin) Valproic acid	Prevents seizures by stabilizing the cell threshold of excitation and inhibiting the spread of impulses to adjacent tissue	CNS depression Cardiovascular collapse Nausea and vomiting Vertigo Ataxia Hypotension Coagulation defects
Acetaminophen	Analgesic and antipyretic	Hemolytic anemia Skin rash Fever Vascular collapse
Aspirin	Analgesic, antiinflammatory, and antipyretic (by altering the temperature regulation center of the hypothalamus)	Interference with synthesis of prothrombin Inhibition of platelet adhesiveness, leading to hemorrhage Tinnitus Hypothrombinemia

Cerebral Embolic Events

There are several types of cerebral embolic events, all of which occur secondarily to disease processes elsewhere in the body. The most frequently seen are thrombi from the heart due to endocardial or valvular disease. The next most frequently occurring emboli are cholesterol and fibrin-platelet formations that disengage from atherosclerotic plaques or discharge cholesterol or lipid composites. Cerebral fat emboli occasionally occur as a complication of crushing injuries and traumatic fractures to long bones. Gaseous and foreign body emboli also occur as a result of traumatic injuries. Tumor cells circulating in the bloodstream, which originate from carcinomas elsewhere in the body, frequently lodge in the brain. They continue to grow and multiply until a full-blown tumor has formed. Finally, septic (or infectious) emboli formed from bacterial endocarditis, pulmonary infections, or infections from contaminated intravenous injections by drug addicts can proliferate in the bloodstream and find their way into the brain. The last two types of embolic events are discussed in depth in the sections addressing the topics of space-occupying lesions and neurological infections, respectively.

Risk factors and precipitating factors and specific pathophysiological processes vary greatly depending on the type of cerebral embolic event. However, the clinical signs and symptoms and the nursing interventions related to the management of such patients do not differ significantly. Therefore, the clinical antecedents and critical referents for each type of cerebral embolic event will be detailed separately, but discussions of signs and symptoms and nursing interventions will be combined.

Cerebral Thrombus

A cerebrovascular accident (CVA), or cerebral thrombus, is characterized by a sudden onset of neurological deficits resulting from a deficiency in the cerebral blood supply. The two major forms of cerebrovascular accident are occlusive and hemorrhagic. The majority of patients with cerebral thrombi (70–80%) have occlusive disease resulting from a thrombus of a cerebral artery or an embolus lodged in a cerebral vessel.

Clinical antecedents

In the United States, occlusive CVA is a major cause of physical disability and ranks as the third leading cause of morbidity and mortality (heart disease and cancer are the top two). The American Heart Association estimates that half a million individuals suffer embolic strokes each year, and it is believed that these persons account for half of all hospitalizations for acute neurological disease.[25] Currently, the relationship between the association of the risk factors and the development of cerebral thrombus is not clearly understood, but it is believed that the best way to prevent cerebral thrombus is to reduce the risks. Since many of these factors also apply to stroke victims, they are referred to as predisposing conditions contributing to the development of disruptions to the cerebrovascular system. Numerous research efforts continue to investigate the risk factors and associated conditions that predispose individuals to occlusive CVA (see Table 3-34).

Hypertension is the single most important risk factor for cerebral thrombus; the degree of risk varies directly with blood pressure. Although cerebral thrombus may occur at any age, it tends to affect a disproportionate percentage of the elderly with multiple health-related problems that include cardiac disease and atherosclerosis. It also appears that the black population tends to be more at risk for cerebral thrombus. This fact may be due to the higher incidence of hypertension in blacks.

Heart disease is also a major risk factor for occlusive CVA. Even when controlling for the effect

Table 3-34 Risk Factors and Predisposing Conditions Associated with Cerebrovascular Accident

Risk Factors	Predisposing Conditions
Cardiac disease	Myocardial infarction
Valvular disease	Atrial fibrillation
Hypertension	Cerebral artery thrombosis
	Previous TIA
	Polycythemia
Atherosclerosis	Open heart surgery
	Fat or air embolism
Congenital heart disease	Endocarditis
Family History	Hyperlipoproteinemia
	Hypertriglyceridemia
	Hypercholesterolemia
	Hypercoagulopathies
Life-style	Smoking
	Physical inactivity
	Oral contraceptives
Diabetes mellitus	Hypertension
Obesity	Physical inactivity
Catastrophe	Trauma

of hypertension, those who experience heart disease are at more than double the risk for cerebral thrombus. Eliminating the risk factors that lead to heart attack (cirgarette smoking, high cholesterol, and hypertension) would in turn help eliminate the risk factors leading to occlusive CVA.

The third major risk factor for cerebral thrombus is the presence of high red blood cell counts. Increased RBCs thicken the blood and predispose the individual to blood clots, resulting in higher embolic incidences.

Critical referents

Thrombotic stroke is primarily associated with valvular and endocardial disease, but can also be associated with atherosclerosis and a progressive narrowing of the lumen of the artery from an accumulation of atheromas (plaques). This type of occlusive thrombi may occur at any age, although it occurs rarely in individuals under the age of 40. Those who have suffered myocardial infarction, especially of an expansive nature (causing heart failure) and involving the anteroseptal wall of the myocardium, are most at risk for blood clots. Atherosclerotic plaques commonly accumulate in larger vessels or branching points such as are found in the internal carotid artery, pulmonary vein, or vertebral arteries. Venous pressure is increased, circulation is decreased, and formation of clots occurs. Figure 3-29 illustrates areas within the cerebral arterial system and the circle of Willis that are most at risk for clot formation.

Although partial compensation through the development of collateral circulation at the circle of Willis provides alternative vascular pathways for cerebral blood flow, a developing thrombus can still interfere with overall flow because perfusion pressure in the vessels distal to the stenosis is altered. The onset of thrombosis is usually slow and occurs over the span of several days. As formation of the thrombus progresses, the lumen of the vessel eventually becomes completely occluded, cerebral blood flow is interrupted, and cerebral infarction results.

Transient Ischemic Attack (TIA)

Transient ischemic attacks are temporary neurological deficits caused by localized cerebral ischemia, which occur only with cerebral thrombosis. TIAs generally last for several minutes to several hours and then clear completely without causing any residual effects. In spite of the innocuous nature of TIAs, patients who experience them should be encouraged

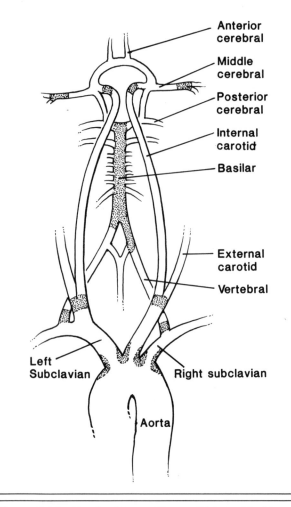

Figure 3-29   Cerebral Artery Sites at Risk for Clot Formation

to seek medical care, for TIAs are precursors of more serious embolic events.

Clinical antecedents

TIAs are thought to be caused by microemboli that have broken off of atherosclerotic plaques located in various regions of the cerebral arterial system. Risk factors associated with TIAs include the commonly known risk factors of atherosclerosis: smoking, obesity, lack of exercise, stress, use of oral contraceptives, diets high in salt and fat, diabetes, hypertension, and family history. TIAs can be considered as clinical antecedents to more serious atherosclerotic disorders, for one-third of those experiencing TIAs who are left untreated eventually suffer cerebral infarction.

Very simply, TIAs occur when very small embolic pieces (microemboli) break off of atherosclerotic plaques formed in very small portions of the cerebral arteries. These microemboli occlude the flow of blood in the affected area, interrupting cerebral oxygenation until they are dislodged or disintegrate.

TIA episodes continue only until the obstruction dissolves or moves and circulation is restored; this usually occurs before permanent damage results. Signs and symptoms exhibited during TIAs vary according to the function of the portion of the brain and the cerebral artery involved. Most commonly, the carotid artery is involved and a temporary inability to speak or loss of vision in one eye occurs. A transient hemiparesis may also occur. If the basilar artery is involved, dizziness and tinnitus are experienced. The symptoms of TIAs are indeed transient, and circulation is restored before permanent damage to the distal brain tissue results. If clinical symptoms persist longer than 24 hours, the syndrome is called reversible ischemic neurological deficit (RIND).

Cerebral Cholesterol, Fibrin, or Lipid Embolus

When fragments of cholesterol, fibrin platelet, or lipid material circulating in the bloodstream get lodged in a cerebral vessel, emboli result. These fragments break off of atherosclerotic plaques that have formed over several years of high-fat and high-cholesterol diet, lack of exercise, smoking, and stress.

Risk factors for individuals who have a tendency for cerebral thrombus formation are consistent for those at risk for cholesterol, fibrin, or lipid embolus. Those who are hypertensive and suffer from heart disease are most at risk for developing this type of embolus. What remains unknown is what event or circumstance serves as the direct precipitant of the actual incidence of the embolus. The one instance documented is the extremely rare but serious complication of administering lipids in conjunction with parenteral nutrition.

A cerebral cholesterol, fibrin, or lipid embolus results when a fragment of cholesterol, fibrin platelet, or lipid material becomes lodged in a cerebral artery and occlusion, ischemia, and infarction occur. Such emboli frequently arise from atherosclerotic plaques that originate in the carotid and vertebrobasilar vessels. The left middle cerebral artery is most commonly affected because of its direct access from the aorta, which facilitates travel of the embolus. As an embolus passes through a cerebral vessel, it may produce varying degrees of neurological deficits, depending on the size and location of the embolus. A sudden onset of a cerebral embolus does not allow collateral circulation to be established, and, therefore, the initial neurological deficits can be severe. When plaques have been formed over the years, neurological damage occurs as a result of obstruction of the artery distal to the embolus that causes cerebral infarction. Prognosis varies, for as the embolus progressively breaks into tiny particles and continues to travel through the artery, severe deficits may improve or at least become temporary.

Fat Embolism

Fat droplets released from the marrow of crushed or fractured bones and circulating in the bloodstream sometimes become lodged in the pulmonary capillaries. Frequently, however, they pass through the vascular bed of the lung into the cerebral circulation and act as fat emboli.

At present, it is not known why some individuals who suffer traumatic injuries experience complications of fat emboli and others suffering similar injuries do not. Identification of risk factors has not been accomplished. Knowledge of precipitating factors is clearer. Crushing injuries and long-bone fractures are the two primary precipitating factors leading to fat emboli.

When circulating fat droplets get lodged in the vascular bed, not only does mechanical obstruction occur, but fat is hydrolyzed by pulmonary lipase to free fatty acids, and these activate clotting factors. Thrombosis occurs in the vessel, and infarction of the area distal to the embolus results.

Gaseous and Foreign Body Embolus

Gaseous or foreign bodies that inadvertently get introduced into the bloodstream may progress into the brain. These materials can be air, nitrogen, bullets, catheter pieces, swabs, or calcium deposits. Like other types of emboli, gaseous or foreign body emboli can obstruct arterial flow, producing signs of neurological compromise.

Clinical antecedents

Risk factors for gaseous and foreign body emboli cannot be detailed because of the inherent characteristics of the event. Precipitating factors leading to this type of embolus range from traumatic injury to the head, heart, lungs, or large arteries to the administration of parenteral nutrition, surgical procedures, and clinical mishaps. The most commonly seen antecedents are surgical procedures involving the dural sinuses and carotid arteries, radical neck procedures, and cardiac surgeries. Also, any time a long-line catheter is inserted, there is a risk of fragments being cut off accidentally. Finally, patients on bypass pumps(which use oxygenators) or intraaortic balloon pump therapy (the balloon is inflated by gas and the balloon can burst) are at risk for gaseous embolus.

Critical referents

Any gaseous or foreign body embolus has the potential to obstruct arteries and cause damage distal to the obstruction. Although all such emboli carry the potential for disastrous effects, some are considered more dangerous than others. The introduction of air into the system is of particular concern, for air binds to hemoglobin very readily and thus can be widely dispersed far into the cerebral arterial circulatory system. Bullets are also of grave concern because so many of them fragment upon impact and are made of materials that are poisonous or are in other ways physiologically detrimental to humans. '

Resulting signs and symptoms

Regardless of the type of cerebral embolic event, the clinical manifestations are sometimes difficult to differentiate. All such events cause signs and symptoms of neurological compromise due to cerebrovascular impairment. Varying degrees of neurological deficits result, ranging from transient and mild to severe and even rapid cerebral deterioration and death. Clinical manifestations reflect the size of the infarct and the vessel involved, as well as the area of the brain it supplies. Table 3-35 lists the neurological deficits associated with embolic stroke according to arterial syndromes. A review of the list will reveal that landmark syndromes do not always surface in isolation and may overlap with each other.

An embolic stroke in evolution is characterized by a progressive deterioration of neurological status lasting for more than 24 hours. In contrast, an embolic stroke is complete when evolution of manifestations has ceased, the patient's condition has stabilized, and neurological deficits remain at status quo. Table 3-36 presents information about the clinical presentation of right and left hemispheric embolic strokes.

The clinical presentation of a TIA varies depending on the arteries involved. Amaurosis fugax is a type of TIA that causes a sudden and transitory blindness in one eye. This visual disturbance results in retinal ischemia and is a manifestation of an internal carotid occlusion. In contrast, involvement of carotid and cerebral arteries is often characterized by headache, aphasia, dysphasia, amaurosis fugax, homonymous hemianopsia, facial paresis or paralysis, hemiparesis or hemiplegia, and hemianesthesia. Vertebrobasilar arterial involvement is characterized by occipital headache, vertigo, nausea, dysarthria, dysphagia, facial weakness, visual disturbances (homonymous hemianopsia, diplopia, flashing lights), tinnitus, global amnesia, ataxia, alternating hemiparesis, and sudden collapse without loss of consciousness (drop attacks). When vertigo or extraocular muscle dysfunction is a component of a TIA, the vertebrobasilar system, rather than the carotid system, is usually the site of the ischemic event.[26]

A fat embolus usually occurs 1 to 3 days after the trauma or surgical repair of traumatic bone injuries. Dyspnea, tachypnea, and cyanosis are almost always experienced by the patient, followed by restlessness and fidgeting (a sign of oxygen deprivation). A differentiating sign of fat embolus is the presence of petechiae across the chest, neck, and shoulders. As with other embolic events, an alteration in the level

Table 3-35 Neurological Deficits Associated with Stroke According to Arterial Syndromes

Artery	Deficits
Common and Internal Carotid Artery	Dysphasia Contralateral sensory deficits and hemiparesis Stenotic bruit from carotid bifurcation Absence of carotid pulse on affected side Headache over ipsilateral eye Ipsilateral amaurosis fugax Homonymous hemianopsia Mild Horner's syndrome
Middle Cerebral Artery	Dysphasia, dyslexia, dysgraphia Hemiparesis, hemiplegia, hemisensory disturbances (upper extremity worse than lower) Homonymous hemianopsia Altered level of consciousness Internal capsule infarct: dense hemoplegia in arm and leg; upper motor neuron facial weakness
Anterior Cerebral Artery	Confusion, mental deterioration, personality change Incontinence Contralateral hemiplegia, hemiparesis, apraxia on side of lesion Expressive dysphasia Eyes and head deviate to opposite side
Lenticulostriate Artery	Hemiplegia, hemisensory disturbances Dysphasia Homonymous hemianopsia Altered level of consciousness
Posterior Cerebral Artery	Hemiplegia with sensory loss and involuntary movement Visual disturbances: homonymous hemianopsia, quadrantanopsia, cortical blindness Dyslexia Hemiballismus
Vertebral-Basilar Artery	Ataxia, vertigo, syncope, drop attacks while still conscious, disorientation Transient global amnesia, loss of memory Dysarthria, dysphagia Tinnitus, sudden deafness Visual disturbances, diplopia, homonymous hemianopsia, nystagmus, ophthalmoplegia, conjugate gaze paralysis Suboccipital headache Nausea Facial weakness, perioral and tongue numbness Alternating hemiparesis Dysmetria Akinetic mutism

Posterior Inferior Cerebellar Artery	General:
	  Ipsilateral facial loss of pain and temperature sensation, abnormal sensation over ipsilateral side of face, paralysis of soft palate and larynx; contralateral body loss of pain and temperature sensation
	  Ipsilateral Horner's syndrome
	  Vertigo, ataxia
	  Dysarthria, dysphagia
	  Hiccoughs
	  Vomiting
	  Nystagmus
	  Dysphonia
	Wallenberg's syndrome:
	  Sudden onset of vertigo, ataxia, falls toward side of lesion without deficit in consciousness
	  Dysphagia
	  Nystagmus
	  Nausea and vomiting
	  Ipsilateral facial loss of pain and temperature sensation and contralateral body loss of same
	Horner's syndrome

Table 3-36 Comparison of Clinical Presentation of Right and Left Hemispheric Stroke

Left Hemispheric Stroke	Right Hemispheric Stroke
Right-sided hemiparesis or hemiplegia	Left-sided hemiparesis or hemiplegia
Expressive aphasia	Denial of deficits (high risk for accidents and physical injury)
Receptive aphasia	
Global aphasia	Impulsive behavior
Slow and cautious behavior	Poor judgment
Intellectual and cognitive impairment	Distractibility
Right visual field defect	Poor concentration
	Spatial/perceptual deficits

of consciousness is the most common neurological effect of a fat embolus, and it may progress to pupillary changes indicating further cerebral damage leading to coma.

If obstruction of neurological vessels by an air or foreign body embolus occurs, classic signs and symptoms of neurological compromises are exhibited. In the event of an air embolus, dyspnea is suddenly experienced in conjunction with chest pain. Frequently, there is a drop in blood pressure. Hemoptysis can also occur. Later, pO_2 and SaO_2 levels may be elevated as a result of the binding of oxygen to hemoglobin in the bloodstream.

Nursing standards of care

Medical management of an acute cerebral embolic event is directed to managing the acute aspects of care, accomplishing accurate diagnosis, reducing or preventing an increase of neurological deficits, and initiating rehabilitative efforts. Without aggressive medical therapy, the patient is placed at increased risk of extending the thrombus or embolus and increasing the neurological deficits arising from the initial insult. Diagnosis is made on the basis of patient history, physical examination, and diagnostic studies. Ascertaining the presence of risk factors for cerebral embolus is important, as is learning the

onset and evolution of symptoms. Diagnostic studies useful in the clinical evaluation include computerized tomography (CT) scan (with or without contrast infusion), magnetic resonance imaging (MRI), cerebral arteriogram, carotid doppler, ECG, lumbar puncture (when hemorrhagic stroke is indicated), hematologic studies (CBC, clotting profiles, electrolytes, cholesterol, and triglycerides), EEG, and echocardiogram (refer to the section on neurological assessment and diagnostics).

Although the beneficial effects of anticoagulation drug therapy in the management of thrombus formation remain controversial, intravenous heparin followed by coumadin is frequently used as one treatment modality for preventing the further progression of occlusive emboli by acting as an anticoagulant and a lipase activator to help reduce circulating triglycerides. Antiplatelet aggregation therapy (enteric-coated aspirin, Persantin, and Anturane) is used to prevent thrombus formation by reducing platelet adhesiveness. Glucose with alcohol is administered for its lipolytic properties. Corticosteroids are given to decrease the inflammatory response that causes edema in the area of embolus formation. Administration of antihypertensive drugs to gradually reduce blood pressure is frequently indicated for severe hypertension that places the patient at higher risk for thrombus formation. Finally, vasodilators may be used to help increase cerebral blood flow and promote collateral circulation.

Surgical interventions to help prevent further progression of embolic events include (1) microvascular (or EC/IC) bypass, or the anastomosis of an extracranial vessel to an intracranial vessel to augment cerebral blood flow to inaccessible areas; (2) excavation of operable emboli and abscesses; and (3) carotid endarterectomy, or the removal of atherosclerotic plaques to allow for improved circulation. It should be noted, though, that the benefits of carotid endarterectomy have been widely debated and are still under clinical investigation and evaluation. The success of an EC/IC bypass depends heavily on appropriate patient selection. Optimally, EC/IC bypass is reserved for those presenting with symptomatic TIA or RIND.

Priorities for nursing the patient experiencing a cerebral embolic event are to support vital functions, to prevent further complications, and to begin rehabilitation. The following nursing care plan outlines the standard critical care practices used in the management of such a patient.

Nursing Care Plan for the Management of the Patient Experiencing a Cerebral Embolic Event

Diagnosis	Signs and symptoms	Intervention	Rationale
Potential for alteration in respiratory function related to: altered level of consciousness, ineffective airway clearance, injury to respiratory center, pulmonary embolus	Abnormal ABGs: $pO_2 < 80$ mm Hg; $pCO_2 < 35$ or > 45 mm Hg; pH < 7.35 or > 7.45; O_2 sat. $< 80\%$; $HCO_3 < 20$ or > 26 mEq/L; BE < 0 or > 3 Dyspnea Hypoxemia Hypercapnia Copious secretions Atelectasis Elevated respiratory rate, wheezing, air hunger, gasping, or asymmetrical expansion of chest wall	Assess breathing pattern frequently	To evaluate respiratory function
		Position to facilitate drainage of oral secretions (HOB at 30–60 degrees); maintain airway and mechanically ventilate as required	To ensure adequate ventilation
		Closely monitor ABGs; closely monitor for absent, unequal, or diminished breath sounds, crackles, wheezing, or asymmetrical chest wall expansion	To assess for ensuing respiratory compromise and/or complications
		Aggressive pulmonary toilet (as neurologically indicated) PRN with chest percussion therapy, incentive spirometry, and hyperinflation using 100% oxygen before and after suctioning; turn and reposition patient every 2 hours (within neurological indications)	To mobilize secretions, provide adequate oxygenation, and open closed alveoli
		Promote extubation as soon as possible by: holding sedation, elevating HOB 30 degrees, incremental weaning (as indicated neurologically)	To assist patient to return to optimal breathing capacity as soon as possible and to prevent atelectasis and secondary infection
Potential for alteration in cerebral perfusion related to: ischemic injury, cerebral edema, increased ICP	Agitation	Control hyper-stimulation from the external environment (noise, temperature, light, and odors) and prevent unnecessary disturbances	Reducing external environmental stimulation may help to decrease patient's activity and startle responses, thus decreasing ICP

Nursing Care Plan for the Management of the Patient Experiencing a Cerebral Embolic Event

Diagnosis	Signs and symptoms	Intervention	Rationale
	Anxiety	Approach patient in a calm and reassuring manner	Nursing activities can lead to anxiety and agitation
	Altered level of consciousness Sensory and motor disturbances	Provide soft stimuli (light touch, soft music, pleasant and familiar sounds)	Calm and quiet environment helps prevent drastic increases in ICP
		Plan activities to allow adequate rest times	Fatigue exacerbates agitation responses
	Higher ICP readings	Monitor increases in ICP to learn what causes them and organize activities to minimize time and intensity of stimulation	To limit activities that challenge (stress) the patient and raise ICP
	Aphasia	Assist family to communicate with patient in a calm and quiet manner and to maintain patience	Education of family may help to prevent unnecessary startles, excessive stimulation, agitation, and frustration when attempting to speak, which can lead to rises in ICP
		Counsel family to avoid emotionally stimulating the patient	
	Headache	Maintain HOB at 30 degrees	Elevation of the head promotes venous drainage and decreases ICP
		Administer pain medication as ordered and provide comfort measures	Alleviating or decreasing pain or discomfort helps to decrease ICP by decreasing MAP; comfort measures decrease agitation and thus ICP
Impaired physical mobility due to motor disturbances	Hemiplegia	Maintain body alignment with assistive devices (pillows, footboard)	To prevent complications of immobility

416

Diagnosis	Signs and symptoms	Intervention	Rationale
	Decreased muscle strength and tone	Maintain splints (especially hand and foot) as ordered	To prevent contractures
	Paresis	Consult with physiotherapist and initiate rehab program when patient's condition is stable	To promote early recovery
	Decreased range of motion	Assist with ROM exercises at least every 2–4 hours, allowing patient to do as much as possible	To maintain joint and muscle mobility and to increase circulation while preventing fatigue
		Try to calm patient during activity	Anxiety increases spasticity
	Signs of impeded circulation in extremities (redness over pressure points)	Apply antiembolism stockings; assess for tenderness, redness, warmth, and pain	To identify and decrease venous stasis and deep vein thrombosis
	Impaired small motor coordination	Assist with required movements	To facilitate patient's movement
Potential for physical injury related to: confusion, sensory-perceptual deficits, seizure activity, altered level of consciousness, emotional lability, possible falls	Confusion	Reorient patient frequently as to surroundings, time, and routine activities	To increase patient's awareness of surroundings
	Seizure activity	Maintain a safe environment by: administering anticonvulsants as prescribed and monitoring therapeutic levels; instituting seizure precautions (padded bed rails, oral airway, suction equipment, and supplemental oxygen)	To help prevent seizures and to decrease risk of physical injury
	Agitation and impulsive behavior	Assess causes of restlessness (hypoxemia, pain, bladder distention) and plan care appropriately	To decrease risk of increased agitation leading to possible accidental injury
	Visual field deficits	Place objects within view and reorient patient to other areas frequently	To increase patient's awareness of surroundings and ability to function within them

Diagnosis	Signs and symptoms	Intervention	Rationale
	Poor judgment and denial of deficit	Increase patient's awareness of deficit and limitations; teach ways to adapt	To help decrease risk of physical injury and increase independent functioning
	Neglect of affected side	Help patient to do passive ROM for extremities of affected side	To prevent complications of immobility and to increase self-care efforts
	Disorientation	Restraints PRN	To remind patient not to get up without assistance and to promote safety
Potential for skin breakdown due to: restriction of movement; pain/discomfort; neuromuscular impairment; depression; diaphoresis or drainage into patient's bed; independent variables such as diabetes, peripheral vascular disease, obesity, etc.; low cardiac output; poor tissue perfusion; altered nutritional status; weakness/fatigue	Restriction of movement, including body mechanics	Place air mattress on bed	To prevent pressure spots on skin
	Impaired coordination or decreased muscle strength preventing independent movement	Assist with required movements; quarter turn every 1–2 hours	To prevent injury and facilitate movement
	Reluctance to attempt movement	Encourage movement within safety parameters	To prevent injury and facilitate movement
	Redness over pressure points	Inspect pressure points, including occiput, sacrum, coccyx, heels, and elbows, every 2 hours	To prevent skin breakdown
		Passive range of motion for all extremities	To prevent pressure spots
		Keep patient dry	To prevent skin breakdown
		Maintain and supplement nutrition as needed	To maintain vital nutrients to skin
		Consult enterostomal therapist	To provide for optimal care planning and intervention and to prevent skin breakdown
	Elevated temperature	Keep patient dry when diaphoretic	To prevent skin breakdown

Diagnosis	Signs and symptoms	Intervention	Rationale
Potential for alteration in bowel function or constipation due to: decreased sensation and muscle tone, altered level of consciousness, decreased mobility, change in eating patterns, side effects of medications, decreased fluid volume	Reports of feeling constipated, "full" feeling in abdomen, inability to move bowels	Assess abdomen for bowel sounds, softness, and appearance and ask patient about discomfort at least every 12 hours	For early diagnosis of constipation in order to prevent Valsalva maneuver and to intervene before serious problems occur
	Decreased or absent bowel soundds	Encourage progressive activity as tolerated	To stimulate peristalsis
	Inadequate oral fluid/food intake as evidenced on I&O records and calorie counts	Reassure patient that constipation is frequently a problem when on fluid restrictions	So patient will not become overly concerned
	Symptoms of dehydration: poor skin turgor, sunken eyes, intake less than output, weight loss	Assess for signs of dehydration and encourage oral intake within fluid restriction limits	Hydration impedes constipation
		Closely monitor electrolytes	Dehydration leads to electrolyte imbalance
	Absence of bowel movement for more than 2 days	Implement bowel regimen as ordered: milk of magnesia 30 mL p.o. every HS; consult with dietician about increased fiber in diet as indicated	Patient may need extra help to have regular bowel movements
Alteration in urinary elimination due to: decreased sensation, impaired muscle tone, altered level of consciousness, urinary tract infection	Urinary retention or incontinence	Assess voiding patterns (I&O, frequency, incontinence, retention)	Evaluation of pattern will help patient to attain optimal functioning
		Foley catheter to be removed as soon as possible	The risk of UTI is greater with indwelling catheter
		Institute a bladder training program as soon as possible	To establish regular bladder function
	Urinary infection: sediment in urine; WBCs in urine; hesitancy, frequency, urgency, burning, difficulty starting stream, or inability to void	Administer antibiotics as ordered	To prevent or fight any infection
		Urine C&S (routine/fungal/gram stain) when indicated or as ordered	To allow early detection and treatment of urinary tract infections
		Routine catheter care every 8 hours	To prevent infection

Nursing Care Plan for the Management of the Patient Experiencing a Cerebral Embolic Event

Diagnosis	Signs and symptoms	Intervention	Rationale
Potential for alteration (decrease) in nutritional status related to: altered level of consciousness, absent gag reflex, dysphagia	Weight loss	Weigh daily	To determine weight losses or gains
	Decreased fluid intake	Assess skin turgor	To assess for dehydration
	Caloric intake less than body's requirements	Consult with dietitian	To determine nutritional needs and plan nutritional support
		Consult with speech pathologist to assist in evaluation of swallowing mechanism	To evaluate ability of patient to swallow (to prevent injury from choking, etc.)
	Inability to feed self	Assist with feeding as appropriate	To facilitate patient's nutritional status
	Complaints of lack of appetite	Assess appetite with patient and family and what is preferred within accepted diet	To facilitate patient's nutritional status
Potential for impaired verbal communication related to decreased LOC, cerebral edema, dysphasia, endotracheal tube, and cerebral injury	Aphasia	Assess patient's ability to hear, understand, and speak	To determine patient's ability to communicate
	Frustration during communication attempts	Teach appropriate strategies to promote communication: using assistive materials such as writing implements and communication board, reducing environmental distractions, decreasing anxiety, decreasing speed of communication, using simple commands with gestures	To help patient identify and use appropriate strategies to facilitate communication
		Face the patient and establish eye contact to provide support and reassurance during communication attempts	To encourage patient's efforts

Diagnosis	Signs and symptoms	Intervention	Rationale
		Consult with speech therapist	To allow for early rehabilitation
	Uneasiness and impatience of family during communication attempts	Teach family successful strategies for communication with patient	To promote family communication and cohesion
Disturbance in body concept related to neurological deficits	Alterations in body concept	Assess patient's and family's interpretation of change in body concept	To establish baseline
	Anxiety during visiting hours	Encourage patient and family to express feelings	To help alleviate feelings of anxiety and promote adjustment
	Inability of family to comfortably and calmly look at and interact with patient	Assist family in adapting to patient's body changes and appearance	To achieve maximal level of self-esteem for patient and acceptance and support from family
	Lack of knowledge of available support services	Consult with hospital and community support services	To help patient and family make use of appropriate resources
Potential for anxiety due to: fear of unknown, fear of death, fear of pain, fear of disability, lack of knowledge regarding hospital procedures and routines	Facial tension Distracting behavior Low attention span Withdrawal Twitching and shaking of extremities Inappropriate laughter or behavior Diaphoresis Tachycardia Nonadherence to treatment plan	Ascertain patient's fears and anxieties	Will allow the nurse to know just what to address
		Ascertain patient's previous hospital experiences (own as well as others')	Will help the nurse to know how to best alleviate anxieties and support positive attitudes
		Ascertain readiness to learn	Need to begin patient and family education when ready
		Teach patient about routines of hospital and care regimen: tubes, lines, ICU routines, visiting hours, pain medication, moving, and deep breathing and coughing; provide patient with educational booklets	To help patient and family be prepared for what is to be experienced
		Sedate as ordered PRN	To help patient relax

Nursing Care Plan for the Management of the Patient Experiencing a Cerebral Embolic Event

Diagnosis	Signs and symptoms	Intervention	Rationale
		Provide emotional support as needed	To help patient and family deal with the situation in the best way possible
		Consult with social worker, chaplain, etc., as needed	Multidisciplinary team effort provides broader, more comprehensive care
Potential for ineffective coping by the patient or family related to: situational crisis, maturational crisis, personal vulnerability, severity and chronicity of impairment	Verbalization of inability to cope	Assess family's usual coping mechanisms	Questions and concerns of patient and family must be answered even if not voiced
	Inability to ask for emotional help	Assist family to identify alternative coping mechanisms; identify and acknowledge family's needs	Optimal coping must be accomplished for maximal healing
	Inability to meet role expectations	Provide information to patient and family regarding diagnosis and supportive services	Patient and family must be helped through role redefinition
	Prolonged progression of disease or disability	Support patient and family through role transition time	To help patient and family make transition
		Encourage open communication among patient, family, and health care team	To facilitate problem solving and care planning
		Reinforce simple explanations to patient and family	During times of crisis, care must be taken not to cause information overload
	Exhaustion	Provide rest periods and offer nutrition; plan visiting schedule to accommodate interventions as well as family's schedule and rest periods; restrict visitors as appropriate	To maximize strength; to improve quality of family time as well as provide for needed rest

Diagnosis	Signs and symptoms	Intervention	Rationale
	Fear and anxiety	Delegate one resource and support person to assist family communication	Consistency in problem solving and care improves quality of decisions
	Inappropriate requests or hypervigilance by patient and/or family	Suggest approaches for family to assist in patient's care	Participatory care decreases family's anxiety
	Inability to solve problems	Assist patient and family to identify problems and work together to solve them	Sometimes patients and families are unable to anticipate possible problems
	Unreasonable and/or excessively frequent requests (excessive use of call light)	Assist family in caring for patient and problem solve about how to continue such care after discharge	Personal involvement in care decreases anxiety while increasing self-confidence and skills
		Encourage progressively independent activities	To avoid rushing patient and family into too much responsibility for care
Potential for self-care deficit due to: sensory and cognitive impairment, muscle deconditioning, disturbance of sleep pattern, fear of overexertion, anxiety, decreased ability and tolerance for activity	Inability to perform daily activities independently	Place assistive equipment within patient's visual field	To allow as much independence as possible
		Instruct patient to turn head to compensate for visual field deficits	To increase awareness of what is in blind spots
	Body neglect	Assist with physical hygiene as needed	To facilitate personal hygiene
	Weak muscles resulting from physical deficits and bedrest	Encourage activities safe to patient: minor self-care, passive ROM	To allow time for patient to regain strength and ability to function
	Fatigue	Assess patient's need for rest and sleep and incorporate rest periods during the day	To allow for maximal rest and strength and decreased ICP

Nursing Care Plan for the Management of the Patient Experiencing a Cerebral Embolic Event

Diagnosis	Signs and symptoms	Intervention	Rationale
	Increased heart rate and respiratory rate upon minimal activity	Progressive activities as tolerated	To prevent anxiety leading to overexertion and stress of activity
		Encourage patient's participation in scheduling and carrying out daily care to decrease anxiety through familiarity	To prevent fatigue, agitation, and discomfort leading to increased ICP
	Unsupervised attempts to get out of bed, etc.	Protect patient from injury	Patient's poor judgment can lead to risky behavior, possibly resulting in injury

Medications Commonly Used in the Care of the Patient Experiencing a Cerebral Embolic Event

Medication	Effect	Major side effects
Heparin	Anticoagulation	Bleeding
Corticosteroids: Dexamethasone Prednisone Hydrocortisone Methylprednisolone	Reduce cerebral edema by stabilizing the capillary endothelial junction and reducing cerebrovascular permeability Promote integrity of cells to inhibit flow of intracellular fluid to extracellular space	Opportunistic infection Cushing's syndrome Nervousness Hyperglycemia Electrolyte imbalances Menstrual irregularities Skin rash Gastric irritation
Antiplatelets: Aspirin Persantin Anturane	Decrease platelet adhesiveness	Bleeding Gastric irritation Tinnitus Hypothrombinemia
Antihypertensives: Nitroprusside Hydralazine	Vasodilation through action on smooth muscle of arterioles Decrease peripheral resistance and blood pressure	Nausea and vomiting Headache Hypotension Angina Muscle twitching Tachycardia Flushing

Neurological Encephalopathy

Neurological encephalopathies are, very simply, disorders of the brain. There are different types of neurological encephalopathies, including hypoxic/ischemic, metabolic, and infectious. These disorders of the brain are consequences of severe problems in other organ systems in the body, and because brain tissue is so sensitive to physiological imbalances, neurological symptoms are sometimes the first indicators of disease processes occurring systemically.

Hypoxic/Ischemic Encephalopathy

Hypoxic/ischemic encephalopathy, the most frequently seen type of encephalopathy, is a neurological disorder caused by deficiencies of oxygen in brain tissue due to occlusion, circulatory failure, or decreases in oxygen saturation of the blood.

Clinical antecedents

Conditions that prevent oxygen supply to brain tissue precipitate hypoxic/ischemic encephalopathy. These conditions are varied and include circulatory collapse, respiratory arrest, drowning, aspiration, strangulation, trauma to the trachea, and carbon monoxide poisoning. In hypoxic encephalopathy, cardiac function is maintained (at least initially), and circulation of blood can continue. In ischemic encephalopathy, circulation (supplying of oxygen to the cells) can be compromised either through obstruction or constriction.

Critical referents

In the event of total hypoxia, brain tissue is depleted of all oxygen reserves within 5 minutes, unless hypothermia or barbiturate-induced coma (which slows down the cellular metabolism rate) is also present. During this very short time period, several compensatory physiological changes occur in an effort to sustain life. First, as cerebral perfusion pressure decreases, vessels compensate by dilating in an effort to maintain constant cerebral blood flow. Even when pressures fall to 60 mm Hg, normal metabolic processes are maintained by increased oxygen extraction. Pressures lower than 60 mm Hg

lead to ischemic injury in a very short time. Simultaneously, when oxygen depletion occurs, cerebral blood flow increases, so much so that when pO_2 has dropped to levels between 24 and 26 mm Hg, cerebral blood flow can increase to up to four times the regular rate.[27] This same mechanism occurs with low hemoglobin levels. Cellular activity continues, and as ischemic necrosis develops, tissue swelling is caused by excessive intracellular and intercellular fluid accumulation. Circulatory oxygenation, already compromised, is further impeded. If the hypoxia is not corrected at this stage, the metabolic processes necessary to sustain the Krebs cycle become impossible, and neurotransmitters fail to operate. Brain neurons, once deprived of their source of oxygen, start to catabolize themselves as they attempt to continue their vital function. Finally, lactic acid produced by this catabolic process leads to parenchymal destruction. Cerebral and cerebellar tissue is damaged, and the progression of injury can extend into the brainstem. At this point, irreversible cerebral damage has occurred, and brain death is near.

Resulting signs and symptoms

As with most neurological diseases, specific neurological compromises accompanying hypoxic/ischemic encephalopathy reflect the severity, location, and size of the occurrence. Headaches, bouts of incoordination, and short spans of attention accompany mild hypoxic incidents. Such is not the case with more advanced degrees of hypoxia/ischemia: consciousness is lost almost immediately, permanent brain damage can occur within 3–5 minutes, and if any more time elapses, death soon follows. Cases have been reported where patients have recovered even after cerebral hypoxia has lasted up to 10 minutes. Usually, if the patient has not lost consciousness, serious damage has not been sustained; but if reflexes and responses are absent after the anoxic period, prognosis is poor. Frequently, brain death, evidenced by an isoelectric EEG recording, will occur. Interpreters of EEGs must be extremely cautious about announcing brain death, for extreme hypothermia, very low serum calcium levels, and some forms of anesthesia and/or drug intoxication can also result in isoelectric EEG tracings.

With severe hypoxic/ischemic episodes not culminating in brain death, clinical presentation becomes more involved. Pupils are reactive although coma is usually present. Extremities can be either completely flaccid or rigid. Immediately after resuscitation, seizure activity frequently occurs; this is particularly dangerous for the patient because it drastically increases the oxygen demand of cerebral tissue. As time progresses and the patient does not regain consciousness, neurological tissue damage can extend into the brainstem. Decerebrate posturing, extremes in core temperature, and positive Babinskis are then seen. Fixed and dilated pupils, absent responses and reflexes, and flattened EEG tracings lasting longer than 4 or 5 days signify cerebral damage of an irreversible nature.

Lesser degrees of hypoxic/ischemic encephalopathy are accompanied by shorter periods of unconsciousness. Some of these patients achieve full recovery; others have lasting neurological compromise. The clinical course exhibited can serve as a rather accurate indicator of recovery. Those who eventually recover usually experience periods of confusion, inability to recognize objects (visual agnosia), and myoclonus. The clinical presentation of those patients who do not fully recover is much more involved and includes one or more of the following posthypoxic syndromes:[28]

Persistent coma or stupor

Dementia

Visual agnosia

Parkinsonian effects

Choreoathetosis (involuntary and irregular movements)

Cerebellar ataxia

Action myoclonus

Amnesia

Seizure activity

Nursing standards of care

Much of the success of the care given to the patient suffering from hypoxic/ischemic encephalopathy depends on accurate diagnosis, which is accomplished primarily by ascertaining the occurrence and history of a hypoxic, anoxic, or ischemic event. Upon confirming the diagnosis, the medical team seeks to prevent further hypoxic injury by supporting basic respiratory and circulatory functions. Making the patient hypothermic is thought by some to decrease the metabolic rate, thus lessening tissue necrosis. Decadron is given to help decrease the swelling that accompanies tissue necrosis, and barbiturates may be given to slow the tissue metabolic rate. Attempts to minimize seizure activity are made (to prevent further oxygen demand in cerebral tissue), and pre-cautions are instituted to prevent physical injury in the event of a seizure.

Metabolic Encephalopathy

Metabolic encephalopathies are those whose etiology is hypoglycemia, hyperglycemia, hepatic failure, or electrolyte imbalance (the latter is discussed in depth in the chapter on renal function).

Hypoglycemic Encephalopathy

Extremely low blood glucose levels can lead to compromises in level of consciousness to the extent of coma, confusion, and seizure activity. Blood glucose levels between 30 and 40 mg/100 mL precipitate a general state of mental confusion and seizure activity; levels nearing the single digits cause unconsciousness and almost always some permanent injury to cerebral tissue. Obviously, the precipitating factor is a significant drop in glucose, and risk factors include diabetes, insulin-secreting pancreatic tumors, alcoholism, and drug addiction.

The specific pathophysiology found in hypoglycemic encephalopathy is as follows. Glucose is metabolized in the brain at rates between 60 and 80 mg/min, and the brain holds between 1000 and 2000 mg of inactive glucose (glycogen) at any given time. When blood glucose is prevented from being delivered to the brain tissue, the brain can sustain regular functioning for up to 90 minutes using the reserve glycogen, until it has been depleted. When glucose stores are drained, oxygen uptake by brain tissue is compromised, compensatory mechanisms increase cerebral blood flow, and blood ammonia levels increase. Concurrently, the adrenal glands and the autonomic nervous system are triggered to cause the liver to form sugar from noncarbohydrates, and this supports regular metabolism for a short while longer. These substrates, though, are unable to provide adequate energy for longer periods of time to prevent damage to the neuron membrane in the face of continued metabolic demand.

Signs and symptoms of hypoglycemic encephalopathy mimic those of anoxia but manifest themselves at a slower rate. Initially, hypoglycemia is evidenced by headache, agitation, nervousness, hunger, facial flushing, diaphoresis, and palpitations. If hypoglycemia progresses, confusion and disorientation occur, followed by motor restlessness and spasm, clutching, and forced sucking. Neuron damage presents clinically as mental confusion progressing to more serious seizure activity. Finally, decerebrate posturing is exhibited, preceded closely by unconsciousness, dilated pupils, shallow respirations, and bradycardia, indicating that the medulla is involved. Once these latter symptoms surface, prospects for recovery begin to wane.

Management of hypoglycemic encephalopathy includes supporting the patient's life systems, correcting the underlining hypoglycemia, and protecting the patient from injury due to complications and seizures. It should be noted that the prompt administration of glucose is not always sufficient treatment. In the case of an overdose of insulin leading to severe hypoglycemia, large quantities of intravenous glucose will not completely remedy the situation; enzymes essential to metabolism are destroyed or depleted with a sudden disappearance of circulating glucose.

Hyperglycemic Encephalopathy

There are two types of hyperglycemic encephalopathy: hyperosmolar nonketotic hyperglycemia and diabetic acidosis.

In hyperosmolar nonketotic hyperglycemia, blood glucose levels reach 1000 mg/100 mL without the characteristic ketoacidosis. At risk for this anomaly is the aged diabetic experiencing a precipitating event such as systemic infection, pancreatitis, or drug interaction that inhibits insulin action. Prognosis for such a patient is poor; as many as 40% die from this syndrome.[29]

Osmolality of the patient reaches levels in the 300s (mOsm/kg serum H_2O), and severe polyuria follows. Severe tissue dehydration occurs, and the brain, in essence, shrinks. If this continues, subdural bleeding can occur as a result of the tearing of the cerebral cortex from the dura.

Clinically, the patient presents in a severe and advanced stage of shock. If the condition is not caught early, seizure activity may develop and unilateral weakness may emerge, accompanied by homonymous visual field defect, such as seen accompanying cerebral vascular accidents. Confusion and agitation are accompanied by psychotic hallucinations, but these symptoms quickly give way to lethargy, leading to coma.

Care is provided to support basic life functions and to correct severe dehydration. Isotonic saline is administered cautiously and slowly. Correction of the high glucose level is also accomplished very carefully, for most of these patients experience hyperglycemia because of reasons other than insulin resistance. Thus, very small doses of insulin prove adequate for bringing blood glucose levels down (once correction of the underlying pathology has been initiated).

Diabetic acidosis is frequently seen and occurs with blood glucose levels of 400 mg/100 mL or higher. This syndrome usually develops when diabetics forget or refuse adequate insulin administration. The blood glucose level increases, and the patient becomes acidotic. Ketone bodies are elevated in the blood and urine, and glycosuria is present.

The patient is characteristically weak and tired, complains of headache and cramping, becomes dehydrated, and experiences Kussmaul breathing. Compromises in level of consciousness progress until unconsciousness is reached.

Care entails support of basic life functions and immediate correction of hyperglycemia and acidosis. Fluid replacement should accompany insulin administration, which reverses cerebral tissue metabolic deficiencies in short order.

Hepatic Encephalopathy

Severe hepatic insufficiency accompanied by portacaval shunting of blood leads to hepatic encephalopathy. Precipitating events in the presence of cirrhosis include excessive protein in the diet, acute inflammation such as pancreatitis (which occurs frequently in patients suffering the effects of alcohol), gastrointestinal hemorrhage (which delivers a large protein load to the intestine), and constipation. It is believed that high levels of blood ammonia caused by hepatic insufficiency precipitate the neurological compromises exhibited by the patient. Hypokalemia and alkalosis can increase renal ammonia, which, in turn, exacerbates hepatic encephalopathy.

The pathophysiological processes underlying this syndrome are not completely understood. Some believe that ammonia ending up in the liver (from urease-producing organisms in the bowel) fails to be converted into urea because of portacaval shunting of blood. This ammonia circulates into the brain and interferes with cerebral metabolism and oxygen uptake. Others believe that hepatic encephalopathy is caused directly by CNS functional disorders stemming from cirrhosis and accompanying short-chain fatty acids.[30]

Clinically, hepatic encephalopathy is a global mental dysfunction evidenced by disorientation as to person, place, and time, developing into compromises in level of consciousness and EEG slowing. There are four stages of hepatic encephalopathy.

Stage 1: In this precoma phase, mental alertness is dimmed, and mild confusion as to time and place occurs. No EEG abnormalities are evident.

Stage 2: Mild EEG slowing begins to be reflected by intermittent muscle contractions and a flapping motion of outstretched hands (asterixis), disorientation as to person, place, and time, and drowsiness (indicating impending coma).

Stage 3: The patient is somnolent and quite disoriented when aroused. Asterixis is present, and EEG tracings slow significantly.

Stage 4: The patient will respond only to deep painful stimuli, sometimes by body and extremity rigidity. Grimacing can be evident. Positive Babinskis are present, and focal and/or generalized seizure activity may occur. Finally, unconsciousness develops, and marked slowing is evident in the EEG tracings.

Care takes the form of assuring basic life support and preventing further occurrence of the syndrome as much as possible. Dietary protein is restricted, and neomycin is administered to suppress urease-producing organisms in the bowel. If these efforts are unsuccessful, surgical exclusion of the bowel may be indicated as a last resort; surgical survival rates of such patients are extremely low, however.

Infectious Encephalopathy

Infectious encephalopathy is epitomized by Guillain-Barré syndrome, which is discussed in detail below. Other infectious encephalopathies include meningitis, encephalitis, and brain abscess, discussed in the section on neurological infections.

Guillain-Barré syndrome (GBS) is an acute, inflammatory, demyelinating polyneuropathy of unknown origin. GBS is characterized by a rapidly progressing weakness, sensory loss, and arreflexia. The illness may progress to respiratory failure in 10–23% of patients, and cardiovascular instability may occur as well. Death follows respiratory or cardiac failure in 2–5% of all patients.[31] Finally, although most patients make a satisfactory recovery, 10–15% remain disabled after one year.[32]

Clinical antecedents

The etiology of GBS is unknown. It is generally believed to be caused by a pathological immune response that is probably triggered by an antecedent condition, most frequently a nonspecific infection of the respiratory or gastrointestinal tract occurring a few weeks earlier. Specific infections by cytomegalovirus, Epstein-Barr virus, and Campalobacter jejuni are commonly, but less frequently, implicated. A variety of other associations have also been made, including recent vaccination, recent surgical procedure, preexisting autoimmune, metabolic, or neoplastic disease, insect bites, and animal bites. One study, in fact, identifies 735 possible associations

with GBS.[33] GBS does not appear to be related to a patient's age, gender, or race.

Critical referents

GBS is characterized by a diffuse inflammatory response in the peripheral nervous system, which causes demyelination of posterior spinal roots, dorsal root ganglia, spinal nerves, and corresponding peripheral and cranial nerves. The pathological process begins (stage I) as lymphocytes migrate from the nerve fiber. This process may occur at one or several points along the nerve. Edema and swelling of the myelin and Schwann cells occur, and segmental demyelination results (stage II). Demyelination may continue distal to the initial lesion (Wallerian degeneration). In more severe cases of GBS, axonal damage may occur (stage III). The exact pathology of this process is, again, unknown. If axonal destruction is severe and in close proximity to the cell body, complete nerve degeneration may occur (stage IV).

As demyelination or axonal damage progresses, nerve conduction slows. As a greater number of neurons become affected, the sensory and motor functions of the entire nerve deteriorate. Severe and widespread muscle weakness and sensory loss occur progressively. The pathological process usually affects pairs of spinal nerves, beginning in the nerves controlling the legs and ascending symmetrically to those for the trunk, arms, and cranial region. Occasionally, the process may begin in other areas, such as the cranial nerves or arms, but usually progresses to include the legs.

The recovery process depends on the severity of the nerve injury as well as the effects of any complications, such as joint contracture, deep venous thrombosis, pulmonary embolus, or respiratory infection. If nerve damage is limited to demyelination, the nerve will fully recover and function will return within weeks to months. If axonal damage occurs, nerve regeneration may take several months to a year or longer.

Resulting signs and symptoms

GBS usually occurs in three clinical phases: an acute phase, a plateau phase, and a recovery phase. The acute phase is generally characterized by an abrupt onset of sensory disturbances and motor deficits that may progress rapidly (in a matter of a few days) or more slowly (over several weeks). Autonomic symptoms may also occur at any time but are usually transient and labile. After the progressive neurological deterioration has ceased, a plateau phase occurs in which the motor and sensory deficits remain stable for a period of time before recovery begins. The plateau and recovery phases last weeks to months. The length of time is dependent on the type and severity of the nerve injury, as previously described.

Variations from the "typical" course of GBS are common. Presenting symptoms in the cranial nerves or arms or asymmetrical symptoms may be seen. Symptoms can progress more slowly, can persist longer, or can recur after recovery. Such variations may not be considered GBS, but "chronic" inflammatory demyelinating polyradiculoneuropathy.

Sensory and motor disturbances typically arise in the lower extremities and ascend symmetrically to the trunk, arms, and head; however, variation of this pattern is quite common. The progression of the disturbance may halt at any level.

Sensory disturbances usually occur first and involve paresthesia (abnormal sensation) in the fingers and feet (the stocking and glove pattern). Sensory involvement may later progress to the trunk. Paresthesia from GBS has been described as hot or cold and tingling or prickly. Hyperesthesia, hypalgesia, or pain may also occur. The pain associated with GBS is often described as burning and constant. Other abnormalities may include pain in the muscles, impaired proprioception (joint sensation), and vibratory perception.

Motor disturbances are usually symmetrical, with weakness followed by flaccid paralysis and areflexia of involved muscles. Weakness often progresses rapidly, and many patients are unable to walk upon admission to the hospital. Movements may be ataxic (uncoordinated). Proximal muscles are usually more greatly affected than distal muscles. Some muscle wasting occurs in most patients.

Weakness or paralysis of the diaphragm and intercostal muscles often occurs and leads to respiratory paralysis in 10–23% of patients.[34] Diaphragmatic weakness can quickly lead to respiratory failure.

Cranial nerve involvement occurs in about one-half to three-quarters of GBS cases.[35] The facial nerve (cranial nerve VII) is most commonly affected, resulting in facial weakness affecting the muscles of expression and eyelid closure. Other cranial nerves that may be affected include the glossopharyngeal (IX), vagus (X), accessory (XI), and hypoglossal (XII). Weakness or paralysis in these nerves affects speaking, swallowing, and chewing. Upper airway obstruction is always a concern in GBS patients who are

not intubated and ventilated, particularly if they are eating or drinking. The acoustic nerve (cranial nerve VIII) is generally not affected. A small number of patients develop weakness or paralysis of the external ocular muscles, which are controlled by the oculomotor (III), trochlear (IV), and abducens (VI) nerves. This may result in diplopia (double vision) and disconjugate eye movements and may progress to complete ophthalmoplegia.

Autonomic symptoms occur frequently with GBS but rarely persist for more than a week or two. Autonomic symptoms usually have a cardiovascular manifestation but endocrine, gastrointestinal, and bowel and bladder function may also be affected. Cardiovascular symptoms may include tachycardia or bradycardia (the latter being less common), vasomotor flushing (especially facial), fluctuating hypotension or hypertension, headache, and fluctuating diaphoresis and loss of sweating. Both dysrhythmias and blood pressure fluctuation can be life threatening. Endocrine, gastrointestinal, bowel, and bladder involvement are less common. Symptoms such as urinary incontinence or retention, paralytic ileus, and bronchial and salivary hypersecretion may occur. Transient SIADH (syndrome of inappropriate ADH) and DI (diabetes insipidus) occur rarely.

Cerebrospinal fluid (CSF) remains under normal pressure and is acellular in most patients. CSF protein begins to elevate several days after the onset of symptoms and reaches a peak in 5–6 weeks, probably as a result of widespread inflammatory disease of the nerve roots.[36] A moderate leukocytosis may be present for a short time early in the illness, but this is not a major factor in diagnosis.

A nerve conduction velocity study is usually performed to confirm a diagnosis of GBS. Nerve conduction slows soon after symptoms appear and worsens with increasing myelin or axonal damage (see Figure 3-30). An EMG may be performed to demonstrate a decrease in motor firing.

Nursing standards of care

Medical intervention for GBS has the goal of arresting the advancement of pathological processes in the immune system. Plasmapheresis with fluid replacement by plasma protein fraction or fresh frozen plasma is generally recognized as a treatment that improves outcomes.[37] Plasmapheresis is theorized to reduce the circulating antibodies or immune complexes thought to be responsible for GBS. The efficacy of corticosteroid therapy in decreasing the inflammatory response of the nerves has not been proven, but such therapy is considered to be helpful in some cases.[38] More recently, intravenous gamma globulin has been suggested as an alternative to plasmapheresis.[39]

The majority of medical care for GBS is supportive (based on symptoms) or prophylactic (to prevent complications). Supportive or prophylactic therapy may include endotracheal intubation or tracheostomy, mechanical ventilation, ECG monitoring, gastric intubation, fluid replacement therapy, urethral catheterization, arterial catheterization, blood pressure monitoring, vasopressor therapy, antiarrhythmic therapy, and prophylactic anticoagulant therapy.

The goals of nursing intervention for the patient with GBS typically include:

1. detecting deterioration in respiratory, swallowing, and autonomic regulatory functions,

2. maintenance of adequate respiration, hydration, nutrition, and elimination,
3. provision for ongoing effective communication,
4. prevention of complications, especially deep venous thrombosis, pressure sores, and joint contractures,
5. stress management, and
6. pain relief.

Nursing care of the patient with GBS involves close monitoring for progression of neurological deficits, rapid treatment of autonomic and respiratory symptoms, and prevention of complications. The patient will require intensive care until the symptoms begin to subside, usually within 2–8 weeks. The following nursing care plan describes standard practices used to care for the patient with Guillain-Barré syndrome and neurological encephalopathy.

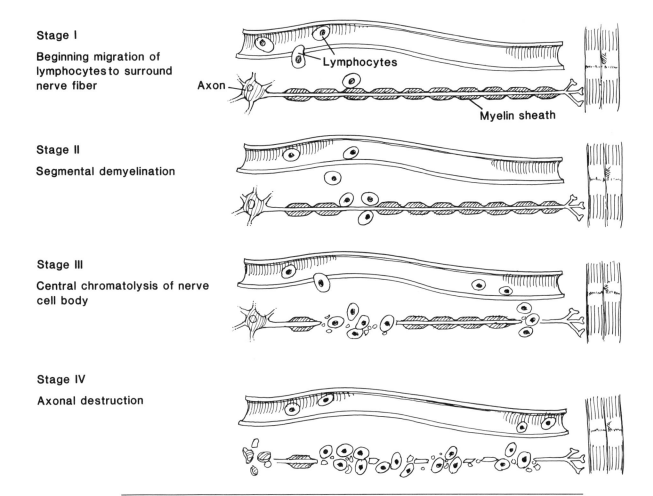

Figure 3-30 Pathogenesis of Guillain-Barré Syndrome

Nursing Care Plan for the Management of the Patient with Neurological Encephalopathy

Diagnosis	Signs and symptoms	Intervention	Rationale
Potential for alteration in respiratory function related to ineffective airway clearance and breathing patterns	Vital capacity below normal for patient	Monitor vital capacity at least every 1–4 hours	Vital capacity decreases with progression of syndrome to level affecting diaphragm and intercostal muscles
	Diminished breath sounds	Assess breath sounds and respiratory rate hourly; monitor ABGs as ordered	To evaluate respiratory and upper airway neuromuscular impairment
		Encourage coughing, deep breathing, and incentive spirometry of unintubated patients; chest physiotherapy and postural drainage as indicated	To provide for maximal pulmonary function and toileting
	Dyspnea (PaO$_2$ < 90)	Maintain intubation equipment near bedside; assist with intubation at first sign of respiratory distress	To support adequate respiratory function and optimal oxygenation
		Give intubated patient routine care for ventilation as indicated	To provide for maximal pulmonary toileting and prevent infection
		Wean patient from ventilator as vital capacity returns to normal	To promote patient's optimal breathing capacity
	Inability to remove secretions	Assess gag, cough, and swallow reflexes frequently and before meals	To decrease risk of aspiration and infection
		Elevate HOB; raise to 90 degrees at meals	To decrease risk of aspiration and infection
		Provide suction equipment at all times; suction ET/oropharynx as indicated	To decrease risk of aspiration and infection

Diagnosis	Signs and symptoms	Intervention	Rationale
Potential for fluid and electrolyte imbalance related to plasmapheresis, inadequate fluid intake, gastrointestinal suctioning, and hyperthermia	Volume excess	Accurately monitor I&O and urine specific gravity	To ascertain fluid balance status
	Volume depletion	Assess for signs of volume depletion or excess	To ascertain fluid balance status
	Electrolyte imbalances	Closely monitor electrolyte status, hematocrit, BUN, creatinine, and serum osmolality	To detect imbalances and determine renal function
		Maintain temperature within normal limits	To prevent excess loss of fluids during diaphoresis
		Assess for presence of bowel sounds and abdominal distention; measure gastric output and test pH every 8 hours; if pH < 5, administer antacids as ordered	Gastric retention and aspiration of gastric contents increase intra-abdominal and intrathoracic pressures
		Consult with dietician and initiate nutritional support as soon as appropriate; initiate tube feeding if needed	Early nutritional support promotes strength leading to recovery
		If patient is on plasmapheresis: obtain serum electrolytes before and after procedure;	Hypokalemia and hypocalcemia are commonly found
		replace volume with NS, fresh frozen plasma, or plasma protein fraction as indicated and ordered;	To maintain fluid and electrolyte balance
		monitor for reaction to transfusion of plasma;	Fever, chills, flushing or urticaria may occur
		administer epinephrine and diphenhydramine as ordered	To counteract allergic reactions

Nursing Care Plan for the Management of the Patient with Neurological Encephalopathy

Diagnosis	Signs and symptoms	Intervention	Rationale
Alteration in cardiac output related to interrupted autonomic regulation	BP > 140/90 or < 90/50 Bradyarrhythmias Tachyarrhythmias	Monitor ECG and BP continuously; monitor cardiac output and CVP when autonomic involvement is apparent	To diagnose autonomic involvement
		Administer vasopressors, hypertensives, antiarrhythmics, and anticholinergics as indicated and prescribed	To prevent life-threatening physiological changes due to autonomic involvement
		Avoid sudden changes of position; raise HOB slowly	Sudden changes of position can disturb autoregulatory balances
		Observe heart rate when suctioning; stop if heart rate decreases	To prevent vagal stimulus
		Use physiologic methods to promote cardiac output (Ace wraps, TED stockings, abdominal binders, etc.)	To maintain adequate cardiac output
Potential for corneal abrasion related to incomplete closure of eyelid	Dry cornea Redness apparent in cornea Complaints of pain in cornea	Use artificial tears as needed; apply eye shield if needed, especially during sleep	To prevent corneal abrasion and/or damage
Potential for infection due to: IV lines, indwelling Foley, endotracheal intubation, stress	Increased temperature WBC > 10,000 mm^3	Tylenol 600 mg every 4 hours PRN as ordered	To alleviate fevers
		Implement thorough hand washing between patient contacts; implement universal isolation precautions if indicated	To prevent spread of infections

Diagnosis	Signs and symptoms	Intervention	Rationale
	Redness, exudate, or increased tenderness at IV insertion site	Routine IV care with povidone-iodine solution, telfa dressing, and foam type	To prevent infections
		Change peripheral IV sites at least every 3 days or with any signs of infection or infiltration; change IV tubing every 48 hours	IV fluid is especially fertile medium for bacterial growth
		Culture suspected origins of infection	To administer antibiotics that bacteria are sensitive to
	Changes in characteristics of sputum: tan, brown, yellow, or green color and/or foul odor	Vigorous pulmonary toilet	To prevent and/or treat pulmonary congestion that can lead to infections (GBS patients are particularly susceptible to respiratory infection)
	Chest x-ray indicative of atelectasis		
	Decreased or absent breath sounds locally		
	Sediment in urine or foul-smelling urine	Routine Foley care every 8 hours; push fluids if taking fluids and not contraindicated	To prevent urinary tract infections
	WBCs in urine; hesitancy, frequency, urgency, burning, difficulty starting stream, incontinence, and/or inability to void		
	Tachycardia and/or decreasing BP		
Potential for alteration in bowel elimination related to paralytic ileus	Gastric distention	Measure abdominal girth every 8 hours and PRN	To monitor intestinal distention
	Absent bowel sounds	Monitor bowel sounds every 8 hours and PRN	To monitor return of peristalsis
	Vomiting or high gastric (NG) output	Maintain NPO until bowel sounds return	To prevent further GI irritation
		Use vented NG tube or place on intermittent suction, as ordered	Appropriate tube or suction minimizes GI irritation

435

Nursing Care Plan for the Management of the Patient with Neurological Encephalopathy

Diagnosis	Signs and symptoms	Intervention	Rationale
		Administer replacement therapy in relation to urine and NG output	To prevent fluid imbalances
		Monitor serum chemistry, especially sodium potassium	High NG output can lead to electrolyte imbalances
		Place rectal tube or suppositories PRN	To prevent rectal distention
Alteration in urinary elimination due to: decreased sensation, impaired muscle tone, altered level of consciousness, urinary tract infection	Urinary retention or incontinence	Assess voiding patterns (I&O, frequency, incontinence, retention)	Evaluation of urinary elimination pattern will help patient to attain optimal functioning
		Foley catheter to be removed as soon as possible	The risk of UTI is greater with indwelling catheter
		Institute a bladder training program as soon as possible	To establish regular bladder function
	Urinary infection: sediment in urine; WBCs in urine; hesitancy, frequency, urgency, burning, difficulty starting stream, or inability to void	Administer antibiotics as ordered	To prevent or fight any infection
		Urine C&S (routine/fungal/gram stain) when indicated or as ordered	For early detection and treatment of urinary tract infections
		Routine catheter care every 8 hours	To prevent infection
Potential for alteration in nutrition due to: dysphagia; NPO status; altered LOC; anorexia and malaise; increased nutritional requirements resulting from physical stress; constipation, diarrhea, abdominal cramping, or flatus	Complaints of lack of appetite	Assess appetite with patient and family and determine what sounds appealing and is allowed	To facilitate patient's nutritional status in any acceptable way
	Eating only small portions	Monitor tray after meals to assess amount eaten	To monitor patient's intake accurately
	Trend for weight loss	Dietary consult	To help meet body's requirement for calories
		Calculate calories	
		Weigh daily	

Diagnosis	Signs and symptoms	Intervention	Rationale
	Decreased fluid intake	Provide preferred food and fluids as much as possible; encourage fluids between meals	To facilitate nutritional status
	GI depression	Progressive diet as tolerated	To prevent GI complications
	Decreased Hgb and Hct	Closely monitor lab data	To achieve accurate picture of patient's status
	Decreased serum albumin and protein		

	Weakness and fatigue	Provide nutritional supplement as needed:
		  iron
		  protein
			GBS accelerates protein catabolism and nutritional demands increase during healing

		Provide smaller, more frequent meals	Will be better tolerated

Potential for alteration in bowel function or constipation due to:
  decreased mobility,
  change in eating patterns,
  side effects of medications,
  decreased fluid volume
	Reports of feeling constipated, "full" feeling in abdomen, inability to move bowels	Assess abdomen for bowel sounds, softness, and appearance and ask patient about discomfort at least every 12 hours	For early diagnosis of constipation in order to intervene before serious problems occur

	Decreased or absent bowel sounds	Encourage progressive activity as tolerated	To stimulate peristalsis
		Reassure patient that constipation is frequently a problem with GBS	So patient will not become overly concerned
	Inadequate oral fluid/food intake as evidenced on I&O records and calorie counts	Assess for signs of dehydration and encourage oral intake within fluid restriction limits	Hydration impedes constipation

	Symptoms of dehydration:
	  poor skin turgor,
	  sunken eyes,
	  intake less than output, weight loss
		Closely monitor electrolytes	Dehydration leads to electrolyte imbalance

	Absence of bowel movement for more than 2 days	Implement bowel regimen as ordered: milk of magnesia 30 mL p.o. every HS; consult with dietician about increased fiber in diet as indicated	Patient may need extra help to facilitate peristalsis

Nursing Care Plan for the Management of the Patient with Neurological Encephalopathy

Diagnosis	Signs and symptoms	Intervention	Rationale
Alteration in comfort related to peripheral nerve damage and denervated muscles	Subjective report of pain or paresthesia	If possible, distinguish between pain, muscle spasm, and paresthesia	To choose appropriate intervention
	Facial grimaces when handled or moved	Administer hot packs, analgesics, or medication for dysesthesia as indicated and ordered	To decrease pain and discomfort during treatments and movement
	Hesitation about moving or being moved	Frequently reposition patient gently using a draw sheet or bed cradle; handle the joints, not the body of the muscle	To promote circulation and prevent contractures in such a way as to avoid unnecessary discomfort
Impaired communication related to: endotracheal tube; respiratory paralysis; facial paralysis	Dysarthria	Listen carefully and allow patient time to speak	To encourage all patient's attempts at communication
	Intubation	Assess patient's ability to hear, understand, and speak	To establish patient's ability to communicate
	Loss of breath control	Teach appropriate strategies to promote communication: using assistive materials such as writing implements and communication board, reducing environmental distractions, decreasing anxiety, decreasing speed of communication, use of simple commands with gestures	To accomplish best level of communication possible
	Frustration during attempts at communication	Face the patient and establish eye contact to provide support and reassurance during communication attempts	To encourage patient's efforts
		Consult with speech therapist	To assist with methods of communication

Diagnosis	Signs and symptoms	Intervention	Rationale
	Frustration and impatience of family during attempts at communication	Teach family strategies for communication with patient	To accomplish maximal interaction of patient and family
	Inability to call for assistance if needed	Check with patient on a regular basis	To assess patient's needs and reassure patient that he or she is not being ignored
Impaired physical mobility due to denervation of skeleton muscle	Decreased muscle strength and tone	Maintain body alignment with assistive devices (pillows, footboard)	To prevent complications of immobility
	Paralysis	Maintain splints (especially hand and foot) as ordered	To prevent contractures
	Decreased range of motion	Consult with physiotherapist and initiate rehab program when condition is stable	To promote early recovery
		Assist with ROM exercises at least every 2–4 hours, allowing patient to do as much as possible	To maintain joint and muscle mobility and increase circulation while preventing fatigue
		Try to calm patient during activity	Anxiety increases spasticity
	Signs of impeded circulation in extremities (redness over pressure points)	Assess for tenderness, redness, warmth, and pain; apply antiembolism stockings	To identify and decrease venous stasis and deep vein thrombosis
	Impaired small motor coordination	Assist with required movements	To facilitate patient's movement
	Backaches	Flex knees PRN	Knee flexion may relieve some back pain
	Physical fatigue	Avoid vigorous movements during acute stage	To prevent fatigue
Potential for altered peripheral and cardiopulmonary tissue perfusion related to disturbance in autonomic nervous control and venous stasis	Signs of altered peripheral perfusion: hypotension; peripheral edema; redness, heat, pain, or tenderness of calf or thigh; asymmetrical calves and thighs	Assess pulses, extremities, and BP every 1–2 hours and as needed	To monitor for deep venous thrombosis or compromised circulation in extremities
		Measure calf and thigh circumference on admission and daily until out of bed at least 6 hours daily	

Nursing Care Plan for the Management of the Patient with Neurological Encephalopathy

Diagnosis	Signs and symptoms	Intervention	Rationale
		Perform ROM to extremities at least four times daily	To prevent venous pooling
		Apply antiembolism stockings, Ace wraps, and/or abdominal binders	To promote venous return
		Administer prophylactic anticoagulant therapy (usually heparin 5,000 U subcutaneously every 12 hours)	To prevent blood clot formation
		Assure proper positioning of the legs	To prevent compression of veins in popliteal space
		Avoid venipuncture in legs	Trauma to veins increases the risk of deep venous thrombosis
	Signs of altered cardiopulmonary perfusion: angina, ischemic changes on ECG, pulmonary embolus, tachypnea or dyspnea, pleural friction rub	Monitor for chest pain	Early detection will help to prevent/allay cardiac complications
		Encourage deep breathing and coughing and turning on a routine schedule	To improve circulation
		Administer supplemental oxygen as needed	To allow for adequate oxygenation to all tissues
Potential for impaired skin integrity related to: decreased sensation, restriction of movement, pain and discomfort, neuromuscular impairment, depression, diaphoresis or drainage into patient's bed	Imposed restriction of movement	Turn and position according to patient's tolerance	To promote circulation and prevent pressure spots on skin
	Impaired coordination	Assist with required movements	To facilitate movement
		Avoid common causes of injury: bedpans, poor transfer techniques, heating appliances, ice packs, injections below injury line	To prevent injury

440

Diagnosis	Signs and symptoms	Intervention	Rationale
	Decreased muscle strength preventing independent movement	Assist with required movements; turn every 1–2 hours; passive ROM exercises as indicated	To facilitate movement
		Maintain and supplement nutrition as needed	To maintain vital nutrients to skin
	Reluctance to attempt movement	Premedicate PRN as ordered to decrease discomfort accompanying movement	To facilitate movement
	Redness over pressure points	Check skin when patient is changing position or increasing time in sitting/lying position, especially at bony prominences and around devices	To ascertain quality of skin and prevent skin breakdown
	Elevated temperature	Keep patient dry	To prevent skin breakdown
	Skin lesions	Consult enterostomal therapist	To provide optimal care planning and intervention
Potential for ineffective coping by the patient or family related to: situational crisis, maturational crisis, personal vulnerability, severity of GBS impairment	Verbalization of inability to cope	Assess family's usual coping mechanisms	Questions and concerns of patient and family must be answered even if not voiced
	Inability to ask for emotional help	Assist family to identify alternative coping mechanisms; identify and acknowledge family's needs	Optimal coping must be accomplished for maximal healing
	Inability to meet role expectations	Provide information to patient and family regarding diagnosis and supportive services	Patient and family must be helped through role redefinition
	Prolonged progression of disease or disability	Support patient and family through role transition time	To help patient and family make transition

Nursing Care Plan for the Management of the Patient with Neurological Encephalopathy

Diagnosis	Signs and symptoms	Intervention	Rationale
		Encourage open communication among patient, family, and health care team	To facilitate problem solving and care planning
		Reinforce simple explanations to patient and family	During times of crisis, care must be taken not to cause information overload
	Exhaustion	Provide rest periods and offer nutrition; plan visiting schedule to accommodate interventions as well as family's schedule and rest periods; restrict visitors as appropriate	To maximize strength; to improve quality of family time as well as provide for needed rest
	Fear and anxiety	Delegate one resource and support person to assist family communication	Consistency in problem solving and care improves quality of decisions
	Inappropriate requests or hypervigilance by patient and/or family	Suggest approaches for family to assist in patient's care	Participatory care decreases family's anxiety
Potential for anxiety due to: lack of knowledge of GBS, fear of unknown, fear of death, fear of pain, fear of disability, lack of knowledge regarding hospital procedures and routines	Verbalizes lack of understanding GBS and resulting physiological processes	Make sure patient understands: effects of GBS rationale for current intervention progression of GBS	To allay patient's fears about prognosis and to attain highest level of understanding of disease and care
	Facial tension Distracting behavior Low attention span Withdrawal Twitching and shaking of extremities Inappropriate laughter or behavior Diaphoresis Tachycardia Nonadherence to treatment plan	Ascertain patient's fears and anxieties	Will allow the nurse to know just what to address
		Ascertain patient's previous hospital experiences (own as well as others')	Will help the nurse to know how to best alleviate anxieties and support positive attitudes
		Ascertain readiness to learn	Need to begin patient and family education when ready

Diagnosis	Signs and symptoms	Intervention	Rationale
		Teach patient about routines of hospital and care regimen: tubes, lines, ICU routines, visiting hours, pain medication, moving, and deep breathing and coughing; provide patient with educational booklets	To help patient and family be prepared for what is to be experienced
		Sedate as ordered PRN	To help patient relax
		Provide emotional support as needed	To help patient and family deal with the situation in the best way possible
		Consult with social worker, chaplain, etc., as needed	Multidisciplinary team effort provides broader, more comprehensive care
Potential for alteration in body temperature and injury due to rapid infusion of solutions during plasmapheresis	Hypothermia Shivering Complaints of feeling cold	Provide blankets; use blood warming coil on return line	To keep patient warm
	Coagulopathy: hemorrhage, increased PT and PTT	Observe puncture sites for bleeding; monitor blood work	To ascertain loss of coagulation factors

Medications Commonly Used in the Care of the Patient with Neurological Encephalopathy

Medication	Effect	Major side effects

Hyperosmotic agents:
  Mannitol
  Glycerol
	Reduce brain water by creating an osmotic gradient between tissue and plasma
	Reduce intracranial pressure within 1–3 hours by rapid diuresis
		Diuresis
		Electrolyte imbalances
		Rebound of increased intracranial pressure

Corticosteroids:
  Dexamethasone
  Prednisone
  Hydrocortisone
  Methylprednisolone
	Reduce cerebral edema by stabilizing the capillary endothelial junction and reducing cerebrovascular permeability
	Promote integrity of cells to inhibit flow of intracellular fluid to extracellular space
		Opportunistic infection
		Cushing's syndrome
		Nervousness
		Hyperglycemia
		Electrolyte imbalances
		Menstrual irregularities
		Skin rash
		Gastric irritation

Diuretics:
  Furosemide
  Ethacrynic acid
	Loop diuretic
	Decrease intracranial pressure within 2–4 hours
		Hypokalemia
		Hypocalcemia
		Hypomagnesemia
		Altered glucose metabolism

Barbiturates:
  Phenobarbital
  Primidone
	Control seizure activity by raising the seizure threshold of cells
	CNS depressant
	Lower cerebral metabolism
		Drowsiness leading to coma
		Confusion
		Respiratory depression
		Hypotension
		Renal failure
		Blood dyscrasias
		Hypocalcemia

Vasopressors:
  Dobutamine
  Dopamine
  Phenylephrine
	Inotropic with alpha-adrenergic stimulant
	Vasoconstriction
	Decrease tissue perfusion
		Headache
		Hypotension
		Dyspnea
		Ectopic arrhythmias

Anticonvulsants:
  Phenytoin (Dilantin)
  Valproic acid
	Prevent seizures by stabilizing the cell threshold of excitation and inhibiting the spread of impulses to adjacent tissue	CNS depression
		Cardiovascular collapse
		Nausea and vomiting
		Vertigo
		Ataxia
		Hypotension
		Coagulation defects

Valium	Decreases force of seizures by relaxing the skeletal muscles and depressing the reticular activating and limbic systems	Respiratory depression Increased frequency of generalized tonic-clonic seizures

Medication	Effect	Major side effects
Carbamazepine	Analgesic Decreases complex partial, simple partial, and generalized tonic-clonic seizures	Nausea and vomiting Vertigo Drowsiness Aplastic anemia Hepatotoxicity Inappropriate secretion of ADH
Antipyretic (Aspirin)	Analgesic Antiinflammatory Antipyretic by altering the temperature regulation center of the hypothalamus	Interference with synthesis of prothrombin Inhibition of platelet adhesiveness leading to hemorrhage Tinnitus Hypothrombinemia
Analgesic (Codeine)	Inhibits transmission of pain impulses at the subcortical level	Respiratory depression Decreased peristalsis Drowsiness Constipation

Seizure Disorders

A seizure disorder is a symptom of a specific pathology and not a disease. Unfortunately, even today a certain social stigma is attached to seizure disorders. The term "seizure disorder" has gained wide acceptance in replacing the word "epilepsy," which tends to have many negative connotations. In this section epilepsy, seizure, and seizure disorder are used interchangeably. Definitions of other terminology used are provided in Table 3-37.

Clinical antecedents

A large segment of the population is at risk for developing seizures, for large numbers of individuals experience antecedents of seizure disorders (listed in Table 3-38). In the United States, approximately 2.5 million Americans suffer from some sort of seizure disorder (1% of the population); 200,000 of these experience seizures more frequently than once a month.[40] People of all ages can be affected, and each condition can vary greatly and require individualized treatment.

Critical referents

The basic pathophysiological process that produces seizures is the recurrent, synchronous, excessive discharge of neurons from a cerebral irritation. Although the exact pathophysiology remains unknown, there is an alteration of the membrane potential, causing certain neurons to become hyperactive and hypersensitive. These abnormal neurons form an epileptogenic focus and fire paroxysmal discharges, thereby producing seizure activity. Abnormal discharges may occur without clinical signs and symptoms; however, some form of seizure activity is more commonly manifested. The abnormal discharge of neurons may be limited to a single focus or may spread throughout the brain hemispheres. The clinical presentation of seizures is as varied as the possible causes leading to different types.

Resulting signs and symptoms

The International Classification of Epileptic Seizures (ICES) is the most universally accepted system of seizure classification. Seizures are classified according to clinical onset. The ICES classification has two major types of seizures: partial seizures, referring to those of local onset; and generalized seizures, referring to bilaterally symmetrical seizures without local onset.[41] Although the ICES classification is widely used, certain traditional terminology continues to be used in the clinical arena (ICES terminology is compared to this terminology in Tables 3-39 and 3-41). The ICES is considered more accurate because it is based on EEG interpretation correlated with clinical findings. Accurate diagnosis of seizure type

Table 3-37   Common Terminology Used for Seizure Disorders

Term	Definition
Aura	Sensory experience (unusual sound, sight, taste, smell) experienced momentarily at the onset of a seizure
Convulsion	Involuntary muscular contraction (tonic-clonic)
Epilepsia partialis contina	Persistent, recurring, simple partial seizures with focal motor signs that may be associated with postictal motor weakness
Ictal	Referring to seizure activity
Ictus	The entire seizure experience
Jacksonian seizures	Simple partial seizures due to focal irritation, which may spread over the adjacent motor cortex to adjacent peripheral areas
Postictal period	Period immediately following a seizure (altered LOC, confusion, motor weakness, fatigue) until the patient returns to baseline neurological status
Prodromal period	Period of emotional or behavior change that precedes a seizure by several hours or days
Todd's paralysis	A residual neurological deficit (severe motor weakness) lasting for up to 24 hours following a seizure

Table 3-38 Precipitating Factors Leading to Seizure Disorders

Precipitating Factor	Examples
Genetic Predisposition	Chromosomal abnormalities
Birth Factors	Birth trauma, anoxia Infection Pharmaceutical agents, drugs
Infectious Disorders	Meningitis Encephalitis Fever Brain abscess
Craniocerebral Trauma	Anoxia Minor head injury Subdural and epidural hematoma
Cerebral Tumors	
Primary Intracranial Tumor	Metastatic tumors
Degenerative Diseases	Cerebellar degeneration Multiple sclerosis

Toxic Disorders	Metallic substances, lead,
	  mercury
	Allergic reaction to drugs,
	  caffeine
	Insulin
	Uremia
	Carbon monoxide

Idiopathic Precipitating Factors	Alcohol withdrawal Sedative withdrawal Anticonvulsant withdrawal Nontherapeutic drug levels Change in medication regimen Nonadherence to prescription Fatigue Physiologic stress Psychological stress Alcohol ingestion Drug abuse
Cerebrovascular Disease	Hemorrhage Thrombosis Embolism Arteriosclerosis Arteriovenous malformation Cerebral aneurysm Vasospasm

Metabolic Dysfunction	Pregnancy
	Fluid and electrolyte
	  imbalance
	Hyponatremia
	Endocrine disorders
	Menstruation
	Vitamin deficiency, pyridoxine
	Acid-base imbalance:
	  hypoxia, acidosis
	Carbohydrate metabolism,
	  hypoglycemia
	Fat and protein metabolism

Table 3-39 ICES and Traditional Classification of Partial Seizures

International Classification of Epileptic Seizures	Traditional

Simple Partial (elementary symptoms)
  motor symptoms
  special sensory/somasensory
    symptoms
  autonomic symptoms
  compound forms
	Focal

Complex Partial Impaired
Consciousness
  impairment of consciousness
  cognitive symptoms
  affective symptoms
  psychosensory symptoms
  psychomotor symptoms
    (automatism)
  compound forms
	Psychomotor or
	Temporal lobe

Partial Seizure Secondarily Generalized	Focal and/or Grand Mal

assists the physician in establishing the appropriate medication treatment program.

Partial seizures Partial seizures arise from localized areas of the cerebral cortex and are associated with focal neurological activity. They are classified as simple, complex, or secondarily generalized. Table 3-39 differentiates the three subtypes.

Clinical manifestations of simple partial seizures reflect the specific area of disturbance in the brain. Partial seizures arising from the motor cortex will stimulate motor activity, commonly manifested as face and hand movements. This motor activity usually consists of clonic, repetitive jerking movements of the limbs. This type of simple partial seizure usually lasts 15–30 seconds, and consciousness is maintained. The Jacksonian seizure can be recognized quickly, for it is a type of simple partial seizure in which the seizure activity spreads to adjacent areas along the same side of the body.

Complex partial seizures may occur in children and adults; however, the onset is usually before the age of 20. This type of seizure is generally accompanied by some degree of impairment of consciousness. The irritable focus is often located in the temporal or frontal lobe. These seizures are also easily recognizable, for they are usually associated with an aura, a sensory experience that immediately precedes the seizure and can serve to alert the individual. A list developed by the Epilepsy Foundation of America of the various types of sensory warnings that can occur is provided in Table 3-40.[42]

Table 3-40 Subjective Descriptions of Experiences During Seizure Auras

Nausea or abdominal discomfort

Faintness or dizziness

Headache

"Funny feeling all over"

Aphasia

Numbness of hands, lips, and/or tongue

Choking or throat sensation

Chest pain or dyspnea

Unpleasant taste

Dread

Dream state

Indescribable feelings

Surroundings appear strange

Vision disturbances

Palpitations

Dejà vu

Recollections

Forced thinking

Auditory disturbances

Olfactory disturbances

Source: Epilepsy Foundation of America. (1981). *How to Recognize and Classify Seizures.* p. 9.

Table 3-41 ICES and Traditional Classification of Generalized Seizures

International Classification of Epileptic Seizure	Traditional Terms
Tonic-clonic seizure	Grand mal
Tonic seizure	Limited grand mal
Clonic seizure	Limited grand mal
Absence seizure	Petit mal
Atonic seizure	Drop attack, minor motor
Myoclonic seizure	Bilateral
Infantile spasms	Massive epileptic

Clinical manifestations of complex partial seizures include alterations in behavior, altered consciousness, automatism, and semipurposeful and inappropriate movements. Examples of behaviors classed under automatism include lip smacking, chewing, facial grimacing, swallowing, staring, fumbling with clothes, and scratching genitalia. These types of seizures last for several minutes and are followed by a postictal period, during which the individual is confused.

Partial seizures become secondarily generalized when the abnormal discharges spread throughout the brain. Potentially, both simple and complex partial seizures may spread throughout the brain and result in generalized tonic-clonic seizures.

Generalized seizures Generalized seizures involve widespread areas of both hemispheres, and consciousness is lost early on. Table 3-41 displays the types of generalized seizures.

Tonic-clonic seizures are the most common type of generalized seizure and affect both children and adults. A prodromal period may occur preceding such a seizure, during which a mood or behavior

persists for several hours or even days. Following a sudden loss of consciousness there are two phases: tonic and clonic. In the tonic phase, the body stiffens, the head and neck rigidly extend, the jaws clamp shut, and the eyes roll up or turn to the side. A characteristic high-pitched cry may be heard as air is forced through the closed vocal cords and the diaphragm and chest muscles contract. The tonic phase usually lasts less than 1 minute, during all of which the patient remains apneic.

The clonic phase is characterized by violent, rhythmic movement of all extremities, which gradually decreases in frequency and intensity. The clinical presentation includes excessive salivation, frothing from the mouth, profuse sweating, dilated and unresponsive pupils, hyperventilation, tachycardia, and elevated blood pressure. Urinary and fecal incontinence may occur as the sphincter muscles relax. Physical injuries may result from a fall at the onset of the seizure. This seizure activity of the clonic phase usually lasts for several minutes and is followed by a postictal period, which also lasts for several minutes. During the postictal period, as arousal from a stuporous state occurs, the individual is lethargic and confused. Those experiencing this state are usually not aware of the seizure but may complain of a headache or generalized muscle discomfort.

Status epilepticus occurs when tonic-clonic seizures are continuous, not allowing the patient to regain consciousness. Status epilepticus may occur with other types of seizure but is extremely dangerous when associated with generalized tonic-clonic seizures.

Absence seizures Absence seizures occur mostly in children between the ages of 4 and 12. The frequency of such seizures varies from occasional to more than 100 per day. This type of seizure is characterized by a brief alteration in consciousness. For example, the child may stare vacantly without speaking or remain motionless in the same position. Previous activities are immediately resumed following the seizure. Automatism or clonic movements may be associated with absence seizures. Absence seizures are not associated with an aura, are brief in duration, and are followed by a prompt recovery.

Nursing standards of care

The optimal medical treatment of seizures requires an accurate diagnosis of the seizure type. The underlying cause of the seizure event will dictate the treatment plan and the choice of diagnostic studies. In addition to a complete history and physical examination, diagnostic evaluation may include EEG, MRI, lab investigations, angiography, CT scan, skull x-ray, PET scan, and simultaneous closed-circuit television electroencephalogram monitoring (CCTV/EEG). (The latter technique compares the clinical manifestations of the seizure to EEG recordings and is reserved for the patient most difficult to diagnose and control.) An EEG provides an analysis of electrical activity in the brain and is very valuable in the diagnosis and treatment of seizures. A description of types of EEG monitoring techniques is given in Table 3-42.

Depending upon diagnostic findings, surgical resection may be recommended if the specific area of the brain responsible for the seizure activity can be localized and removed without significant negative consequences.[43] A temporal lobectomy is most commonly performed to treat partial seizures following a comprehensive evaluation process; 60–90% of those undergoing temporal lobectomy achieve an excellent outcome, with at least a 95% decrease in seizure frequency a year after surgery.[44]

Treatment is aimed at the relief of seizure activity without adverse side effects or complications of drug and surgical therapy. Medical treatment is estimated to be capable of completely controlling seizure activity in more than half of those suffering seizures and partially controlling it in another 20–30%. The remaining 20% of those affected are considered intractable.[45] Monotherapy, the use of a single anticonvulsive medication, is advocated in the pharmacologic management of seizure disorders. After the seizure type is identified, the physician should initiate monotherapy to achieve seizure control with the least toxic effect. Table 3-43 lists common standards by which drug therapy is administered to those suffering seizure disorders. Depending on the ICES class, selected agents are used for monotherapy, including Valium, phenobarbital, Dilantin, valproic acid, paraldehyde, carbamexapine, and ethosuximide. Advantages of monotherapy include greater likelihood of patient adherence, improved seizure control, decreased risk of unpredictable consequences of drug interactions, and better control of side effects.[46]

When initiating monotherapy, an initial loading dose may be administered, at a level considered least

Table 3-42 Types of EEG Monitoring Used for Diagnosis and Classification of Seizure

Technique	Description
Ambulatory Cassette	Ambulatory inpatient and outpatient EEG monitoring
Closed-Circuit Television (CCTV/EEG)	Simultaneous EEG recordings and video monitoring
Depth Electrode Placement	Cranial recordings from probe placed in occipital or mesial temporal lobes, hippocampus, or other intercerebral areas indicated
Neonatal EEG	Extended EEG to document seizure activity in neonates
Nasopharyngeal Access EEG	Mesiotemporal EEG accomplished from leads placed in nasopharynx
Routine Hard Wire EEG	Routine EEG accomplished by routine superficial lead placement
Sleep Deprived EEG	EEG accomplished after sleep depriving patient for more than 24 hours to allow for natural sleep to occur during recording
Sphenoidal Access EEG	Anterior mesial temporal EEG accomplished from leads placed inferior to the zygomatic process in the pterygopalatine fossa
Subdural-Epidural Access EEG	EEG accomplished from leads placed via burr holes or craniectomy to monitor motor and sensory function and areas of speech
Telemetry	Ambulatory EEG accomplished within range of transmitter

Source: Santilli, N., & Sierzant, T. (1987). Advances in the treatment of epilepsy. *Journal of Neuroscience Nursing.* 19(3), p. 145.

Table 3-43 Principles to Apply When Prescribing Antiepilepsy Drugs

1. Purpose
   A. Reduce severity of seizures
   B. Reduce number of seizures
   C. Control seizures
2. Prescription guidelines
   A. Drug indication by type and frequency of seizures
      1. carefully documented description
      2. reported changes in seizure pattern
      3. regularly scheduled EEGs
      4. individual seizure pattern/cycle
         a. maximal effect during periods considered highest risk for seizure activity
            1. time of occurrence
            2. circumstances surrounding occurrence
   B. Consistency in drug serum levels
      1. consideration of specific drug properties
         a. half-life (rate of metabolism)
         b. drug interactions
         c. effects of drug initiation or withdrawal
            1. loading dose
            2. weaning
         d. therapeutic ranges
         e. toxic levels
   C. Patient adherence to drug regimen
      1. patient inability
         a. cognitive
         b. memory
      2. perception of social acceptance
      3. activities of daily living routine
      4. life-style
      5. patient education
         a. what the medication is
         b. when it should be taken
         c. how it should be taken
         d. side effects
         e. instructions for extenuating circumstances
            1. concomitant illness
            2. missed doses
            3. other medical diagnostics, procedures, and interventions
   D. Inherent risk of drug
      1. routine periodic monitoring
         a. CBC
         b. SMAC
         c. platelets
         d. SGOT and SGPT
         e. alkaline phosphatase
      2. monitoring indicated in presence of complicating disease processes
         a. hematological disorders
         b. hepatic diseases
         c. renal deficiencies

Source: Santili, N. & Sierzant, T. (1987). Advances in the treatment of epilepsy. *Journal of Neuroscience Nursing.* 19(3), p. 147.

toxic for optimal seizure control. Serum drug concentrations are monitored to help determine dosages that will maintain serum levels at a steady state within a range considered therapeutic. An acceptable dosage is one at which the patient is seizure-free, does not exhibit serious side effects, and maintains serum drug levels within the therapeutic range.

Dosages may be increased until seizure control is achieved or toxic effects are evident. The introduction of a second drug and tapering of the first drug should be performed cautiously. The first drug may be tapered after seizure control is achieved and a therapeutic serum level is established for the second drug. Drug therapy must be individualized and constantly evaluated in light of factors such as concomitant health problems, age, weight, side effects of therapy, patient adherence, half-life of the drug, and interactions of other drugs. Finally, the long-term effects of a drug are important considerations. Characteristics to be aware of in the long-term administration of medications include dose-related side effects, idiosyncratic reactions to drug therapy, and expected reactions of selected individuals to specific medications.

Prophylactic therapy may need to be continued for several years following a seizure to prevent the risk of recurrent seizures. When indicated, discontinuation of drug therapy is accomplished progressively and slowly, since an abrupt withdrawal of medication may pose further risk in the case of some sensitive and labile seizure disorders.

The treatment of seizure disorders is rapidly taking new directions. Surgical intervention, temporal lobectomy, and stereotaxic procedures are aimed at removing or destroying the epileptogenic area. In the United States an estimated 50,000 to 120,000 people suffer medically refractory partial seizure disorders that are believed to be of a type that could benefit from surgery.[47] Although diagnostic and surgical techniques have improved, surgery continues to remain underutilized in treating seizure disorders. Misconceptions regarding the limited success of medical therapy, limited resources such as equipment and expert care providers, and a lack of widespread dissemination of information are possible reasons for this underutilization.[48]

Nursing management of the patient suffering from seizure disorder is directed to preventing seizure activity, assuring protection from physical injury during a seizure, and preventing complications of seizures and treatments. The primary goals of nursing care are listed below.

1. The prevention of physical injury in the event of a seizure or physical deficit/weakness related to seizure activity.
2. Maintenance of adequate ventilation and circulation.
3. Accurate documentation of seizure events and characteristics.
4. Investigation leading to appropriate treatment of underlying causes of seizure activity.
5. Reduction of seizure severity and frequency.
6. Provision of physical, mental, emotional, and spiritual supportive nursing care while hospitalized.
7. Prevention of complications relating to seizure activity, drug therapy, and medical and nursing interventions.
8. Provision of patient and family education.
9. Planning for rehabilitation and discharge.

The nurse witnessing a seizure may assist the medical team in diagnosing the type of seizure by closely observing and accurately documenting the events surrounding the seizure. Aspects to be observed and documented are listed in Table 3-44. An accurate history of the seizure event, including both its antecedents and its sequelae, is most important to establish diagnosis. A seizure activity sheet such as that shown in Figure 3-31 is a standardized nursing assessment tool used to document information regarding seizures.

The patient suffering recurring seizures (status epilepticus) represents a medical emergency and a great nursing challenge. This patient is at very high risk for respiratory arrest and circulatory collapse. Intensive monitoring and aggressive medical and nursing management are critical to the stabilization of this patient. Intubation, mechanical ventilation, and endotracheal suctioning are usually indicated to maintain a patent airway and ensure adequate ventilation. Maintaining a patent IV access for administration of drugs is often a priority. Nasogastric suctioning may be indicated to prevent vomiting and aspiration. Attempts to identify the underlying cause of the seizures should be pursued while maintaining the above safety measures.

Further details about the standard critical care practices used in the management of a patient suffering from a seizure disorder are presented in the nursing care plan following this section.

Table 3-44 Nursing Considerations When Observing and Documenting Seizure Activity

Category of Observation	Information to Document
Events surrounding the onset of a seizure	Activity of the patient at time of onset Time of day Events surrounding onset Presence of aura Presence of prodromal period Presence of high-pitched epileptic cry
Actual seizure activity	Motor movements such as tremors and tonic and clonic activity Specific types of activity Origin of body movements Type of movements such as progressive, unilateral, or bilateral Presence of automatism (eyelid fluttering, chewing, or lip smacking) Change in level of consciousness Duration of complete loss of consciousness Position of teeth (clenching) Arousability Distractibility Pupillary responses and eye deviations Head movements Respiratory involvement including apnea, shortness of breath, foamy/frothy secretions, or cyanosis Skin color Urine/stool incontinence
Duration of seizure	Length of seizure Time of different phases of seizure process
Events of postictal period	Presence of lethargy, confusion, or other unusual behavior Complaints of headache Level of consciousness Deficits in awareness or memory Complaints of muscle soreness Motor status including transient paralysis or weakness Aphasia Perspiration Vital signs including respiratory patterns Signs of personal injury such as bloody sputum, lacerations, bruises, or head injury Nausea or vomiting Salivation Duration of sleep following seizure

Patient's Name _____

Room No. _____

Physician _____

Age _____

Date	Time	Before		During								After				Nurse's initials
		Warning signs	Part of body where seizure began	General or localized	Type of movement	Duration of each phase		Level of consciousness	Pupils	Other		Behavior	Paralysis	Location of paralysis	Sleep	
						Tonic	Clonic									

Figure 3-31 Seizure Activity Sheet
Source: Hickey, J. (1986). *The clinical practice of neurological and neurosurgical nursing,* (2nd ed.). Philadelphia: J.B. Lippincott Co., p. 536.

Nursing Care Plan for the Management of the Patient with a Seizure Disorder

Diagnosis	Signs and symptoms	Intervention	Rationale
Potential for injury due to seizure activity	Rapid onset of altered level of consciousness and seizure activity	Avoid known precipitating factors that may lead to a seizure (flickering lights, various sounds, and some smells)	Certin factors may trigger seizure activity
		Administer anticonvulsants as prescribed; monitor serum drug levels	To prevent seizure activity as much as possible; to maintain therapeutic drug levels
		Institute seizure precautions: bed in low position; raised and padded rails; only small pillow or folded towel under head; potentially harmful objects removed from proximity; oxygen and suction equipment at hand	To protect patient from injury in the event of a seizure
		Avoid use of physical restraints during seizure activity; if patient is standing or sitting at onset of seizure, assist to the floor and attempt to protect head from injury; loosen restricting clothing (belts, shirt, and collar)	To minimize risk of injury
		Assess the need for oral airway when jaw is relaxed, insert PRN	To maintain adequate ventilation and to facilitate suctioning and oxygenation
		Avoid inserting airway in mouth while teeth are clenched	May break teeth and injure soft tissue

Diagnosis	Signs and symptoms	Intervention	Rationale
		Stay with patient during seizure	To ensure patient's safety and accurate observation of seizure events
		Remain calm and approach patient in a reassuring manner	To keep situation under control and to provide the best care
		Reorient patient following seizure	Confusion following seizures is common
		Turn patient to the side following seizure	To facilitate drainage of oral secretions to prevent aspiration
		Assess patient and document the following during postictal phase: neuro status, respiratory pattern, vital signs, presence of physical injury	To assess the clinical status of the patient to ascertain further need for care and to document characteristics of seizure event, which provide valuable clinical information for accurate classification of seizure disorder
		Immediately alert health care team of medical emergency	To assure appropriate and timely life support if needed
Risk of ineffective airway clearance related to prolonged seizure activity leading to inability to swallow secretions	Seizure activity lasting longer than 30 minutes	Maintain a patent airway	To assure adequate ventilation
	Respiratory compromise	Prepare for intubation, mechanical ventilation, and nasogastric suction	To assure adequate ventilation
	Dyspnea	Administer oxygen therapy and suction PRN	To prevent cerebral hypoxia
	Copious secretions	Establish IV route and administer medication as prescribed	To attempt to stop seizure activity
		Monitor respiratory status closely	To determine complications and intervene as needed
		Implement appropriate seizure precautions	To decrease risk of further injury during seizure event

Nursing Care Plan for the Management of the Patient with a Seizure Disorder

Diagnosis	Signs and symptoms	Intervention	Rationale
Risk of altered level of consciousness related to effects of seizure activity	Confusion	Reorient patient in postictal phase	Patient may not be aware of seizure and is likely to be disoriented during postictal phase
		Establish baseline for neurological functional levels	To compare clinical findings to detect extent of compromise in neurological function
	Altered level of consciousness	Assess for changes by comparing to baseline	To detect extent of compromise in neurological function
		Communicate slowly, using short phrases that are easy to understand	To assist patient to return to previous LOC and alertness
		Gradually resume routine activities	Indicated when patient returns to previous neurological status
Potential for nonadherence to drug therapy and treatment program	Signs of not adhering to prescribed treatment	Explore reasons for nonadherence and individualize regimen to best accommodate patient's needs	An individualized regimen may promote adherence
		Explore new activities that are within those indicated and will be pleasurable and can be used to prevent boredom and sensory deprivation	To be able to offer acceptable activities rather than always denying patient's requests
	Serum drug levels not within therapeutic range	With each medication, explain purpose and importance of accurate administration	To increase patient adherence to drug therapy
		Reiterate information about medications as many times as needed	Attention span and ability to remember may be compromised by seizure activity and effects of ICU stay

Diagnosis	Signs and symptoms	Intervention	Rationale
Alteration in rest/sleep pattern related to continuous environmental stimuli, ICU routine, and interrupted sleep	Disturbances in rest/sleep pattern	Determine the patient's established rest/sleep pattern and organize nursing activities to accommodate it as much as possible	To accommodate to patient's normal pattern
	Exhaustion	Structure nursing activities to provide for fewer interruptions at normal time of sleep; design schedule to balance daytime activities with periods of uninterrupted sleep	To maximize patient's ability to relax, rest, and sleep
	Inability to fall asleep	Provide comfort measures and assistive devices individualized to patient's need; explore the possibility of relaxation therapy	To promote comfort and sleep
	Interrupted rest periods	Plan visiting schedule to accommodate interventions as well as family's schedule and rest periods; restrict visitors as appropriate	To maximize strength; to improve quality of family time as well as provide for needed rest
Potential for anxiety due to: fear of unknown, fear of death, fear of pain, fear of disability, lack of knowledge regarding hospital procedures and routines	Facial tension Distracting behavior Low attention span Withdrawal Twitching and shaking of extremities Inappropriate laughter or behavior Diaphoresis Tachycardia Nonadherence to treatment plan	Ascertain patient's fears and anxieties	Will allow the nurse to know just what to address
		Ascertain patient's previous hospital experiences (own as well as others')	Will help the nurse to know how to best alleviate anxieties and support positive attitudes
		Ascertain readiness to learn	Need to begin patient and family education when ready
		Teach patient about routines of hospital and care regimen: tubes, lines, ICU routines, visiting hours, pain medication, moving, and deep breathing and coughing; provide patient with educational booklets	To help patient and family be prepared for what is to be experienced

457

Nursing Care Plan for the Management of the Patient with a Seizure Disorder

Diagnosis	Signs and symptoms	Intervention	Rationale
		Sedate as ordered PRN	To help patient relax
		Provide emotional support as needed	To help patient and family deal with the situation in the best way possible
		Consult with social worker, chaplain, etc., as needed	Multidisciplinary team effort provides broader, more comprehensive care
Potential for ineffective coping by the patient or family related to: situational crisis, maturational crisis, personal vulnerability	Verbalization of inability to cope	Assess family's usual coping mechanisms	Questions and concerns of patient and family must be answered even if not voiced
	Inability to ask for emotional help	Assist family to identify alternative coping mechanisms; identify and acknowledge family's needs	Optimal coping must be accomplished for maximal healing
	Inability to meet role expectations	Provide information to patient and family regarding diagnosis and supportive services	Patient and family must be helped through role redefinition
	Prolonged progression of disease or disability	Support patient and family through role transition time	To help patient and family make transition
		Encourage open communication among patient, family, and health care team	To facilitate problem solving and care planning
		Reinforce simple explanations to patient and family	During times of crisis, care must be taken not to cause information overload
	Exhaustion	Provide rest periods and offer nutrition; plan visiting schedule to accommodate interventions as well as family's schedule and rest periods; restrict visitors as appropriate	To maximize strength; to improve quality of family time as well as provide for needed rest periods

Diagnosis	Signs and symptoms	Intervention	Rationale
	Fear and anxiety	Delegate one resource and support person to assist family communication	Consistency in problem solving and care improves quality of decisions
	Inappropriate requests or hypervigilance by patient and/or family	Suggest approaches for family to assist in patient's care	Participatory care decreases family's anxiety
	Inability to solve problems	Assist patient and family to identify problems and work together to solve them	Sometimes patients and families are unable to anticipate possible problems
	Unreasonable and/or excessively frequent requests (excessive use of call light)	Assist family in caring for patient and problem solve about how to continue such care after discharge	Personal involvement in care decreases anxiety while increasing self-confidence and skills
		Encourage progressively independent activities	To avoid rushing patient and family into too much responsibility for care
Potential for self-care deficit due to: muscle deconditioning; disturbance of sleep pattern; fear of overexertion; anxiety; decreased tolerance of activity	Weak muscles resulting from bedrest	Encourage activities safe to patient: minor self-care, passive ROM	To allow time for patient to regain strength
	Reports of headaches	Assess discomfort and encourage patient to request medication as appropriate	To allow for maximal rest and decreased ICP
	Fatigue	Assess patient's need for rest and sleep and incorporate rest periods during the day	To allow for needed rest and to promote relaxation and healing
	Increased heart rate and respiratory rate upon minimal activity	Facilitate calm environment (lighting, noise, interruptions, etc.)	To prevent agitation and discomfort, leading to increased ICP
	Repetitive fast speech, indicating anxiety	Encourage patient's participation in scheduling and carrying out daily care to decrease anxiety through familiarity	To prevent anxiety leading to overexhaustion and to facilitate adequate rest

Nursing Care Plan for the Management of the Patient with a Seizure Disorder

Diagnosis	Signs and symptoms	Intervention	Rationale
Potential for alteration in health maintenance due to lack of knowledge of: diagnosis, seizure disorders, medication regimen, activity, medical follow-up, referrals, home management	Inability to describe personal diagnosis and how it relates to prognosis	Instruct patient and family about diagnosis, care, and prognosis with as many repetitions as needed	Patient and family must understand in order to adhere to prescribed regimen, which will promote healing and optimal level of functioning
		Encourage questions and open discussion of problems and concerns	To allow for clear understanding and acceptance
	Inability to describe prescribed regimen and reasons for it	Instruct patient and family about medications, diet, and care arrangements: management of seizures; effectiveness of drug therapy and how to evaluate it; signs of drug toxicity; plan of daily schedule; how to recognize seizure activity and respond appropriately	To assist patient and family to safely manage seizures
	Does not distinguish between permitted and prohibited progression of activities	Include discussion of: activities in routine; balancing rest and activity; progression of activities; resumption of sexual roles and activities	To facilitate progressive resumption of activities without overdoing it and increasing risk of untoward event
	Does not know about followup appointments	Help patient and family to arrange followup plans before discharge	To promote continuity of care
	Lacks information pertaining to home management and followup arrangements	Explore discharge plans and home management with patient and family	To facilitate expeditious discharge

Diagnosis	Signs and symptoms	Intervention	Rationale
	Inability to identify professional and community services available for support	Review patient and family needs and available services and resources	To enable patient and family to utilize available resources and services to attain most comprehensive care possible
		Recommend that patient wear medic alert bracelet or necklace, which identifies medical problem, physician's name and phone number, medications, and allergies	To provide quick access to important information in case of an emergency
		Inform patient, upon discharge, to stick to moderate physical exercise and avoid extreme fatigue, high stress, and intense physical contact of a prolonged nature (contact sports)	To promote a healthy and safe life-style and maximal level of independence
		Refer patient to epilepsy support groups and Epilepsy Foundation of America	Such organizations are committed to assisting those suffering seizure disorders to attain the highest quality of life
Altered self-concept related to fear, social stigma, withdrawal, imposed dependency, life-style changes, and legal implications for persons suffering seizure disorders	Alterations in self-concept Withdrawal Depression	Assess for disturbances in self-concept	To ascertain how and to what extent patient is affected
		Through teaching of patient and family, dispel social myths and stigmas related to seizure disorders	To help remove negative connotations of seizure disorders and promote well-being of patient and family
		Support patient and family in developing positive self-concept	It is important to assist the patient and family in efforts to lead a full and productive life

Nursing Care Plan for the Management of the Patient with a Seizure Disorder

Diagnosis	Signs and symptoms	Intervention	Rationale
Potential for drug toxicity related to change in LOC and nonadherence with medication schedule	Lack of understanding of medication schedule Skin rashes Ataxia Nystagmus, diplopia Lethargy Decreased LOC, confusion Slurred speech Dizziness	Assess for signs of drug toxicity and report to physician possible need for alterations in patient teaching and/or care regimen	To promote patient's adherence to medication schedule
		Assess patient's and family's understanding of medication schedule	To effectively solve problems leading to nonadherence
		Educate patient and family as indicated, using principles of adult learning	To increase level of understanding, which will promote adherence, thus achieving maximal drug effect
		Provide written educational materials for patient and family to refer to as needed	To help patient and family continue regimen independently
		Instruct patient to use frequent preventive care such as oral hygiene	Side effects of drugs may make some patients reluctant to continue them (Dilantin may cause painful gingival membrane damage)

Medications Commonly Used in the Care of the Patient with a Seizure Disorder

Medication	Effect	Major side effects

Hyperosmotic agents:
  Mannitol
  Glycerol
	Reduce brain water by creating an osmotic gradient between tissue and plasma
	Reduce intracranial pressure within 1–3 hours by rapid diuresis
		Diuresis
		Electrolyte imbalances
		Rebound of increased intracranial pressure

Corticosteroids:
  Dexamethasone
  Prednisone
  Hydrocortisone
  Methylprednisolone
	Reduce cerebral edema by stabilizing the capillary endothelial junction and reducing cerebrovascular permeability
	Promote integrity of cells to inhibit flow of intracellular fluid to extracellular space
		Opportunistic infection
		Cushing's syndrome
		Nervousness
		Hyperglycemia
		Electrolyte imbalances
		Menstrual irregularities
		Skin rash
		Gastric irritation

Diuretics:
  Furosemide
  Ethacrynic acid
	Loop diuretic
	Decrease intracranial pressure within 2–4 hours
		Hypokalemia
		Hypocalcemia
		Hypomagnesemia
		Altered glucose metabolism

Barbiturates:
  Phenobarbital
  Primidone
	Control seizure activity by raising the seizure threshold of cells
	CNS depressant
	Lower cerebral metabolism
		Drowsiness leading to coma
		Confusion
		Respiratory depression
		Hypotension
		Renal failure
		Blood dyscrasias
		Hypocalcemia

Vasopressors:
  Dobutamine
  Dopamine
  Phenylephrine
	Inotropic with alpha-adrenergic stimulation
	Vasoconstriction
	Decrease tissue perfusion
		Headache
		Hypotension
		Vasoconstriction
		Dyspnea
		Ectopic arrhythmias

Anticonvulsant:
  Phenytoin (Dilantin)
  Valproic acid
	Prevent seizures by stabilizing the cell threshold of excitation and inhibiting the spread of impulses to adjacent tissue	CNS depression
		Cardiovascular collapse
		Nausea and vomiting
		Vertigo
		Ataxia
		Hypotension
		Coagulation defects

Valium	Decreases force of seizures by relaxing the skeletal muscles and depressing the reticular activating and limbic systems	Respiratory depression Increased frequency of generalized tonic-clonic seizures

Medications Commonly Used in the Care of the Patient with a Seizure Disorder

Medication	Effect	Major side effects
Carbamazepine	Analgesic Decreases complex partial, simple partial, and generalized tonic-clonic seizures	Nausea and vomiting Vertigo Drowsiness Aplastic anemia Hepatotoxicity Inappropriate secretion of ADH
Antipyretic (Aspirin)	Analgesic Antiinflammatory Antipyretic by altering the temperature regulation center of the hypothalamus	Interference with synthesis of prothrombin Inhibition of platelet adhesiveness leading to hemorrhage Tinnitus Hypothrombinemia
Analgesic (Codeine)	Inhibits transmission of pain impulses at the subcortical level	Respiratory depression Decreased peristalsis Drowsiness

CHAPTER 3 POST-TEST

1. An intraventricular catheter is contraindicated for the patient suffering from:
   a. a midline shift.
   b. a fractured cranium.
   c. an enlarged ventricular space.
   d. an intact skull injury.

2. The most important purpose of mechanical hyperventilation of the patient suffering increased intracranial pressure is:
   a. to increase oxygen delivery to brain cells, thus enhancing regeneration.
   b. to eliminate excess carbon dioxide, thus decreasing vasodilation.
   c. to increase intrathoracic pressure, thus decreasing vasodilation.
   d. to hyperoxygenate the patient, thus making it safe to suction him or her.

3. The use of barbiturate therapy leads to all of the following clinical outcomes *except*:
   a. preservation of ischemic cerebral cells from irreversible damage.
   b. vasodilation, and thus increased blood flow to damaged tissues.
   c. decreased cerebral metabolism, and thus stabilization of cell membranes.
   d. decrease of intracranial pressure to acceptable levels.

4. Nursing interventions for the patient in barbiturate coma include:
   a. institution and maintenance of enteral nutrition.
   b. assuring that vasodilator drugs are readily available for emergency use.

   c. maintaining cerebral perfusion in the range 30–40 mm Hg.
   d. assuring that adequate gas exchange is accomplished.

5. Seizure activity causes all of the following physiological changes *except*:
   a. increased cerebral metabolic rate.
   b. increased pCO_2 levels.
   c. decreased pO_2 levels.
   d. decreased bicarbonate levels.

6. The seizure that is typified by a short lapse of consciousness that may or may not be associated with focal myoclonus is referred to as:
   a. petit mal.
   b. akinetic.
   c. Jacksonian.
   d. psychomotor.

7. Which of the following is *not* true of the Jacksonian seizure?
   a. It may be associated with an aura.
   b. It may start with one body part and progress to a generalized state.
   c. It is considered of a focal motor nature.
   d. It usually lasts 2–10 seconds.

8. The grand mal seizure is best described as:
   a. including tonic-clonic symmetric movements involving the whole body.
   b. lasting 2–10 seconds and generally not experienced by individuals older than 12 years.
   c. associated with febrile reactions of core temperature higher than 104°F.
   d. occurring with elaborate behavior.

ENDNOTES

1. Boss, B. (1986). The neuroanatomical and neurophysiological basis of learning. *Journal of Neuroscience Nursing*, 18(5), pp. 256–264.

2. Kunkel, D. (1990). *Core Curriculum for Neuroscience Nursing* (3rd ed.). Chicago: American Association of Neuroscience Nurses, p. Va 1.

3. Hickey, J. (1986). *The clinical practice of neurological and neurosurgical nursing* (2nd ed.). Philadelphia: J.B. Lippincott, p. 132.

4. Ibid., p. 250.

5. Raimond, J., & Taylor, J. (1986). *Neurological Emergencies and Effective Nursing Care*. Rockville, Maryland: Aspen Systems, p. 144.

6. Ausman, J., Diaz, F., Malik, G., Fielding, A., & Son, C. (1985). Current management of cerebral aneurysms: Is it based on facts or myths? *Surgical Neurology*, 24, p. 625.

7. Kassell, N., & Drake, C. (1982). Timing of aneurysm surgery. *Neurosurgery*, 10(4), p. 514.

8. Willis, D. & Drake Harbit, M. (1989). A fatal attraction: Cocaine related subarachnoid hemorrhage. *Journal of Neuroscience Nursing*, 21(3), p. 171; MacDonald, E. (1989). Aneurysmal subarachnoid hemorrhage. *The Journal of Neuroscience Nursing*, 21(5), p. 314.

9. Ausman, J., Diaz, F., Malik, G., Fielding, A., & Son, C., op. cit, p. 626.

10. Kassell, N., Sasaki, T., Colohan, A., & Nazar, G. (1985). Cerebral vasospasm following aneurysmal subarachnoid hemorrhage. *Stroke*, 16(4), p. 562–567.

11. Mitchell, S. & Yates, R. (1986). Cerebral vasospasm: Theoretical causes, medical management and nursing implications. *Journal of Neuroscience Nurses*, 18(6), p. 316.

12. Kassell et al., op. cit., p. 563.

13. Heros, R., & Kistler, P. (1983). Intracranial arterial aneurysms: An update. *Stroke*, 14(4), p. 629.

14. MacDonald, E., op. cit., p. 318.

15. Heros and Kistler, op. cit.

16. Kocan, M. (1988). Electrocardiographic changes following subarachnoid hemorrhage. *Journal of Neuroscience Nursing*, 20(6), p. 363.

17. Heros and Kistler, op. cit., p. 628.

18. Nikas, D. (1985). The neurologic system. In Alspach, J., & Williams, S. (1985). *Core Curriculum for Critical Care Nursing*, Philadelphia: W.B. Saunders, p. 254.

19. Kassell and Drake, op. cit., p. 516.

20. Hummel, S. (1989). Cerebral vasospasms: Current concepts of pathogenesis and treatment. *Journal of Neuroscience Nursing*, 12(4), p. 221.

21. Stover, S., & Fine, P., (Editors). (1986). *Spinal Cord Injury: The Facts and Figures*. Birmingham, Alabama: The National Spinal Cord Injury Statistical Center. University of Alabama at Birmingham.

22. Emhoff, T., Wedel, S., Geisler, F., & Gens, D. (1987). *The Occurrence and Detection of Deep Venous Thrombosis and Pulmonary Embolism in the Spinal Cord Injured Patient: A Prospective Study*. Paper presented at the Society of Critical Care Medicine Meeting, Anaheim, California, May.

23. Zejdlik, C. (1992). *Management of Spinal Cord Injury* (2nd ed.). Boston: Jones and Bartlett Publishers.

24. Hickey, J., op. cit., p. 579.

25. American Heart Association. (1989). *1990 Heart and Stroke Facts*. Dallas, Texas: American Heart Association National Center, p. 2.

26. Sundt, T. (1987). *Occlusive Cerebrovascular Disease Diagnosis and Surgical Management*. Philadelphia: W.B. Saunders, p. 12.

27. Adams, R. & Victor, M. (1985). *Principles of Neurology*. New York: McGraw-Hill, p. 789.

28. Ibid., p. 790.

29. Ibid., p. 794.

30. Ibid., p. 795.

31. McKhann, G., et al. (1988). Plasmapheresis and Guillain-Barré Syndrome: Analysis of prognostic factor and the effect of plasmapheresis. *Annals of Neurology*, 23(4), p. 347–353. Kleyweg, R., et al. (1988). Treatment of Guillain-Barré Syndrome with high-dose gamma globulin. *Neurology*. 38, p. 1639–1641.

32. Kleyweg, R. et al., Ibid; Winer, J. (1988). A prospective study of acute idiopathic neuropathy. I. Clinical features and their prognostic value. *Journal of Neurology, Neurosurgery, and Psychiatry*, 51, p. 605–612.

33. Ibid.

34. McKhann et al., op. cit.; Winer, J., op. cit.

35. Winer, J., op. cit.

36. Adams, R. & Victor, M. (1985). *Principles of Neurology* (3rd ed.). New York: McGraw-Hill.

37. McKhann et al., op. cit.

38. Adams and Victor, op. cit.

39. Kleyweg et al., op. cit.

40. DeVroom, H., & Considine, E. (1987). Advances in the localization of epileptic loci for surgical resection. *Journal of Neuroscience Nursing*, 19(2), p. 77.

41. Epilepsy Foundation of America. (1981). *How to Recognize and Classify Seizures*. Landover, Maryland: Epilepsy Foundation of America, p. 7.

42. Ibid., p. 9.

43. Brewer, K., & Sperling, M. (1988). Neurosurgical treatment of intractable epilepsy. *Journal of Neuroscience Nursing*. 20(6), p. 369.

44. Santilli, N., & Sierzant, T. (1987). Advances in the treatment of epilepsy. *Journal of Neuroscience Nursing*. 19(3), p. 150.

45. Ibid., p. 146.

46. Penry, J. (1986). Epilepsy: Defining the disease and management goals. In Penry, J., (Editor). *Epilepsy: Diagnosis, Management, and Quality of Life*. New York: Raven Press, p. 14.

47. Brewer and Sperling, op. cit., p. 366.

48. DeVroom and Considine, op. cit., p. 78.

The
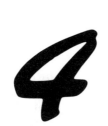
4 Cardiovascular System

CHAPTER 4 PRE-TEST

1. Digitalis:
   a. has a toxic potential unrelated to potassium and calcium levels.
   b. has a negative inotropic effect.
   c. may interfere with AV conduction.
   d. has its effect only on the myocardium.

2. The cardiac action potential:
   a. lacks a relative refractory period.
   b. is dependent on increased permeability to K^+.
   c. is prolonged due to decreased permeability to Na^+.
   d. prevents circus movement in the normal heart.

3. In relating electrical and mechanical events:
   a. the T wave occurs during diastole.
   b. atrial filling initiates the P wave.
   c. ventricular muscle shortening occurs in the P-R interval.
   d. the R-T interval determines the duration of systole.

4. The cardiac index:
   a. tends to remain constant throughout adulthood.
   b. is approximately 1.7 m^2 for a 70-kg human.
   c. is usually reduced during exercise.
   d. provides comparison of cardiac output between different size adults.

5. In cardiogenic shock:
   a. cardiac output is decreased, blood volume is unchanged, and total peripheral resistance is increased.
   b. cardiac output is unchanged, blood volume is decreased, and total peripheral resistance is increased.
   c. cardiac output is decreased, blood volume is decreased, and total peripheral resistance is increased.
   d. cardiac output is decreased, blood volume is unchanged, and total peripheral resistance is decreased.

6. The four most important determinants of myocardial oxygen consumption in a 56-year-old patient with inferior myocardial infarction are:
   a. stroke volume, inotropic state of the heart, heart rate, and myocardial wall tension.
   b. left ventricular stroke work, heart rate, left atrial pressure, and inotropic state.
   c. left ventricular pressure, left ventricular stroke work, inotropic state, and heart rate.

d. cardiac output, total peripheral resistance, subendocardial tissue pressure, and stroke volume.

7. When a patient was admitted for care of a 25% loss in blood volume due to a severed femoral artery, physiological compensatory changes were evidenced by:
   a. increased vasomotor tone, decreased cutaneous blood flow, decreased capillary fluid filtration, and decreased GI blood flow.
   b. increased vasomotor tone, increased cutaneous blood flow, decreased capillary fluid filtration, and decreased GI blood flow.
   c. decreased vasomotor tone, decreased cutaneous blood flow, unchanged capillary fluid filtration, and increased GI blood flow.
   d. increased vasomotor tone, decreased cutaneous blood flow, increased capillary fluid filtration, and increased GI blood flow.

8. The increase in arterial pulse pressure often seen with increasing age is due to:
   a. a decrease in the compliance of the arterial walls combined with the gradual decrease in mean arterial pressure.
   b. a decrease in the compliance of the arterial walls combined with the gradual increase in mean arterial pressure.
   c. an increase in the compliance of the arterial walls combined with the gradual decrease in mean arterial pressure.
   d. an increase in the compliance of the arterial walls combined with the gradual increase in mean arterial pressure.

Please refer to the following graph to answer questions 9 and 10.

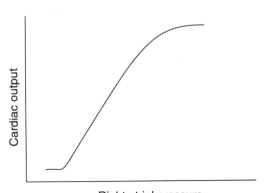

Right atrial pressure

9. Sympathetic stimulation would:
   a. decrease the slope of this curve.
   b. decrease cardiac output at any atrial pressure.
   c. shift this curve to the left.
   d. have a hypoeffective influence on the heart.

10. In a patient experiencing congestive heart failure:
    a. the curve would move to the left.
    b. the curve would move to the right.
    c. the curve would move to the left during vagal stimulation.
    d. none of the above is true.

11. Which of the following can directly depress the pumping function of the heart?
    a. Quinidine, Lidocaine, and Propranolol.
    b. Digitalis, Quinidine, and Lidocaine.
    c. Digitalis, Lidocaine, and Propranolol.
    d. Quinidine, Lidocaine, and calcium.

12. A patient states that he has severe crushing mid-chest pain, which has been present for the last 20 to 30 minutes with no relief from his bedside nitroglycerine tablets. He has a history of angina. His pulse is 110, BP is 110/70 mm Hg when taken twice in a row at 10-minute intervals. He is in a sinus rhythm. The first drug to administer, per orders, is
    a. propranolol 1.0 mg IV every 15 minutes to a maximum of three doses.
    b. morphine sulphate 2–10 mg IV titrated to relieve pain.
    c. prednisone 30 mg IM.
    d. morphine sulphate 15 mg IM.

Please refer to the following clinical vignette to answer questions 13 through 19.

A 60-year-old male presents to the ER because of a "cramping ache in his chest." He reports a 36-hour history of aching chest discomfort with periodic regular palpitations. Having treated his discomfort with soda water to no avail, he drove to the ER.

Past family history: Father died of a "heart arrest" at age 55; two brothers are alive and well at ages 58 and 65.

Past medical history: Denies rheumatic heart disease; (+) for untreated hypertension.

Past surgeries: Unrelated ENT surgeries; cholecystectomy.

Familial support: Lives alone and works 60 hours per week.

Physical Exam: Nonradiating chest pain accompanied by diaphoresis, slight dyspnea, and nausea.

V.S.: 98.6°F; pulse 118/minute; respirations 20/minute, unlabored; BP 148/98.

Neuro: Unremarkable.

CV: No JVD at 30°; grade II/IV holosystolic murmur at apex; no gallop; good peripheral pulses; PMI at sixth ICS to left of sternum along midclavicular line; pulse with normal intensity; no heaves or thrills.

Abdomen: Liver palpated at costal border; abdomen is soft and nontender.

Laboratory: Normal U/A; normal CBC; CPK 164 iu/L; LDH 219 iu/L; SGOT 31 iu/L.

Chemistry: Na = 140; Cl = 99; CO_2 = 22; K = 3.2; glucose = 126; BUN = 18; creatinine = 1.3; osmolarity = 190.

ECG:

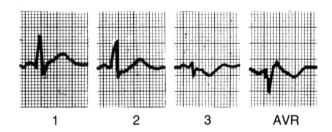

1   2   3   AVR

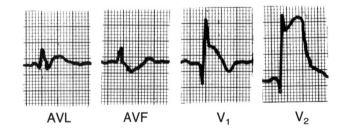

AVL   AVF V_1 V_2

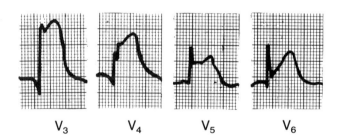

V_3 V_4 V_5 V_6

13. The patient is probably being admitted for:
    a. acute inferior MI.
    b. acute pericarditis with myocardial ischemia.
    c. acute anterior MI.
    d. acute anterolateral MI.

14. The coronary artery(ies) most likely affected is (are):
    a. right coronary artery.

b. left anterior descending artery.

c. left circumflex artery.

d. left anterior descending and circumflex arteries.

15. Based on ECG readings, enzyme reports, and symptoms, the most probable immediate medical action will be to:
    a. bolus and infuse thrombolytic agent.
    b. prophylactically bolus and infuse Lidocaine.
    c. hydrate to prevent MI extension.
    d. monitor and observe.

16. The history of hypertension is most likely a result of:
    a. azotemia.
    b. hyperaldosteronism.
    c. essential hypertension.
    d. congestive heart failure.

17. In teaching this patient about risk factors of cardiovascular disease, special emphasis should be placed on:
    a. stress factors and their control.
    b. low cholesterol and low sodium diets.
    c. family history.
    d. hypertension control.

18. If an S_4 gallop developed, it would most likely indicate:
    a. pulmonary hypertension.
    b. left ventricular failure.
    c. mitral insufficiency.
    d. ischemic damage to the cardiac septum.

19. Which arrhythmia is most likely to be associated with this type of MI?
    a. Wenchebach AV block
    b. multifocal atrial tachycardia
    c. sinus bradycardia
    d. ventricular tachycardia

Please refer to the following cardiac rhythm strip and data to answer questions 20 through 23.

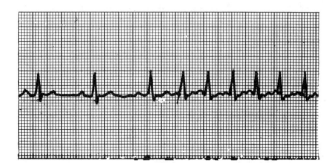

Clinical antecedents: Frequent PACs.

VS before rhythm: Respirations 32/minute; BP 148/88.

ABGs: pH = 7.37; pCO_2 = 43; pO_2 = 84; HCO_3 = 24; O_2 sat. = 98%.

Treatment: O_2 via nasal cannula at 5 L/min.

Clinical course: When the above rhythm started, the patient complained of palpitations and his BP fell to 92/60 within 3 minutes.

20. The most likely interpretation of this rhythm is:
    a. sinus tachycardia.
    b. paroxysmal atrial tachycardia.
    c. multifocal atrial tachycardia.
    d. ventricular tachycardia.

21. The greatest risk of this rhythm for a patient with an acute MI is:
    a. increased risk of myocardial irritability and ventricular tachycardia.
    b. the rapid heart rate will more readily induce left ventricular failure.
    c. decreased myocardial filling time will decrease the amount of oxygenated blood flowing through the coronary arteries.
    d. the heart is more refractory to pharmacologic interventions during the acute stages of MI.

22. The most immediate medical treatment for this patient will probably be:
    a. observe for 5 minutes for spontaneous resolution.
    b. carotid massage.
    c. Inderal 1 mg, intravenous push over 2 minutes.
    d. Verapamil 15 mg, intravenous push over 5–10 minutes.

23. Upon assessment of this rhythm, you would expect to find all *except*:
    a. hepatomegaly and increased peripheral edema.
    b. increased systolic ejection murmur and S_3 gallop after the rhythm is resolved.
    c. weaker, threadier peripheral pulses.
    d. rales in both lungs.

Please refer to the following clinical scenario to answer questions 24 through 27.

A 45-year-old male is admitted after two days of severe retrosternal distress. Four weeks prior, he suffered a mild upper respiratory tract infection with a nonproductive cough, low-grade fever, and myalgias. Although he improved gradually, two days before admission he developed intermittent grabbing pain in the retrosternal region, which worsened with deep respirations and remained unaffected by exertion. Now he complains of an oppressive sensation over the left side of his chest, which is partially relieved in some positions, and dyspnea, which prevents him from sleeping.

Past medical history: Unremarkable.

Physical exam: Moderate respiratory distress with nasal flaring and use of accessory muscles; agitation and restlessness; pale, cool, and diaphoretic skin.

Lungs: Dull to percussion in left base.

PMI: Palpated at fifth ICS left of sternum, shifted laterally from the midclavicular line.

Heart Sounds: Muffled; pericardial friction rub noted only when patient is upright and forward.

Periphery: Trace pedal edema.

JVP at 4 cm above clavicle.

Positive hepatojugular reflex when supine.

VS: T = 100.2°F; P = 94/min; R = 26/min; BP = 108/86 (falling 14 mm upon inspiration).

24. The above physical findings are suggestive of:
    a. acute pericarditis.
    b. hiatal hernia.
    c. angina pectoris.
    d. pericardial effusion.

25. Measures that might relieve the respiratory distress felt by this patient include all *except*:
    a. upright position with arms on pillows.
    b. oxygen therapy.
    c. relaxation exercises.
    d. reduction of preload.

26. ECG changes that might be anticipated with this disorder are:
    a. tented T waves in V4–V6.
    b. ST elevations in precordial leads.
    c. sagging ST segments in precordial leads.
    d. low voltage in limb leads.

27. Abnormal laboratory values that can be anticipated with the above are:
    a. increased CPK, increased creatinine, increased glucose.
    b. decreased pO_2, increased Hct, increased SGPT.
    c. increased WBC, increased SGOT, increased erythrocyte sedimentation rate.
    d. decreased pO_2, increased Hct, increased SGPT.

28. The diagnostic test most commonly indicated when pericarditis or pericardial effusion is suspected is:
    a. muga scan.
    b. chest CT.
    c. chest x-ray.
    d. echocardiogram.

29. A sign that pericarditis is being complicated by pericardial effusion is:
    a. the presence of increased symptoms of right heart failure.
    b. the pericardial friction rub becomes more pronounced.
    c. the pulse pressure widens.
    d. the patient's level of consciousness is altered.

30. Beck's triad of symptoms of impending cardiac tamponade consists of:
    a. arterial hypotension, muffled heart sounds, and elevated JVP.
    b. chest pain, pericardial rub, and dyspnea.
    c. hepatomegaly, pulsus paradoxis, and hypoxemia.
    d. narrowed pulse pressure, ventricular dysrhythmias, and elevated JVP.

31. Medical management of cardiac tamponade is most likely to be:
    a. bedside emergency pericardial tap.
    b. insertion of a pericardial catheter for long-term drainage.
    c. pericardial sclerosis.
    d. pericardial window.

32. What is the mechanism by which R on T phenomenon causes ventricular tachycardia?
    a. Irritable focus overrides the heart's depolarization potential.
    b. A new stimulus to the heart during the relative refractory period can lead to aberrant conduction.
    c. A new stimulus to the heart during the absolute refractory period can lead to aberrant conduction.
    d. An irritable stimulus from the ventricle can override the normal conduction pathways.

33. The mechanism by which atropine works to increase heart rate is:
    a. sympathetic nervous system stimulation.
    b. parasympathetic nervous system stimulation.
    c. vagus nerve inhibition.
    d. direct stimulation of the heart to increase intrinsic rate.

34. When the heart is hypereffective, the cardiac output is shifted upward. Which of the following would cause this to occur?
    a. positive pressure breathing
    b. cardiac tamponade
    c. cardiac anoxia
    d. hypertrophy

35. Which of the following vascular beds has the largest resting blood flow per 100 g of tissue?
    a. renal
    b. cerebral
    c. coronary
    d. salivary glands

36. Which of the following vascular beds has the highest resting resistance?
    a. liver
    b. cerebral
    c. skeletal muscle
    d. renal

37. Which of the following vascular beds has the largest arteriovenous oxygen difference?
    a. myocardial
    b. central nervous system
    c. renal
    d. salivary glands

38. By convention, when connecting the standard limb leads:
    a. the left arm is always negative, and the left leg is always positive.
    b. the right arm is always negative, and the left leg is always positive.
    c. the right arm is always negative, and the nurse can choose polarity for the others.
    d. the left leg is always negative, and the right arm is always positive.

39. Autoregulation of local blood flow is:
    a. the intrinsic tendency of an organ or tissue to maintain a constant resistance despite changes in perfusion pressure.
    b. the intrinsic tendency of an organ or tissue to maintain a constant blood flow despite changes in resistance.
    c. the intrinsic tendency of an organ or tissue to maintain a constant blood flow despite changes in its metabolic rate.
    d. the intrinsic tendency of an organ or tissue to maintain a constant blood flow despite changes in perfusion pressure.

Overview of the Cardiovascular System

The cardiovascular system is composed of the heart and blood vessels. It is a vital transport system responsible for providing nutrients and oxygen to all body cells and for removing metabolic waste products from the cells. This closed system consists of a major pump and conduit and may be further subdivided into the heart, the systemic circulation, and the pulmonary circulation.

The cardiovascular system applies the concept of dynamic equilibrium to maintain homeostasis. Although the actual mechanical function of the pulsating heart maintains the blood flow, the real phenomenon occurs when, upon demand, the cardiovascular system integrates with the nervous, renal, pulmonary, and endocrine systems to adjust blood supply to specific body areas.

Anatomy and Physiology of the Cardiovascular System

The heart, the central organ of the cardiovascular system, is a bioelectrically driven muscular pump. It lies within the mediastinum, between the sternum and the spinal column. It is bordered laterally by the lungs, which overlay most of the heart's anterior surface, and inferiorly by the diaphragm. The heart approximates the size of the person's closed fist and is shaped like a blunt cone. The heart's great vessels suspend the heart, directing the broader end, or base, upward, backward, and to the right. The pointed end, or apex, points downward, forward, and to the left (Figure 4-1).

The heart is enclosed in a tough, fibrous sac—the pericardium—which is divided into two layers: the fibrous pericardium (outer layer), and the serous pericardium. The serous pericardium is further divided into two layers: parietal and visceral. The visceral pericardium is the outer surface layer of the heart. These two layers are separated by a potential space, which is lubricated by approximately 15–20 mL of serous fluid that prevents friction when the surfaces touch during contraction.

The heart is composed of three layers: epicardium, myocardium, and endocardium. The epicardium is the surface layer of the heart and is synonymous with the visceral layer of the serous pericardium. That is, the epicardium is the serous membranous lining of the pericardial sac. There are two sulci, interventricular and coronary, which form indentations on the epicardial surface. The coronary

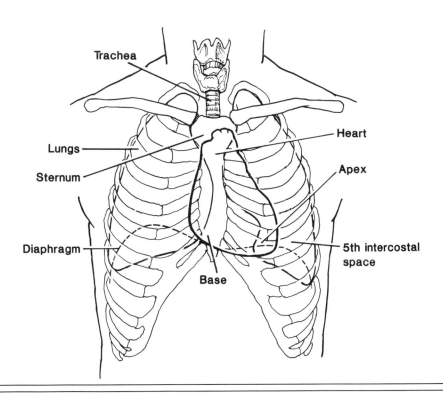

Figure 4-1 Position of the Heart

arteries traverse within these grooves. The myocardium is the major muscle mass of the heart. It is a mass of individual muscle cells that contain actin and myosin protein myofibrils connected by a tubular system (the sarcoplasmic reticulum) and is enclosed in a membranous sheath (the sarcolemma). The endocardium is the innermost layer of the heart. It lines the heart chambers and the valves and is continuous with the lining of the major vessels.

Coronary Chambers

The heart is divided into right and left halves by a muscular partition called the septum (Figure 4-2). The septum extends from the base to the apex of the heart. After birth, there is normally no communication between the left and right sides. The septum and trabeculae divide the heart into four chambers: right atrium, left atrium, right ventricle, and left ventricle.

The atria are reception chambers for blood entering the heart. Both atria are thin-walled structures located behind, slightly above, and to the right of their corresponding ventricles. The trabeculae divide the atria and ventricles.

The right atrium receives unoxygenated (venous) blood from the superior and inferior venae cavae and the coronary sinus. The venae cavae enter the dorsum of the right atrium, and the coronary sinus, which drains blood from the coronary circulation, enters anteriorly and superiorly to the entrance of the inferior vena cava. Also, numerous small thebesian veins drain some of the venous blood from the myocardium directly into the right atrium. The auricle, a small, ear-shaped appendage, opens into the right atrium above and behind the tricuspid valve.

The left atrium receives oxygenated (arterial) blood from the lungs via four pulmonary veins. In contrast to the inner surface of the right atrium, which comprises multiple prominent bands, the interior of the left atrium is smooth, except within its auricle.

The right ventricle is a thin-walled, crescent-shaped musculature, approximately 3–4 mm thick. The inflow tract directs blood to the apex, where it is routed, during contraction, to the outflow tract and through the pulmonic valve. The right ventricle's pumping action is similar to that of a bellows pump.

The left ventricle, with walls approximately 8–14 mm thick, contains approximately three times more muscle mass than the right ventricle. It is cone-shaped and is positioned posteriorly and laterally to the left of the right ventricle. The left ventricle is a high-pressure chamber that pumps (or more appropriately, squeezes) blood into a high-pressure systemic circulation.

Valves

The main purpose of the cardiac valves is to maintain a unidirectional blood flow through the heart chambers. The valves open and close in response to changes in volume and pressure within the heart. Cardiac valves are classified as atrioventricular (AV) valves and semilunar valves.

There are two AV valves: the tricuspid (between right atrium and right ventricle), and the mitral (between left atrium and left ventricle). The tricuspid is formed by three cusps and the mitral by two cusps. In diameter the cusps have greater surface areas than their apertures, so, during closing, there is an overlapping of tissue surfaces. The cusps have tendinous attachments, called chordae tendinae, that are inserted into thick muscle bodies called papillary muscles. Papillary muscles are attached to the ventricular walls and the interventricular septum. The AV valves open on ventricular diastole and close as ventricular pressure increases during systole.

The two semilunar valves that direct blood flow into the pulmonary and systemic circulation are called the pulmonary or pulmonic valve (between the right ventricle and the pulmonary artery) and the aortic valve (between the left ventricle and the aorta). Each valve has three thin, delicate leaflets that are somewhat thickened along their edges. These cusps are attached at the base to a thick fibrous ring. The semilunar valves open when the ventricle contracts and close after ventricular systole, when pressure in the outflow tract is greater than in the ventricle.

Vascular System

The vascular system includes arteries, arterioles, capillaries, venules, and veins. The anatomy of this system is composed of multiple tissue layers that vary as to type and size.

The arteries are composed of three tissue layers: tunica intima, tunica media, and tunica externia (or adventitia). The tunica intima consists of three cell layers: a layer of endothelial cells, a layer of delicate connective tissue that is found only in the larger vessels, and an elastic layer consisting of a membrane or network of elastic fibers. The middle tissue layer of the arteries, or the tunica media, contains mostly smooth muscle fibers and various amounts of elastic and collagenous tissue. In larger arteries, elastic fibers form layers that alternate with the layers of muscle fibers, and some of the larger arteries contain white connective tissue fibers. The structure of this middle layer makes the arteries elastic and extensile, two properties that determine the arteries' proper functioning. The degrees of arterial extensi-

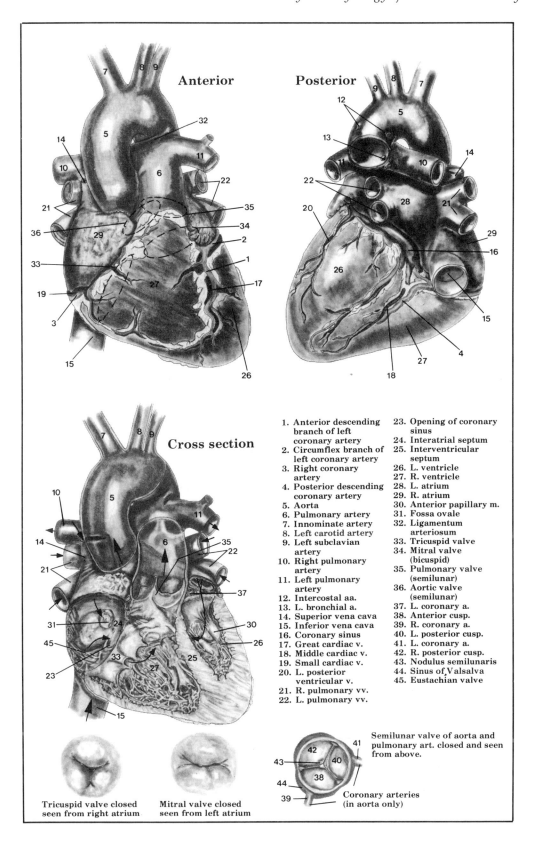

Anterior

Posterior

Cross section

1. Anterior descending branch of left coronary artery
2. Circumflex branch of left coronary artery
3. Right coronary artery
4. Posterior descending coronary artery
5. Aorta
6. Pulmonary artery
7. Innominate artery
8. Left carotid artery
9. Left subclavian artery
10. Right pulmonary artery
11. Left pulmonary artery
12. Intercostal aa.
13. L. bronchial a.
14. Superior vena cava
15. Inferior vena cava
16. Coronary sinus
17. Great cardiac v.
18. Middle cardiac v.
19. Small cardiac v.
20. L. posterior ventricular v.
21. R. pulmonary vv.
22. L. pulmonary vv.
23. Opening of coronary sinus
24. Interatrial septum
25. Interventricular septum
26. L. ventricle
27. R. ventricle
28. L. atrium
29. R. atrium
30. Anterior papillary m.
31. Fossa ovale
32. Ligamentum arteriosum
33. Tricuspid valve
34. Mitral valve (bicuspid)
35. Pulmonary valve (semilunar)
36. Aortic valve (semilunar)
37. L. coronary a.
38. Anterior cusp.
39. R. coronary a.
40. L. posterior cusp.
41. L. coronary a.
42. R. posterior cusp.
43. Nodulus semilunaris
44. Sinus of Valsalva
45. Eustachian valve

Tricuspid valve closed seen from right atrium

Mitral valve closed seen from left atrium

Semilunar valve of aorta and pulmonary art. closed and seen from above.

Coronary arteries (in aorta only)

Figure 4-2   The Heart: Anterior, Posterior, and Coronal Cross-Sectional Views

bility and elasticity enable the arteries to receive the increased blood volume forced into them with each cardiac contraction. If the arteries lack distensibility and elasticity, as in arteriosclerosis, the systolic blood pressure will be markedly increased. The external layer of the arteries, the tunica externia, or the adventitia, comprises loose connective tissue.

The body's arteries vary in size, the largest being the aorta and the pulmonary artery. The smaller arteries are called arterioles. Arterioles are vital to the maintenance of arterial blood pressure. They are well supplied with vasoconstrictor fibers; the autonomic nervous system and autoregulation control arteriolar constriction and dilation. A precapillary sphincter is located on the arteriole just before it enters the capillary network.

The capillaries are exceedingly minute perfusion vessels. They connect the arterioles to the venules (tiny veins), which, like the arterioles, are continuous with the capillaries. The capillary walls consist of a layer of endothelial cells continuous with the layer that lines the arteries, veins, and heart. During periods of rest, approximately 5% of the total blood volume lies in the systemic capillary bed.

Veins and venules carry unoxygenated blood to the heart. The structure of the veins is very similar to that of the arteries. They are composed of three layers: an inner endothelial lining, a middle muscular layer, and an external layer of connective tissue. The walls of the veins have a less-developed middle coat, and veins are therefore not as elastic as arteries. Because their walls are much thinner than those of arteries, veins tend to collapse when not filled with blood. Many veins contain valves that are semilunar folds of the vessel's inner layer and usually consist of two flaps. A valve's convex border is attached to the side of the vein and its free edge points toward the heart. These valves prevent reflux of the blood and keep it flowing toward the heart. Thus, they are most numerous in the veins of the extremities, where reflux is most likely to occur. In an upright individual, gravity alone can cause high pressures in the lower extremities, resulting in edematous tissue; but, normally, pressure in the lower extremities is 25 mm Hg or less.

Coronary Circulation

Coronary circulation is responsible for the nourishment of the heart muscle. The coronary arteries are more variable in anatomical pattern than any other part of the cardiac anatomy. Large arterial branches traverse the epicardium, with subbranches penetrating through to myocardial and subendocardial tissue

layers. Coronary artery perfusion is primarily dependent on pressure in the root of the aorta during diastole. The three major coronary arteries are the right, left, and circumflex arteries.

The right coronary artery (RCA) arises from the right aortic sinus of Valsalva and runs between the right atrium and the right ventricle. It then runs back to the posterior interventricular groove, where it becomes the posterior descending artery, which supplies the right atrium and posterior walls of the right and left ventricles. An anterior right atrial branch frequently arises near the origin of the right coronary artery. A branch of the right coronary artery that arises from the posterior descending branch commonly supplies the atrioventricular node (AV node).

The left main coronary artery arises from the left aortic sinus of Valsalva and generally divides within 1 or 2 cm into the left anterior descending and left circumflex coronary arteries. The left anterior descending artery travels down the anterior surface of the heart in the interventricular sulcus and a few centimeters up the posterior surface of the same groove. Blood is thus supplied to the anterior aspects of the right and left ventricles, the interventricular septum (which contains the ventricular conduction system), and a small posterior portion of both ventricles. The left circumflex artery runs laterally and then posteriorly between the left atrium and ventricle; the obtuse marginal branch breaks off before the artery descends on the posterior surface of the left ventricle. Blood is thus supplied to the lateral and posterior portions of the left ventricle.

Finally, the majority of the coronary veins drain into the coronary sinus. Some veins, such as the thebesian veins, drain directly into the cardiac chambers. The anterior cardiac veins drain the right ventricle.

Physiology of the Cardiac Muscle

The heart is composed of three major types of cardiac muscle: atrial muscle, ventricular muscle, and specialized excitatory and conductive muscle fibers. The atrial and ventricular types of muscle contract in much the same manner as skeletal muscle fibers do. In contrast, the specialized excitatory and conductive fibers contract only feebly because they contain few contractile fibrils; instead they provide an excitatory system for the heart and a transmission system for rapid conduction of electrical impulses throughout the heart.[1]

Cardiac muscle has many similarities to skeletal muscle. Both types of muscle are striated in appearance and contain actin and myosin filaments. Cardiac muscle, however, has no defined tendon and bony attachments, as is characteristic of skeletal muscle. Cardiac muscle contains more mitochondria than does skeletal muscle, which allows the cells to produce more adenosine triphosphate (ATP), which is necessary to fulfill the high energy requirement of the repetitive muscular action specific to the heart.

Cardiac muscle fibers are composed of bundles of muscle cells surrounded by a sarcolemma. Each muscle fiber contains several hundred to several thousand myofibrils. Each myofibril has approximately 1500 myosin filaments and twice that many actin filaments. Myosin is a complex filament that is thicker than actin. Actin, which is equally complex, is composed of three elements: actin, tropomyosin, and troponin. Troponin has a very high affinity for calcium ions. It is believed that the combining of calcium ions with troponin is the trigger that initiates muscle contraction. Thus, myosin and actin filaments interdigitate and slide along each other during the process of contraction. The entire contractile unit is called a sarcomere (Figure 4-3). Calcium alone is not able to cause a contraction. Other ions, such as sodium and potassium, must also be present to cause an action potential. The exchange of ions that causes an action potential will be discussed further in a later section.

Z membranes separate each of the sarcomeres. Striations in the muscle are caused by the overlap of actin and myosin: wide, dark A bands are formed by myosin overlapping with actin; the lighter I bands are seen where only actin is present (Figure 4-4).

Intercalated discs are actually cell membranes that separate individual cardiac muscle cells from one another. Electrical resistance between the intercalated discs is minimal, so electrical impulses are able to travel from one cardiac muscle cell to another

without significant hindrance. In turn, action potentials cause the calcium-rich sarcoplasmic reticulum to release calcium ions, and a contraction is sustained.

This entire arrangement of cardiac cells is known as a syncytium. There are two separate functional syncytiums—the atrial and the ventricular—separated from each other by the fibrous tissue surrounding the valvular rings. Action potentials are conducted between the syncytiums by way of the AV bundle.

Electrical Activity

The pumping action of the heart depends on a specific sequence of electrical activation of all myocardial cells during each beat. This necessary rhythmic excitation is provided by a pathway called the conduction system. The specialized conduction tissue has the following properties: automaticity, rhythmicity, conductivity, and excitability. It is through its electrical action that the pump, via muscular contraction, is effected. The conduction system is composed of the sinoatrial (SA) node, the internodal atrial pathways, the atrioventricular (AV) node, the bundle of His, the right and left bundle branches, and the Purkinje system (Figure 4-5).

The SA node lies at the junction of the superior vena cava and the right atrium. It contains 1.5 cm of conducting tissue that discharges an impulse about 60–100 times per minute. The SA node is referred to as the pacemaker of the heart because it discharges the fastest and strongest impulse of all the pacemakers. The impulse is transmitted through both atria via three internodal pathways (Bachmann's, Wenckebach's, and Thorel's) to the atrioventricular node.

The atrioventricular (AV) node is located in the right posterior portion of the interatrial septum near the base of the tricuspid valve and is continuous with

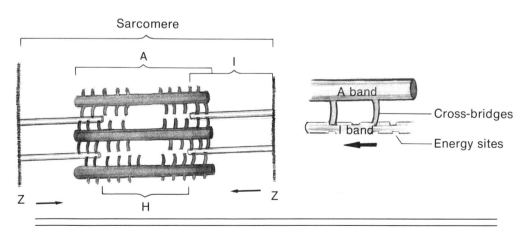

Figure 4-3 Sarcomere as a Contractile Unit

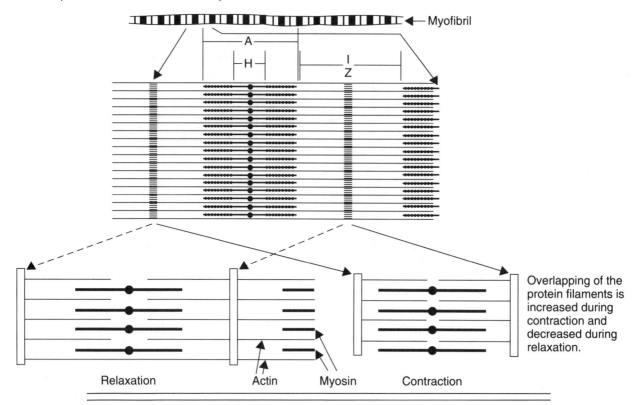

Figure 4-4 Contraction of Myofibril

the bundle of His. It discharges 40 to 60 times per minute, delaying impulses for .08 to .12 second to allow for ventricular filling. The impulse then travels from the AV node to the bundle of His.

The bundle of His, a thick bundle of fibers, runs down the right side of the interventricular septum and divides into right and left bundle branches at the muscular portion of the septum. The right bundle branch continues as a single branch; the left divides into a long, thin branch anteriorly and into a short, thick branch posteriorly, both of which parallel the septum subendocardially and are continuous with the Purkinje system.

The Purkinje system is responsible for transmitting impulses subendocardially into the ventricles. Its firing rate is 20 to 40 times per minute.

Electrophysiology

A voltage can be measured across the cell membrane during the cardiac cycle. This voltage is called the resting membrane potential (RMP), and it measures approximately −85 mV. RMP represents an electrochemical equilibrium that results from the selective permeability of the cell membrane to ions. Potassium has the ability to cross the cell membrane, but it is much less permeable to other ions, such as sodium. It

is thought that RMP is determined primarily by potassium.

Any factor that suddenly increases the permeability of the membrane to sodium is likely to elicit a sequence of rapid changes in membrane potential lasting a minute fraction of a second, followed immediately thereafter by a return of the membrane potential to its resting value. This sequence of potential changes is called the action potential. Various factors can elicit an action potential, including electrical stimulation of the membrane, chemicals, and mechanical damage to the membrane.[2] The action potential is divided into five phases: 0, 1, 2, 3, and 4. The exchange and concentration of the ions varies during each of the phases. The primary ions involved are sodium (Na^+), potassium (K^+), calcium (Ca^{++}), and chloride (Cl^-). In the resting state, there is a greater extracellular concentration of sodium, calcium, and chloride and a greater intracellular concentration of potassium.

Phase 0 is a rapid-rising phase called depolarization. As noted above, sodium is normally found in greater concentration outside the cell, and potassium is normally found in greater concentration inside the cell. Due to changes in the cell's permeability, sodium is able to diffuse intracellularly. At the same time, potassium is able to move extracellularly. The

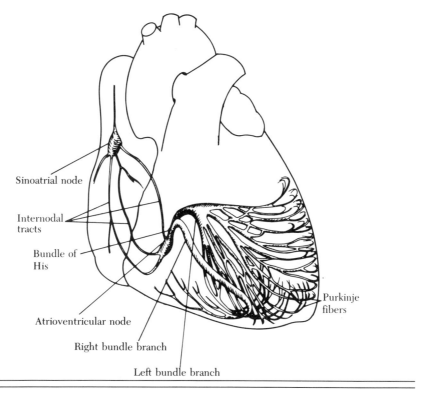

Figure 4-5 Conduction System

cell is actually depolarized at approximately −55 mV. There is an overshoot of sodium influx, however, and the cell becomes electropositive at approximately +20–30 mV.

During phase 0, calcium also moves into the cell carrying positive charges. Unlike sodium, calcium moves slowly, causing a longer lasting positive charge on the cell membrane. Calcium is also believed to play a role in the closure of the sodium gates. Evidence of this is seen when there is a deficiency of calcium ions in the extracellular fluids, which causes the gates to remain leaky to sodium ions to the point of the membrane being continuously depolarized, or fired repetitively. The slow movement of calcium ions begins at membrane potentials less negative than threshold potentials, approximately −35 mV. This can usually be seen in cells where sodium currents are inactivated or where depolarization is slow. These slow-response action potentials are usually found in the SA node, AV node, and AV valve area. How rapidly this phase develops depends on (1) the resting membrane potential (RMP), and (2) during fast response, the equilibrium potential for sodium, and during slow response, the equilibrium potential for calcium.

Phases 1 through 3 are the repolarization phases. Phase 1 is the positive spike on the action potential and is probably due to the influx of chloride ions. The plateau, phase 2, develops slowly as calcium enters the cell via the slow channels and potassium leaves the cell, which balances the electropositive charges. Phase 3 results from inactivation of transmembrane calcium and a rapid increase in potassium efflux from the cell.

Phase 4 is called polarization. The sodium-potassium pumps are most active here in returning the cell membrane to the resting state in anticipation of the onset of phase 0 and another action potential. As is characteristic of all automatic cells, the Purkinje fibers demonstrate automaticity and slow diastolic depolarization during this phase. These features are thought to be related to the constant inward diastolic movement of sodium and the decrease in the movement of potassium. Other pacemaker fibers may not share this phase 4 mechanism. This change may be mediated by a time-dependent increase in the slow inward current carried mainly by calcium. (Figure 4-6 displays phases 0 through 4.)

When the membrane is depolarized, it is almost impossible to elicit an immediate action potential. The membrane is refractory to stimulation. This time period is referred to as the absolute refractory period (ARP). The relative refractory period (RRP) follows, with a voltage-dependent and time-dependent recovery of excitability. Increased current is required to elicit a response. This period ends when excitability reaches a stable value in phase 4 (Figure 4-7).

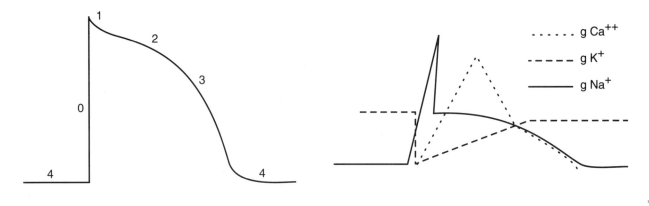

0 = Rapid depolarization with increase in Na$^+$ conductance and decrease in K$^+$

Repolarization

1 = Transmembrane potential returns to zero after overshoot

2 = Plateau; calcium moves

3 = Resting state; decrease in Ca^{++} and increase in K$^+$ conductance

4 = Polarization

Figure 4-6   The Five Phases of Action Potential

The Cardiac Cycle

The cardiac cycle is the time period from the beginning of one heartbeat to the beginning of the next. A normal cardiac cycle lasts 0.8 second. This cycle involves both electrical and mechanical events of the heart, as illustrated in Figures 4-8 and 4-9. As electrical excitation (depolarization) begins, it stimulates the mechanical event (systole). Electrical recovery (repolarization) is followed by muscular relaxation (diastole).

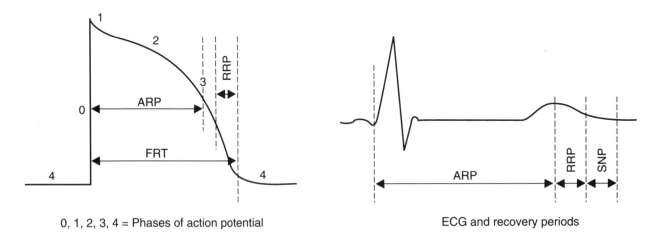

0, 1, 2, 3, 4 = Phases of action potential

ECG and recovery periods

ARP = Absolute refractory period, also called the effective refractory period (ERP)
(no stimulation accepted)

RRP = Relative refractory period
(very strong stimulus accepted)

SNP = Super normal period

FRT = Full recovery time
(closed to threshold potential and any stimulus is accepted)

Figure 4-7   Action Potential and Recovery Periods

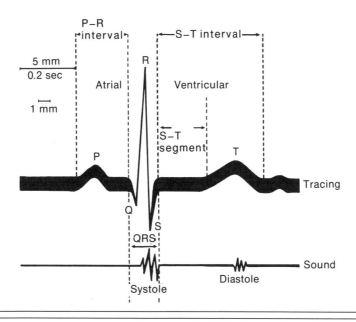

Figure 4-8 Heart Sounds Representing Phases of the Cardiac Cycle

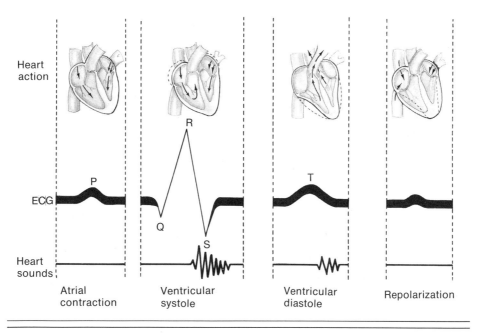

Figure 4-9 Events During the Cardiac Cycle

Figure 4-10 further illustrates the different events during the cardiac cycle. The top three curves show the pressure changes in the aorta, the left atrium, and the left ventricle, respectively. The fourth curve shows the changes in ventricular volume. The fifth curve depicts the electrocardiogram, and the sixth, a phonocardiogram, which is a recording of the sounds produced by the heart as it pumps. Although only the left-side pressures and volume changes are shown, it is important to realize that similar events are occurring nearly simultaneously in the right side of the heart.[3]

The aortic pressure curve in Figure 4-10 is similar to the pressure curve in the pulmonary artery. This pressure curve rises upon the opening of the semilunar valves. Pressure remains high in the aortic/pulmonary artery at the end of ventricular systole because of elastic stretch. The dicrotic notch, caused by back pressure against the semilunar valve, appears at the end of protodiastole. The pressure in the

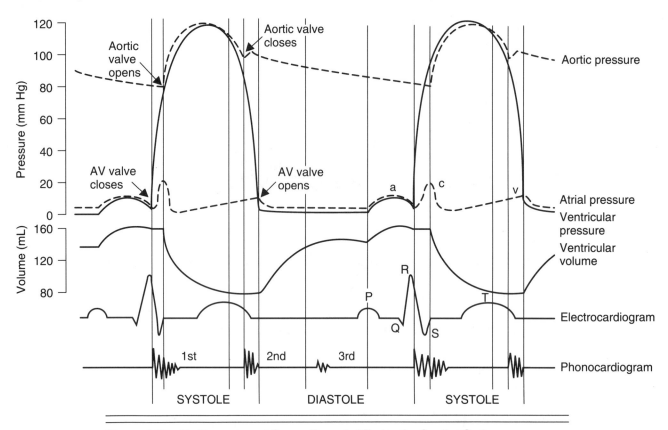

Figure 4-10   Six Measurement Curves Recorded During the Cardiac Cycle

artery continues to fall after this point until the ventricle is ready to contract again.

The atrial pressure curve represents the mechanical event and comprises three waves and two descents. The waves are labeled a, c, and v, and the descents are labeled x and y. These waves and descents can be seen on the cardioscope, should a catheter be introduced into the right or left atrium. (The introduction of catheters into the thoracic cavity will be discussed in a later section.) The a wave represents atrial contraction. Atrial contraction contributes approximately 30% of the ventricular filling. In other words, ventricular filling is primarily due to the passive filling of the ventricles caused by a pressure gradient between the atria and ventricles. This 30% is often referred to as the atrial kick. The c wave occurs during ventricular contraction and is caused by the back pressure of the AV valves toward the atria. The v wave occurs toward the end of ventricular contraction and is caused by atrial filling. The x descent occurs after the a wave and is due to atrial relaxation. The y descent occurs following the v wave and is due to the opening of the semilunar valves.

The ventricular pressure curve in Figure 4-10 also represents a mechanical event and comprises several

stages, occurring during diastole and systole. The first third of ventricular diastole is called rapid inflow and is caused by the opening of the AV valves with a rapid flow of blood from the atria into the ventricles. The second third of diastole is called diastasis and occurs when the inflow of blood into the ventricles is nearly at a standstill. The final third of diastole is due to the atrial contraction emptying into the ventricle. Ventricular systole begins with a period of isometric contraction, during which pressure is maintained on the ventricle, causing an increase in the height of the pressure curve. The semilunar valves are not yet open, however, so there is no ventricular emptying. The second phase of systole is called ejection, which means that the semilunar valves are pushed open, allowing the ventricles to empty. During the third phase, protodiastole, almost no blood flows from the ventricles, yet the ventricles remain contracted. The final phase is called isometric relaxation, which indicates that the ventricles have begun to relax and the pressure in them has begun to fall.

The ventricular volume curve in Figure 4-10 is shown beneath the atrial and ventricular pressure waveforms. Filling of the ventricles during diastole normally increases the volume of each ventricle to about 120–130 mL. This volume is known as the end-diastolic volume. As the ventricles empty during systole, the volume decreases by about 70 mL, and this is called the stroke volume. The remaining volume in each ventricle, about 50–60 mL, is called the end-systolic volume.[4]

Electrical events are recorded on the electrocardiogram, the fifth curve shown in Figure 4-10. The waves that represent electrical activity are

P wave: Atrial depolarization

QRS complex: Ventricular depolarization

T wave: Ventricular repolarization

Atrial repolarization is not normally seen on the surface electrocardiogram because the small voltage elicited by the atrium during repolarization is hidden by ventricular depolarization. It should be noted that the electrical activity precedes the mechanical activity. For example, the P wave on the electrocardiogram begins immediately prior to a rise in atrial pressure; that is, the P wave is caused by the spread of depolarization through the atria, and this is followed by atrial contraction. The same holds true for ventricular activity.[5] The QRS complex, depicting ventricular depolarization, immediately precedes the increase in ventricular pressure caused by systole. The T wave, which represents ventricular repolarization, immediately precedes relaxation and occurs slightly prior to the end of ventricular contraction.

The bottom recording in Figure 4-10 depicts the heart sounds as they occur during the cardiac cycle. The first heart sounds occur as the ventricles contract and are caused by closure of the AV valves. The second heart sounds occur at the end of diastole and are caused by the closure of the semilunar valves. Heart sounds will be discussed in more detail in the section on cardiac auscultation.

Cardiac Output

Cardiac output (CO) is the amount of blood ejected by the heart per unit of time, recorded as liters per minute. The output of both ventricles is usually the same; however, CO measures the volume of blood the left ventricle ejects into the aorta. Normal CO is approximately 4–8 liters per minute in the average 70-kg male.

A more specific parameter is the cardiac index (CI), which is the cardiac output in relation to the person's body surface area (BSA). The BSA is determined using the person's height and weight. Once the BSA is calculated, the CI is calculated by dividing the CO by the BSA. The cardiac index is useful because it provides a standardized range for all persons regardless of size and weight. The normal CI is 2.5-4 liters per minute. Cardiac output, and ultimately the cardiac index, is calculated from the product of heart rate (HR) and stroke volume (SV). Stroke volume is the amount of blood ejected with each heartbeat; that is, as mentioned earlier, it is the difference between the volume of the left ventricle at end diastole (the end of the filling cycle) and the volume remaining in the ventricle at end systole (the end of ejection). The amount of blood ejected with each contraction is approximately 75% of the 100 mL normally contained in the ventricle. Diastolic filling and systolic ejection are the major determinants of stroke volume. For example, if the heart's pumping ability is decreased, as in heart failure, the ejection fraction is reduced. If there is a larger amount of blood in the heart with less forward flow at the end of systole, a marked reduction in the ejection fraction occurs. The pressure during diastole at the end of the filling period is increased as the pump decompensates or as volume increases.

In summary, CO is influenced by five major factors: arterial blood pressure, heart rate, ventricular distensibility, ventricular filling, and myocardial contractile properties. There are three methods used to determine CO. These methods are the Fick method, the indicator-dilution method, and the thermodilution method. Of the three, thermodilution is the most commonly used method.

The Fick Method

The Fick principle states that blood flow through an organ can be determined if a substance is removed from, or added to, the blood during its flow to that organ. When applied to the lung, this principle is used to calculate the volume of blood required to transport the oxygen taken up from the alveoli per unit of time. Because of its accuracy, the Fick method gives an indication of pulmonary status and is relatively reliable in the presence of low output states, cardiac shunts, and valvular insufficiencies. It requires, however, a cooperative patient and a 20-mL sample from both the arterial and venous blood. The administration of oxygen affects the results. It is a time-consuming process that requires at least two people for simultaneous collection of expired air and blood samples. Cardiac output is calculated using a formula that involves measurement of oxygen consumption and arterial and venous oxygen content.

The Indicator-Dilution Method

The indicator-dilution method involves injecting dye into the venous system while arterial blood is steadily withdrawn through an instrument called a densitometer. A time-concentration curve is recorded as the dye passes once through the circulatory system. The concentration of dye peaks after injection and then returns to a baseline until the downward course is interrupted by dye that has been recirculated through the systemic circulation. The CO is calculated using a formula that reflects the time needed for recirculation and reconcentration of dye following the initial circulation time. Although the indicator-dilution method is faster than the Fick method, its results may be skewed, as the time for recirculation is a subjective measure and may vary from one person to another.

The Thermodilution Method

The thermodilution method is a variation of the indicator-dilution theory that requires no blood samples. A solution with a known temperature is injected into the bloodstream, and temperature change is monitored at a point downstream. The temperature changes are recorded on a curve and CO is calculated. Reproducibility is relatively constant because the procedure takes little time and involves minimal recirculation. Readings may be made as frequently as every minute. The thermodilution method is easily performed at the bedside by one person.

Hemodynamic Monitoring

The main factors in hemodynamic monitoring that determine cardiac output are preload, afterload, contractility, and heart rate.

Preload is the amount of tension or load on the muscle prior to contraction. It influences systolic performance. Specifically, preload describes the pressure or quantity of blood in the ventricle at the end of diastole. Remember that diastole is the time cycle when the heart is at rest. End diastole is the point of greatest rest, and there is an end diastolic pressure for each chamber. The clinical practitioner is concerned with ensuring that preload to both sides (or to all chambers) of the heart is maximized without overloading to the point of compromising cardiac function. The heart has an intrinsic ability to adapt to increasing loads of inflowing blood. This ability is described by the Frank-Starling law, which states that the degree of cardiac muscle stretch during diastole (preload) determines the force during systole. In the uncompromised heart, the pressure, volume, and stretch are directly proportional to one another. This form of autoregulation, in which ventricular size changes, is called heterometric autoregulation. Figure 4-11 illustrates this concept. Stated simply, as the filling pressure, or preload, increases, so will the force of contraction, causing the heart to

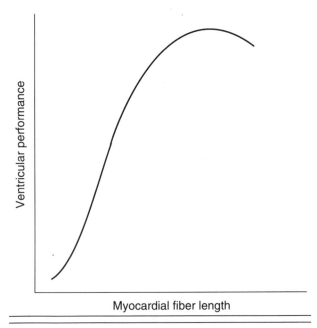

Figure 4-11 Heterometric Autoregulation

pump more blood into the arteries. Thus, cardiac output will increase until it reaches the limit of the heart's ability. Beyond that point, increasing preload will actually cause cardiac output to decrease. Clinically, this condition is often seen as heart failure, in which the heart has been overloaded with fluid. Preload to the right side and the left side of the heart is determined by the central venous pressure reading and the pulmonary capillary wedge pressure reading, respectively. This will be discussed in more detail in the following section.

Afterload is the impedance to ejection of blood from the ventricle. Since there are two sides to the heart, there are actually two areas for resistance to flow. The impedance to flow from the right side of the heart is called pulmonary vascular resistance (PVR), and the impedance to flow from the left side of the heart is called systemic vascular resistance (SVR). Normally the resistance to flow is minimal in the pulmonary vascular bed, but measurement of the SVR is useful in evaluating effectiveness of vasopressor therapy.

Both PVR and SVR can be calculated using the values obtained with the pulmonary artery catheter. The normal values for PVR and SVR are 150–250 dyne-sec/cm^5 and 800–1300 dyne-sec/cm^5, respectively. A low value indicates vasodilitation, and a high value indicates vasoconstriction. Trends are more important than single measurements.

Contractility is the muscle function of the heart and is an inherent property of the myocardium. This function is independent of preload and afterload. Contractility is affected by inotropic agents such as epinephrine or norepinephrine. Independent of the Starling mechanism, contractility allows the heart to increase its effect and force of shortenings. Although contractility is not directly measurable, if the stroke volume increases without a change in preload or afterload, an increase in contractility can be assumed.

The most effective method of altering cardiac output in the normal heart is changing the heart rate. Cardiac output may triple in a healthy individual who can increase his or her rate to approximately 175 beats per minute (bpm). Average heart rates in adults range from 60 to 100 bpm. In the normal heart, maximal cardiac output is reached at approximately 130 bpm. As the rate continues to increase, cardiac output progressively decreases because of a shortening ventricular diastolic filling time. At heart rates less than 120 bpm, the decrease in cardiac output is not proportional to the heart rate, because the degree of filling of the ventricles is enhanced during the prolonged diastolic filling. This increases stroke volume, offsetting the decrease in heart rate. If the heart rate falls below 40 bpm, cardiac output drops drastically in relation to the drop in rate. The ventricles, at this point, have reached maximum stroke volume and compensation.

Hemodynamics

Invasive techniques are frequently used to assess intracardiac pressures. One such device is the Swan-Ganz pulmonary artery pressure catheter, which measures pressures in the right side of the heart and indirectly reflects pressures in the left side of the heart. (Normal hemodynamic pressures are quantified in Figure 4-12, and Figure 4-13 provides examples of pressure tracings corresponding to catheter positioning.)

By obtaining intracardiac pressures, the practitioner can gain information regarding volume status. It is important to remember that pressures do not directly correlate with volumes; factors such as ventricular compliance will affect the measurements. Left-side pressures can be assessed directly with the use of a left atrial pressure catheter. For example, left-side heart pressures are measured during cardiac catheterization and may be measured after cardiac surgery. But one must be alert to the fact that there is a greater risk of complications during catheterization than there is when using the pulmonary artery catheter.

Pulmonary artery catheters contribute a great deal of information about the cardiovascular system. As in any assessment, care must be taken to observe trends rather than just simple numerics. In general,

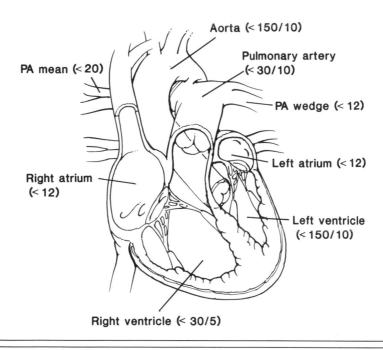

Figure 4-12 Normal Hemodynamic Pressures

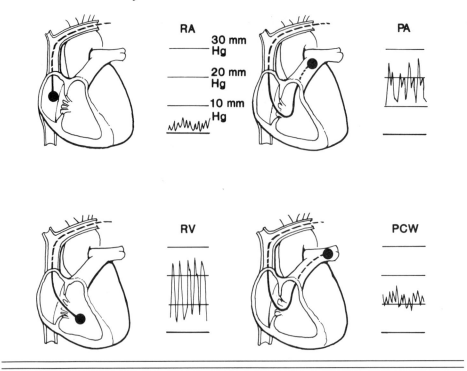

Figure 4-13 Pressure Tracings Corresponding to Catheter Positioning

complications occurring during their use are minimal; however, they can occur and include dysrhythmias, sepsis, clotting, catheter knotting, pulmonary artery perforation, ischemia, and pulmonary emboli.

Pulmonary artery pressure catheters provide several measurements, including central venous pressure (CVP), pulmonary artery pressure (PAP), and pulmonary capillary wedge or occlusion pressure (PCWP or PCOP). In general, measurements of preload that are below the normal range indicate hypovolemia, and measurements that are above the normal range indicate volume overload.

Central Venous Pressure

The CVP reading reflects a low pressure system, indicating the filling pressure (or preload) in the right side of the heart. Since there are no valves between the vena cava and the right atrium, indwelling catheters placed within the intrathoracic cavity will also reflect CVP. Right atrium pressures can be measured in terms of systolic, diastolic, and mean pressures. However, because this is such a low-pressure system with normally only a minimal difference between the systolic and diastolic measurements, it is common to write CVP as the mean right atrial pressure. Certain disorders, such as tricuspid valve disease, will cause a wide pressure difference, necessitating an assessment of systolic/diastolic CVP measurements.

The CVP waveform consists of three distinct waves, discussed earlier in the section on the cardiac cycle. The range of normal values for CVP is 0–6 mm Hg. Central venous pressures may be read using either water manometers (cm H_2O) or transducers (mm Hg). Because 1 mm Hg equals 1.36 cm H_2O, these readings are not interchangeable; one must always state the unit of measurement that is being used. Although the normal values for CVP range from 0 to 6 mm Hg, it is worth noting that CVP is often purposefully maintained at higher levels. Once again, this situation represents application of the Frank-Starling law to clinical practice: it is an attempt to increase cardiac output by maximizing the amount of preload to the heart.

Pulmonary Artery Pressure

Pulmonary artery pressure catheters are not designed to continuously monitor right ventricular pressures. This measurement can be obtained during insertion of the catheter, as it passes through the right ventricle. Right ventricular systolic pressure is much greater than central venous systolic pressure and should be equal to pulmonary artery systolic pressure. Right ventricular diastolic pressure should be equal to the mean right atrial pressure (or CVP), as the ventricle and atrium are a common chamber when the tricuspid valve is open.

The right ventricular waveform begins as a sharp incline caused by ventricular contraction. Initially the pulmonic valve is closed, but once pressure inside the right ventricle exceeds the pressure in the pulmonary artery, that valve opens, allowing blood to flow into the pulmonary artery. The sharp incline in the pressure waveform is followed by a gradual decline that continues until pressure in the pulmonary artery exceeds that in the right ventricle. The pulmonic valve then closes, and there is a gradual decrease in pressure, back to the baseline. The normal right ventricular systolic/diastolic pressure is approximately 20–30/0–6 mm Hg. Although systolic pressure in the pulmonary artery is approximately equal to systolic pressure in the right ventricle, the diastolic pressures will differ: closure of the pulmonic valve allows pressure in the right ventricle to fall while pulmonary artery pressure remains relatively high. The sharp incline in the pulmonary artery pressure waveform represents ejection from the right ventricle. This incline is followed by a gradual decline, until the pulmonic valve closes. This closure creates the dicrotic notch on the pulmonary artery waveform and marks the onset of diastole. The pulmonary artery diastolic pressure is much higher than the systolic pressure, due to the closure of the pulmonic valve (Figure 4-14). The normal values for pulmonary artery systolic/diastolic pressures are 20–30/6–10 mm Hg. The normal mean pressure is less than 20 mm Hg.

Pulmonary Capillary Wedge Pressure

Pulmonary capillary wedge pressure represents the left ventricular end-diastolic pressure (or preload to the left side of the heart). Since the left ventricle is the major pumping chamber of the heart, measurement of the PCWP will provide information regarding overall cardiac function. Left ventricular end-diastolic pressure (LVEDP) reflects the compliance of the left ventricular myocardium during diastole and left atrial filling pressure required to fill the left ventricle with blood prior to systole.[6] These filling pressures in the left side of the heart occur during diastole, when the mitral valve is open. This point in

the cardiac cycle corresponds to the pulmonary artery diastolic pressure, which occurs when the tricuspid valve is open and the pulmonic valve is closed. Therefore, during ventricular diastole, pulmonary artery diastolic pressure should reflect the pressure directed to the left side of the heart as the pressures within the adjoining atrium and ventricle are able to equilibrate. Normally, PCWP should be within 6 mm Hg of and less than the pulmonary artery diastolic pressure. The PCWP reading is obtained by occluding one of the branches of the pulmonary artery, thereby negating the influence of the pulmonary artery compliance that may affect the measurement. In patients with normal pulmonary vasculature, the influence from the pulmonary vascular bed may be negligible. In many patients, however, such as those with obstructive disease or those who are on positive pressure ventilators, PCWP and pulmonary artery diastolic pressure will not be similar. PCWP is therefore a more accurate reflection of left ventricular filling pressures, as it blocks out the influence of the right side of the heart and the pulmonary vascular bed.

The clinical significance of preload in relation to PCWP is as follows:

PCWP	Clinical Status
18–20 mm Hg	Onset of pulmonary congestion
20–25 mm Hg	Moderate pulmonary congestion
25–30 mm Hg	Severe pulmonary congestion
30 mm Hg	Pulmonary edema

The pressures listed above are approximations of pressures used to evaluate a patient's clinical status, considered in addition to the individual's vascular status and degree and chronicity of heart failure. It is possible for a patient to be in pulmonary edema with a pressure reading of less than 30 mm Hg. There are also situations in which PCWP is not an accurate reflection of left ventricular end-diastolic pressure. Some examples include mitral valve disease, high intraalveolar pressure, pulmonary venous obstruction, and left atrial prolapsing tumor.[7]

The PCWP waveform is similar to the right and left atrial waveform tracings (Figure 4-15). Both waveforms have a and v waves; c waves, however, are rarely seen in PCWP waveforms. Like CVP, PCWP has a systolic and a diastolic pressure. Since there is normally minimal difference between the two measurements, it is common practice to write only the mean PCWP reading, which is normally 4–12 mm Hg. However, in clinical practice, one might observe

SCALE=-20/+80 PA =61/25(35)

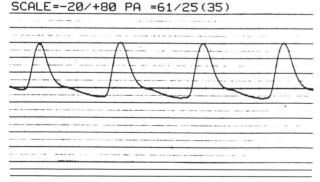

Figure 4-14 Pulmonary Artery Diastolic Pressure Waveform

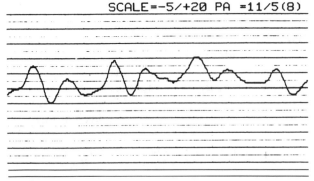

SCALE=-5/+20 PA =11/5(8)

Figure 4-15 Pulmonary Capillary Wedge Pressure Waveform

PCWP measurements that are purposefully maintained at higher than normal levels. Here again, as with the CVP measurements, Frank-Starling's law is applied in an attempt to improve cardiac output via maximization of preload to the left side of the heart.

A useful method for determining whether there is a cardiac or pulmonary component to the pulmonary artery pressure measure is to determine right-left pressure gradients.[8] As noted above, PCWP should be 0 to 6 mm Hg below the pulmonary artery diastolic (PAD) pressure measurement. Measurements within this range indicate minimal pulmonary influence. In other words, if both PAD and PCWP are elevated (above 18 mm Hg) and the difference between the two is within 6 mm Hg, the origin of the abnormality is due to cardiac factors. If PAD is elevated (usually above 18 mm Hg), PCWP is normal (less than 18 mm Hg), and there is a difference greater than 6 mm Hg between the two measurements, then the origin of the disorder is pulmonary. Elevation of both measurements above 18 mm Hg with the difference between the two greater than 6 mm Hg indicates a mixed problem—the presence of both pulmonic and cardiac influences.

Factors Affecting Blood Flow, Pressure, and Distribution

Blood flow is regulated by autoregulation, nervous control, and hormonal responses.

Autoregulation

Autoregulation causes the body to respond to local tissue changes by regulating local blood flow. In most tissues, blood flow is controlled in proportion to nutritional needs, such as the needs for delivery of oxygen and glucose and removal of carbon dioxide and lactic acid.[9] Local blood flow can be regulated to respond to individual needs. This is independent of both the nervous system and the hormonal re-

Table 4-1 Distribution of Circulation

Location	Amount (mL/min)	Percentage of Total
Liver	1350 mL	27%
Portal	1050	21
Arterial	300	6
Kidneys	1100	22
Muscle (resting)	750	15
Brain	700	14
Skin	300	6
Bone	250	5
Tissue	175	3.5
Heart	150	3
Bronchus	150	3
Thyroid gland	50	1
Adrenal gland	25	0.5
Total	5000	

Adapted from Guyton, A. C. (1976). *Textbook of Medical Physiology.* Philadelphia: W. B. Saunders, p. 160.

sponse. Specifically, the arterioles and precapillary sphincters are controlled almost entirely by the local humoral environment of the tissues. Table 4-1 quantifies blood flow to different organs and tissues under basal conditions.

Nervous Control

A second factor affecting blood flow is the nervous regulation of heart action (Figure 4-16). The nervous system plays a key role in maintaining homeostasis whenever there is a massive alteration of the circulation. The sympathetic division of the autonomic nervous system immediately responds to the body's need for increased blood supply. Sympathetic stimulation increases cardiac output and causes vasoconstriction of peripheral vessels, increasing blood pressure and directing blood supply toward major body organs. The sympathetic nervous system controls major organ vessels, increasing blood flow to the brain, heart, and muscles. The parasympathetic division has little effect on blood flow, acting instead as a moderator to prevent overresponse of the sympathetic system and to control the heart rate. Autonomic nervous system (ANS) regulation is effected through intact neural pathways and specialized sensor tissue in the vessels. This specialized sensor tissue may be divided into two types: pressoreceptors (baroreceptors) and chemoreceptors.

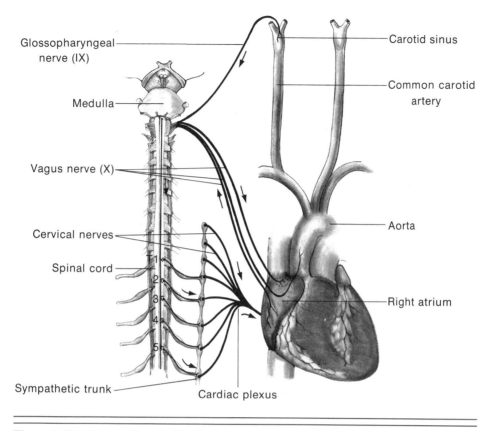

Figure 4-16 Nervous Regulation of Heart Action

Pressoreceptors Pressoreceptors are located in the walls of the aortic arch and at the origin of the internal carotid (carotid sinuses). These sensors respond to stretching of the vessel walls. An increase in blood pressure stretches arterial walls and stimulates the pressoreceptors, which respond by inhibiting the vasomotor center. The pressure returns to normal.

Major adaptive processes take place whenever there is a change in blood volume. As plasma volume decreases, venous pressure and return also decrease. This action is mediated by the pressoreceptors, which cause an increase in cardiac contractility and a vasoconstriction of peripheral blood vessels, thereby raising blood pressure. This response occurs within 1 second of an alteration in blood volume; however, the heart is usually unable to sustain this response for any great length of time. Other adaptive mechanisms—for example, the hormonal response—are required to maintain blood flow and pressure.

Chemoreceptors A second grouping of specialized sensor receptors is located in the bifurcation of the carotid arteries and along the aortic arch. These receptors, called chemoreceptors, are sensitive to changes in arterial oxygen (PaO_2), carbon dioxide ($PaCO_2$), and hydrogen ion concentrations. The carotid bodies send impulses along a tract of nerves called Herings, and the vagus nerve transmits impulses from the aortic bodies. A decrease in PaO_2, an increase in $PaCO_2$, or a decrease in pH stimulates these chemoreceptors and results in sympathetic excitation, stimulation of the vasomotor center, and increased cardiovascular activity (heart rate and blood pressure).

Osmoreceptors A third set of receptors, osmoreceptors, is located in the supraoptic nuclei of the hypothalamus and regulates cardiovascular activity by reflex response. When blood volume is increased, these receptors act by signaling for increased heart rate and diuresis. They respond to changes in the osmolality (sodium concentration) of the extracellular fluid. For example, whenever there is an increase in osmolality, the osmoreceptors increase the rate of impulse discharge. The impulses from the osmoreceptors are transmitted from the supraoptic nuclei through the pituitary stalk into the posterior pituitary gland, where they promote the release of antidiuretic hormone (ADH).

Hormonal Responses

In addition to the above nervous system responses, there are hormonal responses that occur whenever there is a change in blood flow and pressure. Each hormone has a specific effect on cardiovascular activity. The nervous system effect is short-term, but the hormonal response triggers longer-term adaptive mechanisms. The nervous system is able to have a direct effect on the blood vessels and cardiovascular system, but it also causes the adrenal medullae to secrete norepinephrine and epinephrine into the system, which then circulate everywhere in the body fluids and act on all the vasculature. In general, epinephrine and norepinephrine act to increase systemic vasoconstriction, increase the blood pressure, and increase the heart rate.

Angiotensin is the most powerful vasoconstrictor known. Angiotensin is formed by renin, which is secreted from the kidneys whenever there is a drop in arterial pressure or a decrease in osmolality. The renin acts on renin substrate to split away angiotensin. The angiotensin, in turn, has a number of important effects related to arterial pressure control: (1) it causes marked constriction of the peripheral arterioles; (2) it causes moderate constriction of the veins, thereby reducing the vascular volume and also probably decreasing vascular compliance; and (3) it causes constriction of the renal arterioles, thereby causing the kidneys to retain both water and salt, increasing the body fluid volume and helping to raise arterial pressure.[10] Angiotensin is also a precursor of aldosterone, which causes sodium and water retention, thereby increasing arterial pressure. It also causes some peripheral vasoconstriction. Vasopressin is a hormone formed in the hypothalamus and secreted through the posterior pituitary gland. Its effect is similar to that of angiotensin, but it has little effect on the veins.

In addition to the vasoconstrictors, there are a number of vasodilators. Bradykinin causes a very strong vasodilation as well as an increased capillary permeability. Serotonin can have either a vasodilator or vasoconstrictor effect, depending on the condition or the area of circulation. Histamine functions similarly to bradykinin, in that it has a powerful vasodilator effect and can cause increased capillary permeability. The prostaglandins may have either vasoconstrictor or vasodilator effects.

Nervous Control of the Heart

The preceding section discussed the nervous system's responses to changes in blood flow and pressure. Autonomic innervation is extensive in the heart. The ANS is divided into the sympathetic and the parasympathetic systems. The dynamic interplay of the ANS divisions helps to maintain heart function.

Sympathetic nerve fibers are found throughout the atria and ventricles, including both the SA and AV nodes. Parasympathetic fibers, including the SA and AV nodes, are found primarily in the atria but also extend into the ventricles. Regulation and conduction of the excitation impulse throughout the heart are controlled by the autonomic nervous system. Sympathetic innervation arises in the upper thoracic spinal cord and approaches the heart via cervical ganglia. These fibers, composed mostly of adrenergic fibers, exert the dominant influence on ventricular function. Norepinephrine is the sympathetic neurohormone transmitter. It is a vasoconstrictor and has little effect on cardiac function. The effects of sympathetic stimulation are positive chronotropy (increase in heart rate), positive inotropy (increase in contractility), and positive dromotropy (increase in atrioventricular conduction). The sympathetic response is also referred to as the adrenergic response. Alpha and beta receptors within the heart and blood vessels are stimulated by the sympathetic system; alpha receptors respond with vasoconstriction and beta receptors with increased heart rate and increased contractility.

Parasympathetic innervation originates in the medulla oblongata and approaches the heart via the vagus nerve, joining sympathetic fibers in the cardiac plexus. These fibers exert the dominant influence on heart rate. The neurohormone transmitter released is acetylcholine. The parasympathetic system stimulates the beta receptors in the heart. The cardiac effects of parasympathetic (vagal) stimulation are negative chronotropy (decrease in heart rate) and negative chromotropy (decrease in atrioventricular conduction). The parasympathetic response is also called the cholingergic response.

Assessment of the Cardiovascular System

A complete assessment of the cardiovascular system includes the history, a physical assessment, and the interpretation of diagnostic tests.

History

The importance of taking an accurate and thorough history cannot be overemphasized. The history remains the richest source of information concerning a patient's illness. Taking the history also helps to establish a bond with the patient and permits the practitioner to evaluate the results of diagnostic tests that might have a strong subjective component (such as the determination of exercise capacity). Finally, the history permits the practitioner to evaluate the impact of the disease on the patient's and the family's total life and to assess the patient's personality, emotions, and stability.[11]

The primary areas to be addressed in taking the history include dyspnea, chest pain or discomfort, syncope, palpitations, edema, cough, hemoptysis, and excess fatigue.[12]

Dyspnea

Dyspnea is a subjective state that is associated with both cardiac and respiratory disorders as well as anxiety. The sudden onset of dyspnea suggests a pulmonary origin. Slowly developing dyspnea suggests a cardiac abnormality. The sudden occurrence of dyspnea in a patient with a history of rheumatic heart disease, however, suggests the development of atrial fibrillation, rupture of chordae tendineae, or pulmonary embolism.

Chest Pain

In assessing chest pain, the practitioner should use the patient's terminology in describing his or her discomfort. Patients may deny having chest "pain," but in actuality have chest heaviness or "pressure." Chest discomfort should be assessed for quality, location, precipitating factors, successful relief measures, duration, and accompanying symptoms.

Syncope

Syncope is defined as a loss of consciousness and most commonly occurs because of decreased perfusion to the brain. When taking the history, the practitioner should assess for the presence of an aura, associated symptoms such as incontinence and convulsions, length of unconsciousness, precipitating factors such as changes in body position, and family history.

Palpitations

Palpitations alone are rather benign in description and are defined as an unpleasant awareness of the beating of one's heart. Complaints of palpitations should be assessed according to quality (such as "skipped beats" versus "stopped beating"), duration, precipitating factors such as exercise, and associated symptoms such as dizziness or syncope.

Edema

Localization of edema is helpful in determining its etiology. In addition, the time of onset and dura-

tion of the edema should be determined. For example, does the edema occur only at night, or has it been increasing in general over the past several weeks? Associated symptoms, such as dyspnea or jaundice, will be helpful in ascertaining the etiology of the edema. Finally, the type of edema is important to note (pitting, dependent, gradations, etc.).

Cough

Complaints of cough should be assessed according to quality (such as dry or moist), type (spasmodic, nocturnal, wheezing, or intermittent), and associated symptoms (such as expectoration with the cough). In the latter case, a description of the expectorant should be recorded.

Other Symptoms

Other symptoms that should be addressed in taking the history include fatigue, anorexia, nausea, vomiting, visual changes, hoarseness, fever, and chills. In addition to assessing particular symptoms and complaints, the practitioner should assess the patient's history of occupation/work habits, his or her past cardiovascular history, and any environmental factors that may have caused a cardiac disorder. Some specific items to look for include the following:

Rheumatic heart disease
Diabetes mellitus
Hypertension
Hyperlipidemia
Tobacco use
Congenital heart disease
Exposure to environmental toxins
Recent illnesses
Medications, both prescription and nonprescription
Alcohol and social drug use

Physical Assessment

Physical assessment of the patient experiencing cardiovascular disorders is similar to that of the patient experiencing disorders of other body systems; it includes inspection, palpation, percussion, and auscultation. There are several general considerations in the physical examination: (1) the patient should be examined from his or her right side, (2) daytime lighting should be used for inspection of the chest wall, (3) auscultation should take place in a quiet room, (4) the examination should not be rushed and should proceed in an orderly fashion, and (5) abnormalities should be described in terms of timing in the cardiac cycle (systole/diastole) and location.

Inspection

Inspection is the act of looking critically at the patient. Particular attention should be paid to the patient's general appearance as well as to inspection of the chest wall. The patient should be observed for apparent health: handshake, personal appearance, gross deformity, nutrition, posture, and gait. His or her awareness and cooperation should be determined. The skin should be inspected for moisture, temperature, texture, turgor, elasticity, thickness, color, edema, lesions, and superficial vascularity. The nailbeds should be observed for color, size, shape, and clubbing. Precordial pulsations (which may be normal in thin patients) should be checked. The point of maximal intensity (PMI) should be located medial to the left midclavicular line in the fifth intercostal space and covering an area about the size of a nickel. Heaves, thrusts, systolic retractions, and vibrations, which might indicate cardiac enlargement and/or valve dysfunction, should be assessed. Any depression, flattening, or bulging of the precordium should be noted.

Jugular vein distention should be ascertained by positioning the patient at a 45-degree angle. The center of the right atrium lies approximately 5 cm below the sternal angle; therefore, the distance of the column above the sternal angle plus 5 cm equals the central venous pressure (Figure 4-17). The jugular venous pulsations (JVP) should also be ascertained. In normal adults, they can be seen at the base of the neck when the individual is supine. These pulsations consist of a, c, and v waves and x and y troughs, as seen in Figure 4-18. The a wave occurs just before the first heart sound and is identified by palpating the artery. Large a waves will be present in tricuspid stenosis, pulmonary stenosis, right ventricular hypertrophy, and pulmonary hypertension. In contrast, there is no a wave in atrial fibrillation. The c wave is after an S_1 and is rarely observable. The v wave occurs in late systole. It is a sign of tricuspid regurgitation and is also present in atrial fibrillation. The x and y troughs are negative waves; the x wave is produced by atrial diastole and occurs after the c wave, and the y wave occurs with the opening of the tricuspid valve. Large x and y waves are present in pericarditis, pericardial effusion, and severe right heart failure.

Hepatojugular reflex (HJR) should be checked by adjusting the patient so that the highest level of palpation is detectable in the middle of the neck. A hand should be placed over the patient's right upper quadrant and firm pressure applied for 60 seconds. A sustained rise of more than 1 cm in the jugular venous pressure is considered abnormal and indicates inability of the heart to pump the increased venous return.

Palpation

Palpation in the cardiovascular assessment includes palpating both the pulses and the precordium. The pads of the fingers are best for detecting pulsations; the ball of the hand for detecting vibrations and thrills.

Palpation of the pulses should focus on intensity and equality. The following pulses should be palpated: carotid (do not palpate both right and left simultaneously), radial, brachial, femoral, dorsalis

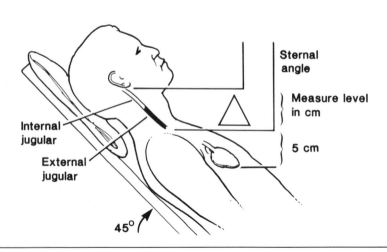

Figure 4-17 Observing for Jugular Vein Distention

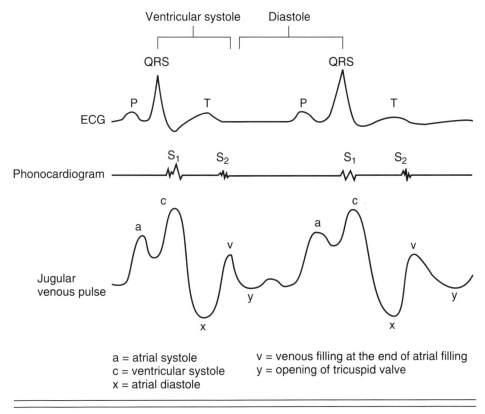

a = atrial systole
c = ventricular systole
x = atrial diastole

v = venous filling at the end of atrial filling
y = opening of tricuspid valve

Figure 4-18 Jugular Venous Pulsations in the Cardiac Cycle

pedis, and posterior tibialis. Pulses are graded according to the following intensity scale.

   0: Absent
+1: Palpable
+2: Normal
+3: Full
+4: Full and bounding

Pulses can also be described according to magnitude and quality. For example, pulsus alternans is felt as a regular beat alternating with an irregular beat. It is not due to electrical (dysrhythmia) abnormality, as might be expected. Instead, it is usually due to poor left ventricular function. Pulsus paradoxus is a physiological response to inspiration that is seen as a drop in cardiac output during inspiration. A drop of 10 mm Hg or more in arterial pressure is abnormal and usually indicates severe left ventricular dysfunction.

The chest wall also should be palpated. The precordium should be checked for thrills (murmurs), precordial friction rubs, and tenderness (usually due to intercostal injury). If a pulsation is felt in the sternoclavicular area, an aneurysm should be ruled out. A slight thrill at the aortic arch may be indicative of dilatation of the aorta. A thrill in the pulmonic area

may be indicative of pulmonary artery stenosis. Other causes of a thrill in this area include anemia, fever, pregnancy, and thin chest walls. Thrills are often felt in children. The epigastric area, inferior to the tip of the xiphoid, should be palpated for vigorous pulsations that may be indicative of an aneurysm.

Percussion

Percussion can be used to determine the size of the cardiac silhouette, although this method is no longer frequently used, since radiographic studies can better indicate cardiac size and placement. The left cardiac border can be percussed for dullness. Abnormalities that may cause changes in the left-border dullness, other than cardiac enlargement, are tumor, pleural effusion, and mediastinal shift.

Auscultation

Auscultation is performed in four major areas. The sites are named according to the underlying valves (see Figure 4-19). The two major characteristics of sound are frequency and pitch. High-frequency vibrations produce high-pitched sounds that are best heard with the diaphragm of the stethoscope. Common high-pitched sounds are S_1, S_2,

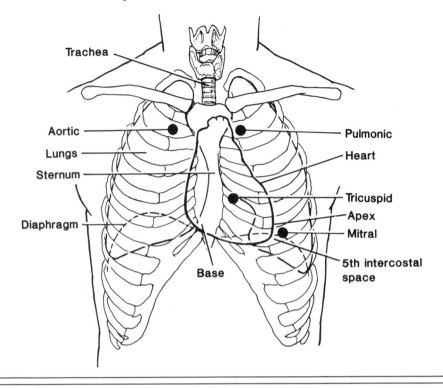

Figure 4-19 Areas of Auscultation

opening snaps, ejection clicks, and murmurs due to stenosis. Low-frequency vibrations are produced by low-pitched sounds that are best heard with the bell of the stethoscope. Common low-pitched sounds are S_3 and S_4. Note that the bell of the stethoscope must be placed lightly on the precordium; otherwise it will function as a diaphragm.

The intensity (or loudness) of the heart sounds is directly proportional to the amount of energy producing the vibration. The quality of sound depends on the loudness and pitch. The duration is the length of time the sound lasts. If the vibrations increase, the sound lasts longer.

S_1 and S_2 are the normal heart sounds (Figure 4-20). S_1 is the first part of the sound (lub). S_1 occurs at the beginning of ventricular systole and is produced by the closing of the mitral and tricuspid valves. The S_1 sound precedes the upstroke of the carotid pulse and coincides with the radial pulse. It is characterized by a low-pitched "lub." When auscultating for S_1, the practitioner should place the diaphragm of the stethoscope at the apex of the heart.

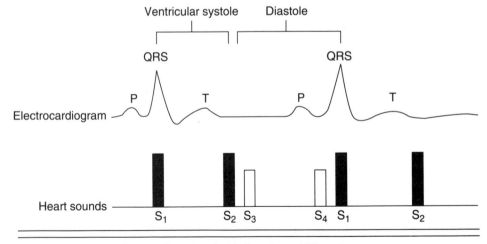

Figure 4-20 Heart Sounds Correlated with Systole and Diastole

S_2 (dub) is the second part of the heart sound and occurs at the end of ventricular systole. It is produced by the closing of the pulmonic and aortic valves. S_2 follows the carotid pulse. It is characterized by a high-pitched "dub," which is louder and shorter than S_1. When auscultating for S_2, the practitioner should place the diaphragm of the stethoscope at the base of the heart.

Physiological splitting of S_2 may occur during inspiration and may be considered normal. This splitting is due to a drop in intrathoracic pressure, which normally occurs during inspiration and causes an increased venous return to the right heart, pooling of blood in the lungs, and decreased venous return to the left heart. This causes a delay in right ventricular ejection and tricuspid valve closing. Wide and persistent splitting of S_2 occurs in right bundle branch block. At times, S_2 is split and does not appear to be affected by respiration. This sound is known as fixed splitting of S_2 and is heard with atrial septal defect.

S_3, the third heart sound, is a ventricular diastolic "gallop" that often occurs because of congestive heart failure. A gallop is an abnormal diastolic event that resembles the sound of a galloping horse. It is characterized by a cadence of extra S_3 (or S_4) sounds. An S_3 may be an intermittent gallop, caused by an unusually large diastolic blood flow into a normal ventricle or a normal blood flow filling an abnormal ventricle. S_3, which is dull and low-pitched, is best heard by using the bell of the stethoscope in the apical area. S_3 may also be caused by an increase in cardiac output due to anemia, hyperthyroidism, ventricular septal defects, exercise, mitral regurgitation, left-to-right shunts, or tricuspid insufficiency.

S_4, the fourth heart sound, is an atrial or presystolic gallop and therefore occurs before S_1. Although it is less common than an S_3, S_4 may be caused by ventricular failure, myocardial infarction, pulmonary hypertension, aortic or pulmonary stenosis, ventricular hypertrophy, and hyperthyroidism. It is produced by increased resistance to ventricular filling following atrial contraction. S_4 is a low-pitched sound and is best heard by placing the bell of the stethoscope medial to the right apex or at the third or fourth intercostal space of the left sternal border.

Summation gallop occurs when both an S_3 and an S_4 are present.

Physiological contraction and filling of the heart create the order in which the sounds are heard. S_4 and S_1 are presystolic and systolic sounds. S_2 and S_3 are prediastolic and diastolic sounds. Therefore, S_4 is heard just before S_1, and S_3 is heard just after S_2 (see Figure 4-20).

In addition to gallops, there are other abnormal extra heart sounds. A "snap" occurs in rheumatic valvular disease, due to the opening of the AV valve, and is heard after S_2. A "click" is a sound heard during systole and is caused by the prolapsed valves. A "rub" is a grating, harsh sound heard over the precordium. It is described as having three components. Rubs sound similar to hair rubbing against the diaphragm of the stethoscope. The time and phase of respiration and posture affect the sound of a rub, and it may be intermittent. A rub is usually indicative of inflammation or irritation to the pericardial sac.

A murmur is a vibration within the heart caused by turbulence around the valve and through abnormal valvular openings. Turbulent blood flow heard through a vessel is called a bruit. Turbulent blood flow felt in a vessel is called a thrill. Murmurs are heard over the auscultatory area of their origin and are classified according to where they occur in the cardiac cycle as systolic, diastolic, or continuous.

Systolic murmurs may be due to aortic stenosis, atrial septal defect, mitral regurgitation, tricuspid regurgitation, and mitral valve prolapse. Sudden onset of a systolic murmur may be due to rupture of the mitral papillary muscle or ventricular septal defect. Systolic murmurs are heard between S_1 and S_2.

Diastolic murmurs may be due to aortic regurgitation, pulmonic regurgitation, mitral stenosis, or tricuspid stenosis. Diastolic murmurs are heard following S_2.

A continuous murmur may be due to patent ductus arteriosus. This murmur also occurs with a shunt surgically created for relief of tetralogy of Fallot and aortopulmonary fistulas.

Murmurs may be described according to timing, location, radiation, and pitch and should be graded in intensity according to the following scale.

Grade I: Very faint, may not be heard in all positions

Grade II: Quiet, heard immediately with the stethoscope

Grade III: Moderately loud, not associated with a thrill

Grade IV: Associated with a thrill

Grade V: Heard with the stethoscope partly off the chest

Grade VI: Heard with stethoscope off the chest

Table 4-2 details the various heart sounds and corresponding causes.

Diagnostic Tests

Diagnostic tests for cardiovascular assessment may include laboratory studies; noninvasive procedures

Table 4-2 Heart Sounds and Corresponding Causes

Terminology	Characteristics	Comments
Third heart sounds in adults (normal in children and young adults) S_1 S_2 S_3 S_1	Occurs about 0.10 sec after aortic component of second sound and is of very low frequency. Best heard in lateral position with bell of stethoscope while client is exhaling.	Caused by sudden distention of ventricular wall when blood flows into ventricle from atrium during period of rapid ventricular filling. May be heard in anemia, hyperthyroidism, ventricular septal defect, mitral regurgitation, constrictive pericarditis.
Fourth heart sound (not always abnormal) S_1 S_2 S_4 S_1	Precedes first heart sound; low frequency; heard best at apex, near xiphoid or in substernal notch.	Often associated with hypertension, aortic insufficiency, aortic stenosis.
Ejection click S_1 E_j S_2	High pitched; caused by sudden dilation of aorta and pulmonary artery. Heard best at base of heart.	Must be differentiated from split S_1. Usually associated with pulmonary hypertension, pulmonary valve stenosis, idiopathic dilation of pulmonary artery.
Midsystolic click S_1 S_2	Sharp clicking sound heard in mid to late systole, often moving with respirations. Click closer to S_1 in inspiration and closer to S_2 in expiration. Heard best over apex.	Floppy mitral valve. Mitral prolapse associated with women more often than men; causes increased risk of bacterial endocarditis.
Gallop rhythms S_4 S_1 S_2 S_3	A dull, low-pitched sequential sound from the intensification of S_3 or S_4; best heard a little below apex but may be heard over entire precordial area.	Not always a sign of heart failure; may occur with rapid heart rate, aortic stenosis, aortic insufficiency.
Protodiastolic gallop S_1 S_2 S_3	Intensification of S_3; has rhythm and accent of word *Ken-tuck-y*.	Position patient on left side. Often accompanied by precardial heave. Seen in ventricular hypertrophy.
Presystolic gallop S_4 S_1 S_2	Intensification of S_4; has rhythm and accent of word *Ten-nes-see*.	Associated with myocardial infarction, excessive blood volume, or rapid blood flow.
Summation gallop S_1 S_2 S_{3-4}	Presence of S_3 and S_4 sounds. Occurs when heart rate becomes rapid.	Seen in hyperdynamic circulation (for example, hyperthyroidism, Cushing's disease).
Fixed split S_1 S_2 S_1 S_2	Split of S_1 or S_2; little or no variation with respirations.	Associated with atrial septal defect, pulmonary stenosis.
Widened split S_2 S_1 S_2 S_1 S_2	Split of S_2; varies with respirations but is more than 0.01 sec on inspiration and less than 0.04 sec on expiration.	Associated with increased pulmonary blood flow (atrial septal defects); decreased pulmonary pressure (pulmonary stenosis); mitral insufficiency.

Table 4-2 *(continued)*

Terminology	Characteristics	Comments
Paradoxical split	Split of S_2 becomes wider and more pronounced on expiration and decreases on inspiration.	Seen in left bundle branch block (LBBB), aortic stenosis, hypertension.
Adventitious sounds: Pericardial friction rub	Scratchy, high-pitched sound heard throughout cardiac cycle. Best heard with client sitting upward and forward at 3ICS to the left of sternum.	Sign of inflammation of pericardium (for example, rheumatic pericarditis).
Venous hum	Turbulent blood flow in internal jugular vein. Continuous, low-pitched humming or roaring sound. Best heard, with client sitting up, above medial one-third of clavicle, especially on the right. Sounds may radiate to first and second ICS.	May occur with anemia, thyrotoxicosis.

such as the electrocardiogram (ECG or EKG), echocardiography, exercise stress testing (EST), and radionuclide techniques; or invasive procedures such as heart catheterization, electrophysiologic studies, and radioisotope scanning.

Laboratory Studies

Laboratory studies include an evaluation of blood enzymes. Enzymes are proteins that alter the speed of chemical reactions and enable coagulation. Most enzymes are found in the intracellular compartment. Elevated serum enzyme levels indicate damage to the cell membrane such as that which occurs in myocardial infarction. The major cardiac enzymes are CPK (creatinine phosphokinase), LDH (lactic dehydrogenase), and SGOT (serum glutamic oxaloacetic transaminase). Enzymes and isoenzymes are discussed in further detail in the section on myocardial infarction.

Another laboratory study that may be performed is a lipid or arterial disease profile. This serum test is used to assess the cholesterol, triglyceride, and phospholipid levels in the bloodstream. Hyperlipidemia is a risk factor for coronary artery disease. A chronically elevated glucose level is also a contributing factor for coronary artery disease.

Prothrombin time (PT) is used to determine anticoagulation status during anticoagulant drug therapy. Usually the prothrombin time is kept within 2 to 2.5 times normal. Partial prothrombin time (PTT) is used to determine anticoagulation status during heparin therapy.

An elevated sedimentation rate may indicate myocardial infarction, bacterial endocarditis, or Dressler's syndrome. A low sedimentation rate may indicate congestive heart failure.

Electrocardiography

The electrocardiogram (ECG or EKG) is a graphic representation of the electrical activity of the heart. The 12-lead ECG is helpful in diagnosing ischemia, infarction, axis deviation, bundle branch blocks, and hypertrophy. The electrical forces are recorded on graph paper that has a horizontal time scale and vertical voltage scale (Figure 4-21). Each horizontal space represents a time interval of .04 second. Every fifth line, both horizontally and vertically, is bold. The time interval between the two bold lines is .20 second. ($.04 \times 5 = .20$ second.) Voltage between two bold lines is 0.5 mV.

The typical ECG represents a cardiac cycle designated by the PQRST waveforms and intervals shown in Figure 4-22. The P wave is the first positive deflection and represents atrial depolarization. It normally appears smoothly rounded and precedes each QRS complex at a specific interval.

The P-R interval represents impulse conduction through the atria and into the AV node. It extends from the beginning of the P wave to the onset of the Q wave. This interval should be no longer than .20 second.

The QRS complex represents ventricular depolarization. It consists of three deflections. The Q wave is the first negative deflection after the P wave. It results from the initial left-to-right septal depolarization. Q waves may also be classified as pathological. The R wave is the first positive deflection after the P wave. The S wave is the negative deflection

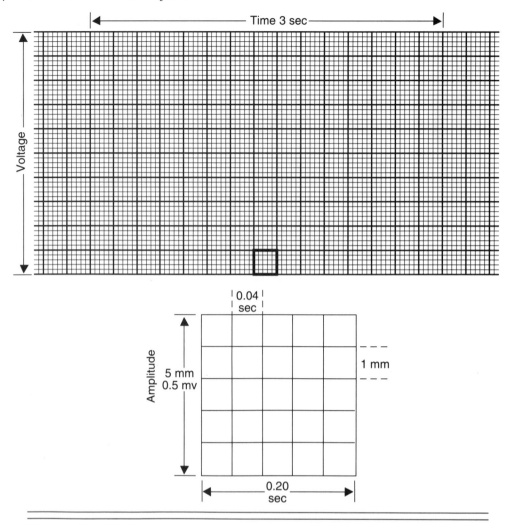

Figure 4-21 ECG Paper

following the R wave. Further deflections following the S wave are classified as R′ and S′, respectively.

The ST segment extends from the end of the S wave to the beginning of the T wave. A normal ST segment is .32 second. ST changes are usually transitory, but they may indicate cardiac abnormalities.

The T wave represents ventricular repolarization. Normally this wave is positive and symmetrical, but drugs, change of position, electrolyte imbalance, and food intake may alter the T wave.

The Q-T interval extends from the beginning of the QRS complex to the end of the T wave. It represents ventricular depolarization and repolarization. It normally measures approximately .36 to .40 second, but this time will vary according to heart rate. Certain drugs—for example, procainamide, quinidine, and disopyramide—will lengthen the Q-T interval. Other drugs, such as digoxin, and certain electrolyte disorders will shorten the interval.

The U wave is a small positive deflection after the T wave. It reflects repolarization of the Purkinje fibers. This wave is not usually visible on the ECG. Some causes of a positive U wave are hypokalemia, thyrotoxicosis, quinidine, and epinephrine.

The electrical forces are transmitted via skin electrodes and leads. A 12-lead electrocardiogram simply looks at the heart from twelve different angles (Figure 4-23). As current moves toward a positive electrode, it produces a positive deflection; as it moves away from a positive electrode, it produces a negative deflection. There are three reference points that are used in performing a 12-lead electrocardiogram: standard bipolar leads, augmented limb leads, and unipolar chest leads.

An equilateral triangle, Einthoven's triangle, is used as a reference for the standard bipolar leads (I, II, and III). Lead I views the heart as current moves from the right arm (RA) to the left arm (LA). Lead II views the heart as current moves from the RA to the left leg (LL). Finally, lead III views the heart as current moves from the LA to the LL. Note in Figure 4-23 that for lead I the LA is positive, but for lead III

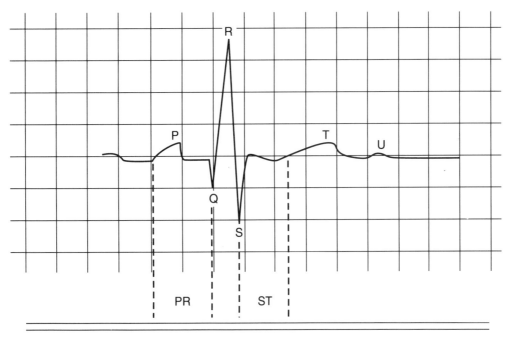

Figure 4-22 Normal Wave Pattern

the LA is negative. The AV node of the heart is actually the focal point for Einthoven's center.

The augmented limb leads and precordial chest leads are unipolar leads. This means that they represent the voltage of the heart in a specific area. In the augmented limb leads (aVR, aVL, and aVF), the positive electrode is the limb and the negative electrode is at an imaginary center of the heart (Figure 4-24). These leads represent the right arm, left arm, and left leg, respectively.

The V leads are unipolar precordial leads. They operate in conjunction with the positive lead (exploring lead), which is placed on the precordium. The common precordial positions are (Figure 4-23):

V_1: Fourth intercostal space at the right sternal border

V_2: Fourth intercostal space at the left sternal border

V_3: Equal distance between V_2 and V_4

V_4: Fifth intercostal space in the left midclavicular line

V_5: Anterior axillary line

V_6: Midaxillary line

Bedside monitors have a three-, a four-, or a five-lead system. In the three-lead system, the reference, or ground, lead is the electrode not being used. For example, for lead II, the electrodes on the right arm and left leg are being used. The left arm electrode becomes the reference lead (Figure 4-24). A modified chest lead (MCL) is a commonly used way of monitoring with a three-lead system. If the exploring electrode (positive) is positioned at the fourth intercostal space, right sternal border, the complex will resemble a V_1 lead. V_1 and V_6 allow for closer scrutiny of ventricular aberrations versus ventricular ectopy. A lead II is best for visualizing P waves.

The four-lead system has an added electrode with no polarity. It is assigned to the right leg. The five-lead system adds a positive electrode, usually attached to the chest. This system allows for monitoring of leads I, II, and III as well as the precordial chest leads.

Electrical axis is the direction in which electrical current flows through the heart. Normally, it flows from the base to apex and from right to left. A vector is a physical force that has both magnitude and direction. Vectors are used to represent electrical activity of the heart. A vector can be plotted for each of the events in the cardiac cycle. The summation of all these events into one vector is known as the electrical axis of the heart.

The QRS complex can give clues to axis deviations and clinical problems. A 12-lead ECG is required to determine axis deviation. To determine the axis, one must look at leads I, II, III, and aVF and identify the QRS complex in these leads as being positive, negative, or bidirectional. Plotting the sum of QRS in millimeters on vector lines determines the axis (Figure 4-25). Table 4-3 summarizes these QRS complex configurations and the type of axis deviation.

Right axis deviation (RAD) has a vector that points toward the positive pole of aVF into the lower

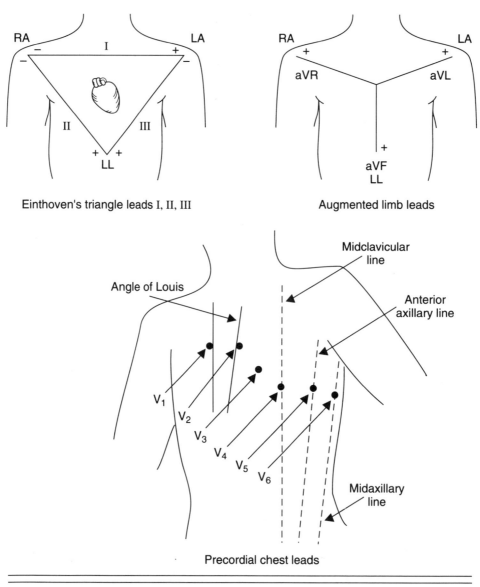

Einthoven's triangle leads I, II, III

Augmented limb leads

Precordial chest leads

Figure 4-23 Electrode Placement for 12-Lead ECG

right quadrant. It is seen in anteriolateral MI, left posterior hemiblock, and right ventricular hypertrophy (Figure 4-26). Left axis deviation (LAD) has a vector that points toward the positive pole of lead I away from the positive pole of aVF and lead II. It is seen clinically in inferior wall MI, left anterior hemiblock, and right ventricular pacing (Figure 4-27). The indeterminate axis has a vector that points away from the positive pole of lead I and aVF and deviates into the upper right quadrant. It is seen in ventricular tachycardia (Figure 4-28).

Echocardiography

Echocardiography refers to a group of tests that utilize ultrasound to examine the heart and record information in the form of echoes, that is, reflected sonic waves. Whereas other methods of examination record the shadow of a structure, ultrasound creates an image using reflected energy. Echocardiography is useful for recording the heart wall thickness, abnormalities in wall motion, valvular abnormalities, blood flow, chamber size, pericardial effusions, septal defects, and ejection fractions.

The M-mode was the first method used in echocardiography. The recording produced by M-mode is sometimes called a one-dimensional, or an "ice pick," view. A transducer is placed on the chest wall and the ultrasonic beam "slices" a view of the heart. Figure 4-29 displays such a cross section of the heart and the cardiac structures transected by the beam, and Figure 4-30 shows a section of an actual echocardiogram strip. As can be seen, M-mode is

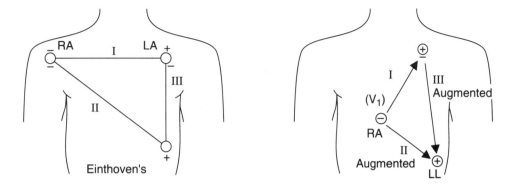

Modified chest lead using monitor with only three-lead capability and three or four electrodes

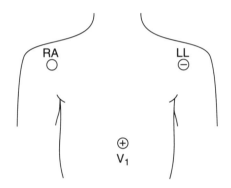

Modified chest lead using monitor with V selection and five-lead electrodes

Figure 4-24 Electrode Placement for Modified Chest Lead

useful for recording the motion of cardiac structures parallel to the ultrasonic beam. It does not permit effective evaluation of the shape of cardiac structures, however, nor can it depict lateral motion, that is, motion perpendicular to the ultrasonic beam.[13]

Another technique, two-dimensional (2-D) echocardiography, is used for recording cardiac shape and lateral motion during real time. With this method the recordings are displayed on video. Instead of an ice pick view, the transducer records an arc-shaped view of the heart using motion from the beam as it is rotated.

There have been various advances in the use of both echocardiography and the adjuncts that can enhance the technique. Color flow is used along with the two-dimensional doppler to better display blood flowing forward and backward through valves and septal wall defects. Echocardiography is being used during exercise stress testing to record cardiac function during increased activity. Esophageal echocardiography, in which the transducer is introduced down the esophagus, is used for better visualization of the heart structures.

Exercise Stress Testing

Exercise stress testing (EST) is a useful noninvasive technique for both diagnosing ischemia and determining heart function during times of high energy requirements. In EST, a 12-lead ECG recording of the heart is made while the patient exercises on a treadmill or bicycle or with an arm ergometer. Various protocols are employed to assess maximum oxygen uptake at different workloads. In addition to the 12-lead ECG, blood pressure and heart rate are recorded at various stages of activity. Table 4-4 lists the indications for noninvasive EST.

EST is used to assess functional ability at certain workloads. Normally, as a person increases exercise, his or her cardiac output will increase proportionally. Cardiac output, in this instance, is determined by blood pressure and heart rate. Failure to increase these two parameters in a stepwise fashion may mean a drop in cardiac output, an indication that the patient should perform activities that require less energy expenditure in order to maintain cardiac output. Thus, with knowledge gained from use of

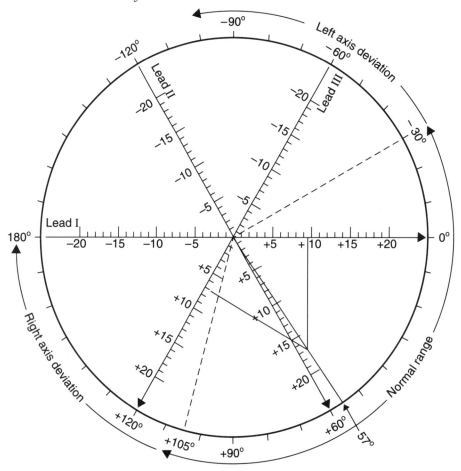

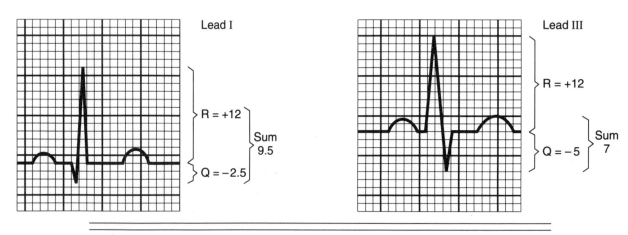

Figure 4-25 Vectorial Axis Determination

EST, the practitioner can prescribe a safe rehabilitation program for the patient.

EST is also used as a diagnostic test for screening high-risk individuals and for interpreting atypical chest pain. A patient is generally exercised to within 90% of his or her predicted maximum heart rate. The 12-lead ECG recording is used to detect ST segment changes. There is much controversy over the sensitivity and accuracy of EST in detecting the presence of coronary artery disease. Given this controversy and the number of false-negative results (meaning a negative test result in an individual who has the disease), EST is often used to ascertain a quantitative risk factor rather than to obtain a simple disease/no disease classification.

EST is a relatively safe procedure. The incidence

Table 4-3 QRS Complexes in Axis Deviations

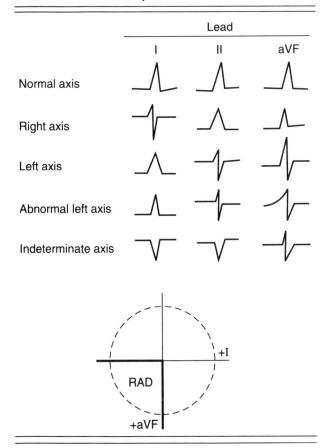

	Lead		
	I	II	aVF
Normal axis			
Right axis			
Left axis			
Abnormal left axis			
Indeterminate axis			

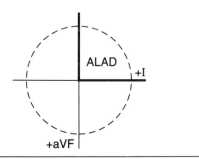

Figure 4-26 Right Axis Deviation

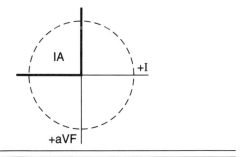

Figure 4-27 Abnormal Left Axis Deviation

Figure 4-28 Indeterminate Axis

Table 4-4 Indications for Exercise Stress Testing (EST)

Safety screening before fitness program
Health screening in preemployment physical
Cardiac risk screening for industry or profession
Diagnostic measure for silent ischemia
Diagnostic measure for angina
Diagnostic measure in CAD risk assessment
Evaluative measure for myocardial efficiency following MI recovery
Evaluative measure for myocardial efficiency during cardiac rehabilitation, following MI recovery
Evaluative measure for myocardial efficiency following medical therapy in CAD
Evaluative measure for myocardial efficiency following angioplasty/coronary bypass

of serious complications during stress testing is less than 1% but several relative contraindications to EST exist (Table 4-5). The test is terminated based on either subjective data (the patient's response) or an objective maximum (heart rate obtained).

Radionuclide Techniques

Radionuclide techniques are noninvasive, requiring only a peripheral intravenous injection, and thus offer distinct advantages over more conventional, invasive methods. They are safe and repeatable and do not induce measurable hemodynamic

Table 4-5 Contraindications for Exercise Stress Testing (EST)

Unstable angina
Unstable and uncontrolled hypertension
Unstable and uncontrolled cardiac arrhythmias
Inability to give informed consent
Acute MI
Recovering from MI
Acute pericarditis, myocarditis, or cardiac contusion
Unstable advanced coronary heart disease
Advanced aortic stenosis
Symptomatic congestive heart failure
Chronic obstructive heart disease
Uncontrolled electrolyte imbalance
Dysfunctional cardiac pacing
Advanced cardiac conduction defect
Other acute illness

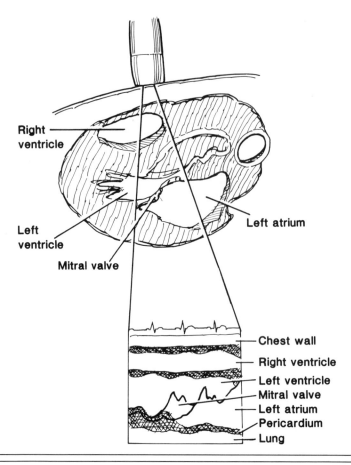

Right ventricle

Left atrium

Left ventricle

Mitral valve

Chest wall
Right ventricle
Left ventricle
Mitral valve
Left atrium
Pericardium
Lung

Figure 4-29   Cardiac Cross-Section (M-mode) Echocardiogram

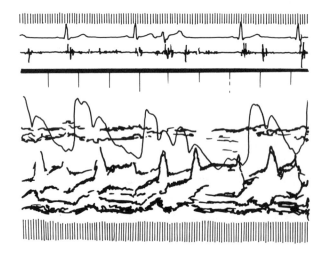

Figure 4-30   Echocardiogram Strip

alterations. In addition, cardiac performance can be studied during a variety of physiological or pharmaceutical interventions.

Radionuclide techniques include methods to assess cardiac performance and those to assess myocardial perfusion. Techniques to assess cardiac performance can be used to measure (1) left and right ventricular ejection fractions; (2) indices of regional ventricular performance; (3) left ventricular cardiac output; (4) end-diastolic and end-systolic ventricular volumes; (5) indices of early systolic and diastolic function; (6) indices of aortic, mitral, and tricuspid regurgitation; (7) indices of asynchrony; (8) transit times within the central circulation; and (9) intracardiac shunts.[14] Radionuclide techniques may be either first-pass studies (from the initial transit of the radiotracer through the heart) or equilibrium studies (the radionuclide reaches equilibration throughout the intravascular system). In first-pass studies, the radiopharmaceutical must be administered each time imaging is to be performed. In equilibrium studies, imaging can be continued for up to four hours after injection of the radiopharmaceutical, allowing imaging in multiple projections and during physiological or pharmacological interventions. Imaging during exercise may be useful in evaluating patients suspected of having coronary disease.

Radionuclide techniques that assess regional perfusion are used to detect and evaluate coronary artery disease and to assess certain therapies. Perfusion is often measured both at rest and during exercise.

One of the more common radiopharmaceuticals is thallium-201, which is used in diagnosing coronary artery diseases. Other indications for the use of thallium-201 include evaluating the functional significance of coronary stenosis, differentiating viable from nonviable myocardium, and determining graft patency following coronary artery bypass graft surgery.[15] Various other radiopharmaceuticals are used to assess myocardial perfusion. Decisions as to type of radiopharmaceutical should be made based on evidence of radiation exposure, half-life, ability to perform subsequent passes or studies, expense, and resolution.

Cardiac Catheterization and Arteriography

Cardiac catheterization is an invasive procedure that involves the percutaneous insertion of a catheter into an artery or vein and advancement of the catheter, with injection of a radiopaque dye, into the right or left side of the heart. It is used to diagnose the presence of coronary artery disease, evaluate therapies such as percutaneous coronary angioplasty and coronary artery bypass graft, and diagnose valvular or congenital heart disease. There are no absolute contraindications to elective cardiac catheterization, but rather a few relative contraindications. Some of these are uncontrolled heart failure, dysrhythmias, electrolyte imbalance, drug toxicity, pregnancy, and infection. The risks are low (morbidity of 1.2% and mortality of 0.1% to 0.2%), and most of the deaths occur in patients with severe coronary artery disease or advanced left ventricular dysfunction.[16]

Right heart catheterization studies consist of right heart hemodynamic pressure readings, angiography of the right side of the heart, oxymetry, hydrogen shunt study, and determination of cardiac output. The left heart catheterization involves hemodynamic pressure readings of the left side of the heart and angiography of the coronary arteries, the aorta, and the left ventricle. Catheterization is usu-

ally performed via the femoral vein or artery, although the brachial vein or artery may also be used. In both right and left heart catheterization, a medium contrast is injected at various positions within the coronary circulation, allowing for multiple images that will later be viewed on a cine film viewer.

Heparin boluses are used during the catheterization to prevent clot formation. Protamine sulfate may be used to reverse the effects of heparin. Atropine sulfate or pacing may be used to reduce the risk of vasovagal reactions that may occur during the catheterization. Nitroglycerin may be used to prevent angina caused by spasm and/or the administration of the medium contrast. Ergonovine, a vasoconstrictor, may be administered to patients suspected of coronary spasm who do not show evidence of coronary artery disease.

Electrophysiologic Studies

Electrophysiologic studies (EPS) are used in the evaluation of a variety of suspected cardiac dysrhythmia disorders. General indications for EPS include unexplained recurrent syncope, recurrent sustained ventricular tachycardia, suspected accessory pathway causing supraventricular tachycardia, and differential diagnosis of wide QRS tachycardia. EPS is a prerequisite to the insertion of automatic implantable cardioverter/defibrillators. EPS is contraindicated for patients with electrolyte disorders, drug toxicities, and active ischemia and for those in whom such a dysrhythmia intentionally induced will be extremely difficult to terminate or will cause severe hemodynamic compromise.

Most EP catheters are inserted via the femoral veins. Heparin may or may not be used. Multiple catheters may be inserted simultaneously and recordings taken from various areas of the right side of the heart, such as the coronary sinus, bundle of His, and right ventricle. Conduction times are recorded as spikes on graph paper and then later interpreted as to potential high-grade versus low-grade blocks.

In addition to the diagnosis of potential blocks, EPS provides a method for simulation of particular dysrhythmias within a controlled environment via stimulation of different areas of the heart. Cardiac pacing is used to assess sinus node recovery time, sinoatrial conduction time, conduction interval through the bundle of His, and refractory times of the AV conduction system.

A left ventricle approach may be required for diagnosing and inducing ventricular tachycardia. The femoral artery is used, and heparin is required.

Mapping refers to tracing the path of a circulating reentrant impulse and is crucial before consideration of surgical interruption of part of the circuit.[17] It is used to evaluate components of the tachycardia circuit and accessory pathways of supraventricular tachycardia.

EPS is also useful in the evaluation of drug therapy. Antiarrhythmic drugs are discontinued prior to all studies. Determination of drug effectiveness includes ascertaining the ability of the drug to prevent initiation of the dysrhythmia, change the dysrhythmia so that it is less hemodynamically compromising, or abolish the dysrhythmia.

Atherosclerosis

The terms "atherosclerosis" and "arteriosclerosis" are often used synonymously, although a slight distinction can be made between the two. Arteriosclerosis is due to the normal aging process and involves minor intimal and medial changes of the arterial wall. Atherosclerosis is a special type of thickening and hardening of medium-sized and large arteries. It accounts for ischemic heart disease, cerebral vascular accidents, peripheral vascular disease, and aneurysms of the lower abdomen.

Clinical antecedents

Heart disease and stroke and related disorders account for almost as many deaths as all other causes of death combined. Almost one out of every two Americans dies of cardiovascular disease. Of the current U.S. population of approximately 243 million, over 67 million suffer some form of this disease—more than one in four Americans.[18] (See Table 4-6 for the estimated deaths due to cardiovascular disease, by major type of disorder.) For 1990, the cost of cardiovascular disease was estimated by the American Heart Association to be $94.5 billion. This figure includes the cost of physician and nursing services, hospital and nursing home stays, the cost of medications, and lost productivity resulting from disability.[19] It is interesting to note that atherosclerosis is limited to the more industrialized nations, such as the United States, Europe, and the Soviet Union, and is rare in Asia, India, Africa, and South and Central America.

Atherosclerotic deposits are most commonly found in the area of a bifurcation, such as in the abdominal aorta. The coronary arteries and thoracic aorta are the second and third most common areas for deposition.

Table 4-6   Estimated Incidence of U.S. Deaths Due to Cardiac Disease, 1987

Disease	Incidence	Percentage of Total U.S. Cardiac Deaths
Heart attack (MI)	513,700	52.6
Other cardiovascular disease	276,800	28.3
Stroke	149,200	15.3
Hypertension	30,900	3.2
Rheumatic fever/heart disease	6100	0.6

Source: National Center for Health Statistics, Department of Health and Human Services.

In the late 1940s and 1950s, several studies investigating the risk factors for atherosclerosis—most specifically, coronary artery disease—were performed. Perhaps the best known of these studies is the Framingham Heart Study. Data from this study are still being collected today, forty years later. The major findings from this study to date conclude that there are major risk factors for coronary artery disease (CAD) as well as contributing risk factors. The major risk factors for CAD can be broken down into modifiable and nonmodifiable factors. The nonmodifiable risk factors are:

Gender   Men have a greater risk of heart attack than women do. Even after menopause, when women's death rate from heart disease increases, it is not as great as men's.

Race   Blacks have almost a 33% greater chance of having high blood pressure than whites. Consequently, their risk of heart disease is greater.

Age   About 55% of all heart attack victims are age 65 or older, and of those who die, almost four out of five are over 65.

Heredity   A tendency toward heart disease or atherosclerosis appears to be hereditary.

The factors that are modifiable include cigarette smoking, high blood pressure, and high blood cholesterol level.

Smoking causes damage to cells of the artery walls from the circulating carbon monoxide. Also, smoking causes an increase in platelet agglutination and an increase in lipid mobilization into the arterial wall. The risk of heart attack for smokers is more than twice that for nonsmokers. In fact, cigarette smoking is the biggest risk factor for sudden cardiac death: smokers run two to four times the risk of nonsmokers. Smoking is also the biggest risk factor for peripheral vascular disease. When people stop smoking, regardless of how long or how much they've smoked, their risk of heart disease rapidly declines.

High blood pressure increases the heart's workload. It causes damage to the inner lining of the blood vessels, which leads to an increase in the permeability of lipids into the arterial wall. Hypertension also causes platelet agglutination, with release of vasoactive amines. Hypertension is most commonly defined as systolic pressure greater than 140 mm Hg and/or diastolic pressure greater than 90 mm Hg. Studies are inconclusive as to which parameter is more important in predicting the development of CAD, but 140/90 is generally the defining point below which a person is considered not at risk.

The risk of CAD is directly related to the concentration of plasma cholesterol. There appears to be no single level that separates risk from no risk. Measuring the cholesterol constituents (lipoproteins) is more accurate and predictive than measuring the total cholesterol level. The major lipoprotein families are chylomicrons, very low-density lipoproteins (VLDL), low-density lipoproteins (LDL), and high-density lipoproteins (HDL). Plasmal concentrations of LDL are most predictive for CAD, because 60–75% of the total plasma cholesterol is normally transported as this type of lipoprotein. Whereas LDL cholesterol is directly related to increased risk, HDL shows an indirect relationship. Chylomicrons are composed primarily of triglycerides. Even marked chylomicronemia has not been associated with premature CAD.[20] However, high triglycerides are usually associated with hypertension, obesity, and glucose intolerance, all of which can contribute to CAD.

Figure 4-31 displays the relationship between the three major modifiable risk factors and the risk for CAD. Note that the risk for CAD increases proportionally to the levels and that the effects are cumulative.

In addition to the major risk factors, there are a number of contributing risk factors.[21] These contributing risk factors, listed below, are not in themselves predictive, but do add to the cumulative effect.

Abnormal glucose intolerance Among adults, both insulin-dependent and non-insulin-dependent diabetics appear to be at increased risk for development of CAD.

Gout Gouty arthritis has been associated with a doubling of the risk of developing CAD.

Menopause and oral contraceptives Women in their forties and fifties who have undergone menopause have been found to have triple the incidence of CAD. The risk of myocardial infarc-

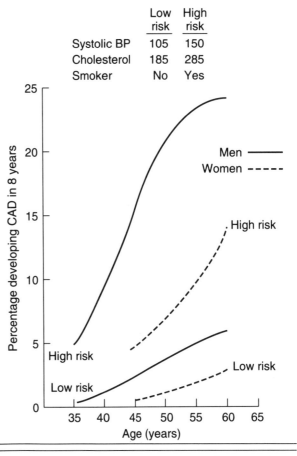

	Low risk	High risk
Systolic BP	105	150
Cholesterol	185	285
Smoker	No	Yes

Figure 4-31 Life-style Risk Factors in Coronary Artery Disease

tion is greatly enhanced in young women using oral contraceptives who have associated adverse risk factors.

Obesity Obese persons also commonly have other associated adverse risk factors such as hypertension and hypercholesterolemia.

Physical activity The benefits of physical activity are becoming more and more evident. A sedentary life-style often enhances risk factors such as hypertension, whereas an active life-style can increase the levels of circulating HDL and lower the blood pressure.

Personality traits There has been identified a "coronary-prone type behavior," often referred to as a Type A personality.

Critical referents

The exact mechanism of atherosclerosis has not yet been identified, but there are basically two theories as to its formation. The encrustation theory states that small white mural thrombi composed of blood elements (platelets, fibrin, and leukocytes) collect on areas of arterial intimal injury (due to hemodynamics and trauma to the arterial wall). The organization of these thrombi by smooth muscle cells and their gradual growth play a definitive role in the progression of the plaque. The insudation theory states that the principal factor in the progression of the plaque is the increased passage and accumulation of plasma constituents from lumen to intima, a type of low-grade inflammatory response.[22] The encrustation theory tends to account for environmental factors, and it accounts for the white thrombi that are often found. The insudation theory, the more predominant theory, accounts for the part played by elevated serum lipoproteins in carrying cholesterol into the arterial wall. There are indications of periods of stability and even regression interspersed with periods of progression, throughout the lifespan, until the plaque becomes clinically evident. Actually, many theorists believe in a convergence of these two theories. That is, the endothelial injury accelerates atherogenesis because it results in encrustation of platelets and passage of lipids into the intimal wall of the artery. Additionally, hypercholesterolemia itself leads to an increase in the endothelial permeability.

Resulting signs and symptoms

Signs and symptoms become evident when the progression of atherosclerosis reaches a clinical state, usually when the vessel is 85–95% occluded. Chronic obstruction of the vessels causes greater and greater compromise in oxygenation of the tissues supplied by the involved arteries. End products of anaerobic cellular metabolism, such as lactic acid that is formed in ischemia, actually cause the physical discomfort experienced clinically. Once the ischemic incident subsides, the metabolites clear, and the pain decreases.

The severity of the pain experienced depends on the site and extent of the occlusion and the amount of collateral circulation the individual has developed. Ischemic pain first appears only during exercise or stress, but as the disease progresses, the pain is soon experienced even during rest.

Nursing standards of care

Treatment for atherosclerosis and CAD must be directed toward reduction of the modifiable risk factors. Medications alone are not successful in halting the progression of the disease. The most successful treatment for CAD continues to be prevention. Preventive measures include education about the etiology of CAD, the risk factors for CAD, and methods to reduce the modifiable risk factors. Dietary modification is required to reduce the cholesterol level (hypercholesterolemia) and to reduce the serum sodium level in order to decrease hypertension. The patient must be encouraged to quit smoking, have frequent blood pressure checks, and take medications as prescribed. Various medications may be prescribed to lower the cholesterol level. These agents work by either decreasing the passage of

Table 4-7 Interventions in Advancing CAD

	Youth	Adult	Middle Age	Elderly
Progression	High cholesterol →	Benign lesion	→ Complex lesion	→ Occlusion
	High fat	High cholesterol		Stroke
	Hypertension	High fat		
	Smoking	Obesity		
		Sedentary life style		
		Stress		
		Hypertension		
		Smoking		
Intervention	Screening	Life-style changes	Coronary artery bypass graft	CPR
	Risk prevention	• lower cholesterol	Angioplasty	Rehabilitation
		• lower dietary fat	Life-style changes	Medication support
		• stop smoking		
		• exercise		
		• lower BP		
		• reduce stress		

cholesterol from the gut into the systemic circulation or by actually lowering the circulating level within the bloodstream. Hypertension may be treated with medication, reduced salt intake, weight reduction, and increased physical activity. Antihypertensives can cause numerous side effects, so during treatment, the patient should be questioned about the occurrence of such effects. Once CAD has developed, methods of intervention must be directed toward retarding or reversing the development of progressive plaques. Invasive techniques may need to be used. These invasive techniques include percutaneous transluminal coronary angioplasty, coronary artery bypass graft surgery, and, recently, laser ablation of the atherosclerotic plaque. Table 4-7 displays the spectrum of available methods of intervention in human atherosclerosis.

The following nursing care plan summarizes the critical care practices used in the management of the patient with atherosclerosis.

Nursing Care Plan for the Management of the Patient with Atherosclerosis

Diagnosis	Signs and symptoms	Intervention	Rationale
Knowledge deficit with respect to diagnostic and follow-up tests and procedures	Patient verbalizes lack of knowledge	Assess patient's understanding of tests	To establish baseline
		Provide information to patient and family on diagnostic tests and procedures: description of procedure, reason for procedure, how it will feel, what is expected of patient, dietary and activity restrictions, follow-up expectations, and final outcome of tests and procedures	Information and patient teaching will help to allay anxiety and increase patient's adherence to regime
Alteration in comfort related to ischemia	Patient describes midsternal chest heaviness, squeezing, crushing, viselike pressure, etc.; may radiate to the jaw, arms, elbows, or between shoulder blades; discomfort occurs more commonly on left side; may also experience epigastric discomfort	Assess for quality and type of discomfort; have patient compare any previous episode of angina to present episode	Angina experience varies greatly among individuals and may be misdiagnosed as GI in origin
		Administer medications such as nitroglycerin and nifedipine SL, as ordered (keep in mind actions and side effects of all drugs given)	Nitroglycerin increases oxygen supply to the arteries by dilating them; nifedipine decreases oxygen demand and increases oxygen supply
		Administer oxygen	Supplemental oxygen will improve oxygen supply to ischemic areas
Knowledge deficit with respect to disease process	Patient verbalizes lack of knowledge; behavior exhibits lack of insight into disease and risk factors	Review etiology and risk factors for CAD	Sound understanding of course and risk factors of CAD aids in adherence to regimen
		Provide information about low-cholesterol, low-fat, and low-salt diet	CAD is directly related to high serum levels of cholesterol and fat and hypertension

Diagnosis	Signs and symptoms	Intervention	Rationale
		Instruct on medications, warning signs and symptoms, and follow-up care	Patients frequently stop taking medications once they feel good or because of multiple side effects; adherence may prevent further complications
Alteration in nutritional status: intake greater than body requirements, leading to high cholesterol, fat, and sodium serum levels	Obesity Elevated cholesterol, sodium, and fat serum levels	Provide instruction on low-cholesterol, low-fat, low-sodium, and reduced calorie diet	Patient understanding of diet will help to improve adherence to regimen
		Instruct patient on importance of periodic cholesterol, sodium, and fat serum screening	
		Provide information on lipid-lowering agents; encourage patient to use bulk laxatives with resin exchange agents	Resin exchange agents frequently cause GI upset and constipation
Anxiety related to newly diagnosed cardiac disorder	Restlessness Withdrawal Denial behavior Acting out	Assess for verbal and nonverbal signs of anxiety	To establish baseline
		Assess anxiety level in relation to episodes of pain	Anxiety may precipitate recurrence of pain
		Provide information regarding CAD to patient and family	Life-style changes will be required of patient and family members
		Encourage questions relating to patient education; set realistic and attainable goals with patient and family	Assurance of patient and family understanding of what is taught and setting realistic, short-term goals increase adherence to regimen

Angina Pectoris

Angina pectoris is a clinical syndrome of ischemic heart disease that is manifested by discomfort in the chest and/or surrounding areas. It was first described by Sir William Heberden as a "disorder of the breast." He continued his description:

> . . . They who are afflicted with it, are seized, while they are walking (more especially if it be uphill and soon after eating) with a painful and most disagreeable sensation in the breast, which seems as if it would extinguish life, if it were to continue, but the moment they stand still, all this uneasiness vanishes.

Angina pectoris can be described in a number of ways. Most commonly, it is distinguished as either stable or unstable. Stable angina is most often caused by an imbalance between supply of and demand for oxygen. It is somewhat predictable, in that similar activities will usually provoke an episode and it can usually be relieved with rest and/or medication. Chronic stable angina may also present with periods of unstable angina. Unstable angina is often due to an underlying process within the lining of the artery. It generally requires further diagnostic testing and medical/surgical intervention. Unstable angina may also be called accelerating angina or unstable rest angina, and the patient suffering this type of angina is usually admitted to the hospital.

Clinical antecedents

In the majority of cases, angina pectoris is caused by atherosclerosis. Mechanisms of atherosclerosis are discussed in the preceding section. Although atherosclerosis is the underlying process, there appear to be a number of factors involved in the clinical presentation of unstable angina. These include the following:

Extracardiac factors These factors are usually those that upset the balance between oxygen supply and oxygen demand, such as tachydysrhythmias, fever, infection, thyrotoxicosis, use of sympathomimetic drugs, anemia, and hypoxia, all of which increase oxygen demand.

Rapid progression of atherosclerosis This may be a cause of unstable angina; however, it is difficult to distinguish between progressive atherosclerosis and incorporation of a thrombus into a plaque. In theory, severe coronary artery stenosis will produce turbulent flow and stasis and may increase local platelet aggregation.[23]

Platelet aggregation in diseased vessels Several studies have shown platelet accumulation at the site of the stenosis. Platelet aggregation has also been shown to release thromboxane and serotonin, which can cause localized vasoconstriction.[24]

Transient coronary artery thrombosis Because it has been shown that patients suffering acute myocardial infarction frequently experience thrombus formation at the site of the stenosis, it is postulated that persons with unstable angina patterns have transient episodes of thrombus formation.

Hemorrhage into an atheromatous plaque This condition is suspected of being a cause of rapid occlusion of a partially obstructed coronary artery. Isolated hemorrhage into a plaque does not seem to be a common mechanism in producing unstable angina, but dissecting hemorrhage and plaque fissuring does.[25]

Abnormal vasoconstriction of a conductive coronary artery A final factor in the unstable angina pattern is abnormal vasoconstriction of a conductive coronary artery. Known as variant or Printzmetal's angina, it is caused by spasm of the coronary artery. Normally, coronary arteries, like other arteries throughout the body, undergo changes in vascularity to meet the heart's demand. In variant angina, there is an area of hyperreactivity that causes the artery to go into spasm, thus diminishing blood supply to an area of the myocardium. This form of angina is most common among young men, especially those who smoke. If prolonged spasm occurs, it can result in permanent damage to the myocardium; prolonged spasm of a major artery may be particularly detrimental because young men usually have not developed the collateral circulation that is commonly seen in the elderly. Thus, a greater area of myocardium is at risk in such cases.

Critical referents

It is proposed that angina is a continually repeating cycle of clinical stability interrupted by acute pathophysiological syndromes. The central idea is that this clinical iteration is driven by two cycles at the endothelial surface, which determine the patient's specific symptomatic presentation.[26] The first cycle consists of stable atheroma, endothelial ulceration, platelet adhesion, and ulcer healing. The coronary arteries in stable angina have smooth, yellow-white atheroma on the endothelial surface. When the atheroma develops an endothelial ulceration, the clinical presentation becomes accelerated angina (increased frequency of angina, without rest pain). Platelet aggregates that form on the ulceration may embolize, causing sudden death or ischemic cardiomyopathy. The ulcer then heals, and there is a rapid progression of the coronary stenosis at the site, but the clinical state returns to chronic stable angina.[27] The second cycle consists of endothelial ulceration, partial thrombosis, thrombus evolution, thrombus incorporation, and stable atheroma, where a partially occlusive thrombosis develops on the endothelial ulcer, and the patient experiences unstable rest angina. The thrombosis may proceed to occlusion and result in an infarction, or the thrombus may be incorporated and cause rapid progression of the coronary stenosis. There is then a return to the chronic stable angina pattern.[28]

Resulting signs and symptoms

Just as the causes of unstable angina pectoris vary, so do the clinical presentations. Descriptions of the pain include "viselike," "squeezing," "strangling," "suffocating," "heavy," "crushing," and "like someone on my chest." The discomfort may even present as a toothache or as numbness in the extremities. The patient may describe chest discomfort while placing a closed fist on the chest. This is known as the Levine sign and is somewhat of a hallmark of descriptors for angina. Angina is not a stabbing, sharp pain, but a continuous mild to severe discomfort, lasting from 3 to 30 minutes or longer, if measures are not taken to relieve it. There is no tenderness to the chest wall, and the discomfort does not abate with change in position. The discomfort may radiate to various areas and, in fact, may not even involve the chest. The most common areas of discomfort are the left inner aspect of the arms, the jaw, between the shoulder blades, the neck, and the elbows. The majority of the radiation is to the left side of the body, frequently to the arm.

Atypical angina has similar precipitating factors but of a different quality (nonanginal discomfort has neither the same precipitating factors nor quality). The patient will often present as anxious, tachypneic or dyspneic, and distressed. The color may be pale, and the patient may be diaphoretic and complain of fatigue. The heart rate and blood pressure may be elevated, either in response to the pain or as a precipitating factor. The physical examination may offer little information. The heart sounds may be normal, unless there is the onset of congestive failure or a ruptured papillary muscle associated with the anginal episode. The most important part of the initial assessment will be ascertaining the history and chief complaint.

In the majority of cases the patient will have a normal initial ECG. When it is abnormal, it may simply show nonspecific ST-T wave changes. The ECG may show ST segment depression or inverted T waves. The patient experiencing variant angina may have ST segment elevation that returns to baseline upon relief of the discomfort. The chest x-ray and serum enzymes (CPK, LDH, and SGOT) will be normal.

Nursing standards of care

Medical interventions are directed toward finding the cause of the patient's chest discomfort. The immediate concern is that it is cardiac-related; once a cardiac origin has been ruled out, other etiologies, such as gastrointestinal, may be investigated. Serial ECGs and serum isoenzymes should be performed to rule out myocardial infarction. If these tests are negative, an exercise stress test, nuclear medicine stress test, or cardiac catheterization may be performed. If a diagnosis of CAD is confirmed, further interventions will depend on the suspected extent and progression of the disease. The patient may be started on a medication regimen of nitrates, beta blockers, and/or calcium channel blockers.

Nitrates work by increasing coronary blood flow and decreasing preload to the heart. Beta blockers decrease the force of contraction and the blood pressure, thereby decreasing the workload and the heart rate. Calcium channel blockers are smooth muscle relaxers that decrease the force of contraction, increase coronary circulation, and can slow SA and AV node conduction. Other interventions include percutaneous transluminal coronary angioplasty (PTCA), coronary artery bypass graft (CABG), and cardiac rehabilitation.

PTCA is an invasive technique that involves dilatation of a stenotic lesion with a balloon on the tip of a catheter. The catheter is inserted in a fashion similar to cardiac catheterization, and the balloon is then inflated for approximately 30 seconds (Figure 4-32). PTCA is indicated for stable angina that is refractory to medical therapy and where there are relatively proximal lesions in one of the major coro-

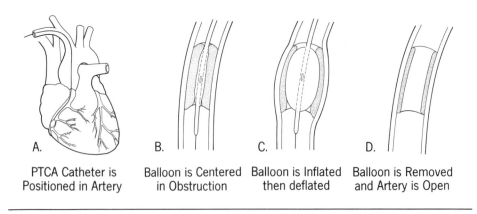

A. PTCA Catheter is Positioned in Artery

B. Balloon is Centered in Obstruction

C. Balloon is Inflated then deflated

D. Balloon is Removed and Artery is Open

Figure 4-32 Angioplasty

nary arteries. Areas of stenosis are usually less than 1 cm in length. The patient with left main stenosis is not a candidate for PTCA since too much of the coronary circulation is involved, but when this procedure is performed it is successful in 60–80% of cases. If the artery reoccludes, it will usually do so within the first 6 weeks following PTCA.

Coronary artery bypass graft (CABG) surgery is indicated for the patient with critical areas of stenosis for which PTCA would not be a viable option. PTCA and CABG are discussed more fully in a later section.

Nursing management of angina should be directed toward actual and potential problems, as identified in the history and risk factor profile. Nursing goals should include (1) promotion of comfort and rest, (2) promotion of health practices through education, and (3) prevention of complications. The following nursing care plan outlines the standards of critical care practice in cases of angina pectoris.

Nursing Care Plan for the Management of the Patient with Angina Pectoris

Diagnosis	Signs and symptoms	Intervention	Rationale
Knowledge deficit with respect to diagnostic and follow-up tests and procedures	Patient verbalizes lack of knowledge	Assess patient's understanding of tests	To establish baseline
		Provide information to patient and family on diagnostic tests and procedures: description of procedure, reason for procedure, how it will feel, what is expected of patient, dietary and activity restrictions, follow-up expectations, and final outcome of tests and procedures	Information and patient teaching will help to allay anxiety and increase patient's adherence to regime
Alteration in comfort related to ischemia	Patient describes midsternal chest heaviness, squeezing, crushing, viselike pressure, etc.; may radiate to the jaw, arms, elbows, or between shoulder blades; discomfort occurs more commonly on left side; may also experience epigastric discomfort	Assess for quality and type of discomfort; have patient compare any previous episode of angina to present episode	Angina experience varies greatly among individuals and may be misdiagnosed as GI in origin
		Administer medications such as nitroglycerin and nifedipine SL, as ordered (keep in mind actions and side effects of all drugs given)	Nitroglycerin increases oxygen supply to the arteries by dilating them; nifedipine decreases oxygen demand and increases oxygen supply
		Administer oxygen	Supplemental oxygen will improve oxygen supply to ischemic areas
		Administer morphine sulfate IV as ordered	To alleviate chest pain promptly
Knowledge deficit with respect to disease process	Patient verbalizes lack of knowledge; behavior exhibits lack of insight into disease and risk factors	Review etiology and risk factors for CAD	Sound understanding of course and risk factors of CAD aids in adherence to regimen
		Provide information about low-cholesterol, low-fat, and low-salt diet	CAD is directly related to high serum levels of cholesterol and fat and hypertension

Nursing Care Plan for the Management of the Patient with Angina Pectoris

Diagnosis	Signs and symptoms	Intervention	Rationale
		Instruct on medications, warning signs and symptoms, and follow-up care	Patients frequently stop taking medications once they feel good or because of multiple side effects; adherence may prevent further complications
Alteration in nutritional status: intake greater than body requirements, leading to high cholesterol, fat, and sodium serum levels	Obesity Elevated cholesterol, sodium, and fat serum levels	Provide instruction on low-cholesterol, low-fat, low-sodium, and reduced calorie diet	Patient understanding of diet will help to improve adherence to regimen
		Instruct patient on importance of periodic cholesterol, sodium, and fat serum screening	
		Provide information on lipid-lowering agents; encourage patient to use bulk laxatives with resin exchange agents	Resin exchange agents frequently cause GI upset and constipation
Anxiety related to newly diagnosed cardiac disorder	Restlessness Withdrawal Denial behavior Acting out	Assess for verbal and nonverbal signs of anxiety	To establish baseline
		Assess anxiety level in relation to episodes of pain	Anxiety may precipitate recurrence of pain
		Provide information regarding CAD to patient and family	Life-style changes will be required of patient and family members
		Encourage questions relating to patient education; set realistic and attainable goals with patient and family	Assurance of patient and family understanding of what is taught and setting realistic, short-term goals increase adherence to regimen

Medications Commonly Used in the Care of the Patient with Angina Pectoris

Medication	Effect	Major side effects
Nitroglycerin Isosorbide	Coronary vasodilation, leading to decreased preload and afterload Increased heart rate and contractility	Hypotension Headache
Propranolol Metoprolol	Beta blockers, leading to decreased heart rate and contractility, thus decreased O_2 demand, and decreased AV conduction time and refractory period	Postural hypotension Dizziness and syncope Palpitations Dry mouth Gastrointestinal upset
Digitalis	Increased contractility Lengthened refractory period of AV node Decreased left ventricular end diastolic pressure Increased ventricular automaticity Decreased atrial automaticity	Tachycardia AV block Bradycardia Gastrointestinal upset Headache Drowsiness Confusion Double vision
Furosemide Ethacrynic acid	Loop diuretic Decreased pulmonary congestion	Hypokalemia Hypocalcemia Hypomagnesemia Altered glucose metabolism
Nifedipine Verapamil	Calcium blocker causing vasodilatation, leading to increased coronary blood supply and decreased myocardial oxygen demands Antidysrhythmia	Hypotension Bradycardia (verapamil) Headache Dizziness Altered glucose tolerance Diarrhea (nifedipine) Constipation (verapamil)
Diazepam	Sedative	Drowsiness Fatigue Ataxia
Morphine sulfate	Analgesia Peripheral vasodilation Sedation Bronchodilation	Hypotension Respiratory depression Nausea and vomiting Constipation Urinary retention

Myocardial Infarction

It is estimated that 513,700 people died of myocardial infarction in 1987 (see Table 4-6). Myocardial infarction (MI) is the result of prolonged ischemia to the myocardium, with resultant necrosis of the cardiac muscle. Like angina pectoris, MI is usually due to the underlying degenerative process of atherosclerosis. MI can present in a number of different ways and with a variety of complications.

Myocardial infarctions are classified according to the amount of myocardium involved. Transmural infarctions involve the full thickness of the myocardial wall, are usually associated with a thrombus, and are frequently localized to the zone of a single coronary artery. A subendocardial infarction involves the inner thickness of the myocardial wall, is frequently due to severely narrowed but not occluded arteries, and usually occurs in the smaller coronary arteries. Infarctions are also classified according to location on the left ventricular wall: anterior, posterior, inferior, lateral, and septal. In the majority of persons, the right coronary artery perfuses the right atrium, right ventricle, the SA and AV nodes, and the posterosuperior intraventricular septum. The left anterior descending artery supplies blood to the anterior two-thirds of the intraventricular septum and the anterior portion of the left ventricle. The circumflex artery supplies the obtuse margin of the heart. In most cases, when discussing an MI, reference is to the left ventricle unless otherwise specified. Most inferior wall MIs, however, also involve portions of the right ventricle. It is rare to have an isolated right ventricle infarct, because the right ventricle has lower oxygen demands, the intercoronary collateral system is richer than the left, and the right wall is thinner and obtains some blood flow from the cavity. Atrial infarctions occur in some patients, most often accompanying left ventricle infarcts.

Clinical antecedents

Risk factors for myocardial infarction are similar to those for angina pectoris, in that both are usually due to the underlying process of atherosclerosis. In most cases, an MI is due to thrombus formation within an atherosclerotic plaque. In addition, a number of nonatheromatous causes account for approximately 4% of the cases. These include (1) trauma to the coronary arteries, (2) emoboli, (3) congenital artery anomalies, (4) aortic stenosis and insufficiency, (5) thyrotoxicosis, (6) blood dycrasias, (7) spasm, (8) dissection, and (9) amyloidosis.

There are very few, if any, immediate precipitating factors that are directly identifiable. In fact, the majority (51%) of MIs occur during rest, as opposed to heavy exertion (13%).[29] Surgical procedures associated with acute blood loss have also been noted as frequent precursors of MI.[30] Different types of MI result because of the fact that different areas of cardiac muscle are oxygenated by the various coronary arteries. Spasm, narrowing, or occlusion of the left circumflex artery can lead to a lateral or posterior MI; right coronary compromise can lead to an inferior MI and possibly left ventricular infarction; and left anterior descending involvement can lead to an anterior, septal, or apical MI.

Critical referents

As was mentioned in the section on angina pectoris, MI may be a consequence of unstable or accelerated angina. In most cases, an MI is due to thrombus formation that occludes the coronary artery. These coronary arterial thrombi are usually superimposed on or adjacent to an atherosclerotic plaque. The precise mechanism that causes the thrombi remains controversial. It has been suggested that degenerative changes occur in the atherosclerotic intima and damage supportive perivascular tissue, with the resultant rupture of a plaque that is sometimes accompanied by intramural hemorrhage.[31] The plaque may then either enlarge and occlude the artery or cause exposure of collagen, which can encourage thrombus formation. Another theory is that ulceration of the atherosclerotic plaque causes platelet adhesion and collagen exposure with resultant thrombus formation. Platelet aggregates also release thromboxane A2, which is a powerful vasoconstrictor.

The amount of myocardium at risk for infarction depends on the amount of myocardium that is supplied by the occluding artery and on the extent of collateral circulation from other arteries into the area of myocardium at risk. Within the first hour following occlusion, blood flow and pressure decrease in some areas, and metabolic stimuli cause collateral vessels to open. Ischemic myocardium gets energy from stored glucose, fatty acids, and glycogen. During an infarction, there is increased availability of glucose and glycogen to the area for energy. There is also an acidosis at the cellular level, with loss of potassium, magnesium, and calcium. Norepinephrine is released, which blocks insulin production, thus creating the high blood sugar levels often seen following infarction. The amount of time until actual necrosis occurs varies. This period may provide the practitioner with a "window of opportunity" to intervene and halt or abate the thrombus formation (see the section on nursing standards of care). Once an MI occurs, it takes from two to three months for scar tissue to be completely formed.

The pathophysiology of right infarct does not always lead to right ventricular failure. When it does, it is similar to left ventricular involvement, except that right ventricular dysfunction, if not appropriately managed, causes shock to the left side of the heart, whereas left ventricular dysfunction causes shock peripherally.

Resulting signs and symptoms

The importance of a careful and thorough history during the initial assessment for MI cannot be overemphasized. With the discovery of thrombolytic agents, determining the actual time of onset is of utmost importance.

The general appearance of a patient experiencing an MI is similar to that of one experiencing unstable or accelerated angina. The patient is anxious and uncomfortable, may be pale, cool, and diaphoretic, is tachypneic or dyspneic, and is restless.

The heart rate may vary from bradycardia to tachycardia. Most commonly, the heart rate is fast, due to the release of epinephrine into the circulation. Infarct in certain areas, however, may involve the conduction system, thus causing bradycardia or AV block. For example, in an inferior MI due to right coronary artery occlusion, the patient may present with bradycardia or high-grade block. In an anterior MI due to left coronary artery occlusion, the patient may present with low-grade (second- and third-degree) block. Regardless of the location of the infarct, more than 90% of patients experience ventricular ectopy.

The patient experiencing an MI is usually normotensive. Hypotension may be seen in inferior MI and right ventricular infarct due to a vasovagal reflex or in a severe case of decreased cardiac output caused by extensive ischemia. Hypertension may be seen in response to the increased circulating epinephrine. Frequently, the individual who is hypertensive before an MI becomes normotensive after an MI, then returns to previous blood pressure measurements after 3 to 6 months.

Fever, caused by the inflammatory response within the damaged cells, may be present, some-times beginning at 4 to 8 hours but most commonly seen at 24 to 48 hours.

The jugular venous pressure is usually normal, unless the patient has a right-side infarct, in which case it will be elevated. This elevation is caused by the decreased pumping ability of the right side of the heart, owing to hypokinesis.

The carotid pulse can provide a clue as to the stroke volume. A small carotid pulse suggests reduced stroke volume. A brief upstroke followed by a crashing pulse may indicate a ruptured septum. Pulsus alternans may be seen in severe left ventricle dysfunction.

The lungs may be clear; in fact, a significant diagnostic sign in the event of right ventricular infarct is the clear status of the lungs, which is in sharp contrast to their status with left ventricular compromise. With extensive infarct, especially of the anterior wall, the patient may be in some degree of failure, however, and present with lung congestion. Chest x-rays usually are not effective at depicting this congestion, because they depict changes occurring at a later or more chronic stage.

Heart sounds are frequently muffled and may be inaudible. (Refer to Table 4-2, pages 496–497.) They are usually easier to hear during recovery. An S_4 is a common finding that provides little diagnostic value. An S_3 is considered a pathological indication, and for the patient who has an S_3, the risk of mortality increases from 15% to 40%.[32]

The patient may complain of abdominal discomfort, especially when experiencing an inferior wall MI. The pain may be localized in the abdomen or right upper quadrant.

Assessment of the extremities affords little diagnostic value. In the patient with decreased cardiac output, the extremities may be cool and the nailbeds cyanotic.

The patient may be confused, especially if there is evidence of decreased cerebral perfusion resulting from decreased cardiac output.

Laboratory tests and ECGs are helpful for diagnosing an MI, but they are less helpful in determining the extent of damage. Laboratory studies will show an increase in serum sedimentation and leukocyte count. Enzyme elevation begins within 2 to 5 hours after onset and may not return to normal for up to 3 weeks. The enzymes include creatinine phosphokinase (CPK), serum glutamic oxaloacetic transaminase (SGOT), and lactic dehydrogenase (LDH). The CPK is the first to rise; it exceeds normal levels at 6 to 8 hours, peaks at 24 hours, and returns to normal at 3 to 4 days. The CPK is made up of three isoenzymes: MM (skeletal muscle), BB (brain and kidney), and MB (cardiac). The percentage of MB isoenzyme to total isoenzyme is calculated. A result greater than 8% is considered to be indicative of infarction. CPK values are the most commonly used. SGOT rises at 8 to 12 hours, peaks at 18 to 36 hours, and returns to normal at 3 to 4 days. The LDH rises at 24 to 48 hours, peaks at 3 to 6 days, and returns to normal at 8 to 14 days. There are five isoenzymes of LDH (named LDH1 through LDH5). Normally LDH2 is greater than LDH1; LDH1 greater than LDH2 indicates infarction. The LDH isoenzyme is the least used because of the length of time required to see a rise in it. Figure 4-33 displays the changes in enzymes that occur during certain time intervals.

Patterns of ischemia, injury, and infarction may be seen on the ECG with transmural infarcts (Figure 4-34). Evolutionary changes on the ECG are seen in the following order of appearance: (1) ST segment elevation, (2) development of pathological Q waves, (3) T wave inversion with return of ST segment to baseline, and (4) continued T wave inversion or return upright. Q waves remain present indefinitely. Abnormal Q waves or altered voltage and morphology of R waves are usually diagnostic. T wave abnormalities may be delayed 2 to 10 days following infarction. In a patient who has suffered a previous MI, diagnosis by ECG may be very difficult, if not impossible. T wave inversion may not appear for 24 hours but may persist for years. ST segment elevation appears immediately and may remain for half a day to 14 days. Table 4-8 displays areas of infarction associated with particular ECG findings.

Hemodynamic findings are also useful when providing care to the MI patient, especially for ascertaining and treating right ventricular infarction ac-

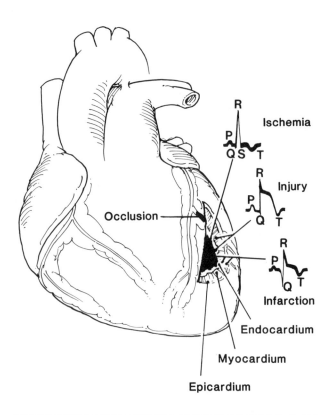

Figure 4-34 ECG Patterns of Ischemia, Injury, and Infarction

companied by failure. When this occurs, hemodynamic findings are (1) normal or slightly decreased pulmonary wedge pressure, (2) right atrial pressure elevation higher than or equal to the wedge pressure, (3) low cardiac output and index, and (4) elevated systemic vascular resistance.

An echocardiogram is often useful for determining the extent of hypokinesis (decreased movement), akinesis (absence of movement), and dyskinesis (paradoxical movement due to aneurysm) as well as other problems of contractility and valve function.

Complications are the most common cause of severe morbidity and death. Dysrhythmias often occur immediately following an MI and may be due to hypotension, hypoxia, ischemia, and hypokalemia or hypomagnesemia. Atrial dysrhythmias are frequently caused by atrial distension secondary to increased left ventricular diastolic pressure. Junctional, first degree, and Wenckebach dysrhythmias are somewhat benign and are seen more often in inferior wall infarctions. Premature ventricular contractions are common and are usually due to ischemic myocardium. Ventricular tachycardia carries a

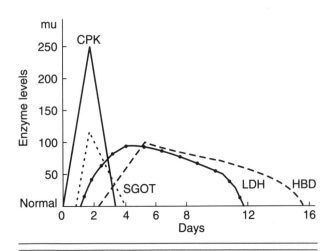

Figure 4-33 Onset and Duration of Cardiac Enzyme Changes

Table 4-8 ECG Characteristics of Myocardial Infarction

Area of Myocardial Infarction	Electrocardiograph Findings
Anteroseptal	Usually, persistent QS; the usual progression in increase in voltage of the R wave will be absent from V_1 through V_3 or V_4.
Anterolateral	Mainly localized to the anterolateral portion of the left ventricle; the greatest ECG changes will be present in leads I, aVL, V_5, and V_6; reciprocal changes may be noted in aVR.
Inferior (diaphragmatic)	Most changes are in limb leads. Minimal changes may appear in V_1 to V_6. Abnormal Q waves are seen in II, III, and aVF. A prominent R wave is seen in I and aVL.
Inferoposterior	A Q wave is seen in II, III, and aVF and prominent R waves in I and aVL; in V_1 through V_4, a tall R and upright T are noted. The usual R/S ratio is reversed.
Posterior	In small infarct, few or no ECG changes are seen. If a large area is involved, a tall R and upright T waves are seen in V_1 through V_4, with a small R in V_6. A Q wave may or may not be present, and T wave inversion is noted in V_5 and V_6. In II, III, and aVF little or no change is noted.
Inferolateral	May produce changes characteristic of anterolateral and inferior infarctions. The greatest change will be noted in II, III, and aVF. There may be only T wave inversions and, possibly, abnormalities in V_5 and V_6.

high mortality rate if seen late in anterior wall infarction. Asystole has an extremely high mortality. Anterior wall infarction may present with Mobitz Type II and complete block and often without previous warning.

Other complications less commonly seen include rupture of the free wall, rupture of the interventricular septum, aneurysm, ventricular thrombus and arterial embolism, rupture of the papillary muscle, cardiogenic shock, and pericarditis. Rupture of the free wall occurs in up to 10% of MI patients who die in hospitals.[33] It leads to hemopericardium and death from cardiac tamponade. Rupture of the interventricular septum is less common and results in extensive hemodynamic deterioration caused by the left-to-right shunt of blood. In such a case the patient presents with a systolic murmur and ventilation/perfusion mismatching. Aneurysms occur most often in an anterior wall infarction and are usually located at the apex of the heart. A ventricular aneurysm is a noncontractile outpouching that causes paradoxical movement of the myocardium wall during systole. This results in a stealing of some of the left ventricle's stroke volume and may result in thrombus formation because of the stasis of blood. Ventricular aneurysms may need to be surgically repaired. Rupture of the papillary muscle is a rare but often fatal consequence of MI. The patient presents with a sudden onset of heart failure coupled with a systolic murmur. Cardiogenic shock and pericarditis are not uncommon complications of an MI and are discussed in another section.

Nursing standards of care

The most recent and dramatic medical interventions for MI have been the development of agents that cause lysis of the thrombus and salvage of the myocardium. These agents, known as thrombolytics or fibrinolytics, act as catalysts in converting plasminogen to plasmin, which then dissolves the thrombus. Thrombolytics are administered during the window of opportunity (the period of time before actual necrosis occurs) to revascularize an occluded coronary artery.

Streptokinase, the first of these agents to be introduced, has several undesirable effects, including systemic anticoagulation, a long half-life, and potential antigenic effects such as anaphylactic reactions. Urokinase does not cause antigenic effects, but it is much more expensive. Tissue plasminogen activator (t-PA) is the most recently introduced thrombolytic agent. It is also called a fibrinolytic because it is clot-specific; that is, it causes lysis only at the thrombus formation. It is superior to the other agents in that it has a short half-life (approximately 2 minutes) and does not cause an antigenic reaction. Relative contraindications to the use of t-PA include a recent history of surgery, significant trauma, pregnancy, cerebrovascular accident, bleeding disorders, and significant gastrointestinal bleeding.

Evidence of reperfusion following thrombolytic therapy include (1) CPK washout (early or markedly elevated peak noted in the CPK isoenzyme), (2) return of ST segment elevation to baseline without development of pathological Q waves, and (3) reperfusion dysrhythmia, often difficult to distinguish from that caused by ischemia and irritability. Cardiac catheterization is essential after thrombolytic therapy.

Therapy in the event of a right ventricular infarct is different from that for left side involvement. Cardiac output and peripheral perfusion must be improved; thus left ventricular filling must be improved. This is accomplished by fluid loading in the presence of high right atrial pressures, rather than fluid restricting. Afterload must also be decreased, and, as usual, this is accomplished by administration of nipride or dopamine.

Other medical interventions in treatment of the MI patient include the following:

Beta blockers Beta blockers are used to decrease the demand for oxygen and decrease the workload of the heart. They are best suited for the patient presenting in hyperdynamic states with tachyarrhythmias.

Nitrates Nitrates are used, especially if the patient is in heart failure. Nitroglycerin IV has a short half-life (2 minutes) and should be titrated rapidly. If the patient is not in failure, the venous pressure may need to be maintained with fluids.

Glucose/insulin/potassium The combination of glucose, insulin, and potassium, at least in theory, is thought to decrease ischemia because increasing the potassium levels intracellularly acts as a protective mechanism.

Morphine sulfate Pain relief is of primary concern in management of the MI patient. Morphine sulfate is the drug of choice because it reduces anxiety, decreases the heart's metabolic activity, diminishes sympathetic tone, and decreases pulmonary congestion.

Adequate oxygenation Coronary arteries must deliver adequate oxygen to the cardiac muscle to prevent further ischemic injury leading to tissue necrosis

Limitation of physical activity Physical activity increases the workload (and thus oxygen demand) of the heart. The patient must be encouraged to rest to allow for maximal oxygenation.

Dietary restrictions Diets must be low in sodium so as not to exacerbate fluid retention, leading to fluid overload (increasing work demands) and congestive failure.

Anticoagulant or antiplatelet agents These agents are used to revascularize an occluded coronary artery to facilitate adequate oxygenation of cardiac tissue.

Nursing interventions for the patient experiencing MI are directed toward actual problems, such as pain and dysrhythmias, and toward potential problems, such as patient nonadherence. The goals of these interventions should include (1) achievement of a pain-free state, (2) achievement of hemodynamic stability, (3) decreased risk of complications, and (4) education about the disease process, risk factors, and medical regime. The following nursing care plan outlines the standards of critical care practice for cases of MI.

Nursing Care Plan for the Management of the Patient with Myocardial Infarction

Diagnosis	Signs and symptoms	Intervention	Rationale
Potential for alteration in cardiac output related to electrical, mechanical, and structural cardiac factors	Decreased cardiac output, as measured with pulmonary artery catheter	Continuous monitoring utilizing V_1 or V_6 and lead II	Most patients will have dysrhythmias following MI; V_1 and V_6 are best for viewing ventricular ectopy; lead II is best for monitoring P waves
		Monitor changes in ST segment elevation	May indicate early extension of MI
		Monitor vital signs with changes in rhythm	May cause hemodynamic changes
		Maintain a patent IV at all times	In emergencies, quickest route and fastest action is via IV
	Decreased BP, sluggish capillary refill, lethargy, and dyspnea	Monitor for signs and symptoms of heart failure	Occurs most commonly in anterior MI but may occur in any type
		Have patient rest and avoid isometric movement/activities; use bedside commode, if stable, rather than bedpan; avoid Valsalva maneuver	Isometrics increase peripheral vascular resistance, thereby increasing the workload of the heart
		Check for capillary refill and pulses every 4 hours and PRN	Sluggish refill indicates decreased perfusion
		Monitor BP and heart rate every 2 hours and PRN	Compromises in BP and heart rate are early signs of decreased cardiac output
	Evidence of dysrhythmia, papillary muscle rupture, septal defect, or aneurysm	Assess heart sounds for sudden onset of systolic murmur	May indicate papillary muscle tear or ventricular septal defect

Nursing Care Plan for the Management of the Patient with Myocardial Infarction

Diagnosis	Signs and symptoms	Intervention	Rationale
	Symptoms of cardiogenic shock: systolic BP < 90; pallor and cyanosis; weak and thready pulse; cool and clammy skin; altered mental states; decreased urinary output; pulsus alternans	Monitor left ventricular function with pulmonary artery catheter	PAD or PCWP > 18 mm Hg indicates onset of pulmonary congestion
		Administer inotropics as ordered (dopamine, dobutamine, amrinone)	To increase myocardial contractility
		Maintain fluid and electrolyte balance using volume expanders	PAD or PCWP < 10 mm Hg may indicate volume deficit
		Anticipate the use of intraaortic balloon pump counterpulsation	To decrease afterload and improve cardiac perfusion
		Administer afterload reduction agents as ordered (nitroprusside, 0.5–1.0 mcg/kg/min)	Reducing the SVR to normal range decreases the workload of the heart
		Administer drugs, as ordered, to maintain normal sinus rhythm	Dysrhythmias can decrease filling time, thus decreasing cardiac output
		Insert Foley catheter; maintain accurate I&O records	Need to monitor output accurately
		Anticipate the administration of other agents to salvage myocardium, such as thrombolytics, propanolol, and glucose/insulin/K^+	Providing nutrients and oxygen, improving circulation, and decreasing myocardial oxygen demand help to salvage myocardium
Potential for alteration in cerebral, peripheral, and cardiopulmonary tissue perfusion	Signs of venous thromboembolism: mottled extremities; edema	Monitor for signs and symptoms of altered stasis	Thromboembolism is a potential complication of bedrest

Diagnosis	Signs and symptoms	Intervention	Rationale
	Signs of pulmonary emboli: sudden onset of chest pain; V/Q mismatch; bloody sputum; dyspnea; very rapid, shallow breathing	Use elastic antiembolism stockings; remove every 8 hours for 10 minutes	To improve venous return
		Check all pulses; compare for bilateral strength of pulse every 8 hours	Diminished pulses are indicative of arterial perfusion alteration
	Signs of arterial thromboembolism: loss of pulses; pain in calf on dorsiflexion (Homan's sign); pale, cool extremities	Check for Homan's sign every 8 hours	A positive Homan's sign indicates arterial thromboembolism
		Do not allow knee gatch of bed to be elevated	Gatching the knee in bed causes pooling of blood in lower extremities
	Signs of cerebrovascular accident: weakness or paralysis on one side of body; altered level of consciousness	Check capillary refill every 4 hours	Indicates the quality of arterial perfusion
		Check breath sounds every 4 hours	Diminished breath sounds may indicate pulmonary emboli
		Check neurological status every 4 hours	Alterations in mental status may indicate altered cerebral blood flow
Potential for complications from pulmonary artery catheter	Infection Balloon rupture Kinking and/or dislodgement of catheter Dysrhythmia Pulmonary artery perforation	Assess temperature and catheter insertion site every 4 hours	Temperature elevation is sign that infection may be at IV site
		Discontinue use of IV as soon as possible; change site after 3–5 days.	Decreases chance of infection at site (per Centers for Disease Control standards)
		Inflate balloon with 1.5 cc or less of air	Overinflation may cause balloon rupture
		Check balloon lumen for presence of blood	Indicates balloon rupture
		Monitor for PVCs, especially right side (appear with same deflection as normal beats)	May indicate irritation from catheter
		Continuously monitor PA waveform for continued wedge shape	Catheter expands after insertion due to body temperature, so it may extend into occluded position

Nursing Care Plan for the Management of the Patient with Myocardial Infarction

Diagnosis	Signs and symptoms	Intervention	Rationale
		Monitor for RV waveform	May indicate kinking or knotting of catheter, which requires repositioning
		Monitor for dampening of PA waveform	May indicate that a blood clot is forming, that the tip is against the arterial wall, or that the pressure bag is not inflated to 300 mm Hg
		Monitor for sudden onset of dyspnea, cough, or bloody expectorant	May indicate perforation of pulmonary artery
Potential for complications related to thrombolytic therapy	Excessive bleeding, reperfusion Dysrhythmias Bruising Decreased hemoglobin and hematocrit	Monitor for signs of bleeding and unexplained bruising	Thrombolytics cause anticoagulation, either on-site (t-PA) or systemic (streptokinase)
		Insert IV lines prior to initiation of thrombolytic therapy	Insertion after thrombolytic therapy is started may cause excessive bleeding at insertion site
		Hold all venipuncture for 30 minutes; avoid arterial punctures during therapy	Thrombolytics break down clotting factors and inhibit clot formation
		Monitor coagulation studies as ordered, specifically PTT and thrombin time; keep level at 2.5 times normal	2.5 times normal is considered optimal anticoagulation state for MI patients on bedrest
		Monitor ECG continuously; treat dysrhythmias per protocol	Risk of reperfusion dysrhythmia is increased with thrombolytic therapy
		Place heparin lock with three-way stopcock for drawing blood	Venipuncture should be avoided as much as possible

Diagnosis	Signs and symptoms	Intervention	Rationale
		Anticipate steroid administration if streptokinase is used	To decrease the risk of anaphylactic reactions
		Monitor 12-lead ECG for ST changes	Return of ST elevation indicates obstruction and possible need for readministering of thrombolytic
		Check all stools, emesis, and urine for blood	Can be an indication of internal bleeding
		Anticipate institution of heparin infusion	To maintain anticoagulation therapy once thrombolytic is discontinued
Impaired physical mobility related to bedrest	Orthostatic hypotension Weakness and fatigue	Assist patient to turn every 2 hours while on bedrest	To promote circulation
		Initiate extremity flexion/extension exercises while patient is on bedrest and patient is free of pain	To promote venous return and decrease risk of complications
		Use bedside commode when patient is free of pain	To minimize patient's expension of energy
		Use antiembolism stockings; remove every 8 hours for 10 minutes	To promote venous return
		Check BP, lying, sitting, and standing	To monitor for orthostatic hypotension
		Encourage patient's involvement in activities of daily living within prescribed MET level: 2 METS (wash face and hands, perineal care, brush teeth); 3 METS (partial bath with assistance, out of bed for meals); 4–5 METS (complete bath, ambulation)	It is important to start cardiac rehab process as soon after patient is free of pain as possible

Nursing Care Plan for the Management of the Patient with Myocardial Infarction

Diagnosis	Signs and symptoms	Intervention	Rationale
Potential for alteration in GI status and bowel elimination	Nausea Constipation	Monitor I&O	To optimize nutritional status and fluid and electrolyte balances
		Provide a liquid diet during first 24 hours after MI, or until patient is free of pain for 24 hours	To decrease the amount of perfusion required by GI tract so that it can be directed elsewhere, especially to the heart; to allay nausea, common with infarction
		Encourage activity when patient is free of pain	To improve GI motility
		Monitor frequency of bowel movements	Constipation is common complaint, due to physical inactivity; Valsalva maneuver and straining during bowel movements are contraindicated
		Administer stool softeners and bulk laxatives as ordered	To provide bulk to GI tract, thereby decreasing constipation
		Administer drugs for the treatment of nausea and vomiting as ordered	Patient should be as calm and relaxed as possible; vomiting precipitates further electrolyte imbalances
Alteration in comfort related to ischemia or infarction	Midsternal chest discomfort that may radiate to one or both arms, elbows, jaw, or neck, or between shoulder blades	Assess for type and quality of discomfort, utilizing scale from 0 (no pain) to 10 (most pain bearable)	To help to evaluate effectiveness of therapy
		Administer nitroglycerin drip as ordered; titrate to control pain while monitoring BP	Nitroglycerine IV increases oxygen supply, but also lowers BP (volume expansion may be necessary)
		Administer analgesics, usually morphine sulfate, as ordered	To lower anxiety, diminish pain, and relieve pulmonary congestion

Diagnosis	Signs and symptoms	Intervention	Rationale
		Assist patient to position of comfort, usually with HOB elevated	To enhance breathing patterns and relaxation
		Monitor for related signs and symptoms such as nausea, vomiting, and hiccoughing	Treatment of symptoms enhances comfort and relaxation
		Assess for pain caused by pericarditis	Pericarditis may occur 24–48 hours after an MI
		Monitor vital signs before and after administering narcotics	Narcotics may cause hypotension due to venous pooling of blood
Anxiety related to ICU experiences and hospitalization	Expression of fears Evidence of inability to concentrate Denial Restlessness	Explain activity levels, monitoring, ICU care routine, diet, and all tests	Not knowing about procedures and routine is common source of anxiety
		Reinforce progress frequently	Patients progress at various rates
		Provide information and educational materials according to patient's needs	Unnecessary information may only increase anxiety
		Assist in techniques of relaxation and imagery; administer anxiolytics, as prescribed	To help to decrease anxiety reactions
Knowledge deficit with respect to disease process and prescribed regimes	Patient verbalizes lack of knowledge	Assess patient's present knowledge level	To establish baseline
		Evaluate patient's readiness to learn	Information will not be assimilated until patient is ready to learn

		Institute teaching program based on patient's needs and covering:
		    normal heart function;
		    MI;
		    risk factors;
		    activity regulation;
		    warning signs;
		    medication
			Presenting to patient only what is applicable increases retention of information; using principles of adult learning helps to increase knowledge retention

Nursing Care Plan for the Management of the Patient with Myocardial Infarction

Diagnosis	Signs and symptoms	Intervention	Rationale
		Evaluate patient's understanding of information and correct as appropriate	Simply providing information does not assure that learning is attained
		Assess patient's potential adherence to regimen following discharge	Nonadherence to required changes in life-style is potential problem; alterations in plan of care may be needed
		Encourage enrollment in rehab program	Six weeks are required for myocardial recovery; significant changes in life-style will be necessary
Alteration in family process	Patient verbalizes stressors in family process	Assess present processes and status of family	To establish baseline
	Ineffective coping mechanisms exhibited by patient and/or family	Encourage family's participation in learning opportunities	Life-style adjustments will be required of all family members
		Consult with social worker and other health care personnel, as indicated	A collaborative team approach increases quality of problem solving and care planning
Anticipatory grieving related to diagnosis and requisite alteration in life-style	Signs of depression Withdrawal Inappropriate behavior: denial; aggressiveness; passive-aggressiveness; extreme anger; flat affect Altered communication patterns	Assess patient's present understanding of disease and its management	Patient may have exaggerated perception
		Encourage patient and family to vent feelings	To provide outlet for stress
		Assess for anticipated changes in life-style	Patient will need much guidance in reordering life-style
		Consult with appropriate health personnel (social workers, home health care workers, nutritionists, psychotherapists)	Multidisciplinary team is most effective and efficient in providing wide range of support services

Medications Commonly Used in the Care of the Patient with Myocardial Infarction

Medication	Effect	Major side effects
Nitrates (nitroglycerine, isosorbide)	Vasodilatation, leading to increased coronary blood supply and decreased myocardial oxygen demand	Hypotension Headache
Beta blockers (nadolol, propranolol, metoprolol)	Blocked beta adrenergic stimulation, leading to decreased myocardial oxygen demand	Hypotension Bradycardia Heart failure Bronchoconstriction Elevated cholesterol Altered glucose metabolism
Calcium channel blockers (nifedipine, diltiazem, verapamil)	Vasodilatation, leading to increased coronary blood supply and decreased myocardial oxygen demand Antidysrhythmia	Hypotension Bradycardia (verapamil and diltiazem) Headaches Dizziness Altered glucose tolerance Diarrhea (nifedipine) Constipation (verapamil)
Morphine sulfate	Analgesia Peripheral vasodilation Sedation Bronchodilation	Hypotension Respiratory depression Nausea and vomiting Constipation Urinary retention
Lidocaine	Decreased ventricular ectopy	In toxicity: disorientation, slurred speech, and seizures
Furosemide	Diuresis Decreased pulmonary congestion	Hypokalemia Hypocalcemia Hypomagnesemia Altered glucose metabolism
Thrombolytics	Lyses intracoronary thrombi, leading to increased coronary artery blood supply and decreased size of infarct area	Bleeding
ASA	Decreased platelet aggregation, leading to decreased thrombosis	GI upset Bleeding

Acute Cardiac Inflammatory Disease

Cardiac inflammatory disease includes three major disorders of the heart: endocarditis, pericarditis, and myocarditis.

Endocarditis

Endocarditis is, very simply, inflammation of the endocardium, usually occurring in the membranous lining of the heart valves.

Clinical antecedents

At risk for endocarditis is the individual who has already experienced damage to the heart valves. Valvular congenital malformations and other preexisting disorders, such as damage caused by rheumatic heart disease, predispose the patient to infections at the site of damage. Valvular structural abnormalities seem to be particularly at risk for bacterial, viral, or fungal opportunistic growth. Invasive occurrences, including dental procedures, surgery, and injury, are precipitating events to endocarditis, as are systemic infections affecting other areas of the body, including the respiratory, genitourinary, and gastrointestinal systems.

Critical referents

Once infectious agents have nestled into the recesses of structural irregularities in the cardiac valves, lesions begin to form as a result of vegetative growth. With the inflammatory process, irregular nodules called verrucae develop at the site of inflammation. These nodules contain bacteria, blood cells, fibrin, collagen, necrotic tissue, and cell material. This mass of growth expands as the inflammation continues, and either emboli form and break off from the parent growth or hemorrhage occurs in the vicinity of the tissue necrosis. Either occurrence leads to extremely serious complications. If left unchecked, the spreading infection will cause extensive destruction to the valve leaflets, as illustrated in Figure 4-35.

Resulting signs and symptoms

The most common symptom seen with endocarditis is, as expected, fever. However, the fever may be extremely high or may be low grade; it may be continuous or intermittent, depending on the infecting agent's clinical characteristic presentation. Regardless, the presence of any fever in an individual who has a history of some abnormality in heart valves, especially in the wake of some other infectious or inflammatory precipitator, should be cause to suspect endocarditis. Other nonspecific complaints such as malaise, fatigue, and general aches and pains also surface in the patient suffering this inflammatory disorder. Physiologically, anemia, a high number of circulating monocytes, and the appearance of petechiae can be indicators of endocarditis. Finally, the presence of a newly developed murmur or the worsening of a preexisting murmur also points to the possibility of endocarditis. As the in-

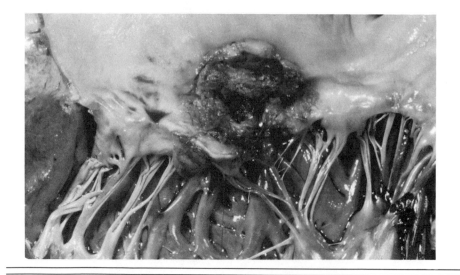

Figure 4-35 Valve Leaflet Damage Caused by Severe Endocarditis

flammation progresses and further damage to the heart occurs, congestive heart failure develops rapidly. This is the leading cause of death for the endocarditis patient.

Nursing standards of care

The most important medical intervention is trying to prevent endocarditis from occurring in the first place. Prophylactic antibiotic treatment is recommended for the individual at risk for endocarditis before any dental procedure or urethral, gynecologic, or abdominal invasive procedure. In the event of actual endocarditis, however, prompt diagnosis leading to appropriate medical therapy is crucial to the successful care of the patient. Blood cultures allow physicians to ascertain the infectious agent and thus to prescribe the correct antibiotic therapy. Echocardiography, doppler imaging, and x-rays also aid in the diagnosis of endocarditis. If the endocarditis proves resistant to aggressive medical therapy or worsens to the point of causing congestive heart failure, surgical valve replacement is indicated.

Nursing priorities are planned in concert with the medical regimen and entail preventing the occurrence of further complications. Fever is treated, and measures are taken to promote healing through facilitating rest and comfort. Further nursing responsibilities are outlined in the care plan presented at the end of this section.

Pericarditis

Pericarditis is an inflammation of the lining of the heart. The incidence of pericardial inflammation detected in several autopsy series ranges from 2 to 6%, whereas pericarditis is diagnosed clinically in only about 1 out of 1000 hospital admissions.[34] Pericarditis is classified according to the acuity of the disease, with most cases being acute. A less common presentation, Dressler's syndrome, or post–myocardial infarction syndrome, also occurs, and is often difficult to differentiate from the acute form of pericarditis. Dressler's syndrome usually occurs 2 to 10 weeks after an infarction and is probably the result of an autoimmune antibody response to certain pericardial and myocardial antigens released at the time of infarction.[35]

Clinical antecedents

Unlike many of the other cardiac disorders, pericarditis does not appear to have an underlying disease process. It is caused by any of a number of problems affecting or involving the cardiac system that may result in inflammation. The most common causes include viral pericarditis, uremia, bacterial infection, acute MI, tuberculosis, neoplasm, and trauma.[36] Table 4-9 lists some common antecedents of pericarditis. Although pericarditis is more common in men than women, the syndrome does not appear to have other risk factors.

Critical referents

The pathophysiology of acute pericarditis is like that of any other type of inflammation, including increased number of leukocytes, increased vascularity, exudation of fluid, and deposition of fibrin. Pericarditis will most often resolve without complication. In a small portion of cases, however, a pericardial effusion can develop and possibly cause a cardiac tamponade. This is a greater risk if the patient is on anticoagulants (for example, post MI). The most common complication is a recurrence of the inflammation. This is more common if the cause of pericarditis is some agent such as a bacteria, virus, or fungus. A final complication that can occur is calcification or fibrosis of the pericardium, leading to constrictive disease.

Table 4-9 Antecedents of Pericarditis

Acute myocardial infarction

Autoimmunity (Dressler's syndrome, postpericardiotomy syndrome)

Drug-related responses (procainamide, hydralazine, penicillin, isoniazid, methysergide, anticoagulants, and daunorubicin)

Infection (bacterial, viral, fungal, parasitic, and tuberculous)

Neoplasms (pericardial tumors and metastatic involvement)

Radiation

Rheumatology (rheumatic fever and arthritis, lupus, and scleroderma)

Trauma (wounds and contusions, angiography, dissecting aortic aneurysm, and pacemaker insertion)

Uremia

Miscellaneous (myxedema and chylopericardium; or condition may be idiopathic or cholesterol related)

Source: Braunwald, E. (1984). *Heart Disease: A Textbook of Cardiovascular Medicine.* Philadelphia: W. B. Saunders, p. 1474.

Resulting signs and symptoms

Pericarditis is diagnosed from complaint of chest pain, ECG changes, laboratory tests, physical examination, and past history. Clinically, the patient frequently complains of severe chest pain that is different from the pressure-type discomfort of angina or MI. The location of the pain may be similar to that of ischemia; that is, it is retrosternal and may radiate down the left arm, into the shoulders, or into the abdomen. Changes of position usually affect the pain, however; the patient is more comfortable sitting upright or forward. The pain is aggravated by coughing, deep breathing, and hiccoughing and may mimic pain that is pleuritic in origin. In addition, the patient may complain of dyspnea.

The most common finding on physical examination is the presence of a pericardial rub. Pericardial rub is caused by friction between the pericardial sac and the epicardium and has a scratching, grating sound. It may be intermittent, and it is best heard at the left sternal border when the patient leans forward or turns to the left side. Classically, a pericardial rub is described as having three components: before S_1, before S_2, and after S_2.

The ECG is helpful in the diagnosis of pericarditis, and the changes in it occur several hours to days following the onset. The changes are seen in most of the leads on the ECG rather than within one area. ST segment elevation is seen but differs from that of an MI in that the elevation is concave upward. The T waves become inverted, but not before the ST segment returns to baseline. There is no loss of R waves or development of Q waves, as is typical of MI. Another change that may occur is P-R segment flattening. Table 4-10 summarizes ways in which the ECG and other characteristics help the diagnostician differentiate pericarditis from pericardial effusion and tamponade.

Laboratory tests such as sedimentation and white blood cell count (WBC) will aid in the diagnosis of pericarditis. The sedimentation and WBC will both be elevated, indicating inflammation.

Table 4-10   Differentiation of Pericarditis, Pericardial Effusion, and Tamponade

Characteristic	Pericarditis	Pericardial Effusion	Tamponade
Etiology	Infection Inflammation	Malignancy Hypothyroidism Renal failure	Cardiac surgery Trauma Excessive effusion
Pain	Severe discomfort upon deep inspiration, relieved by leaning forward	Less intense discomfort of a dull and aching nature, does not respond well to positional changes	Very slight discomfort, if any
Respiratory	No cough Dyspnea	Increased cough	No cough Shortness of breath occurs in advanced stages
Heart sounds	Pericardial rub	PMI displaced Heart sounds may be faint and are heard better when patient is leaning forward or lying on left side	Heart sounds are muffled in all positions
Pulses	Normal	Weak and thready	Faint, especially in lower extremities
JVP	Normal	Slightly increased	Very distended Cannon A waves may be present
Hemodynamics	Narrow pulse pressure Mild hypotension	Pulsus paradox	Arterial hypotension Very narrow pulse pressure High PCWP, LAP, and CVP
ECG	ST elevation in 2–3 limb leads and precordial leads ST depression in V_1 and aVR T wave inversion after ST is isoelectric	ST elevation in precordial leads Low voltage Bradycardia upon inspiration	Low voltage Electrical alternans (especially QRS) Heart block Asystole

Nursing standards of care

Medical management of the patient with pericarditis includes measures to decrease the inflammation and discomfort. Nonsteroidal antiinflammatory agents are usually sufficient to decrease the inflammation, although steroids will occasionally have to be employed. The institution of these agents will also usually resolve the pain. Treatment of the underlying problem is indicated, because pericarditis in most cases is related to some other cardiac disorder.

Nursing management of the patient with pericarditis includes interventions to alleviate the presenting problems (pain and anxiety) and to monitor for complications such as dysrhythmias. The nursing care plan outlines these standards of care.

Myocarditis

Myocarditis is the inflammation of the heart muscle, the myocardium. Myocarditis occurs in association with systemic inflammatory disorders, usually of an infectious nature.

Clinical antecedents

Infectious disorders such as pericarditis, collagen diseases such as lupus, and rheumatic fever are precipitating factors of myocarditis. The infectious agent active in myocarditis may be bacterial, viral, or fungal in nature, but viruses are the most commonly seen.

Critical referents

As with endocarditis or pericarditis, infectious and inflammatory processes overcome normal, healthy tissue to cause serious damage to the heart. These processes are almost always in association with infections and inflammations occurring elsewhere in the body. As in other inflammatory responses, leukocytes rush to the site and fluid exudate increases. As the infectious process progresses, tissue damage occurs and, if left unchecked, will worsen.

Resulting signs and symptoms

The usual signs and symptoms of infection occur with myocarditis: fever, fatigue, and general aches and pains are common. If the myocarditis has progressed, signs of congestive heart failure are evident. Dyspnea on exertion, dependent edema, the presence of an S_3 heart sound, and tachycardia are all symptoms indicating serious damage to the cardiac muscle. Further damage is indicated by the occurrence of chest pain and a pericardial friction rub. X-rays will reveal cardiomegaly, and ECG changes such as ST elevation or depression occur. Depending on the area of the myocardium involved, cardiac arrhythmias and conduction disturbances may be exhibited.

Nursing standards of care

The primary objective of medical care in myocarditis is diagnosing and treating the underlying causes. If the infection has progressed to the point of causing congestive heart failure, the treatment given is that indicated in the care of the patient suffering congestive heart failure. If arrhythmias are present, they must be treated so as to prevent life-threatening cardiac rhythms. Frequently, antiarrhythmics are found to be ineffective, and temporary pacing or elective cardioversion is indicated. As is the case with patients with endocarditis, the patient with myocarditis is at risk for emboli formation, so anticoagulant therapy is indicated. Finally, appropriate antibiotic or antiviral therapy is prescribed, appropriate to culture, sensitivity, and viral screening results.

Nursing care is targeted at protecting the patient from complications of the infection and prohibiting further spread of the inflammatory process. Basic life support is provided, and rest and comfort measures are supplied. The standard practices are outlined in the following nursing care plan.

Nursing Care Plan for the Management of the Patient with Acute Cardiac Inflammatory Disease

Diagnosis	Signs and symptoms	Intervention	Rationale
At risk for complications related to cardiac inflammatory process	Signs of cardiac tamponade: narrowed pulse pressure; low voltage ECG pattern; muffled heart sounds; widening of mediastinum; decrease in cardiac output; distended neck veins	Monitor BP and check for pulsus paradoxus by noting inspiratory drop in systolic blood pressure	Difference greater than 10 mmHg indicates presence of exaggerated pulsus paradoxus and should be reported to physician; may indicate decreased ability of the heart to fill
	ECG changes suggestive of cardiac tissue inflammation: diffuse changes; ST elevation without T-wave inversion; PR segment depression	Prepare patient for echocardiogram	To check the extent of pericardial effusion
		Prepare patient for pericardiocentesis	To remove blood or fluid from pericardial sac to prevent cardiac tamponade
		Avoid the use of anticoagulants in the presence of pericarditis	Anticoagulants can lead to cardiac tamponade
		Obtain 12-lead ECG	Monitor for ECG changes indicative of pericarditis
		Maintain patent IV	To allow for emergency access
		Be prepared for potential complications	Cardiac tamponade can easily recur after pericardiocentesis
Alteration in cardiac output related to myocardial failure	Signs of low cardiac output: decreased BP; increased SVR; increased PAP and PCWP	Anticipate insertion of pulmonary artery catheter	Provides more accurate measure of cardiac function
	Signs of high cardiac output: increased cardiac output measures; decreased BP; decreased SVR; increased PAP and PCWP	Administer preload-reducing agents (nitroglycerin) as ordered, to maintain PAD/PCWP < 18 mm Hg	To decrease venous return
		Administer afterload-reducing agents (nitroprusside) as ordered, to maintain SVR at 800–1300 dyne-sec/cm^5	To reduce SVR

Diagnosis	Signs and symptoms	Intervention	Rationale
		Administer inotropics (dopamine, dobutamine) as ordered	To improve contractility
		Administer drugs, as indicated and ordered, to maintain normal sinus rhythm	To maintain cardiac efficiency and output
		Administer digoxin as ordered	To improve cardiac contractility and control tachycardia
		Monitor BP closely	To assess for hypotension and pulsus alternans
		Participate in identification and correction of aggravating factors	It is most important to correct the underlying cause rather than just treating the symptoms
Potential for alteration in cardiac output related to dysrhythmia	Decreased BP Chest discomfort Dyspnea Palpitations	Check patient's vital signs upon changes in rhythm	Hemodynamic compromise depends on patient's intrinsic state rather than on dysrhythmia alone
		Administer drugs and perform measures, as ordered	As per ACLS standards
		For symptomatic bradycardia and heart blocks: atropine, 0.5–1 mg; repeat in 5 minutes, up to 2 mg; anticipate pacemaker and/or isoproterenol drip at 2–10 mcg/min	
		For ventricular ectopy and tachycardia: lidocaine, 1 mg/kg; repeat in 8 minutes, up to 3 mg/min, followed by infusion at 2–4 mg/min; cardioversion; procainamide at 20 mg/min; bretylium 5 mg/kg, repeat after 8 minutes, up to 30 mg/kg	

Nursing Care Plan for the Management of the Patient with Acute Cardiac Inflammatory Disease

Diagnosis	Signs and symptoms	Intervention	Rationale
		For ventricular fibrillation: defibrillation; epinephrine 0.5–1 mg; repeat every 5 minutes; lidocaine and/or bretylium, as for tachycardia	
		For SVT: carotid massage and/or Valsalva maneuver; verapamil 5 mg IV; repeat in 10–15 minutes; synchronized cardioversion	
		Monitor electrolytes (K^+, Mg^+, and Ca^{++})	Need to correct underlying electrolyte disorder, which may exacerbate dysrhythmias
		Monitor drug levels	To maintain doses in therapeutic range
Potential for alteration in cerebral, cardiopulmonary, renal, and/or peripheral tissue perfusion	Signs of altered cerebral perfusion: mental confusion; dizziness; syncope; convulsions and/or seizures; TIA; yawning	Rule out noncardiac causes of altered cerebral perfusion	Could be due to lidocaine toxicity, neurological disorders, etc.
	Signs of altered cardiopulmonary perfusion: angina; ischemic changes	Monitor for chest pain	Early detection will help to prevent and allay cardiac complications
	Signs of altered renal perfusion: oliguria; anuria	Check urine output every 8 hours, or every hour if oliguria occurs	May indicate onset of prerenal failure from decreased renal perfusion

538

Diagnosis	Signs and symptoms	Intervention	Rationale
	Sign of altered peripheral perfusion: hypotension	Monitor BUN, creatinine, and K^+	A BUN:creatinine ratio greater than 10:1 is indicative of prerenal failure; patient may become hyperkalemic
		Check pulses and BP every 1–2 hours or as needed	Dysrhythmias may cause decrease in cardiac output to periphery
Alteration in fluid volume (excess)	Weight gain Elevated PAD and PCWP Edema Decreased urinary output	Maintain accurate I&O records	To ascertain presence and cause of fluid imbalance
		Limit salt intake as ordered	Excess sodium causes fluid retention
		Restrict fluids to 1500 cc/day if PAD and PCWP are elevated	To prevent fluid overload, which can lead to congestive failure
		Administer diuretics as ordered	Prerenal failure may develop as a result of decreased renal perfusion
		Monitor BUN and creatinine	
		Anticipate low-dose (2–5 mcg/kg/min) dopamine infusion	To provide increased renal perfusion
		Monitor weight daily	Weight change is best indicator of excess fluid loss
		Monitor for crackles (rales) and presence of S_3 heart sounds every 4 hours or as needed	Warn of heart failure and pulmonary edema
		Anticipate need for salt-poor albumin administration	Chronic heart failure predisposes patient to loss of protein, leading to edema; albumin provides mechanism for returning interstitial fluid to intravascular space
		Apply elastic antiembolism stockings	To promote venous return and prevent edema

539

Nursing Care Plan for the Management of the Patient with Acute Cardiac Inflammatory Disease

Diagnosis	Signs and symptoms	Intervention	Rationale
Potential for alteration in gas exchange and ineffective breathing pattern	Dyspnea Decreased O_2 levels on ABGs Change in mental status Fluid overload	Monitor ABGs closely	Problems with oxygenation are commonly seen
		Assist to position of comfort (semi- or high Fowler's position is best)	To improve breathing patterns and lower diaphragm
		Assess for crackles (rales), S_3, and increased JVP every 4 hours or as needed	Signs of heart failure, with resultant pulmonary edema
		Administer oxygen as ordered	To counter problems with oxygenation
		Monitor heart rhythm	Tachycardia is commonly seen
		Review chest x-ray for signs of pulmonary edema	Pulmonary congestion can be clinically delayed up to 24 hours
Potential for infection related to pulmonary congestion, indwelling lines, and Foley catheter	Elevated temperature	Encourage coughing and deep breathing; turn patient in bed every 2 hours while on bedrest	Help to prevent atelectasis, blood clots in legs, and pressure sores
		Change respiratory tubing every 24 hours	Per CDC specifications
		Increase activity as soon as indicated	To promote healing
		Monitor temperature every 4 hours	Sign of infection
	Increased WBCs	Assess WBC count	Sign of infection
		Maintain strict aseptic technique with invasive lines and indwelling catheters; change lines unless contraindicated: PAP every 72 hours, arterial lines every 7 days, tubing every 48 hours, IV bags every 24 hours; provide Foley care every 8 hours	Per Centers for Disease Control recommendation

Diagnosis	Signs and symptoms	Intervention	Rationale
		Assist in identifying source of infection: collect cultures; note atelectasis on chest x-ray; note sputum and urine characteristics; check insertion site for redness every 8 hours	Sites at risk of infection must be kept clean with aseptic technique; appropriate antibiotic therapy must be chosen
		Administer antibiotics as ordered	To combat infectious process
Potential for alteration in body temperature	Elevated core body temperature Tachycardia	Monitor temperature every 4 hours or as needed	Temperature elevation 48 hours after surgery or infarction may indicate pericarditis, myocarditis, or endocarditis
	Diaphoresis	Obtain sedimentation rate and WBC count	Elevated levels indicate pericarditis, myocarditis, or endocarditis
		Administer antipyretics as ordered	To lower temperature
		Keep patient on bedrest until afebrile and chest pain is relieved	To decrease metabolic needs
Alteration in comfort related to inflammatory process	Patient describes severe, stabbing chest pain, altered by changes in body position	Assess for type of discomfort	May be mistaken for extension of MI or vice versa
		Assess heart sounds for pericardial rub (best heard when patient leans forward or turns to left side)	Commonly heard with pericarditis and myocarditis
		Administer aspirin as ordered	Normally sufficient to relieve chest discomfort; also has antiinflammatory effect
		Assist to position of comfort	Sitting in high Fowler's position or leaning forward is usually most comfortable

Nursing Care Plan for the Management of the Patient with Acute Cardiac Inflammatory Disease

Diagnosis	Signs and symptoms	Intervention	Rationale
Anxiety or fear related to onset of chest discomfort	Nervous and restless facial expressions Verbalization of anxiety or fear	Confirm and then intervene for chest discomfort	Prompt intervention may help to allay anxiety
		Differentiate the causes of new chest discomfort versus angina	Patient may be reliving the experience of an MI and fear that this is another "heart attack"
		Administer anxiolytics as ordered	Anxiety increases heart rate and BP
Potential for impaired skin integrity	Redness on pressure points	Assess skin integrity every 2–4 hours	To prevent skin breakdown
		Note redness on pressure points	Early signs of skin breakdown
		Use egg crate or air mattress	To relieve pressure on bony prominences
		Assist patient to turn every 2 hours	To improve circulation
		Institute skin care regimen	Dryness predisposes skin to break down

Patient lacks knowledge of disease process and prescribed regimen	Patient does not adhere to care plan
	
	Patient verbalizes lack of knowledge and understanding or exhibits anxiety and apprehension, especially during procedures and treatments
		Assess patient's present understanding
		
		Institute teaching program for patient and family:
		    normal lung
		    function,
		    pathology,
		    risk factors,
		    control of
		    precipitating and
		    aggravating factors,
		    activity,
		    diet,
		    medications,
		    weight monitoring,
		    signs and symptoms
		    of recurring
		    respiratory failure,
		    follow-up care
			Provides baseline
			
			Increasing knowledge, understanding, and thus potential ability to adhere to regimen may prevent unnecessary rehospitalization

Diagnosis	Signs and symptoms	Intervention	Rationale
		Allow patient and family to ask questions and verify understanding of information	Patient may need reinforcement and several repetitions of information before it is fully understood and integrated
Decreased tolerance of activity related to dyspnea	Dyspnea on exertion Fatigue Exaggerated increase in heart rate and BP on exertion	Assess level of activity tolerance (should be related to the New York Heart Association's classification for consistency)	Provides a baseline
		Assist patient to change position every 2 hours while on bedrest	To decrease risk of complications and promote venous return
		Check BP with patient in horizontal, sitting, and standing positions	To monitor for orthostatic hypotension
		Avoid activity for a half-hour to an hour after meals	May decrease chance of hypoxia due to increased blood flow to GI tract
		Monitor heart rate and BP with activity increases	To maintain heart rate within 10 bpm of resting heart rate and maintain systolic BP within 20 mm Hg of resting BP; if a drop occurs, it may indicate a drop in cardiac output
		Anticipate institution of progressive rehab	To provide controlled mechanism for increasing activity
		Encourage frequent rest periods	To prevent excessive fatigue
Anxiety related to: palpitations; fear of consequences; monitoring equipment; special diagnostic procedures	Restlessness Frequent questioning Withdrawn behavior	Assess level of anxiety	To establish baseline
		Encourage patient and family to verbalize fears	Helps to allay exaggerated concerns
		Explain symptoms in terms of dysrhythmia	Patient may be more aware of heart beating because of diagnosis

Nursing Care Plan for the Management of the Patient with Acute Cardiac Inflammatory Disease

Diagnosis	Signs and symptoms	Intervention	Rationale
		Educate patient and family about etiology and process of dysrhythmia, purpose and procedure of diagnostic studies and interventions, and follow-up care	Lack of knowledge and understanding may increase anxiety and decrease adherence to care regimen
		Administer anxiolytics as ordered	To decrease anxiety
Knowledge deficit with respect to use of antidysrhythmic drugs	Patient verbalizes lack of knowledge and understanding	Assess present understanding of dysrhythmias and drug therapy	To establish baseline
	Nonadherence to care regimen	Instruct on medications and side effects and how to deal with them	Antidysrhythmics commonly have side effects, and patient may stop taking them as a result
		Assess patient's and family's ability to adhere to care regimen	To adapt teaching to status of patient and family in order to maximize adherence to regimen
Knowledge deficit with respect to inflammatory process and follow-up care	Patient verbalizes lack of knowledge	Assess patient's understanding	To establish baseline
	Nonadherence to care regimen	Institute teaching program based on patient's and family's knowledge and needs and covering: signs of recurrence; nature of disorder; taking temperature; chest pain; activity levels	Pericarditis, often in the form of Dressler's syndrome, may recur after discharge; risk of recurrence of myocarditis and endocarditis is also high
		Provide discharge information covering all of the above as well as medications, if applicable	Follow-up care, including medications, is crucial

Medications Commonly Used in the Care of the Patient with Acute Cardiac Inflammatory Disease

Medication	Effect	Major side effects
ASA	Decreased platelet aggregation, leading to decreased thrombosis	GI upset Bleeding
Corticosteroids	Inhibit inflammatic release of proteolytic enzymes to alter acute injury	Hypertension Impaired glucose metabolism Osteoporosis Peptic ulcer Hypokalemia Increased risk for infection
Furosemide Ethacrynic acid	Loop diuretic Decreased pulmonary congestion	Hypokalemia Hypocalcemia Hypomagnesemia Altered glucose metabolism
Antibiotics	Bacteriostatics and bactericidals	As per specific drug
Analgesics	Kinin release inhibitor, to relieve pain and discomfort	As per specific drug

Hypertensive Shock

Hypertensive shock is a sudden and significant rise in blood pressure, producing a crisis situation. Hypertension is a major risk factor for coronary artery disease, and it is prevalent in approximately 25–39% of U.S. adults.[37] Hypertensive shock occurs much less frequently than in the past because of the advances that have been made in antihypertensive therapy. Hypertensive shock is an emergency situation requiring immediate intervention. The patient will most likely present with specific signs and symptoms; hypertension, in contrast, is usually diagnosed by simple blood pressure measurement.

Clinical antecedents

Any patient with hypertension can experience a hypertensive crisis. Although advances in antihypertensive medications and therapy have made hypertensive crises rare, hypertension remains idiopathic in over 90% of the cases. Therefore, the vast majority of patients presenting with an episode of rapidly increased blood pressure will have a diagnosis of unknown etiology.

Hypertension afflicts an estimated 57,710,000 Americans age 6 and older.[38] The frequency of hypertension is greater in men. The life expectancy for a 45-year-old male with a blood pressure of 140/100 is 20 years.[39] Blacks experience almost twice the incidence of hypertension of whites, and, interestingly, Black females have the highest frequency of hypertension in the United States (Table 4-11). There is also an increase in the incidence of hypertension with increasing age. Elderly persons tend to have a greater increase in systolic blood pressure than in diastolic blood pressure. The significance of this occurrence,

which is largely due to decreased aortic distensibility, is unclear.

Salt intake appears to play a role in the development of hypertension. Populations with an overall higher level of salt intake (such as Japan's) have a higher incidence of hypertension than those with a lesser salt intake level.

Heredity also appears to be a factor in hypertension; it is three to four times more common in siblings of hypertensive individuals than in siblings of normotensive individuals.

Obese persons and smokers also tend to have higher blood pressures. The mechanism of these relationships is unclear but may have something to do with increased cardiac output and decreased arterial capacitance. Smoking, for instance, is known to cause vasoconstriction and increased release of catecholamines, both of which cause blood pressure to rise.

Stress is another factor involved in the development of hypertension. Stress causes an increase in the release of epinephrine, mineralocorticoids, and glucocorticoids, all of which cause a rise in blood pressure.

As stated previously, most cases of hypertension are caused by unknown factors. In a smaller percentage of cases, a cause can be found. The most frequent antecedents are listed in Table 4-12. Most theorists

Table 4-11   Incidence of Hypertension by Gender and Race

Race	Gender	Incidence
Black	Female	39%
Black	Male	38%
Caucasian	Male	33%
Caucasian	Female	25%

Source: National Health & Nutrition Survey, 1976–1980, Department of Health and Human Services.

Table 4-12   Antecedents of Hypertension

System or Type	Precipitating Factor
Neurological	Increased intracranial pressure Brain stem encephalitis
Cardiovascular	Aortic atherosclerosis Aortic coarctation
Renal	
Parenchymal disease	Diabetic nephropathy Glomerulonephritis
Renal artery stenosis	Fibromuscular hyperplasia Atheroma
Trauma	Perinephric hematoma
Endocrine	
Adrenal cortex	Cushing's syndrome Primary aldosteronism
Gender-related	Toxemia of pregnancy
Drug side effect	Oral contraceptive Na^+-retaining drugs, for renal patients
Essential hypertension	Unknown

Source: Guenter, C. A. (ed.). (1983). *Internal Medicine.* New York: Churchhill Livingstone.

agree that the causes of hypertension are too diverse to be related to one hypothesis. The most widely accepted theories about the causes of hypertension recognize the effect of salt intake, autoregulation, heredity, calcium regulation, and pressure-natriuresis. But, regardless of the etiological theory, there appears to be an underlying pattern of increased cardiac output and peripheral vascular resistance.

The physiological response first involves an increase in salt intake and/or a decrease in salt excretion. It has been proposed that certain individuals have a decreased ability to excrete sodium. This decreased ability, coupled with an increased salt intake, causes volume expansion, which, by itself, will lead to an increase in the pressure. This increase in intracellular sodium enhances a sodium-calcium exchange mechanism and thereby increases intracellular calcium. An increase in intracellular calcium is known to increase the resting tone of vascular smooth muscle, thereby increasing the pressure.[40] The body normally responds to an acute increase in pressure and volume by increasing renal blood flow and diuresis. It has been proposed that this process might be defective in hypertensives and that this mechanism is somehow reset in these individuals. Another process, known as autoregulation, which attempts to maintain a stable blood flow to the tissues, causes vasoconstriction within resistance vessels to avoid overperfusion whenever the pressure and volume increase beyond certain levels. Increased sympathetic response causes an increase in arteriolar and venous constriction, cardiac output, and salt and fluid retention. It also causes an increase in renin to be released from the kidneys. Renin causes decreased perfusion to the kidneys and leads to the conversion of angiotensin, a powerful vasoconstrictor. Angiotensin is a precursor of aldosterone, which is also a powerful vasoconstrictor and causes sodium retention and potassium excretion.

A final point concerns the role of heredity. Certain individuals are more prone to these maladaptive mechanisms and therefore are at greater risk for the development of hypertension. Figure 4-36 summarizes these hypotheses for the pathogenesis of essential hypertension.

Critical referents

In hypertensive crisis, two processes usually occur. The first involves dilatation of the cerebral arteries, which allows excessive cerebral blood flow, which leads to hypertensive encephalopathy. Normally, cerebral arterial constriction occurs with increased pressure and dilatation occurs with decreased pressure. Once the pressure exceeds a certain level, however, the arteries are no longer able to autoregulate the blood flow by constricting, so instead they become dilated. This dilation leads to leakage of fluid and resultant cerebral edema. The second process involves damage to the arteriolar wall. The precise mechanism, which causes end-organ damage and involves necrosis of the arterial wall, is turbulent blood flow with resultant thickening of the arteriolar wall. This mechanism provides a medium for atherosclerotic change to develop, which then leads to stenosis of the artery and/or weakening of the arterial wall. Thrombus formation occurs when the arterial wall disrupts. This process is discussed in further detail in the section on atherosclerosis.

Hypertension eventually affects other body systems in numerous ways. These effects include left ventricular enlargement, congestive heart failure, angina, myocardial infarction, valve disorders, renal failure, lacunar infarctions in the brain, aneurysms, and encephalopathy.

Resulting signs and symptoms

The signs and symptoms of hypertensive crisis are dramatic and evident. An altered level of consciousness results from cerebral manifestations of increased pressure and resultant cerebral edema. Retinal hemorrhages, exudates, and papilledema can be seen at diastolic pressures greater than 140 mm Hg. Impairment of vision may also occur.

Lacunar infarctions may develop in the brain and are almost exclusively the result of a sudden rise in blood pressure. These lesions may have no clinical manifestations, or they may cause mild focal neurological deficits that are often heralded by a few days of transient symptoms. Symptoms can include motor hemiplegia, unilateral ataxia, dysarthria and upper limb ataxia, and unilateral sensory loss. There is often complete clinical recovery.[41] The patient may complain of headache, be restless, convulse, or exhibit a decreased level of responsiveness including somnolence, stupor, or coma.

Acute oliguric renal failure and elevated levels of renin may occur. The elevated renin levels may exacerbate the hypertension and cause a cyclical process of renin release, angiotensin, and hypertension. Along with renal dysfunction, urine specific gravity may be low, and urine protein and RBCs may be present. Serum BUN and creatinine will rise as a result of the azotemia. Hypokalemia will be present

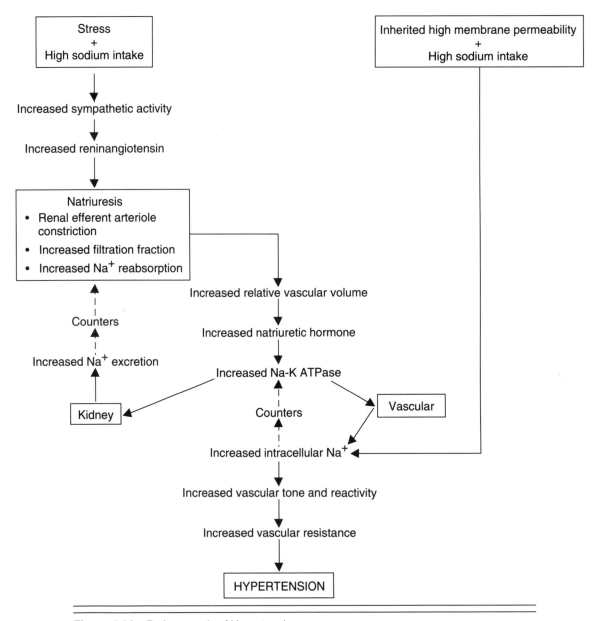

Figure 4-36 Pathogenesis of Hypertension

because of the elevated plasma renin and secondary aldosteronism. Because of the electrolyte imbalance caused by renal disfunction, the ECG may show signs of hypokalemia and left ventricular hypertrophy.

Cardiac changes also include a prominent apical impulse, cardiac enlargement, and congestive failure. The patient will often present with nausea and/or vomiting. Evidence of left ventricular hypertrophy may be noted as a left ventricular heave that does not displace to the left unless cardiac failure is present. The thickness of the left ventricle produces an S_4 heart sound, indicating decreased left ventricular compliance.

Sometimes the patient may evince hemolytic anemia with deformed red blood cells. In addition, the patient may show evidence of intravascular coagulation with increased fibrin split products, thrombocytopenia, and reduced fibrinogen.

Nursing standards of care

Medical management of the patient in hypertensive crisis consists of immediate lowering of the blood pressure. If left untreated, the patient will die of neural or renal damage. Pharmacological management is instituted, and the medication of choice is usually a vasodilator such as nitroprusside. Nitroprusside is administered by intravenous infusion at a dosage between 0.5 and 1.0, initially, to 10 mcg/kg/min. Its half-life is 1 minute, which allows minute-to-minute titration. It acts primarily as an arteriolar vasodilator. Another drug that is less commonly used is diazoxide. It is given by intravenous injection push and repeated every 5 to 15 minutes. It also acts as an arteriolar dilator, but its half-life is considerably longer, and it may cause some reflex tachycardia as well as salt and water retention.

Further medical management includes the use of diuretics and sympathetic nervous system inhibitors and interventions directed toward the resulting renal failure and congestive failure. The major nursing goal is reducing the blood pressure through administration of antihypertensive medications and prevention of complications. Nursing standards of care are outlined in the following care plan.

Nursing Care Plan for the Management of the Patient with Hypertensive Shock

Diagnosis	Signs and symptoms	Intervention	Rationale
Potential for alteration in cerebral, cardiopulmonary, renal, and peripheral tissue perfusion	Signs of alteration in cerebral tissue perfusion: altered sensorium; headache; lethargy; nausea and vomiting; visual disturbances; seizures	Perform neurological assessment every hour; report changes	Change in level of consciousness is first indication of increasing intracranial pressure
		Monitor BP continuously and anticipate arterial line insertion	For closer and more accurate monitoring of BP
		Position head of bed elevated, as ordered	To increase orthostatic effect
		Provide calm, quiet environment	To decrease noxious stimuli
		Don't cluster care; turn patient slowly; avoid Valsalva maneuver; suction only when necessary; institute seizure precautions	To help to maintain more constant intracranial pressure levels
		Monitor CO_2 levels	Elevated levels enhance cerebral edema
		Anticipate CT head scan	To determine degree of cerebral edema
	Signs of alteration in cardiopulmonary tissue perfusion: heart failure	Assess breath sounds every 4 hours and PRN	To assess for crackles (rales)
		Assess jugular venous pressure every 4 hours	Elevation indicates fluid overload
		Obtain 12-lead ECG	To check for evidence of hypertrophy
		Monitor dysrhythmias	Elevated ICP can cause decrease in heart rate leading to ischemia
	Signs of alteration in renal tissue perfusion: oliguria; anuria	Monitor I&O every hour; insert Foley catheter	To assess for effective diuresis
		Administer diuretics as ordered	May experience hypertensive shock due to fluid overload

Diagnosis	Signs and symptoms	Intervention	Rationale
		Monitor K^+, BUN, and creatinine	Assess for renal failure; watch K^+ with diuresis and hyperkalemia with renal failure
		Weigh patient daily	To assess for weight gain due to excess fluid
	Signs of alteration in peripheral tissue perfusion: cool, cyanotic periphery; sluggish capillary refill	Monitor all pulses every 2–4 hours and PRN	Aneurysm can occur from prolonged hypertension
		Administer antihypertensives as ordered (usually nitroprusside at 0.5–1.0 mcg/kg/min)	To alleviate hypertension
		Titrate nitroprusside closely	Half-life of nitroprusside is 2 minutes
		Monitor thiocyanate levels with continued administration of nitroprusside	Indicates signs of toxicity
Alteration in fluid volume (excess)	Elevated BP Edema Increased jugular venous pressure	Administer diuretics as ordered	To decrease fluid retention, thereby decreasing BP
		Follow low-sodium diet when food is tolerated	Additional salt increases fluid retention
Impaired gas exchange related to altered CNS, ineffective airway clearance, and pulmonary edema	Altered ABGs, oxygenation, and respiratory patterns	Monitor respiratory patterns	Cheyne-Stokes respiration and periods of apnea may occur with increased BP
		Assess breath sounds every 4 hours and PRN	Pulmonary edema and/or atelectasis may occur from increased fluid and decreased respiratory effort
		Monitor tidal and minute volumes	Decreasing volumes warn of atelectasis and consolidation
		Assess ABGs as indicated	To check for oxygenation and carbon dioxide elimination

Nursing Care Plan for the Management of the Patient with Hypertensive Shock

Diagnosis	Signs and symptoms	Intervention	Rationale
		Provide humidified oxygen and maintain patent airway	To maintain moist air passages and oxygenation
Potential for alteration in thought processes	Confusion Inability to concentrate	Provide protective environment: side rails up and bed in low position	Patient may become restless and may be unsteady when getting up alone
		Reorient patient to environment	Frequent reminders of place and time help to improve orientation
		Explain all procedures	Familiarity with surroundings, expectations, and various sensory experiences helps to reduce mental confusion
Knowledge deficit with respect to disease process, complications, and treatment	Patient verbalizes lack of understanding Nonadherence to prescribed therapy	Review etiology and complications of hypertension with patient	Episodes of hypertensive crisis are frequently due to patient's nonadherence to therapy
		Instruct about low-salt diet	High salt intake is one risk factor of hypertension
		Instruct on importance of frequent BP checks	To assess early signs of hypertension and prevent reoccurrence of hypertensive crisis
		Educate patient on medications, emphasizing their side effects and how to effectively deal with them	Antihypertensives frequently have side effects that discourage patients from continuing to take them
Potential for alteration in nutritional status due to nausea and vomiting	Nausea	NPO until BP is stable	Retching can increase BP; should not exacerbate nauseous state
	Vomiting	Maintain accurate I&O records	To assess fluid depletion from vomiting
		Administer antiemetics as ordered and PRN	Retching also increases ICP

Medications Commonly Used in the Care of the Patient with Hypertensive Shock

Medication	Effect	Major side effects
Nitroprusside	Vasodilation with direct action on vascular smooth muscle	Nausea and vomiting Muscle twitching Hypotension
Nitroglycerin	Vasodilation, leading to increased coronary blood supply and decreased myocardial oxygen demand	Hypotension Headache
Hydralazine Minoxidil Diazoxide	Vasodilation with direct action on vascular smooth muscle, leading to relaxed arterioles, decreased vascular resistance, and increased cardiac output	Angina Nausea and vomiting Tachycardia Headache Flushing Hypotension
Furosemide Ethacrynic acid	Loop diuretic Decreased pulmonary congestion	Hypokalemia Hypocalcemia Hypomagnesemia Altered glucose metabolism
Trimethaphan Phentolamine	Ganglionic blocker, inhibiting the peripheral sympathetic nervous system	Orthostatic hypotension Ileus Urinary retention Blurred vision Dry mouth
Reserpine Guanethidine	Peripheral adrenergic antagonist, inhibiting peripheral sympathetic nervous system	Drowsiness Nausea and vomiting Tremors Bradycardia Dyspnea Fatigue
Methyldopa Clonidine	Centrally stimulates alpha-adrenergic receptors, leading to decreased peripheral vascular resistance	Drowsiness Dry mouth Vertigo Depression GI upsets
Atenolol Propranolol Timolol	Beta-adrenoreceptor antagonist	Postural hypotension Dizziness and syncope Palpitations Dry mouth

Heart Failure and Pulmonary Edema

Heart failure is a potential complication of nearly every form of heart disease. It is defined as the inability of the heart to pump enough blood to meet the metabolic needs of the tissues. The clinical presentation and prognosis of heart failure varies widely among patients and depend on the patient's underlying disease and risk factors, the etiology, the rate and development of the heart failure, the precipitating factors, and the chambers involved in the failure.

Heart failure may be classified in a number of ways that include high versus low output states (Figure 4-37), forward versus backward failure (Figure 4-38), and left versus right heart failure (Figure 4-39). In addition, heart failure may be either acute or chronic (chronic cases may have episodes of acute heart failure due to, for example, a high output state). Cases of acute heart failure do not necessarily become chronic; for instance, there may be some underlying pathology, such as papillary muscle rupture, that can be remedied surgically.

Most cases of heart failure are caused by low output states. A low output state is defined as decreased pumping of the heart and is characterized by vasoconstriction and cold, pale, and cyanotic extremities, decreased stroke volume, and a narrowed pulse pressure. A high output state is defined as increased pumping of the heart, which still does not provide enough blood to meet the metabolic needs of the tissues. This inefficiency is due to shunting of the blood away from the tissues and is characterized by warm, flushed extremities, a widened pulse pressure, and a cardiac output that is elevated but still

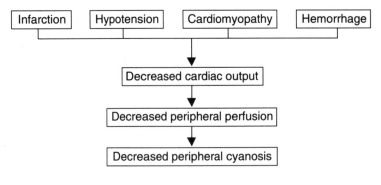

GENESIS OF LOW OUTPUT FAILURE

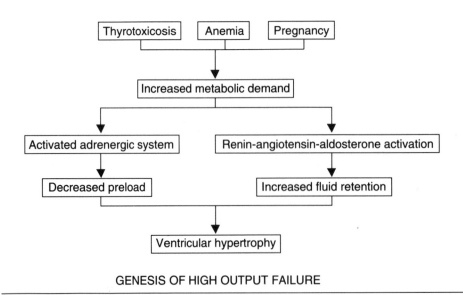

GENESIS OF HIGH OUTPUT FAILURE

Figure 4-37   Low Output and High Output Heart Failure

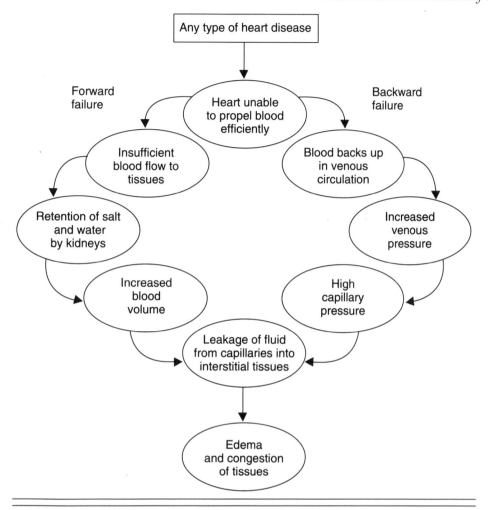

Figure 4-38 Forward and Backward Heart Failure

remains less than it was prior to the onset of heart failure. A low output state may involve the left or right side or both sides of the heart, whereas a high output state usually causes both sides of the heart to fail.

Left or right heart failure simply refers to the side of the heart that caused the failure. Over time, however, problems involving only one chamber will lead to biventricular failure, because both chambers share a common wall (the interventricular septum) and because hemodynamic alterations in one chamber will ultimately cause an alteration in the other. For example, left heart failure can eventually lead to right heart failure if the fluid in the left chambers backs up into the pulmonary bed and into the right chambers.

Clinical antecedents

Heart failure does not have one specific etiology but is a manifestation of other cardiac disorders.

Heart failure can be caused by underlying conditions such as structural defects, physiological events such as increased hemodynamics, and/or precipitating factors such as thyrotoxicosis. Table 4-13 lists specific examples of each of these factors.

Structural defects may cause either a sudden onset of heart failure, such as when the papillary muscle of the mitral valve ruptures, or a slow progression of failure, such as when aortic stenosis is present. Most commonly, these defects cause either a pressure or a volume overload that progresses slowly over time and causes heart dilatation and hypertrophy. A pressure overload is caused by an obstruction to outflow, whereas a volume overload is caused by an increased volume of blood to the ventricle. Aortic and pulmonary stenosis both cause pressure overloads. In contrast, rupture of the papillary muscle or chordae tendineae of the mitral valve or rupture of the interventricular septum will cause an acute volume overload. Arteriovenous malformation will cause both a pressure and a volume overload.

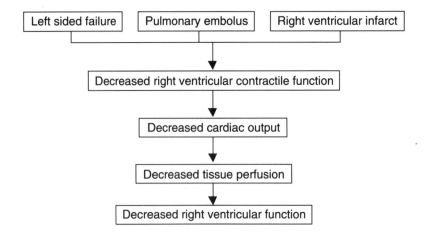

GENESIS OF RIGHT VENTRICULAR FAILURE

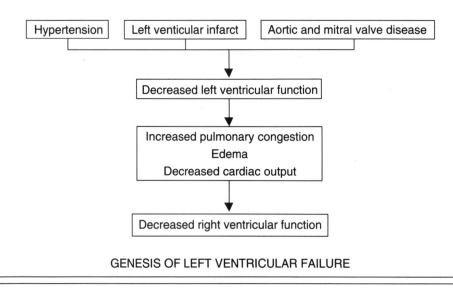

GENESIS OF LEFT VENTRICULAR FAILURE

Figure 4-39 Right and Left Heart Failure

Underlying physiological causes involve factors that either increase the hemodynamic burden or reduce the oxygen delivery to the myocardium. Either situation results in an impairment of myocardial contraction and, over time, results in dilatation, hypertrophy, and stiffness of the ventricle. Systemic hypertension and pulmonary hypertension increase the hemodynamic burden on the heart. MI causes both an alteration in the hemodynamics and a decreased oxygen supply to the myocardium; thus, areas of the myocardium become hypokinetic and akinetic, and cardiac output decreases. Ventricular aneurysm causes a dyskinesis (outpouching of the ventricular wall) of the myocardium, which also results in decreased cardiac output and eventual pressure overload and hypertrophy. Myocardial and endocardial fibrosis result in an overall stiffening of

the myocardium, which decreases contractility and causes decreased oxygen supply.

In order for the heart to meet the metabolic needs of the body, it must have a controlled rhythm, sufficient volume, good contractility, and a properly functioning outflow. Precipitating factors will cause an alteration in one or more of these variables and frequently result in the onset of acute heart failure. The most common precursor to heart failure in a previously compensated patient is inappropriate relaxation of the treatment regimen—dietary sodium restriction, reduced physical activity, a drug regimen, or, most commonly, a combination of these measures.[42] Dysrhythmias can cause a reduction in filling time, decreased cardiac output, and loss of the atrial kick. Systemic infection can lead to heart failure in an already compromised heart, because it causes

Table 4-13 Antecedents of Heart Failure

Type	Antecedents
Structural risk factors	Aortic stenosis AV fistula Interventricular septum rupture Mitral papillary muscle rupture Pulmonary stenosis Ventricular aneurysm
Physiological risk factors	Cardiomyopathy Endocardial fibrosis Hypertension Myocardial infarction Pulmonary embolism Pulmonary hypertension
Clinical precipitating factors	Anemia Bacterial endocarditis Beriberi Cardiac-depressant drug therapy Dysrhythmias Inappropriate reduction of cardiac medical therapy Infection Thyrotoxicosis

increased metabolism and places an increased hemodynamic burden on the heart. Pulmonary emboli also increase the hemodynamic burden through elevation of right ventricular systolic pressure. Bacterial endocarditis and cardiac infection directly impair the myocardium, causing decreased contractility. Thyrotoxicosis, pregnancy, anemia, and beriberi do not in and of themselves cause heart failure but can lead to heart failure in an already diseased heart. These precipitating factors cause a hyperkinetic condition because the peripheral tissues require increased oxygen. If the heart is already compromised, it is unable to meet these increased demands. Finally, cardiac depressant drugs such as beta blockers and calcium channel blockers cause decreased contractility of the myocardium. Other drugs such as nonsteroidal anti-inflammatory agents can cause increased salt and water retention, which increases the volume load to the heart.

Critical referents

Although many of the cases of heart failure seen in critical care are due to precipitating factors, the majority of the patients will also have some form of myocardial heart failure. Myocardial heart failure is the result of specific pathology of the myocardium. Therefore, a distinction needs to be made between myocardial failure and circulatory failure. In myocardial failure, there is an abnormality of myocardial function; circulatory failure entails an abnormality of some part of the circulation, for example, salt and water retention. Myocardial failure, when sufficiently severe, always produces heart failure, but the converse is not necessarily the case: a number of conditions in which the heart is suddenly overloaded can produce heart failure in the presence of normal myocardial function.[43]

Myocardial heart failure is caused by permanent changes to the myocardium. These permanent changes are the result of the prolonged use of compensatory mechanisms that develop over an extended period of time and that are similar to those that occur during times of increased stress, such as (1) an increase in heart rate, (2) an increase in stroke volume, (3) hypertrophy of cardiac tissue mass, (4) an increase in sodium and water retention, (5) renal artery vasoconstriction, (6) dilation of the cardiac chamber, (7) lengthening of the sarcomeres to accommodate the increased preload, and (8) release of catecholamines both directly from the nerves, and indirectly from the adrenal medulla.

All of the above responses work to increase cardiac output. Increases in heart rate and stroke volume directly increase cardiac output because cardiac output is a product of heart rate times stroke volume. Hypertrophy of cardiac tissue mass yields an increase in the number of contractile units. An increase in sodium and water retention and the renal artery vasoconstriction result in an increase in preload to the heart. Dilatation of the cardiac chamber and lengthening of the sarcomeres provide increased contractile force according to the Starling principle of increased preload. The catecholamines released include norepinephrine, angiotensin, and aldosterone. Norepinephrine causes peripheral vasoconstriction and an increase in heart rate, angiotensin is a powerful vasoconstrictor, and aldosterone produces both vasoconstriction and sodium and water retention.

Over time, these responses are limited in their ability to sustain cardiac output, and heart failure ensues. The heart remains enlarged and/or dilated but works inefficiently to pump out the increased venous return. This inability to "keep up" results in an increase in end-diastolic volume, which eventually causes pulmonary or systemic venous congestion and promotes pulmonary or peripheral edema. Other changes include a redistribution of peripheral blood flow in order to maintain the necessary level of oxygen delivery to the vital organs. Increased sodium and water retention causes an increase in interstitial pressure, which then leads to stiffening, thickening, and compression of the blood vessel walls. Lactic acidemia results from inadequate perfusion of skeletal muscle. Because of an increase in 2,3-diphosphoglycerate (DPG) and tissue acidosis, there is a decline in the affinity of hemoglobin for oxygen, which causes a rightward shift in the oxyhemoglobin dissociation curve. Therefore, an increased supply of oxygen is required to bind with the hemoglobin. Contractility becomes further depressed as a result of a defect in the myocardium caused by these compensatory mechanisms. This depression further exacerbates the already existing failure and produces a downward cycle of decreased cardiac output, ineffective compensatory mechanisms, and depressed contractility. These changes may affect only one ventricle, but over time they will cause decreased cardiac output of both ventricles. In left heart failure, the diseased myocardium fails to pump blood from the lungs into the systemic circulation, which results in increased pulmonary venous pressure, left atrial pressure, and left ventricular diastolic pressure. Cardiac output is decreased, and an accumulation of blood increases lung pressure, engorging pulmonary capillaries. If pulmonary capillary hydrostatic pressure is allowed to exceed 30 mm Hg, fluid leaks into the pulmonary interstitial spaces. This influx leads to pulmonary edema and impedes oxygen–carbon dioxide exchange.

Right heart failure is a direct result of an increase in lung pressure. The right side fails to pump blood to the lungs and impedes venous return. As pressure continues to build, fluid accumulates in organs, producing engorgement of liver and spleen, neck vein distention, and edema of the extremities. Liver failure occurs as a result of increased hepatic pressure.

Resulting signs and symptoms

The clinical presentation of the patient in heart failure will depend on both the side (or sides) affected and the extent of underlying pathology. Some underlying pathologies of left and right heart failure are presented in Table 4-14, and assessment differentiators of each are given in Table 4-15.

Left heart failure   Left heart failure presents as dyspnea, orthopnea, paroxysmal nocturnal dyspnea, acute pulmonary edema, fatigue, nocturia, elevated PAD and PCWP, S_3 and/or S_4 heart sounds and crackles (rales), dysrhythmias, and pulsus alternans.

Dyspnea is a chief complaint of the patient in failure. Breathing becomes difficult as the lungs be-

Table 4-14   Underlying Pathologies of Left and Right Heart Failure

Left Heart Failure	Right Heart Failure
Atherosclerotic heart disease	Atherosclerotic heart disease
Acute myocardial infarction	Acute myocardial infarction
Tachycardia/bradycardia	Tachycardia/bradycardia
Myocarditis	Left heart failure
Increased circulating volume	Fluid overload/excess Na^+ intake
Valvular disease	Valvular disease
	Pulmonary embolism
	COPD

come stiffer. Dyspnea first occurs on exertion and then eventually occurs at rest. Fluid in the alveolar spaces causes a cough upon exertion. Symptoms usually develop slowly.

Orthopnea is described as shortness of breath while horizontal and is relieved by a semi-Fowler's or high Fowler's position. As venous return from the lower extremities increases, a greater force of contraction is needed, but contractility cannot increase sufficiently to compensate for the greater venous return.

Paroxysmal nocturnal dyspnea (PND) is characterized by the patient waking suddenly in the night

Table 4-15   Assessment Differentiators of Left and Right Heart Failure

Left Heart Failure	Right Heart Failure
Anxiety	Dependent pitting edema
Air hunger	Na^+ water retention
Dyspnea (nocturnal, exertional, or orthopnea)	Jugular venous distention
Cough	Bounding pulses
Tachycardia	Oliguria
Fatigue	Increased CVP
Increased jugular venous pressure	Right upper quadrant pain
	Anorexia and nausea
Crackles (rales) at bases	Normal PAP and PCWP
Increased PAD and PCWP	Low ejection fraction
Decreased SV	Increased inspiratory phase
Displaced PMI	Widely split S_2
Decreased pH and increased pCO_2 on ABG	Right-sided S_3 or S_4

with complaints of shortness of breath. It is the result of fluid flowing from the interstitial spaces into the intravascular compartment, which occurs when the patient reclines. PND is an exaggerated form of orthopnea and may be seen with expiratory and inspiratory wheezing due to bronchospasm. It generally dissipates when the patient sits or stands, but it may progress to acute pulmonary edema.

Acute pulmonary edema occurs when rising pulmonary capillary pressure causes a massive influx of fluid into the alveoli. The patient presents with cold, pale skin; anxiety; tachypnea; and diaphoresis. Expectorated sputum is white or pink-tinged.

Fatigue on exertion and moderate-to-severe weakness from reduced cardiac output are common complaints and may disappear with rest. This fatigue with severe weakness is due to several factors, including decreased cardiac output, decreased oxygenation of skeletal muscles, and a sustained increase in circulating catecholamines.

Nocturia results when accumulated fluid shifts into the intravascular space, and the resting heart's decreased burden allows for its excretion.

Elevated PAD and PCWP are evidence of increased volume to the left side of the heart. This occurs at pressures greater than 18 mm Hg, although clinical signs and symptoms may not be apparent until pressures reach 25 mm Hg or higher.

The S_3 heart sound in adults almost always indicates left ventricular heart failure. The S_4 heart sound is not a definitive sign of heart failure but does indicate a noncompliant left ventricle. As the degenerative process progresses, crackles (rales)—an indication of left heart failure—may be heard. Crackles (rales) are caused by an accumulation of fluid in the alveoli and are heard in the most dependent portion of the lung fields. Therefore, a patient in the recumbent position will have scattered crackles (rales), whereas a patient sitting up will have crackles (rales) that are prominent in the bases of the lungs.

A variety of dysrhythmias may be present in the patient with left heart failure. Most patients will present with tachycardia due to the increased preload and decreased cardiac output, as well as the increased presence of circulating catecholamines.

Atrial dysrhythmias may be present due to atrial distension caused by volume overload. Ventricular dysrhythmias may occur as the myocardium becomes ischemic.

Pulsus alternans results when the left ventricle becomes unable to eject its end-diastolic volume in the presence of a regular rhythm. A bigeminal pattern of decreased arterial pressure is seen and is almost exclusively a sign of left ventricular failure (Figure 4-40).

Radiographic findings in left heart failure usually reveal changes in the blood vessels of the lungs due to pulmonary engorgement. It should be noted, though, that these changes may not be immediate and that the absence of these changes does not rule out left ventricular failure. A chest roentgenogram may also show an enlarged cardiac silhouette, if the patient has developed left ventricular hypertrophy.

Right heart failure   Right heart failure can occur independently, but it is usually secondary to left heart failure. The prime symptom is systemic venous congestion. Pulmonary symptoms are rare, unless left heart failure is present, but may include edema, liver engorgement, anorexia, extra heart sounds, dysrhythmias, and jugular venous distention. Fatigue results from the decreased cardiac output, and the patient complains of weakness, lethargy, and heaviness.

Edema of the lower extremities and ankles occurs when the patient ambulates. If the patient is on bedrest, fluid accumulates in the sacrum, flank, and thighs. Abdominal girth increases, and weight gain is experienced; the patient may complain of discomfort when wearing clothing and shoes that used to fit.

Liver engorgement occurs as the capsule around the liver becomes distended with fluid. When this symptom occurs, it is good to ascertain any other indices of cardiac failure, because one symptom alone may be mistaken as a sign of another disease process. For example, right upper quadrant pain is often misdiagnosed as cholecystitis.

Gastrointestinal symptoms such as anorexia, bloating, and other nonspecific symptoms occur as hepatic visceral engorgement raises the venous pres-

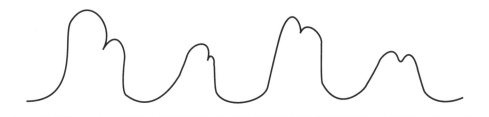

Figure 4-40   Bigeminal Pulsus Alternans

sure. The patient suffering right heart failure has a typical cachexic appearance.

As in left heart failure, right heart failure may present with right-side S_3 or S_4. The dysrhythmias exhibited are the same as those found in left heart failure. Jugular venous distention is common in the patient with right heart failure. In addition, a hepatojugular reflex is generally present, usually due to the inability of the right chambers to accommodate the increased venous return. A similar reflex is seen when the patient performs a Valsalva maneuver.

A chest roentgenogram will have minimal diagnostic value unless there is underlying pulmonary disease or left heart involvement. The diaphragm may be upwardly displaced, owing to the enlarged liver.

Nursing standards of care

Medical management is directed in stepwise fashion and depends on the extent of myocardial failure as well as presenting signs and symptoms. Medical approaches in treating heart failure will include a reduction or elimination of underlying and precipitating causes, reduction of myocardial workload, improvement of myocardial contractility, and reduction of excess salt and fluid. A useful method for assessing the extent of failure is the Killip classification, developed to classify failure accompanying MIs but readily applied to all heart failure (Table 4-16).

As with any medical approach, treatment of the underlying cause or precipitating factor should be instituted as soon as feasible. This may involve, for example, surgical correction of a diseased valve, ischemic myocardium, or ruptured interventricular septum or medical treatment of precipitating causes such as infection, dysrhythmias, and anemia.

Cardiac contractility may be improved by the administration of positive inotropic agents such as digoxin, dopamine, dobutamine, and amrinone. Digitalis glycosides are also useful in controlling the tachyarrhythmias that exacerbate heart failure. Dopamine's effect depends on the dosage administered. Dosages of 2–5 mcg/kg/min will cause increased renal perfusion, with resultant elimination of excess fluids. At dosages of 5–10 mcg/kg/min, the primary effect is beta stimulation of the heart, which causes a positive inotropic and chronotropic effect. Dosages greater than 10 mcg/kg/min cause alpha stimulation, which results in peripheral vasoconstriction. Dobutamine is a synthetic catecholamine that is generally infused at dosages of 5–15 mcg/kg/

Table 4-16   Killip Classification of Myocardial Infarction in CCU

Class	Signs and Symptoms	Percentage of Patients Presenting	Mortality Rate
I	Clear lungs S_1 S_2	30–40	8%
II	Crackles (rales) in less than 50% of lung fields S_3	30–50	30%
III	Crackles (rales) in more than 50% of lung fields Frequent pulmonary edema	5–10	44%
IV	Cardiogenic shock	10	80–100%

Source: Adapted from Killip, T., and Kimball, J. T. (1967). Treatment of myocardial infarction in a coronary care unit: A two-year experience with 250 patients. *American Journal of Cardiology.* 20:457.

min. Within this range it causes a positive inotropic effect. Unlike dopamine, it has little effect on heart rate or peripheral vascular resistance. Amrinone does not stimulate alpha or beta receptors but appears to work by increasing intracellular calcium concentration. It produces a positive inotropic effect (with a less pronounced chronotropic effect) as well as a powerful vasodilator effect. It is generally administered at dosages of 5–10 mcg/kg/min, at which rates it increases cardiac output, stroke volume, and contractility and decreases systemic vascular resistance.

Diuretics are useful in reducing increased levels of salt and fluid and may be instituted as a first-step therapy. Both thiazide and loop diuretics are used. Other measures to decrease the excess volume include thoracentesis, paracentesis, dialysis, and phlebotomy.

Vasodilators may be administered to decrease either the preload or the afterload of the heart. The most commonly used are nitrate preparations, which are used with the patient in whom diuretic therapy does not completely reduce to normal the venous return to the heart; they are also desirable for the patient suffering pulmonary congestion caused by increased left ventricular filling pressures. Afterload reducing agents are used for the patient with increased systemic vascular resistance, and they include nitroprusside as well as the ACE inhibitors (for example, Captopril). By reducing afterload to within normal range, these agents allow the heart to pump more easily, thus decreasing the pressure overload.

Table 4-17 Rate of Use of Selected Therapies in the Treatment of Heart Failure

	Functional Class			
	I	II	III	IV
Health promotion	Heavy	Heavy	Heavy	Heavy
Restriction of physical activity	Very light	Light	Moderate	Heavy
Digitalis	Rare	Light	Light	Moderate
Restriction of sodium intake	Very light	Light	Light	Moderate to heavy
Diuretics	Rare	Light	Moderate	Heavy
Vasodilators	Rare	Rare	Light	Moderate
Inotropic agents	Rare	Rare	Rare	Light

Dysrhythmias should be controlled to allow for maximum filling time and ejection of blood from the ventricle. A pacemaker may be required in cases of bradycardia or AV dissociation.

Other measures to reduce heart failure include dietary restrictions on salt and fluids, rest, weight reduction, and oxygenation. Also, cardiac performance must be improved; treatments to accomplish this include intraaortic balloon pump therapy, which is discussed in the section that addresses cardiogenic shock. Table 4-17 outlines rates of use of the various treatments used at the four stages of heart failure.

Nursing management of the patient suffering heart failure is directed toward alleviating precipitating factors, reducing myocardial workload, and observing and treating current and potential problems. Education of the patient and family is crucial to reducing the unnecessary complications that lead to readmissions. The following nursing care plan outlines standard critical care practices used in treating heart failure.

Nursing Care Plan for the Management of the Patient with Heart Failure and Pulmonary Edema

Diagnosis	Signs and symptoms	Intervention	Rationale
Alteration in cardiac output related to myocardial failure	Signs of low cardiac output: decreased BP; increased SVR; increased PAP and PCWP Signs of high cardiac output: increased cardiac output measures; decreased BP; decreased SVR; increased PAP and PCWP	Anticipate insertion of pulmonary artery catheter	Provides more accurate measure of cardiac function
		Administer preload-reducing agents (nitroglycerin) as ordered, to maintain PAD/PCWP < 18 mm Hg	To decrease venous return
		Administer afterload-reducing agents (nitroprusside) as ordered, to maintain SVR at 800–1300 dyne-sec/cm^5	To reduce SVR
		Administer inotropics (dopamine, dobutamine) as ordered	To improve contractility
		Administer drugs, as indicated and ordered, to maintain normal sinus rhythm	To maintain cardiac efficiency and output
		Administer digoxin as ordered	To improve cardiac contractility and control tachycardia
		Monitor BP closely	To assess for hypotension and pulsus alternans
		Participate in identification and correction of aggravating factors	It is most important to correct the underlying cause rather than just treating the symptoms
Alteration in fluid volume (excess)	Weight gain Elevated PAD and PCWP Edema Decreased urinary output	Maintain accurate I&O records	To ascertain presence and cause of fluid imbalance
		Limit salt intake as ordered	Excess sodium causes fluid retention
		Restrict fluids to 1500 cc/day if PAD and PCWP are elevated	To prevent fluid overload, which can lead to congestive failure

Diagnosis	Signs and symptoms	Intervention	Rationale
		Administer diuretics as ordered	Prerenal failure may develop as a result of decreased renal perfusion
		Monitor BUN and creatinine	
		Anticipate low-dose (2–5 mcg/kg/min) dopamine infusion	To provide increased renal perfusion
		Monitor weight daily	Weight change is best indicator of excess fluid loss
		Monitor for crackles (rales) and presence of S_3 heart sounds every 4 hours or as needed	Warn of heart failure and pulmonary edema
		Anticipate need for salt-poor albumin administration	Chronic heart failure predisposes patient to loss of protein, leading to edema; albumin provides mechanism for returning interstitial fluid to intravascular space
		Apply elastic antiembolism stockings	To promote venous return and prevent edema
Potential for alteration in gas exchange and ineffective breathing pattern	Dyspnea Decreased O_2 levels on ABGs Change in mental status Fluid overload	Monitor ABGs closely	Problems with oxygenation are commonly seen
		Assist to position of comfort (semi- or high Fowler's position is best)	To improve breathing patterns and lower diaphragm
		Assess for crackles (rales), S_3, and increased JVP every 4 hours or as needed	Signs of heart failure, with resultant pulmonary edema
		Administer oxygen as ordered	To counter problems with oxygenation
		Monitor heart rhythm	Tachycardia is commonly seen
		Review chest x-ray for signs of pulmonary edema	Pulmonary congestion can be clinically delayed up to 24 hours

Nursing Care Plan for the Management of the Patient with Heart Failure and Pulmonary Edema

Diagnosis	Signs and symptoms	Intervention	Rationale
Potential for infection related to pulmonary congestion, indwelling lines, and Foley catheter	Elevated temperature	Encourage coughing and deep breathing; turn patient in bed every 2 hours while on bedrest	Help to prevent atelectasis, blood clots in legs, and pressure sores
		Change respiratory tubing every 24 hours	Per CDC specifications
		Increase activity as soon as indicated	To promote healing
		Monitor temperature every 4 hours	Sign of infection
	Increased WBCs	Assess WBC count	Sign of infection
		Maintain strict aseptic technique with invasive lines and indwelling catheters; change lines unless contraindicated: PAP every 72 hours, arterial lines every 7 days, tubing every 48 hours, IV bags every 24 hours; provide Foley care every 8 hours	Per Centers for Disease Control recommendation
		Assist in identifying source of infection: collect cultures; note atelectasis on chest x-ray; note sputum and urine characteristics; check insertion site for redness every 8 hours	Sites at risk of infection must be kept clean with aseptic technique; appropriate antibiotic therapy must be chosen
		Administer antibiotics as ordered	To combat infectious process

Diagnosis	Signs and symptoms	Intervention	Rationale
Decreased tolerance of activity related to dyspnea	Dyspnea on exertion Fatigue Exaggerated increase in heart rate and BP on exertion	Assess level of activity tolerance (should be related to the New York Heart Association's classification for consistency)	Provides a baseline
		Assist patient to change position every 2 hours while on bedrest	To decrease risk of complications and promote venous return
		Check BP with patient in horizontal, sitting, and standing positions	To monitor for orthostatic hypotension
		Avoid activity for a half-hour to an hour after meals	May decrease chance of hypoxia due to increased blood flow to GI tract
		Monitor heart rate and BP with activity increases	To maintain heart rate within 10 bpm of resting heart rate and maintain systolic BP within 20 mm Hg of resting BP; if a drop occurs, it may indicate a drop in cardiac output
		Anticipate institution of progressive rehab	To provide controlled mechanism for increasing activity
		Encourage frequent rest periods	To prevent excessive fatigue
Potential for impaired skin integrity	Redness on pressure points	Assess skin integrity every 2–4 hours	To prevent skin breakdown
		Note redness on pressure points	Early signs of skin breakdown
		Use egg crate or air mattress	To relieve pressure on bony prominences

Nursing Care Plan for the Management of the Patient with Heart Failure and Pulmonary Edema

Diagnosis	Signs and symptoms	Intervention	Rationale
		Assist patient to turn every 2 hours	To improve circulation
		Institute skin care regimen	Dryness predisposes skin to break down
Patient lacks knowledge of disease process and prescribed regimen	Patient does not adhere to care plan	Assess patient's present understanding	Provides baseline
	Patient verbalizes lack of knowledge and understanding or exhibits anxiety and apprehension, especially during procedures and treatments	Institute teaching program for patient and family: normal lung function; pathology; risk factors; control of precipitating and aggravating factors; activity; diet; medications; weight monitoring; signs and symptoms of recurring respiratory failure; follow-up care	Increasing knowledge, understanding, and thus potential ability to adhere to regimen may decrease unnecessary rehospitalization
		Allow patient and family to ask questions and verify understanding of information	Patient may need reinforcement and several repetitions of information before it is fully understood and integrated

Medication	Effect	Major side effects
Digitalis	Increases contractility Lengthens refractory period of AV node Decreases left ventricular end diastolic pressure Increases ventricular automaticity Decreases atrial automaticity	Tachycardia AV block Bradycardia GI upset Headache Drowsiness Confusion Double vision
Furosemide Ethacrynic acid	Loop diuretic Decreases pulmonary congestion	Hypokalemia Hypocalcemia Hypomagnesemia Altered glucose metabolism
Morphine sulfate	Analgesia/sedation Peripheral vasodilation Decreases systemic venous return Bronchodilation Relief of cardiac dyspnea	Hypotension Respiratory depression Nausea and vomiting Constipation Urinary retention
Nitroprusside	Vasodilation, with direct action on vascular smooth muscle that decreases afterload, thus causing greater ejection fractions, stroke volume, and cardiac output	Gastrointestinal upset Muscle twitching Hypotension Confusion
Nitrates	Vasodilation leading to increased coronary blood supply and decreased myocardial oxygen demand	Hypotension Headache
Hydralazine Minoxidil Diazoxide	Vasodilation with a direct action on vascular smooth muscle, leading to relaxed arterioles, decreased vascular resistance, and increased cardiac output	Angina Nausea and vomiting Tachycardia Headache Flushing Hypotension
Dobutamine Dopamine	Inotropic with alpha-adrenergic stimulant Increases myocardial contractility, output, and stroke volume Dilates renal and mesenteric vessels in low doses	GI upset Angina Dyspnea Headache Hypotension Ectopic arrhythmias Palpitations Vasoconstriction

Medications Commonly Used in the Care of the Patient with Heart Failure and Pulmonary Edema

Medication	Effect	Major side effects
Captopril	Angiotensin-converting enzyme that decreases vasoconstriction, decreases circulating aldosterone, and suppresses renin-angiotensin system	Hypotension Renal impairment Vertigo Rash
Aminophylline	Bronchodilator Increases renal blood flow Positive inotropic effect on heart	Cardiac arrhythmias Gastrointestinal upset

Myocardial Conduction Defects

Myocardial conduction defects are disorders in conduction of electrical impulses through the normal pathways of the heart. These include problems of aberrant conduction, heart blocks, and preexcitation. Most commonly, they are due to pathology of conducting fibers, and most patients with heart disease (or pulmonary disease) will exhibit some form of dysrhythmia and/or conduction defect. The significance of the disorder will depend on the rate of development, the extent of the underlying cardiac disease, and the hemodynamic consequence.

Clinical antecedents

Conduction defects are most commonly caused by ischemia and/or necrosis of portions of the myocardium, drug effects, or congenital defects. Any disorder that affects oxygen supply can potentially cause abnormalities in the conduction of electrical impulses through the normal pathways of the heart. Some specific examples include myocardial infarction and/or ischemia, cardiomyopathy, and heart failure. Cardiac surgery is a frequent cause of conduction disturbances because it involves direct manipulation of the coronary arteries and resultant irritability.

The majority of conduction defects can be traced to anatomical abnormalities (see Figure 4-41). For example, since the right coronary artery supplies the SA node and portions of the AV node in the majority of individuals, ischemia in this artery will primarily affect the normal initiation of impulse formation. This is seen most often with inferior and posterior wall infarctions. Conversely, in the majority of individuals, the left coronary artery supplies portions of the bundle branch fascicles. Disease within this artery commonly causes disorders in the conduction through the fascicles. Hypertrophy of the myocardium can cause alteration in conduction due to dilation of the coronary arteries. Heart failure, as well, can cause conduction disturbances, because it can lead to ischemia and hypertrophy of the myocardium.

Bundle branch block is the most common form of intraventricular block and is caused by disease of one of the branches of the bundle of His. The most common cause of bundle branch block is ischemic heart disease. Other causes are rheumatic disease, syphilis, trauma, tumors, cardiomyopathy, and congenital lesions.[44] Transient bundle branch block may occur in acute heart failure, acute myocardial infarction, acute coronary insufficiency, and acute infections.[45] But bundle branch block may also be seen in patients with normal hearts.

Antidysrhythmic drugs can both annihilate and cause cardiac dysrhythmias. Drugs with the capability of inducing dysrhythmias are known as proarrhythmics. Class 1A antidysrhythmics (disopyramide, procainamide, and quinidine) increase the QT interval and may widen the QRS complex, even when given in therapeutic dosages. They can also cause reentrant-type tachycardias as a result of prolonged repolarization in the normally conducted beats. Other drugs that increase the refractory tone through the normal AV node include digitalis and propranolol. Psychotherapeutic medications can also cause a widening of the QRS complex.

Congenital defects in conduction may or may not be associated with other congenital defects. The most common congenital defects involve conduction through accessory pathways, as in Wolff-Parkinson-White syndrome (WPW). WPW is classified as a problem of preexcitation, or the premature depolarization of ventricular myocardium by a supraventricular impulse. This defect is found more commonly in males (1 per 1000 population).[46] Other forms of preexcitation include Lown-Ganong-Levine syndrome and conduction over Mahaim fibers.

Critical referents

Bundle branch blocks and hemiblocks may indicate coronary artery pathology. They are commonly associated with fibrosis of the conduction system and anterior wall MIs. In the majority of cases, the three fascicles that conduct stimuli to the ventricles are supplied by the left coronary artery (there are variations, however, owing to the differences in anatomical origin of the coronary arteries). Normally, conduction through the branches occurs simultaneously, but when there is a block in one of the branches, the impulse travels to one of the ventricles before the other. After activating the first ventricle, the impulse spreads to the other ventricle and, in turn, activates it. Since the impulse travels more slowly through the myocardium than it does down the normal conduction pathway, the QRS interval is prolonged. The right bundle is more vulnerable than the left because of its shorter length and single blood supply. The left bundle branch (LBB) is divided into two fascicles: the anterior and the posterior. If one of these fascicles is disturbed, the conduction disturbance is known as a hemiblock. Left anterior

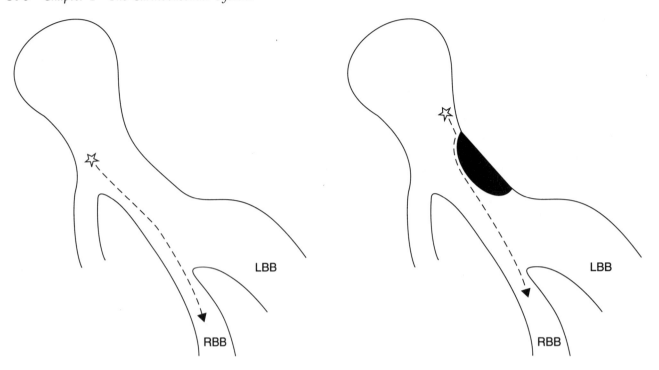

AV junctional impulse down through ipsilateral bundle branch

Junctional impulse deflected by diseased tissue

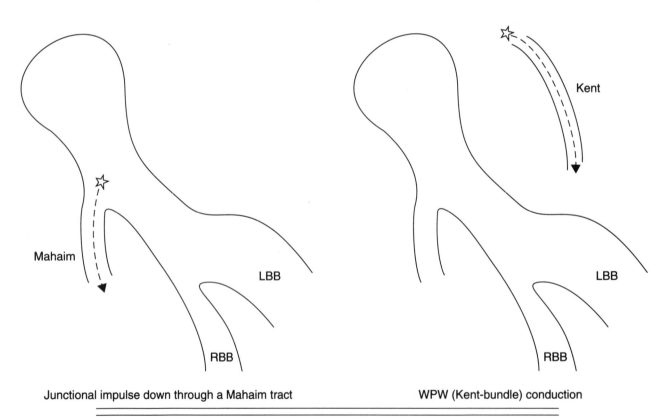

Junctional impulse down through a Mahaim tract

WPW (Kent-bundle) conduction

Figure 4-41 Type B Abberations

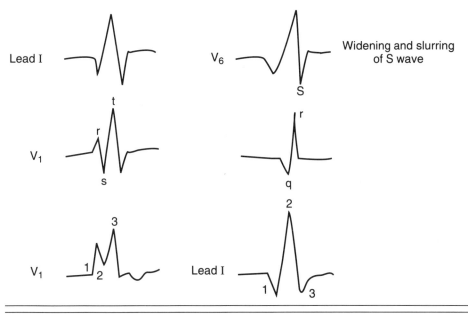

Figure 4-42 ECG Changes Indicating Right Bundle Branch Block

hemiblock results from blocked impulse conduction in the left anterior division of the left bundle branch, the most vulnerable part of the conduction system. Left posterior hemiblock occurs when the posterior division of the left bundle branch is blocked. The combination of right bundle branch block (RBBB)

with either left anterior or left posterior hemiblock is called bifascicular block. When bifascicular block is combined with either first-degree or second-degree block, it is known as trifascicular block. Trifascicular block has a high probability of leading to complete heart block. The clinical significance of bundle branch blocks lies in the number of fascicles involved. Monofascicular blocks may be relatively benign in origin, whereas a trifascicular block almost always indicates a need for a cardiac pacemaker.

In addition to bundle branch blocks, there are intraventricular conduction delays, which are most commonly caused by detours around necrotic or ischemic areas of the myocardium, administration of certain drugs, or electrolyte disorders such as hyperkalemia, hypercalcemia, and hypermagnesemia.

Aberrant ventricular conduction is an abnormal intraventricular conduction of supraventricular impulses. What is important about this aberrancy is not its hemodynamic compromise but that it is frequently misdiagnosed as ventricular in origin, because of the differences in refractoriness of the two bundle branches. Aberrant ventricular conduction is most frequently due to alterations in the R-R interval and heart rate. As heart rate slows (that is, R-R interval increases), there is a proportional lengthening of repolarization time. Aberrancy most frequently follows a prolonged R-R interval, since portions of the ventricle are still depolarized, and there is a delay in depolarization caused by the preceding beat. Most aberrant beats favor a right bundle branch appearance, as the right fascicle normally has a longer refractory period. Aberrant beats do not al-

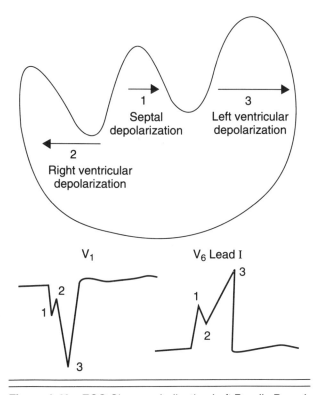

Figure 4-43 ECG Changes Indicating Left Bundle Branch Block

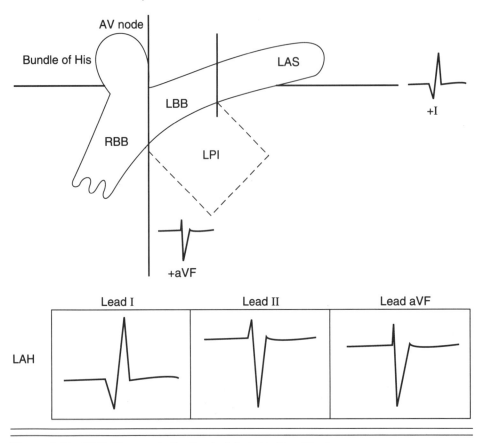

Figure 4-44 ECG Changes Indicating Left Anterior Hemiblock

ways follow prolonged R-R intervals. Some aberrant beats occur as the sinus rhythm gradually accelerates. At increased rates, it may be difficult to differentiate aberrancy from ventricular ectopy.

Preexcitation is the premature depolarization of the ventricles by a supraventricular impulse, which occurs via an accessory pathway. As was noted earlier, the most common such condition is Wolff-Parkinson-White syndrome (WPW). Normally, there is an area of tissue between the atria and the ventricles that prevents premature spreading of supraventricular impulses into the ventricles. In preexcitation conduction disturbances, however, there is an accessory pathway that allows the normally conducted impulse to travel down into the ventricles and reenter the atria in retrograde fashion. This transmission sets up a circus movement of impulse formation (Figure 4-41), and the heart rate is greatly accelerated. In most cases, these conduction disturbances cause great hemodynamic compromise as a result of the decreased filling time caused by the increased heart rate and subsequent decreased cardiac output.

Resulting signs and symptoms

Diagnosis of conduction disturbances is made with the 12-lead ECG. The precordial leads are most helpful in distinguishing RBBB from LBBB. ECG changes that indicate right bundle branch block are (1) wide QRS, measuring 0.12 second or more in width, (2) QRS showing RSR' configuration in lead V_1, (3) inverted T wave in V_1, and (4) QRS showing late, prolonged S wave that is slurred in V_6. In contrast, left bundle branch block is identified by (1) wide QRS, measuring 0.12 second or more in width, (2) V_1 and V_2 precordial leads showing wide, deep S wave, (3) wide, notched R wave in leads V_5 and V_6, and (4) notched T waves in leads V_5 and V_6. Figures 4-42 and 4-43 display right and left bundle branch block changes in leads V_1 and V_6.

Hemiblocks are usually diagnosed in the frontal leads. Left anterior hemiblock (LAH) is diagnosed by axis shift. The QRS does not widen. Characteristics of LAH include (1) left axis deviation, (2) small initial

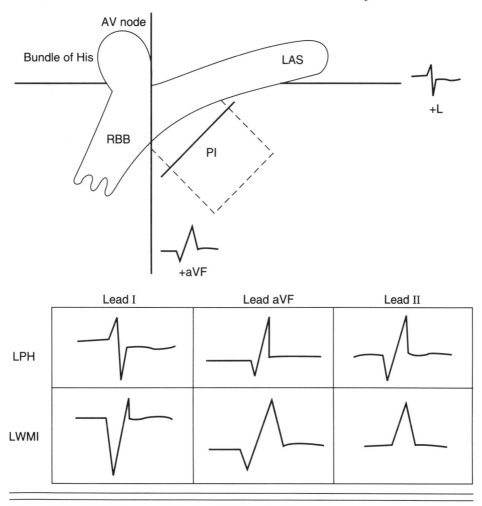

Figure 4-45 ECG Changes Indicating Left Posterior Hemiblock

R wave followed by deep S wave in leads II, III, and aVF, and (3) small Q and tall R waves in leads I and aVL, as illustrated in Figure 4-44.

Left posterior hemiblock (LPH) is characterized by (1) right axis deviation, (2) regular QRS segments, (3) small initial R wave followed by deep S wave in leads I and aVL, and (4) small initial Q wave followed by tall R wave in leads II, III, and aVF, as illustrated in Figure 4-45.

Aberrancy is diagnosed from two indications: QRS morphology and Ashman's phenomenon. QRS morphology is viewed in leads V_1 and V_6. Table 4-18 summarizes the factors to consider when distinguishing aberrant beats from ectopics. Ashman's phenomenon refers to a coupling mechanism of R-R intervals. Stated simply, a long pause followed by a short coupling interval favors aberrancy. This rule does not always hold true, however, since many ventricular ectopic beats also have long pauses preceding them. Other clues that may help with the

Table 4-18 Morphology of Aberrancies Versus Ectopics

Factor	Aberrancy	Ectopy
P wave	Yes	No
Initiating event:		
Atrial beat	Yes	Very rare
PVC	Rare	Frequent
Coupling interval compared to previous cycle	Shorter	Equal
Notched QRS	—	Taller left rabbit ear
qRs segment	QRS in V_6	rS in V_6 or QS in V_6

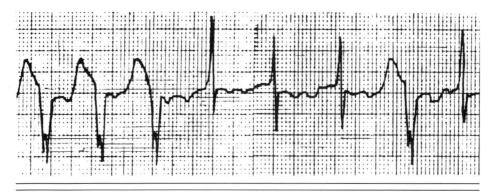

Figure 4-46   Ashman's Phenomenon

differentiation include (1) the presence of a longer returning cycle (favors ventricular origin), (2) the absence of a longer preceding cycle (favors ventricular origin), (3) the identification of a longer preceding cycle followed by a shorter succeeding with a normal beat (favors ventricular ectopy), and (4) a regular repeating pattern of long-short intervals, called fixed coupling (favors ventricular ectopy). Figure 4-46 shows an example of Ashman's phenomenon.

Preexcitation is usually diagnosed with the 12-lead ECG; however, there are cases in which electrophysiological studies are needed to confirm or differentiate the diagnosis. ECG changes characteristic of WPW, as illustrated in Figure 4-47, include (1) shortened PR interval, (2) delta wave, and (3) abnormally wide QRS complex. During episodes of accelerated rate through the accessory pathway, however, the QRS will widen and look bizarre and will give the impression of ventricular tachycardia. A definitive diagnosis of WPW may not be obtainable until the

rate is slowed and further investigational studies are performed.

Other signs and symptoms of conduction defects will depend on the degree of hemodynamic compromise. The clinical presentation of a patient with a compromised hemodynamic pattern will be the same as one presenting with decreased cardiac output; that is, decreased BP, diaphoresis, cool and clammy skin, tachypnea, and weakness will be evident. These symptoms are determined by the ventricular rate and decreased stroke volume.

Nursing standards of care

Medical management of the patient suffering conduction defects is directed toward both actual problems such as deterioration in hemodynamic stability and potential problems such as the potential for

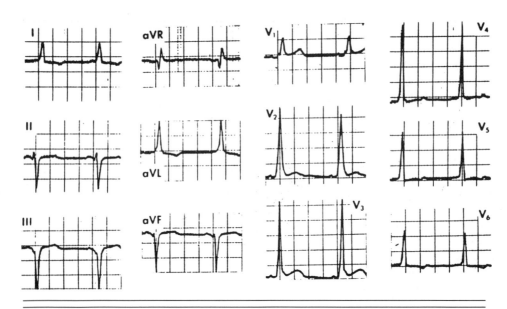

Figure 4-47   ECG Changes Characteristic of WPW (Type A)

progression to further degree of block. Monofascicular block does not, in itself, require direct intervention, and the likelihood of progression to further block is not great. Bifascicular block also does not necessarily pose an actual threat to the patient's hemodynamic stability. In the presence of ischemia, however, it may progress to further block and slowing of the heart rate. Trifascicular block yields a high risk for progression to complete heart block and, therefore, almost always requires cardiac pacing. The presence of pathology in two of the fascicles increases the likelihood of trifascicular block. Aberrant conduction does not require direct intervention. The danger of aberrancy, however, lies in the difficulty in distinguishing it from tachycardias that are ventricular in origin.

Medical management of the patient with a preexcitation conduction defect, such as WPW, must begin with electrophysiological studies if the patient presents with recurrent episodes of tachyarrhythmias. Termination of these episodes must be accomplished

as soon as possible, and verapamil is the drug of choice for doing so. However, verapamil is contraindicated in the patient with WPW accompanied by atrial fibrillation. Lidocaine does not appear to affect WPW. Digitalis is generally not used to slow an episode of tachyarrhythmia, especially if it is atrial fibrillation. Carotid massage and cardioversion are other measures that may be instituted.

Drugs that prolong refractoriness (such as procainamide and quinidine) are most useful for preventing recurrence of tachyarrhythmic episodes. Surgical ablation may be required if tachyarrhythmias persist.

Nursing management of the patient with myocardial conduction defects is directed toward actual and potential problems. Prioritization of the nursing goals should reflect (1) maintenance of hemodynamic stability and (2) prevention of complications. The following nursing care plan presents standard critical care practices followed for the patient with myocardial conduction defects.

Nursing Care Plan for the Management of the Patient with Myocardial Conduction Defects

Diagnosis	Signs and symptoms	Intervention	Rationale
Alteration in cardiac output related to tachydysrhythmias	ECG monitor shows SVT Hypotension Dyspnea Chest discomfort Palpitations	If patient is stable, attempt to obtain history of WPW or preexcitation conduction abnormality	For atrial fibrillation with history of WPW, verapamil is contraindicated
		Attempt vagal maneuver or carotid massage	Per ACLS standards
		Administer verapamil 5 mg IV; repeat every 10–15 minutes; monitor BP	Risk of hypotension with verapamil
		If patient is stable, prepare for synchronized cardioversion: explain procedure to patient; administer sedation; have emergency drugs readily available; remove dentures; secure electrodes to chest and turn defibrillator to sync mode; deliver shock while applying firm pressure and utilizing conductive material or gel; obtain 12-lead ECG and continue to monitor rhythm, respirations, and BP	To attempt to cardiovert to NSR under nonemergent circumstances
Potential for complications related to myocardial conduction defects	Bifascicular and trifascicular blocks Signs of low cardiac output	Anticipate insertion of temporary and/or permanent pacemaker	Bifascicular and trifascicular blocks on ECG indicate high risk for complete heart block

Diagnosis	Signs and symptoms	Intervention	Rationale
		If temporary pacemaker is to be inserted: explain procedure; obtain permit; assist with procedure using sterile technique	
		After pacemaker insertion: evaluate pacemaker's functioning and patient's rhythm; observe for complications and document strips every 2 hours or as needed	Complications may occur due to local inflammation and irritability
		Be aware of electrical hazards: use appropriate grounding; secure all wires and pacer connections; use nonelectrical bed; use gloves when working with wires and pacer connections	There is a risk of microshock, even from static electricity
		Monitor hemodynamic stability	Ventricular pacemaker insertion may cause retrograde conduction, with decreased cardiac output
		Check threshold every 24 hours	Indicates minimum amount of voltage required for pacemaker to cause myocardial capture; higher thresholds may indicate need for repositioning
		Monitor for failure of pacemaker to sense patient's intrinsic rhythm	May need to increase sensitivity of pacemaker, administer antidysrhythmias, or turn off pacemaker

Nursing Care Plan for the Management of the Patient with Myocardial Conduction Defects

Diagnosis	Signs and symptoms	Intervention	Rationale
		Monitor catheter sites for signs of infection: redness; drainage; tenderness; fever	Invasive lines pose high risk of infection
		Monitor for dysrhythmias, expecially PVCs	May occur due to irritability caused by insertion or presence of wires
		Administer lidocaine as ordered	To prevent or decrease incidence of dysrhythmias
Knowledge deficit with respect to diagnostic tests such as electrophysiological (EP) studies and drug therapies	Patient verbalizes lack of understanding	Assess patient's present understanding	To establish baseline
	Nonadherence to care regimen	Discontinue all antiarrhythmic drugs prior to EP studies	To assess effectiveness of each drug as well as interactive effects
		Instruct patient about EP study or other procedure patient is undergoing	To allay patient's anxiety
		Monitor BP and heart rhythm after any diagnostic procedure, especially EP studies	To discover any hypotension and/or return of dysrhythmia
		Provide instruction on drug therapies and importance of following prescription closely	Understanding and adherence to a regular medication schedule promote optimum therapeutic drug levels
		Identify methods of controlling or terminating dysrhythmia during EP study: pacing; cardioversion	Will help to control complications and allay anxiety

Diagnosis	Signs and symptoms	Intervention	Rationale
Anticipatory grieving related to diagnosis and requisite alteration in life-style	Signs of depression Withdrawal Inappropriate behavior: denial; aggressiveness; passive-aggressiveness; extreme anger; flat affect Altered communication patterns	Assess patient's present understanding of disease and its management Encourage patient and family to vent feelings Assess for anticipated changes in life-style Consult with appropriate health personnel (social workers, home health care workers, nutritionists, psychotherapists)	Patient may have exaggerated perception To provide outlet for stress Patient will need much guidance in reordering life-style Multidisciplinary team is most effective and efficient in providing wide range of support services

Medications Commonly Used in the Care of the Patient with Myocardial Conduction Defects

Medication	Effect	Major side effects
Isoproterenol	Stimulates beta receptor sites and relaxes smooth muscle, leading to: increased myocardial contractility; increased heart rate; increased myocardial oxygen demand; and decreased peripheral vascular resistance	Tachycardia Ventricular irritability Hypotension Headache Flushing Angina GI upset Dizziness Weakness Tremors
Atropine	Parasympatholytic Decreases refractory period Increases SA node discharge and conduction through AV node	Dry mouth Ventricular irritability Difficulty in voiding
Calcium chloride	Increases myocardial contractility Increases ventricular excitability	Mild hypotension Hypercalcemia Local necrosis upon extravasation

Dysrhythmias

Recognition of dysrhythmia is vital in the nursing assessment of the patient with cardiovascular problems. Dysrhythmias may be classified by origin as sinus rhythms, atrial dysrhythmias, junctional dysrhythmias, AV blocks, or ventricular dysrhythmias.

Sinus Rhythms

Normal Sinus Rhythm (NSR)

Normal sinus rhythm (NSR) is illustrated in Figure 4-48. NSR is the normal, healthy rhythm, so no pathophysiology is involved. There are no signs and symptoms of NSR other than what is seen in a healthy heart. The ECG configuration is as follows:

P waves: normal (upright, smoothly rounded)

QRS: normal (less than 0.12 second in duration)

Conduction: each QRS is preceded by a P wave; each P wave is followed by one QRS complex

Rate: 60–100 bpm

Rhythm: regular

Sinus Bradycardia (SB)

Sinus bradycardia is illustrated in Figure 4-49.

Clinical antecedents

Sinus bradycardia may be normal, and it is common in athletes and in the general population during sleep.

Critical referents

Drugs used to slow the conduction system may produce the SB rhythm, which is caused by decreased impulse formation in the SA node.

Resulting signs and symptoms

ECG characteristics of SB are the same as those of NSR, except that the rate is slower—less than 60 bpm.

Nursing standards of care

Care of the individual with a sinus bradycardic rhythm involves continuing to monitor and check

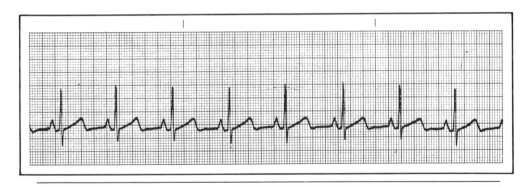

Figure 4-48 Normal Sinus Rhythm

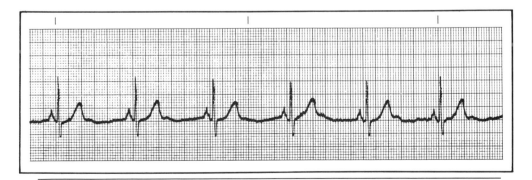

Figure 4-49 Sinus Bradycardia

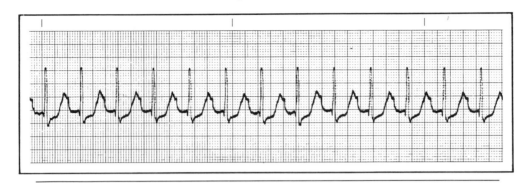

Figure 4-50   Sinus Tachycardia

the hemodynamic status of the patient. In the presence of deteriorating clinical states, atropine is the treatment of choice.

Sinus Tachycardia (ST)
Figure 4-50 illustrates sinus tachycardia.

Clinical antecedents

Sinus tachycardia is usually secondary to sympathetic stimulation. It may be triggered by fear, caffeine, fever, decreased cardiac output, or increased metabolic demand.

Critical referents

Sinus tachycardia is caused by increased impulse formation within the SA node.

Resulting signs and symptoms

ECG characteristics of ST are the same as those of NSR, except that the rate is faster—usually about 100 bpm but generally less than 160 bpm.

Nursing standards of care

The objective of nursing care in cases of sinus tachycardia is to continue to monitor and check the hemodynamic status of the patient. The underlying problem needs to be treated.

Sinus Arrhythmia
A sinus arrhythmia is illustrated in Figure 4-51.

Clinical antecedents

Sinus arrhythmias are commonly seen in children and athletes. However, they may also be due to factors that increase vagal tone.

Critical referents

Impulse formation in sinus arrhythmias is normal and originates from the SA node. The arrhythmias are caused by changes in intrathoracic pressure due to respirations. Thus, respirations are the con-

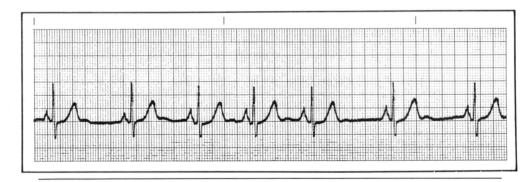

Figure 4-51   Sinus Arrhythmia

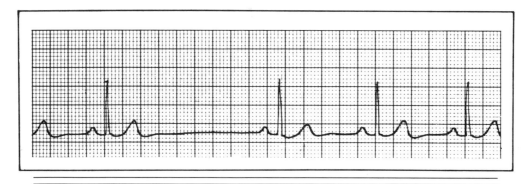

Figure 4-52 Sinus Block

trolling factor of the rhythm, which increases on inspiration and decreases on expiration.

Resulting signs and symptoms

ECG characteristics of sinus arrhythmias appear the same as those for NSR, except that the rhythm varies.

Nursing standards of care

Treatment is usually not required in the case of a sinus arrhythmia. This is a benign rhythm that does not decrease cardiac output. However, in the patient with cardiac disease, continued slowing may occur, which can then lead to an escape rhythm.

Sinus Block

Figure 4-52 illustrates a sinus block.

Clinical antecedents

Sinus blocks may be due to vagal stimulation and are also frequently seen with digitalis intoxication.

Critical referents

Sinus blocks are due to decreased impulse formation within the SA node.

Resulting signs and symptoms

The patient suffering a sinus block may or may not be aware of the pause in rhythm. If the blocks become increasingly frequent, clinical presentation may include dizziness, feelings of faintness, and syncope. The following outlines the ECG patterns:

P wave: normal (upright, smoothly rounded)
QRS: normal (less than 0.12 second in duration)
Conduction: each QRS is preceded by a P wave; each P wave is followed by one QRS complex
Rhythm: One complete P wave, QRS complex, and T wave cycle is dropped; there is no interruption in the timing cycle
Rate: the underlying rate is between 60 and 100 bpm

Nursing standards of care

If clinical symptoms are present, the patient should be treated with atropine, isoproterenol, or a pacemaker.

Sinus Arrest

An example of sinus arrest is shown in Figure 4-53.

Clinical antecedents

The factors leading up to a sinus arrest are the same as those for a sinus block.

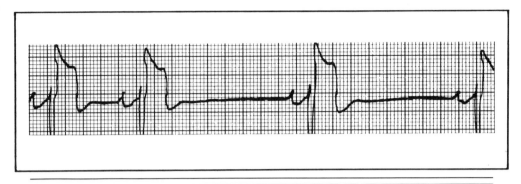

Figure 4-53   Sinus Arrest

Critical referents

The specific pathophysiology for sinus arrest is also the same as for sinus block.

Resulting signs and symptoms

If clinical symptoms are present, they will be similar to those found with sinus blocks, but they may be more prominent. The ECG patterns accompanying sinus arrest are:

P wave: normal (upright, smoothly rounded)

QRS: normal (less than 0.12 second in duration)

Conduction: each QRS is preceded by a P wave; each P wave is followed by one QRS complex

Rhythm: one or more complexes drop, and the timing cycle is interrupted

Rate: the underlying rate is normal; however, the rate will be slowed during the sinus arrest

Nursing standards of care

Nursing intervention for sinus arrest is the same as for sinus block.

Atrial Dysrhythmias

Premature Atrial Contraction (PAC)

An example of premature atrial contraction can be seen in Figure 4-54.

Clinical antecedents

PACs are caused by irritation of the atrial tissue and may be a warning of more serious atrial dysrhythmias. They can occur in a normal heart in times of emotional stress or anxiety, or if the individual is particularly sensitive to tobacco, alcohol, or caffeine. In disease states, PACs may occur with the increased stretching of the atrium commonly seen in heart failure, thyrotoxicosis, or rheumatic heart disease.

Critical referents

A PAC is a cardiac contraction that originates somewhere in the atrium other than the SA node. The ectopic foci within the atrium fire before the regular electrical impulse from the SA node does.

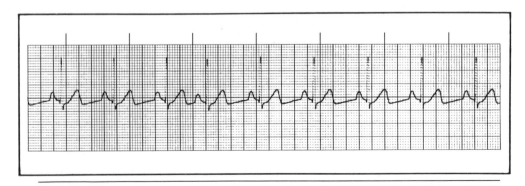

Figure 4-54   Premature Atrial Contractions

Resulting signs and symptoms

The patient may or may not be aware of palpitations. Characteristics of the ECG pattern are:

P wave: The morphology of the premature beat is different from normally conducted P waves. It is seen as a notch on the preceding T wave or is hidden in the preceding T wave.

QRS: The QRS is usually normal but may be conducted with aberration through the ventricles.

Conduction: There is usually one P wave preceding each QRS complex.

Rate: The rate varies.

Rhythm: The underlying rhythm is regular, but the beats are irregular. Because PACs cause less than a full compensatory pause, the R-R interval is disrupted.

Nursing standards of care

The first priority is to monitor for increasing frequency of PACs, because they may be a warning sign of other atrial dysrhythmias. If it is believed that use of stimulants, alcohol, or tobacco is the cause, ingestion of the substance should be stopped. If the PACs become frequent enough for the patient to become symptomatic (shortness of breath, anxiety, dizziness, fatigue and/or syncope), medical treatment with an antidysrhythmic drug such as digoxin, quinidine, propranolol, procainamide, or verapamil is instituted.

Blocked Premature Atrial Contraction

Figure 4-55 provides an example of a blocked PAC.

Clinical antecedents

The clinical antecedents for a blocked PAC are the same as for PACs.

Critical referents

The specific pathophysiology of blocked PACs is the same as that for PACs, except that when the electrical impulse reaches the AV node, it is stopped and thus is not conducted down through the ventricles.

Resulting signs and symptoms

The patient is usually unaware of blocked PACs, and there is no hemodynamic compromise. What differentiates these dysrhythmias from PACs is the conduction changes that are usually seen during an NSR: an ectopic focus originates from the atria, but is not conducted through the AV node. Consequently, there is a premature P wave of unusual morphology, but with no ventricular response. Blocked PACs are the most common cause of a pause in NSR.

Nursing standards of care

Nursing interventions for the patient with blocked PACs are the same as those for the patient with PACs.

Paroxysmal Atrial Tachycardia (PAT)

An example of paroxysmal atrial tachycardia is provided in Figure 4-56.

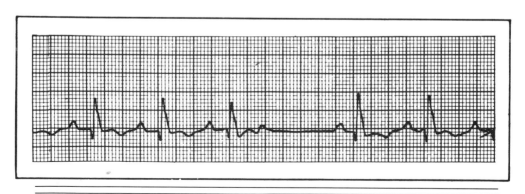

Figure 4-55 Blocked Premature Atrial Contraction

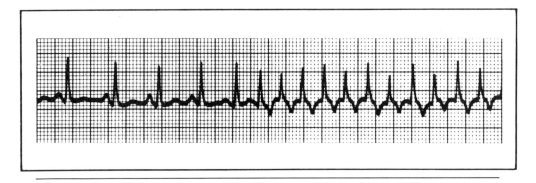

Figure 4-56 Paroxysmal Atrial Tachycardia

Clinical antecedents

Paroxysmal atrial tachycardia is frequently seen with rheumatic heart disease, WPW, pulmonary edema, and digitalis toxicity, but may also be seen when overdistension has caused irritability within the atrium. In normal hearts, PAT can be caused by deep emotional stress, overexertion, stimulants such as tobacco and coffee, and/or ingestion of extremely heavy meals.

Critical referents

PAT is a tachycardia with an abrupt onset and termination (usually with a regular rate) that originates somewhere within the atrium and above the bundle of His. Specifically, the result is the action relating to the very rapid, spontaneous depolarization of the atrial ectopic foci. PAT may also be due to the reentry phenomenon.

Resulting signs and symptoms

As the word "paroxysmal" indicates, this dysrhythmia starts and stops suddenly. The underlying rhythm is usually a sinus rhythm. PAT may cause hemodynamic compromise because of diminished cardiac output in the face of such rapid heart beats. The ECG characteristics are:

P waves: usually hidden in previous T waves

QRS: usually normal but may become aberrantly conducted

Conduction: a sudden onset of atrial discharge that may be so rapid as to cause some atrial impulses to be blocked at the AV node

Rhythm: Usually regular, may continue or terminate suddenly

Rate: ranges from 160 to 240 bpm

Nursing standards of care

Reducing the causative factors (if apparent) is the primary objective in the treatment of PAT. For those who become increasingly symptomatic or suffer a compromise in cardiac function, vagal stimulation should be attempted. The Valsalva maneuver increases intrathoracic pressure and decreases venous return, which raises blood pressure and slows the pulse. But care should be taken in employing this action, because stimulating the vagal nerve may produce dangerous slowing or even cardiac arrest. The patient must be constantly monitored, and advanced life support equipment should always be available. Clinical cardioversion, using conduction-depressing drugs such as verapamil, digitalis, procainamide, and propranalol, may be used. If this fails and the PAT is sustained and heart failure is imminent, electrical cardioversion may be necessary.

Paroxysmal Atrial Tachycardia with Block

An example of PAT with block is featured in Figure 4-57.

Clinical antecedents

Precipitating factors for PAT with block are the same as those for PAT.

Critical referents

The pathophysiological process involved in PAT with block is the same as for PAT.

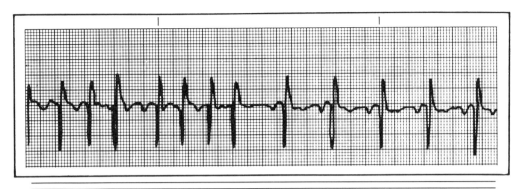

Figure 4-57 Paroxysmal Atrial Tachycardia with Block

Resulting signs and symptoms

Signs and symptoms of PAT with block are also the same as for PAT, except that some of the P waves are not conducted. A PAT with block, though, must be differentiated from second-degree Mobitz II by checking the atrial rate; a rapid atrial rate is diagnostic for PAT with block.

Nursing standards of care

Nursing management for the individual suffering PAT with block is the same as for PAT. The patient requires continuous monitoring. Usually, a digitalis level is taken, since this dysrhythmia is frequently caused by digitalis toxicity.

Atrial Flutter

An example of atrial flutter is provided in Figure 4-58.

Clinical antecedents

Atrial flutter is frequently due to heart failure, hypertension, overdistensibility of the atrium, pul-

monary disease, thyroid toxicosis, or rheumatic heart disease. It can also be a side effect of a drug such as digitalis, quinidine, or epinephrine.

Critical referents

Atrial flutter is seen as a fluttering caused by a circadian depolarization of the atrium, at times associated with a slower ventricular contraction rate.

Resulting signs and symptoms

Clinical signs of atrial flutter may not be evident unless there is (1) increased or decreased ventricular response that causes hemodynamic compromise or (2) decreased cardiac output caused by the loss of the atrial kick. The patient with atrial flutter is at risk for thrombus formation within the atrium due to diminished emptying of the atrium. Other risks include increased ventricular rate or slowing of the ventricular response. ECG characteristics of atrial flutter are as follows:

P waves: regular, sawtoothed in configuration, at approximately 300 bpm, and known as F waves; there is no P-R interval.

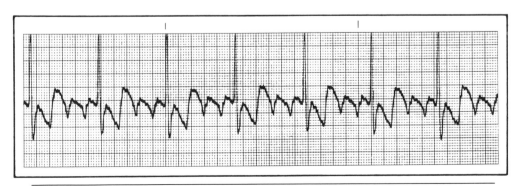

Figure 4-58 Atrial Flutter

QRS: normal, although the flutter waves may distort the T wave

Conduction: the AV node generally does not conduct each wave, so any of a number of flutter waves may reach the ventricle. Conduction is described as the ratio of the number of F waves to each QRS complex—for example, 2:1, 3:1, or 4:1.

Rhythm: regular or irregular, depending on the regularity of the blocked F waves

Rate: ventricular rate can vary greatly, depending on the degree of AV block. A ventricular rate of 150 bpm is a reliable indicator of atrial flutter, since conduction is 2:1 and the flutter waves may not be identifiable.

Nursing standards of care

Attempts are usually made to convert the patient to an NSR or at least to control the ventricular rate. Commonly used pharmacological agents include quinidine, procainamide, propranolol, digitalis, and verapamil. Cardioversion may also be used, starting at lower voltages (for example 25 joules).

Atrial Fibrillation

Figure 4-59 is an example of atrial fibrillation.

Clinical antecedents

Precipitating factors for atrial fibrillation are the same as those for atrial flutter.

Critical referents

The most common of all supraventricular tachyarrhythmias, atrial fibrillation is due to an irregular fibrillating mass of atrial muscle, which does not produce a coordinated atrial contraction. The ventricular response is also irregular.

Resulting signs and symptoms

The clinical presentation of atrial fibrillation is the same as that of atrial flutter. ECG characteristics include the following:

P waves: there are no true P waves but, rather, irregular F waves that may be very coarse or fine.

QRS: of normal shape and duration and occurring without a preceding P wave, so the rate is irregularly irregular

Conduction: conduction from the atria to the AV junction is bizarre, but becomes normal beyond the AV junction; there is no P-R interval.

Rhythm: irregularly irregular

Rate: varies, according to ventricular response, from very slow to very fast. New onsets of atrial fibrillation frequently occur at greatly accelerated rates, and it may be difficult to determine irregularity.

Nursing standards of care

Nursing care for cases of atrial fibrillation is the same as that for atrial flutter.

Junctional Dysrhythmias

Junctional dysrhythmias are rhythms that arise within the AV junction. High nodal, midnodal, or low nodal is used to identify the location of the P wave with respect to the QRS complex, but these terms do not represent the origin of the impulse

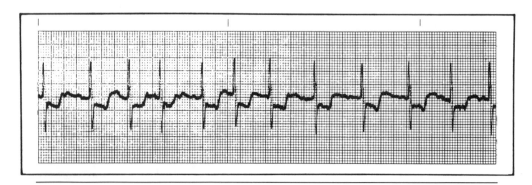

Figure 4-59 Atrial Fibrillation

within the AV node. In general, junctional dysrhythmias are identified by an inverted P wave caused by the retrograde conduction from the AV node. It is sometimes difficult to differentiate a junctional dysrhythmia from an atrial dysrhythmia that arises low within the atrium. One distinguishing factor is that junctional rhythms usually have a shortened P-R interval (of less than 0.12 second). This differentiation is not usually clinically significant, however.

Premature Junctional Contraction (PJC)

Figure 4-60 is an example of premature junctional contractions.

Clinical antecedents

PJCs are usually due to irritation within the AV nodal tissue. They may, however, occur in normal individuals, especially in well-trained athletes with sinus bradycardia. In the diseased heart, PJCs may be seen with MI (especially an inferior MI), increased vagal tone, digitalis toxicity, and rheumatic heart fever. They also frequently occur after cardiac surgery, when the cardiac tissue is especially irritable.

Critical referents

Impulse formation leading to a PJC occurs prematurely within the AV node. The impulse may either move up through the atrium in a retrograde fashion (thus the name, retrograde P wave) or move along other electrical pathways, which results in P waves that occur just before, in, or after the QRS complex. Once the impulse reaches the ventricles, it progresses normally, giving rise to a normal-appearing QRS.

Resulting signs and symptoms

The ECG configuration is the most reliable way to detect PJCs since there are usually no clinical signs and symptoms.

P wave: P waves are usually normal, except for premature beats, but can be upright or inverted; they may precede, follow, or be hidden in the QRS. The P-R interval is less than 0.12 second.

Conduction: Premature ectopic discharge occurs at the AV junction. Conduction through the ventricles is normal; retrograde conduction occurs through the atria.

Rhythm: regular, except for PJCs

Rate: depends on the underlying rhythm

Nursing standards of care

Usually no treatment is necessary for PJCs unless it is to alleviate the underlying cause, such as digitalis toxicity.

Junctional Rhythm

Figure 4-61 shows an example of a junctional rhythm.

Clinical antecedents

As with a PJC, a junctional rhythm may occur in a healthy individual. However, it may be caused by

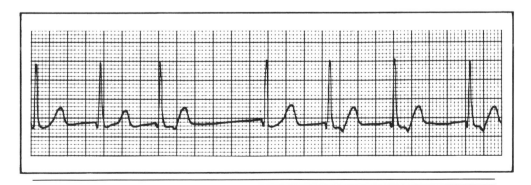

Figure 4-60 Premature Junctional Contraction

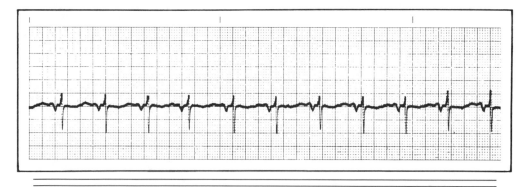

Figure 4-61   Junctional Rhythm

excessive slowing of the sinus node, in which case the AV node takes over pacemaker activity.

Critical referents

Frequently, junctional rhythm is a compensatory mechanism for bradycardia and may be considered an indication that there is something seriously wrong with the SA node. The electrical pathway taken to produce a junctional rhythm is the same as that described for PJCs.

Resulting signs and symptoms

Depending on the degreee of slowing and the cardiac status of the patient, clinical signs and symptoms may be evident. If the rhythm is slow enough, signs of diminished cardiac output may occur. The ECG signs of junctional rhythm are as follows:

P waves: usually inverted and with a shortened P-R interval

QRS: usually normal

Conduction: same as for PJC

Rhythm: regular

Rate: between 40 and 60 bpm

Nursing standards of care

The nursing care priority is the need to continually monitor and check the hemodynamic stability of the patient. If the patient becomes symptomatic, medical treatment with atropine, isoproterenol, or a temporary pacemaker is indicated.

Junctional Tachycardia

Junctional tachycardia is an accelerated junctional rhythm that originates from the AV node. Frequently it is extremely difficult to distinguish between a PAT and a junctional tachycardia; therefore, the term "supraventricular tachycardia" can be used in both instances.

Clinical antecedents

Junctional tachycardia may be seen with digitalis toxicity or MI.

Critical referents

Junctional tachycardia is due to an accelerated junctional rhythm and, again, serves as an indication that there is something seriously wrong with the SA node.

Resulting signs and symptoms

Signs and symptoms exhibited with junctional tachycardia are the same as those for junctional rhythm, except that the rate can be greater than 60 bpm. Some classifications define a tachycardia as a rate greater than 100 bpm; other classifications describe a tachycardia as any rate greater than the upper limit of normal.

Nursing standards of care

The nursing objective is to monitor the patient. Usually no treatment is necessary unless there are symptoms of compromised cardiac output, in which case measures to alleviate the condition must be instituted. Once again, the underlying cause must be treated.

AV Blocks

An AV block may be either a delay or a total block in the intraventricular conduction system. AV dissociation is a term commonly used to describe a total block in the conduction system; however, AV dissociation is a symptom that may be present in a number of different dysrhythmias and does not represent a block per se.

First-Degree Block

Figure 4-62 is an example of a first-degree heart block, which is a type of AV block. It is a slowing of the conduction of the electrical impulse from the SA node as it passes through the AV node down to the ventricles.

Clinical antecedents

First-degree block may be seen in healthy individuals as well as in those with coronary artery disease or degenerative disease of the conduction system. It may also be seen with rheumatic fever, acute MI, vagal stimulation, and hyperthyroidism and as a side effect of drugs such as digitalis and propranolol.

Critical referents

First-degree block only slows the progress of the impulse, because it is due to a delay rather than an actual block in the intraventricular conduction system.

Resulting signs and symptoms

First-degree block rarely produces any clinical signs or symptoms. It is the same as an NSR, except that the P-R interval is lengthened to greater than 0.20 second.

Nursing standards of care

The patient with first-degree block is usually clinically asymptomatic, and no treatment is needed.

Second-Degree Block Type I (Wenckebach or Mobitz I)

Figure 4-63 presents an example of second-degree block, type I (Wenckebach or Mobitz I).

Clinical antecedents

A type I second-degree block (Wenckebach) is rarely seen in normal individuals. It may be caused by coronary artery disease, acute inferior MI, digitalis toxicity, or degenerative disease of the intraventricular conduction system.

Critical referents

This type of dysrhythmia is due to a delay in the conduction of impulses from the SA node to the AV node that increases until, eventually, the next impulse fails to conduct to the AV node. That is, following the previous delay, each impulse from the SA node arrives earlier and earlier in the refractory period of the AV node until an impulse is eventually

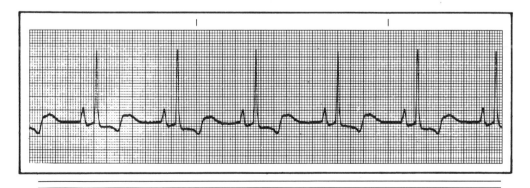

Figure 4-62 First-Degree AV Block

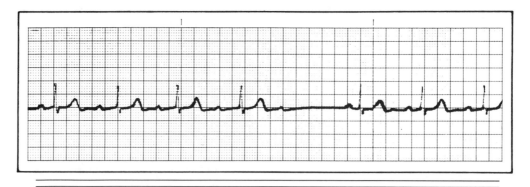

Figure 4-63   Second-Degree AV Block, Type I (Mobitz I)

completely impeded, which results in the absence of a ventricular beat. Once this occurs, the whole process is reiterated.

Resulting signs and symptoms

Usually a type I second-degree block is self-limiting, and the patient is not symptomatic. However, such a dysrhythmia may be a warning of an impending greater degree of heart block. The ECG has the following characteristics:

P waves: usually normal and regular

QRS: usually normal

Conduction: a progressively prolonged impulse at the AV junction results in a gradual lengthening of the P-R interval and successive R-R interval shortening until a P wave is dropped in the refractory period of the ventricle. Therefore, there is no QRS or ventricular depolarization. The rhythm is identified by the ratio of P waves to QRS complexes (for example, 4:3 or 3:2 conduction).

Rhythm: P-P is regular, R-R is irregular

Rate: varies

Nursing standards of care

The nurse's primary responsibility is to monitor the patient. If the patient becomes symptomatic of compromised cardiac functioning, medical treatment with atropine, isoproterenol, or a pacemaker is indicated.

Second-Degree Block, Type II

Figure 4-64 provides an example of a second-degree block, type II (Mobitz II).

Clinical antecedents

Type II second-degree block may be seen following an MI (particularly an anterior wall MI), with digitalis toxicity, with rheumatic heart disease, or during episodes of ischemia.

Critical referents

Type II second-degree block is almost always associated with disease of the ventricular conduction

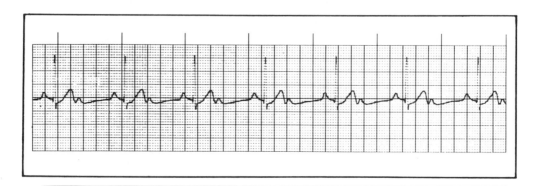

Figure 4-64   Second-Degree AV Block, Type II (Mobitz II)

system. A type II block cannot be distinguished from a type I block if 2:1 conduction is present. Type II second-degree block is due to blocking of sinus impulses at or below the level of the AV node.

Resulting signs and symptoms

The patient with this rhythm may be clinically symptomatic, depending on the ventricular response. This block is more likely than a type I block to progress to complete heart block. In addition, depending on the ventricular response rate, cardiac output may be compromised and symptoms of that will appear. The ECG pattern of type II second-degree block is:

P waves: usually normal and regular

QRS: normal

Conduction: sudden block at or below the AV junction; the P-R interval is constant for conducted beats and may or may not be prolonged.

Rhythm: P-P is regular; R-R is regular or irregular; a nonconducted QRS may occur in a cyclic pattern; blocks may be 2:1, 3:1, or greater.

Rate: varies

Nursing standards of care

The patient with type II second-degree block must be monitored closely for progression to complete heart block, especially if ischemia is present. If the patient is symptomatic, medical treatment with atropine, isoproterenol, or a pacemaker should be instituted.

Complete Heart Block

Figure 4-65 illustrates a complete heart block (third-degree AV block).

Clinical antecedents

Complete heart block is almost always caused by underlying pathology such as ischemia, infarction, or disease of the intraventricular conduction system. It is frequently seen with acute MI, rheumatic heart disease, and atherosclerotic heart disease.

Critical referents

Complete heart block is a complete block in the conduction system separating atrial activity from ventricular activity. As a result, ventricular beats do not occur or, more frequently, occur independently of atrial activity. Ventricular activity may originate high in the conduction system close to the AV node or low in the bundle of His.

Resulting signs and symptoms

The patient with a complete heart block will usually be symptomatic because of the decreased cardiac output from the slowed ventricular response, although some patients may be able to tolerate complete heart block indefinitely. The ECG pattern includes the following:

P waves: usually normal and regular

QRS: will look normal if the ventricular impulse originates near the AV node; will be widened if the impulse originates lower in the bundle of His

Conduction: atrial impulses are completely blocked at the AV junction or below; ventricles are paced independently of the atria by an ectopic focus; P-R interval varies

Rhythm: P-P is regular, R-R is regular; P waves and R waves are completely independent of one another

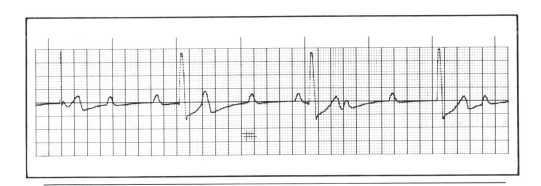

Figure 4-65 Third-Degree AV Block (Complete Heart Block)

Rate: Ventricular rates will be regular. Ventricular impulses originating near the AV node will usually conduct at 40 to 60 bpm; those originating lower in the conduction system will conduct at 20 to 40 bpm

In the event of complete heart block, the practitioner must continuously monitor the patient and check for hemodynamic compromise. Complete heart block that occurs at the time of MI is usually transitory and will resolve itself. Temporary medical treatment includes atropine 0.5 mg to 1.0 mg and isoproterenol infusion at 2 to 10 mcg/min. The maximum dose of atropine is 2.0 mg. Doses of less than 0.5 mg should not be given, because they can cause a paradoxical slowing of the heart rate.

Ventricular Dysrhythmias

Ventricular dysrhythmias may be caused by irritation, ischemia, and/or electrolyte disorders. They frequently cause an alteration in the cardiac output, which may be hazardous to a patient with active ischemia or cardiac disease. A careful and accurate assessment is necessary to avoid serious complications.

Electromechanical dissociation (EMD) is a symptom and not a dysrhythmia. The patient will present with a rhythm (sometimes even an NSR on the ECG), but will not have the responding mechanical component (or contraction). The patient presenting with EMD has an extremely high mortality rate. Treatment involves interventions directed toward the underlying cause. Causes of EMD include tension pneumothorax, pulmonary emboli, acidosis, hypocalcemia, hypoxia, cardiac tamponade, and hypovolemia.

Premature Ventricular Contraction (PVC)

Premature ventricular contractions are contractions that originate in the ventricles rather than in the SA node. Figure 4-66 presents an example of premature ventricular contraction.

PVCs may be caused by a number of factors, including fatigue, caffeine, alcohol, anxiety, irritation, hypokalemia, cardiomyopathy, and ischemia/infarction. They may also be side effects of drugs such as epinephrine, isoproterenol, aminophylline, and digitalis.

PVCs occur as a result of overexcitability of the ventricular myocardium. Simply stated, impulse formation arises before a sinus beat. An irritable focus in the ventricle discharges an impulse before the SA node initiates the next regular beat.

Clinical signs and symptoms of PVCs will depend on the extent of hemodynamic compromise they cause. In a healthy person, PVCs are not usually considered threatening. The ECG strip has the following configuration:

P waves: absent (may be hidden in the QRS)

QRS: usually wide, bizarre, and different from normal; duration is usually greater than 0.12

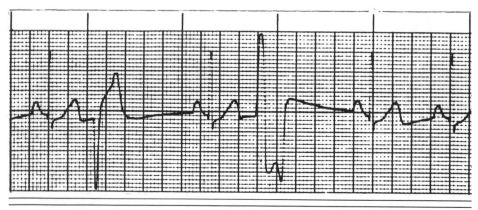

Figure 4-66   Premature Ventricular Contraction

second; T wave is usually opposite the deflection of the QRS.

Conduction: may cause retrograde conduction to the atrium

Rhythm: irregular; a full compensatory pause is usually observed after a PVC (a compensatory pause refers to the time between the beat preceding and the beat subsequent to the PVC, equal to two R-R cycles).

Rate: varies

Nursing standards of care

Treatment of PVCs involves both careful determination of the type of dysrhythmia as well as assessment of the hemodynamic compromise and underlying disease process. The patient with cardiac disease should be treated if any of the following conditions are observed: (1) more than 6 PVCs per minute, (2) coupled PVCs, (3) multifocal PVCs, and (4) R-on-T firing of the PVC. The drug of choice is lidocaine, given as a bolus followed by a maintenance infusion. Normally, a bolus of 1 mg/kg is given, up to a total of 3 mg/kg if necessary. A drip is infused at 2–4 mg/min. Lidocaine levels may need to be checked, especially at infusion rates of 3 mg/min and higher. Signs of lidocaine toxicity include lethargy, tinnitus, altered vision, and confusion.

Idioventricular Rhythm

An example of an idioventricular rhythm is shown in Figure 4-67.

Clinical antecedents

An idioventricular rhythm is compensatory for an extreme bradycardia that would otherwise occur.

Critical referents

An idioventricular rhythm is produced by the inherent automaticity of a pacemaking cell in the His bundle system.

Resulting signs and symptoms

Idioventricular rhythms are usually seen in cases of complete heart block. They tend to be unstable dysrhythmias that require cardiac pacing. The ECG characteristics of idioventricular rhythms are as follows:

P waves: absent or not related

QRS: wide, bizarre, and of greater than 0.12 second in duration

Conduction: stimulus occurs from an ectopic focus in the ventricles

Rhythm: regular

Rate: 20 to 60 bpm; sometimes increasing to 60 to 100 bpm

Nursing standards of care

Medical treatment with atropine, isoproterenol, and/or cardiac pacing is required. An accelerated idioventricular rhythm occurs at rates of 60 to 100 bpm. An idioventricular rhythm is an escape rhythm caused by slowing of the sinus rate and should not be treated with lidocaine.

Ventricular Tachycardia

An example of ventricular tachycardia is presented in Figure 4-68. Ventricular tachycardia is the

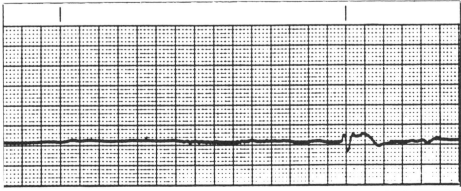

Figure 4-67 Idioventricular Rhythm

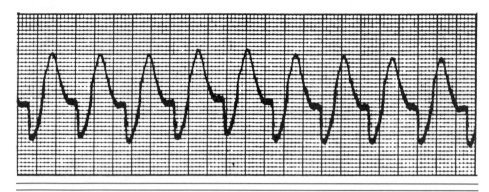

Figure 4-68 Ventricular Tachycardia

repetitive firing of an ectopic ventricular focus that is acting as pacemaker instead of the SA node.

Clinical antecedents

Ventricular tachycardia is most frequently seen with sudden cardiac death, myocardial irritability, and MI. It may also result from respiratory acidosis, hypokalemia, digitalis toxicity, and irritation caused by intracardiac catheters and pacing wires.

Critical referents

Ventricular tachycardia results when an ectopic impulse formed within the ventricles travels through the ventricles and atria in pathways not taken by regularly fired impulses from the SA node.

Resulting signs and symptoms

A frequent mistake in diagnosing ventricular tachycardia occurs in defining it according to hemodynamic stability. Ventricular tachycardia often presents with minimal hemodynamic compromise. But a severe decrease in cardiac output due to inadequate time for ventricular chamber filling usually occurs. Signs of congestive heart failure, shock, and cerebral insufficiency frequently surface. Sudden death may occur. ECG characteristics are as follows:

P waves: may be buried in the QRS complex if retrograde conduction occurs; are not related to the QRS complex

QRS: greater than 0.12 second in duration. A 12-lead ECG will show indeterminate axis (either extreme right or left axis) and concordant QRS deflection in the precordial leads; the initial deflection is greater than 0.04 second.

Conduction: ectopic focus stimulates the ventricles independently of the atria

Rhythm: usually regular

Rate: between 100 and 300 bpm

Nursing standards of care

Much time may be spent trying to distinguish ventricular tachycardia from supraventricular tachycardia with aberrancy. In the presence of hemodynamic instability, however, time should not be wasted in attempting to distinguish these two dysrhythmias; immediate cardioversion should be performed. A bizarre, wide tachyrhythmia should be considered ventricular tachycardia until determined otherwise.

The patient who is hemodynamically stable may be treated with lidocaine. Dosage administration is the same as that for PVCs. Other drugs that may be used include procainamide and bretylium. Of the three drugs, procainamide has the slowest onset. It can be given in doses of 20 mg/min up to a total dose of 1 g. When administering procainamide, though, the practitioner must be aware that it can cause QRS widening and hypotension. Procainamide should not be given to the patient with prolonged Q-T intervals, as it can further lengthen the segment, which can then potentiate the ventricular tachycardia. Should the QRS complex widen by 50% or more, procainamide therapy should be stopped. Bretylium was originally used as an antihypertensive. It initially causes an increase in blood pressure due to catecholamine release, but after approximately 20 minutes, there will be a drop in BP. Bretylium may be useful for multiform (Torsades de Pointes) ventricular tachycardia, which is usually refractory to lidocaine. Other agents that may be used include magnesium and phenytoin.

Ventricular Fibrillation

Figure 4-69 illustrates ventricular fibrillation.

Clinical antecedents

Most frequently, ventricular fibrillation is preceded by ventricular tachycardia. Specific antecedents may include electrocution and hyperkalemia, and cardiac disease represents the primary risk factor.

Critical referents

Ventricular fibrillation occurs when multiple ventricular ectopic foci stimulate the cardiac muscle, producing chaotic ventricular activity with no demonstrable coordinated contraction. The fibrillating cardiac muscle resembles a quivering bowl full of Jello, because the multiple foci are stimulating the heart in many directions.

Resulting signs and symptoms

Ventricular fibrillation results in complete loss of cardiac output. It may appear either fine or coarse, referring to the characteristics of the baseline. This rhythm results in death within 3 to 4 minutes.

Nursing standards of care

Immediate intervention is indicated. Defibrillation is the therapy of choice and CPR is performed.

Administration of epinephrine at doses of 0.5–1.0 mg should follow and may be repeated every 5 minutes. Other antiarrhythmics such as lidocaine and bretylium may also be used.

Asystole

Asystole is the cessation of electrical impulses in the cardiac muscle. The ECG strip displays a straight line.

Clinical antecedents

Most frequently, asystole is preceded by ventricular fibrillation. It may be mistaken for very fine ventricular fibrillation, so it should be confirmed in two leads. In any event, intervention should not be delayed.

Critical referents

Asystole is the complete cessation of myocardial activity.

Resulting signs and symptoms

The result of asystole is imminent death, if the process is not reversed.

Nursing standards of care

Asystole requires immediate CPR. Incidences of asystole carry very high mortality rates. After CPR is

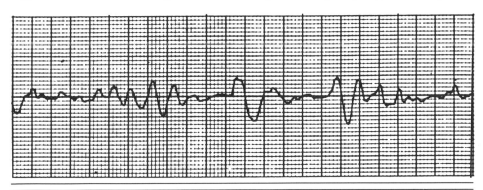

Figure 4-69   Ventricular Fibrillation

Table 4-19   Indications for and Limitations of Selected Pacemakers

Type	Indications	Limitations
VVI Ventricular demand	Complete or intermittent AV block Rhythms needing support when in and out of SR	Does not vary with metabolic needs 10% decreased cardiac output Atrial activity not synchronized to ventricular filling Tricuspid or mitral regurgitation occurs due to asynchrony
AAI Atrial demand	Sick sinus without His-Purkinje disease Atrial escape arrhythmias (PAT)	Atrial fibrillation renders ineffective Contraindicated with AV block

DVI
  AV sequential
  Committed
  Noncommitted
	Sick sinus with His-Purkinje disease
	AV synchrony when needed to enhance cardiac output
	AV synchrony; AV block overdrive
		Does not help in atrial fibrillation
		May needlessly fire for ventricle that is functional
		Potentially self-inhibiting

VAT Atrial synchronous	Complete AV block with normal sinus function	Does not sense intrinsic ventricular activity
VDD	Same as VAT	Contraindicated with intermittent AV block or ventricular ectopy
DDD Universal	AV block	Must rule out retrograde VA conduction or tachyarrhythmias

Note: Pacemaker three-letter code describes, respectively, 1) chamber(s) paced, 2) chamber(s) sensed, and 3) mode of response to sensed potentials. A: atrium; D: double; I: inhibited; R: reverse; T: triggered; V: ventricle; and 0: none.

instituted, epinephrine and atropine, 0.5 to 1.0 mg, may be given.

Use of Pacemakers in the Management of Dysrhythmias

Cardiac pacing may be required as part of the medical management of certain dysrhythmias. Table 4-19 provides a description of various types of pacemakers available today, the limitations of each, and indications for their use.

Pacemakers are either external (temporary) or implantable (permanent). They consist of a pulse generator, a lead, and electrodes. There are two types of electrodes. A unipolar electrode, which is connected to another (indifferent) electrode located elsewhere and produces a large pacemaker spike on the ECG. Bipolar electrodes are positive and negative electrodes placed on the anterior surface of the heart or within the chamber. A small pacemaker spike appears on the ECG. If one electrode fails, bipolar electrodes can become a unipolar system by the addition of a skin electrode.

Figure 4-70 displays the pattern of a normally functioning ventricular pacemaker. Note the pacemaker spike and the widened QRS complex, indicating that the origin of the impulse is in the ventricle.

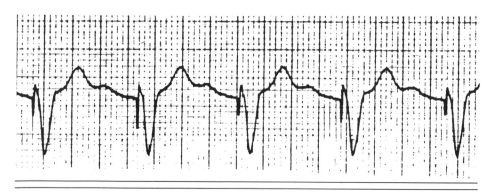

Figure 4-70   VVI Pacemaker Pattern

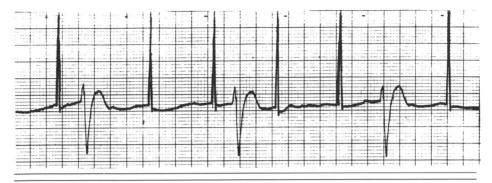

Figure 4-71 Non-Sensing Pacemaker

One of three techniques is used for inserting a temporary pacemaker: transvenous endocardial, epicardial, or transthoracic technique.

Transvenous endocardial is the most common technique. The catheter is inserted via a percutaneous route or venous cutdown (subclavian, antecubital, femoral, and jugular veins are common sites). Electrocardiogram or fluoroscopy is used during insertion. Electrodes are placed in the right ventricle or atrium or both and are then attached to the external pulse generator. The generator is set with respect to electrical output, rate, and ability to sense the patient's intrinsic rhythm.

The epicardial technique is routinely used following heart surgery. The wires are placed through the thorax and are easily removed once the patient's condition has stabilized.

The transthoracic technique is used in an emergency situation. The electrodes are placed via a needle inserted directly through the thorax into the myocardium. Possible complications include coronary artery laceration and cardiac tamponade.

A fourth method is external pacing, which involves two electrodes placed on the patient's chest and back. This method requires much larger voltages of electricity (50 to 150 V) than the others do and thus causes pain and burns on the skin.

Following the insertion of a pacemaker, the patient must be continuously monitored for signs that the pacemaker is not sensing the patient's own rhythm (Figure 4-71) or not capturing (Figure 4-72).

Electrical hazards (including static electricity) must be avoided, and the catheter and its site will need to be protected from dislodgement, kinking, disconnection, and infection.

The following nursing care plan outlines standard critical care practices for cases of dysrhythmias.

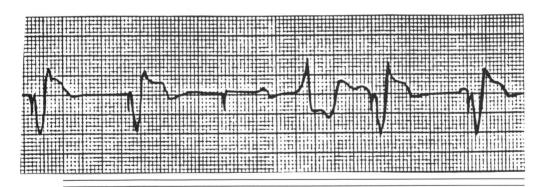

Figure 4-72 Non-Capturing Pacemaker

Nursing Care Plan for the Management of the Patient with Dysrhythmias

Diagnosis	Signs and symptoms	Intervention	Rationale
Potential for alteration in cardiac output related to dysrhythmia	Decreased BP Chest discomfort Dyspnea Palpitations	Check patient's vital signs upon changes in rhythm	Hemodynamic compromise depends on patient's intrinsic state rather than on dysrhythmia alone
		Administer drugs and perform measures, as ordered	As per ACLS standards
		For symptomatic bradycardia and heart blocks: atropine, 0.5–1 mg; repeat in 5 minutes, up to 2 mg; anticipate pacemaker and/or isoproterenol drip at 2–10 mcg/min	
		For ventricular ectopy and tachycardia: lidocaine, 1 mg/kg; repeat in 8 minutes, up to 3 mg/min, followed by infusion at 2–4 mg/min; cardioversion; procainamide at 20 mg/min; bretylium 5 mg/kg, repeat after 8 minutes, up to 30 mg/kg	
		For ventricular fibrillation: defibrillation; epinephrine 0.5–1 mg; repeat every 5 minutes; lidocaine and/or bretylium, as for tachycardia;	

Diagnosis	Signs and symptoms	Intervention	Rationale
		For SVT: carotid massage and/or Valsalva maneuver; verapamil 5 mg IV; repeat in 10–15 minutes; synchronized cardioversion	
		Monitor electrolytes (K^+, Mg^+, and Ca^{++})	Need to correct underlying electrolyte disorder, which may exacerbate dysrhythmias
		Monitor drug levels	To maintain doses in therapeutic range
Potential for alteration in cerebral, cardiopulmonary, renal, and/or peripheral tissue perfusion	Signs of altered cerebral perfusion: mental confusion; dizziness; syncope; convulsions and/or seizures; TIA; yawning	Rule out noncardiac causes of altered cerebral perfusion	Could be due to lidocaine toxicity, neurological disorders, etc.
	Signs of altered cardiopulmonary perfusion: angina; ischemic changes	Monitor for chest pain	Early detection will help to prevent and allay cardiac complications
	Signs of altered renal perfusion: oliguria; anuria	Check urine output every 8 hours, or every hour if oliguria occurs	May indicate onset of prerenal failure from decreased renal perfusion
	Sign of altered peripheral perfusion: hypotension	Monitor BUN, creatinine, and K^+	A BUN:creatinine ratio greater than 10:1 is indicative of prerenal failure; patient may become hyperkalemic
		Check pulses and BP every 1–2 hours or as needed	Dysrhythmias may cause decrease in cardiac output to periphery

Nursing Care Plan for the Management of the Patient with Dysrhythmias

Diagnosis	Signs and symptoms	Intervention	Rationale
Anxiety related to: palpitations; fear of consequences; monitoring equipment; special diagnostic procedures	Restlessness	Assess level of anxiety	To establish baseline
	Frequent questioning	Encourage patient and family to verbalize fears	Helps to allay exaggerated concerns
	Withdrawn behavior	Explain symptoms in terms of dysrhythmia	Patient may be more aware of heart beating because of diagnosis
		Educate patient and family about etiology and process of dysrhythmia, purpose and procedure of diagnostic studies and interventions, and follow-up care	Lack of knowledge and understanding may increase anxiety and decrease adherence to care regimen
		Administer anxiolytics as ordered	To decrease anxiety
Knowledge deficit with respect to use of antidysrhythmic drugs	Patient verbalizes lack of knowledge and understanding	Assess present understanding of dysrhythmias and drug therapy	To establish baseline
		Instruct on medications and side effects and how to deal with them	Antidysrhythmics commonly have side effects, and patient may stop taking them as a result
	Nonadherence to care regimen	Assess patient's and family's ability to adhere to care regimen	To adapt teaching to status of patient and family in order to maximize adherence to regimen

Medications Commonly Used in the Care of the Patient with Dysrhythmias

Medication	Effect	Major side effects
Atropine	Parasympatholytic Decreases refractory period Increases SA node discharge and conduction through AV node	Dry mouth Ventricular irritability Difficulty in voiding
Verapamil	Calcium channel blocker	Headache Dizziness GI upset Dyspnea Skin rashes
Digitalis	Increases contractility Lengthens refractory period of AV node Decreases left ventricular end-diastolic pressure Increases ventricular automaticity Decreases atrial automaticity	Tachycardia AV block Bradycardia GI upset Headache Drowsiness Confusion Double vision
Propranolol	Beta blocker leading to decreased heart rate and contractility, thus decreased oxygen demand and decreased AV conduction time and refractory period	Bradycardia or heart block Hypotension Fatigue Dizziness GI upset
Quinidine	Increases refractory period Decreases excitability Decreases myocardial contractility Increases conduction time Decreases automaticity of pacemaker cells	Nausea and vomiting Heart block Ventricular irritability Hypotension Thrombocytopenia Vertigo Tinnitus
Lidocaine	Decreases automaticity, conduction velocity, and refractory period of Purkinje fibers	Lethargy/slurred speech Confusion and disorientation Hypotension Heart block or bradycardia Convulsions
Procainamide	Increases refractory period Decreases excitability	GI upset CNS depression/convulsions Hypotension AV block
Bretylium	Increases contractility Increases refractory period of Purkinje fibers and ventricle	Postural hypotension GI upset Angina

Cardiac Trauma

Cardiac trauma is damage to the heart or the great vessels caused directly or indirectly by external forces. Direct trauma can be penetrating or nonpenetrating; indirect trauma affects the heart through hemorrhage and shock.

Clinical antecedents

Penetrating wounds result when foreign objects (knives, ice picks, bullets, etc.) pierce the heart or great vessels, either directly through the chest wall or diaphragm or indirectly through the esophagus or bronchial tree. Nonpenetrating injuries can result from a blow to the chest wall or a compression caused by force, deceleration, or increases in intravascular pressure. The right ventricle is most frequently involved because of its anterior position in the chest, the left ventricle and right atrium are next in frequency of incidence, and the left atrium is the least often involved because of its posterior position in the chest cavity. The prognosis for victims of penetrating and nonpenetrating wounds has become quite favorable (usually 90% of those reaching the hospital survive) with the advanced surgical corrective techniques available today.

Critical referents

A penetrating injury can sometimes cause a laceration of the pericardium deep enough to involve the myocardium. Depending on the site of injury, one, two, or all chambers may be involved, and if more than one chamber has been damaged, there is usually septal injury as well. Most diffuse injurious assaults (gunshots) not only damage the myocardium, but cause injury to the valves and their papillary muscles and chordae tendinea. A nonpenetrating wound usually results in myocardial contusion or, if serious enough, myocardial infarction or rup-

ture. Again, injury may occur to the valves and their papillary muscles and chordae tendinea.

Resulting signs and symptoms

Complications of penetrating and nonpenetrating wounds are similar and are evidenced according to the region involved. Generalized complications are frequent, too; these include bleeding to the point of tamponade, pneumopericardium, pericardial effusion, massive hemorrhage and shock, infection, aneurysm, and thrombosis. Hypotension almost always occurs, and arrhythmias (frequently of a life-threatening nature) are very common because of irritation of impulse origin or interruption in conduction pathways. Hypoxia is almost always a problem, and agitation and delirium commonly result. Finally, persistent pain is experienced by the patient.

Signs of cardiac tamponade include hypotension, muffled or indiscernible heart sounds, increased jugular venous pressure (caused by impaired ventricular filling), and the presence of a paradoxical pulse. These signs must be differentiated from those of intrapleural hemorrhage, which are the same except for the increased jugular venous pressure. Delayed signs and symptoms that may occur include recurrent pericardial effusion, retrosternal chest pain, fever, cardiac enlargement, and congestive heart failure.

Nursing standards of care

Treatment is aimed at supporting life processes of the patient and alleviating life-threatening complications such as tamponade and arrhythmias. Immediate interventions indicated are thoracotomy for relief of tamponade and surgical repair of lacerations, aneurysms, and valve and septal defects. On a long-term basis, the patient requires care similar to that given the MI and cardiac surgery patient.

Nursing care is provided in concert with the medical regimen. The following highlights the nursing care provided to individuals suffering cardiac trauma.

Diagnosis	Signs and symptoms	Intervention	Rationale
Potential for fluid volume deficit due to: estimated blood loss not fully replaced; bleeding due to thrombocytopenia, elevated clotting time, increased afterload, or hypertension; suboptimal preload status from OR; increased afterload when patient is still hypothermic from OR; vasodilation in response to warming or to nitroglycerine or Nipride; postoperative diuresis	LAP < 6–10 mm Hg CVP < 6 mm Hg PAD < 10 mm Hg SBP < 100 mm Hg HR > 120 bpm Urine output > intake or: > 500 cc after 1 hour; > 800 cc after 2 hours; > 900 cc after 3 hours; > 1000 cc after 4 hours; > 1200 cc after 5 hours Sudden increase in chest tube drainage SVR < 800 or > 1200 dyne-sec/cm^5 Weight loss	Monitor VS closely: TPR; ECG; LAP; arterial BP; PA pressures; I&O Blood replacement, as ordered, for chest tube drainage > 200 cc/hr with LAP < 16 mm Hg; IV infusions, as ordered, for LA < 10 or PAD < 14 Administer fresh frozen platelets or packed cells during rewarming Monitor effects of vasodilating agents (NTG, dobutamine, Inocor, MSO$_4$, renal dose dopamine) Monitor PT, PTT, platelets, and Hct closely; be prepared to administer protamine sulfate, cryoprecipitate, FFP, PC, platelets, or Amicar for abnormally elevated clotting time, bleeding, or reduced platelet count	To ascertain trends by which to establish medication regimen To maintain volume and cardiac function and efficiency and to maintain patency of grafts To counteract vasodilation effect of rewarming To prevent early volume insufficiency To prevent or treat early bleeding complications
Potential for decreased cardiac output from arrhythmias; fluid volume deficit; fluid volume overload; hypothermia; hypertension; hypotension; tamponade; increased afterload	CO < 3 L/min CI < 2 L/min/m^2 Reduced peripheral tissue perfusion evidenced by decreased distal pulses and cool extremities	Monitor CO and CI closely Administer vasoactive medications as ordered (dobutamine, Inocor)	To facilitate early intervention To maintain adequate perfusion in vital organs and periphery

*Care plan adapted from plan provided by the Georgetown University Hospital Department of Nursing.

Nursing Care Plan for the Management of the Patient with Cardiac Trauma

Diagnosis	Signs and symptoms	Intervention	Rationale
	Arrhythmias, such as PVCs, heart blocks, SVT, PAT, AF, AFL, MAT related to edematous suture line, ventricular tachycardia, ventricular fibrillation	Administer antiarrhythmias as ordered and PRN	To allow for adequate cardiac function and prevention of life-threatening rhythms
		Assess and treat ABGs and K^+ in relation to PVCs	Potassium imbalance and compromised ABGs can cause PVCs
		Serial ECGs	To allow early recognition of ischemia, injury, or arrhythmia
		Maintain stable heart rhythm, as ordered: atrially paced to keep heart rate at 60–100; ventricularly paced for second- and third-degree heart blocks; cardioversion for ventricular tachycardia or fibrillation; verapamil for SVT; digoxin	To maintain normal sinus rhythm and stable hemodynamics
Fluid volume deficit		Correct fluid volume deficit, as ordered	To maintain cardiac function and output
Ischemia: CPK > 180 IU/L; MBs > 15 IU/L; new ECG ischemic changes		Serial ECGs Maintain oxygenation	To facilitate early recognition of ischemia and prevent further cellular damage from lack of oxygenation
Hypothermia		Administer $NaHCO_3$ for base deficit > −3 when hypothermic	Acid-base imbalance is exacerbated by hypothermia
		Warm with warming blankets or lights	To return patient to normal core temperature

Diagnosis	Signs and symptoms	Intervention	Rationale
	Hypertension	Administer antihypertensives, as ordered, to keep SBP > 100 and < 150 mm Hg (MSO$_4$, nitroprusside 0.5–8.0 mcg/kg/min, nitroglycerin up to 200–300 mcg/min)	Fast-acting or short-lasting medications for hypertensive events
		Taper vasoconstrictive meds to maintain SBP > 100 and < 160 mm Hg (epinephrine, Levophed, dobutamine 2–10 mcg/kg/min, dopamine 2–10 mcg/kg/min, neosynephrine)	To maintain safe blood pressure levels
	Tamponade: elevation and equalization of filling pressures (CVP + PAD = LAP = 20–30); reduction in SBP to less than 100 mm Hg; abrupt cessation of CT drainage; widening of mediastinum on x-ray; increased jugular venous pressure; cool, clammy skin; reduced peripheral pulses; muffled heart sounds; pulsus paradoxus > 10	Immediate medical intervention, including extracting clot from mediastinal tube with Fogarty catheter, open chest procedure, and/or return to OR	Cardiac tamponade presents a high risk of death if not treated immediately

	Increased SVR
	
	Crackles (rales)
		Reduce SVR, as ordered, by:
		    warming patient;
		    administering vasodilators (Inocor, dobutamine, nitroglycerine, MSO$_4$);
		    restricting fluids;
		    administering diuretics
			To maintain hemodynamic stability

Nursing Care Plan for the Management of the Patient with Cardiac Trauma

Diagnosis	Signs and symptoms	Intervention	Rationale
Alteration in cardiac output related to myocardial failure	Signs of low cardiac output: decreased BP; increased SVR; increased PAP and PCWP Signs of high cardiac output: increased cardiac output measures; decreased BP; decreased SVR; increased PAP and PCWP	Anticipate insertion of pulmonary artery catheter	Provides more accurate measure of cardiac function
		Administer preload-reducing agents (nitroglycerin) as ordered, to maintain PAD/PCWP < 18 mm Hg	To decrease venous return
		Administer afterload-reducing agents (nitroprusside) as ordered, to maintain SVR at 800–1300 dyne-sec/cm^5	To reduce SVR
		Administer inotropics (dopamine, dobutamine) as ordered	To improve contractility
		Administer drugs, as indicated and ordered, to maintain normal sinus rhythm	To maintain cardiac efficiency and output
		Administer digoxin as ordered	To improve cardiac contractility and control tachycardia
		Monitor BP closely	To assess for hypotension and pulsus alternans
		Participate in identification and correction of aggravating factors	It is most important to correct the underlying cause rather than just treating the symptoms
Potential for alteration in cardiac output related to electrical, mechanical, and structural cardiac factors	Decreased cardiac output, as measured with pulmonary artery catheter	Continuous monitoring utilizing V_1 or V_6 and lead II	Most patients will have dysrhythmias following MI; V_1 and V_6 are best for viewing ventricular ectopy; lead II is best for monitoring P waves

Diagnosis	Signs and symptoms	Intervention	Rationale
		Monitor changes in ST segment elevation	May indicate early extension of MI
		Monitor vital signs with changes in rhythm	May cause hemodynamic changes
		Maintain a patent IV at all times	In emergencies, quickest route and fastest action is via IV
	Decreased BP, sluggish capillary refill, lethargy, and dyspnea	Monitor for signs and symptoms of heart failure	Occurs most commonly in anterior MI but may occur in any type
		Have patient rest and avoid isometric movement/activities; use bedside commode, if stable, rather than bedpan; avoid Valsalva maneuver	Isometrics increase peripheral vascular resistance, thereby increasing the workload of the heart
		Check for capillary refill and pulses every 4 hours and PRN	Sluggish refill indicates decreased perfusion
		Monitor BP and heart rate every 2 hours and PRN	Compromises in BP and heart rate are early signs of decreased cardiac output
	Evidence of dysrhythmia, papillary muscle rupture, septal defect, or aneurysm	Assess heart sounds for sudden onset of systolic murmur	May indicate papillary muscle tear or ventricular septal defect
	Symptoms of cardiogenic shock: systolic BP < 90; pallor and cyanosis; weak and thready pulse; cool and clammy skin; altered mental states; decreased urinary output; pulsus alternans	Monitor left ventricular function with pulmonary artery catheter	PAD or PCWP > 18 mm Hg indicates onset of pulmonary congestion
		Administer inotropics as ordered (dopamine, dobutamine, amrinone)	To increase myocardial contractility
		Maintain fluid and electrolyte balance using volume expanders	PAD or PCWP < 10 mm Hg may indicate volume deficit
		Anticipate the use of intraaortic balloon pump counterpulsation	To decrease afterload and improve cardiac perfusion

Nursing Care Plan for the Management of the Patient with Cardiac Trauma

Diagnosis	Signs and symptoms	Intervention	Rationale
		Administer afterload reduction agents as ordered (nitroprusside, 0.5–1.0 mcg/kg/min)	Reducing the SVR to normal range decreases the workload of the heart
		Administer drugs, as ordered, to maintain normal sinus rhythm	Dysrhythmias can decrease filling time, thus decreasing cardiac output
		Insert Foley catheter; maintain accurate I&O records	Need to monitor output accurately
		Anticipate the administration of other agents to salvage myocardium, such as thrombolytics, propanolol, and glucose/insulin/K^+	Providing nutrients and oxygen, improving circulation, and decreasing myocardial oxygen demand help to salvage myocardium
Potential for alteration in cardiac output related to dysrhythmia	Decreased BP Chest discomfort Dyspnea Palpitations	Check patient's vital signs upon changes in rhythm	Hemodynamic compromise depends on patient's intrinsic state rather than on dysrhythmia alone
		Administer drugs and perform measures, as ordered	As per ACLS standards
		For symptomatic bradycardia and heart blocks: atropine, 0.5–1 mg; repeat in 5 minutes, up to 2 mg; anticipate pacemaker and/or isoproterenol drip at 2–10 mcg/min	
		For ventricular ectopy and tachycardia: lidocaine, 1 mg/kg; repeat in 8 minutes, up to 3 mg/min, followed by infusion at 2–4 mg/min;	

Diagnosis	Signs and symptoms	Intervention	Rationale
		cardioversion; procainamide at 20 mg/min; bretylium 5 mg/kg, repeat after 8 minutes, up to 30 mg/kg	
		For ventricular fibrillation: defibrillation; epinephrine 0.5–1 mg; repeat every 5 minutes; lidocaine and/or bretylium, as for tachycardia	
		For SVT: carotid massage and/or Valsalva maneuver; verapamil 5 mg IV; repeat in 10–15 minutes; synchronized cardioversion	
		Monitor electrolytes (K^+, Mg^+, and Ca^{++})	Need to correct underlying electrolyte disorder, which may exacerbate dysrhythmias
		Monitor drug levels	To maintain doses in therapeutic range
Potential for alteration in cerebral, cardiopulmonary, renal, and/or peripheral tissue perfusion	Signs of altered cerebral perfusion: mental confusion; dizziness; syncope; convulsions and/or seizures; TIA; yawning	Rule out noncardiac causes of altered cerebral perfusion	Could be due to lidocaine toxicity, neurological disorders, etc.
	Signs of altered cardiopulmonary perfusion: angina; ischemic changes	Monitor for chest pain	Early detection will help to prevent and allay cardiac complications

Diagnosis	Signs and symptoms	Intervention	Rationale
	Signs of altered renal perfusion: oliguria; anuria	Check urine output every 8 hours, or every hour if oliguria occurs	May indicate onset of prerenal failure from decreased renal perfusion
	Sign of altered peripheral perfusion: hypotension	Monitor BUN, creatinine, and K^+	A BUN:creatinine ratio greater than 10:1 is indicative of prerenal failure; patient may become hyperkalemic
		Check pulses and BP every 1–2 hours or as needed	Dysrhythmias may cause decrease in cardiac output to periphery
Potential for alteration in cerebral, peripheral, and cardiopulmonary tissue perfusion	Signs of venous thromboembolism: mottled extremities; edema	Monitor for signs and symptoms of altered stasis	Thromboembolism is a potential complication of bedrest
	Signs of pulmonary emboli: sudden onset of chest pain; V/Q mismatch; bloody sputum; dyspnea; very rapid, shallow breathing	Use elastic antiembolism stockings; remove every 8 hours for 10 minutes	To improve venous return
		Check all pulses; compare for bilateral strength of pulse every 8 hours	Diminished pulses are indicative of arterial perfusion alteration
	Signs of arterial thromboembolism: loss of pulses; pain in calf on dorsiflexion (Homan's sign); pale, cool extremities	Check for Homan's sign every 8 hours	A positive Homan's sign indicates arterial thromboembolism
		Do not allow knee gatch of bed to be elevated	Gatching the knee in bed causes pooling of blood in lower extremities
	Signs of cerebrovascular accident: weakness or paralysis on one side of body; altered level of consciousness	Check capillary refill every 4 hours	Indicates the quality of arterial perfusion
		Check breath sounds every 4 hours	Diminished breath sounds may indicate pulmonary emboli
		Check neurological status every 4 hours	Alterations in mental status may indicate altered cerebral blood flow

Diagnosis	Signs and symptoms	Intervention	Rationale
Potential for alteration in gas exchange and ineffective breathing pattern	Dyspnea Decreased O_2 levels on ABGs Change in mental status Fluid overload	Monitor ABGs closely	Problems with oxygenation are commonly seen
		Assist to position of comfort (semi- or high Fowler's position is best)	To improve breathing patterns and lower diaphragm
		Assess for crackles (rales), S_3, and increased JVP every 4 hours or as needed	Signs of heart failure, with resultant pulmonary edema
		Administer oxygen as ordered	To counter problems with oxygenation
		Monitor heart rhythm	Tachycardia is commonly seen
		Review chest x-ray for signs of pulmonary edema	Pulmonary congestion can be clinically delayed up to 24 hours
Decreased tolerance of activity related to dyspnea	Dyspnea on exertion Fatigue	Assess level of activity tolerance (should be related to the New York Heart Association's classification for consistency)	Provides a baseline
		Assist patient to change position every 2 hours while on bedrest	To decrease risk of complications and promote venous return
		Check BP with patient in horizontal, sitting, and standing positions	To monitor for orthostatic hypotension
		Avoid activity for a half-hour to an hour after meals	May decrease chance of hypoxia due to increased blood flow to GI tract
	Exaggerated increase in heart rate and BP on exertion	Monitor heart rate and BP with activity increases	To maintain heart rate within 10 bpm of resting heart rate and maintain systolic BP within 20 mm Hg of resting BP; if a drop occurs, it may indicate a drop in cardiac output

Nursing Care Plan for the Management of the Patient with Cardiac Trauma

Diagnosis	Signs and symptoms	Intervention	Rationale
		Anticipate institution of progressive rehab	To provide controlled mechanism for increasing activity
		Encourage frequent rest periods	To prevent excessive fatigue
At risk for complications related to cardiac inflammatory process	Signs of cardiac tamponade: narrowed pulse pressure; low voltage ECG pattern; muffled heart sounds; widening of mediastinum; decrease in cardiac output; distended neck veins	Monitor BP and check for pulsus paradoxus by noting inspiratory drop in systolic blood pressure	Difference greater than 10 mmHg indicates presence of exaggerated pulsus paradoxus and should be reported to physician; may indicate decreased ability of the heart to fill
	ECG changes suggestive of cardiac tissue inflammation: diffuse changes; ST elevation without T-wave inversion; PR segment depression	Prepare patient for echocardiogram	To check the extent of pericardial effusion
		Prepare patient for pericardiocentesis	To remove blood or fluid from pericardial sac to prevent cardiac tamponade
		Avoid the use of anticoagulants in the presence of pericarditis	Anticoagulants can lead to cardiac tamponade
		Obtain 12-lead ECG	Monitor for ECG changes indicative of pericarditis
		Maintain patent IV	To allow for emergency access
		Be prepared for potential complications	Cardiac tamponade can easily recur after pericardiocentesis

Diagnosis	Signs and symptoms	Intervention	Rationale

Potential for infection due to:
  IV lines;
  indwelling Foley catheter;
  chest tubes;
  endotracheal intubation;
  stress of surgery (in the event of trauma)
	Increased temperature
	
	Tachycardia and/or decreasing BP
	
	WBC > 10,000 mm^3
		Tylenol 600 mg every 4 hours or PRN, as ordered	To alleviate fevers

	Redness, exudate, increased tenderness, and/or induration of surgical incisions, IV insertion site, pacer wire sites, or chest tube sites	Implement thorough hand washing between patient contacts; implement universal isolation precautions if indicated	To prevent spread of infections
		Routine incision care with povidone-iodine solution, Telfa dressing, and foam tape	To prevent incisional infections
		Change peripheral IV sites at least every 3 days or with any signs of infection or infiltration; change IV tubing every 48 hours	IV fluid is especially fertile medium for bacterial growth
	Changes in characteristics of sputum: tan, brown, yellow, or green color and/or foul odor	Culture suspected origins of infection	To administer antibiotics that bacteria are sensitive to
	Chest x-ray indicative of atelectasis Decreased or absent breath sounds locally	Vigorous pulmonary toilet	To prevent and/or treat pulmonary congestion leading to infections
	Sediment in urine or foul-smelling urine	Routine Foley care every 8 hours	To prevent urinary tract infections
	WBCs in urine Hesitancy, frequency, urgency, burning, difficulty starting stream, incontinence, and/or inability to void	If patient is taking fluids, push fluids, unless contraindicated by cardiac condition	To flush urinary tract
Potential for alteration in GI status and bowel elimination	Nausea Constipation	Monitor I&O	To optimize nutritional status and fluid and electrolyte balances
		Provide a liquid diet during first 24 hours after injury, or until patient is free of anginal pain for 24 hours	To decrease perfusion required by GI tract so that it can be directed elsewhere, especially to the heart; to allay nausea, common with anginal pain

Nursing Care Plan for the Management of the Patient with Cardiac Trauma

Diagnosis	Signs and symptoms	Intervention	Rationale
		Encourage activity when patient is free of anginal pain	To improve GI motility
		Monitor frequency of bowel movements	Constipation is common complaint, due to physical inactivity; Valsalva maneuver and straining during bowel movements are contraindicated
		Administer stool softeners and bulk laxatives as ordered	To provide bulk to GI tract, thereby decreasing constipation
		Administer drugs for the treatment of nausea and vomiting as ordered	Patient should be as calm and relaxed as possible; vomiting precipitates further electrolyte imbalances
Potential for skin breakdown due to: restriction in movement; pain or discomfort; drug-induced neuromuscular or musculoskeletal impairment; depression; stiffness from extended catheterization time and/or time on operating table; diaphoresis or drainage into patient's bed; independent variables such as diabetes, peripheral vascular disease, obesity, etc.	Imposed restriction of movement due to body mechanics, medical protocol, etc.	Put air mattress on all postoperative beds	To prevent pressure spots on skin
	Impaired coordination or decreased muscle strength preventing independent movement	Assist patient with required movements and with a quarter turn every 1–2 hours	To prevent injury and facilitate movement
	Reluctance to attempt movement	Premedicate PRN or as ordered to decrease discomfort accompanying movement	To facilitate movement
	Redness over pressure points	Inspect skin pressure points, including occiput, sacrum, coccyx, heels, and elbows, every 2 hours	To prevent skin breakdown
		Passive range of motion to all extremities	To prevent pressure spots and improve circulation without increasing oxygen demand

Diagnosis	Signs and symptoms	Intervention	Rationale
		Keep patient dry	To prevent skin breakdown
		Maintain and supplement nutrition as needed	To maintain vital nutrients to skin
		Consult enterostomal therapist for actual breakdown	For optimal care planning and intervention
	Elevated temperature	Keep patient dry when diaphoretic	To prevent skin breakdown
Potential for alteration in health maintenance due to knowledge deficit concerning: diagnosis; surgical procedure; medications; diet; activity; medical follow-up; referrals; when to notify MD; self-monitoring	Inability to describe personal diagnosis and how it relates to type of surgery	Instruct patient and family about diagnosis and surgery	Patient and family must understand what is being done and why
		Encourage questions and discussion of problems and concerns	To allow for greatest learning
	Inability to identify medications and their schedules	Instruct patient about medications: what they look like; names and doses; indications; side effects and what can be done; daily schedule; standard drug information and complete medication schedule	Safe and accurate medication regimen is necessary
	Inability to list foods appropriate for personal diet	Provide instruction on low-sodium, modified-fat/cholesterol diet; consult with dietician	To facilitate healing and prevent complications arising from incorrect diet
	Inability to distinguish between permitted and prohibited progression of activities	Discuss activity instructions: activities in routine; balancing rest and activity; progressive walking schedule; no lifting more than 20 pounds; no driving for 6 weeks;	To allow for progressive resumption of activities without risk of overdoing it and precipitating an untoward event In the event of an accident, steering wheel may crush incompletely healed sternum

Diagnosis	Signs and symptoms	Intervention	Rationale
		stopping every hour for a short walk when taking long car trips; resumption of sexual activities	To increase circulation and prevent prolonged venous pooling
	Lack of knowledge about follow-up appointments	Help patient and family to arrange follow-up appointments	Plans for follow-up care must be initiated as soon as possible
	Inability to identify professional services available for support	Advise patient and family of services and resources available	To provide most comprehensive and effective services to patient and family
	Inability to explain when to notify MD or seek emergency assistance	Review with patient and family when to notify MD: angina, SOB, dizziness, or nausea during or following activity; weight gain of more than 1 lb/day; signs of infected incision, including redness, swelling, increased tenderness, drainage; temperature > 101°F; irregular/fast heart rate	Patient and family need to know what to do in the case of an untoward event
	Inability to properly count pulse, assess weight fluctuations, and/or take temperature	Instruct patient and family and require return demonstration: weighing self and recording weight; taking temperature and pulse and recording them	Patient and family need to increase self-help abilities
	Inability to verbalize significance of weight changes	Instruct patient on meaning of weight gain and what to do in its event	To increase patient's self-help abilities in preventing congestive failure

618

Diagnosis	Signs and symptoms	Intervention	Rationale
Potential for ineffective individual or family coping related to: situational crisis; maturational crisis; personal vulnerability	Verbalization of inability to cope Inability to ask for emotional help	Assess family's usual coping mechanisms	Questions and concerns of patient and family must be answered even if not voiced
		Assist family to identify alternative coping mechanisms; identify and acknowledge family's needs	Optimal coping must be accomplished for maximal healing
	Inability to meet role expectations	Provide information to patient and family regarding diagnosis and purpose of supportive services	Patient and family must be helped through role redefinition
	Prolonged progression of disease or disability	Support patient and family through role transition	To facilitate necessary role changes
		Encourage open communication among patient, family, and health care team	To facilitate problem solving and care planning
		Reinforce simple explanations to patient and family	During times of crisis, care must be taken not to cause information overload
	Exhaustion	Provide rest periods and offer nutrition to family; plan visiting schedule to accommodate interventions as well as family schedule and rest periods; restrict visitors as appropriate	To maximize quality family time as well as allow for needed rest
	Fear and anxiety	Delegate one resource and support person to assist family through this very critical time	Consistency in problem solving and care improves quality of decisions
	Inappropriate requests or hypervigilance by patient and/or family	Suggest ways for family to assist in patient's care	Participatory care decreases anxiety

Nursing Care Plan for the Management of the Patient with Cardiac Trauma

Diagnosis	Signs and symptoms	Intervention	Rationale
	Inability to solve problems	Assist patient and family to identify problems and work together to solve them	Sometimes patients and families are unable to anticipate possible problems
	Unreasonable and/or excessively frequent requests (excessive use of call light)	Assist family in caring for patient and problem solve about how to continue such care following discharge	Personal involvement in care decreases anxiety while increasing self-confidence and skills
		Encourage progressively independent activities	To avoid rushing patient and family into too much responsibility for care
Potential for self-care deficit due to: muscle deconditioning; postoperative incisional discomfort; sleep pattern disturbance; fear of overexertion; anxiety; decreased activity tolerance	Weak muscles resulting from bedrest	Encourage progressive activities: self-care, ambulation, active ROM	To allow time for patient to regain strength
	Reports of postoperative pain Fatigue	Assess discomfort and encourage patient to request medication as appropriate	To allow for maximal activities
	Slow movement, ambulating with caution, refusal to participate in daily care routine	Reassure patient that postoperative pain is expected and teach patient how to minimize discomfort while moving, deep breathing, coughing, etc.	To minimize effects of pain
	Increased heart rate and respiratory rate upon minimal activity	Assess patient's need for rest and sleep and incorporate rest periods during the day	To prevent overexhaustion
	Repetitive fast speech, indicating anxiety	Maintain calm environment (lighting, noise, interruptions, etc.)	To facilitate adequate rest
	Inability to concentrate on activities required	Encourage patient's participation in scheduling and carrying out daily care	To accommodate routines to patient's ability to progress
		Praise patient's progress in activities	Encouragement is a good motivator

Medications Commonly Used in the Care of the Patient with Cardiac Trauma

Medication	Effect	Major side effects
Metaraminol	Adrenergic receptor stimulation, which causes vasoconstriction Increases myocardial contractility Increases rate of myocardial contractility	Bradycardia Oliguria CNS depression
Dopamine	Inotropic with alpha-adrenergic stimulant Increases myocardial contractility, output, and stroke volume Dilates renal and mesenteric vessels in low doses	GI upset Angina Dyspnea Headache Hypotension Ectopic arrhythmias Palpitations Vasoconstriction
Methoxamine	Alpha-adrenergic receptor stimulation, causing vasoconstriction	Cardiac arrhythmias Bradycardia
Isoproterenol	Stimulates beta receptor sites and relaxes smooth muscle, leading to increased myocardial contractility, increased heart rate, increased myocardial oxygen demand, and decreased peripheral vascular resistance	Tachycardia Ventricular irritability Hypotension Headache Flushing Angina GI upset Dizziness Weakness Tremors
Phentolamine Phenoxybenzamine Chlorpromazine	Alpha-adrenergic blockers, causing vasodilation	Cardiac arrhythmias Tachycardias Orthostatic hypotension
Calcium chloride	Replaces calcium depletion	Hypercalcemia
Corticosteroids	Inhibits inflammatic release of proteolytic enzymes to alter acute injury Potentiates vasoconstrictor effect of norepinephrine Increases sodium retention to increase blood volume	Hypertension Impairéd glucose metabolism Osteoporosis Peptic ulcer Hypokalemia Increased risk for infection

Medications Commonly Used in the Care of the Patient with Cardiac Trauma

Medication	Effect	Major side effects
Digitalis	Increases contractility Lengthens refractory period of AV node Decreases left ventricular end-diastolic pressure Increases ventricular automaticity Decreases atrial automaticity	Tachycardia AV block Bradycardia GI upset Headache Drowsiness Confusion Double vision
Morphine sulfate	Analgesia/sedation Peripheral vasodilation Decreases systemic venous return Bronchodilation Relief of cardiac dyspnea	Hypotension Respiratory depression Nausea and vomiting Constipation Urinary retention
Nitroprusside	Vasodilator with a direct action on vascular smooth muscle to decrease afterload, causing greater ejection fractions, stroke volume, and cardiac output	GI upset Muscle twitching Hypotension Confusion
Nitrates	Vasodilation, leading to increased coronary blood supply and decreased myocardial oxygen demand	Hypotension Headache
Hydralazine Minoxidil Diazoxide	Vasodilator with a direct action on vascular smooth muscle, leading to relaxed arterioles, decreased vascular resistance, and increased cardiac output	Angina Nausea and vomiting Tachycardia Headache Flushing Hypotension
Lidocaine	Decreased ventricular ectopy	In toxicity: disorientation, slurred speech, and seizures
Furosemide	Diuresis Decreased pulmonary congestion	Hypokalemia Hypocalcemia Hypomagnesemia Altered glucose metabolism

Cardiomyopathy

Cardiomyopathy is a disorder of the heart muscle that destroys the endocardium and, sometimes, the pericardium. There are different types of cardiomyopathy, classified according to precipitating factors; congestive, hypertrophic (idiopathic hypertrophic subaortic stenosis), and restrictive cardiomyopathy are three such classifications.

Clinical antecedents

No specific etiology can be clearly identified for cardiomyopathy. The individual who appears to hold greater risk for this type of cardiomyopathy is the one who suffers from diabetes, alcoholism, cancer, muscular dystrophy, and diseases of the thyroid. The individual who suffers other types of cardiac disease sometimes presents with congestive and restrictive cardiomyopathies. Black males between 40 and 60 years of age have been found to be the most frequently affected group of individuals.

Critical referents

Cardiomyopathy, which causes permanent damage to the myocardium, is sometimes of an idiopathic nature but is usually caused by various stressors on the heart, including hypertrophy of cardiac tissue, release of catecholamines from both nerves, increases in sodium and fluid retention, and dilatation of the cardiac chamber. The heart becomes enlarged from trying to compensate for loss of cardiac output and efficiency by working harder to increase stroke volume and heart rate. Increased venous return is handled inefficiently, causing an increase in end-diastolic volume, eventually leading to pulmonary congestion. Cardiac muscle contractility becomes compromised as a result of overexertion of the cardiac muscle in its compensatory effort. A vicious circle of decreased cardiac output, ineffective compensatory mechanism, and depressed contractility finally causes serious damage to the left ventricle and, if not checked, eventually leads to right heart failure as well.

Resulting signs and symptoms

Congestive cardiomyopathy is characterized by congestive heart failure, arrhythmias, murmurs, em-

bolus formation, and cardiomegaly. Hypertrophic cardiomyopathy can be identified by the presence of myocardial hypertrophy in the absence of ventricular dilatation. Frequently, if left ventricular flow is not affected, this type of cardiomyopathy may remain asymptomatic until its very late stages, when serious arrhythmias, chest pain, and congestive heart failure are present. In contrast, if left ventricular flow is compromised, mitral regurgitation may occur, and angina, dyspnea, edema, arrhythmias, and syncope are present. Restrictive cardiomyopathy involves extensive compromises in ventricular filling ability, resulting in chest pain, slowly progressing congestive heart failure, peripheral edema and ascites, dyspnea, and diarrhea (caused by protein malabsorption from lymphatic drainage, originating from increased portal pressure).

Nursing standards of care

Care of the individual suffering cardiomyopathy is oriented toward symptom relief. Treatment is offered to overcome congestive failure, but the prognosis is poor. Nursing care revolves around protecting the patient from further complications and relieving the discomfort accompanying congestive heart failure.

Cardiac Surgery and Angioplasty

Cardiac surgeries and invasive interventions seen most frequently by critical care nurses include coronary artery bypass grafts (CABG), percutaneous transluminal coronary angioplasty (PTCA), surgeries for correction of valvular disorders, ventricular septal defect repairs, and cardiac transplantation. By far, the most widely used interventions are those for the treatment of coronary artery disease caused by atherosclerosis. As discussed in the section on atherosclerosis, many experts are of the opinion that life-style risk factors hold much of the blame for the rate of incidence of the disease in the United States. As documented in cardiovascular research reports, about 66–75% of the American population begin to develop atherosclerosis in their teens.[47] Much of the progression of the disease can be retarded and even reversed if personal habits concerning exercise, diet, smoking, and stress are changed.

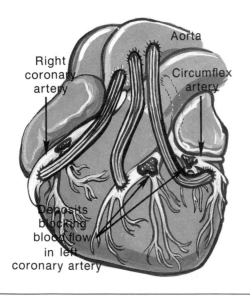

Figure 4-73 Coronary Artery Bypass Grafting

Coronary Artery Bypass Grafting (CABG)

Coronary artery bypass grafting is the surgical intervention devised to improve blood supply to the segments of heart muscle that have become ischemic because atherosclerotic lesions are occluding one or more of the coronary arteries. Grafts made from sections of the patient's saphenous veins (from the legs) or internal mammary artery are used to bypass an occluded coronary artery (Figure 4-73). The number of coronary arteries bypassed depends on the number that are severely obstructed as well as the viability and patency of the distal vessels and myocardium. There are surgeons who believe that complete revascularization is the treatment of choice and who will perform as many as fifteen bypasses in one operation, but generally the surgery involves two to five bypasses. The procedure is performed while the patient is on cardiopulmonary bypass, graphically illustrated in Figure 4-74.

Clinical antecedents

The purposes of coronary artery bypass grafting are to alleviate angina and to improve the quality of life of the patient with CAD. The procedure has not been found to significantly lengthen the lives of those with the disease. Indications for CABG can be divided into three categories: definite, probable, and questionable.[48] The indications in each category are listed in Table 4-20.

Critical referents

The specific pathophysiological process experienced by the patient in need of CABG is the same as that of atherosclerosis. Simply, it is characterized as the development of plaque deposits on the inner lining of large coronary arteries, which partially or completely block the flow of blood. Plaque develops from an initial injury to the endothelium followed by build-up of fatty substances, cholesterol, calcium, fibrin, and cellular waste products via diffusion from the bloodstream. If hemorrhage or thrombus occurs in or around the plaque formation, infarction or stroke results.

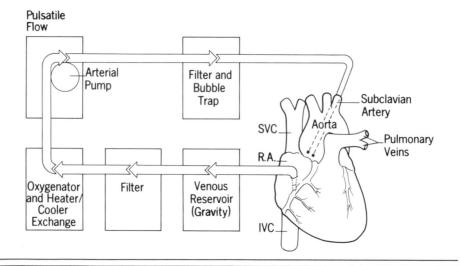

Figure 4-74 Cardiopulmonary Bypass

Table 4-20   Indications for CABG

Candidacy Status for CABG	Indicator
Definite	Multivessel disease with stable but medically uncontrollable angina
	Multivessel disease with unstable and medically uncontrollable angina
	Symptomatic and significant (greater than 50%) lesion of the left main coronary artery
Probable	Symptomatic triple-vessel disease with moderate to severe left ventricular dysfunction
	Symptomatic multivessel disease in addition to high risk for one of the following reasons:
	older age
	history of anterior MI
	history of MI with congestive heart failure
	conduction defects
	ejection fraction less than 30%
	complex ventricular arrhythmias
	abnormal response to low-level exercise testing within 3 weeks post MI
	Severe ischemic left ventricular dysfunction
	Asymptomatic severe left main CAD
	Multivessel disease with survival of ventricular fibrillation
	Severely symptomatic CABG occlusion
	Noncoronary cardiac surgery with CAD conducive to CABG
Questionable	Mildly to moderately symptomatic triple-vessel disease with normal left ventricular function
	Asymptomatic triple-vessel disease
	High-risk recent MI
Contraindicated	Severe left ventricular dysfunction
	Severe diffuse distal CAD
	Mildly symptomatic or asymptomatic one- or two-vessel disease
	Ability to qualify for PTCA
	Noncardiac contraindications for surgery

Resulting signs and symptoms

The primary symptom experienced by the candidate for CABG is angina during physical exertion, during intensely emotional times, following heavy meals, in cold weather, during and immediately after sexual activity, and when smoking cigarettes. Shortness of breath may occur simultaneously. Ischemic changes indicative of compromised oxygenation to segments of the heart distal to lesion formation are evident on an ECG, especially during exercise stress testing.

Nursing standards of care

Nursing management of the patient undergoing CABG closely follows the medical care plan and is directed toward promoting recovery and preventing complications during the very critical period immediately following surgery. The following care plan details the responsibilities of the critical care nurse in the care of the individual undergoing CABG.

Nursing Care Plan for the Management of the Patient with Coronary Artery Bypass Graft*

Diagnosis	Signs and symptoms	Intervention	Rationale
Potential for fluid volume deficit due to: estimated blood loss not fully replaced; bleeding due to thrombocytopenia, elevated clotting time, increased afterload, or hypertension; suboptimal preload status from OR; increased afterload when patient is still hypothermic from OR; vasodilation in response to warming or to nitroglycerine or Nipride; postoperative diuresis	LAP < 6–10 mm Hg CVP < 6 mm Hg PAD < 10 mm Hg SBP < 100 mm Hg HR > 120 bpm Urine output > intake or: > 500 cc after 1 hour; > 800 cc after 2 hours; > 900 cc after 3 hours; > 1000 cc after 4 hours; > 1200 cc after 5 hours Sudden increase in chest tube drainage SVR < 800 or > 1200 dyne-sec/cm^5 Weight loss	Monitor VS closely: TPR; ECG; LAP; arterial BP; PA pressures; I&O Blood replacement, as ordered, for chest tube drainage > 200 cc/hr with LAP < 16 mm Hg; IV infusions, as ordered, for LA < 10 or PAD < 14 Administer fresh frozen platelets or packed cells during rewarming Monitor effects of vasodilating agents (NTG, dobutamine, Inocor, MSO$_4$, renal dose dopamine) Monitor PT, PTT, platelets, and Hct closely; be prepared to administer protamine sulfate, cryoprecipitate, FFP, PC, platelets, or Amicar for abnormally elevated clotting time, bleeding, or reduced platelet count Assess operative leg drainage frequently Administer antihypertensive medication, as ordered, to keep SBP < 150 mm Hg	To ascertain trends by which to establish medication regimen To maintain volume and cardiac function and efficiency and to maintain patency of grafts To counteract vasodilation effect of rewarming To prevent early volume insufficiency To prevent or treat early bleeding complications To completely assess total body output To prevent hypertensive crisis and protect graft patency

*Care plan adapted from plan provided by the Georgetown University Hospital Department of Nursing.

Diagnosis	Signs and symptoms	Intervention	Rationale
Potential for decreased cardiac output from arrhythmias; fluid volume deficit; fluid volume overload; ischemia from graft occlusion, spasm, intraoperative MI; hypothermia; hypertension; hypotension; tamponade; increased afterload	CO < 3 L/min CI < 2 L/min/m^2	Monitor CO and CI closely	To facilitate early intervention
	Reduced peripheral tissue perfusion evidenced by decreased distal pulses and cool extremities	Administer vasoactive medications as ordered (dobutamine, Inocor)	To maintain adequate perfusion in vital organs and periphery
	Arrhythmias, such as PVCs, heart blocks, SVT, PAT, AF, AFL, MAT related to edematous suture line, ventricular tachycardia, ventricular fibrillation	Administer antiarrhythmias as ordered and PRN	To allow for adequate cardiac function and prevention of life-threatening rhythms
		Assess and treat ABGs and K$^+$ in relation to PVCs	Potassium imbalance and compromised ABGs can cause PVCs
		Serial ECGs	To allow early recognition of ischemia, injury, or arrhythmia
		Maintain stable heart rhythm, as ordered: atrially paced to keep heart rate at 60–100; ventricularly paced for second- and third-degree heart blocks; cardioversion for ventricular tachycardia or fibrillation; verapamil for SVT; digoxin	To maintain normal sinus rhythm and stable hemodynamics
	Fluid volume deficit	Correct fluid volume deficit, as ordered	To maintain cardiac function and output
	Ischemia: CPK > 180 IU/L; MBs > 15 IU/L; new ECG ischemic changes	Serial ECGs Maintain oxygenation	To facilitate early recognition of ischemia and prevent further cellular damage from lack of oxygenation
	Hypothermia	Administer NaHCO$_3$ for base deficit > −3 when hypothermic	Acid-base imbalance is exacerbated by hypothermia
		Warm with warming blankets or lights	To return patient to normal core temperature

Nursing Care Plan for the Management of the Patient with Coronary Artery Bypass Graft

Diagnosis	Signs and symptoms	Intervention	Rationale
	Hypertension	Administer antihypertensives, as ordered, to keep SBP > 100 and < 150 mmHg (MSO_4, nitroprusside 0.5–8.0 mcg/kg/min, nitroglycerin up to 200–300 mcg/min)	Fast-acting or short-lasting medications for hypertensive events
		Taper vasoconstrictive meds to maintain SBP > 100 and < 160 mm Hg (epinephrine, Levophed, dobutamine 2–10 mcg/kg/min, dopamine 2–10 mcg/kg/min, neosynephrine)	To maintain safe blood pressure levels
	Tamponade: elevation and equalization of filling pressures (CVP + PAD = LAP = 20–30); reduction in SBP to less than 100 mm Hg; abrupt cessation of CT drainage; widening of mediastinum on x-ray; increased jugular venous pressure; cool, clammy skin; reduced peripheral pulses; muffled heart sounds; pulsus paradoxus > 10	Immediate medical intervention, including extracting clot from mediastinal tube with Fogarty catheter, open chest procedure, and/or return to OR	Cardiac tamponade presents a high risk of death if not treated immediately
	Increased SVR	Reduce SVR, as ordered, by: warming patient; administering vasodilators (Inocor, dobutamine, nitroglycerine, MSO_4); restricting fluids; diuretics	To maintain hemodynamic stability and graft patency
	(Crackles) rales		

Diagnosis	Signs and symptoms	Intervention	Rationale
Potential for impaired gas exchange due to: fluid volume overload; ineffective airway clearance, atelectasis, or effusion; bronchospasm; inadequate supplemental oxygen; inadequate tidal volume; low hematocrit and hemoglobin levels; low cardiac output; excessive pulmonary vascular resistance; malpositioned ETT or inadequate cuff volume; pneumothorax or hemothorax	Abnormal ABGs: $pO_2 < 80$ mm Hg; $pCO_2 < 35$ or > 45 mm Hg; pH < 7.35 or > 7.45; O_2 sat. $< 80\%$; $HCO_3 < 20$ or > 26 mEq/L; BE < 0 or > 3 Cyanosis ETT cuff leak Lowered peak pressure Inadequate volume exchange Chest x-ray indicates atelectasis, effusion, pneumothorax, or hemothorax Copious secretions Elevated respiratory rate, wheezing, air hunger, gasping, or asymmetrical expansion of chest wall	Mechanically ventilate for 8–12 hours postoperatively, as ordered Closely monitor for absent, unequal, or diminished breath sounds, crackles, wheezing, or asymmetrical chest wall expansion; closely monitor ABGs PRN and after ventilator changes; obtain chest x-ray immediately and PRN postoperatively and examine for ETT placement, lung expansion (pneumothorax), width of mediastinal shadow, presence of pleural fluid, and presence of foreign body Aggressive pulmonary toilet PRN with chest percussion therapy, incentive spirometry, and hyperinflation using 100% O_2 before and after suctioning; turn and reposition patient every 2 hours	Ventilation support is needed until stabilization To discover early indications of ensuing respiratory compromise and/or complications To mobilize secretions, provide adequate oxygenation, and open closed alveoli
		If patient is stable, promote extubation by: holding sedation after midnight on day of surgery; elevating HOB 30 degrees; decreasing IMV by increments of 2–4 breaths/min if $pO_2 > 90$, pH 7.35–7.45, and O_2 sat. 90–100%	To assist patient to return to optimal breathing capacity as soon as possible (to prevent atelectasis, secondary infection, etc.)
	Hematocrit level less than 30 with abnormal ABGs	Administer packed cells as ordered	To improve hematocrit and oxygen-carrying ability

Nursing Care Plan for the Management of the Patient with Coronary Artery Bypass Graft

Diagnosis	Signs and symptoms	Intervention	Rationale
	Cardiac index < 2.5 L/min/m^2	Correct low cardiac output	To maintain adequate cardiac function and tissue perfusion and oxygenation
	Excessive PVR (>120 dyne-sec/cm^5)	Administer prostaglandin E or thomboxine as ordered	To counteract excessive PVR
	Copious secretions Respirations > 30 bpm	Administer theophylline by infusion and bronchodilator (Alupent, Bronchosol) through ventilator or increase FIO$_2$ as ordered	To improve breathing capacity
	Signs of fluid overload: crackles on auscultation; pO$_2$ < 90 mm Hg; chest x-ray indicative of fluid overload; PAD > 20 mm Hg; LAP > 20 mm Hg; urine output < 30 cc/hr; weight gain > 5 kg; frothy sputum	Administer diuretics PRN or as ordered	To facilitate diuresis of extra fluid volume
Potential for skin breakdown due to: restriction in movement; pain or discomfort; drug-induced neuromuscular or musculoskeletal impairment; depression; stiffness from extended catheterization time and/or time on operating table; diaphoresis or drainage into	Imposed restriction of movement due to body mechanics, medical protocol, etc.	Put air mattress on all postoperative beds	To prevent pressure spots on skin
	Impaired coordination or decreased muscle strength preventing independent movement	Assist patient with required movements and with a quarter turn every 1–2 hours	To prevent injury and facilitate movement
	Reluctance to attempt movement	Premedicate PRN or as ordered to decrease discomfort accompanying movement	To facilitate movement

Diagnosis	Signs and symptoms	Intervention	Rationale
patient's bed; independent variables such as diabetes, peripheral vascular disease, obesity, etc.	Redness over pressure points	Inspect skin pressure points, including occiput, sacrum, coccyx, heels, and elbows, every 2 hours	To prevent skin breakdown
		Passive range of motion to all extremities	To prevent pressure spots and improve circulation without increasing oxygen demand
		Keep patient dry	To prevent skin breakdown
		Maintain and supplement nutrition as needed	To maintain vital nutrients to skin
		Consult enterostomal therapist for actual breakdown	For optimal care planning and intervention
	Elevated temperature	Keep patient dry when diaphoretic	To prevent skin breakdown
Potential for infection due to: IV lines; indwelling Foley catheter; chest tubes; endotracheal intubation; stress of surgery (in the event of trauma)	Increased temperature Tachycardia and/or decreasing BP WBC > 10,000 mm^3	Tylenol 600 mg every 4 hours or PRN, as ordered	To alleviate fevers
	Redness, exudate, increased tenderness, and/or induration of surgical incisions, IV insertion site, pacer wire sites, or chest tube sites	Implement thorough hand washing between patient contacts; implement universal isolation precautions if indicated	To prevent spread of infections
		Routine incision care with povidone-iodine solution, Telfa dressing, and foam tape	To prevent incisional infections
		Change peripheral IV sites at least every 3 days or with any signs of infection or infiltration; change IV tubing every 48 hours	IV fluid is especially fertile medium for bacterial growth

Nursing Care Plan for the Management of the Patient with Coronary Artery Bypass Graft

Diagnosis	Signs and symptoms	Intervention	Rationale
	Changes in characteristics of sputum: tan, brown, yellow, or green color and/or foul odor	Culture suspected origins of infection	To administer antibiotics that bacteria are sensitive to
	Chest x-ray indicative of atelectasis Decreased or absent breath sounds locally	Vigorous pulmonary toilet	To prevent and/or treat pulmonary congestion leading to infections
	Sediment in urine or foul-smelling urine	Routine Foley care every 8 hours	To prevent urinary tract infections
	WBCs in urine Hesitancy, frequency, urgency, burning, difficulty starting stream, incontinence, and/or inability to void	If patient is taking fluids, push fluids, unless contraindicated by cardiac condition	To flush urinary tract
Potential for alteration in bowel function (constipation) due to: decreased mobility; change in eating patterns; side effects of medications; postoperative paralytic ileus; decreased fluid volume	Reports of feeling constipated, "full" feeling in abdomen, inability to move bowels Decreased or absent bowel sounds Inadequate oral fluid/food intake as evidenced on I&O records and calorie counts	Assess abdomen for bowel sounds, softness, and appearance and ask patient about discomfort at least every 12 hours	To allow for early diagnosis of constipation, in order to intervene before problems become serious
		Encourage progressive ambulation and activity, as tolerated	To stimulate peristalsis
		Reassure patient that constipation is frequently a problem postoperatively	So patient will not become overly concerned

	Symptoms of dehydration:
	    poor skin turgor;
	    sunken eyes;
	    intake < output;
	    weight loss
		Assess for signs of dehydration and encourage oral fluid intake, unless patient is on fluid restriction	Hydration impedes constipation

		Closely monitor electrolytes	Dehydration leads to electrolyte imbalance

Diagnosis	Signs and symptoms	Intervention	Rationale
	Absence of bowel movement for more than 2 days	Implement bowel regimen as ordered: milk of magnesia 30 mL PO every h.s.; consult with dietician about increased fiber in diet; rehydrate patient, as ordered, via IV or oral fluids	Patient may need extra help to start peristalsis postoperatively
		Reduce narcotic consumption when feasible	Narcotics inhibit bowel activity
Potential for alteration in bowel function (diarrhea) due to: side effects of cardiac medications and/or antibiotics; bacterial infections; change in eating patterns	Diarrhea or frequent liquid stools Hyperactive bowel sounds	Assess abdomen for hyperactive bowel sounds	To allow for early intervention
		Educate patient about medications that may cause diarrhea	To help patient understand cause
		Assess fluid status in attempt to avoid dehydration and monitor electrolytes	Diarrhea quickly leads to dehydration and electrolyte imbalance
		Implement treatment as ordered: antidiarrheal medication; rehydration; change of cardiac medications or antibiotics if possible, to relieve diarrhea	To prevent further systemic complications
		Culture for clostridia difficile, as ordered	High risk for diarrhea; should be treated as soon as possible
Potential for alteration in health maintenance due to knowledge deficit concerning: diagnosis; surgical procedure; medications;	Inability to describe personal diagnosis and how it relates to type of surgery	Instruct patient and family about diagnosis and surgery	Patient and family must understand what is being done and why
		Encourage questions and discussion of problems and concerns	To allow for greatest learning

Nursing Care Plan for the Management of the Patient with Coronary Artery Bypass Graft

Diagnosis	Signs and symptoms	Intervention	Rationale
diet; activity; medical follow-up; referrals; when to notify MD; self-monitoring	Inability to identify medications and their schedules	Instruct patient about medications: what they look like; names and doses; indications; side effects and what can be done; daily schedule; standard drug information and complete medication schedule	Safe and accurate medication regimen is necessary
	Inability to list foods appropriate for personal diet	Provide instruction on low-sodium, modified-fat/cholesterol diet; consult with dietician	To facilitate healing and prevent complications arising from incorrect diet
	Inability to distinguish between permitted and prohibited progression of activities	Discuss activity instructions: activities in routine; balancing rest and activity; progressive walking schedule; no lifting more than 20 pounds; no driving for 6 weeks; stopping every hour for a short walk when taking long car trips; resumption of sexual activities	To allow for progressive resumption of activities without risk of overdoing it and precipitating an untoward event In the event of an accident, steering wheel may crush incompletely healed sternum; walking increases circulation and prevents prolonged venous pooling
	Lack of knowledge about follow-up appointments	Help patient and family to arrange follow-up appointments	Plans for follow-up care must be initiated as soon as possible
	Inability to identify professional services available for support	Advise patient and family of services and resources available	To provide most comprehensive and effective services to patient and family

Diagnosis	Signs and symptoms	Intervention	Rationale
	Inability to explain when to notify MD or seek emergency assistance	Review with patient and family when to notify MD: angina, SOB, dizziness, or nausea during or following activity; weight gain of more than 1 lb/day; signs of infected incision, including redness, swelling, increased tenderness, drainage; temperature > 101°F; irregular/fast heart rate	Patient and family need to know what to do in the case of an untoward event
	Inability to properly count pulse, assess weight fluctuations, and/or take temperature	Instruct patient and family and require return demonstration: weighing self and recording weight; taking temperature and pulse and recording them	Patient and family need to increase self-help abilities
	Inability to verbalize significance of weight changes	Instruct patient on meaning of weight gain and what to do in its event	To increase patient's self-help abilities in preventing congestive failure
Potential for anxiety due to: fear of unknown; fear of death; fear of disfigurement; fear of pain; fear of disability; lack of knowledge regarding hospital and/or operative procedures, routines	Facial tension Distracted behavior Low attention span Withdrawal Twitching and shaking of extremities Inappropriate laughter or behavior Diaphoresis Tachycardia PVCs Other arrhythmias Nonadherence to treatment plan	Ascertain patient's fears and anxieties	Will allow the nurse to know just what to address
		Ascertain patient's previous hospital experiences (own as well as others')	Will help the nurse to know how to best alleviate anxieties or support positive attitudes
		Ascertain patient's and family's readiness to learn	Need to begin patient and family education when ready
		Teach patient about: routine of lab, radiology, ECG, house staff; surgery, donor sites, incisions, tubes, lines, operation	To help patient and family be prepared for what is to be experienced

Diagnosis	Signs and symptoms	Intervention	Rationale
		length, ICU routine, visiting hours, pain medication, and deep breathing and coughing; provide patient with educational booklets	
		Give ICU tour, if desired	To familiarize patient with environment
		Sedate patient, as ordered or PRN	To help patient relax
		Provide emotional support as needed	To help patient and family deal with the situation in the best way possible
		Consult with social worker, chaplain, etc., as needed	Multidisciplinary team effort provides broader, more comprehensive care
Potential for ineffective individual or family coping related to: situational crisis; maturational crisis; personal vulnerability	Verbalization of inability to cope Inability to ask for emotional help	Assess family's usual coping mechanisms	Questions and concerns of patient and family must be answered even if not voiced
		Assist family to identify alternative coping mechanisms; identify and acknowledge family's needs	Optimal coping must be accomplished for maximal healing
	Inability to meet role expectations	Provide information to patient and family regarding diagnosis and purpose of supportive services	Patient and family must be helped through role redefinition
	Prolonged progression of disease or disability	Support patient and family through role transition	To facilitate necessary role changes

Diagnosis	Signs and symptoms	Intervention	Rationale
		Encourage open communication among patient, family, and health care team	To facilitate problem solving and care planning
		Reinforce simple explanations to patient and family	During times of crisis, care must be taken not to cause information overload
	Exhaustion	Provide rest periods and offer nutrition to family; plan visiting schedule to accommodate interventions as well as family schedule and rest periods; restrict visitors as appropriate	To maximize quality family time as well as allow for needed rest
	Fear and anxiety	Delegate one resource and support person to assist family through this very critical time	Consistency in problem solving and care improves quality of decisions
	Inappropriate requests or hypervigilance by patient and/or family	Suggest ways for family to assist in patient's care	Participatory care decreases anxiety
	Inability to solve problems	Assist patient and family to identify problems and work together to solve them	Sometimes patients and families are unable to anticipate possible problems
	Unreasonable and/or excessively frequent requests (excessive use of call light)	Assist family in caring for patient and problem solve about how to continue such care following discharge	Personal involvement in care decreases anxiety while increasing self-confidence and skills
		Encourage progressively independent activities	To avoid rushing patient and family into too much responsibility for care
Potential for self-care deficit due to: muscle deconditioning; postoperative incisional discomfort; sleep pattern disturbance; fear of overexertion; anxiety; decreased activity tolerance	Weak muscles resulting from bedrest	Encourage progressive activities: self-care; ambulation; active ROM	To allow time for patient to regain strength
	Reports of postoperative pain	Assess discomfort and encourage patient to request medication as appropriate	To allow for maximal activities
	Fatigue		

Nursing Care Plan for the Management of the Patient with Coronary Artery Bypass Graft

Diagnosis	Signs and symptoms	Intervention	Rationale
	Slow movement, ambulating with caution, refusal to participate in daily care routine	Reassure patient that postoperative pain is expected and teach patient how to minimize discomfort while moving, deep breathing, coughing, etc.	To minimize effects of pain
	Increased heart rate and respiratory rate upon minimal activity	Assess patient's need for rest and sleep and incorporate rest periods during the day	To prevent overexhaustion
		Maintain calm environment (lighting, noise, interruptions, etc.)	To facilitate adequate rest
	Repetitive fast speech, indicating anxiety Inability to concentrate on activities required	Encourage patient's participation in scheduling and carrying out daily care	To accommodate routines to patient's ability to progress
		Praise patient's progress in activities	Encouragement is a good motivator

Percutaneous Transluminal Coronary Angioplasty (PTCA)

Percutaneous transluminal coronary angioplasty (PTCA) is a technique similar to coronary angiography. The procedure is usually performed in the cardiac catheterization lab with the cardiac surgery team on standby. During heparinization and platelet-inhibiting infusion, a guiding catheter is introduced through a large artery (usually in the leg), threaded into the lesioned artery, and positioned directly at the site of the lesion. The balloon catheter is then inserted through the guide catheter until the balloon lies in the resulting narrowing. When the balloon is accurately positioned, the surgeon inflates it to a very high pressure (8–15 atmospheres) for up to 1 minute. Proximal and distal pressures are taken before and after each dilatation to evaluate the success of that attempt. This process may be repeated several times if necessary. The process compresses the plaque, pushing it into the wall of the vessel, and thus relieves the obstruction. The lumen of the artery is dilated, and blood flow to the myocardium is restored.

Clinical antecedents

Risk factors and precipitating factors leading to the need for PTCA are similar (but not as severe) to those leading to the need for CABG. Indications for PTCA are classified as those for CABG: definite, probable, and questionable.[49] The indications in each category are listed in Table 4-21.

In light of the criteria presented in Table 4-21, 10–15% of patients who undergo angiography for diagnosis of CAD become suitable candidates for PTCA. It is important to note, though, that all considered for PTCA should be considered appropriate for CABG in the emergency event of unsuccessful, complicated PTCA.

Critical referents

The specific pathophysiology leading to the need for PTCA is the same as that leading to the need for CABG.

Resulting signs and symptoms

Signs and symptoms leading to the need for PTCA are similar to those leading to the need for CABG.

Table 4-21 Indications for PTCA

Candidacy Status for PTCA	Indicator
Definite	Severe angina with a single high-grade proximal lesion in a coronary artery (other than the left main), which is concentric, short, and noncalcified Symptomatic restenosis of a previous PTCA site
Probable	Angina with dilatable lesions in a single vessel Angina with multiple-vessel disease in which only one vessel is high-grade and dilatable Angina with multivessel disease with dilatable lesions in the presence of other medical problems contraindicating CABG Angina with post CABG with high-grade stenosis of the distal graft at the anastomosis of the vessel Angina with recent (up to a month) total occlusion of a single proximal artery
Questionable	Mild to moderate angina with a dilatable single-vessel lesion High-grade, single-vessel dilatable lesion with silent ischemia Post CABG angina with dilatable lesion in the graft CABG candidate with angina in the presence of double- or triple-vessel dilatable lesions High-grade dilatable lesion in the presence of infarction after successful streptokinase treatment
Contraindicated	Left main coronary artery lesion Calcified, very long, or inaccessible lesions Lesions involving the origin of one or more significant branch vessels Patient's refusal to consent to CABG

Nursing standards of care

Although it was common when PTCA was originally introduced to medical centers for the patient to spend time in the critical care unit, today the procedure is usually performed in a step-down unit with monitoring capabilities. However, the critical care nurse should still know the appropriate nursing interventions in case of untoward complications. Most serious complications require immediate and direct surgical intervention, and nursing care in such cases is as detailed as for any cardiac surgery. The most frequently seen complication of the procedure is a dissection of the artery (9% incidence), necessitating immediate surgical repair. The following nursing care plan details the responsibilities of nurses in the care of a patient after a successful PTCA.

Diagnosis	Signs and symptoms	Intervention	Rationale
Potential for decreased cardiac output from complications of PTCA procedure: dysrhythmias during catheter installation; coronary artery spasm during balloon dilation; reaction to dye; decrease in blood flow during balloon dilation; thrombosis; dissection of atheroma; myocardial infarction/ischemia; hemorrhage	Reduced peripheral tissue perfusion as evidenced by decreased distal pulses, mottling, cool extremities Arrhythmias or palpitations Decreased BP Chest discomfort Dyspnea	Closely monitor VS, ECG, and peripheral pulses during and after procedure Assess patient's level of consciousness frequently Maintain patency of IV lines Assess frequently for chest discomfort Have immediate accessibility to arrest cart with emergency drugs, defibrillator, and temporary pacemaker and have OR on standby Have immediate accessibility to drugs and administer, as ordered, to prevent coronary artery spasm and clotting (nifedipine, nitroglycerin, heparin, and dipyridamole) Provide supplemental oxygen as necessary	To assess and treat quickly all untoward events during and immediately following procedure Indication of ischemia and cardiac compromise For fast access to bloodstream in the event of an emergency Indication of cardiac ischemia To be prepared for an emergency In case of vessel spasm or thrombosis To maintain adequate oxygenation to tissues and vital organs
Potential alteration in tissue perfusion related to hematoma, blood loss, thrombus, or infection at site of cannulation, from invasive procedure	Hematoma, ecchymosis, erythema, swelling, warmth, and/or tenderness at cannulation site	Maintain sterile pressure dressing for at least 6 hours following procedure and as necessary	To decrease incidence of bleeding complications

*Care plan adapted from care plan provided by the Georgetown University Hospital Department of Nursing.

Nursing Care Plan for the Management of the Patient with Percutaneous Transluminal Coronary Angioplasty

Diagnosis	Signs and symptoms	Intervention	Rationale
		Assess for cyanosis, coolness, sensation, movement, numbness, tingling, and/or diminished pulses in affected extremity	Signs of impaired peripheral perfusion
		Keep affected extremity straight for at least 6 hours following procedure	So as not to reopen cannulation site
		Use sandbag over cannulation site as necessary	For better pressure dressing
	Inflammation, swelling, warmth, redness, and/or extreme discomfort at cannulation site	Assess for signs of impending infection at cannulation site	To allow for early detection of infection
		Keep dressing dry and intact and provide routine sterile wound care as needed; maintain sterile technique during dressing changes	To prevent serious infectious complications
	Fever	Administer Tylenol as ordered	Aspirin will further compound risk for bleeding
		Administer antibiotics as ordered	To prevent serious infectious complications
Potential for impaired gas exchange from sedation and immobilization during procedure	Diminished breath sounds	Encourage patient to perform deep breathing and coughing	To prevent atelectasis and pulmonary complications
	Shortness of breath Compromised ABGs	Supply supplemental oxygen as indicated and ordered	To allow for continued oxygenation and gas exchange
Potential for alteration in fluid volume due to sensitivity to contrast medium	Urine output < 30 cc/hr	Administer IV fluids as ordered	To flush out system as thoroughly as possible
	Weight gain Elevated BUN and creatinine	Closely monitor for signs of renal dysfunction, volume overload, and/or dehydration	To help prevent serious renal complications

Diagnosis	Signs and symptoms	Intervention	Rationale

Potential for anxiety due to:
  fear of unknown;
  fear of death;
  fear of disfigurement;
  fear of pain;
  fear of disability;
  lack of knowledge regarding hospital and/or angioplasty procedures, routines
	Facial tension
	Distracted behavior
	Low attention span
	Withdrawal
	Twitching and shaking of extremities
	Inappropriate laughter or behavior
	Diaphoresis
	Tachycardia
	PVCs
	Other arrhythmias
	Nonadherence to treatment plan
		Ascertain patient's fears and anxieties	Will allow the nurse to know just what to address

		Ascertain patient's previous hospital experiences (own as well as others')	Will help the nurse to know how to best alleviate anxieties or support positive attitudes
		Ascertain patient's and family's readiness to learn	Need to begin patient and family education when ready

		Teach patient about:
		  routine of lab, radiology, ECG, house staff;
		    information about the procedure, lines, length of time on table, unit routine, visiting hours, pain medication, and deep breathing and coughing; provide patient with education booklets
			To help patient and family be prepared for what is to be experienced

		Sedate patient, as ordered or PRN	To help patient relax
		Provide emotional support as needed	To help patient and family deal with the situation in the best way possible
		Consult with social worker, chaplain, etc., as needed	Multidisciplinary team effort provides broader, more comprehensive care

Potential for ineffective individual or family coping related to:
  situational crisis;
  maturational crisis;
  personal vulnerability
	Verbalization of inability to cope
	
	Inability to ask for emotional help
		Assess family's usual coping mechanisms	Questions and concerns of patient and family must be answered even if not voiced

Nursing Care Plan for the Management of the Patient with Percutaneous Transluminal Coronary Angioplasty

Diagnosis	Signs and symptoms	Intervention	Rationale
		Assist family to identify alternative coping mechanisms; identify and acknowledge family's needs	Optimal coping must be accomplished for maximal healing
	Inability to meet role expectations	Provide information to patient and family regarding diagnosis and purpose of supportive services	Patient and family must be helped through role redefinition
	Prolonged progression of disease or disability	Support patient and family through role transition	To facilitate necessary role changes
		Encourage open communication among patient, family, and health care team	To facilitate problem solving and care planning
		Reinforce simple explanations to patient and family	During times of crisis, care must be taken not to cause information overload
	Exhaustion	Provide rest periods and offer nutrition to family; plan visiting schedule to accommodate interventions as well as family schedule and rest periods; restrict visitors as appropriate	To maximize quality family time as well as allow for needed rest
	Fear and anxiety	Delegate one resource and support person to assist family through this very critical time	Consistency in problem solving and care improves quality of decisions
	Inappropriate requests or hypervigilance by patient and/or family	Suggest ways for family to assist in patient's care	Participatory care decreases anxiety

Mitral Commissurotomy and Valvular Replacement

Surgeries for correction of valvular disorders include mitral commissurotomy and mitral, aortic, and tricuspid valve replacements. Any other valvular surgeries are extremely rare and generally have to do with repairing congenital defects or traumatic wounds.

Mitral commissurotomy involves splitting fused valve leaflets. A commissurotomy may be either closed or open. A closed commissurotomy is performed by guiding a dilator through the apex of the left ventricle to then break apart the fused valve segments. The surgeon inserts a finger through the mitral orifice to guide the instrument. In contrast, an open commissurotomy requires the support of cardiopulmonary bypass, and a knife is used to incise the commissures. Commissurotomy is indicated only when there is a documented absence of calcification and thrombus or embolus.

Usually, valvular heart disease—be it mitral, aortic, or tricuspid stenosis (incomplete opening) or insufficiency (incomplete closing)—has progressed rather extensively if valvular replacement or valvuloplasty (repair) is required. (The pulmonic valve is almost never affected.) Nearly all such surgeries require cardipulmonary bypass, and about 43,000 valvular surgeries were conducted in 1987, down from 46,000 the previous year.[50]

Clinical antecedents

The primary precipitating factor leading to valvular heart disease is the presence of rheumatic fever and then rheumatic heart disease, resulting in scarring of the valves upon healing of the antibody-induced inflammation. Usually the valves on the left side of the heart are affected, and cardiac function is increasingly impaired. When the valve is stenosed, the heart must work harder to force circulation through the narrowed valve opening; during incomplete closing, ventricular output lessens, for the heart must repump the regurgitated blood to maintain cardiac output to the periphery. If allowed to advance, valvular heart disease will lead to heart failure.

Also, fibrosis and calcification of valves may progress in a degenerative manner in the elderly, sometimes to the extent that the valve is unable to open due to valvular rigidity. If this occurs in the aortic valve, severe stress is placed on the left ventricle which, in turn, leads to heart failure.

Critical referents

Simply described, mitral stenosis impedes the flow of blood into the left ventricle, resulting in left atrial hypertrophy and pulmonary congestion. Mitral regurgitation allows a backflow of blood into the left atrium, resulting eventually in its dilation but not to the extent of the hypertrophy seen in mitral stenosis. Left ventricular failure occurs in the long term, and blood flow into the aorta is compromised. Simultaneously, the pulmonary vasculature is compromised due to back flow from the left atrium.

Aortic stenosis leads to significant left ventricular hypertrophy. Eventually, left atrial hypertrophy occurs as a result of the constant atrial effort to increase ventricular filling at the end of diastole. Aortic regurgitation allows a back flow of blood from the aorta into the left ventricle, leading to its hypertrophy.

Tricuspid stenosis leads to increased blood pressure in the right atrium, which results in increased pressure in the right side of the heart and the systemic circulation. Tricuspid regurgitation occurs late in the disease process of left ventricular failure, so it is difficult to describe the specific pathophysiology of tricuspid regurgitation alone.

Rheumatic heart disease is a type of hypersensitivity reaction induced by antigens present in streptococcus. An antibody against the antigens is formed, and inflammation and injury occur to the connective tissue, although signs of fever and inflammation subside. Scar tissue is formed during healing, and the complication is exacerbated, becoming even more damaging if another streptococcus infection occurs.

Degenerative stenosis occurs in a manner similar to the atherosclerotic process: the valve gradually becomes thickened and eventually calcified. In contrast, however, although the pathology is not yet understood, the degenerative process may result in a floppy valve (prolapse). One or more leaflets eventually become enlarged and redundant, and margins of the valve fail to proximate. Not only does blood reflux into the left atrium, but this condition tends to place excessive strain on the chordae and papillary muscles, causing rupture or cardiac arrhythmia.

Resulting signs and symptoms

The primary signs and symptoms of the above valvular diseases all lead to progressing congestive heart failure. Left-side (mitral and aortic) valve abnormalities cause symptoms earlier in the course of

Table 4-22 Clinical Manifestations of Selected Valvular Disorders

Type of Disorder	Symptoms	Signs

Aortic regurgitation	Syncope
	Angina
	Dyspnea on exertion
		Diastolic and systolic murmur
		Palpitations
		Congestive heart failure
		  Weakness
		  Peripheral edema
		  Increased JVP
		  Hepatomegaly
		  Jaundice
		  Liver tenderness
		  High CVPs

Aortic stenosis	Syncope
	Angina
	Fatigue
	Dyspnea
		Systolic murmur
		Left ventricular failure
		  Pulmonary congestion
		  Edema
		  Low cardiac output

Mitral regurgitation	Weakness Fatigue Dyspnea on exertion	Murmur throughout systole Palpitations
Mitral stenosis	Dyspnea on exertion Weakness Fatigue Paroxysmal nocturnal dyspnea Hemoptysis	Diastolic murmur Predisposition to respiratory infections Orthopnea Palpitations (usually atrial fibrillation)

Tricuspid regurgitation	Peripheral edema
	Weakness
	Dyspnea on exertion
	Fatigue
		Murmur throughout systole
		Right ventricular failure
		  Weakness
		  Peripheral edema
		  Hepatomegaly
		  Increased JVP
		  Jaundice
		  Liver tenderness
		  High CVPs

Tricuspid stenosis	Peripheral edema
	Weakness
	Dyspnea on exertion
	Fatigue
		Diastolic murmur
		Right ventricular failure
		  Weakness
		  Peripheral edema
		  Hepatomegaly
		  Increased JVP
		  Jaundice
		  Liver tenderness
		  High CVPs

the illness than do right-side ones. Table 4-22 outlines the signs and symptoms of the various valvular disorders. Diagnostic findings indicating valvular disorders are detailed in Table 4-23.

Nursing standards of care

As in the care of all cardiac surgical interventions, nursing management after valvular surgery is directed toward the prevention and early detection of postoperative complications. Complications most likely to occur as a result of surgery range from low output syndrome, possible MI, embolism, and hemorrhage to cardiac arrhythmias, renal failure, and wound infection. The following care plan details the responsibilities of the critical care nurse in providing service to the patient who has undergone valvular surgery.

Table 4-23 Diagnostic Findings Indicating Valvular Disorders

Disorder Type	EOG	X-Ray	Catheterization	Other
Aortic regurgitation	Left ventricular hypertrophy	Aortic valve calcification Left ventricular enlargement Ascending aortic dilatation	Increased pulse pressure Diastolic pulse slope increase Reflux through aortic valve	Left ventricular dilatation Diastolic fluttering of anterior leaflet
Aortic stenosis	Left ventricular hypertrophy	Poststenotic aortic dilatation Aortic valve calcification	Pressure gradient across aortic valve in systole Increased diastolic ventricular pressure Normal left atrial and pulmonary pressures	Increased echoes Left ventricular wall thickening Restricted movement of aortic valve
Mitral regurgitation	P mitrale Left ventricular hypertrophy Atrial fibrillation	Left atrial enlargement Left ventricular enlargement Pulmonary vascular congestion	Regurgitation	Left atrial enlargement Hyperdynamic left ventricle
Mitral stenosis	Left atrial enlargement Prolonged P mitrale Right ventricular hypertrophy	Left atrial enlargement Pulmonary venous congestion Interstitial pulmonary edema Right ventricular enlargement	High pressure across valve High left atrial pressure High pulmonary capillary wedge pressure Low cardiac output	Decreased excursion of leaflets Diminished EF slope
Tricuspid regurgitation	Tall, peaked P waves	Right atrial enlargement Right ventricular enlargement	Reflux into right atrium	
Tricuspid stenosis	Tall, peaked P waves	Right atrial enlargement Right ventricular enlargement	Pressure gradient across valve High right atrial pressure	

Nursing Care Plan for the Management of the Patient with Mitral Commissurotomy and Valvular Replacement*

Diagnosis	Signs and symptoms	Intervention	Rationale
Potential for viral, bacterial, and/or prosthetic valve infection	Increased sedimentation rate	Administer antimicrobial therapy as ordered	For prevention or treatment of microbial infection
	Fever	Tylenol 600 mg every 4 hours or PRN as ordered	To alleviate fever
	WBCs > 8,000	Implement thorough hand washing between patient contacts; implement universal isolation precautions if indicated	To prevent the spread of infection
	Redness, exudate, increased tenderness, and/or induration of surgical incision, IV insertion site, pacer wire sites, or chest tube sites	Routine incision care with povidone-iodine solution, Telfa dressing, as indicated; change peripheral IV sites at least every 3 days or with any signs of infection or infiltration; change IV tubing every 72 hours	To prevent incisional infections, leading to valvular vegetative growth
		Culture suspected origins of infection	To determine correct antibiotic therapy
	Sediment in urine or foul-smelling urine; hesitancy, frequency, urgency, burning, difficulty starting stream, incontinence, and/or inability to void	Routine Foley care every 8 hours; push fluids if not contraindicated	To prevent urinary tract infections, leading to valvular vegetative growth
	Fatigue	Assess patient's need for rest and sleep and incorporate rest periods during the day; maintain calm environment (lighting, noise, interruptions, etc.)	To allow patient time to rest adequately, to prevent overexhaustion, and to help patient regain strength to combat infections

*Care plan adapted from care plan provided by the Georgetown University Hospital Department of Nursing.

Diagnosis	Signs and symptoms	Intervention	Rationale
	Palpitations	Assess vital signs, especially for pulse > 100	For early detection and treatment of developing complications
	Precordial discomfort	Medicate, as ordered	To keep patient pain-free
	Abnormal heart sounds from aortic valve indicate: left ventricular hypertrophy; sinus tachycardia; first degree atrioventricular block; bundle branch block; intraventricular conduction disturbances; atrial arrhythmias	Assess heart sounds for gallop rhythm, murmur, and/or pericardial friction rub, and administer cardiac medications as ordered	For early detection and treatment of developing complications
		Assess for symptoms of digitalis toxicity	So as not to mistake digitalis toxicity for signs of infection, and vice versa
		Monitor for evidence of arrhythmias	May be signs of valvular involvement and compromise
	Abnormal heart sounds from mitral valve indicate: left atrial hypertrophy; sinus tachycardia; widened P waves, due to left atrial enlargement; atrial fibrillation	Assess extremities for pulse, color, and temperature changes	Indicate anoxia or decreased perfusion
Potential for fluid volume excess due to: fluid imbalance; dysfunctional valve; infection	Increased pedal edema	Administer diuretics as ordered	To draw off excess fluid
	Intake > output	Limit oral intake; introduce low-sodium diet	To decrease fluid retention
	Increased pulmonary congestion	Vigorous pulmonary toilet	To facilitate clearing of lungs
	Labored respirations	Ascertain amount of activity patient can tolerate	To prevent progressive episodes of SOB, tachycardia, and/or hypoxemia
	Tachycardia		
	Hypoxemia		

Nursing Care Plan for the Management of the Patient with Mitral Commissurotomy and Valvular Replacement

Diagnosis	Signs and symptoms	Intervention	Rationale
Potential for decreased cardiac output from arrhythmias; fluid volume deficit; fluid volume overload; ischemia from intraoperative MI; hypothermia; hypertension; hypotension; tamponade; increased afterload	CO < 3 L/min CI < 2 L/min/m^2	Monitor CO and CI closely	To facilitate early intervention
	Reduced peripheral tissue perfusion evidenced by decreased distal pulses and cool extremities	Administer vasoactive medications as ordered (dobutamine, Inocor)	To maintain adequate perfusion in vital organs and periphery
	Arrhythmias, such as PVCs, heart blocks, SVT, PAT, AF, AFL, MAT related to edematous suture line, ventricular tachycardia, ventricular fibrillation	Administer antiarrhythmias as ordered and PRN	To allow for adequate cardiac function and prevention of life-threatening rhythms
		Assess and treat ABGs and K$^+$ in relation to PVCs	Potassium imbalance and compromised ABGs can cause PVCs
		Serial ECGs	To allow early recognition of ischemia, injury, or arrhythmia
		Maintain stable heart rhythm, as ordered: atrially paced to keep heart rate at 60–100; ventricularly paced for second- and third-degree heart blocks; cardioversion for ventricular tachycardia or fibrillation; verapamil for SVT; digoxin	To maintain normal sinus rhythm and stable hemodynamics
	Fluid volume deficit	Correct fluid volume deficit, as ordered	To maintain cardiac function and output
	Ischemia: CPK > 180 IU/L; MBs > 15 IU/L; new ECG ischemic changes	Serial ECGs Maintain oxygenation	To facilitate early recognition of ischemia and prevent further cellular damage from lack of oxygenation

Diagnosis	Signs and symptoms	Intervention	Rationale
	Hypothermia	Administer NaHCO$_3$ for base deficit > -3 when hypothermic	Acid-base imbalance is exacerbated by hypothermia
		Warm with warming blankets or lights	To return patient to normal core temperature
	Hypertension	Administer antihypertensives, as ordered, to keep SBP > 100 and < 150 mm Hg (MSO$_4$, nitroprusside 0.5–8.0 mcg/kg/min, nitroglycerin up to 200–300 mcg/min)	Fast-acting or short-lasting medications for hypertensive events
		Taper vasoconstrictive meds to maintain SBP > 100 and < 160 mm Hg (epinephrine, Levophed, dobutamine 2–10 mcg/kg/min, dopamine 2–10 mcg/kg/min, neosynephrine)	To maintain safe blood pressure levels
	Tamponade: elevation and equalization of filling pressures (CVP + PAD = LAP = 20–30); reduction in SBP to less than 100 mm Hg; abrupt cessation of CT drainage; widening of mediastinum on x-ray; increased jugular venous pressure; cool, clammy skin; reduced peripheral pulses; muffled heart sounds; pulsus paradoxus > 10	Immediate medical intervention, including extracting clot from mediastinal tube with Fogarty catheter, open chest procedure, and/or return to OR	Cardiac tamponade presents a high risk of death if not treated immediately

Diagnosis	Signs and symptoms	Intervention	Rationale
	Increased SVR Crackles (rales)	Reduce SVR, as ordered, by: warming patient; administering vasodilators (Inocor, dobutamine, nitroglycerine, MSO$_4$); restricting fluids; administering diuretics	To maintain hemodynamic stability
Potential for impaired gas exchange due to: fluid volume overload; ineffective airway clearance, atelectasis, or effusion; bronchospasm; inadequate supplemental oxygen; inadequate tidal volume; low hematocrit and hemoglobin levels; low cardiac output; excessive pulmonary vascular resistance; malpositioned ETT or inadequate cuff volume; pneumothorax or hemothorax	Abnormal ABGs: pO$_2$ < 80 mm Hg; pCO$_2$ < 35 or > 45 mm Hg; pH < 7.35 or > 7.45; O$_2$ sat. < 80%; HCO$_3$ < 20 or > 26 mEq/L; BE < 0 or > 3 Cyanosis ETT cuff leak Lowered peak pressure Inadequate volume exchange Chest x-ray indicates atelectasis, effusion, pneumothorax, or hemothorax Copious secretions Elevated respiratory rate, wheezing, air hunger, gasping, or asymmetrical expansion of chest wall	Mechanically ventilate for 8–12 hours postoperatively, as ordered Closely monitor for absent, unequal, or diminished breath sounds, crackles, wheezing, or asymmetrical chest wall expansion; closely monitor ABGs PRN and after ventilator changes; obtain chest x-ray immediately and PRN postoperatively and examine for ETT placement, lung expansion (pneumothorax), width of mediastinal shadow, presence of pleural fluid, and presence of foreign body Aggressive pulmonary toilet PRN with chest percussion therapy, incentive spirometry, and hyperinflation using 100% O$_2$ before and after suctioning; turn and reposition patient every 2 hours	Ventilation support is needed until stabilization To discover early indications of ensuing respiratory compromise and/or complications To mobilize secretions, provide adequate oxygenation, and open closed alveoli

Diagnosis	Signs and symptoms	Intervention	Rationale
		If patient is stable, promote extubation by: holding sedation after midnight on day of surgery; elevating HOB 30 degrees; decreasing IMV by increments of 2–4 breaths/min if $pO_2 > 90$, pH 7.35–7.45, and O_2 sat. 90–100%	To assist patient to return to optimal breathing capacity as soon as possible (to prevent atelectasis, secondary infection, etc.)
	Hematocrit level less than 30 with abnormal ABGs	Administer packed cells as ordered	To improve hematocrit and oxygen-carrying ability
	Cardiac index < 2.5 $L/min/m^2$	Correct low cardiac output	To maintain adequate cardiac function and tissue perfusion and oxygenation
	Excessive PVR (>120 dyne-sec/cm^5)	Administer prostaglandin E or thromboxine as ordered	To counteract excessive PVR
	Copious secretions Respirations > 30 bpm	Administer theophylline by infusion and bronchodilator (Alupent, Bronchosol) through ventilator or increase FIO_2 as ordered	To improve breathing capacity
	Signs of fluid overload: crackles on auscultation; $pO_2 < 90$ mm Hg; chest x-ray indicative of fluid overload; PAD > 20 mm Hg; LAP > 20 mm Hg; urine output < 30 cc/hr; weight gain > 5 kg; frothy sputum	Administer diuretics PRN or as ordered	To facilitate diuresis of extra fluid volume

Nursing Care Plan for the Management of the Patient with Mitral Commissurotomy and Valvular Replacement

Diagnosis	Signs and symptoms	Intervention	Rationale
Potential for skin breakdown due to: restriction in movement; pain or discomfort; drug-induced neuromuscular or musculoskeletal impairment; depression; stiffness from extended catheterization time and/or time on operating table; diaphoresis or drainage into patient's bed; independent variables such as diabetes, peripheral vascular disease, obesity, etc.	Imposed restriction of movement due to body mechanics, medical protocol, etc.	Put air mattress on all postoperative beds	To prevent pressure spots on skin
	Impaired coordination or decreased muscle strength preventing independent movement	Assist patient with required movements and with a quarter turn every 1–2 hours	To prevent injury and facilitate movement
	Reluctance to attempt movement	Premedicate PRN or as ordered to decrease discomfort accompanying movement	To facilitate movement
	Redness over pressure points	Inspect skin pressure points, including occiput, sacrum, coccyx, heels, and elbows, every 2 hours	To prevent skin breakdown
		Passive range of motion to all extremities	To prevent pressure spots and improve circulation without increasing oxygen demand
		Keep patient dry	To prevent skin breakdown
		Maintain and supplement nutrition as needed	To maintain vital nutrients to skin
		Consult enterostomal therapist for actual breakdown	For optimal care planning and intervention
	Elevated temperature	Keep patient dry when diaphoretic	To prevent skin breakdown

Diagnosis	Signs and symptoms	Intervention	Rationale
Potential for alteration in bowel function (constipation) due to: decreased mobility; change in eating patterns; side effects of medications; postoperative paralytic ileus; decreased fluid volume	Reports of feeling constipated, "full" feeling in abdomen, inability to move bowels Decreased or absent bowel sounds Inadequate oral fluid/food intake as evidenced on I&O records and calorie counts	Assess abdomen for bowel sounds, softness, and appearance and ask patient about discomfort at least every 12 hours Encourage progressive ambulation and activity, as tolerated Reassure patient that constipation is frequently a problem postoperatively	To allow for early diagnosis of constipation, in order to intervene before problems become serious To stimulate peristalsis So patient will not become overly concerned
	Symptoms of dehydration: poor skin turgor; sunken eyes; intake < output; weight loss	Assess for signs of dehydration and encourage oral fluid intake, unless patient is on fluid restriction Closely monitor electrolytes	Hydration impedes constipation Dehydration leads to electrolyte imbalance
	Absence of bowel movement for more than 2 days	Implement bowel regimen as ordered: milk of magnesia 30 mL PO every h.s.; consult with dietician about increased fiber in diet; rehydrate patient, as ordered, via IV or oral fluids Reduce narcotic consumption when feasible	Patient may need extra help to start peristalsis postoperatively Narcotics inhibit bowel activity
Potential for alteration in bowel function (diarrhea) due to: side effects of cardiac medications and/or antibiotics; bacterial infections; change in eating patterns	Diarrhea or frequent liquid stools Hyperactive bowel sounds	Assess abdomen for hyperactive bowel sounds Educate patient about medications that may cause diarrhea Assess fluid status in attempt to avoid dehydration and monitor electrolytes	To allow for early intervention To help patient understand cause Diarrhea quickly leads to dehydration and electrolyte imbalance

Diagnosis	Signs and symptoms	Intervention	Rationale
		Implement treatment as ordered: antidiarrheal medication; rehydration; change of cardiac medications or antibiotics if possible, to relieve diarrhea	To prevent further systemic complications
		Culture for clostridia difficile, as ordered	High risk for diarrhea; should be treated as soon as possible
Potential for alteration in health maintenance due to knowledge deficit concerning: diagnosis; surgical procedure; medications; diet; activity; medical follow-up; referrals; when to notify MD; self-monitoring	Inability to describe personal diagnosis and how it relates to type of surgery	Instruct patient and family about diagnosis and surgery	Patient and family must understand what is being done and why
		Encourage questions and discussion of problems and concerns	To allow for greatest learning
	Inability to identify medications and their schedules	Instruct patient about medications: what they look like; names and doses; indications; side effects and what can be done; daily schedule; standard drug information and complete medication schedule	Safe and accurate medication regimen is necessary
	Inability to list foods appropriate for personal diet	Provide instruction on low-sodium, modified-fat/cholesterol diet; consult with dietician	To facilitate healing and prevent complications arising from incorrect diet

Diagnosis	Signs and symptoms	Intervention	Rationale
	Inability to distinguish between permitted and prohibited progression of activities	Discuss activity instructions: activities in routine; balancing rest and activity; progressive walking schedule; no lifting more than 20 pounds; no driving for 6 weeks; stopping every hour for a short walk when taking long car trips; resumption of sexual activities	To allow for progressive resumption of activities without risk of overdoing it and precipitating an untoward event In the event of an accident, steering wheel may crush incompletely healed sternum; walking increases circulation and prevents prolonged venous pooling
	Lack of knowledge about follow-up appointments	Help patient and family to arrange follow-up appointments	Plans for follow-up care must be initiated as soon as possible
	Inability to identify professional services available for support	Advise patient and family of services and resources available	To provide most comprehensive and effective services to patient and family
	Inability to explain when to notify MD or seek emergency assistance	Review with patient and family when to notify MD: angina, SOB, dizziness, or nausea during or following activity; weight gain of more than 1 lb/day; signs of infected incision, including redness, swelling, increased tenderness, drainage; temperature > 101°F; irregular/fast heart rate	Patient and family need to know what to do in the case of an untoward event
	Inability to properly count pulse, assess weight fluctuations, and/or take temperature	Instruct patient and family and require return demonstration: weighing self and recording weight; taking temperature and pulse and recording them	Patient and family need to increase self-help abilities

Nursing Care Plan for the Management of the Patient with Mitral Commissurotomy and Valvular Replacement

Diagnosis	Signs and symptoms	Intervention	Rationale
	Inability to verbalize significance of weight changes	Instruct patient on meaning of weight gain and what to do in its event	To increase patient's self-help abilities in preventing congestive failure
Potential for anxiety due to: fear of unknown; fear of death; fear of disfigurement; fear of pain; fear of disability; lack of knowledge regarding hospital and/or operative procedures, routines	Facial tension Distracted behavior Low attention span Withdrawal Twitching and shaking of extremities Inappropriate laughter or behavior Diaphoresis Tachycardia PVCs Other arrhythmias Nonadherence to treatment plan	Ascertain patient's fears and anxieties	Will allow the nurse to know just what to address
		Ascertain patient's previous hospital experiences (own as well as others')	Will help the nurse to know how to best alleviate anxieties or support positive attitudes
		Ascertain patient's and family's readiness to learn	Need to begin patient and family education when ready
		Teach patient about procedure, lines, length of time on table, unit routine, visiting hours, pain medication, and deep breathing and coughing	
		Provide patient with educational booklets	
		Teach patient about: routine of lab, radiology, ECG, house staff; surgery, incisions, tubes, lines, operation length, ICU routine	To help patient and family be prepared for what is to be experienced
		Give ICU tour, if desired	To familiarize patient with environment
		Sedate patient, as ordered or PRN	To help patient relax
		Provide emotional support as needed	To help patient and family deal with the situation in the best way possible

658

Diagnosis	Signs and symptoms	Intervention	Rationale
		Consult with social worker, chaplain, etc., as needed	Multidisciplinary team effort provides broader, more comprehensive care
Potential for ineffective individual or family coping related to: situational crisis; maturational crisis; personal vulnerability	Verbalization of inability to cope Inability to ask for emotional help	Assess family's usual coping mechanisms	Questions and concerns of patient and family must be answered even if not voiced
		Assist family to identify alternative coping mechanisms; identify and acknowledge family's needs	Optimal coping must be accomplished for maximal healing
	Inability to meet role expectations	Provide information to patient and family regarding diagnosis and purpose of supportive services	Patient and family must be helped through role redefinition
	Prolonged progression of disease or disability	Support patient and family through role transition	To facilitate necessary role changes
		Encourage open communication among patient, family, and health care team	To facilitate problem solving and care planning
		Reinforce simple explanations to patient and family	During times of crisis, care must be taken not to cause information overload
	Exhaustion	Provide rest periods and offer nutrition to family; plan visiting schedule to accommodate interventions as well as family schedule and rest periods; restrict visitors as appropriate	To maximize quality family time as well as allow for needed rest
	Fear and anxiety	Delegate one resource and support person to assist family through this very critical time	Consistency in problem solving and care improves quality of decisions
	Inappropriate requests or hypervigilance by patient and/or family	Suggest ways for family to assist in patient's care	Participatory care decreases anxiety

Nursing Care Plan for the Management of the Patient with Mitral Commissurotomy and Valvular Replacement

Diagnosis	Signs and symptoms	Intervention	Rationale
	Inability to solve problems	Assist patient and family to identify problems and work together to solve them	Sometimes patients and families are unable to anticipate possible problems
	Unreasonable and/or excessively frequent requests (excessive use of call light)	Assist family in caring for patient and problem solve about how to continue such care following discharge	Personal involvement in care decreases anxiety while increasing self-confidence and skills
		Encourage progressively independent activities	To avoid rushing patient and family into too much responsibility for care
Potential for self-care deficit due to: muscle deconditioning; postoperative incisional discomfort; sleep pattern disturbances; fear of overexertion; anxiety; decreased activity tolerance	Weak muscles resulting from bedrest	Encourage progressive activities: self-care; ambulation; active ROM	To allow time for patient to regain strength
	Reports of postoperative pain Fatigue	Assess discomfort and encourage patient to request medication as appropriate	To allow for maximal activities
	Slow movement, ambulating with caution, refusal to participate in daily care routine	Reassure patient that postoperative pain is expected and teach patient how to mini-mize discomfort while moving, deep breath-ing, coughing, etc.	To minimize effects of pain
	Increased heart rate and respiratory rate upon minimal activity	Assess patient's need for rest and sleep and incorporate rest periods during the day	To prevent overexhaustion
	Repetitive fast speech, indicating anxiety	Maintain calm environ-ment (lighting, noise, interruptions, etc.)	To facilitate adequate rest
	Inability to concentrate on activities required	Encourage patient's participation in scheduling and carrying out daily care	To accommodate routines to patient's ability to progress
		Praise patient's progress in activities	Encouragement is a good motivator

Acquired and Congenital Structural Heart Defects

Acquired structural defects usually affect the valves in some way and occur as a result of rheumatic heart disease, infective endocarditis, pericarditis, myocardial infarction, and trauma. The primary structural defects found are aortic, pulmonic, or mitral stenosis and aortic, tricuspid, or mitral regurgitation. Table 4-24 provides an overview of these different types of valvular disorders, their etiologies and accompanying pathophysiology, and their clinical manifestations.

Structural defects found in adults include the following congenitally originating disorders:

Ventricular septal defect: an opening in the septum separating the two ventricles

Bicuspid aortic valve: an aortic valve with only two cusps

Atrial septal defect: an opening in the septum separating the two atria

Aortic stenosis: narrowing of the aortic valve

Pulmonic stenosis: narrowing of the pulmonic valve

Coarctation of the aorta: narrowing of the aorta caused by the wall of the vessel curving inward

The critical care nurse usually sees the patient with structural heart defects only when the disorder has progressed so far that congestive heart failure has developed or after surgical correction of the defect. Thus, care provided is consistent with that provided in the event of congestive heart failure or that provided postoperatively. The care plan highlights the standards of care for such a patient.

Table 4-24 Acquired Valvular Defects: Their Etiology, Pathophysiology, and Clinical Manifestations

Type	Etiology	Pathophysiology	Clinical Manifestations

Aortic stenosis	Congenital, or acquired from rheumatic endocarditis or atherosclerosis	Left ventricular hypertrophy
		Aortic valve calcification
		Increased diastolic ventricular pressure (up to 300 mm Hg)
		Normal left atrial and pulmonary pressures
		Poststenotic aortic dilatation
		Increased myocardial oxygen demand
			Angina
			Extreme weakness
			Fatigue
			Debilitation
			Venous hypertension
			Edema
			Hepatomegaly
			Ascites
			Congestive heart failure
			Diagnostic indicators:
			  medium-pitched heart sound, best heard in 2nd right interspace
			  thrill palpated over precordium
			  diminished S_2
			  early ejection click
			  narrow pulse pressure

Pulmonic stenosis	Congenital defect, usually associated with other defects such as ventricular septal or atrial septal defect	Chamber enlargement
		Right ventricular hypertrophy
		Left parasternal lift
		Narrowing of pulmonic passageway with resulting murmur and blood turbulence
			Congestive heart failure
			Diagnostic indicators:
			  medium- to high-pitched heart sound
			  thrill palpated over pulmonic area
			  widely split S_2
			  early ejection click

(continued)

Table 4-24 Acquired Valvular Defects: Their Etiology, Pathophysiology, and Clinical Manifestations (*continued*)

Type	Etiology	Pathophysiology	Clinical Manifestations
Mitral stenosis	Acquired from rheumatic heart disease and endocarditis	Pulmonary edema Left atrial enlargement Right ventricular hypertrophy Pulmonary venous congestion Interstitial pulmonary edema Atrial dilation Increased pulmonary wedge pressure Increased left atrial pressure Right heart failure	Fatigue Shortness of breath, orthopnea Bronchitis, cough Cyanosis Diagnostic indicators: rumbling, low-pitched sounds with patient in left lateral position and stethoscope held lightly to skin accentuated S_1 in mitral area
Aortic regurgitation	Congenital, or acquired from rheumatic endocarditis or syphilis	Left ventricular hypertrophy Aortic valve calcification Dilatation of ascending aorta Increased pulse pressure Increased diastolic pulse slope Aortic valve reflux	Syncope Dyspnea Angina Pulmonary congestion Sinus tachycardia Diagnostic indicators: diastolic and systolic murmurs heard with patient leaning forward and on forced expiration blowing, high-pitched heart sound S_3
Tricuspid regurgitation	Acquired from right ventricular failure resulting from left ventricular failure or pulmonary hypertension	Increased circulatory volume in right atrium leading to enlargement Right-sided heart failure Venous engorgement Hepatojugular reflex	Tricuspid murmur throughout systole Diastolic murmur Peripheral edema Hepatomegaly Ascites Slate-colored complexion Diagnostic indicators: regurgitation heard in tricuspid soft, blowing, high-pitched heart sound, increasing with respiration systolic thrill can be palpated over right ventricle
Mitral regurgitation	Acquired from rheumatic fever, bacterial endocarditis, or aortic valvular disease, or may be congenital anomaly	Left atrial enlargement Left ventricular hypertrophy Pulmonary vascular congestion	Fatigue, weakness Dyspnea, cough Murmur throughout systole Palpitations, atrial fibrillation Diagnostic indicators: regurgitation at apex and back of left side, preceded by a click soft, blowing, high-pitched sound S_3, decreased S_1

Nursing Care Plan for the Management of the Patient with Structural Heart Defects

Diagnosis	Signs and symptoms	Intervention	Rationale
Alteration in cardiac output related to myocardial failure	Signs of low cardiac output: decreased BP; increased SVR; increased PAP and PCWP Signs of high cardiac output: increased cardiac output measures; decreased BP; decreased SVR; increased PAP and PCWP	Anticipate insertion of pulmonary artery catheter	Provides more accurate measure of cardiac function
		Administer preload-reducing agents (nitroglycerin) as ordered, to maintain PAD/PCWP < 18 mm Hg	To decrease venous return
		Administer afterload-reducing agents (nitroprusside) as ordered	To maintain SVR at 800–1300 dyne-sec/cm^5
		Administer inotropics (dopamine, dobutamine) as ordered	To improve contractility
		Administer drugs, as indicated and ordered, to maintain normal sinus rhythm	To maintain cardiac efficiency and output
		Administer digoxin as ordered	To improve cardiac contractility and control tachycardia
		Monitor BP closely	To assess for hypotension and pulsus alternans
		Participate in identification and correction of aggravating factors	It is most important to correct the underlying cause rather than just to treat the symptoms
Potential for decreased cardiac output from arrhythmias; fluid volume deficit; fluid volume overload; hypothermia; hypertension; hypotension; tamponade; increased afterload	CO < 3 L/min CI < 2 L/min/m^2 Reduced peripheral tissue perfusion evidenced by decreased distal pulses and cool extremities	Monitor CO and CI closely	To facilitate early intervention
		Administer vasoactive medications as ordered (dobutamine, Inocor)	To maintain adequate perfusion in vital organs and periphery

Diagnosis	Signs and symptoms	Intervention	Rationale
	Arrhythmias, such as PVCs, heart blocks, SVT, PAT, AF, AFL, MAT related to edematous suture line, ventricular tachycardia, ventricular fibrillation	Administer antiarrhythmias as ordered and PRN	To allow for adequate cardiac function and prevention of life-threatening rhythms
		Assess and treat ABGs and K^+ in relation to PVCs	Potassium imbalance and compromised ABGs can cause PVCs
		Serial ECGs	To allow early recognition of ischemia, injury, or arrhythmia
		Maintain stable heart rhythm, as ordered: atrially paced to keep heart rate at 60–100; ventricularly paced for second- and third-degree heart blocks; cardioversion for ventricular tachycardia or fibrillation; verapamil for SVT; digoxin	To maintain normal sinus rhythm and stable hemodynamics
	Fluid volume deficit	Correct fluid volume deficit, as ordered	To maintain cardiac function and output
	Ischemia: CPK > 180 IU/L; MBs > 15 IU/L; new ECG ischemic changes	Serial ECGs Maintain oxygenation	To facilitate early recognition of ischemia and prevent further cellular damage from lack of oxygenation
	Hypothermia	Administer $NaHCO_3$ for base deficit > -3 when hypothermic	Acid-base imbalance is exacerbated by hypothermia
		Warm with warming blankets or lights	To return patient to normal core temperature
	Hypertension	Administer antihypertensives, as ordered, to keep SBP > 100 and < 150 mm Hg (MSO_4, nitroprusside 0.5–8.0 mcg/kg/min, nitroglycerin up to 200–300 mcg/min)	Fast-acting or short-lasting medications for hypertensive events

Diagnosis	Signs and symptoms	Intervention	Rationale
		Taper vasoconstrictive meds to maintain SBP > 100 and < 160 mm Hg (epinephrine, Levophed, dobutamine 2–10 mcg/kg/min, dopamine 2–10 mcg/kg/min, neosynephrine)	To maintain safe blood pressure levels
	Tamponade: elevation and equalization of filling pressures (CVP + PAD = LAP = 20–30); reduction in SBP to less than 100 mm Hg; abrupt cessation of CT drainage; widening of mediastinum on x-ray; increased jugular venous pressure; cool, clammy skin; reduced peripheral pulses; muffled heart sounds; pulsus paradoxus > 10	Immediate medical intervention, including extracting clot from mediastinal tube with Fogarty catheter, open chest procedure, and/or return to OR	Cardiac tamponade presents a high risk of death if not treated immediately
	Increased SVR Crackles (rales)	Reduce SVR, as ordered, by: warming patient; administering vasodilators (Inocor, dobutamine, nitroglycerine, MSO_4); restricting fluids; administering diuretics	To maintain hemodynamic stability
Alteration in fluid volume (excess)	Weight gain Elevated PAD and PCWP Edema Decreased urinary output	Maintain accurate I&O records	To ascertain presence and cause of fluid imbalance
		Limit salt intake as ordered	Excess sodium causes fluid retention
		Restrict fluids to 1500 cc/day if PAD and PCWP are elevated	To prevent fluid overload, which can lead to congestive failure

Nursing Care Plan for the Management of the Patient with Structural Heart Defects

Diagnosis	Signs and symptoms	Intervention	Rationale
		Administer diuretics as ordered Monitor BUN and creatinine	Prerenal failure may develop as a result of decreased renal perfusion
		Anticipate low-dose (2–5 mcg/kg/min) dopamine infusion	To provide increased renal perfusion
		Monitor weight daily	Weight change is best indicator of excess fluid loss
		Monitor for crackles (rales) and presence of S_3 heart sounds every 4 hours or as needed	Warn of heart failure and pulmonary edema
		Anticipate need for salt-poor albumin administration	Chronic heart failure predisposes patient to loss of protein, leading to edema; albumin provides mechanism for returning interstitial fluid to intravascular space
		Apply elastic antiembolism stockings	To promote venous return and prevent edema
Potential for viral, bacterial, and/or prosthetic valve infection	Increased sedimentation rate	Administer antimicrobial therapy as ordered	For prevention or treatment of microbial infection
	Fever	Tylenol 600 mg every 4 hours or PRN as ordered	To alleviate fever
	WBCs > 8,000	Implement thorough hand washing between patient contacts; implement universal isolation precautions if indicated	To prevent the spread of infection

Diagnosis	Signs and symptoms	Intervention	Rationale
	Redness, exudate, increased tenderness, and/or induration of surgical incision, IV insertion site, pacer wire sites, or chest tube sites	Routine incision care with povidone-iodine solution, Telfa dressing, as indicated; change peripheral IV sites at least every 3 days or with any signs of infection or infiltration; change IV tubing every 24 hours	To prevent incisional infections, leading to valvular vegetative growth
		Culture suspected origins of infection	To determine correct antibiotic therapy
	Sediment in urine or foul-smelling urine; hesitancy, frequency, urgency, burning, difficulty starting stream, incontinence, and/or inability to void	Routine Foley care every 8 hours; push fluids if not contraindicated	To prevent urinary tract infections, leading to valvular vegetative growth
	Fatigue	Assess patient's need for rest and sleep and incorporate rest periods during the day; maintain calm environment (lighting, noise, interruptions, etc.)	To allow patient time to rest adequately, to prevent overexhaustion, and to help patient regain strength to combat infections
	Palpitations	Assess vital signs, especially for pulse > 100	For early detection and treatment of developing complications
	Precordial discomfort	Medicate, as ordered	To keep patient pain-free
	Abnormal heart sounds from aortic valve indicate: left ventricular hypertrophy; sinus tachycardia; first degree atrioventricular block; bundle branch block; intraventricular conduction disturbances; atrial arrhythmias	Assess heart sounds for gallop rhythm, murmur, and/or pericardial friction rub, and administer cardiac medications as ordered	For early detection and treatment of developing complications
		Assess for symptoms of digitalis toxicity	So as not to mistake digitalis toxicity for signs of infection, and vice versa

Nursing Care Plan for the Management of the Patient with Structural Heart Defects

Diagnosis	Signs and symptoms	Intervention	Rationale
	Abnormal heart sounds from mitral valve indicate: left atrial hypertrophy; sinus tachycardia; widened P waves, due to left atrial enlargement; atrial fibrillation	Monitor for evidence of arrhythmias Assess extremities for pulse, color, and temperature changes	May be signs of valvular involvement and compromise Indicate anoxia or decreased perfusion
Potential for impaired gas exchange due to: fluid volume overload; ineffective airway clearance, atelectasis, or effusion; bronchospasm; inadequate supplemental oxygen; inadequate tidal volume; low hematocrit and hemoglobin levels; low cardiac output; excessive pulmonary vascular resistance; malpositioned ETT or inadequate cuff volume; pneumothorax or hemothorax	Abnormal ABGs: $pO_2 < 80$ mm Hg; $pCO_2 < 35$ or > 45 mm Hg; pH < 7.35 or > 7.45; O_2 sat. $< 80\%$; $HCO_3 < 20$ or > 26 mEq/L; BE < 0 or > 3 Cyanosis ETT cuff leak Lowered peak pressure Inadequate volume exchange Chest x-ray indicates atelectasis, effusion, pneumothorax, or hemothorax Copious secretions Elevated respiratory rate, wheezing, air hunger, gasping, or asymmetrical expansion of chest wall	Mechanically ventilate for 8–12 hours postoperatively, as ordered Closely monitor for absent, unequal, or diminished breath sounds, crackles, wheezing, or asymmetrical chest wall expansion; closely monitor ABGs PRN and after ventilator changes; obtain chest x-ray immediately and PRN postoperatively and examine for ETT placement, lung expansion (pneumothorax), width of mediastinal shadow, presence of pleural fluid, and presence of foreign body Aggressive pulmonary toilet PRN with chest percussion therapy, incentive spirometry, and hyperinflation using 100% O_2 before and after suctioning; turn and reposition patient every 2 hours	Ventilation support is needed until stabilization To discover early indications of ensuing respiratory compromise and/or complications To mobilize secretions, provide adequate oxygenation, and open closed alveoli

Diagnosis	Signs and symptoms	Intervention	Rationale
		If patient is stable, promote extubation by: holding sedation after midnight on day of surgery; elevating HOB 30 degrees; decreasing IMV by increments of 2–4 breaths/min if $pO_2 > 90$, pH 7.35–7.45, and O_2 sat. 90–100%	To assist patient to return to optimal breathing capacity as soon as possible (to prevent atelectasis, secondary infection, etc.)
	Hematocrit level less than 30 with abnormal ABGs	Administer packed cells as ordered	To improve hematocrit and oxygen-carrying ability
	Cardiac index < 2.5 $L/min/m^2$	Correct low cardiac output	To maintain adequate cardiac function and tissue perfusion and oxygenation
	Excessive PVR (>120 $dyne\text{-}sec/cm^5$)	Administer prostaglandin E or thomboxine as ordered	To counteract excessive PVR
	Copious secretions Respirations > 30 bpm	Administer theophylline by infusion and bronchodilator (Alupent, Bronchosol) through ventilator or increase FIO_2 as ordered	To improve breathing capacity
	Signs of fluid overload: crackles on auscultation; $pO_2 < 90$ mm Hg; chest x-ray indicative of fluid overload; PAD > 20 mm Hg; LAP > 20 mm Hg; urine output < 30 cc/hr; weight gain > 5 kg; frothy sputum	Administer diuretics PRN or as ordered	To facilitate diuresis of extra fluid volume
Potential for infection related to pulmonary congestion, indwelling lines, and Foley catheter	Elevated temperature	Encourage coughing and deep breathing; turn patient in bed every 2 hours while on bedrest	Help to prevent atelectasis, blood clots in legs, and pressure sores

Nursing Care Plan for the Management of the Patient with Structural Heart Defects

Diagnosis	Signs and symptoms	Intervention	Rationale
		Change respiratory tubing every 24 hours	Per CDC specifications
		Increase activity as soon as indicated	To promote healing
		Monitor temperature every 4 hours	Sign of infection
	Increased WBCs	Assess WBC count	Sign of infection
		Maintain strict aseptic technique with invasive lines and indwelling catheters; change lines unless contraindicated: PAP every 72 hours, arterial lines every 7 days, tubing every 48 hours, IV bags every 24 hours; provide Foley care every 8 hours	Per CDC recommendation
		Assist in identifying source of infection: collect cultures; note atelectasis on chest x-ray; note sputum and urine characteristics; check insertion site for redness every 8 hours	Sites at risk of infection must be kept clean with aseptic technique; appropriate antibiotic therapy must be chosen
		Administer antibiotics as ordered	To combat infectious process
Potential for skin breakdown due to: restriction in movement; pain or discomfort; drug-induced neuromuscular or musculoskeletal impairment; depression; stiffness from extended catheterization time and/or time on operating table;	Imposed restriction of movement due to body mechanics, medical protocol, etc.	Put air mattress on all postoperative beds	To prevent pressure spots on skin
	Impaired coordination or decreased muscle strength preventing independent movement	Assist patient with required movements and with a quarter turn every 1–2 hours	To prevent injury and facilitate movement
	Reluctance to attempt movement	Premedicate PRN or as ordered to decrease discomfort accompanying movement	To facilitate movement

Diagnosis	Signs and symptoms	Intervention	Rationale
diaphoresis or drainage into patient's bed; independent variables such as diabetes, peripheral vascular disease, obesity, etc.	Redness over pressure points	Inspect skin pressure points, including occiput, sacrum, coccyx, heels, and elbows, every 2 hours	To prevent skin breakdown
		Passive range of motion to all extremities	To prevent pressure spots and improve circulation without increasing oxygen demand
		Keep patient dry	To prevent skin breakdown
		Maintain and supplement nutrition as needed	To maintain vital nutrients to skin
		Consult enterostomal therapist for actual breakdown	For optimal care planning and intervention
	Elevated temperature	Keep patient dry when diaphoretic	To prevent skin breakdown
Potential for alteration in bowel function (constipation) due to: decreased mobility; change in eating patterns; side effects of medications; postoperative paralytic ileus; decreased fluid volume	Reports of feeling constipated, "full" feeling in abdomen, inability to move bowels Decreased or absent bowel sounds Inadequate oral fluid/food intake as evidenced on I&O records and calorie counts	Assess abdomen for bowel sounds, softness, and appearance and ask patient about discomfort at least every 12 hours	To allow for early diagnosis of constipation, in order to intervene before problems become serious
		Encourage progressive ambulation and activity, as tolerated	To stimulate peristalsis
		Reassure patient that constipation is frequently a problem postoperatively	So patient will not become overly concerned
	Symptoms of dehydration: poor skin turgor; sunken eyes; intake < output; weight loss	Assess for signs of dehydration and encourage oral fluid intake, unless patient is on fluid restriction	Hydration impedes constipation

Nursing Care Plan for the Management of the Patient with Structural Heart Defects

Diagnosis	Signs and symptoms	Intervention	Rationale
		Closely monitor electrolytes	Dehydration leads to electrolyte imbalance
	Absence of bowel movement for more than 2 days	Implement bowel regimen as ordered: milk of magnesia 30 mL PO every h.s.; consult with dietician about increased fiber in diet; rehydrate patient, as ordered, via IV or oral fluids	Patient may need extra help to start peristalsis postoperatively
		Reduce narcotic consumption when feasible	Narcotics inhibit bowel activity
Potential for alteration in bowel function (diarrhea) due to: side effects of cardiac medications and/or antibiotics; bacterial infections; change in eating patterns	Diarrhea or frequent liquid stools Hyperactive bowel sounds	Assess abdomen for hyperactive bowel sounds	To allow for early intervention
		Educate patient about medications that may cause diarrhea	To help patient understand cause
		Assess fluid status in attempt to avoid dehydration and monitor electrolytes	Diarrhea quickly leads to dehydration and electrolyte imbalance
		Implement treatment as ordered: antidiarrheal medication; rehydration; change of cardiac medications or antibiotics if possible, to relieve diarrhea	To prevent further systemic complications
		Culture for clostridia difficile, as ordered	High risk for diarrhea; should be treated as soon as possible

Diagnosis	Signs and symptoms	Intervention	Rationale
Decreased tolerance of activity related to dyspnea	Dyspnea on exertion Fatigue Exaggerated increase in heart rate and BP on exertion	Assess level of activity tolerance (should be related to the New York Heart Association's classification for consistency)	Provides a baseline
		Assist patient to change position every 2 hours while on bedrest	To decrease risk of complications and promote venous return
		Check BP with patient in horizontal, sitting, and standing positions	To monitor for orthostatic hypotension
		Avoid activity for a half-hour to an hour after meals	May decrease chance of hypoxia due to increased blood flow to GI tract
		Monitor heart rate and BP with activity increases	To maintain heart rate within 10 bpm of resting heart rate and maintain systolic BP within 20 mm Hg of resting BP; if a drop occurs, it may indicate a drop in cardiac output
		Anticipate institution of progressive rehab	To provide controlled mechanism for increasing activity
		Encourage frequent rest periods	To prevent excessive fatigue
Potential for alteration in health maintenance due to knowledge deficit concerning: 　diagnosis; 　surgical procedure; 　medications; 　diet; 　activity; 　medical follow-up; 　referrals; 　when to notify MD; 　self-monitoring	Inability to describe personal diagnosis and how it relates to type of surgery	Instruct patient and family about diagnosis and surgery	Patient and family must understand what is being done and why
		Encourage questions and discussion of problems and concerns	To allow for greatest learning
	Inability to identify medications and their schedules	Instruct patient about medications: 　what they look like; 　names and doses; 　indications; 　side effects and what can be done; 　daily schedule; 　standard drug information and complete medication schedule	Safe and accurate medication regimen is necessary

Nursing Care Plan for the Management of the Patient with Structural Heart Defects

Diagnosis	Signs and symptoms	Intervention	Rationale
	Inability to list foods appropriate for personal diet	Provide instruction on low-sodium, modified-fat/cholesterol diet; consult with dietician	To facilitate healing and prevent complications arising from incorrect diet
	Inability to distinguish between permitted and prohibited progression of activities	Discuss activity instructions: activities in routine; balancing rest and activity; progressive walking schedule; no lifting more than 20 pounds; no driving for 6 weeks; stopping every hour for a short walk when taking long car trips; resumption of sexual activities	To allow for progressive resumption of activities without risk of overdoing it and precipitating an untoward event In the event of an accident, steering wheel may crush incompletely healed sternum; walking increases circulation and prevents prolonged venous pooling
	Lack of knowledge about follow-up appointments	Help patient and family to arrange follow-up appointments	Plans for follow-up care must be initiated as soon as possible
	Inability to identify professional services available for support	Advise patient and family of services and resources available	To provide most comprehensive and effective services to patient and family
	Inability to explain when to notify MD or seek emergency assistance	Review with patient and family when to notify MD: angina, SOB, dizziness, or nausea during or following activity; weight gain of more than 1 lb/day;	Patient and family need to know what to do in the case of an untoward event

Diagnosis	Signs and symptoms	Intervention	Rationale
		signs of infected incision, including redness, swelling, increased tenderness, drainage; temperature > 101°F; irregular/fast heart rate	
	Inability to properly count pulse, assess weight fluctuations, and/or take temperature	Instruct patient and family and require return demonstration: weighing self and recording weight; taking temperature and pulse and recording them	Patient and family need to increase self-help abilities
	Inability to verbalize significance of weight changes	Instruct patient on meaning of weight gain and what to do in its event	To increase patient's self-help abilities in preventing congestive failure
Potential for anxiety due to: fear of unknown; fear of death; fear of disfigurement; fear of pain; fear of disability; lack of knowledge regarding hospital and/or operative procedures, routines	Facial tension Distracted behavior Low attention span Withdrawal Twitching and shaking of extremities Inappropriate laughter or behavior Diaphoresis Tachycardia PVCs Other arrhythmias Nonadherence to treatment plan	Ascertain patient's fears and anxieties	Will allow the nurse to know just what to address
		Ascertain patient's previous hospital experiences (own as well as others')	Will help the nurse to know how to best alleviate anxieties or support positive attitudes
		Ascertain patient's and family's readiness to learn	Need to begin patient and family education when ready
		Teach patient about: routine of lab, radiology, ECG, house staff; procedure, lines, length of time on table, unit routine, visiting hours, pain medication, and deep breathing and coughing; Provide patient with educational booklets	To help patient and family be prepared for what is to be experienced
		Give ICU tour, if desired	To familiarize patient with environment

Nursing Care Plan for the Management of the Patient with Structural Heart Defects

Diagnosis	Signs and symptoms	Intervention	Rationale
		Sedate patient, as ordered or PRN	To help patient relax
		Provide emotional support as needed	To help patient and family deal with the situation in the best way possible
		Consult with social worker, chaplain, etc., as needed	Multidisciplinary team effort provides broader, more comprehensive care
Potential for ineffective individual or family coping related to: situational crisis; maturational crisis; personal vulnerability	Verbalization of inability to cope

Inability to ask for emotional help | Assess family's usual coping mechanisms | Questions and concerns of patient and family must be answered even if not voiced |
		Assist family to identify alternative coping mechanisms; identify and acknowledge family's needs	Optimal coping must be accomplished for maximal healing
	Inability to meet role expectations	Provide information to patient and family regarding diagnosis and purpose of supportive services	Patient and family must be helped through role redefinition
	Prolonged progression of disease or disability	Support patient and family through role transition	To facilitate necessary role changes
		Encourage open communication among patient, family, and health care team	To facilitate problem solving and care planning
		Reinforce simple explanations to patient and family	During times of crisis, care must be taken not to cause information overload

Diagnosis	Signs and symptoms	Intervention	Rationale
	Exhaustion	Provide rest periods and offer nutrition to family; plan visiting schedule to accommodate interventions as well as family schedule and rest periods; restrict visitors as appropriate	To maximize quality family time as well as allow for needed rest
	Fear and anxiety	Delegate one resource and support person to assist family through this very critical time	Consistency in problem solving and care improves quality of decisions
	Inappropriate requests or hypervigilance by patient and/or family	Suggest ways for family to assist in patient's care	Participatory care decreases anxiety
	Inability to solve problems	Assist patient and family to identify problems and work together to solve them	Sometimes patients and families are unable to anticipate possible problems
	Unreasonable and/or excessively frequent requests (excessive use of call light)	Assist family in caring for patient and problem solve about how to continue such care following discharge	Personal involvement in care decreases anxiety while increasing self-confidence and skills
		Encourage progressively independent activities	To avoid rushing patient and family into too much responsibility for care
Potential for self-care deficit due to: muscle deconditioning; postoperative incisional discomfort; sleep pattern disturbances; fear of overexertion; anxiety; decreased activity tolerance	Weak muscles resulting from bedrest	Encourage progressive activities: self-care; ambulation; active ROM	To allow time for patient to regain strength
	Reports of postoperative pain Fatigue	Assess discomfort and encourage patient to request medication as appropriate	To allow for maximal activities
	Slow movement, ambulating with caution, refusal to participate in daily care routine	Reassure patient that postoperative pain is expected and teach patient how to minimize discomfort while moving, deep breathing, coughing, etc.	To minimize effects of pain

Nursing Care Plan for the Management of the Patient with Structural Heart Defects

Diagnosis	Signs and symptoms	Intervention	Rationale
	Increased heart rate and respiratory rate upon minimal activity	Assess patient's need for rest and sleep and incorporate rest periods during the day	To prevent overexhaustion
	Repetitive fast speech, indicating anxiety	Maintain calm environment (lighting, noise, interruptions, etc.)	To facilitate adequate rest
	Inability to concentrate on activities required	Encourage patient's participation in scheduling and carrying out daily care	To accommodate routines to patient's ability to progress
		Praise patient's progress in activities	Encouragement is a good motivator
Knowledge deficit concerning disease process and prescribed regimen	Displays nonadhering behavior during care	Assess patient's present understanding	To establish baseline
	Verbalizes lack of knowledge and understanding	If heart failure requires chronic management, teach patient and family about:	Life-style changes will be required
	Anxiety and apprehension, especially during procedures and treatments	normal heart function; pathology; risk factors; control of precipitating and aggravating factors; allowed activity; diet; medications; weight monitoring; signs and symptoms of recurring heart failure; follow-up care	Increasing patient's family's knowledge, understanding, and ability to adhere to regimen may eliminate unnecessary rehospitalization
		Allow patient and family to ask questions and verify their understanding of information	Patient and family may need reinforcement and several repetitions of information in order to fully understand it

Medications Commonly Used in the Care of the Patient with Structural Heart Defects

Medication	Effect	Major side effects
Digitalis	Increases contractility Lengthens refractory period of AV node Decreases left ventricular end-diastolic pressure Increases ventricular automaticity Decreases atrial automaticity	Tachycardia AV block Bradycardia GI upset Headache Drowsiness Confusion Double vision
Furosemide Ethacrynic acid	Loop diuretic Decreases pulmonary congestion	Hypokalemia Hypocalcemia Hypomagnesemia Altered glucose metabolism
Morphine sulfate	Analgesia/sedation Peripheral vasodilation Decreases systemic venous return Bronchodilation Relief of cardiac dyspnea	Hypotension Respiratory depression Nausea and vomiting Constipation Urinary retention
Nitroprusside	Vasodilator with a direct action on vascular smooth muscle, leading to decreased afterload, causing greater ejection fractions, stroke volume, and cardiac output	GI upset Muscle twitching Hypotension Confusion
Nitrates	Vasodilation, leading to increased coronary blood supply and decreased myocardial oxygen demand	Hypotension Headache
Hydralazine Minoxidil Diazoxide	Vasodilators with a direct action on vascular smooth muscle, leading to relaxed arterioles, decreased vascular resistance, and increased cardiac output	Angina Nausea and vomiting Tachycardia Headache Flushing Hypotension
Dobutamine Dopamine	Intropics with alpha-adrenergic stimulant Increases myocardial contractility, cardiac output, and stroke volume Dilates renal and mesenteric vessels in low doses	GI upset Angina Dyspnea Headache Hypotension Ectopic arrhythmias Palpitations Vasoconstriction

Medications Commonly Used in the Care of the Patient with Structural Heart Defects

Medication	Effect	Major side effects
Captopril	Angiotensin-converting enzyme that decreases vasoconstriction, decreases circulating aldosterone, and suppresses renin-angiotensin system	Hypotension Renal impairment Vertigo Rash
Aminophylline	Bronchodilator Increases renal blood flow Positive inotropic effect on heart	Cardiac arrhythmias GI upset

Cardiac Transplantation

For the patient who suffers from idiopathic cardio-myopathy that is unresponsive to all other available treatment or is of the inoperable stage IV (end-stage) type of coronary artery disease, cardiac or cardiopul-monary transplantation is the only hope for survival. Cardiac transplantation is recognized as a proven procedure for treatment of the appropriately screened patient. Since the first transplant in 1968, the number of transplants performed in the United States has steadily grown; in 1988 it reached 1,640.[51] Survival rates after one year range from 60% to 80%, and expected five-year survival rates are in the 30–50% range.[52]

Clinical antecedents

Severe ischemic heart disease that persists de-spite aggressive medical and/or surgical treatment and idiopathic cardiomyopathy are the two primary antecedents to cardiac transplantation. The cardio-myopathy may be due to a suddenly occurring virus-like infection, complicated congenital heart disease, or even, although extremely rarely, postpartum car-diomyopathy. Regardless, the candidate for trans-plantation has a life expectancy of only six months without a transplant. These are the criteria a patient must meet in order to be considered an appropriate candidate for transplantation:

1. Between 20 and 50 years of age
2. Duration of illness is less than 5 years
3. Pulmonary artery mean pressure < 40 mm Hg
4. Pulmonary vascular resistance < 10 units
5. No severe renal dysfunction secondary to cardiac decompensation
6. No active infection or dental abcesses
7. No muscle wasting, hepatomegaly, or ascites
8. No insulin-dependent diabetes
9. Strong psychosocial support system

Finally, donor hearts must be tissue and type matched to the recipient's so as not to be rejected after the transplant has been performed.

Critical referents

End-stage cardiac disease progresses in the transplant candidate until the left ventricular ejection fraction ranges from 0.4 down to 0.2. Congestive heart failure occurs despite maximal therapy with digoxin and diuretics, afterload reduction, and re-striction of physical activity. The patient has a very large, dilated heart and is prone to develop left ventricular mural thrombosis and, consequently, systemic emboli. The patient also tends to develop pulmonary emboli, probably from venous stasis re-sulting from low cardiac output. Angina, alone, has never been an indication for heart transplantation.[53]

There are two techniques for cardiac transplanta-tion, although the second is rarely used anymore. Regardless of the procedure chosen, the patient, obviously, is first placed on cardiopulmonary bypass after central cannulation of the venae cavae and aorta. The most widely used (and safest) technique is the orthotopic procedure, in which the donor heart is placed in the recipient's heart's former position. This is accomplished after the recipient's heart is excised by severing the atria in a plane just posterior to the bases of both atrial appendages and by cutting the great vessels just above the semilunar valves. Four anastomoses are then performed in order: the left atrial cuffs, the right atrial cuffs, the aortas, and, last, the main pulmonary arteries.[54] The other procedure is the heterotopic, or piggyback, procedure, in which the donor heart is placed parallel to the recipient's. The recipient's heart may become a source for throm-boembolism as well as lung volume compromise, however, because it occupies a very large space in the mediastinum while not functioning efficiently.

Resulting signs and symptoms

Signs and symptoms indicative of the need for cardiac transplantation are those of cardiomyopathy and severe ischemic heart disease and include all the classic signs of severe congestive heart failure. Right and left failure are seen, and, generally, the heart is rendered ineffective and serious cardiac decompen-sation is experienced.

Nursing standards of care

Nursing care in managing the cardiac transplant patient emphasizes the prevention of infection and tissue rejection, the maintenance of cardiopulmo-nary function, and the support of other organ sys-tems. Critical care nurses work closely with the medical team to assess and intervene in the case of rejection, infection, and/or complication of treatment and/or medications. Furthermore, nurses serve as primary providers of patient teaching and prepare the patient for long-term self-care demands. Follow-ing is an outline of the care to be provided for the cardiac transplant patient.

Nursing Care Plan for the Management of the Patient Undergoing Cardiac Transplantation*

Diagnosis	Signs and symptoms	Intervention	Rationale
Potential for fluid volume deficit caused by: bleeding (estimated blood loss not fully replaced); postoperative bleeding (thrombocytopenia, elevated clotting time, increased afterload, or hypertension); suboptimal preload status from OR; vasodilation (when on Nipride or warmed); postoperative diuresis > 200 cc/hr	LAP < 6–10 mm Hg CVP < 6 mm Hg PAD < 10 mm Hg SBP < 100 mm Hg HR > 130 bpm Urine output < 30 cc/hr Output > input Chest tube drainage: > 500 cc after 1 hour > 800 cc after 2 hours > 900 cc after 3 hours > 1000 cc after 4 hours > 1200 cc after 5 hours Sudden increase in drainage amount SVR < 800 and > 1200 dyne-sec/cm^5	Monitor VS every 15 minutes for first 4 hours, then every hour for 24 hours or until stable, including: ECG; LAP; arterial BP; HR; TPR; pulmonary artery pressures	Early assessment and intervention will facilitate optimal fluid volume balance
		Replace blood, as ordered, for chest tube drainage > 200 cc/hr with LAP < 16 mm Hg; have at least 4 units of whole blood on hand to infuse if needed	To prevent fluid volume deficit
		Administer volume (500 mL D$_5$W/m^2/24 hrs or 20 cc/m^2/hr and greater if LA < 10 or PAD < 14)	To maintain adequate cardiac output
		Be prepared to administer SPA, Ringers lactate, FFP, or PC, especially during rewarming	Rewarming has a vasodilating effect
		Monitor effects of vasodilating agents (NTG, dobutamine, Inocor, MSO$_4$, and/or renal dose dopamine), and be prepared to reduce dose, as ordered	To maintain SVR between 800 and 1200 dyne-sec/cm^5 and to prevent peripheral edema

*Care plan adapted from care plan provided by the Georgetown University Hospital Department of Nursing.

Diagnosis	Signs and symptoms	Intervention	Rationale
		Monitor PT, PTT, platelet count, and HCT closely	Need to intervene quickly in the event of bleeding disorders
	Abnormal clotting/bleeding studies	Administer protamine sulfate, cryoprecipitate, FFP, PC, platelets, and/or Amicar, as ordered	For abnormally elevated clotting studies, bleeding, or reduced platelets
		Administer antihypertensives (Nipride, NTG) to keep SBP < 150	To prevent high pressures from causing more bleeding
	Weight imbalance	Closely monitor weight	Weight provides an accurate reflection of fluid loss or gain
Potential for tissue rejection relating to: donor graft; reactive antibody greater than 20%; positive antibodies produced by recipient when crossed with donor lymphocytes	Malaise, anorexia	Closely monitor patient for acute rejection first 5–7 days, when immunosuppressive therapy is being adjusted	Patient is particularly susceptible to rejection during this time
	Decreased cardiac output and biventricular failure: malaise, lethargy; weight gain; peripheral edema; ascites; distended neck veins; anorexia; nausea and vomiting; low urine output; fever; diaphoresis; confusion; decreased peripheral pulses; crackles (rales); S_3 upon auscultation	Administer immunosuppressive drugs, as ordered, following results of endomyocardial biopsy	To prevent rejection, leading to cardiac compromise
		Closely monitor efficacy of immunosuppressive therapy ($T_3 < 5\%$ while on OKT3; $T_{11} < 5\%$ while on ALG; cyclosporine serum levels between 200 and 300 mg/mL); closely monitor for low cardiac output states and/or biventricular failure	To immunosuppress while supporting optimal cardiac function
	Decreased voltage, right axis deviation, poor R wave progression, atrial arrhythmias	Closely monitor ECG findings	Early assessment of impending cardiac compromise allows for early intervention

Nursing Care Plan for the Management of the Patient Undergoing Cardiac Transplantation

Diagnosis	Signs and symptoms	Intervention	Rationale
Potential for decreased cardiac output due to: arrhythmias; fluid volume deficit; global ischemia related to organ storage, preservation, transport time > 4 hours and/or acute rejection; hypothermia; hypertension; hypotension; increased afterload; fluid volume overload; lack of autonomic response (denervated heart does not produce catecholamines that increase heart rate to repair low output states); biventricular failure; enlarged pericardial sac due to cardiomegaly; tamponade; ventricular perforation, post biopsy	CO < 3 L/min CI < 2 L/min/m^2 Decreased distal pulses Cool extremities Arrhythmias: PVCs; heart block; SVT, PAT, atrial fibrillation, or atrial flutter (related to edematous suture line in atria); ventricular tachycardia; ventricular fibrillation	Closely monitor CO and CI every hour for first 6 hours, then every 2 hours for next 6 hours, then every 4 hours for next 12 hours	To allow for early detection and treatment of compromised cardiac output
		Administer vasoactive meds (dobutamine, Inocor) as ordered	To increase cardiac index
		Closely monitor PVCs, multifocal PVC, etc., and treat as ordered with Lidocaine bolus and infusion	Frequent PVCs lead to compromised cardiac output and efficiency
		Closely monitor ABGs and potassium in relation to PVCs and treat as ordered (KCl for K$^+$ < 3.5, sodium bicarbonate for base deficit > −3 when hypothermic)	Blood gas and electrolyte imbalances exacerbate cardiac irritability, which in turn compromises cardiac output
		Monitor sources of potassium depletion (NG, urine output, diarrhea)	To allow for correction of hypokalemia
		Atrially pace, as ordered, to keep heart rate between 80 and 120 bpm; closely monitor underlying rhythm, obtaining a strip with pacer off at least daily	To ascertain underlying rhythm and maintain adequate heart rate and rhythm
		Emergent cardioversion and/or defibrillation for ventricular tachycardia or fibrillation or decompensating atrial flutter	May be life-threatening rhythms

Diagnosis	Signs and symptoms	Intervention	Rationale
		Administer verapamil as ordered (0.075 to 0.15 mg/kg IV over 2–3 minutes)	To treat SVT
		Administer digoxin as ordered	To enhance cardiac contractility
	Fluid volume deficit: LAP < 6 mm Hg; PAD < 10; SBP < 100; urine output < 60 cc/hr during first 6 hours; excessive chest tube output; systemic bleeding; hypotension	Correct fluid volume deficit	To facilitate optimal fluid volume balance in order to maintain adequate cardiac output
		Be aware of main and interactive effects on cardiac output of selected drugs, especially atropine, tensilon, aramine, digoxin, verapamil, nifedipine, beta-blockers, and quinidine	Patient faces risk of compromised cardia rhythm and output from combinations of drugs
	Ischemia: CPK > 180 IU/L; MBs > 15 IU/L; ECG ischemic changes such as ST changes or new bundle branch block	Closely monitor serial ECGs	To ascertain any ischemic changes that may occur
		Infuse NTG, as ordered	Has a venodilating effect and decreases myocardial oxygen requirements
	Hypothermia	Monitor patient's temperature continuously via pulmonary artery catheter; apply warmed blankets and/or lights, as needed	To return patient to normothermia as soon as possible
	Hypertension (SBP > 160 mm Hg)	Administer antihypertensives (MSO_4 2–4 mg IV every 2 hours PRN; nitroprusside 0.5–8.0 mcg/kg/min; NTG 200–300 mcg/min) as ordered	To keep SBP > 100 and < 150 mm Hg

Nursing Care Plan for the Management of the Patient Undergoing Cardiac Transplantation

Diagnosis	Signs and symptoms	Intervention	Rationale
		Taper vasoconstrictive meds (epinephrine, Levophed, dobutamine, dopamine, neosynephrine) as ordered	To keep SBP > 100 and < 160 mm Hg
	Pericardial effusion on chest x-ray	Observe x-ray for effusion, and follow up	To ascertain presence of and treat pericardial effusion
	Tamponade: elevation and equalization of filling pressures (CVP = PAD = LAP = 20–30); SBP < 100 mm Hg; widening of mediastinum on chest x-ray; increased jugular venous pressure; cool and clammy skin; reduced peripheral pulses; muffled heart sounds; pulsus paradoxus > 10;	Be prepared to supply open-chest tray and/or return patient to OR	Tamponade is life-threatening and must be treated immediately
		Calculate SVR with each CO and CI	To ascertain hemodynamic status
	abrupt cessation of chest tube drainage	Be prepared to supply Fogarty catheter to physician to extract clot from chest tube	To restore patency of chest tube in a timely fashion
	Anaphylaxsis, rejection, and/or side effects of antilymphocyte therapy: increased temperature; nausea and/or vomiting; diaphoresis; bone or joint pain; rash; hypotension	Administer premedications as ordered with antilymphocyte preparation, for example: 1. with OKT3: Solucortef 100 mg IV; Benadryl 50 mg IV; Ranitidine 100 mg IV; Tylenol 650 mg PO;	To prevent or reduce side effects, anaphylaxsis, and/or rejection due to antilymphocyte therapy to maintain adequate cardiac output

30 minutes after
dose give Solucortef
100 mg IV;
at 6, 12, and 18 hrs
give:
Benadryl 25 mg IV;
Ranitidine 25 mg IV;
Tylenol 650 mg PO
2. with rabbit
antithymocyte serum
(ATS):
Tylenol 650 mg PO
every 3 hrs during
infusion
3. with equine
antilymphocyte (ALG)
Solucortef 25 mg IV;
heparin 500 units IV;
use 5-micron filter;
skin test prior to
drug administration
4. Minnesota ALG
0.02 cc of each test
allergen I.D. (rabbit
in right arm; equine
in left arm);
observe arm for 20
min for wheal and/or
flare reaction;
do not administer
product if there is
wheal and/or flare
reaction;
Tylenol 650 mg PO;
Benadryl 50 mg
PO/IM 30 min prior
to med;
repeat Tylenol and
Benadryl in 4 hrs;
Persantine 75 mg PO
qid;

With all of the above,
keep at bedside:
adrenaline 1:10,000
IV;
Benadryl 50 mg IV;
Solucortef 100 mg
IV;
microfilter on IV
tubing

Nursing Care Plan for the Management of the Patient Undergoing Cardiac Transplantation

Diagnosis	Signs and symptoms	Intervention	Rationale
		Check VS every 15 min × 4, then every 1 hr during all infusions; MD to remain at bedside 15–30 min (during peak times for anaphylaxsis) during all infusions; If anaphylaxsis develops: discontinue infusion; administer adrenalin 1:10,000/2 cc IV, Benadryl 50 mg IV, Solucortef 100 mg IV, O$_2$ by 50 percent face mask, and get help STAT	
	Perforation and/or tamponade following endomyocardial biopsy: elevated heart rate; decreased BP; increased filling pressures; widening mediastinum on chest x-ray	Monitor VS every 15 minutes for first hour after biopsy, then every 30 minutes for next hour, then per routine and as needed	To prevent and/or treat complications of biopsy that would lead to decreased cardiac output
		Institute care regimen for tamponade if it occurs	Tamponade must be treated immediately
Potential for impaired gas exchange due to: fluid volume overload; ineffective airway clearance, atelectasis, or effusion; bronchospasm; inadequate supplemental oxygen; inadequate tidal volume; low hematocrit and	Abnormal ABGs: pO$_2$ < 80 mm Hg; pCO$_2$ < 35 or > 45 mm Hg; pH < 7.35 or > 7.45; O$_2$ sat. < 80%; HCO$_3$ < 20 or > 26 mEq/L; BE < 0 or > 3 Cyanosis ETT cuff leak Lowered peak pressure	Mechanically ventilate for 8–12 hours postoperatively, as ordered Closely monitor for absent, unequal, or diminished breath sounds, crackles, wheezing, or asymmetrical chest wall expansion; closely monitor ABGs PRN and after ventilator	Ventilation support is needed until stabilization To discover early indications of ensuing respiratory compromise and/or complications

Diagnosis	Signs and symptoms	Intervention	Rationale
hemoglobin levels; low cardiac output; excessive pulmonary vascular resistance; malpositioned ETT or inadequate cuff volume; pneumothorax or hemothorax	Inadequate volume exchange Chest x-ray indicates atelectasis, effusion, pneumothorax, or hemothorax Copious secretions Elevated respiratory rate, wheezing, air hunger, gasping, or asymmetrical expansion of chest wall	changes; obtain chest x-ray immediately and PRN postoperatively and examine for ETT placement, lung expansion (pneumothorax), width of mediastinal shadow, presence of pleural fluid, and presence of foreign body Aggressive pulmonary toilet PRN with chest percussion therapy, incentive spirometry, and hyperinflation using 100% O_2 before and after suctioning; turn and reposition patient every 2 hours	To mobilize secretions, provide adequate oxygenation, and open closed alveoli
		If patient is stable, promote extubation by: holding sedation after midnight on day of surgery; elevating HOB 30 degrees; decreasing IMV by increments of 2–4 breaths/min if $pO_2 > 90$, pH 7.35–7.45, and O_2 sat. 90–100%	To assist patient to return to optimal breathing capacity as soon as possible (to prevent atelectasis, secondary infection, etc.)
	Hematocrit level less than 30 with abnormal ABGs	Administer packed cells as ordered	To improve hematocrit and oxygen-carrying ability
	Cardiac index < 2.5 $L/min/m^2$	Correct low cardiac output	To maintain adequate cardiac function and tissue perfusion and oxygenation
	Excessive PVR (>120 dyne-sec/cm^5)	Administer prostaglandin E or thomboxine as ordered	To counteract excessive PVR
	Copious secretions Respirations > 30 bpm	Administer theophylline by infusion and bronchodilator (Alupent, Bronchosol) through ventilator or increase FIO_2 as ordered	To improve breathing capacity

Nursing Care Plan for the Management of the Patient Undergoing Cardiac Transplantation

Diagnosis	Signs and symptoms	Intervention	Rationale
	Signs of fluid overload: crackles on auscultation; $pO_2 < 90$ mm Hg; chest x-ray indicative of fluid overload; PAD > 20 mm Hg; LAP > 20 mm Hg; urine output < 30 cc/hr; weight gain > 5 kg; frothy sputum	Administer diuretics PRN or as ordered	To facilitate diuresis of extra fluid volume
Potential for infection due to: immunosuppressive therapy; invasive hemodynamic lines; indwelling urinary catheter; endotracheal tube; intravenous catheters; surgical drains; surgical incisions; poor nutritional state; stress of surgery	Incisional infection: elevated temperature, elevated WBCs, redness, exudate, increased tenderness, induration of surgical incision	Inspect incisions, catheter or line insertion sites, wire insertion site every 8 hours for erythema, inflammation, or drainage and paint with povidone-iodine solution followed by dry, sterile, occlusive dressing every day and PRN	To keep patient free from infection
		Monitor VS closely	To watch for signs of infection
		Utilize and teach family about protective isolation: 3-minute handwash with povidone-iodine scrub; wear disposable mask, gloves, gown, and hair cover; absolutely no personnel/visitors with infectious process in room (sore throat, cold sores, cough, etc.); restrict visitors to immediate family only; no children under 12 years old to visit	Isolation minimizes risk of infection

Diagnosis	Signs and symptoms	Intervention	Rationale
		Use TBQ solution (or equivalent) and change solution every 4 days: clean *all* equipment entering room; maintain all housekeeping routines	To destroy bacteria
		No personnel caring for infected patients may cross over to heart transplant proximity	To prevent spread of infection
		Replace bath basin and slippers weekly; change all equipment (respiratory tubing, face mask, nasal cannula, suction cannister, etc.) daily; maintain clean and tidy patient care room	To keep patient free from infection To prevent bacteria from colonizing on heated, moist surfaces of respiratory equipment
	Infection from intravenous lines: redness, induration, pain, exudate at line insertion site	Change IV site every 48 hours; IV site care every day	To prevent infection from IV site
		Change IV tubing and solutions every 24 hours	
		Discontinue IV ASAP	
	Pulmonary infection: changes in characteristics of sputum (tan, brown, yellow, or green color or foul odor), chest x-ray indicative of atelectasis, decreased or absent breath sounds locally	Inspect mouth for thrush and/or ulcerations t.i.d. prior to Mycostatin mouthwash	To prevent and treat any fungal or viral infection in mouth
		Instill NS, hyperventilate, and suction ET tube using sterile technique every 2–3 hours while patient is intubated	
		Assess sputum for amount and character and get culture and sensitivity, as ordered or PRN	
		Closely monitor chest x-rays for evidence of atelectasis and/or infiltrates	

Diagnosis	Signs and symptoms	Intervention	Rationale
		Auscultate lung fields every 6 hours and PRN	
		CPT every 4–6 hours	
		Incentive spirometry every 1–2 hours while patient is awake (post extubation); assist patient to cough and deep breathe after incentive spirometry	
		Assist patient to change positions from side to side every 2–3 hours	To prevent atelectasis, which can serve as an antecedent to respiratory infection
		Assess need for pain medication prior to coughing and deep breathing and/or activities of daily living	Effort will be stronger if patient is not impeded by discomfort
		Administer antibiotics, as ordered	To prevent or fight any beginning infection
	Urinary infection: sediment in urine, WBC in urine, hesitancy, frequency, urgency, burning, difficulty starting stream, inability to void	Urine culture and sensitivity (routine/fungal/gram stain) every day while Foley is in place; urine for CMV	To allow for early detection and treatment of urinary tract infections
		Routine catheter care every 8 hours	To prevent infection
		Low-bacteria diet (no unpeeled fruit, fresh lettuce, garnishes, etc.)	To minimize bacterial intake
		Use paper services for 2 weeks postoperatively	To decrease the chance of spread of infection
Potential for liver, renal, gastrointestinal, cardiac, and/or pulmonary dysfunction due to: immunosuppressive drug therapy; administration of	Renal dysfunction: urine output < 30 cc/hr and/or rising BUN and creatinine	12-hour urine for creatinine clearance every other day; guaiac test urine as needed; check urine for glucose while patient is on steroids	To allow for early diagnosis and treatment of renal complications and injury

Diagnosis	Signs and symptoms	Intervention	Rationale
corticosteroids; ischemic time of transplanted heart more than 4 hours	Liver dysfunction: elevated LFTs (LDH > 180 IU/L, SGOT > 42 IU/L, SGPT > 60 IU/L, T bili > 1.5 mg/dL)	Closely monitor and report lab levels; check for bleeding gums; guaiac test all stools	To allow for early diagnosis and treatment of hepatic complications and injury
	Cardiac dysfunction: ECG changes (new Q waves, ST segment elevation and/or depression), elevated MB/CPK, clinical signs of decreased cardiac output	CPK-MB every 8 hours	To allow for early diagnosis and treatment of cardiac complications and injury
	Gastric dysfunction: guaiac-positive stools, lack of bowel sounds, distended abdomen, cramping, decreased Hct, upper and lower GI bleeding	Guaiac test all stools Progress diet as tolerated	To allow for early diagnosis and treatment of gastric complications and injury
	Pulmonary dysfunction: increase in rate and amount of sputum, increase in congestion, compromised ABGs	Mechanical ventilator support as needed; vigorous pulmonary toilet	To allow for early diagnosis and treatment of pulmonary complications and injury
Potential for alteration in bowel function (constipation) due to: decreased mobility; change in eating patterns; side effects of medications; postoperative paralytic ileus; decreased fluid volume	Reports of feeling constipated, "full" feeling in abdomen, inability to move bowels Decreased or absent bowel sounds Inadequate oral fluid/food intake as evidenced on I&O records and calorie counts	Assess abdomen for bowel sounds, softness, and appearance and ask patient about discomfort at least every 12 hours Encourage progressive ambulation and activity, as tolerated Reassure patient that constipation is frequently a problem postoperatively	To allow for early diagnosis of constipation, in order to intervene before problems become serious To stimulate peristalsis So patient will not become overly concerned
	Symptoms of dehydration: poor skin turgor; sunken eyes; intake < output; weight loss	Assess for signs of dehydration and encourage oral fluid intake, unless patient is on fluid restriction Closely monitor electrolytes	Hydration impedes constipation Dehydration leads to electrolyte imbalance

Nursing Care Plan for the Management of the Patient Undergoing Cardiac Transplantation

Diagnosis	Signs and symptoms	Intervention	Rationale
	Absence of bowel movement for more than 2 days	Implement bowel regimen as ordered: milk of magnesia 30 mL PO every h.s.; consult with dietician about increased fiber in diet; rehydrate patient, as ordered, via IV or oral fluids	Patient may need extra help to start peristalsis postoperatively
		Reduce narcotic consumption when feasible	Narcotics inhibit bowel activity
Potential for alteration in bowel function (diarrhea) due to: side effects of cardiac medications and/or antibiotics; bacterial infections; change in eating patterns	Diarrhea or frequent liquid stools Hyperactive bowel sounds	Assess abdomen for hyperactive bowel sounds	To allow for early intervention
		Educate patient about medications that may cause diarrhea	To help patient understand cause
		Assess fluid status in attempt to avoid dehydration and monitor electrolytes	Diarrhea quickly leads to dehydration and electrolyte imbalance
		Implement treatment as ordered: antidiarrheal medication; rehydration; change of cardiac medications or antibiotics if possible, to relieve diarrhea	To prevent further systemic complications
		Culture for clostridia difficile, as ordered	High risk for diarrhea; should be treated as soon as possible
Potential for alteration in nutritional status due to: anorexia and malaise during rejection;	Complaints of lack of appetite	Assess patient's appetite with patient and family and decide which allowable foods sound appealing	To facilitate patient's healthy nutritional status in any way acceptable

Diagnosis	Signs and symptoms	Intervention	Rationale
nausea and vomiting associated with rejection or steroid therapy; increased nutritional requirements due to surgical stress; less appealing taste of food, related to low-sodium and low-bacteria diet; constipation, diarrhea, abdominal cramping, or flatus	Patient eats only small portions on tray	Monitor tray after meals for amount eaten	To ascertain type and amount of food intake for calorie counts
		Calculate calorie intake	To ensure adequate calorie intake for healing
	Trend toward weight loss	Weigh patient daily	To ensure patient compliance with prescribed diet
	Decreased fluid intake	Consult with dietician about food preferences and review low-bacteria diet	
		Provide as much preferred food as possible	To provide for as much calorie intake as possible
		Assess lab data	To ascertain nutritional status and evaluate patient's adherence to diet
	Pain or discomfort	Medicate 30 minutes before meal to alleviate pain, which reduces appetite	To provide for as good an appetite as possible
Potential for skin breakdown due to: restriction in movement; pain or discomfort; drug-induced neuromuscular or musculoskeletal impairment; depression; stiffness from extended catheterization and/or time on operating table; diaphoresis or drainage into patient's bed; independent variables such as diabetes, peripheral vascular disease, obesity, etc.	Imposed restriction of movement due to body mechanics, medical protocol, etc.	Put air mattress on all postoperative beds	To prevent pressure spots on skin
	Impaired coordination or decreased muscle strength preventing independent movement	Assist patient with required movements and with a quarter turn every 1–2 hours	To prevent injury and facilitate movement
	Reluctance to attempt movement	Premedicate PRN or as ordered to decrease discomfort accompanying movement	To facilitate movement
	Redness over pressure points	Inspect skin pressure points, including occiput, sacrum, coccyx, heels, and elbows, every 2 hours	To prevent skin breakdown

Nursing Care Plan for the Management of the Patient Undergoing Cardiac Transplantation

Diagnosis	Signs and symptoms	Intervention	Rationale
		Passive range of motion to all extremities	To prevent pressure spots and improve circulation without increasing oxygen demand
		Keep patient dry	To prevent skin breakdown
		Maintain and supplement nutrition as needed	To maintain vital nutrients to skin
		Consult enterostomal therapist for actual breakdown	For optimal care planning and intervention
	Elevated temperature	Keep patient dry when diaphoretic	To prevent skin breakdown
Potential for alteration in health maintenance due to knowledge deficit concerning: diagnosis; surgical procedure; medications; diet; activity; medical follow-up; referrals; when to notify MD; self-monitoring	Inability to describe personal diagnosis and how it relates to type of surgery	Instruct patient and family about diagnosis and surgery	Patient and family must understand what is being done and why
		Encourage questions and discussion of problems and concerns	To allow for greatest learning
	Inability to identify medications and their schedules	Instruct patient about medications: what they look like; names and doses; indications; side effects and what can be done; daily schedule; standard drug information and complete medication schedule	Safe and accurate medication regimen is necessary
	Inability to list foods appropriate for personal diet	Provide instruction on low-sodium, modified-fat/cholesterol diet; consult with dietician	To facilitate healing and prevent complications arising from incorrect diet

Diagnosis	Signs and symptoms	Intervention	Rationale
	Inability to distinguish between permitted and prohibited progression of activities	Discuss activity instructions: activities in routine; balancing rest and activity; progressive walking schedule; no lifting more than 20 pounds; no driving for 6 weeks; stopping every hour for a short walk when taking long car trips; resumption of sexual activities	To allow for progressive resumption of activities without risk of overdoing it and precipitating an untoward event

In the event of an accident, steering wheel may crush incompletely healed sternum; walking increases circulation and prevents prolonged venous pooling |
	Lack of knowledge about follow-up appointments	Help patient and family to arrange follow-up appointments	Plans for follow-up care must be initiated as soon as possible
	Inability to identify professional services available for support	Advise patient and family of services and resources available	To provide most comprehensive and effective services to patient and family
	Inability to explain when to notify MD or seek emergency assistance	Review with patient and family when to notify MD: angina, SOB, dizziness, or nausea during or following activity; weight gain of more than 1 lb/day; signs of infected incision, including redness, swelling, increased tenderness, drainage; temperature > 101°F; irregular/fast heart rate	Patient and family need to know what to do in the case of an untoward event
	Inability to properly count pulse, assess weight fluctuations, and/or take temperature	Instruct patient and family and require return demonstration: weighing self and recording weight; taking temperature and pulse and recording them	Patient and family need to increase self-help abilities

697

Nursing Care Plan for the Management of the Patient Undergoing Cardiac Transplantation

Diagnosis	Signs and symptoms	Intervention	Rationale
	Inability to verbalize significance of weight changes	Instruct patient on meaning of weight gain and what to do in its event	To increase patient's self-help abilities in preventing congestive failure

Potential for anxiety due to:
  fear of unknown;
  fear of death;
  fear of disfigurement;
  fear of pain;
  fear of disability;
  lack of knowledge regarding hospital and/or operative procedures, routines
	Facial tension
	Distracted behavior
	Low attention span
	Withdrawal
	Twitching and shaking of extremities
	Inappropriate laughter or behavior
	Diaphoresis
	Tachycardia
	PVCs
	Other arrhythmias
	Nonadherence to treatment plan
		Ascertain patient's fears and anxieties	Will allow the nurse to know just what to address

		Ascertain patient's previous hospital experiences (own as well as others')	Will help the nurse to know how to best alleviate anxieties or support positive attitudes
		Ascertain patient's and family's readiness to learn	Need to begin patient and family education when ready

		Teach patient about:
		  routine of lab, radiology, ECG, house staff;
		  surgery, isolation techniques, incisions, tubes, lines, operation length, ICU routine, visiting hours, pain medication, and deep breathing and coughing; provide patient with educational booklets
			To help patient and family be prepared for what is to be experienced

		Give ICU tour, if desired	To familiarize patient with environment
		Sedate patient, as ordered or PRN	To help patient relax
		Provide emotional support as needed	To help patient and family deal with the situation in the best way possible
		Consult with social worker, chaplain, etc., as needed	Multidisciplinary team effort provides broader, more comprehensive care

Medications Commonly Used in the Care of the Patient Undergoing Cardiac Transplantation

Medication	Effect	Major side effects
Acetaminophen (Tylenol)	Analgesic Antipyretic	Hemolytic anemia Skin rash Fever Vascular collapse
Aminophylline	Bronchodilator Pulmonary vasodilator Relaxes smooth muscles of bronchial airways and pulmonary blood vessels Cardiac stimulant	Gastrointestinal upset, nausea and vomiting Dizziness, vertigo Headache Tachycardias, extrasystoles
Aminocaproic acid (Amicar)	Fibrinolysis inhibitor to enhance hemostasis	Nausea Cramps and diarrhea Hypotension Dizziness Tinnitus Headache Nasal stuffiness Skin rash
Amrinone lactate (Inocor)	Cardiac inotropic Vasodilator Increases cardiac output	Thrombocytopenia Gastrointestinal upset, nausea and vomiting Arrhythmias Hypotension
Antiarrhythmias (as per dysrhythmia section)	As per specific medication	As per specific medication
Antibiotics	As per specific drug	As per specific drug
Atropine	Increased myocardial contractility Increased ventricular excitability	Dry mouth Ventricular irritability Difficulty in voiding
Beta blockers (nadolol, propranolol, metaprolol)	Blocked beta adrenergic stimulation leading to decreased myocardial oxygen demand	Hypotension Bradycardia Heart failure Bronchoconstriction Elevated cholesterol Altered glucose metabolism
Bronchosol Theophylline Alupent	Bronchodilator Increased renal blood flow Positive inotropic effect on heart	Cardiac arrhythmias Gastrointestinal upset

Medications Commonly Used in the Care of the Patient Undergoing Cardiac Transplantation

Medication	Effect	Major side effects
Calcium channel blockers (nifedipine, diltiazem, verapamil)	Vasodilation leading to increased coronary blood supply and decreased myocardial oxygen demands Antidysrhythmia	Hypotension Bradycardia (verapamil and diltiazem) Headaches, dizziness Altered glucose tolerance Diarrhea (nifedipine) Constipation (verapamil)
Calcium chloride	Increased myocardial contractility Increased ventricular excitability	Mild hypotension Hypercalcemia Local necrosis upon extravasation
Diazepam (Valium)	Sedative	Drowsiness Fatigue Ataxia
Digitalis (Digoxin)	Increased contractility Lengthened refractory period of AV node Decreased left ventricular end diastolic pressure Increased ventricular automaticity Decreased atrial automaticity	Tachycardias AV blocks Bradycardias Gastrointestinal upset Headache Drowsiness Confusion Double vision
Diphenhydramine hydrochloride (Benedryl)	Antihistamine Anticholinergic	Hypotension, dizziness Headache Tachycardias, extrasystoles Epigastric distress Sedation Thickening of bronchial secretions
Dipyridamole (Persantin)	Platelet adhesion inhibitor Decreased thromboembolic events	Dizziness Abdominal distress, diarrhea, vomiting Headache Rash

Diuretics
  Furosemide (Lasix)
  Ethacrynic acid
	Diuresis
	Decreased pulmonary congestion
		Hypokalemia
		Hypocalcemia
		Hypomagnesemia
		Altered glucose metabolism

Dobutamine Dopamine	Inotropic with alpha-adrenergic stimulant Increased myocardial contractility, output, and stroke volume Dilator of renal and mesenteric vessels in low doses	Gastrointestinal upset Angina Dyspnea Headache Hypotension Ectopic arrhythmias Palpitations Vasoconstriction

Medication	Effect	Major side effects
Docusate sodium (Colace)	Stool softener	Bitter taste Nausea Throat irritation
Edrophonium (Tensilon)	Short- and rapid-acting cholinergic Curare antagonist	Convulsions Increased tracheobronchial secretions Laryngospasm Bronchoconstriction Arrhythmias (bradycardias) Hypotension Nausea and vomiting Diarrhea and cramping Urinary frequency
Epinephrine	Stimulates alpha and beta receptor sites causing increased heart rate, myocardial contractility, systemic vascular resistance, automaticity, and myocardial oxygen consumption	Headache Anxiety Palpitations Hyperglycemia
Heparin	Anticoagulant	Bleeding
Hydrocortisone sodium succinate (Solu-Cortef)	Anti-inflammatory adrenocortical steroid	Sodium retention Fluid retention leading to congestive failure Hypokalemic alkalosis Hypertension Muscle weakness Peptic ulcer Convulsions Headache, vertigo
Hydralazine Minoxidil Diazoxide	Vasodilator with a direct action on vascular smooth muscle leading to relaxed arterioles, decreased vascular resistance, and increased cardiac output	Angina Nausea and vomiting Tachycardia Headache Flushing Hypotension
Immunosuppressants (Imuran)	Immunosuppressive metabolite	Secondary infections Leukopenia Nausea and vomiting, diarrhea Skin rash
Isopreoterenol (Isuprel)	Stimulates beta receptor sites and relaxes smooth muscle leading to increased myocardial contractility, heart rate, and myocardial oxygen demand and decreased peripheral vascular resistance	Tachycardias Ventricular irritability Hypotension Headache, flushing Angina Gastrointestinal upset Dizziness, weakness, tremors

Medications Commonly Used in the Care of the Patient Undergoing Cardiac Transplantation

Medication	Effect	Major side effects
Laxatives	Promote bowel function	Diarrhea Electrolyte imbalance
Metaraminal bitartrate (Aramine)	Potent sympathomimetic amine with increased systolic and diastolic blood pressure Positive inotropic effect on heart Peripheral vasoconstrictor	Arrhythmias Ventricular tachycardias
Methoxamine (Vasoxyl)	Vasoconstriction Alpha adrenergic receptor stimulator	Cardiac arrhythmias Bradycardias
Morphine sulfate	Analgesia Peripheral vasodilation Sedation Bronchodilation	Hypotension Respiratory depression Nausea and vomiting Constipation Urinary retention
Neosynephrine (phenylephrine hydrochloride)	Sympathomimetic Alpha-adrenergic Potent vasoconstrictor and pressor	Headache Bradycardias Arrhythmias Excitability, restlessness
Nitroglycerin	Vasodilation leading to increased coronary blood supply and decreased myocardial oxygen demand	Hypotension Headache
Nitroprusside (Nipride)	Vasodilator with a direct action on vascular smooth muscle	Nausea and vomiting Muscle twitching Hypotension
Nystatin (Mycostatin)	Antifungal antibiotic	Oral irritation (rarely)
Prostaglandin E	Arteriolar and bronchiolar dilation Inhibition of platelet aggregation	Flushing Apnea Bradycardia Hypotension Fever Seizures
Protamine sulfate	Anticoagulant when administered alone; in the presence of heparin it is inactivated (as is heparin)	Hypotension Bradycardia Pulmonary hypertension, dyspnea Flushing

Medication	Effect	Major side effects
Quinidine	Increased refractory period Decreased excitability Decreased myocardial contractility Increased conduction time Decreased automaticity of pacemaker cells	Nausea and vomiting Heart blocks Ventricular irritability Hypotension Thrombocytopenia Vertigo Tinnitus
Ranitidine hydrochloride (Zantac)	Histamine inhibitor Basal gastric acid secretion inhibitor	Pain and burning at site of IM or IV injection Vertigo Tachyarrhythmias and bradyarrhythmias Nausea and vomiting Constipation Diarrhea Hepatic compromise
Sodium bicarbonate	Alkaline buffer that corrects metabolic acidosis	Metabolic alkalosis Hypernatremia Fluid overload
Warfarin (Coumadin)	Anticoagulant by inhibiting vitamin K synthesis	Hemorrhage Tissue necrosis GI upset Fever

Vascular Disorders

Arterial disease due to atherosclerosis may present in three ways: coronary artery disease, cerebrovascular accident, and aortic or peripheral disease. It is difficult to estimate the number of persons afflicted with aortic or peripheral vascular disease since many never experience an acute episode of the disease and are able to tolerate it without medical or surgical intervention. Nevertheless, 1,493,000 surgical procedures, excluding cardiac, were performed in the United States in 1987, an increase from the 1,370,000 performed in 1986.[55]

This section will focus on diseases of the arterial circulation because this system is involved in the cases of the majority of patients admitted to critical care following surgical intervention. Arterial circulation problems may be occlusive or aneurysmal in nature and interventions include surgery on the aorta, lower and upper extremity reconstruction, and renovascular bypass.

Clinical antecedents

The majority of arterial disease is due to atherosclerosis. As described in the earlier section that addresses CAD, the exact mechanism of atherosclerosis is not known, but two theories predominate. The insudation (lipid) theory proposes that high levels of circulating LDL infiltrate arterial walls, stimulating smooth muscle cell production and the deposition of lipids within and amongst these cells. The encrustation theory proposes that atherosclerosis is due to endothelial injury of the arterial wall caused by turbulent blood flow. This promotes platelet aggregation and the release of growth factors, which leads to smooth muscle cell proliferation.

Risk factors for atherosclerosis of the aorta and extremities are the same as for CAD, the three major modifiable risk factors being cigarette smoking, hypertension, and hypercholesterolemia; family history, or heredity, is a nonmodifiable risk factor. Contributing factors include diabetes mellitus, hypertriglyceridemia, obesity, hyperuricemia, sedentary life-style, and stress.

There are a number of other disorders that comprise a small portion of vascular disease. Raynaud's phenomenon includes a vasospastic disorder most commonly affecting women. The patient tends to have normal vessels but exhibits hypersensitive vasoconstrictive responses to cold and stress. Other disorders involve arterial compression by an abnormal muscle or fibrous band, as in thoracic outlet syndrome, in which the brachial plexus, subclavian vein, or artery is compressed as it passes between the rib and clavicle.

Arterial trauma and resultant compartment syndrome are also known to cause arterial disruption. Blunt or penetrating trauma may result in direct injury to the artery. Damage to the artery following trauma is, however, most frequently due to fractured bones, particularly in the area of joints, where the vessels are in a more fixed position. Compartment syndrome results from increased pressure within the muscular compartment. It first involves decreased perfusion of the capillary bed and occurs at intracompartmental pressures of 30–40 mm Hg or even less. Arterial involvement and loss of pulses is a late sign.

Arterial emboli may occur and cause occlusion of a peripheral artery. These emboli commonly arise from mural thrombi within the heart. Unlike arteriosclerotic occlusions, arterial emboli result in an acute episode of ischemia, with resultant hemodynamic alterations.

Congenital anomalies may also be a cause of arterial disease. These include both gross defects, such as coarctation of the aorta or anomalous arterial branches, and histological changes due to, for example, Marfan's syndrome.

Patients with renovascular hypertension have disruption in the perfusion of the kidney, which results in activation of the renin-angiotensin system. Ninety percent of all renal artery lesions in hypertensive patients are caused by either atherosclerosis or fibromuscular dysplasia. Other, much less common, etiologies include renal artery thrombosis or embolism, dissection, neoplasm, trauma, or extrinsic compression.[56]

Critical referents

As noted previously, alterations in the arterial circulation will most likely present as occlusions or aneurysms. Less likely is the development of an arteriovenous malformation or vasospasm.

Vessels are composed of three layers; the tunica intima, tunica media, and tunica adventitia. The intima is the innermost layer and is composed primarily of endothelial cells. The media is the middle layer and is made up mostly of smooth muscle cells, collagen, and elastic fibers. The outermost layer, the adventitia, is composed of connective tissue and provides strength to the arterial wall. The vasa vasorum are small blood vessels that provide nutrients to the adventitia and portions of the media. The intima and inner portion of the media receive nutrition directly from the blood flowing through the artery.

Arteries may be classified by their function as conductive or distributive. Conductive arteries follow relatively straight courses, have few branches, and are most severely affected by atherosclerosis.[57] Examples include the aorta and superficial femoral arteries. Distributive arteries are smaller. They arise from conductive arteries and divide into numerous smaller arteries. Examples include the splenic and mesenteric arteries. In addition, arteries vary in composition according to their size and distribution. For example, the aortic arteries, in contrast to the peripheral arteries, contain very little smooth muscle, although there is a network of some smooth muscle and collagen between the elastic membranes.[58] Occlusions of conductive arteries are more likely to require surgical intervention as they supply a greater

area and are less influenced by collateral circulation. Figure 4-75 displays the arterial circulation.

Histological changes that occur in atherosclerosis may cause either occlusion or aneurysm formation. In general, alterations in the intimal lining of the artery result in occlusion, whereas damage to the medial layer results in aneurysm formation. However, certain areas are more prone to one condition than the other. For example, the lack of vasa vasorum in the abdominal aorta may promote aneurysm formation, because inadequate nutrition weakens the vessel wall. Areas of high turbulence at bifurcations are more prone to damage of the intimal lining.

Changes within the vessel may begin in childhood and are described as a fatty streak. Some of these fatty streaks may develop into fibrous plaques composed of smooth muscle cells. These fibrous plaques may lead to a more complicated lesion due to

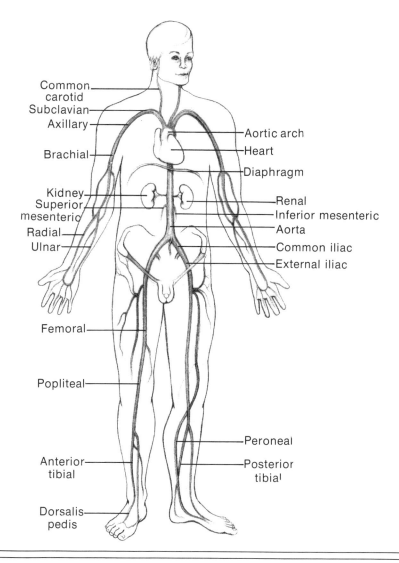

Figure 4-75   Arterial Circulation

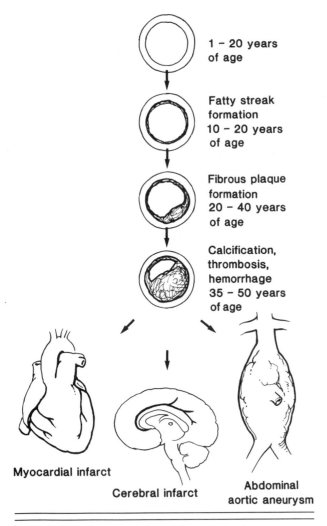

1 – 20 years
of age

Fatty streak
formation
10 – 20 years
of age

Fibrous plaque
formation
20 – 40 years
of age

Calcification,
thrombosis,
hemorrhage
35 – 50 years
of age

Myocardial infarct

Cerebral infarct

Abdominal
aortic aneurysm

Figure 4-76   Genesis of Atherosclerotic Lesions

in the aortic arch, where it may dissect back into the aortic valve and cause cardiac ischemia.

Approximately three-quarters of all arteriosclerotic aortic aneurysms are confined to the abdominal aorta.

The atherosclerotic process erodes the aortic wall, destroying the medial elastic elements. This causes weakening of the aortic wall and eventually leads to aneurysm formation. In the thorax, saccular aneurysms are more common, while in the abdomen, a fusiform aneurysm is more common. As the aorta widens, tension in the wall of the aorta rises in accordance with Laplace's law, which states that tension is proportional to the product of pressure and radius. Further widening results in greater tension, which in turn leads to acceleration in the rate of enlargement of the aneurysm. A vicious circle is thus established, which produces dilatation that is often rapidly progressive. Hypertension may also contribute to the pathogenesis of these aneurysms.[59]

Erosion of adjacent organs may occur and may be a physical finding on examination. This erosion may also result in arteriovenous malformation.

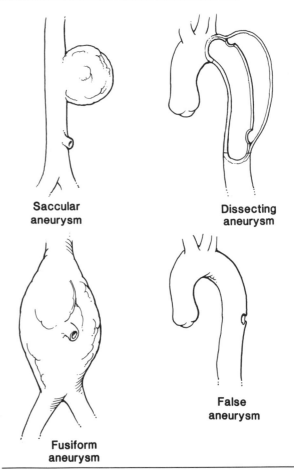

Saccular
aneurysm

Dissecting
aneurysm

Fusiform
aneurysm

False
aneurysm

Figure 4-77   Aneurysm Types

hemorrhage, ulceration, or thrombus within the plaque. Figure 4-76 diagrams the history of the atherosclerotic lesion.

An aneurysm is a bulging of the arterial wall with resultant tearing and blood accumulation. It can continue to enlarge or become chronic, with eventual calcification. Aneurysms may be classified as true or false (Figure 4-77). False aneurysms involve a complete tear in all three arterial layers. The sac is composed of connective tissue, and this generally is considered the more stable of the aneurysms. True aneurysms involve tearing into the layers of the arterial wall; they are called fusiform, saccular, or dissecting. A fusiform aneurysm is a circumferential enlargement surrounding a segment of the artery. A saccular aneurysm is a bulbular pouch of the artery. A dissecting aneurysm occurs when blood follows the cavity between the arterial layers. It may dissect antegrade or retrograde and most commonly occurs

Arterial disease may be diagnosed in a variety of ways, from secondary findings during a routine physical examination to hemorrhagic emergency caused by a ruptured aneurysm. The signs and symptoms will depend on the size and location of the process as well as the progression of the disease. Assessment of a patient with suspected arterial disease includes history and physical examination, radiologic and Doppler examination, digital subtraction angiography, CAT scan or MRI, and arteriography.

Aneurysms Aneurysms are considered significant when they measure 4 cm or greater or when they produce symptoms. Serial monitoring of aneurysms is important in order to note the progression of the arterial disease. Aneurysms larger than 6 cm carry a much greater risk of rupture.

The history and physical examination include identifying the patient's chief complaint. The patient presenting with thoracic aneurysms may complain of wheezing, cough, dyspnea, hemoptysis, hoarseness, dysphagia, and atypical chest discomfort. The chest discomfort is usually different from angina in that it feels as though it is boring or stabbing and may be pulsatile. However, the patient may be asymptomatic. Physical findings may include deviation of the trachea or a pulsatile mass above the clavicle. The patient with an abdominal aneurysm is usually asymptomatic but may occasionally complain of back discomfort that is not affected by movement. In the thin person, a pulsatile mass may be felt or a bruit may be heard on auscultation. Spontaneous rupture into an adjacent vein may occur and result in a cardiac output failure.

The patient presenting with a ruptured thoracic or abdominal aneurysm is at increased risk for complications in the postoperative period or death. In fact, death may ensue before surgery can be attempted, as a result of tremendous blood loss from the aorta. The patient undergoing emergency aortic aneurysm repair is at increased risk for complications such as disseminated intravascular coagulation (DIC) and renal failure. DIC may be due to tremendous blood loss and the need for massive blood transfusions. Acute tubular necrosis occurs because the renal arteries are more likely to be cross-clamped due to the lack of time available to perform an adequate preoperative assessment and diagnostic work-up. Massive blood transfusions also add to the cellular debris that can potentiate acute tubular necrosis.

A dissecting thoracic aneurysm may involve the aortic valve. In this case, the coronary arteries are no longer perfused and myocardial infarction ensues. Heart failure and tamponade may arise as consequences of the MI and dissection. If the dissection moves distally, there may be an occlusion of one or more of the branches of the aorta, resulting in differential arm pressures, stroke, renal failure, bowel ischemia, or even limb loss.[60]

Chest roentgenograms and fluoroscopy may be helpful in identifying thoracic aneurysms. Aortic angiography is the definitive procedure for outlining an aneurysm, making a diagnosis, and revealing the anatomical features of the aneurysm.[61] However, it carries many risks, such as embolization of the thrombus as well as dissection. Digital subtraction angiography may be of use since it eliminates the need for arterial injection and thus decreases some of the risks. Ultrasound is generally not used for thoracic aneurysms because it is not sufficiently accurate, but it is frequently used for suspected abdominal aneurysms or to view portions of the aortic arch, especially in suspected dissection. Angiography, on the other hand, may not be as accurate in the abdomen because of possible calcification of adjacent organs. CAT scan with contrast medium and magnetic resonance imaging are useful for identifying both thoracic and abdominal aneurysms, including their size and any retroperitoneal bleeds.

Occlusions The patient with occlusive disease may present with a variety of symptoms depending on the disease's onset and the existence of collateral circulation. The patient may complain of pain, parathesis, faint pulse, and coolness of the extremity. Intermittent claudication, which causes pain on exertion that disappears with rest, may occur. An acute embolic episode frequently results in excruciating pain unless it is superimposed on existing arterial disease. In that case, the patient may have developed collateral circulation within the area of narrowing. The extremity is usually pale or cyanotic and has sluggish capillary refill. Relief of pain occurs when the extremity is in a dependent position.

Doppler examination is most commonly used for examination of the extremity. Flow velocity waveforms are obtained by placing the Doppler at various pulse points along the extremity. Normally, the waveform is triphasic (Figure 4-78). In the presence of arterial disease, this waveform becomes dampened. Both extremities are evaluated, for comparison. Segmental lower-extremity BP measurements are useful in evaluating occlusive disease. Through calculations, an index is derived that compares lower-

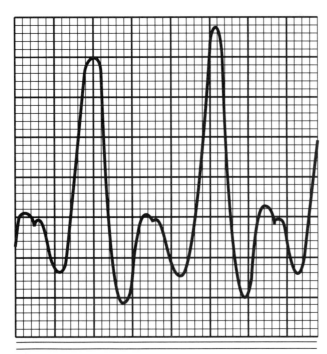

Figure 4-78   Doppler Triphasic Waveform

extremity BP to brachial BP. Arteriography is useful for both upper-extremity and lower-extremity occlusions. Digital subtraction angiography is of limited usefulness as it provides a minimal view of the arterial fields.

The patient with distal occlusion to small arteries is less likely to be a surgical candidate. The diabetic tends to have an increased incidence of diffuse distal disease. The majority of diabetics have vascular disease, and this accounts for 75% of their deaths.[62] Unfortunately, diabetic patients also experience a higher amputation rate, despite revascularization surgery. The exact reason for this is not known.

Renovascular hypertension   The patient with renovascular hypertension will present with severe hypertension that may be acute in onset. Since 90% of all cases of hypertension are essential in nature, renovascular hypertension should be suspected in the following cases:

1. Hypertension before age 25, especially with DBP > 110 mm Hg
2. Hypertension that is of sudden onset and is labile
3. Recent onset of hypertension after age 50
4. Hypertension accompanied by retinal changes.[63]

Renovascular hypertension is due to both the vasoconstriction caused by the renin-angiotensin activat-

ing system and the activation of aldosterone production, resulting in sodium and fluid overload. This discovery was made by Goldblatt, who experimentally tied off the renal arteries in dogs to induce hypertension, then subsequently released the arteries and recorded a resultant decrease in blood pressure.[64] Diagnostic studies for renovascular hypertension include renal vein renin assays, rapid-sequence intravenous pyelography, isotope renography, and renal arteriography.[65]

Nursing standards of care

Management of the patient with arterial disease involves both surgical and medical interventions. Surgical interventions include arterial bypass grafting, endarterectomy, percutaneous transluminal angioplasty, and resection.

The most common approaches for arterial occlusion are either to open the artery and remove the obstruction via endarterectomy or to bypass the obstruction via an end-to-end or end-to-side anastomosis graft. End-to-end anastomosis involves total bypass of the occluded areas and thus does not allow for perfusion to side arteries that branch off close to the occluded area. End-to-side anastomosis allows blood flow around the occluded area as well as through it. Partial occlusions may benefit from this procedure. Indications include symptomatic limb ischemia that causes the patient a life-style or occupational disability. Bypass grafting for renovascular disease is indicated for the patient with severe hypertension and significant lesions. Selection of the most appropriate route for a bypass graft is individualized to the patient and dependent on history, physical examination, and diagnostic findings. The choice of bypass graft material also varies from patient to patient. Autologous grafts, such as saphenous vein grafts, are most successful, but often the material is not readily available. This type of grafting involves reversal of the vein so that blood may flow unimpeded by the valves within the vein. Figure 4-79 illustrates an end-to-end and an end-to-side bypass graft using the saphenous vein. In-situ bypass grafting may also be performed using this vein; it uses the vein in its natural position, without reversal. It involves interruption of the valves within the vein, however. In-situ vein grafts have the advantage of allowing the saphenous vein to retain its own blood supply, since the vein is never removed from the subcutaneous tissue.

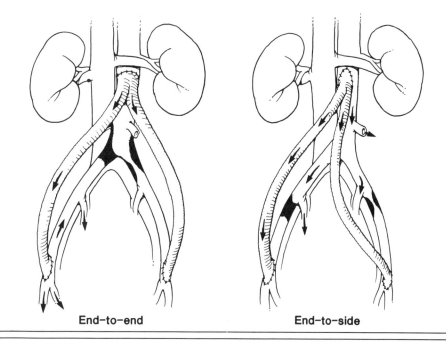

End-to-end   End-to-side

Figure 4-79 Bypass Grafts

Synthetic grafts may be used, the most common material being polytetrafluorethylene (PTFE). These grafts are best used to bypass obstructions in the upper extremities and obstructions above the popliteal artery. Endarterectomy involves opening the artery and gently removing the diseased inner layer. It is a very delicate type of surgery that is most often used for localized, single obstructions on the carotid artery.

Percutaneous transluminal angioplasty may be useful for certain types of stenotic lesions such as renovascular or lower-extremity occlusions. A guide catheter is inserted into the artery and positioned within the stenotic lesion. The balloon catheter is threaded through the guide catheter, and the balloon is inflated several times; pressure measurements proximal and distal to the lesion are taken. The patient who is a poor surgical risk may benefit from this procedure. Laser angioplasty is an experimental approach showing great promise.

Resection of the artery is most commonly performed for aneurysms. The procedure involves clamping of the artery proximal and distal to the aneurysm, opening the artery, and removing the aneurysm. A synthetic graft that may be preclotted with the patient's blood is inserted and sewn to either end of the resected artery. The old aneurysm wall is then sewn over the new graft and is used as a cover. This helps to prevent the erosion of adjacent organs that might occur should they come into contact with the synthetic graft. Of prime concern during this procedure is maintenance of blood flow to distal arteries and organs. Cross-clamping time is monitored closely in an attempt to keep it under 45 minutes. Hypothermia and shunt bypass may be used during the procedure if lengthy cross-clamping times are anticipated. Cardiopulmonary bypass is used for repair of thoracic aneurysms. The clamps are released slowly, at regular intervals, to prevent the hypotension that might otherwise ensue. Heparin may be used during the procedure to prevent clot formation and Lasix or mannitol may be used to promote renal perfusion, which may be diminished because of cross-clamping and/or hypotensive episodes.

Medical management of the patient with arterial disease is directed toward control of modifiable risk factors such as cigarette smoking, hypertension, and hypercholesterolemia. Medications such as heparin may be used to control acute arterial thrombosis or emboli and following certain types of arterial surgery. Intraarterial infusion of streptokinase may be useful for embolic occlusions of the extremities. Oral anticoagulants may be given following the administration of heparin. Antiplatelet agents are indicated for graft occlusion following peripheral arterial surgery and following carotid endarterectomy. Low-molecular-weight dextran, a polysaccharide, may be used as an antithrombotic agent, since it improves the impaired blood flow and volume that are secondary to decreased blood viscosity and platelet aggregation. Calcium channel blockers may be useful in preventing vasospasm.

Nursing management of the patient with arterial disease is directed toward care of the patient before and after surgery as well as education of the patient and family regarding follow-up care and reduction of modifiable risk factors. The following care plan outlines the standards of critical care practice for such a case.

Nursing Care Plan for the Management of the Patient with Vascular Disorder

Diagnosis	Signs and symptoms	Intervention	Rationale
Potential for fluid volume deficit due to: estimated blood loss not fully replaced; bleeding due to thrombocytopenia, elevated clotting time, increased afterload, or hypertension; suboptimal preload status from OR; increased afterload when patient is still hypothermic from OR; vasodilation in response to warming or to nitroglycerine or Nipride; postoperative diuresis; third spacing	LAP < 6–10 mm Hg CVP < 6 mm Hg PAD < 10 mm Hg SBP < 100 mm Hg HR > 120 bpm Urine output > intake or > 500 cc after 1 hour > 800 cc after 2 hours > 900 cc after 3 hours > 1000 cc after 4 hours > 1200 cc after 5 hours Sudden increase in chest tube drainage SVR < 800 or > 1200 dyne-sec/cm^5 Weight loss	Monitor VS closely: TPR; ECG; LAP; arterial BP; PA pressures; I&O	To ascertain trends by which to establish medication regimen
		Blood replacement, as ordered, for chest tube drainage > 200 cc/hr with LAP < 16 mm Hg; IV infusions, as ordered, for LA < 10 or PAD < 14	To maintain volume and cardiac function and efficiency and to maintain patency of grafts
		Administer fresh frozen platelets or packed cells during rewarming	To counteract vasodilation effect of rewarming
		Monitor effects of vasodilating agents (NTG, dobutamine, Inocor, MSO$_4$, renal dose dopamine)	To prevent early volume insufficiency
		Monitor PT, PTT, platelets, and Hct closely; be prepared to administer protamine sulfate, cryoprecipitate, FFP, PC, platelets, or Amicar for abnormally elevated clotting time, bleeding, or reduced platelet count	To prevent or treat early bleeding complications
		Assess incisional drainage frequently	To allow for complete assessment of body output
		Administer antihypertensive medication as ordered, to keep SBP < 150 mm Hg	To prevent hypertensive crisis

Nursing Care Plan for the Management of the Patient with Vascular Disorder

Diagnosis	Signs and symptoms	Intervention	Rationale
Potential for alteration in peripheral tissue perfusion related to graft thrombosis or embolization	Cool extremities Decreased or absent distal pulses Sluggish capillary refill Discomfort in extremity	Monitor VS and peripheral pulses and capillary refill closely, especially distal to surgical site	Need to monitor all extremities because patient may embolize to other areas
		Monitor sensation and motor function distal to surgical site	For purposes of comparison
		Administer heparin and vasoactive medications (dobutamine, etc.) as ordered	To prevent thrombosis and increase peripheral circulation and perfusion
Potential for alteration in perfusion to vital organs due to cross-clamping time, embolization, and/or hypotension	Postoperative complications of ileus or renal failure	Observe patient for abdominal distention, pain, bowel sounds, increased NG tube drainage, and/or diarrhea	Ileus may develop due to manipulation of bowel or graft erosion into bowel
		Advance patient to clear liquid diet upon peristalsis	To return patient to optimal nutritional state
		Observe urine output every hour and specific gravity every 8 hours; check for hematuria; monitor BUN and creatinine	For early detection and treatment of renal complications caused by hypotension, cross-clamping ischemia, or acute tubular necrosis
		Weigh patient daily	To monitor fluid balance
Potential for complications related to hemodynamic instability	SBP < 100 or > 160 DBP < 60 or > 90 MAP < 80 or > 100	Closely monitor with A-line, as needed	
		Administer nitroprusside for hypertensive episodes and initiate antihypertensives as indicated and ordered	Risk of graft rupture increases with hypertensive episodes

Diagnosis	Signs and symptoms	Intervention	Rationale
		Administer colloids and/or blood for hypotensive episodes	Risk of embolization and decreased perfusion increases with hypotensive episodes

Potential for infection due to
    IV lines;
    indwelling Foley catheter;
    chest tubes;
    endotracheal intubation;
    stress of surgery (in the event of trauma)
	Increased temperature
	
	Tachycardia and/or decreasing BP
	
	WBC > 10,000 mm^3
		Tylenol 600 mg every 4 hours or PRN, as ordered	To alleviate fevers

	Redness, exudate, increased tenderness, and/or induration of surgical incisions, IV insertion site, pacer wire sites, or chest tube sites	Implement thorough hand washing between patient contacts; implement universal isolation precautions if indicated	To prevent spread of infections
		Routine incision care with povidone-iodine solution, Telfa dressing, and foam tape	To prevent incisional infections
		Change peripheral IV sites at least every 3 days or with any signs of infection or infiltration; change IV tubing every 24 hours	IV fluid is especially fertile medium for bacterial growth
	Changes in characteristics of sputum: tan, brown, yellow, or green color and/or foul odor	Culture suspected origins of infection	To administer antibiotics that bacteria are sensitive to
	Chest x-ray indicative of atelectasis Decreased or absent breath sounds locally	Vigorous pulmonary toilet	To prevent and/or treat pulmonary congestion leading to infections
	Sediment in urine or foul-smelling urine	Routine Foley care every 8 hours	To prevent urinary tract infections
	WBCs in urine Hesitancy, frequency, urgency, burning, difficulty starting stream, incontinence, and/or inability to void	If patient is taking fluids, push fluids, unless contraindicated by cardiac condition	To flush urinary tract

Nursing Care Plan for the Management of the Patient with Vascular Disorder

Diagnosis	Signs and symptoms	Intervention	Rationale
Potential for impaired gas exchange due to: fluid volume overload; ineffective airway clearance, atelectasis, effusion; bronchospasm; inadequate supplemental O_2; inadequate tidal volume; low hematocrit and hemoglobin; low cardiac output; incisional discomfort; immobility; general anesthesia	Abnormal ABGs: $pO_2 < 80$ mm Hg; $pCO_2 < 35$ or > 45 mm Hg; pH < 7.35 or > 7.45; O_2 sat. $< 80\%$; $HCO_3 < 20$ or > 26 mEq/L; BE < 0 or > 3 Cyanosis Inadequate volume exchange Chest x-ray indicates atelectasis or effusion Copious secretions Elevated respiratory rate, wheezing, air hunger, gasping, or asymmetrical expansion of chest wall Difficulty weaning from ventilator	Mechanically ventilate as ordered Closely monitor for absent, unequal, or diminished breath sounds, crackles, wheezing, or asymmetrical chest wall expansion; closely monitor ABGs PRN and after ventilation changes if intubated; obtain chest x-ray immediately and PRN postoperatively and examine for ETT placement, lung expansion (pneumothorax), width of mediastinal shadow, presence of pleural fluid, and presence of foreign body	Ventilation support is needed until stabilization To discover early indications of ensuing respiratory compromise and/or complications
		Aggressive pulmonary toilet PRN with chest percussion therapy, incentive spirometry, and, when intubated, hyperinflation using 100% O_2 before and after suctioning; turn and reposition patient every 2 hours	To mobilize secretions, provide adequate oxygenation, and open closed alveoli
		If patient is stable, promote extubation by: holding sedation after midnight on day of surgery; elevating HOB 30 degrees; decreasing IMV by increments of 2–4 breaths/min if $pO_2 > 90$, pH 7.35–7.45, and O_2 sat. 90–100%	To assist patient to return to optimal breathing capacity as soon as possible (to prevent atelectasis, secondary infection, etc.)

Diagnosis	Signs and symptoms	Intervention	Rationale
Alteration in comfort related to surgical procedure	Restlessness	Assess level and type of pain or discomfort	To differentiate from potential complications of surgical procedure
	Complaints of discomfort	Medicate, as ordered and indicated	To minimize and alleviate discomfort
	Guarding of incision	Assist patient to position of comfort	To facilitate rest
		Elevate affected extremities on pillows	To promote arterial circulation
		Reassure patient and provide reinforcement	To help to decrease anxiety, which can potentiate sense of pain
Potential alteration in neurological function related to emboli and/or hemodynamic instability	Altered level of consciousness	Closely monitor neurological signs	To discover alterations from preoperative assessment
	Decreased movement on one side	Maintain hemodynamic stability: SBP 100–160 mm Hg, DBP 60–80 mm Hg, MAP 80–100 mm Hg	To decrease the risk of embolization
	Disorientation		
		Maintain adequate cardiac output and tissue perfusion	To ensure adequate supply of oxygenated blood to the brain
Potential for anxiety due to: fear of unknown; fear of death; fear of disfigurement; fear of pain; fear of disability; lack of knowledge regarding hospital and/or operative procedures, routines	Facial tension Distracted behavior Low attention span Withdrawal Twitching and shaking of extremities Inappropriate laughter or behavior Diaphoresis Tachycardia PVCs Other arrhythmias Nonadherence to treatment plan	Ascertain patient's fears and anxieties	Will allow the nurse to know just what to address
		Ascertain patient's previous hospital experiences (own as well as others')	Will help the nurse to know how to best alleviate anxieties or support positive attitudes
		Ascertain patient's and family's readiness to learn	Need to begin patient and family education when ready
		Teach patient about: routine of lab, radiology, ECG, house staff; surgery, donor sites, incisions, tubes, lines, operation length, ICU routine, visiting hours, pain medication, and deep breathing and coughing; provide patient with educational booklets	To help patient and family be prepared for what is to be experienced

Nursing Care Plan for the Management of the Patient with Vascular Disorder

Diagnosis	Signs and symptoms	Intervention	Rationale
		Give ICU tour, if desired	To familiarize patient with environment
		Sedate patient, as ordered or PRN	To help patient relax
		Provide emotional support as needed	To help patient and family deal with the situation in the best way possible
		Consult with social worker, chaplain, etc., as needed	Multidisciplinary team effort provides broader, more comprehensive care
Knowledge deficit with respect to risk factors and pathophysiology	Patient verbalizes lack of understanding	Assess patient's and family's present level of knowledge	To establish baseline
	Nonadherence in regard to risky behavior Evidence of denial	Assist patient and family in identifying personal risk factors; develop plan of action to moderate or eliminate risk factors	Lack of knowledge regarding risk factors results in nonadherence to medical regimen; planning facilitates needed changes in the patient's lifestyle
		Provide information on pathophysiology and consequences of ignoring disease	To facilitate patient's understanding of disease and importance of care regimen
		Provide information on medications, their mechanisms and actions, and their side effects	To help patient realize the need for and importance of prescribed medications and prepare for side effects, if any
		Have patient and family confirm their understanding of instructions	To ensure complete understanding and prevent miscommunication of instructions

Diagnosis	Signs and symptoms	Intervention	Rationale
Lack of knowledge of operative procedure and postoperative care	Patient and family verbalize lack of understanding	Assess patient's and family's present level of knowledge	To establish baseline
	Fear, anxiety, acting out behavior	Apply principles of adult learning to patient teaching strategies	Application of principles of adult learning in patient teaching increases amount of learning
	Nonadherence to medical regimen		
		Use diagrams and analogies to demonstrate operative procedures	To improve understanding
		Allow practice time for postoperative care such as incentive spirometry, etc.	To improve skills and thus adherence

Medications Commonly Used in the Care of the Patient with Vascular Disorder

Medication	Effect	Major side effects
Morphine sulfate	Analgesia Peripheral vasodilation Sedation Bronchodilation	Hypotension Respiratory depression Nausea and vomiting Constipation Urinary retention
Nitrates (nitroglycerine, isosorbide)	Vasodilation, leading to increased coronary blood supply and decreased myocardial oxygen demand	Hypotension Headache
Dobutamine Dopamine	Inotropics with alpha-adrenergic stimulant Increase myocardial contractility, cardiac output, and stroke volume Dilate renal and mesenteric vessels in low doses	GI upset Angina Dyspnea Headache Hypotension Ectopic arrhythmias Palpitations Vasoconstriction
Protamine sulfate	Fibrin split product binding to facilitate clotting	Coagulation
Antiarrhythmics	As per specific medication	As per specific medication
Digitalis	Increases contractility Lengthens refractory period of AV node Decreases left ventricular end-diastolic pressure Increases ventricular automaticity Decreases atrial automaticity	Tachycardia AV block Bradycardia GI upset Headache Drowsiness Confusion Double vision
Sodium bicarbonate	Alkaline buffer that corrects metabolic acidosis	Metabolic alkalosis Hypernatremia Fluid overload
Nitroprusside	Vasodilator with a direct action on vascular smooth muscle	Nausea and vomiting Muscle twitching Hypotension
Hydralazine Minoxidil Diazoxide	Vasodilator with a direct action on vascular smooth muscle, leading to relaxed arterioles, decreased vascular resistance, and increased cardiac output	Angina Nausea and vomiting Tachycardia Headache Flushing Hypotension

Medication	Effect	Major side effects
Furosemide Ethacrynic acid	Loop diuretics Decrease pulmonary congestion	Hypokalemia Hypocalcemia Hypomagnesemia Altered glucose metabolism
Trimethaphan Phentolamine	Ganglionic blockers, inhibiting the peripheral sympathetic nervous system	Orthostatic hypotension Ileus Urinary retention Blurred vision Dry mouth
Reserpine Guanethidine	Peripheral adrenergic antagonists, inhibiting peripheral sympathetic nervous system	Drowsiness Nausea and vomiting Tremors Bradycardia Dyspnea Fatigue
Methyldopa Clonidine	Centrally stimulate alpha-adrenergic receptors, leading to decreased peripheral vascular resistance	Drowsiness Dry mouth Vertigo Depression GI upsets
Atenolol Propranolol Timolol	Beta adrenoreceptor antagonists	Postural hypotension Dizziness and syncope Palpitations Dry mouth
Epinephrine	Stimulates alpha and beta receptor sites, causing increased heart rate, myocardial contractility, systemic vascular resistance, automaticity, and myocardial oxygen consumption	Headache Anxiety Palpitations Hyperglycemia
Levarterenol	Stimulates alpha and beta receptors, causing increased peripheral vasoconstriction and myocardial contractility	Bradycardia Hypertension Headache
Prostaglandin E	Arteriolar and bronchiolar dilation Inhibition of platelet aggregation	Flushing Apnea Bradycardia Hypotension Fever Seizures
Theophylline Alupent Bronchosol	Bronchodilators Increase renal blood flow Positive inotropic effect on heart	Cardiac arrhythmias GI upset

Medications Commonly Used in the Care of the Patient with Vascular Disorder

Medication	Effect	Major side effects
Acetaminophen	Analgesic Antipyretic	Hemolytic anemia Skin rash Fever Vascular collapse
Milk of magnesia	Laxative	Diarrhea Electrolyte imbalance
Pyridamole	Antiplatelet action	Bleeding
Heparin	Anticoagulation	Bleeding

Cardiogenic and Hemorrhagic Shock

Shock is the rapidly developing and severe pathophysiological syndrome associated with inadequate cellular metabolism caused by poor tissue perfusion. Shock is further classified into five categories, only two of which will be addressed in this chapter: cardiogenic shock and hemorrhagic shock. Simply described, cardiogenic shock is the shock resulting from impaired functioning of the heart as a pump, and hemorrhagic shock is the shock associated with a drastic decrease of intravascular volume relative to vascular capacity.

Cardiogenic Shock

The patient experiencing cardiogenic shock is the one who experiences a significant decrease in cardiac output. The syndrome is extremely serious, for it is estimated that 10–15% of hospital admissions for myocardial infarction result in cardiogenic shock, and, of those patients, approximately 80% die.[66]

Clinical antecedents

Cardiogenic shock is brought on by a serious compromise in cardiac output resulting from acute MI, tamponade, pulmonary embolus, arrhythmias, or congestive heart failure. Regardless of origin, pump failure occurs, and the failure usually is related to extreme inefficiency of the left ventricle or, more directly, extensive loss (at least 40%) of the myocardium. The following is a list of antecedents of cardiogenic shock:

1. Myocardial infarction
2. Severe congestive heart failure
3. Tamponade
4. Contusion
5. Papillary muscle rupture and/or severe valvular dysfunction
6. Acute ventricular septal defect
7. End-stage cardiomyopathy
8. Pulmonary embolism
9. Valvular or septal disruption
10. Drug ingestion

Critical referents

In cardiogenic shock, the tissue oxygen demands of the body are not met because of cardiac failure of some origin. As a result, tissue deteriorates rapidly, and death ensues quickly if the process is not reversed. Sometimes death occurs in less than an hour; at other times it follows a more extended period of up to several days. For this reason, four different stages of cardiogenic shock have been identified: initial, compensatory, progressive, and refractory.[67]

Initial stage   The initial stage of cardiogenic shock is when cardiac output begins to decrease but not to the extent that tissue perfusion is compromised. The metabolic needs of the body continue to be met.

Compensatory stage   When cardiac output decreases to the point where a compromise to cellular metabolism begins, the body attempts to maintain homeostasis by mediating the sympathetic nervous system in order to increase cardiac output. Baroreceptors are stimulated, as are alpha- and beta-adrenergic receptors, which, respectively, cause selective vasoconstriction and increased heart rate and contraction. Simultaneously, because of decreased perfusion to the kidneys, secretion of renin-angiotensin occurs. Aldosterone is released to facilitate sodium and water reabsorption in an effort to increase total fluid volume, which, in turn, enhances venous return and cardiac output.

Progressive stage   If the causative factors are not eliminated during the compensatory stage of cardiogenic shock, it is only a matter of time until the described compensatory mechanisms become ineffective in maintaining homeostasis. In the progressive stage, these same mechanisms perpetuate the shock cycle by placing increased demand on an already compromised heart, to the point of cardiac decompensation. Furthermore, resulting changes in cellular metabolism (ATP reduction and anaerobic cellular metabolism) cause the development of metabolic acidosis, which occurs first intracellularly, then in the capillaries, and, finally, venously. Sustained vasoconstriction and fluid shifts out of the capillaries into third spaces result in decreased intravascular circulation and increased blood viscosity, which only exacerbates the decompensatory cycle.

Refractory stage   If the patient in severe progressive shock lives long enough, a combined respiratory and metabolic acidosis develops. The chances for survival once this refractory stage is reached are extremely poor. Cardiac failure becomes irreversible, and therapy is generally found useless. Inadequate cerebral perfusion occurs, and multisystem shutdown develops, followed by cardiopulmonary arrest, and, finally, death.

Resulting signs and symptoms

Signs and symptoms of each stage of cardiogenic shock are listed in Table 4-25.

Nursing standards of care

Medical management of cardiogenic shock is directed toward maintaining adequate perfusion. A secondary goal is decreasing myocardial oxygen demand and increasing ventricular efficiency. When cardiogenic shock is caused by a mechanical defect, such as rupture of the intraventricular septum or papillary muscle, immediate surgical correction is

indicated. If surgery cannot be attempted, the insertion of an intraaortic balloon counterpulsation device, or intraaortic balloon pump (IABP), the use of mechanical ventilation for adequate oxygenation, and the use of venovasodilators and arterial vasodilators to decrease preload and afterload, respectively, are indicated for life support.

The use of the IABP has been found to be most beneficial in treating (1) severe left ventricular failure, (2) acute MI associated with prolonged ischemic pain (usually occurring with sustained, irreversible myocardial damage of 40–50%), or (3) cardiogenic shock caused by acute mechanical defects such as a ruptured ventricular septum or papillary muscle. An IABP works to improve myocardial oxygenation and reduce cardiac workload by use of a balloon placed directly below the left subclavian artery and directly above the renal arteries, as illustrated in Figure 4-80. The balloon is inflated during diastole, thus augmenting coronary flow, and then deflated at the end of diastole, creating a decrease in the arterial pressure, which effectively reduces the workload of the left ventricle.

Table 4-25　Clinical Manifestations of the Four Stages of Cardiogenic Shock

Stage	Signs and Symptoms
Initial	Decreased cardiac output
Compensatory	Sinus tachycardia Rapid, deep ventilations Respiratory alkalosis Altered level of consciousness PAW > 18 mm Hg Urine output < 20 cc/hr Hyperglycemia Hypernatremia Decreased urinary sodium Increased urinary osmolarity Cold and clammy skin Decreased bowel sounds
Progressive	Sinus tachycardia Weak and thready pulse Complaints of chest pain and palpitations Nausea and vomiting Rapid and shallow respirations Signs of peripheral vasoconstriction Elevated pulmonary artery pressures Metabolic acidosis
Refractory	Signs of cardiac failure Highly elevated pulmonary artery pressures Metabolic and respiratory acidosis Disseminated intravascular coagulation (DIC) Severe mental obtundation Cardiopulmonary arrest Death

Source: Thelan, L. A., Davie, J. K., and Urden, L. D. (1990). *Textbook of Critical Care Nursing: Diagnosis and Treatment.* St. Louis: C. V. Mosby Company, p. 282.

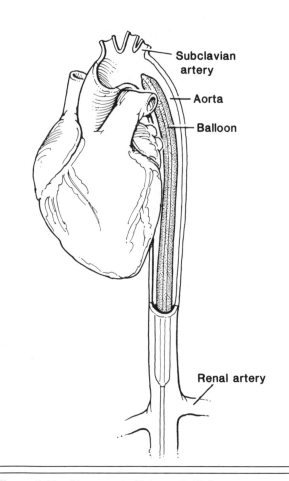

Figure 4-80　Placement of Intraaortic Balloon

The use of the IABP is contraindicated in the following conditions:

1. Severe aortic insufficiency or dissection
2. Compromised neurological status
3. Absent femoral pulses
4. Trauma accompanied by internal bleeding
5. Active bleeding ulcers or other bleeding/blood dyscrasias
6. Dysrhythmias resulting in rates of over 150 bpm

Nursing responsibilities toward the patient with an IABP include adjusting balloon timing using the arterial wave form, as illustrated in Figure 4-81, assessing for malpositioning of the balloon, continu-ally monitoring hemodynamic and cardiovascular function, and watching for and responding to complications such as balloon rupture or catheter fracture. Preventing thrombus or emboli through measures such as antiembolism stockings and other routine nursing care practices for the bedrest patient and preventing infection are also important concerns. Simultaneously, care of the patient experiencing cardiogenic shock also includes attention to respiratory function, skin integrity, nutrition, and fluid and electrolyte balances. But nursing care is primarily focused on the continuous assessment and support of tissue and organ perfusion conducted in concert with medical management. The following care plan outlines the nursing practices to be followed in the event of cardiogenic shock.

AUGMENTED BEAT

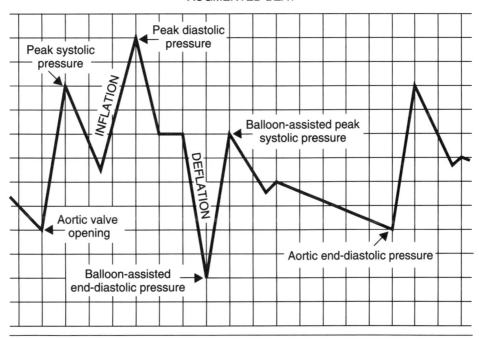

Figure 4-81   Synchronized Balloon Inflation and Deflation Tracings

Nursing Care Plan for the Management of the Patient with Cardiogenic Shock

Diagnosis	Signs and symptoms	Intervention	Rationale
Alteration in cardiac output related to myocardial failure (impaired ventricular contractility)	Signs of low cardiac output: decreased CVP; decreased BP; increased SVR; increased PAP and PCWP; CO < 5; CI < 2.5; tachycardia; S_3 heart sounds; urine output < 30 cc; pale, cool, and clammy skin; bibasilar fluid crackles (rales); faint peripheral pulses	Administer inotropics (dopamine, dobutamine) as ordered	To improve contractility
		Administer digoxin as ordered	To improve cardiac contractility and control tachycardia
		Monitor VS closely	To discover early signs of further failure
		Restrict fluids and double concentrate IV infusions when possible	To decrease amount of fluid volume infused and thus decrease cardiac load
		Position patient with extremities dependent	To pool blood in extremities, which decreases preload
		Administer diuretics as ordered	To draw off all excess circulating fluid
		Limit patient's physical activity	To decrease metabolic demand, which would place greater demands on heart
		Administer preload-reducing agents (nitroglycerin) as ordered, to maintain PAD/PCWP < 18 mm Hg	To reduce venous return
		Administer afterload-reducing agents (nitroprusside) as ordered	To maintain SVR 800–1300 dynes-sec/cm^5
Alteration in fluid volume (excess)	Weight gain Elevated PAD and PCWP Edema Decreased urinary output	Maintain accurate I&O records	To ascertain presence and cause of fluid imbalance
		Limit salt intake as ordered	Excess sodium causes fluid retention
		Restrict fluids to 1500 cc/day if PAD and PCWP are elevated	To prevent fluid overload, which can lead to congestive failure

Diagnosis	Signs and symptoms	Intervention	Rationale
		Administer diuretics as ordered	Prerenal failure may develop as a result of decreased renal perfusion
		Monitor BUN and creatinine	
		Anticipate low-dose (2–5 mcg/kg/min) dopamine infusion	To provide increased renal perfusion
		Monitor weight daily	Weight change is best indicator of excess fluid loss
		Monitor for crackles (rales) and presence of S_3 heart sounds every 4 hours or as needed	Warn of heart failure and pulmonary edema
		Anticipate need for salt-poor albumin administration	Chronic heart failure predisposes patient to loss of protein, leading to edema; albumin provides mechanism for returning interstitial fluid to intravascular space
		Apply elastic antiembolism stockings	To promote venous return and prevent edema
Potential for alteration in gas exchange and ineffective breathing pattern	Dyspnea Decreased O_2 levels on ABGs	Assist to position of comfort (semi- or high Fowler's position is best)	To improve breathing patterns and lower diaphragm
		Assess for crackles (rales), S_3, and JVP every 4 hours or as needed	These are signs of heart failure, with resultant pulmonary edema
		Administer oxygen, as ordered	To counter problems with oxygenation
		Monitor heart rhythm	Tachycardia is commonly seen
	Fluid overload	Review chest x-ray for signs of pulmonary edema	Pulmonary congestion can be clinically delayed by up to 24 hours
	Change in mental status	Monitor level of consciousness closely	Change in mental status may be one of the first signs of anoxia

Nursing Care Plan for the Management of the Patient with Cardiogenic Shock

Diagnosis	Signs and symptoms	Intervention	Rationale
Potential for infection related to pulmonary congestion, indwelling lines, and Foley catheter	Elevated temperature	Encourage coughing and deep breathing; turn patient in bed every 2 hours while on bedrest	Help to prevent atelectasis, blood clots in legs, and pressure sores
		Change respiratory tubing every 24 hours	Per CDC specifications
		Increase activity as soon as indicated	To promote healing
		Monitor temperature every 4 hours	Sign of infection
	Increased WBCs	Assess WBC count	Sign of infection
		Maintain strict aseptic technique with invasive lines and indwelling catheters; change lines unless contraindicated: PAP every 72 hours, arterial lines every 7 days, tubing every 48 hours, IV bags every 24 hours; Provide Foley care every 8 hours	Per CDC recommendation
		Assist in identifying source of infection: collect cultures; note atelectasis on chest x-ray; note sputum and urine characteristics; check insertion site for redness every 8 hours	Sites at risk of infection must be kept clean with aseptic technique; appropriate antibiotic therapy must be chosen
		Administer antibiotics as ordered	To combat infectious process
Decreased tolerance of activity related to dyspnea	Dyspnea on exertion Fatigue Exaggerated increase in heart rate and BP on exertion	Assess level of activity tolerance (should be related to the New York Heart Association's classification for consistency)	Provides a baseline

Diagnosis	Signs and symptoms	Intervention	Rationale
		Assist patient to change position every 2 hours while on bedrest	To decrease risk of complications and promote venous return
		Check BP with patient in horizontal, sitting, and standing positions	To monitor for orthostatic hypotension
		Avoid activity for a half-hour to an hour after meals	May decrease chance of hypoxia due to increased blood flow to GI tract
		Monitor heart rate and BP with activity increases	To maintain heart rate within 10 bpm of resting heart rate and maintain systolic BP within 20 mm Hg of resting BP; if a drop occurs, it may indicate a drop in cardiac output
		Anticipate institution of progressive rehab	To provide controlled mechanism for increasing activity
		Encourage frequent rest periods	To prevent excessive fatigue
Potential for impaired skin integrity	Redness on pressure points	Assess skin integrity every 2–4 hours	To prevent skin breakdown
		Note redness on pressure points	Early signs of skin breakdown
		Use egg crate or air mattress	To relieve pressure on bony prominences
		Assist patient to turn every 2 hours	To improve circulation
		Institute skin care regimen	Dryness predisposes skin to break down

Nursing Care Plan for the Management of the Patient with Cardiogenic Shock

Diagnosis	Signs and symptoms	Intervention	Rationale
Patient lacks knowledge of disease process and prescribed regimen	Patient does not adhere to care plan	Assess patient's present understanding	Provides baseline
	Patient verbalizes lack of knowledge and understanding or exhibits anxiety and apprehension, especially during procedures and treatments	Institute teaching program for patient and family: normal lung function; pathology; risk factors; control of precipitating and aggravating factors; activity; diet; medications; weight monitoring; signs and symptoms of recurring respiratory failure; follow-up care	Increasing knowledge, understanding, and thus potential ability to adhere to regimen may decrease unnecessary rehospitalization
		Allow patient and family to ask questions and verify understanding of information	Patient may need reinforcement and several repetitions of information before it is fully understood and integrated

Medications Commonly Used in the Care of the Patient with Cardiogenic Shock

Medication	Effect	Major side effects
Morphine sulfate	Analgesia Peripheral vasodilation Sedation Bronchodilation	Hypotension Respiratory depression Nausea and vomiting Constipation Urinary retention
Sodium bicarbonate	Alkaline buffer that corrects metabolic acidosis	Metabolic alkalosis Hypernatremia Fluid overload
Furosemide Ethacrynic acid	Loop diuretics Decrease pulmonary congestion	Hypokalemia Hypocalcemia Hypomagnesemia Altered glucose metabolism
Dobutamine Dopamine	Inotropics with alpha-adrenergic stimulant Increase myocardial contractility, cardiac output, and stroke volume Dilates renal and mesenteric vessels in low doses	GI upset Angina Dyspnea Headache Hypotension Ectopic arrhythmias Palpitations Vasoconstriction
Digitalis	Increases contractility Lengthens refractory period of AV node Decreases left ventricular end-diastolic pressure Increases ventricular automaticity Decreases atrial automaticity	Tachycardia AV block Bradycardia GI upset Headache Drowsiness Confusion Double vision
Adrenal glucocorticoid hormone (ACTH)	Inhibits inflammatic release of proteolytic enzymes in order to alter acute ischemic injury and decrease size of infarct Potentiates vasoconstrictor effect of norepinephrine Increases sodium retention in order to increase blood volume	Hypertension Impaired glucose metabolism Osteoporosis Peptic ulcer Hypokalemia Increased risk for infection
Heparin	Anticoagulant	Bleeding
Antiarrhythmics	As per specific medication	As per specific medication
Methoxamine	Vasoconstriction Alpha-adrenergic receptor stimulator	Cardiac arrhythmias Bradycardia

Nursing Care Plan for the Management of the Patient Undergoing Intraaortic Balloon Pump Therapy

Diagnosis	Signs and symptoms	Intervention	Rationale

Potential alteration in peripheral tissue perfusion on IABP insertion side, related to risk of vessel obstruction, hemorrhage from arterial wall dissection, and/or thrombus	Very distant or absent peripheral pulses on affected leg
	
	Paleness of affected leg
	
	Motor deficits and/or tingling on affected leg
		Monitor affected leg for:
		    pulses;
		    temperature;
		    color;
		    sensation;
		    mobility
			To monitor circulation of affected leg

	Bleeding at insertion site Abdominal pain Prolonged PT or PTT	Instruct patient about signs of impaired circulation and need to notify staff of occurrences	Patient can help in monitoring affected leg
	Hematocrit less than 37% in females or less than 40% in males	Pad heel of affected foot protectively; separate toes with lambswool	To protect heel and toes of affected foot from effects of compromised circulation due to balloon placement
		Assist patient with passive ROM, without bending leg at the hip	To enhance circulation and perfusion in affected leg
		Keep HOB at less than 30 degrees	To prevent upward migration of balloon, resulting in occlusion of subclavian artery
		Administer heparin as ordered; maintain adequate hydration	To prevent clot formation about balloon

	Signs of balloon migration:
	    distant/absent left radial pulse;
	    sudden decrease in urine output;
	    flank pain;
	    dizziness
		Closely monitor patient for signs of balloon migration	To facilitate detection of complications from balloon therapy

		When balloon is no longer needed, maintain inflation rate until removed	To prevent clot formation while balloon is still in place

Diagnosis	Signs and symptoms	Intervention	Rationale
Potential for impaired tissue integrity related to prolonged bedrest, compromised circulation, and decreased protein intake	Skin redness Interruption of skin integrity	Institute progressive skin care and use of protective bed	To reduce capillary pressure to less than closing pressure, enhancing blood flow to dependent areas
		Reposition patient every 2 hours using log roll method and keeping affected leg extended	To prevent pressure spots
		Keep skin clean and dry; use occlusive dressing on skin over bony prominences if it becomes reddened	To prevent skin breakdown
		Provide high-protein, high-calorie diet, as tolerated	To promote nitrogen balance
		As patient improves, teach patient how to move in bed in ways that do not risk affected leg	To prevent complications due to immobility in ways that are safe for balloon therapy
Potential for hemorrhage secondary to mechanical coagulopathy and IV anticoagulants	Evidence of bleeding: frank bleeding; hematoma; skin is hot and inflamed; hardened area (induration) around affected site Secretions and excretions are positive for frank or occult blood Abdominal pain Drop in hematocrit level Prolonged PT and/or PTT Decreased platelet count	Closely monitor PT, PTT, ACT, platelets, and HCT; test secretions and excretions for frank and occult blood	To facilitate detection of bleeding
		Use extra care not to bump or injure patient during moving and/or turning	To protect patient from injury that may cause hemorrhage
		Use special care with oral care (toothettes, etc.)	To avoid instigating bleeding
		Test gastric pH every 4 hours and maintain pH > 5.0	To prevent increased gastric acidity

Hemorrhagic Shock

Hemorrhagic shock is the most frequently occurring of all the different types of shock. It results when drastic reductions in circulating blood volume leave the body's metabolic needs unmet. Circulating fluid losses constituting hemorrhagic shock range from 10% to 50% (2500 mL) and lead to severe hypotension, peripheral vasoconstriction, obtundation, and anuria.

Clinical antecedents

Hemorrhagic shock is caused by direct internal or external bleeding. Traumatic injuries such as long-bone fractures and skin cuts, lesions, and lacerations are frequent antecedents to this type of shock. Other precipitating factors include severe diarrhea and/or vomiting, loss of plasma from burns, hemorrhagic pancreatitis, severe sodium depletion, ruptured spleen, and hypopituitarism. Hypovolemic shock, which is very similar to hemorrhagic shock, involves loss of fluid other than circulating blood, such as third spacing due to capillary permeability or decreased colloidal osmotic pressure.

Critical referents

Loss of circulating volume causes a decrease in preload (venous return), cardiac filling pressure, and stroke volume, leading to lower cardiac output and, eventually, decreased tissue perfusion. In response, the body activates the sympathetic nervous system followed by the renin-aldosterone system, which leads to antidiuretic hormone being secreted in a compensatory effort. The three stages of shock relate directly to the amount of fluid loss: mild shock involves a 10–25% loss of volume, moderate shock involves from 25% to 35% fluid loss, and severe shock occurs when 35–50% of the total volume is lost.

Resulting signs and symptoms

Mild hemorrhagic shock (500–1200 mL fluid loss) results in the patient's becoming pale, hypotensive, and possibly tachycardic. Other cardiac symptoms are rare, but signs of hemorrhage may be obvious or hidden, depending on whether the bleeding is external or internal.

Moderate shock occurs with a 1200–1800 mL loss and leads to marked hypotension and inadequate cardiac output. Extremities become cool, and signs of decreased capillary refill are evident. Kidney function decreases, as does gastrointestinal activity, and the patient becomes anxious and restless. Pulses become weak and thready, and the skin becomes diaphoretic.

If not tended to, moderate shock becomes severe shock, with a loss of 1800–2500 mL of circulating blood. As in all advanced shock, both respiratory and metabolic acidosis develop due to ischemia. The patient becomes severely hypotensive and diaphoretic, and obtundation and anuria result.

Nursing standards of care

Medical and nursing management of the patient with hemorrhagic shock involves control of the underlying cause, basic support of oxygenation, rapid administration of fluids to restore intravascular volume, close monitoring of cardiovascular status, and treatment to restore and maintain homeostasis. The rapid infusion of electrolyte solutions (crystalloids such as lactated Ringers solution, in the case of hypovolemia) or blood products (colloids, in the case of hemorrhage) is instituted as soon as possible and 3 parts replacement solution is usually given for every 1 part fluid loss. Frequently, the patient is placed in pneumatic antishock garments, which externally constrict extremities to help increase venous return. Vasopressors are administered to help maintain perfusion pressures, but these can only be started after fluid resuscitation is well underway. The following nursing care plan summarizes the usual critical care practices for the individual suffering from hemorrhagic shock.

Nursing Care Plan for the Management of the Patient with Hemorrhagic Shock

Diagnosis	Signs and symptoms	Intervention	Rationale
Alteration in cardiac output related to decreased preload caused by fluid volume deficits	Signs of hypovolemia: CO < 5; CI < 2.5; decreased PAWP, PADP, and/or CVP; tachycardia; narrow pulse pressure; MAP < 80; urine output < 30 cc/hr; decreased BP; cool and clammy skin; pale color; apprehensiveness and agitation	Position patient supine with extremities elevated, or in pneumatic antishock garment	To increase preload (venous return) and eventually, cardiac output
		Avoid placing patient in Trendelenburg position	That position inhibits optimal diaphragmatic function
		Administer colloids (in the case of hemorrhage) and/or crystalloids (in the case of hypovolemia) at 3 parts infusion to 1 part loss	To remedy compromises in capillary permeability, colloidal osmotic pressure, and circulating volume
		Closely monitor patient for signs of fluid overload	In compromised states, fluid overload leading to congestive problems can occur very quickly
		Replace fluids before administering vasopressors	Coronary perfusion is compromised by fluid deficit; vasopressors increase oxygen demand in the heart, so perfusion must be adequate before demand is increased
		Move patient as little as possible	To limit tissue oxygen demand caused by physical activity
		Keep patient as free of anxiety as possible	To limit tissue oxygen demand caused by anxiety
Alteration in peripheral tissue perfusion related to vasopressor therapy	Distant peripheral pulses	Closely monitor peripheral pulses and capillary refill	To allow for early detection and intervention
	Pale or cyanotic fingers and/or slowed capillary refill	Avoid therapy until tissue is adequately perfused with circulating fluids	Vasopressors decrease peripheral circulation and increase central circulation
	Complaints of ischemic pain and/or tingling in extremities		

Nursing Care Plan for the Management of the Patient with Hemorrhagic Shock

Diagnosis	Signs and symptoms	Intervention	Rationale
Decreased tolerance of activity related to dyspnea	Dyspnea on exertion Fatigue Exaggerated increase in heart rate and BP on exertion	Assess level of activity tolerance (should be related to the New York Heart Association's classification for consistency)	Provides a baseline
		Assist patient to change position every 2 hours while on bedrest	To decrease risk of complications and promote venous return
		Check BP with patient in horizontal, sitting, and standing positions	To monitor for orthostatic hypotension
		Avoid activity for a half-hour to an hour after meals	May decrease chance of hypoxia due to increased blood flow to GI tract
		Monitor heart rate and BP with activity increases	To maintain heart rate within 10 bpm of resting heart rate and maintain systolic BP within 20 mm Hg of resting BP; if a drop occurs, it may indicate a drop in cardiac output
		Anticipate institution of progressive rehab	To provide controlled mechanism for increasing activity
		Encourage frequent rest periods	To prevent excessive fatigue
Potential for alteration in gas exchange and ineffective breathing pattern	Dyspnea Decreased O_2 levels on ABGs	When patient is able, assist to position of comfort (semi- or high Fowler's position is best)	To improve breathing patterns and lower diaphragm
		Administer oxygen as ordered	To counter problems with oxygenation
		Monitor rhythm	Tachycardia is commonly seen

Diagnosis	Signs and symptoms	Intervention	Rationale
	Change in mental status	Monitor level of consciousness closely	Change in mental status may be one of the first signs of anoxia
Potential for infection due to IV lines; indwelling Foley catheter; chest tubes; endotracheal intubation; stress of surgery (in the event of trauma)	Increased temperature Tachycardia and/or decreasing BP WBC > 10,000 mm^3	Tylenol 600 mg every 4 hours or PRN, as ordered	To alleviate fevers
	Redness, exudate, increased tenderness, and/or induration of surgical incisions, IV insertion site, pacer wire sites, or chest tube sites (if present)	Implement thorough hand washing between patient contacts; implement universal isolation precautions if indicated	To prevent spread of infections
		Routine incision care with povidone-iodine solution, Telfa dressing, and foam tape	To prevent incisional infections
		Change peripheral IV sites at least every 3 days or with any signs of infection or infiltration; change IV tubing every 24 hours	IV fluid is especially fertile medium for bacterial growth
	Changes in characteristics of sputum: tan, brown, yellow, or green color and/or foul odor	Culture suspected origins of infection	To administer antibiotics that bacteria are sensitive to
	Chest x-ray indicative of atelectasis Decreased or absent breath sounds locally	Vigorous pulmonary toilet	To prevent and/or treat pulmonary congestion leading to infections
	Sediment in urine or foul-smelling urine	Routine Foley care every 8 hours	To prevent urinary tract infections
	WBCs in urine Hesitancy, frequency, urgency, burning, difficulty starting stream, incontinence, and/or inability to void	If patient is taking fluids, push fluids, unless contraindicated by cardiac condition	To flush urinary tract

Medications Commonly Used in the Care of the Patient with Hemorrhagic Shock

Medication	Effect	Major side effects
Metaraminol	Stimulates adrenergic receptor, which causes vasoconstriction Increases myocardial contractility Increases rate of myocardial contractility	Bradycardia Oliguria CNS depression
Dopamine	Inotropic with alpha-adrenergic stimulant Increases myocardial contractility, cardiac output, and stroke volume Dilates renal and mesenteric vessels in low doses	GI upset Angina Dyspnea Headache Hypotension Ectopic arrhythmias Palpitations Vasoconstriction
Methoxamine	Stimulates alpha-adrenergic receptor, causing vasoconstriction	Cardiac arrhythmias Bradycardia
Isoproterenol	Stimulates beta receptor sites and relaxes smooth muscle, leading to increased myocardial contractility, increased heart rate, increased myocardial oxygen demand, and decreased peripheral vascular resistance	Tachycardia Ventricular irritability Hypotension Headache Flushing Angina GI upset Dizziness Weakness Tremors
Phentolamine Phenoxybenzamine Chlorpromazine	Alpha-adrenergic blockers, causing vasodilation	Cardiac arrhythmias Tachycardias Orthostatic hypotension
Calcium chloride	Replaces depleted calcium	Hypercalcemia
Corticosteroids	Potentiate vasoconstrictor effect of norepinephrine Increase sodium retention to increase blood volume	Hypertension Impaired glucose metabolism Osteoporosis Peptic ulcer Hypokalemia Increased risk for infection

CHAPTER 4 POST-TEST

1. As the mean pressure within a distensible artery increases, the resistance to blood flow through the blood vessel:
   a. increases, because as the pressure increases, it is approaching the critical closing pressure.
   b. decreases, because as pressure increases, the radius tends to increase.
   c. increases, because the increased pressure causes an increase in viscosity.
   d. decreases, because the velocity of blood flow increases with increasing pressure.

2. The vascular tone in tissue is primarily determined by:
   a. the radius of the precapillary resistance, which is controlled by the tension in the vascular smooth muscle.
   b. the frequency of vibrations caused by turbulent flow through the capillaries.
   c. its resting metabolic rate.
   d. the total length of all the vessels in the tissue divided by the mean vessel diameter plus viscosity.

3. Increased sympathetic nerve activity to the heart:
   a. decreases heart rate while increasing contractility.
   b. causes both negative chronotropic and negative inotropic actions.
   c. shortens ventricular filling time but lengthens coronary perfusion time.
   d. causes both positive chronotropic and positive inotropic effects.

4. Depolarization through the heart:
   a. can be blocked at the AV node by left vagal stimulation.
   b. must begin at the SA node.
   c. cannot occur after a myocardial infarction.
   d. travels at a relatively constant rate from start to finish.

5. Pulmonary artery pressure is much lower than pressure in the systemic arteries because:
   a. right atrial pressure is lower than left atrial pressure.
   b. right ventricular mass is less than left ventricular mass.
   c. resistance in the pulmonary vasculature is substantially less than that in the systemic vasculature.
   d. the volume of the lungs is much less than that of the entire circulation system.

6. For a patient suffering chronic congestive heart failure, which of the following is true?
   a. Total peripheral resistance is increased because of increased sympathetic tone, circulating plasma levels of norepinephrine and vascular stiffness.
   b. The lymphatic circulation is minimally affected by CHF.
   c. Distribution of cardiac output systemically remains normal during exercise and rest.
   d. Increased precapillary resistance throughout the body increases mean capillary hydrostatic pressure, causing edema and ascites.

7. An increase in venous return can be caused by:
   a. an increase in sympathetic vasomotor tone.
   b. an increase in venous vascular compliance.
   c. an increase in right atrial pressure.
   d. a decrease in blood volume.

8. The vasomotor center:
   a. controls sympathetic outflow.
   b. receives impulses directly from the arterial baroreceptors.
   c. overrides control in the feedback loop.
   d. produces afferent impulses.

9. In a case of hemorrhagic shock, the following physiological changes could be expected:
   a. decreased cardiac output, decreased circulating volume, and increased peripheral resistance.
   b. decreased cardiac output, constant circulating volume, and increased peripheral resistance.
   c. decreased cardiac output, decreased circulating volume, and decreased peripheral resistance.
   d. decreased cardiac output, constant circulating volume, and decreased peripheral resistance.

10. In a case of cardiogenic shock, the following physiological changes could be expected:
    a. increased cardiac output, constant circulating volume, and decreased peripheral resistance.
    b. increased cardiac output, decreased circulating volume, and decreased peripheral resistance.
    c. decreased cardiac output, decreased circulating volume, and increased peripheral resistance.
    d. decreased cardiac output, constant circulating volume, and increased peripheral resistance.

11. In a case of severe congestive heart failure, vascular tone:
    a. will remain unchanged in the heart and brain and will decrease in the kidney.
    b. will remain unchanged in the brain and kidney and will decrease in the heart.
    c. will remain unchanged in the kidney and heart and will decrease in the brain.
    d. will remain unchanged in the heart and brain and will increase in the kidney.

12. Increased arterial pulse pressure in the elderly is probably due to:
    a. decreased arterial wall compliance and mean arterial pressure.
    b. increased arterial wall compliance and decreased mean arterial pressure.
    c. increased arterial wall compliance and mean arterial pressure.
    d. decreased arterial wall compliance and increased mean arterial pressure.

13. Which of the following is the patient suffering intermittent atrial fibrillation at highest risk for?
    a. pulmonary embolism
    b. coronary artery embolism
    c. cerebral embolism
    d. peripheral vascular thrombus

Please refer to the following clinical vignettes to answer questions 14 through 23.

A 73-year-old female with a history of severe CAD and a four-vessel coronary bypass 6 years ago is admitted for treatment of increasing unstable angina pectoris uncontrolled by medication. Arteriography shows partial occlusion of two of the existing grafts and a new RCA lesion. The patient is scheduled for another coronary bypass procedure.

14. Preoperative assessment of the CABG patient includes all of the following *except*:
    a. ascertaining the patient's and family's fears and concerns.
    b. checking the results of coagulation studies.
    c. checking for indicators of renal dysfunction.
    d. checking enzyme levels for recent myocardial damage.

15. The patient's history of CAD and surgery most strongly predispose her to which of the following intraoperative and postoperative complications?
    a. ventricular aneurysm
    b. dependence on intraaortic balloon pump
    c. coagulopathy
    d. MI

16. Bleeding problems immediately postoperatively may be a result of any of the following *except*:
    a. hypothermia-induced platelet dysfunction.
    b. excessive fibrinolysis.
    c. over-heparinization.
    d. vitamin K deficiency from hepatic congestion.

The patient could not be weaned from the intraaortic balloon pump due to left ventricular failure after grafts were placed to the right coronary artery and from the aorta to the obtuse marginal and circumflex branches of the left coronary artery. She returned to the ICU on the pump at a 2:1 ratio, intubated and mechanically ventilated and with a pulmonary artery line, left atrial line, and arterial line in place.

17. The *primary* mechanism by which the IABP reduces left ventricular failure is by:
    a. reducing preload.
    b. reducing afterload.
    c. augmenting cardiac contractility.
    d. increasing stroke volume.

18. Signs that the IABP requires adjustment include all of the following *except*:
    a. asynchronous balloon and ECG rhythms.
    b. presence of V waves on pulmonary artery tracing.
    c. significant decreases in urinary output with weaning efforts.
    d. patient's complaints of new chest pain.

19. Independent nursing care of the patient on IABP therapy includes all of the following *except*:
    a. maintaining the patient in proper position, with the head of the bed at 45° or less with no flexion at the groin.
    b. regularly checking the temperature and pulses of the involved extremity.
    c. adjusting the balloon in response to dysrhythmias.
    d. monitoring for thromboembolic complications.

20. A significant finding with regard to the patient's chest tubes that should be reported immediately is:
    a. 400 cc of blood from the mediastinal chest tube within the first 4 hours postoperatively.
    b. fluctuations in the pleural chest tube coinciding with respirations.
    c. an air leak in the mediastinal chest tube.
    d. 50 cc/hr of serosanguinous fluid draining from the pleural chest tube.

21. The bleeding disorder the patient is most likely to develop is:
    a. heparin overdose.
    b. coagulopathy related to hepatic congestion.
    c. IABP-induced thrombocytopenia.
    d. disseminated intravascular coagulation.

22. Bypass surgery differs from valvular surgery in all of the following *except*:
    a. those undergoing valvular surgery are more likely to become balloon-dependent.
    b. valvular surgery is a longer procedure, accompanied by more pump-related complications.
    c. bypass procedures are more vascular in nature and usually require more blood replacement.
    d. morbidity statistics are higher for bypass surgery than for valvular surgery.

23. Long-term postoperative medications for the bypass patient are likely to include:
    a. nitrates and calcium channel blockers.
    b. beta blockers and antianginal agents.
    c. digoxin and anticoagulants.
    d. antiplatelet medications and antianginal agents.

24. Which of the following ECG changes indicate right ventricular hypertrophy?
    a. right axis deviation and R wave voltage greater than S wave voltage in right precordial leads
    b. RSR' in lead V_6
    c. left axis deviation and a widened QRS segment
    d. left axis deviation and R wave voltage greater than S wave voltage in right precordial leads

25. A right bundle branch block is evidenced by a split S_2 because:
    a. the closing of the aortic valve occurs earlier than normal.
    b. the closing of the aortic valve occurs later than normal.
    c. the closing of the pulmonic valve occurs later than normal.
    d. the closing of the pulmonic valve occurs earlier than normal.

26. Why would dopamine and nipride be administered simultaneously to a patient immediately after CABG?
    a. to increase cardiac output while maintaining adequate blood pressure
    b. to decrease peripheral vascular resistance while maintaining mean arterial pressure
    c. to decrease cardiac output while maintaining peripheral vasoconstriction
    d. to increase renal perfusion while maintaining adequate blood pressure

27. A patient with a history of COPD suffering an acute MI has a pulmonary capillary wedge of 12 mm Hg and a pulmonary artery pressure of 40/20 mm Hg. The severe dyspnea the patient experiences is most likely caused by:
    a. left ventricular failure.
    b. a pericardial effusion.
    c. the longstanding lung disease.
    d. increased afterload.

28. The presence of a large V wave on a pulmonary capillary wedge pressure tracing after a newly developed murmur has been discovered most likely indicates that:
    a. a papillary muscle has ruptured.
    b. the patient is suffering pericarditis.
    c. the patient is cardiac tamponading.
    d. a ventricular septal defect is forming.

29. To lower an extremely elevated serum K^+ level, which of the following would be administered?
    a. glucose and insulin
    b. Lasix
    c. sodium chloride
    d. calcium gluconate

30. If a postoperative aorto-femoral bypass patient complains of shortness of breath one day after surgery, which of the following should the nurse do?
    a. increase the FIO_2 and suction the patient
    b. assess the lung sounds, raise the head of the bed only slightly, and obtain an ABG
    c. administer Lasix
    d. perform chest percussion, and have the patient breathe and cough after premedication with morphine sulfate

31. The care plan for a postoperative aorto-femoral bypass patient who complains of shortness of breath would include:
    a. performing chest percussion t.i.d., keeping the grafted leg dependent.
    b. keeping the grafted leg in flexion and ordering physical therapy once a day.
    c. monitoring for signs of thrombus and preventing flexion of the grafted leg.
    d. keeping the grafted leg in flexion and administering prescribed antihypertensives.

32. Which of the following is responsible for recurrent chest pain in the case of Prinzmetal's angina?
    a. coronary artery spasms
    b. 75% occlusion of the circumflex artery
    c. complete occlusion of the left anterior descending artery

d. a coronary embolic event

33. Which of the following signs would alert the nurse of right-side failure in a patient suffering an acute MI?
    a. lung crackles and an elevated wedge pressure
    b. the development of hypertension
    c. distended neck veins and hypotension
    d. hypotension and paradoxical pulses

34. In which of the following types of MI does the heart block that develops carry a very high risk of mortality?
    a. inferior
    b. anterior
    c. posterior
    d. subendocardial

35. An embolic event in the mesenteric artery is likely to cause ischemia to which of the following?
    a. stomach
    b. small bowel
    c. trachea
    d. large bowel

36. A patient admitted for acute MI exhibits an abnormal ECG reading: the ST segment is greatly elevated in the V leads 1–4 and depressed in leads II, III, and aVF, and the T wave is inverted in leads II, III, and aVF. This suggests that the patient has suffered:

a. an anterior MI.
b. an inferior MI.
c. a posterior MI.
d. left ventricular hypertrophy.

37. Which of the following has occurred if a nurse observes elevation of the ST segment on a 12-lead ECG?
    a. Restoration of circulation to that specific area of the heart
    b. Injury to the heart muscle
    c. Ischemia to the heart muscle
    d. Necrosis of that area of the heart muscle

38. The drug of choice to be administered in the treatment of atrial fibrillation is:
    a. Pronestyl.
    b. Procardia.
    c. quinidine.
    d. Inderal.

39. Two weeks following a CABG, a patient is admitted with high fevers accompanied by chills. She is hypotensive and in severe respiratory distress. Blood cultures are positive for bacteremia. The patient also begins to exhibit signs of disseminated intravascular coagulation. Antecedents that would indicate a true case of DIC would include:
    a. respiratory insufficiency.
    b. documentation of septic shock.
    c. renal insufficiency.
    d. COPD.

ENDNOTES

1. Guyton, A. C. (1976). *Textbook of Medical Physiology*, (5th Edition). Philadelphia: W. B. Saunders Company, p. 160.
2. Ibid., p. 116.
3. Ibid., p. 164.
4. Ibid., p. 166.
5. Ibid., p. 164.
6. Bustin, D. (1986). *Hemodynamic Monitoring for Critical Care*. Norfolk, Conn.: Appleton-Century-Crofts, p. 6.
7. Ibid., p. 17.
8. Ibid., p. 18.
9. Guyton, op. cit., p. 250.
10. Ibid., p. 262.
11. Braunwald, E. (1984). *Heart Disease: A Textbook of Cardiovascular Medicine*. Philadelphia: W. B. Saunders Company, p. 250.
12. Ibid., p. 2.
13. Ibid., p. 93.
14. Ibid., p. 356.
15. Ibid., p. 374.
16. Tilkian, A. G., Daily, E. K. (1986). *Cardiovascular Procedures. Diagnostic Techniques and Therapeutic Procedures*. St. Louis, Mo.: C. V. Mosby Company, p. 119.

17. Ibid., p. 213.
18. American Heart Association (1989). *1990 Heart and Stroke Facts*. Dallas: American Heart Association National Center, p. 1.
19. Ibid., p. 3.
20. Braunwald, op. cit., p. 1210.
21. Ibid., p. 1217.
22. Ibid., p. 1188.
23. Conti, C. R. (1986). Unstable Angina Before and After Infarction: Thoughts on Pathogenesis and Therapeutic Strategies. *Heart and Lung* 15(4): 361.
24. Ibid., p. 361–388.
25. Ibid., p. 364.
26. Forrester, J. S., Litvach, F., Grundfest, W., Hickley, A. (1987). A Perspective of Coronary Disease Seen Through the Arteries of Living Man. *Circulation* 75(3): 505–513.
27. Ibid.
28. Ibid.
29. Braunwald, op. cit., p. 1277.
30. Ibid.
31. Ibid., p. 1265.
32. Ibid., p. 1281.

33. Ibid., p. 1269.

34. Ibid., p. 1474.

35. Ibid., p. 1272.

36. Ibid., p. 1474.

37. American Heart Association, op. cit., p. 10.

38. Guenter, C. A. (Editor) (1983). *Internal Medicine.* New York: Churchhill Livingston, p. 55.

39. Ibid., p. 53.

40. Braunwald, op. cit., p. 865.

41. Guenter, op. cit., p. 60.

42. Braunwald, op. cit., p. 491.

43. Ibid., p. 447.

44. Marriott, H. J. L. (1983). *Practical Electrocardiography* (7th Edition). Baltimore: Williams & Wilkens, p. 78.

45. Ibid., p. 78.

46. Sweetwood, H. M. (1983). *Clinical Electrocardiography for Nurses.* Rockville, Md.: Aspen, p. 161.

47. Castelli, W. P. (1989). *Reversing the Course of Atherosclerosis: A View from Framingham.* Kalamazoo, Mich.: Upjohn Company, p. 43.

48. Davidson, R. (1985). *Coronary Heart Disease.* New York: Medical Examination Publishing Company, p. 144–145.

49. Ibid., p. 161–162.

50. American Heart Association, op. cit., p. 15.

51. Ibid., p. 34.

52. Copeland, J. G. (1984). "Cardiac Transplantation Today." *Journal of Cardiovascular Medicine*, 9: 528–534.

53. Ibid.

54. Ibid., p. 531–532.

55. American Heart Association, op. cit.

56. Fahey, V. A. (Editor) (1988). *Vascular Nursing.* Philadelphia: W. B. Saunders Company.

57. Ibid.

58. Braunwald, op. cit.

59. Braunwald, op. cit., p. 1542.

60. Fahey, op. cit.

61. Braunwald, op. cit.

62. Moore, W. S. (Editor) (1983). *Vascular Surgery: A Comprehensive Review.* Orlando, Florida: Grune & Stratton.

63. Fahey, op. cit.

64. Goldblatt, H. (1934). "Studies on Experimental Hypertension." *Journal of Experimental Medicine*, 59: 347–379.

65. Fahey, op. cit.

66. Lewis, S. M., Collier, I. C. (1983). *Medical-Surgical Nursing: Assessment and Management of Clinical Problems.* New York: McGraw-Hill Book Company, p. 663.

67. Thelan, L. A., Davie, J. K., Urden, L. D. (1990). *Textbook of Critical Care Nursing.* St. Louis, Mo.: C. V. Mosby Company, p. 281–282.

The
5 Renal
System

CHAPTER 5 PRE-TEST

1. The kidneys are perfused with blood at the rate of:
   a. 1200 mL/min.
   b. 10,000 mL/hr.
   c. 600 mL/min.
   d. 6000 mL/hr.

2. ECG symptoms of hyperkalemia include:
   a. decrease in all depolarization waves.
   b. peaked T waves, tall RS wave, and decreased P-R interval.
   c. depressed T wave, increased P-R interval, and development of RS wave.
   d. peaked T wave, increased P-R interval, and broadened QRS complex.

3. A patient with a labile low blood pressure who experiences renal failure with mild to moderate azotemia is most likely to be dialyzed via:
   a. SCUF.
   b. CAVHD.
   c. hemodialysis.
   d. peritoneal dialysis.

Refer to the following clinical vignette to answer questions 4 through 6.

J.W. is a 29-year-old Caucasian male who is admitted with an initial diagnosis of septicemia incurred as a result of IV drug abuse. He is emaciated, pale, and anxious, although oriented and behaving appropriately. He has tremors of all extremities and a nonproductive cough he claims to have had for 2 weeks. His admission vital signs are: blood pressure, 132/92; pulse, 114/minute; respirations, 32/minute; temperature 102°F by mouth. His laboratory values are as follows:

Na: 138 mEq/L

K: 5.2 mEq/L

Cl: 107 mEq/L

BUN: 80 mg/dL

Creatinine: 4.8 mg/dL

Ca: 7 mg/dL

Phos: 6 mg/dL

Uric acid: 7 mg/dL

Mg: 2 mEq/L

CO_2: 15 mEq/L

Alkaline phosphatase: 16 units

Osmolality: 307 mOsm/L

4. The most likely clinical findings to expect at this time include:
   a. hyper-reflexia and hyperactivity.

   b. premature ventricular contractions and bradycardia.
   c. muscle flaccidity and bruising.
   d. hypoactive bowel sounds and polydipsia.

5. Urinalysis and analysis of electrolytes reveal the following:

   Na: 145 mEq/L
   K: 10 mEq/L
   Casts: Positive
   Urine osmolality: 800 mOsm/L
   Specific gravity: 1.012
   Protein: Negative

   These findings are indicative of:
   a. glomerulonephritis.
   b. acute tubular necrosis.
   c. post-renal obstruction.
   d. dehydration.

6. Medical interventions that may be initiated to reverse the process identified above are:
   a. steroid therapy and fluid restrictions.
   b. use of immunosuppressive drugs and hydration.
   c. use of osmotic diuretics and colloids.
   d. loop diuretics and dialysis.

7. A nephron is composed of:
   a. Bowman's capsule and afferent and efferent arterioles.
   b. renal pyramid, calyx, and glomerulus.
   c. glomerulus, proximal tubule, Henle's loop, distal tubule, and collecting tubule.
   d. glomerulus, juxtaglomerular apparatus, and Henle's loop.

8. A patient is admitted for mental status changes and has a phosphate level of 6.2 mg %. Which of the following is true?
   a. ECG changes may include a depressed ST segment and development of a U wave.
   b. This condition can be treated with aluminum hydroxide gels.
   c. The patient will be hypercalcemic as well.
   d. Seizures may be anticipated, given this laboratory value.

9. L.J. is a 60-year-old man admitted with lethargy, nausea, vomiting, and dehydration. He has a primary diagnosis of small-cell lung cancer and is currently undergoing chemotherapy. Pertinent lab values include:

   Ca: 13.4 mg % (normal is 9–11)
   Albumin: 2.0 mg % (normal is 3.5–5)

The corrected calcium is:
a. 11.4 mg %.
b. 12.2 mg %.
c. 14.6 mg %.
d. 15.8 mg %.

10. The first treatment of choice for the patient described in question 9 will be:

a. fluid restrictions and calcitonin.
b. hydration and diuretics.
c. glucose and insulin.
d. phosphate and bicarbonate infusions.

Renal Anatomy and Physiology

Introduction

Smaller than an adult's fist and weighing approximately 4–6 ounces, the kidneys perform the remarkable job of regulating and maintaining the life-sustaining internal environment of the body. One major function performed by the kidneys is the regulation of body fluid. Each kidney receives approximately 1200 mL of blood per minute. Together the kidneys filter 180 L of fluid within a 24-hour period. Under normal conditions most of this fluid is reabsorbed back into the body, leaving 1–1.5 L to be excreted as urine per day. Under abnormal conditions, such as dehydration, the kidneys either concentrate or dilute urine, based on the composition and volume of the extracellular fluid. The kidneys have the unique capacity to adjust urine production from as little as 400 mL to as much as 25 L a day to meet changing physiologic needs.

Another major role of the kidneys is electrolyte regulation. Through the process of filtration and selective reabsorption, the kidneys maintain the delicate balance within the body of electrolytes such as sodium, potassium, calcium, and phosphorus. Controlling this balance is crucial for the maintenance of many normal body processes.

In addition to electrolyte regulation, the kidneys eliminate from the body over 200 metabolic waste products such as blood urea nitrogen (BUN) and creatinine. They also eliminate foreign chemicals such as food additives and pharmaceuticals.

The body maintains an acid-base equilibrium through the integration of processes involving the kidneys, lungs, and pH buffers such as bicarbonate, calcium, and plasma proteins. The kidneys work in conjunction with the respiratory system and the blood buffer system to regulate pH; however, only the kidneys can eliminate hydrogen ions from the body.

In addition to the excretory functions discussed above, the kidneys perform at least three vital endocrine functions. Through the release of renin and the renin-angiotensin mechanism, the kidneys are able to regulate blood pressure and maintain the body's circulating blood volume. A second endocrine function involves the kidneys' role in the production of erythropoietin. Erythropoietin stimulates the bone marrow to increase red blood cell production, a critical mechanism for the anemic or hypoxic patient. Third, the activation of vitamin D takes place in the kidneys. This process is an essential component of the calcium metabolism necessary for the maintenance and normal functioning of the body's neuro-muscular, skeletal, and vascular systems.

An Overview of the Urinary Tract

The urinary system is composed of the kidneys, ureters, bladder, and urethra, which are depicted in Figure 5-1. The major filtration functions occur within the kidneys, and the other structures serve as passageways for the removal of urine.

The kidneys are located on either side of the spinal column, just below the diaphragm in the retroperitoneal space. They extend from the eleventh or twelfth thoracic vertebra to the second lumbar vertebra. They are each approximately 11 cm ($4\frac{1}{4}$ inches) long, 7 cm (2–3 inches) wide, and 2.5 cm (1 inch) thick. The right kidney is positioned lower than the left kidney because the liver is just above it. As a result, in the absence of disease only the lower border of the right kidney is palpable upon physical exam. Alterations in the size and shape of the kidneys are common sequelae in disease and injury to the renal system. Located on top of each kidney are the adrenal glands.

The ureters exit from the medial borders of each kidney. They are 28–36 cm (11–14 inches) in length and provide a conduit between the kidneys and the bladder. The ureters measure only 2–8 mm (0.1–0.3 inches) in diameter, which makes them highly susceptible to obstruction. Normally, however, urine produced in the kidney is propelled by peristaltic contractions through the ureters into the bladder.

The bladder is an ovoid hollow organ approximately 10 cm (3 inches) in length. Normally the bladder holds 200–300 cc of urine; however, its capacity is several times greater. When empty, the bladder is located under the symphysis pubis; but if it is distended, it can be readily palpated and percussed above the symphysis pubis.

The urethra carries urine from the bladder to outside of the body. In males the urethra is about 6.5 cm (2.5–3 inches) long, and in females the urethra is 2.5–4 cm (1–1.5 inches) long. Because their urethras are shorter, women are more prone to bladder/urinary infections than men.

The Kidney

The gross structure of the kidneys is such that filtration and waste removal occur in the outer portions of the kidney (renal cortex) and final excretory products are collected centrally near the renal pelvis before exiting the kidney to be excreted from the body.

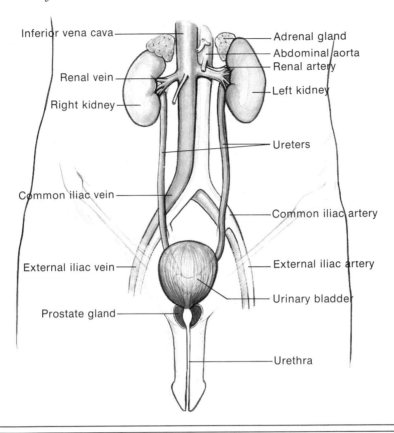

Inferior vena cava

Renal vein

Right kidney

Common iliac vein

External iliac vein

Prostate gland

Adrenal gland

Abdominal aorta

Renal artery

Left kidney

Ureters

Common iliac artery

External iliac artery

Urinary bladder

Urethra

Figure 5-1   Gross Anatomy of the Urinary System

Important anatomic structures of the kidneys are shown in Figure 5-2.

The Renal Fascia

The kidney's outermost covering is composed of a thin membrane known as the renal fascia. The renal fascia forms a sheet of tissue that surrounds the kidney and the layer of adipose tissue, the perirenal fat, directly adjacent to the kidney. The function of the renal fascia and the perirenal fat is to provide protection from trauma (mechanical blows) and to limit blood loss when injury is sustained. The kid-

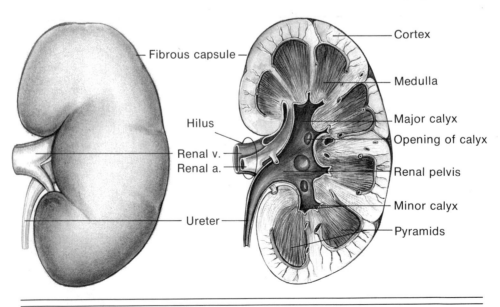

Fibrous capsule

Hilus

Renal v.

Renal a.

Ureter

Cortex

Medulla

Major calyx

Opening of calyx

Renal pelvis

Minor calyx

Pyramids

Figure 5-2   Internal Anatomy of the Kidney

neys are also protected by the intestines, which provide a thick cushion anteriorly, and by the ribs, which provide protection from the back.

The renal capsule is a thin, fibrous innermost covering which is loosely attached to the kidney. This tough, nonelastic structure provides protection and holds the organ together. However, when the kidney becomes edematous as a result of injury or disease, the capsule resists expansion, thereby increasing the renal interstitial pressure. This increased pressure subsequently contributes to reduced intrarenal filtration, further renal injury and symptomatic dysfunction.

The Hilum

The hilum is the indented or concave portion of the medial surface of the kidney. It is through the hilum that blood vessels, lymphatic vessels, and nerves enter and exit each kidney. The ureters are also connected to the kidneys at the hilum.

The Renal Cortex

Immediately under the capsule lies the renal cortex, comprising the outer third of the kidney. It is reddish-brown in color because of its large blood supply. It is mainly composed of thousands of capillary tufts called glomeruli. The distal and proximal convoluted tubules of the nephrons (to be discussed later in this section) are located in the cortex. These glomeruli and tubular systems perform the functions of filtration and reabsorption; thus injuries to the renal cortex are of major concern and significantly decrease renal function. The cortex extends from the renal capsule to the medulla and down between the renal pyramids toward the renal pelvis. These columns of cortical tissue are referred to as the renal columns.

The Renal Medulla

The middle third of the kidney is the renal medulla. It is lighter in color than the cortex because of its decreased blood supply. The renal medulla contains 8–10 cone-shaped structures called renal pyramids. The pyramids are composed of thousands of collecting tubules from the nephrons. At the apex of each pyramid is the papilla. The papilla, which has a perforated opening, serves to funnel urine from the pyramids into the renal pelvis.

The Renal Pelvis

The renal pelvis is the inner third of the kidney and primarily serves as a collecting reservoir for urine. The urine, which is funneled through the papillae, is first collected in a short, cuplike tubule called the calyx. From the calyx, the urine then collects in the renal pelvis, which has a capacity of approximately 3–5 cc. The urine is then propelled via peristalsis down the ureters to the bladder.

The Nephron

The functional unit of the kidney is the nephron. Each kidney contains more than a million of these tiny, urine-producing structures. The millions of nephrons combined have the ability to function as a composite unit. In fact, 70–75% of the kidneys' nephrons can be destroyed, and adequate renal function will still be maintained. Unfortunately, renal disease can be difficult to diagnose, since signs and symptoms may not appear until 90–95% of the nephrons are destroyed, making recovery unlikely.

Anatomically, the nephron can be divided into two components, a vascular component and a tubular component, as depicted in Figure 5-3.

The Vascular Component

The vascular component of the nephron consists of the glomerulus and the peritubular capillary network. The glomerulus is a unique high-pressure system that is located between two arterioles.[1] The looped or tufted structure of the glomerulus is important to renal function in that it provides a large, porous surface area for the filtration of fluids and solutes.

The blood in the glomerular capillaries is separated from the tubular component of the nephron by a single-cell capillary lining. The layer of basement membrane and the single-cell lining is called Bowman's capsule.

The peritubular capillaries are a low-pressure, reabsorptive system originating from the efferent arteriole.[2] These capillaries closely surround the remaining tubular portions of the nephron and provide for rapid movement of solutes and water between the capillary and tubular lumens. Most of the peritubular capillary network lies in the renal cortex; however, long, straight capillary loops called the vasa recta extend downward into the medulla.[3] The vasa recta wrap around and run parallel to the long thin loops of Henle and play a role in the concentration of urine.[4]

The Tubular Component

The initial portion of the tubular component of the nephron is Bowman's capsule. Bowman's capsule is a thin-walled membrane that supports and surrounds the glomerulus. One side of the capsule is intimate with the capillary tuft, and the other opens into the proximal convoluted tubule.

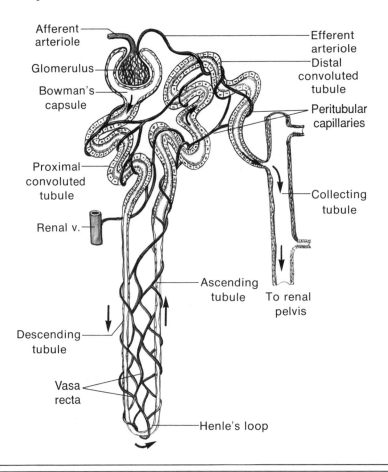

Figure 5-3 The Nephron

The proximal convoluted tubule (PCT) receives glomerular filtrate (water and solutes), which has been filtered through the glomerulus into Bowman's capsule. The primary function of the PCT is to further process the glomerular filtrate. Approximately 65% of all reabsorptive and secretory processes in the kidney take place in the PCT.

The proximal convoluted tubule ends at the loop of Henle. The loop of Henle is composed of a thin-walled descending limb, a sharp hairpin turn, and a thick-walled ascending limb. The configuration and the length of this loop play a vital role in the kidney's ability to concentrate and dilute urine.

The distal convoluted tubule (DCT) is the portion of nephron following the loop of Henle. The DCT further refines the glomerular filtrate. It plays a major role in the reabsorption of water, sodium, chloride, and sodium bicarbonate into the body and the excretion of potassium, ammonia, and hydrogen ions out of the body.

The final portion of the nephron is the collecting duct. The collecting duct joins with the papilla, emptying filtrate in its final form, urine, into the renal pelvis. The major function of the collecting duct is to finely adjust the dilution or concentration of urine, based on the physiologic needs of the body.

Renal Blood Flow

The kidneys are perfused with 1200 mL of blood per minute, which constitutes 20–25% of the cardiac output. About 90% of the renal blood flow (RBF) perfuses the cortex and the remaining 10% perfuses the medulla. A mean arterial pressure (MAP) of 80–100 mm Hg is considered essential for the maintenance of renal function.[5] Reductions in MAP will result in compromised renal function and reduced urine output. If the MAP drops below 60 mm Hg for over 40 minutes, ischemic injury will occur.[6]

Blood is supplied to the kidney by means of the renal artery, which arises from the abdominal aorta. The normal flow of blood through the kidney and its related structures is illustrated in Figure 5-4.

The renal artery is the initial vascular access into all parts of the kidney. Once inside the kidney, the renal artery divides into a series of arterial branches known as segmental arteries. The segmental arteries further divide into interlobar arteries and then into

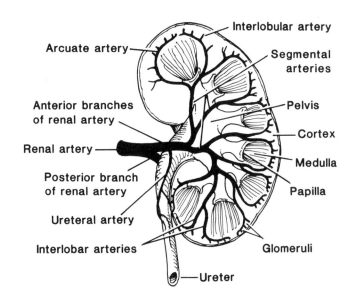

Figure 5-4 Blood Supply to the Kidney

arcuate arteries. The arcuate arteries divide into smaller interlobular arteries, which give rise to the afferent arterioles that enter the nephrons. Each afferent arteriole supplies blood to an individual glomerulus. When exiting the glomeruli, the glomerular capillaries come together again to form the efferent arterioles. The efferent arterioles then split to form the peritubular capillary network, which surrounds the tubular portion of the nephron. Blood from the peritubular capillaries returns to the venous system through the interlobular veins, followed by the arcuate veins and the interlobar veins. The interlobar veins and segmental veins then return blood to the renal vein. Both right and left renal veins empty into the inferior vena cava, which returns the blood to the heart.

Urine Formation

The three major steps in urine formation are glomerular filtration, tubular reabsorption, and tubular secretion. These are shown in Figure 5-5.

Glomerular filtration is the initial step in the formation of urine, by which protein-free plasma is filtered through the glomeruli into Bowman's capsule. Tubular reabsorption is the transfer of solutes from the filtrate inside the renal tubules into the peritubular capillaries; from there it is reabsorbed back into the body. Tubular secretion is the transfer of solutes from the peritubular capillaries into the filtrate within the renal tubules. Substances secreted into the tubule lumen will eventually be excreted in urine when they reach the end of the collecting duct of a nephron.

Glomerular Filtration

The capillaries in the glomerulus, like other capillaries in the body, are freely permeable to water and solutes of small molecular weight, such as electrolytes and end products of protein metabolism. These capillaries are relatively impermeable to substances of large molecular weight, such as plasma proteins, white blood cells, and red blood cells. As blood enters the normal glomerulus and is filtered into Bowman's capsule, the resultant glomerular filtrate is essentially protein-free and isotonic with plasma (specific gravity 1.010). In reality, the glomerulus is not a perfect sieve, and a small amount (less than 1%) of plasma proteins may be accidentally filtered through Bowman's capsule. Normally, however, this small amount of protein is reabsorbed, and therefore is not detectable in the urine. In cases of renal disease or injury, the membrane of the glomerulus may become leaky, allowing large quantities of proteins and red blood cells to be excreted in the urine.

As mentioned earlier, the glomerulus is a high-pressure capillary system because it is located between two arterioles. Since these arterioles are innervated by the sympathetic nervous system, they have the ability to constrict or dilate, thereby regulating the pressure in the glomerulus to meet physiologic

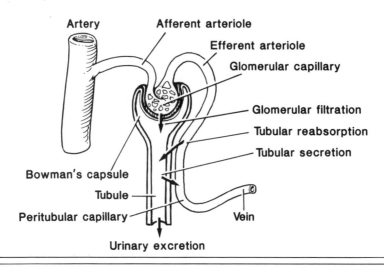

Artery   Afferent arteriole
Efferent arteriole
Glomerular capillary
Glomerular filtration
Tubular reabsorption
Tubular secretion
Bowman's capsule
Tubule
Peritubular capillary
Vein
Urinary excretion

Figure 5-5   Steps in Urine Formation

demands. The efferent arteriole, which is highly sensitive to sympathetic stimulation, has the ability to constrict in response to a decrease in renal blood flow. This constriction causes blood to back up in the glomerulus, restoring the glomerular blood pressure to a normal range. It is believed that a decrease in sodium and chloride concentrations within the renal tubules, often seen in hypovolemia, also stimulates constriction of the efferent arterioles. It is also believed that this decrease in ion concentration stimulates the dilation of the afferent arterioles, allowing for an even greater increase in glomerular blood flow and glomerular pressure.[7] The afferent arteriole can also constrict in hypervolemic states, thereby decreasing blood flow and glomerular pressure. The ability of the kidney to control renal blood flow and maintain glomerular pressure is known as autoregulation. This fine control over glomerular pressure allows renal blood flow and glomerular filtration to remain relatively constant in the face of mean arterial pressure fluctuations between 80 and 180 mm Hg.[8]

How does pressure affect glomerular filtration? Normally the pressure within the glomerular capillaries is about 50 mm Hg. This is at least twice as high as the pressure in other capillary systems. This high pressure favors the movement of plasma from the glomerular capillaries into Bowman's capsule. However, this pressure does not remain unopposed. Opposing filtration is the pressure of fluid already within Bowman's capsule, which is approximately 10 mm Hg. In addition, since plasma proteins (colloids) do not filter into Bowman's capsule but remain in the capillaries, they exert an opposing osmotic pressure of approximately 25 mm Hg. Water (in body fluids) has the tendency to move from areas of low solute concentration to areas of high solute concentration to

establish a concentration equilibrium. Osmosis is the movement of water across a semipermeable membrane in response to a concentration gradient. Osmotic pressure is the amount of pressure that must be applied to a solution in order to stop osmosis. The osmotic pressure created by the presence of proteins is referred to as oncotic pressure. The net result, as Table 5-1 illustrates, is a 15 mm Hg pressure difference favoring glomerular filtration.

The kidneys filter approximately 180 L of glomerular filtrate per day at a rate of 125 mL/min. This rate of flow per minute is commonly referred to as the glomerular filtration rate (GFR). As the filtrate passes through the remaining portions of the tubular nephron, all but 1–1.5 L a day will be returned to the bloodstream via the peritubular capillary network.

In summary, the factors that can affect the glomerular filtration rate are changes in glomerular capillary pressure, changes in osmotic pressure, or alterations in pressure within Bowman's capsule. Changes in glomerular pressure can arise secondary to radical changes in the systemic blood pressure. For

Table 5-1   Net Filtration Pressure in the Kidneys

Type of Pressure	Normal Level
Favoring filtration: Glomerular capillary pressure	+50 mm Hg
Opposing filtration: Fluid pressure in Bowman's capsule	−10 mm Hg
Opposing filtration: Colloid oncotic pressure	−25 mm Hg
Net pressure favoring filtration	+15 mm Hg

example, patients experiencing profound shock (mean arterial pressure less than 60 mm Hg) will experience decreased renal blood flow and blood pressure, producing a decrease in the GFR. A decreased GFR ultimately results in decreased urine output. Alterations in the body's circulating protein levels (for example, an increase due to dehydration or a decrease due to hypoproteinemia) can subsequently decrease or increase the GFR as a result of osmotic changes. Finally, alterations in Bowman's capsule pressure (such as increased pressure due to urinary obstruction, nephron destruction, renal interstitial edema, or renal diseases) can severely decrease the GFR, resulting in little or no urine output.

Tubular Reabsorption and Secretion

The renal tubules reabsorb over 99% of the glomerular filtrate the kidneys produce. Both active and passive transport mechanisms play a role in the reabsorption and secretion of substances in the renal tubules. Solutes such as sodium, chloride, and bicarbonate have a tendency to move from an area of high concentration to an area of lower concentration. This process is known as diffusion. Diffusion is a passive process—it does not require the use of energy. Active transport occurs when a substance is transported by a carrier molecule against a concentration gradient, which requires the use of energy. The reabsorption

of sodium from the renal tubules is one of the major energy-consuming processes occurring within the renal epithelial cells. This process (to be discussed later in this chapter) is thought to facilitate the passive movement of water, chloride, and other solutes such as potassium. The substances reabsorbed and the location of the reabsorption are diagrammed in Figure 5-6.

Sixty to eighty percent of the glomerular filtrate is reabsorbed in the proximal convoluted tubule. The majority of sodium, calcium, potassium, phosphate, and magnesium ions, uric acid, glucose, and amino acids are reabsorbed by active transport within the PCT. Ninety-nine percent of sodium and ninety percent of sodium bicarbonate are reabsorbed into the body. Urea diffuses passively from the tubules into the peritubular capillaries. Fifty-six percent of all urea is reabsorbed back into the body. Chloride is passively reabsorbed as it follows the positively charged sodium ions through the tubular lumens. Hydrogen ions are passively secreted within the proximal tubule. Pharmaceutical products are also actively secreted in the proximal convoluted tubule. Glucose and amino acids are completely reabsorbed in the PCT unless their serum concentrations exceed the renal threshold. Substances such as glucose require active transport systems to facilitate their reabsorption back into the bloodstream. The renal threshold is reached when the amount of solute exceeds the

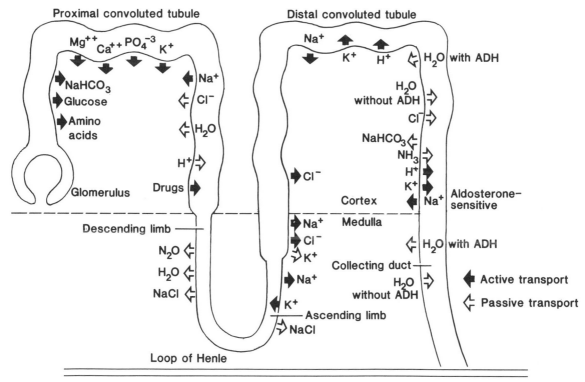

Figure 5-6 Absorption and Secretion in the Renal Tubules

capacity of the transport carrier molecule system within the tubule cells. When this happens, the substance that is in excess is excreted in urine. A patient with uncontrolled diabetes mellitus, for example, may have such a high serum glucose level that the amount of glucose filtered through the glomerulus exceeds the capacity of the glucose transport system (320 mg/min). As a result, glucose spills into the urine, where it can be readily detected.

The rate of reabsorption depends upon the length of time the filtrate remains within the renal tubules. In a hypovolemic patient, the GFR decreases, allowing the filtrate to remain within the tubules for a longer period of time. As a result, there is more time for reabsorption to occur, so urine output decreases. Conversely, in hypervolemia, the GFR increases and tubular reabsorption decreases, resulting in an increased urine output. The water reabsorption process is mediated by aldosterone and antidiuretic hormone (ADH), which will be discussed later in more detail.

The primary role of the loop of Henle is the reabsorption of sodium and chloride, providing a mechanism for the concentration of urine. The descending limb of the loop of Henle is freely permeable to both water and ions, allowing for the passive reabsorption of sodium, chloride, and water into the renal interstitium. The ascending limb is impermeable to water and ions, but contains active transport systems that pump large quantities of sodium chloride into the interstitium.

The selective process of reabsorption and secretion is completed in the distal convoluted tubule (DCT) and the collecting tubule or duct. Sodium is actively reabsorbed in the DCT, and uric acid, hydrogen, and potassium are secreted. Water reabsorption is a primary function of the collecting tubule. The reabsorption of solute-free water from the collecting tubule is dependent upon the reabsorption of sodium ions into the renal interstitium and the activity of antidiuretic hormone (ADH). Potassium, hydrogen ions, and ammonia are also secreted into the collecting tubules.

Regulation of Water Balance

Regulation of water balance is achieved by both internal mechanisms (shifts between intracellular and extracellular fluids) and external mechanisms (fluid intake and excretion). The cardiovascular system provides the flow of blood to the microcirculation so that essential nutrients, gases, products of cell metabolism, and cellular wastes may be exchanged between the plasma and the intracellular fluid (ICF). The body's exchange vessels are capillaries and venules. Exchanges between the cellular and vascular areas regulate the cellular environment. All capillaries are permeable to oxygen, carbon dioxide, and glucose. Capillaries differ in their permeability to other substances, such as proteins, electrolytes, and complexes such as bicarbonate. This selective permeability aids each type of body tissue in regulating its internal environment to perform necessary functions.

Water balance in the body is achieved by a complex set of interactions between the lungs, the cardiovascular system, the gastrointestinal system, and the renal system. The kidneys, however, play the major role in fluid volume regulation.

The body maintains a fluid balance that is largely governed by fluid shifts dictated by specific cellular needs. In general, the body's total fluid intake should equal its total fluid output. Average daily values for intake and output of water in the body are noted in Table 5-2.

Three mechanisms are responsible for the regulation of water balance in the body: thirst, which regulates the intake of fluid; the release of antidiuretic hormone (ADH), which mediates the reabsorption of water back into the body in response to increased serum osmolality; and the loop of Henle countercurrent mechanism, which plays a role (in conjunction with ADH) in the dilution or concentration of urine.

Thirst

Thirst is the primary regulator of the intake of water in the conscious individual. In order to under-

Table 5-2   Average Daily Intake and Output
of Water

Route	Average Value, mL
Intake:	
Beverages	1100
Food	950
Metabolism	350*
Output:	
Insensible	800*
Sweat	50*
Feces	150
Urine	1400

*These values vary considerably with activity, temperature, and humidity. In addition, individuals can vary their intake of food and water over a wide range of values and still remain in water balance.
Source: Keyes, J. L. (1990). *Fluid, Electrolyte, and Acid-Base Regulation.* Boston: Jones and Bartlett Publishers, p. 30.

stand how this powerful mechanism works, one must first realize that the kidneys are continually execreting water. In fact, 90% of all excreted urine is water. In addition to urine production, water is lost through evaporation from the skin and lungs. Therefore, the body is continually being dehydrated, causing the volume of extracellular fluid to decrease and the concentration of sodium and other osmotic elements to rise. Normally the osmolality of body fluids is maintained at approximately 285–295 mOsm/L (milliosmoles/liter). Slight increases in this value have the ability to trigger the thirst response; thus, this value is sometimes referred to as the threshold for drinking. Once the thirst response is stimulated, a person will usually drink precisely the amount of fluid required to bring the extracellular and intracellular fluids back to normal, that is, to reach a satiety state.

The thirst center is located slightly anterior to the supraoptic nuclei in the lateral preoptic area of the hypothalamus. The cells within the thirst center function very much the way osmoreceptors do. An increase in osmotic pressure within the cerebrospinal fluid or the circulating extracellular fluid promotes the sensation of thirst. Factors that contribute to increased osmolality are dehydration and increased sodium concentrations. However, another important cause is excessive potassium loss from the body.[9] Excessive potassium loss reduces the intracellular potassium of the cells of the thirst center and therefore decreases their volume. This decrease in intracellular fluid volume creates the desire to drink.

Release of Antidiuretic Hormone

Antidiuretic hormone (ADH) is synthesized in the hypothalamus and is then stored and released from the posterior pituitary gland. There are essentially five physiologic factors that promote the release of ADH.

By far the main stimulant for the release of ADH is an increase in extracellular fluid (ECF) osmolality. This increase in osmotic pressure stimulates the osmoreceptors located in the hypothalamus to release ADH from the posterior pituitary gland. When ADH is released, it acts on the distal convoluted and collecting tubules, causing water to be reabsorbed, thereby concentrating the urine. Conversely, when the ECF osmolality falls below normal, less ADH will be released. As a result, the kidneys will conserve less water in an attempt to decreased the ECF volume, producing a more dilute urine. A diagram of this relationship is shown in Figure 5-7.

ADH is also released in response to stimulation of the baroreceptors (stretch receptors) located in the atria and blood vessels. In the case of hypovolemia,

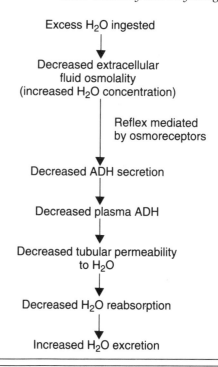

Figure 5-7 Mechanism of Stimulation of ADH

the baroreceptors sense the decrease in blood volume and stimulate the release of ADH. The release of ADH facilitates the reabsorption of water in the kidneys and reduces the hypovolemic state, as shown in Figure 5-8. The release of ADH is inhibited by this mechanism in instances of hypervolemia, allowing the kidneys to excrete more water, which increases the urine output.

The release of ADH is stimulated through several other mechanisms. These include pain and stress; certain drugs, such as morphine sulfate and diabinese; and the use of positive pressure stimulation of the alveolar ADH receptors, such as occurs with IPPB (intermittent positive pressure breathing) or mechanical ventilation.

The Loop of Henle Countercurrent System

The ability of the kidneys to concentrate urine is the major determinant of human beings' ability to survive for moderate periods of time without water. The loop of Henle countercurrent system allows the kidney to adjust urine concentration from a very dilute 50 mOsm/L to a very concentrated 1200 mOsm/L. The dynamics of this mechanism are highly dependent on the structure of the loop of Henle. Recall that the loop is positioned between the proximal and distal convoluted tubules. The loop itself extends deep into the medulla. The deeper the loop extends into the medulla, the greater the ability

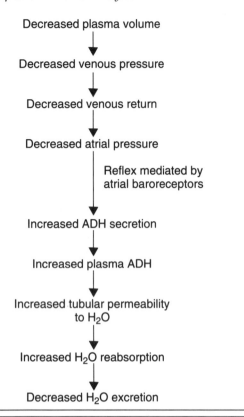

Figure 5-8 Mechanism of Inhibition of ADH

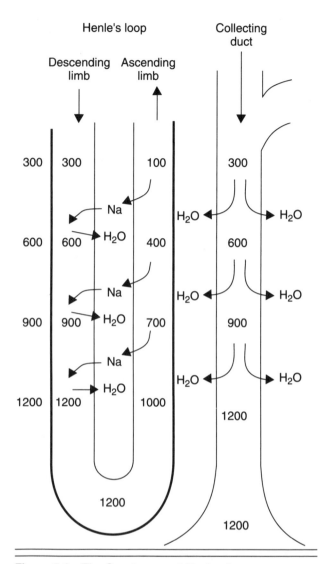

Figure 5-9 The Countercurrent Mechanism

of the nephron to concentrate urine. Within the loop itself, filtrate travels down the descending limb toward the medulla, makes a hairpin turn, and progresses up the ascending limb. Therefore, the filtrate is moving in opposite directions within the medulla—giving rise to the name *countercurrent system.*

The diagram in Figure 5-9 shows that as filtrate flows from the proximal tubule into the descending limb and progresses downward toward the medulla, the osmolality of the filtrate increases progressively from 300 mOsm/L to 1200 mOsm/L. Also, note that the osmolality of the filtrate and the osmolality of the renal interstitium are essentially the same. This occurs because the cells in the descending limb are freely permeable to both water and ions. As a result, passive fluxes of fluid and ions occur in this limb until the interstitial fluid and the intratubular fluids equilibrate. Therefore, since the interstitial fluid of the medulla is extremely concentrated, the deeper the nephron loop extends into the medulla, the more concentrated the filtrate inside the descending limb becomes, to a maximum of 1200 mOsm/L.

As the filtrate rounds the hairpin turn and travels up the thicker ascending limb of the loop of Henle, the osmolality of the filtrate inside the tubule immediately decreases, causing the filtrate to become more

and more dilute. This phenomenon occurs as a result of the ascending loop's impermeability to water and ions and its ability to actively transport or pump sodium chloride into the renal interstitium. As the filtrate moves up the ascending limb, it becomes progressively more dilute as sodium chloride is actively transported out of the tubule. By the time the filtrate enters the distal tubule, it is very dilute, approximately 100 mOsm/L. Since the filtrate is so dilute when it reaches the distal tubule, how does the kidney have the ability to concentrate urine?

What is actually accomplished as the filtrate progresses through the loop of Henle is the concentration or increase in osmolality of the fluid in the renal interstitium. This interstitial concentration plays a key role in enabling water to be reabsorbed back into the body. The final adjustments to urine concentration do not occur until the urine reaches the collecting tubule. It is the lining of the collecting tubule that is responsive to ADH. In the presence of ADH, the tubules become permeable to water, allowing water to rapidly diffuse out of the collecting duct into the interstitium as a result of the pressure gradient caused by the high interstitial concentration. It is important to note that ADH, through the mechanism described above, closely controls the amount of water that is excreted as urine. An increase in the release of ADH causes a proportional decrease in urine excretion; a decrease in the release of ADH causes a proportional increase in urine excretion.

The Vasa Recta

The vasa recta is the capillary network that extends deep into the medulla, surrounding and running parallel to the descending and ascending limbs of the loop of Henle. This specialized vascular system enables the fluid in the renal interstitium to remain concentrated. The two side-by-side streams of moving fluid and solutes within the capillary and the tubular systems prevent the washout of solutes from the interstitium. This, combined with the very small blood flow within the medulla (only 1–2%), allows for the concentration of sodium and chloride at the tip of the loop, facilitating the kidneys' ability to concentrate urine.

Blood Pressure Regulation

An adequate circulating blood volume is essential for the maintenance of tissue perfusion. The kidneys play an important role in blood pressure regulation through their renal endocrine functions, which are mediated by the renin-angiotensin mechanism.

Renin is released from the kidneys in response to a decrease in blood pressure, a decrease in sodium in the distal tubule, and/or an increase in sympathetic nervous stimulation mediated by the release of circulating catecholamines. Renin is secreted from the juxtaglomerular cells located within a specialized group of renal cells known as the juxtaglomerular apparatus (JGA). A portion of the JGA, the macula densa, maintains contact with the afferent and efferent arterioles and the distal convoluted tubule. It is these cells that are able to detect changes in arterial blood pressure. It is also believed that the macula densa responds to decreases in sodium and chloride and an increase in potassium within the renal tubules.[10]

When the macula densa registers a decrease in blood pressure and/or a decrease in sodium and chloride in the renal tubules, it stimulates the release of renin from the juxtaglomerular cells. Renin then converts angiotensinogen, a plasma protein pro-

duced by the liver, to angiotensin I. Angiotensin I (a mild vasoconstrictor) is converted to angiotensin II by a pulmonary enzyme as it circulates through the pulmonary system. Angiotensin II has very strong vasoconstricting properties, which create an increase in systemic blood pressure. Angiotensin II also stimulates the adrenal glands to release the hormone aldosterone from the adrenal cortex. The secretion of aldosterone causes the reabsorption of sodium in the renal tubules. As a result of sodium reabsorption, additional water is passively reabsorbed, thereby increasing the extracellular fluid volume. This process is diagrammed in Figure 5-10.

Erythropoiesis

Although the role of the kidneys in erythropoietin production is not fully understood, it is believed that the kidneys produce a hormone activator, which interacts with a plasma substrate to produce an erythropoietic hormone. This hormone, erythropoietin, acts to increase the rate of red blood cell production and the rate of red blood cell release from the bone marrow. There are at least two erythropoietin-mediated stimuli that have been shown to increase the rate of erythrocyte production. These are a reduction in inspired oxygen (pO_2) and anemia. For example, patients with chronic hypoxia, such as those with congestive heart failure or chronic obstructive pulmonary disease, often develop polycythemia (excessive red cell production). On the other hand, patients who suffer from acute or chronic renal failure are often anemic as a result of decreased erythropoietin production.

Regulation of Electrolytes

Regulation of electrolytes via renal excretory mechanisms is one of the major functions of the renal system. The electrolytes of importance to bodily functions that are regulated by the kidneys include sodium, potassium, calcium, phosphate, magnesium, and chloride. A summary of these electrolytes and their major functions in the body is given in Table 5-3.

Regulation of electrolytes involves a complex process of osmosis and active transport in the proximal tubule, descending or ascending loop of Henle, and the distal tubule. (Review Figure 5-6 for the location of reabsorption or excretion of the electrolytes.)

Sodium

Sodium is the major extracellular cation. The normal serum sodium concentration is 135–145

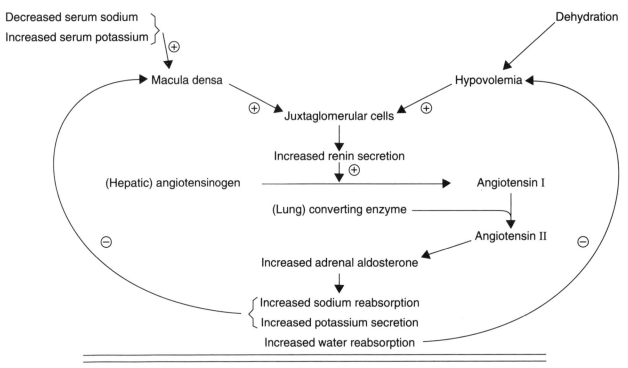

Figure 5-10　The Renin-Angiotensin Mechanism
Source: Pagana, K. D. and Pagana, T. J. (1982). *Diagnostic Testing and Nursing Implications.* St. Louis: C.V. Mosby Co.

mEq/L. Because sodium is osmotically active, its reabsorption promotes the reabsorption of water. Thus, sodium plays a major role in the maintenance of both the extracellular and intracellular fluid volumes. Ninety-nine percent of filtered sodium is reabsorbed by the nephron. The proximal tubule actively reabsorbs approximately 65%, the loop of Henle reabsorbs 25%, the distal tubule 6%, and the remaining 3–4% is reabsorbed via the collecting duct. The amount of sodium excreted in the urine normally varies from 40 to 80 mEq/L, depending on the physiological needs of the body.

There are two major factors determining the amount of sodium that is reabsorbed or excreted. These factors are the glomerular filtration rate (GFR) and the renin-angiotensin-aldosterone mechanism.

When the GFR is decreased, tubular reabsorption is increased, reducing the amount of sodium that is excreted in the urine. In this instance, the urine sodium may be reduced to 10–20 mEq/L. The decrease in sodium excretion is directly attributable to two factors. When the GFR is decreased (in states of renal hypoperfusion), less sodium is filtered into the renal tubules; therefore, less sodium is excreted. In addition, as a result of the decreased GFR, the filtrate remains in the tubules longer, thereby increasing the length of time available for tubular reabsorption. Conversely, increases in GFR deliver larger quantities of sodium to the renal tubules and

decrease reabsorption time. The result is an increase in urine sodium and a decrease in the amounts of sodium and water reabsorbed back into the body.

The renin-angiotensin-aldosterone mechanism also regulates sodium and water. When a decrease in renal blood flow is registered by the macula densa, renin is released from the juxtaglomerular cells, initiating the renin-angiotensin-aldosterone mechanism (discussed previously). The release of aldosterone from the adrenal glands causes the reabsorption of sodium and the secretion of potassium in the distal convoluted tubule. In the presence of large quantities of aldosterone, almost all of the sodium in the distal tubule will be reabsorbed. In addition, aldosterone is released in response to a decrease in sodium within the distal tubule. This response is also mediated through the macula densa and the release of renin. A decrease in the glomerular filtration rate, as seen in hypovolemia, causes a decrease in sodium and chloride within the renal tubules. Theoretically, this decrease stimulates the release of renin, triggering the renin-angiotensin-aldosterone mechanism.[11] The release of aldosterone facilitates the reabsorption of both sodium and water, thereby restoring both sodium and fluid volume to the body.

Potassium

Potassium is the major intracellular cation. The body's serum potassium concentration normally

Table 5-3 Major Electrolytes and Their Functions

Electrolyte/Normal Value	Function
Sodium 135–145 mEq/L	Major extracellular cation Regulates volume of fluid compartments Increases cell membrane permeability Maintains acid-base balance Involved in nerve impulse conduction Involved in muscle contraction
Potassium 3.5–5.0 mEq/L	Major intracellular cation Allows for proper smooth and skeletal muscle contraction Involved in depolarization and repolarization of heart Involved in nerve impulse conduction Assists in maintenance of acid-base balance
Calcium 8.5–10.5 mg/dL (mg %)	Involved in nerve impulse transmission Essential for cellular permeability Involved in bone/teeth formation Involved in muscular contraction Involved in blood coagulation
Phosphorus 3–4.5 mg/dL (mg %)	Principle intracellular anion Involved in metabolic functions: acid-base homeostasis, bone formation, nerve/ muscle activity, cell division, and metabolism of carbohydrates, protein, and fat Has inverse relationship with calcium
Magnesium 1.5–2.5 mEq/L	Enhances neuromuscular function Stimulates parathyroid secretion of parathormone Involved in enzyme activation Regulates skeletal muscle function
Chloride 96–106 mEq/L	Involved in digestion Maintenance of acid-base balance Maintains body water balance Influences osmolality and toxicity of ECF (Renal chloride loss always accompanies sodium loss; sodium cannot be reabsorbed without chloride)

Source: M. J. Holechek. (1990). *Acute Renal Failure.* Baltimore: The Johns Hopkins Hospital Department of Medical Nursing.

ranges from 3.5 to 5.0 mEq/L. The body maintains a constant balance between the potassium in the intracellular fluid and that in the extracellular fluid. Since dietary intake of potassium is variable, internal mechanisms are responsible for reducing the extracellular concentration of potassium. These mechanisms include alterations in the cells' uptake of potassium and variations in excretion. Cellular uptake of potassium is regulated by osmolar properties and insulin levels. Excretion of excessive potassium is stimulated by increased aldosterone levels and the sodium-potassium balance and accomplished by excretion by the distal convoluted tubule. Potassium is actively reabsorbed in the proximal tubule, but it is actively and passively secreted into the distal tubule so that the body achieves homeostasis. Generally speaking, 10–15% of the filtered potassium is excreted in the urine, in comparison to the 1–2% of filtered sodium excreted.

At least three factors influence the amount of potassium excreted. These factors are the serum potassium level, pH, and the urine output.

An elevation in serum potassium, hyperkalemia, directly stimulates the release of aldosterone. As a result, an exchange of sodium and potassium ions occurs in the distal convoluted tubule and the collecting duct. In the presence of aldosterone, sodium is reabsorbed and potassium is excreted. In hypokalemia, the kidney tries to reabsorb potassium. However, the amount of potassium excreted is influenced by the GFR and urine output. An increase in GFR and urine output will ultimately result in an increased potassium excretion even in the presence of hypokalemia.

The hydrogen ion concentration also plays a role in potassium excretion. Within the distal tubule cells, there is an inverse relationship between the hydrogen ion and the potassium ion. When there is an increase in hydrogen ion excretion (for example, in states of acidemia), potassium and hydrogen ions exchange across the cell membrane. Potassium is shifted from the intracellular fluid into the extracellular fluid, thereby increasing serum potassium levels. Normal renal mechanisms will ensure that the

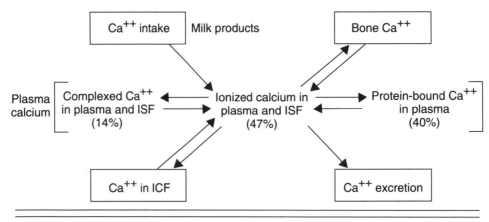

Figure 5-11 Factors Affecting Calcium Regulation

excess potassium ions are excreted via the urine, but in cases of renal failure, potassium ions accumulate in the serum and lead to hyperkalemia. In alkalotic states, the kidney responds by secreting potassium ions, but unless the alkalosis is severe, the serum potassium levels will not drop below normal limits.

Calcium and Phosphate

Calcium is an important cation within the body, as it is necessary for the transmission of nerve and muscle impulses, the coagulation of blood, the formation of bones, and the maintenance of cellular permeability. Less than 1% of total body calcium is found in the serum; most is located in the bones. The complex relationship among the various forms of calcium and the factors affecting its concentration are diagrammed in Figure 5-11.

A normal serum calcium level is a count of the total amount of calcium in the body in all of its forms. Normal levels are 8.5–10.5 mg/dL (4.5–5.5 mEq/L). About 40% of the body's plasma calcium is bound to proteins such as albumin, 14% is complexed with other ions such as citrate or phosphate, and about 47% is freely ionized and available for chemical and biological reactions.[12] Ionized calcium levels are normally 2–2.5 mEq/L.[13] The relationship between calcium and serum proteins is such that for every 1 g/dL decrease in albumin (the major serum protein) there is an 0.8 mg/dL increase in available ionized and active calcium.[14] It is therefore necessary to correct serum calcium levels, since a decrease in protein will cause more calcium to be available to the tissues.

An example of how to compute correct serum calcium levels based on protein levels is given in Table 5-4. In this example, the patient's original calcium level is within normal limits; however, once the albumin level changes, the patient's calcium level is elevated, and may be reflected in the patient's symptoms. The calculation of calcium levels is im-

portant with patients who are severely hypoalbuminemic, those who may appear slightly hypocalcemic, or those who are already hypercalcemic.

About 98% of calcium is reabsorbed, primarily in the proximal convoluted tubule. In general, calcium levels are regulated downward by thyrocalcitonin (or calcitonin, CT) and upward by parathyroid hormone (PTH). Vitamin D plays a role in permitting PTH to resorb calcium from the bone, and increases calcium absorption from the intestine.

A decrease in ionized serum calcium levels stimulates the secretion of PTH from the parathyroid glands. The PTH functions to increase the reabsorption of calcium at the distal tubule to replenish serum calcium levels. In exchange for calcium ions, PTH causes the excretion of phosphate. PTH also liberates calcium from the bones.

Vitamin D is necessary for the absorption of calcium from the small intestines; however, it must first be activated by both the liver and the kidneys. Cholecalciferol, vitamin D_3, is hydroxylated in the liver to form 25-hydroxycholecalciferol. This is then converted to 1,25-dihydroxycholecalciferol (the activated form of vitamin D) in the kidneys. This process is diagrammed in Figure 5-12.

Patients who suffer from chronic renal failure do not have the ability to activate vitamin D in the

Table 5-4 Correction of Serum Calcium Levels Based on Albumin Levels

(Initial) Serum calcium	9 mg/dL (normal = 8.5–10.5)
Serum albumin	4 g/dL (normal = 3.5–5)
(Later) Serum albumin	1 g/dL (4 − 1 = 3)
Corrected calcium	3 × 0.8 = 2.4
	9.0 (initial) + 2.4 = 11.4 mg/dL

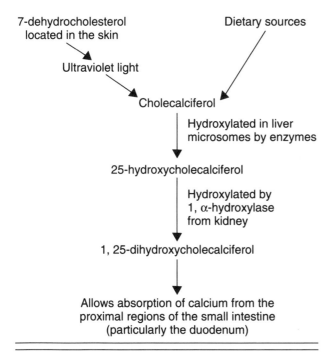

7-dehydrocholesterol located in the skin

Dietary sources

Ultraviolet light

Cholecalciferol

Hydroxylated in liver microsomes by enzymes

25-hydroxycholecalciferol

Hydroxylated by 1, α-hydroxylase from kidney

1, 25-dihydroxycholecalciferol

Allows absorption of calcium from the proximal regions of the small intestine (particularly the duodenum)

Figure 5-12 Vitamin D Activation

kidneys. As a result, they are unable to maintain serum calcium levels through the absorption of ingested calcium. Their bones may become extremely brittle and fragile as the PTH-mediated release of calcium from the bones continues in the body's futile attempt to maintain calcium within normal limits.

Increasing concentrations of ionized calcium in the plasma stimulates the release of thyrocalcitonin, which lowers the plasma concentration by limiting the resorption of calcium from the bones and increasing urinary excretion.

It was once believed that calcium and phosphorus were in a reciprocal relationship whereby increases in one ion led to decreases in the other ion. It is now known that the relationship is far more complex.[15] Sudden increases in phosphate can lead to decreased calcium levels as a result of increased renal excretion of calcium, but the reverse is not true. Mechanisms for phosphate regulation are not fully understood, but it does require active transport. Phosphate is the major buffer excreted in the urine. The rate of excretion of phosphate depends upon oral intake and levels of PTH. The normal serum concentration of phosphate is 3.0–4.5 mg/dL. Phosphate ions are found in the bone and are necessary for intracellular energy-producing reactions.

Active phosphate reabsorption takes place in the PCT. Phosphate reabsorption depends upon the sodium concentration and is inversely related to the GFR. Increased GFR results in decreased reabsorption; decreased GFR results in increased

reabsorption. As discussed above, PTH inhibits the reabsorption of phosphate. As the kidney is the primary excretory organ for phosphate, in acute or chronic renal failure, phosphate is not removed from the body. Such an increase in serum phosphate level perpetuates the body's inability to maintain an adequate serum calcium level by inhibiting the resorption of calcium from the bones.[16]

Excretion of Waste Products

The kidneys excrete over 200 different waste products. Two waste products that are readily measured and used as an indication of renal function are blood urea nitrogen (BUN) and creatinine.

BUN is a nitrogenous waste product of muscle or protein metabolism. Its normal serum concentration is 12–25 mg/dL. Urea is filtered at the glomerulus and reabsorbed throughout the nephron. In renal failure the BUN is elevated, but it can be elevated in other circumstances as well, which makes it an unreliable indicator of renal function. Since urea is an end product of protein metabolism, serum levels can be elevated by a high-protein diet, catabolic states (bleeding, infection, disease processes), steroids, changes in protein metabolism, and changes in GFR. It is essential to look at BUN in conjunction with the creatinine level to determine if true renal failure has occurred.

Creatinine is a very reliable indicator of renal function. Creatinine is the waste product of muscle metabolism. Since the body's muscle mass does not radically change from day to day, creatinine production remains fairly constant. The normal serum concentration ranges between 0.4 and 1.5 mg/dL. The kidneys normally excrete creatinine at a rate approximately equal to the GFR. Since creatinine is produced at a constant rate and is freely filtered and not reabsorbed or excreted anywhere along the tubule, creatinine levels can be directly related to renal function. For example, when the serum creatinine levels and BUN levels of a patient with intrarenal deterioration are compared the BUN and creatinine often rise proportionately (in a 10:1 ratio of BUN to creatinine). In cases in which the BUN is elevated but the creatinine is not, renal failure may not be the cause of the increase in BUN.

Thus, it should be obvious why creatinine is one of the substances used to calculate the GFR. The clearance rate is the amount of a substance cleared by the kidney in a 1-minute period. The formulas for calculating clearance rates are shown in Table 5-5.

Creatinine clearance is normally 115–125 mL/min; a given value must be corrected for body surface area (reflecting muscle mass). The test is performed

Table 5-5 Formulas for Calculation of Creatinine Clearance Rates

$$C = \frac{U \times V}{P}$$

$$GFR = \frac{U_x \times V}{P_x}$$

C = clearance rate
U = urine concentration
V = urine volume (mL/min)*
P = plasma concentration

U_x = urine concentration of *x*, any substance
    freely filtered but not reabsorbed or secreted,
    in this case, creatinine
V = urine volume (mL/min)
P_x = plasma concentration of *x*

*Urine volume in mL/min is obtained by dividing the total volume of urine (in mL) for a 24-hour period by 1440 (the number of minutes in 24 hours).

on a 24-hour urine specimen, with blood drawn for serum creatinine at intervals during the 24-hour period that depend on the practices of the institution.

The creatinine clearance rate (that is, GFR) is a valuable clinical assessment tool used to determine renal function. In particular, decreases in the creatinine clearance rate can indicate serious renal pathology such as urinary tract obstruction, nephron destruction (acute tubular necrosis) or glomerular/capsular inflammation (glomerulonephritis).

Acid-Base Balance

The body is maintained in a state of acid-base balance through the combined efforts of the respiratory, buffer, and renal systems. The kidneys normally excrete approximately 50–90 mEq of acid per day. Although slow to respond to states of acidosis and alkalosis, the kidneys are very effective at accurately correcting changes in pH. Unlike the respiratory system, however, which responds to changes in pH within minutes, the kidneys take up to 24–48 hours to effect change. This response may continue over a period of several days.

Three basic mechanisms enable the kidneys to maintain acid-base balance. These include the regulation of bicarbonate, the ability to excrete hydrogen ions directly, and the ability to neutralize acids.

Bicarbonate and Hydrogen Ion Regulation

Bicarbonate, sodium, chloride, and phosphate are filtered in Bowman's capsule.[17] Ninety percent of all filtered bicarbonate (HCO_3^-) is reabsorbed in the proximal tubule in an exchange process involving sodium (Na^+) and hydrogen (H^+) ions. This process is begun within the cells of the proximal convoluted tubule (PCT). Inside the cells carbon dioxide (CO_2) combines with water (H_2O) and forms carbonic acid (H_2CO_3). Carbonic anhydrase (CA), an enzyme found on the luminal borders of the proximal tubule cells, is needed to catalyze or speed up the process.[18]

$$CO_2 + H_2O \xrightarrow{CA} H_2CO_3$$

The carbonic acid then dissociates into hydrogen ions and bicarbonate.

$$H_2CO_3 \longrightarrow H^+ + HCO_3^-$$

The newly formed bicarbonate is reabsorbed into the plasma and the hydrogen ions are actively secreted into the tubular lumens in exchange for sodium. In cases of decreased extracellular fluid volume, when sodium reabsorption is increased, the secretion of hydrogen ions is enhanced. Although the mechanism is not fully understood, the release of aldosterone also stimulates hydrogen ion secretion and sodium reabsorption.

Once inside the tubular lumen, the secreted hydrogen ions combine with the filtered bicarbonate ions to form carbonic acid.[19]

$$H^+ + HCO_3^- \longrightarrow H_2CO_3$$

The carbonic acid then dissociates into water and carbon dioxide.

$$H_2CO_3 \xrightarrow{CA} H_2O + CO_2$$

The carbon dioxide is reabsorbed into the tubular cells, and the water is either excreted or reabsorbed, depending upon the fluid needs of the body.

This process continues throughout the length of the nephron. About 2% of the filtered bicarbonate is reabsorbed in the loop of Henle, about 8% in the distal tubule, and the remainder in the collecting duct. For every filtered bicarbonate ion that combines with a secreted hydrogen ion, a new bicarbonate ion is generated within the tubular cells. These bicarbonate ions are also reabsorbed, replenishing the body's bicarbonate (buffer) stores.

Phosphate and Renal Buffers

A very small amount of free hydrogen ions is present in the urine at any given time. The amount directly excreted is less than 1 mEq/day. In the tubular lumen the hydrogen ions are buffered or combined with several substances. A small amount of filtered bicarbonate escapes tubular reabsorption and buffers hydrogen ions in the distal portion of the nephron. Titratable acids, however, buffer a sizable percentage of hydrogen ions.

The filtered phosphate (HPO_4) is delivered to the distal portion of the nephron. The phosphate combines with hydrogen and sodium to form monosodium acid phosphate (NaH_2PO_4):[20]

$$HPO_4^{2-} + H^+ + Na^+ \longrightarrow NaH_2PO_4$$

The monosodium acid phosphate is then excreted as a titratable acid in the urine. Several other titratable acids act to a lesser extent to buffer hydrogen ions; however, titratable acids have a limited usefulness in correcting pH imbalances. Substances such as phosphate are filtered at a fairly constant rate despite changes in pH.

Ammonia Secretion

Ammonia (NH_3) is produced by the distal tubular cells. It passively diffuses into the tubular lumen and attaches to hydrogen ions, forming ammonium (NH_4^+):

$$NH_3 + H^+ \longrightarrow NH_4^+$$

Since ammonia is a neutral substance, it does not affect the pH of the urine. The kidneys can increase the production of ammonium, thereby buffering approximately 30–250 mEq of hydrogen ions per day, depending upon the body's requirements.[21]

Acidosis

In response to increased secretion of hydrogen ions into the tubular lumen during cellular acidosis, all bicarbonate and sodium are reabsorbed back into the plasma. An increase in the excretion of phosphate and an increase in the production of ammonia occur, buffering excess hydrogen ions and allowing more acid to be excreted into the urine. The urine pH will be less than 5.0 because of the higher than usual concentration of hydrogen ions being excreted. The

plasma pH will slowly be returned to normal as a result of the reabsorption of bicarbonate and the excretion of hydrogen ions.

Alkalosis

In a patient in an alkalotic state, fewer hydrogen ions are secreted and excess amounts of bicarbonate ions are excreted in the urine, resulting in a urine pH greater than 7.0. The retention of hydrogen ions and the excretion of bicarbonate will slowly decrease the plasma pH to normal.

Assessment of Renal Function

Renal assessment includes historical, physical, and laboratory examination of fluid and electrolyte balances and actual kidney function. Important factors to consider when evaluating a patient with a possible renal or fluid disorder are listed in Table 5-6.

The assessment of patients with suspected fluid and electrolyte disturbances involves the evaluation of several factors known to influence body needs for water: body surface area, percentage of body fat (fat holds water), body and environmental temperatures (increased heat requires additional fluid), exercise or activity, and general health status. Physical exam of the patient with a potential fluid or renal problem should involve a complete head-to-toe assessment, as all body systems may be implicated. Pertinent assessment parameters are shown in Figure 5-13.

Table 5-6 Important Factors in Assessment of Renal Status

Personal Practices	Recent Changes in Health Status
Bowel routines	Increased thirst
Urination routines	Excessive perspiration
Daily fluid intake	Increased or decreased urinary output
Dietary restrictions	Chronic diarrhea
Exercise routines	Weakness
	Dizziness
	Fatigue
	Weight loss
	Nausea/vomiting
	Anorexia
	Cramps (legs, abdomen)
	Muscle tremors or twitches
	Fever
	Palpitations
	Irritability

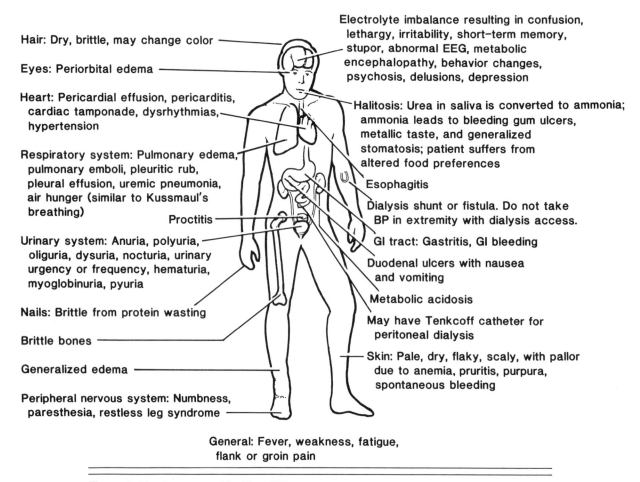

Hair: Dry, brittle, may change color

Eyes: Periorbital edema

Heart: Pericardial effusion, pericarditis, cardiac tamponade, dysrhythmias, hypertension

Respiratory system: Pulmonary edema, pulmonary emboli, pleuritic rub, pleural effusion, uremic pneumonia, air hunger (similar to Kussmaul's breathing)

Proctitis

Urinary system: Anuria, polyuria, oliguria, dysuria, nocturia, urinary urgency or frequency, hematuria, myoglobinuria, pyuria

Nails: Brittle from protein wasting

Brittle bones

Generalized edema

Peripheral nervous system: Numbness, paresthesia, restless leg syndrome

Electrolyte imbalance resulting in confusion, lethargy, irritability, short-term memory, stupor, abnormal EEG, metabolic encephalopathy, behavior changes, psychosis, delusions, depression

Halitosis: Urea in saliva is converted to ammonia; ammonia leads to bleeding gum ulcers, metallic taste, and generalized stomatosis; patient suffers from altered food preferences

Esophagitis

Dialysis shunt or fistula. Do not take BP in extremity with dialysis access.

GI tract: Gastritis, GI bleeding

Duodenal ulcers with nausea and vomiting

Metabolic acidosis

May have Tenkcoff catheter for peritoneal dialysis

Skin: Pale, dry, flaky, scaly, with pallor due to anemia, pruritis, purpura, spontaneous bleeding

General: Fever, weakness, fatigue, flank or groin pain

Figure 5-13   Assessment for Renal Disease

Intake and output measurement is the most common method of assessing fluid balance in the critically ill. Unfortunately many losses are unaccounted for in these measurements. Nurses may increase the accuracy of intake and output records by establishing standards of care addressing such measurements or using the clearance mechanism on intravenous pumps to determine accurate intake. Another helpful practice is to recognize obscure but sometimes appreciable losses caused by blood drawing (possible 100–200 cc/day), invasive monitoring of fluid intake, or loss of fluid with rapid ventilation. A conversion that may be helpful in calculating less definitive losses is the milliliter-to-kilogram metric conversion: approximately 1000 cc is equal to 1 kilogram (0.1 kg = 100 cc). This conversion may be helpful in assessing anticipated weight gains from 24-hour intake and output comparisons or drainage output. Dressings, linen, or dialysis bags can be weighed dry, then saturated, and approximate losses calculated. Fluids may be lost from many drainage devices and orifices. Characteristic fluid losses are listed in Table 5-7.

Insensible losses are estimated to be about 200 cc per day, but patients with diaphoresis, tachypnea, or skin breakdown will lose more fluid through the skin or lungs. Overall fluid balance can be assessed through various means, but body weight is the most accurate reflection of net gain or loss of fluid. Again, a fluid excess of 1000 cc will produce approximately 1 kilogram of weight gain. When insensible losses are incalculable, or patients have very labile fluid problems, weighing the patient several times a day may guide clinicians in maintaining a goal weight.

Assessment of the circulating blood volume, or intravascular volume, will assist the nurse in deter-

Table 5-7 Expected Drainage from Tubes and Catheters

Type of Device	Measures	Potential Fluid Loss	Normal Appearance of Fluid	Normal Smell of Fluid	Normal Consistency of Fluid
Foley catheter	Urine	500–700 mL for first 2 postop days; 1500–2500 mL normal	Clear, yellow	Ammonia	Watery
Gastrostomy tube	Gastric fluid	Up to 1500 mL	Pale, yellow-green	Sour	Watery
Hemovac	Wound drainage	Varies with procedure	Varies with procedure	Like wound dressing	Variable
Ileal conduit	Urine	500–2500 mL	Clear, yellow	Ammonia	Watery (with mucus and blood initially)
Ileostomy	Small bowel contents	Up to 4000 mL in first 24 hr; then less than 1000 mL	Brown	Sour, fecal	Initially serous with mucus; brown liquid stool when peristalsis resumes
Miller-Abbott tube	Intestinal contents	Up to 3000 mL	Dark green or brown	Neutralized acid; fecal	Thick
Nasogastric tube	Gastric contents	Up to 1500 mL	Pale, yellow-green	Sour	Watery
T tube	Bile	500 mL	Bright yellow to dark green	Acrid	Thick
Suprapubic catheter	Urine	500–2500 mL	Clear, yellow	Ammonia	Watery
Ureteral catheter	Urine	250–1250 mL	Clear, yellow	Ammonia	Watery

Source: Bellack, J. P., and Edlun, B. J. (1992). *Nursing Assessment and Diagnosis.* Second edition. Boston: Jones and Bartlett Publishers, p. 594.

mining whether the fluid volume reflected by the patient's weight is in the vascular space or elsewhere. Blood pressure readings and pulse measurement with evaluation for orthostatic changes may be helpful but not necessarily sensitive approaches to intravascular volume assessment, since other factors may cause alterations. The most accurate measures of vascular volume are central venous pressures or pulmonary artery pressures. Factors that interfere with the accuracy of these measurements include heart failure, pulmonary disease, vasoconstriction, and vasodilation.

Assessment of fluid in the tissues is achieved by evaluating the patient for edema. Edema reflects the movement of fluid from intravascular and intracellu-

lar locations to interstitial spaces. Edema may be caused by inflammatory stimulation, hypoproteinemia, and hypernatremia. Although assessment of peripheral cutaneous edema can reveal the existence of a fluid imbalance, peripheral edema is not always present when venous congestion and organ edema are occurring. Symptoms of fluid overload without peripheral edema include dyspnea, hypertension, jugular vein pulsations, and hepatomegaly.

Laboratory evaluation of fluid balance is best achieved by reviewing the serum osmolality in the context of the electrolyte and blood chemistry values. When other solutes are not proportionately high or low, the plasma osmolality reflects the solute concentration of the blood. Normal serum osmolality is

Table 5-8 Laboratory Tests for Evaluation of Fluid, Electrolytes, and Renal Status

Lab Test	Normal Value	Significance
Hematological		
Hematocrit	Female: 37–47 mL/100 mL	Increases with dehydration
	Male: 40–54 mL/100 mL	Decreases with hypervolemia
Serum Chemistry		
Serum osmolality	280–295 mOsm/kg	Increases with dehydration
		Decreases with hypervolemia
Blood urea nitrogen (BUN)	12–25 mg/100 mL	Increases with protein breakdown or renal dysfunction
Creatinine (Creat)	0.5–1.5	Elevated with excessive muscle breakdown or when 50% or more of kidney nephrons are destroyed
Sodium (Na)	135–145 mEq/L	Increases with dehydration and decreases with fluid overload and with SIADH
Chloride (Cl)	98–106 mEq/L	
Potassium (K)	3.5–5.0 mEq/L	Increases with crush injuries, hemolysis, renal failure, or overutilization of K^+ sparing diuretics
Calcium (Ca)	8.5–10.5 mg/100 mL (4.5–5.5 mEq/100 mL)	Potential decreases with multiple banked blood transfusions and in oncologic tumor lysis syndrome
Phosphate (PO_4)	3.0–4.5 mg/100 mL	Increases in oncologic tumor lysis syndrome, renal failure, or antacid overdose/abuse
Magnesium (Mg)	1.5–2.0	May decrease with use of nephrotoxic agents, diuretics
Urine chemistry		
24-hour-urine creatinine clearance	115–125 mL/min	Decreases with inadequate fluid intake, hypotension, or renal dysfunction
Urine osmolality	50–1200 mOsm/L	Should be 1½ times serum osmolality
Urine electrolytes	Na: 40–80 mEq/L K: 20–40 mEq/L	Selective excretion of electrolytes with specific medications or types of renal failure
Urine specific gravity	1.010–1.030	Increases with dehydration or kidney hypoperfusion and decreases in diuretic phase of recovery from renal failure
Urine pH	4.6–6.0	

Source: B. K. Shelton (1991). Electrolyte disturbances. Baltimore: The Johns Hopkins Oncology Center.

between 280 and 295 mOsm. This narrow margin is achieved by renal excretion or reabsorption of solutes. This value will not be an accurate reflection of the patient's clinical condition when the patient has abnormally high or low serum levels of high-molecular-weight substances such as glucose, BUN, sodium, or proteins.

Laboratory studies of renal disease are addressed extensively in the sections of this chapter that cover electrolyte disorders and acute renal failure. Common laboratory assessment parameters for evaluation of renal or fluid status are listed in Table 5-8. Radiologic and diagnostic procedures for evaluating the kidneys, ureters, bladder, urethra, and related vessels are summarized in Table 5-9.

Assessment of patients at risk for fluid, electrolyte, and renal problems can be a complex task. Many presenting symptoms overlap and point to various etiologies. The following sections outlining the major renal disorders should help clarify the finer points of renal assessment.

Electrolyte Imbalances

Electrolytes are the essential anions and cations that act within the body to regulate various homeostatic functions such as maintenance of blood volume, glomerular filtration rate, toxic waste removal, muscular contractility, and nerve conduction. Imbalances of these electrolytes can result from (1) external losses, (2) excessive intake, (3) improper excretion, or (4) inefficient usage. Such imbalances may lead to physical disorders and symptomatology. The major electrolytes and the associated disorders likely to be encountered by the critical care nurse are described within this section.

Sodium

Adults have approximately 60 mEq of sodium per kilogram of body weight. Forty percent of this sodium is found in bone, 50% in the extracellular fluid, and the remaining 10% in the intracellular fluid. The normal serum level of sodium is 135–145 mEq/L. About 80% of these stores is available for replacement of some sodium lost in normal body processes such as excretion, diaphoresis, and gastrointestinal secretion.

Sodium is the chief extracellular cation. It has several important roles, including (1) maintenance of the distribution of fluids in the body, (2) promotion of osmotic pressures, (3) regulation of acid-base balance, (4) conduction and alteration of cell permeability, and (5) promotion of cell irritability (which assists in electrical conduction of impulses).[22]

Table 5-9 Radiologic and Invasive Renal Diagnostic Studies

Study	Purpose	Procedure	Patient Care
KUB x-ray (kidneys, ureters, bladder)	To visualize size, shape, position and number of renal, ureteral, and bladder structures; will locate objects, foreign bodies, calculi or neoplasms	x-ray is taken of patient	Before: Explain procedure to the patient During: None After: None
Renal ultrasound	To identify gross renal anatomy and depth; will detect obstruction, hydronephrosis, tumors and cysts; can differentiate tumors and cysts	Mineral oil is applied over the kidneys; inaudible, nonharmful sound waves are reflected off the kidneys and photographs are taken; a hand-held transducer is moved over the mineral oil	Before: Explain the procedure. Let patient know he or she will have to lie prone for 30 min and that a transducer will be applied with some pressure During: Provide comfort measures After: Ensure all mineral oil has been removed
Renal scan	To reveal renal anatomy, function, and perfusion	A radionuclide is given IV; serial x-rays are taken	Before: Explain the procedure During: None After: None
Intravenous pyelogram (IVP)	To visualize size, shape and position of urinary tract and renal excretory function; not useful if creatinine >3 mg/dL	A radiopaque dye is given IV and x-rays are taken at intervals; use with care in patients with impaired renal function or iodine allergy	Before: Explain the procedure; NPO after midnight; bowel preparation (enema and laxatives); ensure patient has no allergies to sulfa or shellfish; hydration During: Assess patient for anaphylaxis and have emergency drugs (Benadryl, epinephrine, steroids) and equipment on hand After: Hydration to facilitate dye excretion
CT scan	To create an image of the kidney and calculate its density; allows visualization of masses, vascular disorders, and filling defects of the collecting system	Multiple x-rays are taken 10 min. apart and transmitted to a computer, which creates an image of the kidney; can be done with or without dye	Before: Explain procedure; ensure that patient has no dye allergies; let patient know that he or she will have to be still in a confined space for 40 min. During: Observe patient for anaphylaxis After: None

(continued)

Table 5-9   Radiologic and Invasive Renal Diagnostic Studies (*continued*)

Study	Purpose	Procedure	Patient Care
Renal arteriogram	To outline renal vasculature and differentiate renovascular disorders	Dye is injected through an arterial catheter (femoral, usually) and numerous x-rays are taken; use with caution in renal failure patients	Before: Explain procedure; let patient know dye can cause a bad taste and/or a burning sensation; ensure patient has no allergies; NPO after midnight; IV hydration; pretest sedation During: Provide comfort measures; keep cannulated limb immobile; apply pressure dressing after catheter removed After: Check patient's vital signs frequently; assess site for hematoma; peripheral pulse checks; hydration; bedrest for 24 hr; maintain immobility of affected extremity
Renal venogram	To outline venous system	Dye is injected through a venous catheter and numerous x-rays are taken	Care as above
Cystoscopy	To visualize ureteral opening, bladder wall, and urethra	Fiberoptic light and lens are inserted via the urethra into the bladder	Before: Explain procedure; pretest sedation During: Provide comfort measures After: Observe for urinary retention, excess hematuria, or bladder infection or abnormalities
Renal biopsy	To determine the nature and extent of renal disease for diagnosis, treatment, and prognosis from a histologic sample	A needle is inserted through the patient's back while the patient holds his breath. Two or three samples are usually needed; an open renal biopsy can be done in the OR; the tissue samples are removed with direct visualization of the kidney	Before: Explain procedure; check clotting times; pretest sedation During: Help patient maintain prone position; provide supportive care and pressure dressing After: Check patient's vital signs frequently; assess biopsy site; assess hematuria; bedrest, prone for 8 hr, then bedrest till morning; hydration

Source: M. J. Holechek. (1990). Acute renal failure. Baltimore: The Johns Hopkins Hospital Department of Medical Nursing.

Hyponatremia

Hyponatremia is a deficit of sodium in the extracellular fluid, for instance, when the serum concentration of sodium is below 135 mEq/L.[23] Severity of hyponatremia is determined based on serum sodium, which can provide clues regarding anticipated symptoms. The serum levels and symptoms are summarized in Table 5-10.

Table 5-10 Clinical Symptoms and Severity of Hyponatremia

Serum Sodium Level (mEq/L)	Classification	Symptoms
125–135	Mild	Possibly none or confusion, fatigue
118–124	Moderate	Weakness, short-term memory loss, inappropriate behavior, lethargy
112–117	Severe	Coma, seizures

Source: B. K. Shelton (1991). Electrolyte disturbances. Baltimore: The Johns Hopkins Oncology Center.

Clinical antecedents

Hyponatremia can be categorized as being associated with varying levels of extracellular fluid (ECF) volume and renal versus nonrenal etiologies. A list of clinical antecedents of hyponatremia is given in Table 5-11.

Critical referents

The list of precipitating factors for hyponatremia identifies three possible causes. The first includes renal and nonrenal disorders that result in extracellular fluid and electrolyte excretion. When hyponatremia results from renal losses, the sodium excreted with free water cannot be reabsorbed in the loop of Henle or the distal tubule. With nonrenal losses, sodium is lost through gastrointestinal secretions or the loss of skin integrity. The second category involves the factors that increase the loss of salt with no change in the water volume. The third category involves the factors that increase the water volume relative to the sodium content, which produces a dilutional effect.

Extracellular fluid volume may be reduced with a normal resultant diuresis and sodium loss. When fluid volume is lost, the osmolality of the plasma is increased, leading to release of the antidiuretic hormone (ADH). This hormone stimulates the body to retain replacement fluid, enhancing the appearance of hypovolemia with hyponatremia. Fluid and sodium losses are common with excessive excretion of body fluids (diarrhea, vomiting, nasogastric suction, profuse diaphoresis) and may vary in severity. Renal causes include excessive use of diuretics, renal disease, and hypoaldosteronism associated with adrenal insufficiency (refer to Chapter 7 on endocrine function for a discussion of the actions of aldosterone). One unusual etiology of hyponatremia is starvation, but this etiology is commonly associated with only mild to moderate sodium reductions (122–133 mEq/L). Retention of hyperosmolar substances such as lipids and glucose can lead to an intracellular shift of sodium and serum hyponatremia.

ECF may remain stable in another type of hyponatremia when hormonal influences are interfering with the regulation of sodium, such as with glucocorticoid deficiency (hypoglycemia) or syndrome of inappropriate antidiuretic hormone (SIADH). In these instances, sodium is truly lost, and low serum levels are not a reflection of osmolality; therefore, ECF volume remains the same.

Hyponatremia may also occur with excessive fluid and sodium retention, as seen with disorders such as congestive heart failure and cirrhosis. In these disorders, fluid is retained in greater quantity than sodium, with a resulting hyponatremia.

Resulting signs and symptoms

The clinical presentation of a patient with hyponatremia is the same regardless of the etiology. Most critical symptoms involve the neuromuscular and gastrointestinal systems and range in severity from mild to life-threatening. Such symptoms are listed in Tables 5-10 and 5-12.

Laboratory data is essential to document hyponatremia. The characteristic pattern is a decreased serum sodium level (below 135 mEq/L), a lowered serum chloride level (less than 96 mEq/L), a urine sodium level of less than 100 mOsm/L, and a decreased urine specific gravity (less than 1.010).[24]

Nursing standards of care

The medical management of hyponatremia focuses on two goals. The first goal is to determine the cause of the sodium deficiency and correct it. Symptomatic presentation may dictate the decision to treat the disorder aggressively, which will require nursing assessment and evaluation of patient responses. In less severe cases, symptomatic support during conservative management will be the priority of nursing

Table 5-11   Clinical Antecedents of Hyponatremia

Decreased ECF Volume		Normal ECF Volume	Increased ECF Volume (Generalized Edema)
Renal Losses	Nonrenal Losses		
Diuretics	Upper gastrointestinal: Excessive GI irrigations, infusion or ingestion of electrolyte substances, GI suctioning, vomiting	SIADH	Cirrhosis
Adrenal insufficiency		Glucocorticoid deficiency	Congestive heart failure
Renal disease		"Reset" osmoreceptors	Renal disease
	Lower gastrointestinal: Diarrhea, excessive enemas or laxatives		Excessive IV fluids
	Third-space sequestration		Water intoxication (i.e., manic-depression)
	Hypoalbuminemia		
	Septicemia		
	Biologic therapy		
	Burns		
	Certain medications		
	Starvation hyponatremia (imprudent dieting with loss of 15% of body weight)		
	Skin (sweating)		
	Hyperosmolar hyponatremia (hyperlipidemia, hypoproteinemia, hyperglycemia)		

care. The second goal is to control the environment, provide appropriate orientation and stimulation, and maximize the patient's safety and comfort.

Nursing management should focus on the complete assessment of the patient, but particular attention should be directed to the neurological and gastrointestinal symptoms. The patient should be monitored for changes in level of consciousness and orientation. Inappropriate behavior or inability to follow complex commands and answer questions may be early symptoms of the neurologic effects of hyponatremia. Special measures should be taken to protect the patient during seizures.

Fluid balances should be assessed by daily weights, strict intake and output measurements, urine specific gravity measurements, and frequent vital sign checks. Edema and poor skin turgor predispose these patients to skin problems at pressure areas. Good skin integrity can be promoted by frequent position changes and skin care. Dietary restrictions should include increased amounts of food and fluid high in sodium content. Table 5-13 lists foods and medications with high sodium content.

The medical interventions are influenced by the cause of the problem. Differential diagnosis of inappropriate levels of antidiuretic hormone is desirable prior to treatment decisions. If the problem is due to sodium loss, replacement therapy is indicated if the underlying cause cannot be corrected. A diet high in sodium with fluid restrictions should be instituted. Oral sodium supplements may include various formulations of sodium chloride. Special electrolyte solutions used by athletes may also be used. If the imbalance is due to overhydration or hormonal hyponatremia, aggressive use of diuretics may be implemented.[25] Isotonic sodium chloride solutions, sodium bicarbonate solution, or Ringer's lactate may be given parenterally for a reliable and steady replenishment regimen, although replacement should not exceed 1–2 mEq/hr. Too rapid replacement may cause congestive heart failure or cerebral hemorrhage.[26] When life-threatening neurologic symptoms are present, more aggressive sodium replenishment may be necessary. Hypertonic saline solutions (3% or 5%) may be administered cautiously. Sodium needs can be calculated using the following formula:

Na requirement = (140 − patient's serum sodium level)(0.6)(body weight in kilograms)

Table 5-12 Signs and Symptoms to Hyponatremia and Hypernatremia

	Hyponatremia	Hypernatremia
Neuromuscular	Fatigue Weakness Lethargy Confusion Tremors Seizures	Tremors Mental irritability Seizures
Cardiovascular	Orthostatic hypotension Tachycardia	Hypertension Tachycardia
Respiratory	Inability to protect airway	Inability to protect airway
Gastrointestinal	Anorexia Nausea Vomiting Diarrhea	Rough and dry tongue Thirst Anorexia Foul taste in mouth
Renal	Oliguria Dry mucous membranes Cool, clammy skin	Oliguria Weight gain Poor skin turgor Fever

Source: Shelton, B. K. (1991). Electrolyte disturbances. Baltimore: The Johns Hopkins Oncology Center.

Half of the calculated need should be replaced within 8–12 hours.[27] Neurologic symptoms should resolve within 24–96 hours of sodium correction.[28]

Patient education on hyponatremia will depend greatly upon the etiology. Potential causes of hyponatremia specific to the patient's risk factors should be emphasized. Although it is important to teach the patient about warning signals, it is imperative that family members or significant others be made aware of these symptoms, as the patient is frequently neurologically impaired and unable to remember what has been taught.

Hypernatremia

Hypernatremia is an excess of sodium in the extracellular fluid. In hypernatremia the serum concentration of sodium is greater than 145 mEq/L.[29] This high value is usually due to a loss of ECF, not a true rise in sodium.

Clinical antecedents

Hypernatremia is likely to result from reduced fluid intake, excessive fluid losses, or increased so-

Table 5-13 Selected Foods and Over-the-counter (OTC) Medications with High Sodium Content

Foods	Over-the-Counter (OTC) Medications
Salted snack foods	Antacids: Maalox and Maalox Plus, Gaviscon, Alka-Seltzer, Mylanta
Dried fruits	Laxatives/stool softeners: Colace, MOM, Senokot, Ducolax, Metamucil
Canned soups or vegetables	Cough medications: Robitussin, Vick's Formula 44, Coricidin
Lunch meat and delicatessen foods	
Items preserved in brine (pickles, olives)	
Cheeses	
Gatorade	

dium retention. Some clinical antecedents of hypernatremia are listed in Table 5-14.

Critical referents

Precipitating factors for hypernatremia fall into two classes. The first group of factors involves a decrease in total body fluid in relationship to the quantity of body sodium. Body fluid may be decreased because of inadequate intake to meet body needs, as in the case of excessive sweating without fluid replacement. Body fluid is also reduced with diuresis (hyperglycemia, diuretic therapy, diabetes insipidus) and through such fluid losses as gastrointestinal excretions. Some types of fluid losses may involve loss of sodium; others do not. When fluid is lost without sodium, hypernatremia occurs more quickly. The second group of precipitating factors involves an absolute increase of sodium in the extracellular fluid. This occurs with increased intake and unnatural retention of sodium. Retention can occur when hormones influence sodium excretion or when the resorptive properties of the kidneys fail, as in acute renal failure.

Resulting signs and symptoms

A hypernatremic patient will present with signs and symptoms that closely resemble those of a patient with hyponatremia, potentially making the differential diagnosis a difficult one. (Refer to Table 5-12 for a comparison of presenting signs and symptoms.) The outstanding differences between hyponatremia

and hypernatremia include a tendency toward weight gain, edema, and increased skin turgor in hypernatremia.

The laboratory data is essential in documenting hypernatremia. Laboratory evidence of hypernatremia will usually include the following:[30]

Serum sodium > 145 mEq/L

Urine sodium < 50 mEq/L

Urine osmolarity > 800 mOsm/L

Serum chloride > 106 mEq/L

Urine chloride < 50 mEq/L

Urine specific gravity > 1.030

Nursing standards of care

The first goal in the treatment of the patient with hypernatremia is to determine the cause of the sodium excess, correct it, and treat the symptoms. The second goal is to control the environment, provide appropriate orientation and stimulation, and maximize the patient's safety and comfort.

Nursing management is determined by the results of the total physical assessment. Maintaining fluid balance by recording daily weights, monitoring accurate intake and output, assessing skin turgor, temperature, and color, checking vital signs frequently, and assessing mucous membranes is vital. Assessment of the patient's neurological status should note any changes in the level of consciousness, orientation, or irritability. Comfort measures should be instituted to provide relief from water retention or dehydration, muscle weakness, or pain.

The medical interventions for hypernatremia revolve around treating the cause and correcting the

Table 5-14 Clinical Antecedents of Hypernatremia

Decreased ECF Volume		
Reduced Fluid Intake	Excessive Fluid Loss	Increased Sodium Retention
Decreased oral intake: Swallowing disorders, decreased sense of thirst, unconsciousness	GI distress: Vomiting, diarrhea	Hyperaldosteronism
Unavailability of fluids	GI drains: NG tube, Cantor tube, wound drains, bili stints	Increased sodium in diet
	Fever or profuse diaphoresis	Renal dysfunction
	Heat stroke	Excessive use of steroids
	Dialysis therapy	
	Diabetes	
	Hyperventilation	

imbalance. If the imbalance is due to the loss of body fluids, intravenous isotonic saline solutions can be administered. If the imbalance is due to sodium excess, the sodium intake will be restricted.[31]

Patient education should focus on the causes of hypernatremia and key reportable symptoms. It is particularly important for patients to recognize that fluid losses can be monitored and fluids replenished. Most hypernatremia is a result of secretion losses from vomiting, diarrhea, or wounds. Symptoms such as thirst, poor skin turgor, and muscle weakness can be addressed immediately when patients recognize the danger they exhibit.

Potassium

Potassium is the major intracellular cation; its normal concentration is 140 mEq/L. The extracellular serum concentration of potassium is 3.5–5.0 mEq/L.[32] Small deviations in either direction can have disastrous consequences, particularly for individuals who are already ill. Virtually all of the potassium in the body is exchangeable, making it difficult at times to assess potassium balance. Serum potassium levels are easily altered by acidosis, alkalosis, hyperglycemia, hypoglycemia, and cell lysis. Normally the kidneys will rapidly shift these levels to regulate serum potassium and excrete excesses. When these homeostatic processes fail or clinical disorders persist for long periods of time, altered serum potassium levels will be seen. Potassium is important in several physiologic functions, including (1) maintaining osmotic pressure within the cell, (2) protecting the resting membrane potential, (3) securing the acid-base balance, (4) promoting protein synthesis, and (5) promoting glycogen synthesis and carbohydrate metabolism.[33]

Hypokalemia

Hypokalemia is a deficit of potassium in the extracellular fluid. In hypokalemia the serum concentration of potassium is below 3.5 mEq/L.[34] The most significant clinical effects of hypokalemia relate to its effects on electrical conduction.

Clinical antecedents

Precipitating factors for hypokalemia may be grouped into five classifications. They are (1) low intake, (2) increased intracellular shifts of potassium, (3) increased renal loss, (4) gastrointestinal losses, and (5) increased integumentary loss.[35] A summary of the clinical antecedents of hypokalemia is given in Table 5-15.

Table 5-15 Clinical Antecedents of Hypokalemia

Type of Antecedent	Possible Sources
Low potassium intake	
Increased cellular uptake of potassium	Excess insulin Pancreatic abscess or pseudocyst Alkalosis Excess glucose DKA Hyperalimentation
Excess renal excretion of potassium	Hyperaldosteronism due to volume depletion, mineralocorticoid-secreting tumors, or steroid therapy Increased sodium to nephrons resulting from use of diuretics, certain antibiotics (carbenecillin) Acid-base disturbances: metabolic acidosis/alkalosis or respiratory acidosis/alkalosis
Excessive gastrointestinal loss	Hypersalivation GI lavage Vomiting Diarrhea Malabsorption Excessive use of laxatives
Excessive integumentary loss	Burns (after third day) Profuse diaphoresis

Critical referents

Potassium's highly exchangeable status can lead to many difficulties in accurately assessing potassium balance. Potassium will often shift between intracellular and extracellular spaces when other solute imbalances occur. Hypokalemia occurs when the extracellular (intravascular) potassium is low. Low intake leads to reduction of total body stores. Potassium will return to the inside of cells under any of the following conditions: hyperglycemia, increased insulin levels, and alkalosis.

Excessive renal excretion can occur by various mechanisms. In conditions in which excessive aldosterone is present, potassium is secreted in the distal tubule and more sodium is reabsorbed. This can lead to serum hypokalemia. Because volume depletion is a powerful stimulator of aldosterone secretion (through the renin-angiotensin mechanism), volume depletion can lead to potassium loss. Excess mineralocorticoid (aldosterone) also leads to sodium retention, thus contributing to potassium excretion.

Diuretics, other medications (carbenecillin, amphotericin, ticarcillin) and acid-base disturbances (for example, in diabetic ketoacidosis) cause hypokalemia by increasing fluid and sodium flowing to the distal nephron. This change in the concentration gradient makes the distal nephron more electronegative, favoring potassium secretion.[36]

Excessive body secretions that are high in potassium—saliva, gastric juice, ileal fluid, and colonic fluid—will also lead to hypokalemia.

Resulting signs and symptoms

The clinical presentation of the hypokalemic patient involves every body system. Table 5-16 compares the observable effects of hypokalemia and hyperkalemia. The primary symptoms result from dysfunction of excitable membranes of muscle and neural tissue. Excitable cells possess membranes that respond to stimuli in an all-or-nothing fashion; that is, they generate action potentials. To generate an action potential, the cell must depolarize from a resting state to an electrically active state. In hypokalemia, the potassium concentration outside the cell (in the ECF) decreases and the resting potential is raised, inhibiting electrical impulse conduction. This decreases the cell's excitability because more electrical activity is required for the cell membrane to reach threshold and generate an action potential. This leads to the classic muscle weakness reported with hypokalemia. Certain electrocardiogram changes are

Table 5-16 Signs and Symptoms of Hypokalemia and Hyperkalemia

Body System	Signs and Symptoms of Hypokalemia	Signs and Symptoms of Hyperkalemia
Neuromuscular	Drowsiness, confusion, apathy, irritability, coma, muscle weakness, paresthesia, muscle pain, muscle cramps, muscle tenderness, hyporeflexia, tetany, paralysis	Mental confusion, weakness, extremity numbness, paresthesias, flaccid paralysis, muscle irritability, hyperreflexia
Cardiovascular	Weak pulse, bradycardia, hypotension, ECG changes (including a depressed ST segment, flattened, inverted T waves, and prominent U waves), cardiac arrest, enhanced digitalis effect	Cardiac dysrhythmias (PVBs, ventricular tachycardia or fibrillation, cardiac arrest), ECG changes (including peaked T waves, flattened P waves, prolonged P-R interval, broadened QRS, suppressed ST segment), reduced cardiac contractility
Respiratory	Muscle weakness, hypoventilation (respiratory arrest)	Muscle weakness, hypoventilation (respiratory arrest)
Gastrointestinal	Anorexia, nausea, vomiting, abdominal distention, abdominal cramps, diminished bowel sounds leading to paralytic ileus or perforated bowel	Anorexia, nausea, vomiting, diarrhea, hyperactive bowel sounds
Endocrine	Polydipsia, hyperglycemia, and in some cases negative nitrogen balance	Hypoglycemia
Renal	Polyuria, nocturia	Oliguria

Source: Adapted from Kinney, M., Packa, D. R., and Dunbar, S. B. (1988). *AACN's Clinical Reference for Critical Care Nursing.* 2nd edition. New York: McGraw-Hill Book Company.

also typical of the presentation of hypokalemia. An inverted T wave and prominent U waves indicate its presence.[37] Figure 5-14 illustrates these changes. Part (a) of Figure 5-14 shows a normal ECG (labeled A) and several ECGs that illustrate the characteristic flattening of the T wave, development of U waves, and depression of the S-T segment. Overall, ECG changes with hypokalemia are nonspecific, but the diagnosis should be strongly considered if U-wave amplitude ever exceeds T-wave amplitude. Part (b) of the figure illustrates the changes on a larger scale. Ventricular dysrhythmias are common in patients with hypokalemia and may be treated with antidysrhythmics while correcting potassium levels. A particularly chaotic type of ven-

tricular tachycardia called torsades de pointes is common with hypokalemia and is resistant to standard therapy.

Renal function is also altered with hypokalemia. Hypokalemia leads to decreases in glomerular filtration, reduced ability to concentrate urine (fixed normal or low specific gravity), and increased bicarbonate production.[38]

Laboratory data is essential when assessing the patient for hypokalemia. A serum potassium level of 3.5 mEq/L or less, an elevated plasma bicarbonate, and increased pH are characteristic findings. In addition, a decreased osmolality, decreased pH, normal potassium, and increased phosphate level in the urine may be found.[39]

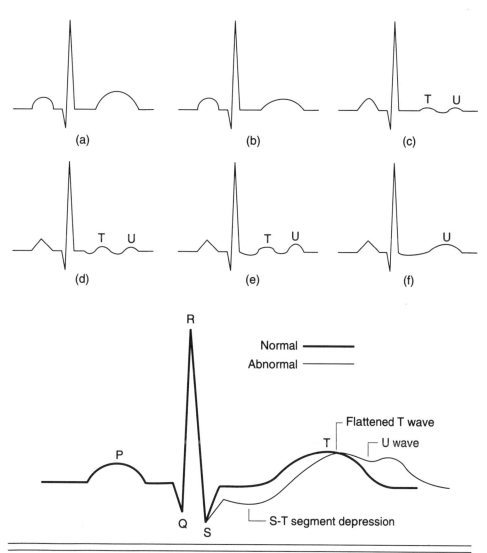

Figure 5-14 ECG Changes Associated with Hypokalemia
Source: Adapted from Grauer, K. and Curry, W. (1988). *Clinical Electrocardiography.* Oradell, NJ: Medical Economics Books.

Nursing standards of care

Care of the patient with hypokalemia focuses on several goals. The first goal is to determine the cause of the deficiency and treat it. A decreased potassium level has an effect on all body systems. Therefore, all body systems must be assessed and symptoms must be treated as a second goal. The third goal is to control the environment, provide appropriate orientation and stimulation for the patient, and maximize the patient's safety and comfort. The fourth goal is to prevent the complications that may arise from a decreased potassium level. As the list of symptoms is evaluated, particular attention should be given to the neurological, cardiovascular, and respiratory systems. Any symptom in one of these systems is likely to lead to life-threatening events.

The medical interventions to be implemented focus on replacement therapy. If oral replacement is a possibility, the diet should be enhanced with high-potassium foods (fruits and vegetables) or potassium supplements. Oral potassium supplementation through foods can be expected to produce changes in potassium levels in 24–36 hours. Intravenous replacement increases potassium levels immediately. Oral supplements are absorbed with effective increases in potassium levels in 1–2 hours. If potassium supplements are prescribed, administer them with large amounts of fluid or food to decrease mucosal irritations.[40] When potassium preparations are given orally, the chances of rebound hyperkalemia are decreased. Oral potassium supplements come in many forms; some are enteric-coated, and others are timed-release. Practitioners must pay careful attention to the manufacturer's recommendations for use and necessary precautions. Intravenous potassium chloride is another alternative. Generally, with this approach, potassium chloride is infused into a peripheral vein at a rate of 10–20 mEq/hour. Different settings and patient populations may cause policies to differ from one institution to another; dosages may range from 10 to 30 mEq/hr, diluted in from 100 to 500 cc of fluid.[41] Rapid infusion may be life-threatening, causing vessel necrosis, rebound hyperkalemia, or induction of ventricular fibrillation. If the patient experiences pain at the infusion site, a slower rate of infusion, ice, or a local anesthetic will provide relief. The amount of supplement given should be calculated based on the severity of hypokalemia and the presence of other potassium-depleting substances. The frequency with which potassium levels should be checked will depend on the amount replenished during a particular time. Some patients require potassium evaluations three or four times per day until a pattern of loss and replenishment is established.

Patients with hypokalemia who take digitalis are prone to digitalis toxicity. The nurse must remember to monitor this closely and provide adequate potassium supplements before administering the digitalis.

Hyperkalemia

Hyperkalemia is an excess of potassium in the extracellular fluid. In hyperkalemia the serum concentration of potassium is greater than 5.0 mEq/L.[42] Moderately elevated levels (up to 6 mEq/L) may be treated conservatively, but levels greater than 6 mEq/L are considered life-threatening and call for immediate intervention.

Clinical antecedents

The precipitating factors found to provoke hyperkalemia include (1) increased potassium intake, (2) altered cellular uptake, (3) increased cell lysis, and (4) decreased renal excretion. There are a few factors that can create falsely high potassium levels. These factors include hemolyzed blood caused by venipuncture, increased leukocyte counts, or a difficult blood draw that requires the use of a tourniquet.[43] A comprehensive listing of the clinical antecedents of hyperkalemia can be found in Table 5-17.

Critical referents

As Table 5-17 shows, the causative factors of hyperkalemia fall into four groupings. The first group consists of those factors that contribute to an increased intake of potassium. The second group consists of conditions in which potassium may be shifted from the intracellular to the intravascular space. Potassium shifts into the intravascular fluid occur in disorders such as acidosis, when hydrogen ion concentrations rise. In addition, lack of insulin in diabetics slows the cellular uptake of potassium, and hyperkalemia may result if glucose levels are corrected at the same time that potassium supplements are administered. The third group of causative factors includes disorders in which cells are lysed and the internal components (which include large amounts of potassium) are spilled into the intravascular space. When cells are rapidly destroyed (in tumor lysis syndrome, hemolytic transfusion reaction, sepsis, catabolic states), the cellular compo-

Table 5-17 Clinical Antecedents of Hyperkalemia

Type of Antecedent	Possible Sources
Increased potassium intake	Ingestion or intravenous administration Massive RBC transfusions
Altered cellular uptake of potassium	Acidosis Diabetes mellitus
Increased cell lysis	Cardiac arrest Sepsis/catabolic state Cancer chemotherapy Burns (early) Trauma Intravascular hemolysis
Decreased renal excretion	Renal failure Adrenal insufficiency Potassium-sparing diuretics

nents are spilled into the circulating bloodstream.[44] This most often results in hyperkalemia and acidosis. The last group of factors consists of those that decrease renal function, which leads to decreased renal excretion from the distal tubule. (This fourth category is sometimes described as renal excretion problems.)

Resulting signs and symptoms

Table 5-16 contrasts the clinical symptoms of a hyperkalemic patient with those of a person suffering from hypokalemia. With hyperkalemia, membrane thresholds are increased in excitable tissues, leading to automaticity of contractile tissues. This translates into muscle irritability, tremors, and ectopic or chaotic cardiac rhythms. The cardiac involvement varies according to the degree of hyperkalemia. With levels of 5.0–6.0 mEq/L, the dysfunction begins with tall, peaked, tented T waves and a depressed ST segment. As the hyperkalemia progresses to levels of 6.1–6.8 mEq/L, the P waves decrease in size and the P-R interval is prolonged.[45] If hyperkalemia persists and worsens, atrial asystole with a widened QRS complex merges with the T wave. These changes are depicted in Figure 5-15. Part (a) of Figure 5-15 shows a normal ECG (labeled A) and several ECGs that illustrate the characteristic changes in the amplitude of the T-wave and the P-wave and in the length of the PR and QRS intervals. Part (b) of the figure illustrates the changes on a larger scale.

Ventricular dysrhythmias and cardiac arrest may occur at any time with hyperkalemia, regardless of the baseline changes.[46] No matter what the symptoms are, the patient's serum potassium level must be assessed. Dangerous hyperkalemia is usually defined as a level greater than 5.5 mEq/L.

Nursing standards of care

There are two goals associated with the treatment of hyperkalemia. The first goal is to correct the potassium imbalance, and the second is to prevent the complications associated with the imbalance.

Keen assessment skills are required when managing a patient with hyperkalemia. It is necessary to monitor the status of all body systems. This includes level of consciousness, pulse rate and rhythm, muscle strength and movement, and gastrointestinal and genitourinary characteristics. Additional nursing interventions should include (1) reducing potassium intake, (2) administering proper medications (being careful to evaluate the use of potassium-sparing diuretics), (3) providing a safe and comfortable environment, and (4) assisting the patient with range-of-motion exercises and activities of daily living.

The medical interventions involved in the treatment of hyperkalemia focus on several factors. The first intervention is to reduce potassium intake. This is accomplished by evaluating the dietary intake, the medication intake, or the amount infused via intravenous therapy. A daily intake of 40 mEq of potassium is normal, but intake must be evaluated according to the needs of each patient.

The second intervention is to introduce agents to facilitate the shift of potassium into the cell. Possible agents include glucose and insulin infusion. Hypertonic dosages of glucose (such as 500 cc of 10% glucose or 50 cc of 50% dextrose) are given with 10 units of regular insulin over 30 minutes. This is a temporary measure used to treat emergent potassium levels and is not viewed as curative. This solution will alter the serum potassium level but will have no effect on the total body potassium.

Bicarbonate solution is often given to induce an alkalosis and hypertonic sodium load that leads to potassium excretion via the urine. Unless given as a bolus infusion, this intervention may take hours to effect changes in potassium levels.

Administration of calcium salts by slow intravenous infusion can counteract potassium's effects on the neuromuscular membranes and antagonize the cardiotoxocity of hyperkalemia. The effects of calcium are rapid but transient and limited, so it is generally accepted that calcium infusions should not exceed 70 mEq/day.[47] All measures such as glucose,

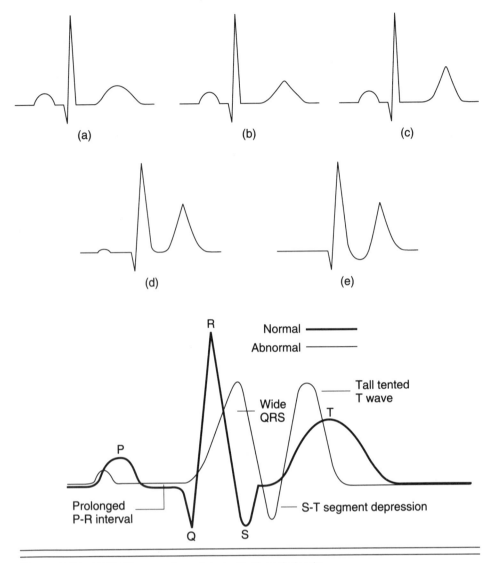

Figure 5-15   ECG Changes Associated with Hyperkalemia
Source: Adapted from Grauer, K. and Curry, W. (1988). *Clinical Electrocardiography.*
Oradell, NJ: Medical Economics Books.

insulin, bicarbonate, and calcium are temporary, and it is necessary to follow them with a more permanent intervention to rid the body of potassium.

The last and most commonly used interventions assist with the removal of potassium from the body. The administration of sodium polystyrene sulfonate (Kayexalate) and sorbitol will cause an exchange process of one sodium ion for one potassium ion in the bowel wall. Sorbitol is a sugar that induces diarrhea. The two substances are given in a solution that may be administered orally or rectally. If the patient's renal function is normal, potassium-wasting diuretics may be used. In patients with renal dysfunction, dialysis offers an alternative for potas-

sium removal. In any situation, potassium levels must be monitored frequently to document the trends.[48]

Calcium

Calcium is the most abundant cation in the body. Normal serum calcium concentrations range from 8.5 to 10.5 mg/dL, or 4.5 to 5.5 mEq/dL.[49] Most clinical laboratories report calcium levels in mg/dL. Calcium is found in several forms: freely ionized and available for activity, bound to protein, and stored in bones. The serum calcium balance is affected by three factors: deposition and resorption of bone, absorption of calcium from the gastrointestinal tract, and excretion of calcium in urine and feces. Bone-deposited calcium comprises the majority of the body's calcium stores and provides strength and structure to the bones.[50] Absorption of calcium via the gastrointestinal tract is facilitated by dietary vitamin D and phosphates. Calcium excretion is primarily regulated by parathormone, a parathyroid hormone. Calcium's most important role is in bone formation and metabolism. But it also influences synaptic transmission and function, blood coagulation, muscle contraction, exocrine and endocrine gland secretion, and cardiac cell action potentials.

Hypocalcemia

Hypocalcemia is a deficit of calcium in the extracellular fluid. In hypocalcemia, the concentration of total serum calcium is less than 8.5 mg/100 dL.

Clinical antecedents

The etiology of hypocalcemia may be reduced availability of any of calcium's major regulators (bone storage, parathormone, vitamin D, or phosphates) or a change in the way that calcium binds to protein. Clinical antecedents of hypocalcemia are listed in Table 5-18.

Critical referents

A decrease in serum calcium may result from abnormal regulation of serum calcium, a calcium intake deficiency, or an increase in calcium losses. Thyroid surgery, in which all or part of the parathyroid gland is removed (resulting in a parathormone deficiency), is the major contributor to the abnormal regulation of calcium. Other causes of hypocalcemia include parathormone deficiency, hyperphosphatemia, hypomagnesemia, burns, sepsis, and pancreatitis.[51]

A deficient intake of calcium or vitamin D may cause hypocalcemia but most often causes osteoporosis. This is because the largest amount of body calcium is stored in bones. When intake of calcium decreases, feedback mechanisms cause the release of calcium bone stores to replenish serum levels rather than altering resorption.[52] Removing large quantities of calcium from bones helps maintain a steady state of serum calcium but depletes bone stores and leads to bone breakdown—osteoporosis. Vitamin D is a fat-soluble vitamin ab-

Table 5-18 Clinical Antecedents of Hypocalcemia

Type of Antecedent	Possible Sources
Reduced bone storage	Osteomalacia Malignant disease metastatic to bone Medication-induced bone breakdown (e.g., steroids)
Decreased parathormone	Hypoparathyroidism
Reduced vitamin D	Relative dietary deficiency Intestinal malabsorption syndromes: small bowel resections, short bowel syndrome, GI infections, Crohn's disease, cystic fibrosis, sprue
Decreased protein binding of calcium	Hypoalbuminemia Citrate intoxication: dialysis, pheresis, massive blood transfusions
Abnormal calcium regulation	Hyperphosphatemia Hypomagnesemia Renal dysfunction Alkalosis Pancreatitis

sorbed from the intestine and necessary for calcium absorption. Absolute deficits resulting from poor dietary intake of dairy products may cause a calcium deficiency, but fat absorption problems such as sprue or general diarrhea may also contribute to this syndrome.

An increase in calcium losses may occur in patients suffering burns, acute pancreatitis, renal failure, massive blood transfusions, and peritonitis.[53] In acute pancreatitis, the inflamed pancreas releases proteolytic and lypolytic enzymes. It is thought that free calcium binds with the free fatty acids produced and is then excreted. Some authors even consider the degree of hypocalcemia to be an indicator of the severity of pancreatitis.[54] Hypocalcemia from acute renal failure is usually related to the combined effects of hypoparathyroidism and high phosphate levels, which drive calcium out of the serum and into the bone for storage. Hypocalcemia in the patient with renal failure may be enhanced when citrate preservative is used with hemodialysis procedures. Citrate binds with free calcium, reducing the ionized calcium available to participate in homeostatic functions. Red blood cells packed for use in transfusions are preserved in citrate solution, predisposing patients receiving massive transfusions to hypocalcemia. Hypocalcemia may present as a secondary problem of many other disorders that affect the body's major regulators of calcium; thus, it should be monitored for in all critically ill patients with compromised renal, nutritional, and gastrointestinal systems.

Resulting signs and symptoms

The clinical symptoms exhibited by a person suffering from hypocalcemia are primarily neuromuscular in nature. The calcium deficit causes neuromuscular membranes to become partially charged. This increased irritability causes the transmission of repetitive impulses that create muscular spasms seen as tetany, carpopedal spasm (Trousseau's sign), and Chvostek's sign (see Figure 5-16). Other signs and symptoms of neuromuscular dysfunction include numbness and tingling of the extremities, circumoral tingling, muscle cramps, facial grimacing, increased deep tendon reflexes, and seizures. General signs and symptoms of this syndrome include abdominal pain, nausea and vomiting, diarrhea, cardiac arrest, and pathologic fractures.[55] The signs and symptoms of both hypercalcemia and hypocalcemia are summarized in Table 5-19.

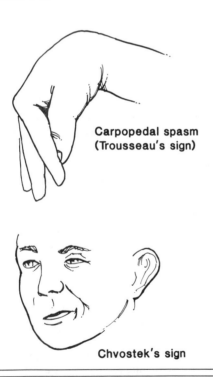

Carpopedal spasm
(Trousseau's sign)

Chvostek's sign

Figure 5-16   Clinical Symptoms of Hypocalcemia: Chvostek's and Trousseau's Signs

A lengthened Q-T interval is a characteristic ECG abnormality associated with hypocalcemia, whereas hypercalcemia produces a shortened Q-T interval. These ECG patterns are illustrated in Figure 5-17.[56] The figure shows a normal ECG (labeled a), an ECG illustrating hypercalcemia (labeled b), and one illustrating hypocalcemia (labeled c). Premature ventricular beats may also occur as a result of cardiac irritability.

Laboratory diagnostic tests that should be considered when assessing the presence and severity of hypocalcemia include tests of serum calcium, ionized calcium, serum phosphate, and serum albumin levels. The important interactive effects of these factors have been discussed earlier in this chapter.

Nursing standards of care

Nursing care will focus on assisting with identification of the causes of the hypocalcemia and promoting the patient's comfort and safety. Thorough neurological assessment is essential, as even slightly reduced calcium levels will cause neuromuscular irritability such as cramping or tremors. Seizure and safety precautions may be indicated.

Because dietary intake is one of the regulators of calcium levels, it is necessary to assess phosphate intake and note those foods high in calcium content and vitamin D. Gastrointestinal and genitourinary assessment should include monitoring the feces for amount, color, consistency, and frequency. Diarrhea may indicate a predisposition for hypocalcemia.

It is imperative when managing a hypocalcemic patient that the underlying causes be discovered and corrected. If the calcium imbalance is part of an acute process, intravenous therapy of calcium chloride, calcium gluconate, or calcium gluceptate may be used. The decision of which calcium supplement to use may be based on other electrolyte values, such as chloride levels, or upon the amount of calcium to be replaced. An ampule of calcium chloride contains 15 mEq of calcium, whereas an ampule of calcium gluconate or gluceptate contains 4.5 mEq of calcium. Except with a life-threatening event, calcium infusions should be diluted in solution and administered very slowly (one ampule in 50 cc of dextrose solution over 20–60 minutes).[57] Calcium infusions given too quickly will cause bradycardia or heart block. The nurse must remember that calcium is a medication that is incompatible with many other substances, such as epinephrine, sodium bicarbonate, and phosphate. If the calcium imbalance is part of a chronic

Table 5-19 Signs and Symptoms of Hypercalcemia and Hypocalcemia

Body System	Signs and Symptoms of Hypocalcemia	Signs and Symptoms of Hypercalcemia
Neurological	Confusion Anxiety Emotional lability Paresthesias (peripheral)	Apathy Lethargy Depression Coma Fatigue Dizziness
Muscular	Muscle aches and spasms Seizures	Excessive thirst Muscle weakness and atrophy Flaccidity
Skeletal	Pathological fractures	Porous, cystic bone Tenderness, pain
Cardiovascular	Dysrhythmias Hypotension Lengthened Q-T interval	Dysrhythmias Hypertension Widened T waves (shortened Q-T interval)
Renal	Decreased tubular resorption of Ca Increased phosphate clearance	Polyuria Dehydration Nephrolithiasis
Gastrointestinal	Increased motility (nausea, vomiting, diarrhea)	Decreased motility (anorexia, constipation) Ulcers Pancreatitis

Source: Walpert, N. (1990). Calcium, metabolism disorders. *Nursing* 90 (7): pp. 60–64.

process, daily doses of calcium and vitamin D preparations with an increase in dietary calcium can correct the calcium depletion. In either event, serum calcium and phosphorus levels should be monitored.[58] Phosphorus levels need to be monitored because hypocalcemia is often accompanied by hyperphosphatemia. Although the two electrolytes do not have a true inverse relationship, rapid changes in calcium levels will affect the phosphate level.

Patient education should focus on the warning signs of neuromuscular involvement, such as tremors or tetany. The patient is instructed to notify the appropriate health care provider at the onset of these symptoms. Monitoring and intervention for more severe manifestations such as seizures and tetany are also recommended.

Hypercalcemia

Hypercalcemia is an excess of calcium in the extracellular fluid. In hypercalcemia, the concentration of total serum calcium is greater than 10.5 mg/100 mL.[59] Most clinicians consider absolute serum calcium levels when making a diagnosis of hypercalcemia. But the relationship of calcium to albumin (described earlier in the discussion of renal anatomy and physiology) is such that actual ionized levels are

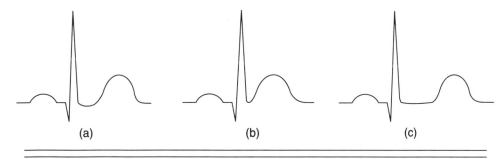

(a)　　　　　(b)　　　　　(c)

Figure 5-17 ECG Changes Associated with Hypercalcemia and Hypocalcemia
Source: Adapted from Grauer, K. and Curry, W. (1988). *Clinical Electrocardiography.* Oradell, NJ: Medical Economics Books.

more accurate reflections of the degree of elevation of calcium levels.

Clinical antecedents

There are a variety of precipitating factors that can cause hypercalcemia. The most prevalent etiology is malignant tumors; in fact, 10–20% of all patients with cancer will experience hypercalcemia.[60] Tumors generate hypercalcemia by (1) ectopic production of calcium or (2) promotion of intravascular shifts of calcium stores (such as from bones when bone metastases occur). Malignancies most likely to cause a primary hypercalcemia include leukemia, lymphoma, multiple myeloma, lung cancer, carcinoma of the thyroid or parathyroids, other endocrine tumors, and renal cancer. Other tumors treated with the hormones estrogen and androgen (prostate cancer and breast cancer) can predispose individuals to hypercalcemia.[61]

Hypercalcemia may be the result of an abnormal regulation of calcium levels, as in hyperparathyroidism. Major differences between hypercalcemia of malignancy and primary hyperparathyroidism are highlighted in Table 5-20. These distinctions may be helpful in clinical diagnosis, as many patients with malignancies will present with symptoms of hypercalcemia as their chief complaint, even prior to a cancer diagnosis.

Other etiologies of hypercalcemia include increased mobilization of calcium from the bones as a consequence of prolonged bedrest, fractures, or bone tumors; decreased renal calcium excretion, as in renal failure; and increased intestinal reabsorption of calcium or vitamin D due to increased dietary intake.[62] Adrenal insufficiency and thiazide diuretic therapy are known precipitators as well.[63]

Critical referents

Pathophysiological effects of hypercalcemia are the opposite of those produced by hypocalcemia. Neuromuscular function and automaticity are reduced, and all electrical conduction within the body is slowed. Excessive calcium availability enhances all processes that calcium influences; therefore, effects of hypercalcemia include an increased propensity for coagulation, bone abnormalities, and renal calcium deposits with possible formation of kidney stones.

Resulting signs and symptoms

The clinical signs and symptoms that may be present in the patient suffering from hypercalcemia

Table 5-20 Comparison of Primary Hyperparathyroidism and Hypercalcemia of Malignancy

Feature	Hypercalcemia of Cancer	Primary Hyperparathyroidism
History	Short, rapidly progressive	Long, fluctuating, slowly progressive
Major symptoms of diagnostic value	Moderate to severe weight loss, no renal calculi, pancreatitis rare	Minimal weight loss, renal calculi, pancreatitis and peptic ulcer common
Serum calcium concentration	Usually high (14 mg/dL or 3.5 mmol/L in 75% of cases)	Variable (14 mg/dL or 3.5 mmol/L in 25% of cases)
Serum phosphate concentration	Increased, normal, or decreased	Normal or decreased
Serum alkaline phosphatase concentration	Elevated in more than 50% of cases	Significantly elevated only in patients with gross bone disease
Serum chloride concentration	Low (usually < 102 mmol/L)	High (usually >102 mmol/L)
Serum bicarbonate concentration	Elevated or normal	Normal or low
Erythrocyte sedimentation rate	Usually elevated	Normal
Roentgenogram	Normal or shows metastatic disease	May show subperiosteal erosions in hands
Steroid suppression	Serum calcium concentration is often decreased	Serum calcium concentration is rarely decreased

are varied. (These symptoms are listed in Table 5-19.) Cardiac dysrhythmias are common, particularly bradycardia or heart block, which may progress to cardiac arrest. Hypercalcemia is evidenced by a shortened Q-T interval on the ECG, as shown in Figure 5-17. It is important to note that a patient taking digitalis may experience an effect that can contribute to dysrhythmias and cardiac arrest.[64]

Characteristic laboratory findings reveal an increased serum calcium greater than 10.5 mg/100 mL, increased urine calcium, and a decrease in urine osmolality and specific gravity.[65]

Nursing standards of care

The major goal of treatment of hypercalcemia is to correct the imbalance of calcium in the body. Nurses play an essential role in implementing a care plan that includes neurological assessment, cardiac assessment, and monitoring of fluid balances and calcium levels. Nursing interventions include assessing the patient's level of consciousness, evaluating muscle strength and coordination, assessing the pulse rate and rhythm, assessing bowel sounds and stools, accurate recording of intake and outputs, straining the urine for possible kidney stones, and monitoring all laboratory data.[66]

Additional nursing measures specific to hypercalcemia patients focus on decreasing calcium intake and maximizing safety. To reduce the likelihood of pathological fractures, the nursing staff provides a safe environment by padding bedrails, maintaining quiet rooms, and moving the patient gently when necessary. The patient should perform range-of-motion excercises whenever possible. To decrease intravascular calcium concentrations, fluids are pushed. Calcium-restricted diets and acid-ash fluids such as cranberry juice are provided.

Calcium levels may be lowered in several ways. The most common and easily implemented strategy is administration of an IV saline flush, which dilutes the intravascular calcium concentration. The amount of normal saline needed will vary from one patient to another, but the standard dose is 1000 cc every 4–6 hours until the calcium level is observed to decrease.[67] The success of this treatment is dependent upon adequate calcium excretion through the urine, so intact and efficient renal function is a prerequisite. Fluid is given in combination with a loop diuretic, which increases the glomerular filtration rate for calcium.

Various medications with different mechanisms are used to lower calcium levels. These are listed and contrasted in Table 5-21. Mithracin (Plicamycin) is one of the oldest and most rapid-acting of antihypercalcemic agents. It is used to stimulate calcium uptake by the bones. Calcitonin (Calcimar) is an external supplement that enhances the body's existing mechanism of calcium regulation by inhibiting bone lysis and increasing renal excretion of calcium. Oral phosphate binders will bind with calcium for elimination. In some cases, dialysis may be initiated for rapid removal of excessive amounts of calcium. Above all, the major cause of the elevated calcium must be corrected first before therapeutic measures can have any long-lasting effect.[68]

Education of patients at risk for hypercalcemia must include information regarding the specific etiology and chosen therapy and the neuromuscular symptoms that can be life-threatening. Patients need to be made aware of the likelihood that this problem will become chronic and of the potential for long-term therapy. Patients with long-term hypercalcemia may have to learn to cope with bone deformities, repeated renal calculi, and chronic bone pain.

Phosphate

Phosphate is an important electrolyte often omitted from discussions of major electrolytes. It is a major anion in the extracellular fluid, where it is bound in organic and inorganic compounds. The normal serum concentration of phosphate has a very narrow range, from 3.0 to 4.5 mg/dL, as most of the phosphate in the body is intracellular. Serum phosphate levels do not adequately reflect total body stores of phosphate; thus, symptoms are not necessarily reflective of serum levels. This is exemplified by the malnourished patient who depletes his or her body's stores of phosphate, yet has a normal serum phosphate. When such a patient receives proper nourishment, the tissue repair and anabolism that take place deplete all available phosphate, leading to hypophosphatemia.

Phosphate ions in the body are used in a variety of ways. Seventy-five percent of phosphate is combined with calcium in the bone structure. Phosphate is also an active ingredient in the metabolism of carbohydrates and lipids and is the body's primary source of energy for the active transport system. Phosphates act as buffers for hydrogen ions, assisting in metabolic acid-base balance. Phosphate's effects on the hematologic system are multiple and involve all three blood components. Phosphate also influences several intracellular energy-producing reactions and assists in maintaining the structural integrity of cell walls.[69]

Table 5-21   Treatment of Hypercalcemia

Agent	Mechanism	Administration	Side Effects	Comments
Hydration with isotonic solution; dose: 3–6 L/day	Restores extracellular volume, diluting Ca^+	IV; takes about 24–48 hr to see benefit	Hypervolemia Dilutional decreases in other electrolytes	Observe for heart failure and edema; maximum benefit is about 1 mg/dL
Loop diuretics (e.g., Furosemide); dose: up to 100 mg every 2 hr	Enhances renal excretion of Ca^+; blocks Ca^+ reabsorption in ascending loop	IV or PO PRN	Hypokalemia Hypomagnesemia	Monitor fluids and electrolytes for depletion; may only be effective for short time
Mithracin (Plicamycin); dose: 25 mcg/kg	Increases bone reabsorption of Ca^+ through osteoclast destruction	Single-dose IV (look for dramatic decrease in Ca^+ in 24–48 hr)	Neutropenia Vesicant Renal impairment Hepatic dysfunction Increased PT Thrombocytopenia Nausea and vomiting	Is a vesicant (give cautiously); antineoplastic agent (handle with precautions); potential for over-correction due to delayed onset activity
Calcitonin (Calmar); single dose: 3–8 U/kg (may repeat every 4–8 hr)	Thyroid hormone causes bone resorption of Ca^+	Skin test for reaction (dramatic decrease in Ca^+ within 8–24 hr)	Development of tolerance Nausea Flushing Fevers	Produces 1–4 mg/dL decrease in Ca^+ over short time; monitor for tetany
Glucocorticoids (Prednisone 50–100 mg/day, Decadron 24 mg/day)	Uncertain; possible direct antitumor effects, inhibition of vitamin absorption, or blockage of osteo-clast activation	IV in divided daily doses	Cushing's syndrome Adrenal insufficiency Hypernatremia Hyperglycemia	Often given in conjunction with Calcitonin; may produce 1–2 mg/dL decrease in Ca^+
Didronel (Etidronate); dose: 7 mg/kg/day for 4–7 days	Inhibits Ca^+ release from bone	IV or PO infusion (4–5 hr)	Mild to moderate renal dysfunction Diarrhea Nausea Bone pain	Usually produces about 2 mg decrease in Ca^+; therapy should not exceed 3 months; reduced absorption with food or milk
Ganite (gallium nitrate); dose: 200 mg/m²/day for up to 5 days	Inhibits bone Ca^+ release by reducing bone turnover	IV (continuous infusion for 5 days)	Hypocalcemia Renal dysfunction Decreased bicarbonate Anemia Asymptomatic mild hypotension	Onset of primary Ca^+ reducing effect occurs about 72–90 hr after treatment
Pamidronate diphosphonate (Aredia); dose: 60–90 mg/day IV or 250–1200 mg/day orally	Inhibits bone Ca^+ release without decreasing bone growth	IV; single dose lasts weeks to months; oral (investiga-tional)	Bone pain Thrombophlebitis Transient rigors at beginning of therapy Retinitis	More potent than Etidronate; high or long-term doses may cause gastric irritation

Source: Shelton, B. K. (1991). *Hypercalcemia*. Baltimore: Johns Hopkins Oncology Center.

Hypophosphatemia

Hypophosphatemia is a reduced level of phosphate in the extracellular fluid. In hypophosphatemia, the serum phosphate concentration is less than 3.0 mg/dL.[70]

Clinical antecedents

The precipitating factors of hypophosphatemia fall into the categories of inadequate intake and abnormal regulation of phosphate. The list of specific factors ranges from inadequate dietary intake of phosphate to vascular fluid expansion with dilution. Hyperparathyroidism, malnutrition, malabsorption, decreased vitamin D metabolism, and increased growth hormone are among the most common causes.[71] Hypophosphatemia may be a result of decreased phosphate absorption by the bowel or increased phosphate excretion from the kidneys.

Critical referents

The regulation of phosphate levels and subsequent disorders is a complex process involving parathormone, calcitonin, vitamin D, glucose, and insulin.

Respiratory alkalosis is known to promote glycolysis, which requires that phosphate be extracted from the cells and results in hypophosphatemia. For this reason, patients who hyperventilate for a prolonged period of time will have hypophosphatemia.

Phosphate is used during the metabolic breakdown for excretion of ketoacids by the kidney. Diabetic ketoacidosis leads to catabolism and generation of phosphate from cells, followed by acidosis. As normal compensatory mechanisms or medical intervention correct this acidosis, the remaining phosphate, which was not excreted, is returned to the cells to promote anabolism, resulting in hypophosphatemia.[72]

Hypophosphatemia is a common complication of liver disease (relating to the chronic use of antacids common in liver patients), malnutrition, and metabolic acidosis. Hypophosphatemia's effects on hematologic components are profound: decreased oxygen-carrying capacity, thrombocytopenia, and reduced neutrophil activity against bacteria. If hypophosphatemia is permitted to continue, the decreased phosphate levels may result in decreased calcification of bones and bone deformities may develop.[73]

Resulting signs and symptoms

The clinical presentation of a patient experiencing hypophosphatemia may include such symptoms as lethargy, mental confusion, muscle weakness, cardiac dysrhythmias, hemolytic anemia, metabolic acidosis, anorexia, bone pain, and pathologic fractures. In prolonged hypophosphatemia, platelet production and phagocytic activity of the white blood

cells are also inhibited. Hypophosphatemia has been noted to cause or complicate congestive heart failure by reducing the ATP available for contraction of the myocardium.[74]

The most critical laboratory value to assess is the serum phosphorus level, which in hypophosphatemia has a value of less than 3.0 mg/dL. An additional symptom that may be observed is evidence of calcium in the urine.[75]

Nursing standards of care

There are two goals associated with the management of hypophosphatemia. The first goal is to correct the low phosphate level and possible hypercalcemia. It is essential to correct the underlying cause of hypophosphatemia, as it will adversely affect cell growth and repair if it persists. The lack of energy available for these processes may lead to malnutrition, poor wound healing, and general muscle atrophy.

The second goal is promotion of the patient's safety by monitoring for neuromuscular changes, level of consciousness, and coagulopathies. It is necessary to recognize that neuromuscular involvement affects the patient's psychosocial being as well as his or her physical being. When there is a change in normal muscular function, the patient's ability to perform the activities of daily living is affected, and his or her participation in health care is limited. It is beneficial to assess the following: (1) the patient's activities of daily living, (2) the patient's safety, (3) exercise, and (4) the patient's mental orientation. Because of the potential anxiety and depression that can occur with hypophosphatemia, it is imperative to assess the patient's psychosocial adjustment and provide counseling as needed.

The replacement of phosphate is usually done by administering an oral or intravenous preparation. Intravenous phosphate is often given in the form of potassium phosphate, which should be given conservatively. Foods high in phosphate are encouraged. These include shellfish, red meat, organ meat, and dairy products. Administration of phosphate-binding gels should be discontinued. Phosphate and calcium levels are monitored throughout the therapy.[76]

Hyperphosphatemia

Hyperphosphatemia is an excess of phosphate in the extracellular fluid. In hyperphosphatemia, the serum phosphate concentration is greater than 4.5 mg/dL.[77]

Major etiologies of hyperphosphatemia include (1) increased phosphate intake through intravenous administration, laxative abuse, or excessive dietary intake through meats and dairy products; (2) acute and chronic renal disease; and (3) neoplastic disease.

Increased intake is considered the most common etiology, but generally the kidneys are able to excrete some excess phosphate, so levels must be very high over a short time frame to exceed this compensatory ability. Infants given cow's milk can develop hyperphosphatemia, as the amount of phosphate in it is excessive for an infant's body weight. Most laxatives and antacids contain large quantities of phosphate; overuse of these products can lead to excess phosphate levels.

Hyperphosphatemia is common with neoplastic disease. Malignancies destroy normal tissue or bone and lead to the release of intracellular substances. Phosphate is found in large amounts within tumor cells and the bony structure; therefore, phosphate levels increase when cell breakdown occurs. As might be expected, cytotoxic therapy such as chemotherapy or radiation therapy accelerates the destruction of tumor cells and may enhance the risks of elevating phosphate to levels beyond the capacity of the kidneys to excrete.

Indirect hormonal influences can contribute to hyperphosphatemia if calcium regulation is disturbed by imbalances in parathyroid or thyroid hormones. Hypoparathyroidism is unusual but can lead to hyperphosphatemia related to reduced calcium levels. Hyperthyroidism resulting in the release of calcitonin and hypocalcemia can also lead to hyperphosphatemia.

Hyperphosphatemia commonly occurs as a result of the inability of the kidney to excrete phosphate. This is usually due to renal failure, when the body's excretory ability is greatly compromised.

Hyperphosphatemia can indirectly affect renal function by increasing the amount of phosphate to be excreted and thereby damaging renal tubules. Although renal failure may cause the syndrome, renal failure can also be a result of it. High phosphate levels will alter enzymatic reactions and the active transport systems. Although phosphate is necessary for these functions, excessive levels can hinder their actions.

Because of the phosphorus-calcium relationship, hyperphosphatemia often mirrors the clinical symptoms of hypocalcemia: tetany, cardiac irritability, hyperreflexia, tremors, seizures, and GI distress. These symptoms are directly attributable to the low calcium rather than to the high phosphate.[78] High phosphate levels are most likely to have effects on glucose utilization and active transport at the cellular level and to create vague general clinical symptoms. As a result, the general clinical presentation of the patient suffering hyperphosphatemia can vary; muscle wasting, bony deposits, bone pain, anorexia, and GI distress are all possible. Poor wound healing and inability to adjust to hormonal or infectious challenges may be apparent.

Symptoms related to renal failure may be evident if hyperphosphatemia is prolonged or extremely severe. These are described in detail later in this chapter.

Essential laboratory data reveals an elevated serum phosphorus level greater than 4.5 mg/100 mL and usually a decreased serum calcium level.[79]

Since the clinical presentation of a patient with hyperphosphatemia is very similar to that of a patient with hypocalcemia, the nursing management is also similar. Many times the hyperphosphatemic patient is relatively asymptomatic.

The actual treatment of hyperphosphatemia involves eliminating the cause and treating the symptoms. The process may include restricting the intake of phosphates, using aluminum-hydroxide gels, phosphate-binding agents, or diuretics (which increase renal excretion of phosphates), and subjecting the patient to dialysis when other measures fail.[80]

Magnesium

Magnesium is the second major intracellular cation. It plays a significant role in initiating multiple essential enzyme systems and biochemical reactions. ATP synthesis is dependent upon magnesium to assist in the maintenance of intracellular sodium-potassium pumps, muscle contractions, and carbohydrate utilization. Sixty percent of the body's magnesium is a structural element of bone. Magnesium influences the secretion of parathyroid hormone. Magnesium is regulated by intestinal absorption and secretion exchange between bone and extracellular fluid and by renal excretion. The normal serum concentration of magnesium ranges from 1.5 to 2.0 mEq/L.[81]

Hypomagnesemia

Hypomagnesemia is a deficit of magnesium in the extracellular fluid. In hypomagnesemia, the serum concentration of magnesium is less than 1.5 mEq/L.[82] This disorder frequently occurs concomitantly with hypokalemia and hypocalcemia. Clinicians often find that the persistent symptoms that occur even after correction of the potassium and calcium disorders reflect hypomagnesemia.

Clinical antecedents

The precipitating factors of hypomagnesemia in Table 5-22 may be grouped into two classifications that involve (1) low intake or reduced intestinal absorption of magnesium, and (2) excessive loss of magnesium from body fluids, in the urine, or from miscellaneous causes.

Critical referents

Only about 1% of the body's magnesium is found in the extracellular fluid, but it is essential for

Table 5-22 Clinical Antecedents of Hypomagnesemia

Type of Antecedent	Possible Sources
Impaired intake or absorption	Malnutrition Prolonged IV therapy without Mg$^+$ supplementation Malabsorption syndromes: sprue, cystic fibrosis, enema or laxative abuse, diarrhea, ulcerative colitis, Crohn's disease Chronic alcoholism Acute and chronic pancreatitis
Excessive renal excretion or ECF loss	Acute renal failure Diuretic therapy Diabetic ketoacidosis Excessive steroid administration Secretion of inappropriate ADH Cancer chemotherapeutic agents Hyperthyroidism Toxemic pregnancy Hypercalcemia Cardiac glycosides Aminoglycosides Intestinal drains and fistulas Nasogastric suctioning

active transport systems and can affect both calcium and potassium levels. Calcium and magnesium compete for absorption in the GI tract, and when gastrointestinal calcium levels are high, that cation is preferentially absorbed by the small intestine, which leads to hypomagnesemia. Hypomagnesemia causes both hypocalcemia and hypokalemia when the lack of magnesium causes the movement of these electrolytes into the extracellular fluid and their subsequent excretion. The pathophysiologic effects of hypomagnesemia are similar to those of hypophosphatemia, although they are often not visible clinically.

Resulting signs and symptoms

The signs and symptoms of magnesium deficiency reflect those of hypocalcemia and hypokalemia. The characteristic symptom of hypomagnesemia is tetany, with its muscle tremors, weakness alternating with cramping, and seizures. Other symptoms include Chvostek's and Trousseau's signs, apathy, coma, confusion, anorexia, nausea, vomiting, and dysrhythmias.[83] An electrocardiogram may show a prolonged Q-T interval and broadened, flat, or inverted T waves.[84] Hypomagnesemia enhances the effects of digitalis; therefore, digitalis toxicity may be present.[85] Digitalis toxicity results in cardiac dysrhythmias, blurred vision or diplopia, tinnitus, and gastrointestinal distress. Many of these symptoms will be masked by the symptoms of the electrolyte deficiency. The clinical manifestations of hypomagnesemia are listed in Table 5-23.

Laboratory data is essential when assessing hypomagnesemia. The serum magnesium level is likely to be less than 1.5 mEq/L. The serum calcium and potassium levels, as well as the urine magnesium and calcium levels, will be low.[86]

Nursing standards of care

The goals of nursing management of hypomagnesemia focus on three aspects of treatment. The first is the need to manage the environment and promote the patient's safety and comfort. This is particularly important because of the extensive neuromuscular involvement. Symptom management is the second nursing goal. The third is to assist in correction of the underlying problem.

As in the management of hypocalcemia, the patient's environment must be monitored, with par-

Table 5-23 Signs and Symptoms of Hypomagnesemia

Body System	Signs and Symptoms
Neuromuscular	Insomnia Muscle irritability and tetany Muscle weakness Flapping tremors Ataxia Vertigo Personality changes such as apathy or psychoses Nystagmus
Cardiovascular	Cardiac dysrhythmias (PVBs, VT, VF) Sinus tachycardia ECG changes including broadened Q-T interval and T waves and shortened ST segment
Respiratory	Usually none
Gastrointestinal	Anorexia, nausea and vomiting
Renal	Usually none

ticular attention to stimulation and safety. Seizure precautions should be instituted, and patients should not be allowed out of bed unless they are able to support themselves.

The patient should be assessed through physical examination, analysis of laboratory data, and ECG analysis. Symptomatic support of gastrointestinal symptoms may be provided with antiemetics or parenteral nutrition. Cardiac dysrhythmias are transient, but may indicate the need for antiarrhythmic therapy until magnesium is replaced. Acute myocardial ischemia with failure has been noted in patients with hypomagnesemia, but since hypomagnesemia often occurs in conjunction with hypocalcemia and hypokalemia, this problem cannot be attributable to a specific electrolyte deficiency.

Replacement therapy for hypomagnesemia involves the administration of magnesium sulfate intravenously or intramuscularly. There are several considerations to note when replacement therapy begins. If magnesium is to be given to patients with renal insufficiency, it should be given very cautiously, as they are unable to excrete excesses.[87] Some postulate that too rapid an infusion of magnesium will result in renal excretion of the excess and will nullify the attempt to correct the hypomagnesemia.[88] Calcium gluconate may be given adjunctively to act as a retardant to sudden hypermagnesemia or kept on standby to treat magnesium

intoxication.[89] The dangers of respiratory depression or heart block during infusion necessitate careful consideration of the patient's need for the therapy and the staff's ability to monitor it.[90] Magnesium is also a vessel irritant, and when given intravenously, it should be diluted to a concentration of 20% or less and administered no faster than 150 mg/min.[91] Magnesium sulfate may be ordered by grams (g) or by milliequivalents (mEq); 1 g is equal to 8.12 mEq. The usual replacement intravenous dose is 1–4 g (8–32 mEq).[92] However, dosages of up to 6 g (48 mEq) may be given if the patient is having seizures.[93] Dosages should be reduced if the patient is also receiving central nervous system depressants or neuromuscular blocking agents.[94] Rapid infusion can cause the patient to experience a feeling of flushing, hypoventilation, and bradyarrhythmias. For fewer potential side effects, magnesium supplements can be included in hyperalimentation solutions or given by intramuscular injection. Precautions should be taken when infusing magnesium, as it is incompatible with phenothiazines, calcium, phosphate, and bicarbonate solutions.[95]

Oral magnesium supplements or magnesium in the form of antacids have laxative effects. The loose stools are best treated with bulking agents such as Metamucil. Intestinal malabsorption syndromes known to cause hypomagnesemia may also inhibit the absorption of these supplements; therefore, intake and output as well as stool assessments are important nursing care measures. Magnesium supplements have also been noted to interfere with absorption of some antibiotics and anticonvulsants, so precautions should be taken to avoid giving these medications at the same time.[95]

Patient education about potential causes and symptoms of hypomagnesemia is important for the patient who is receiving chemotherapy or diuretics, since symptoms such as vision changes and muscle weakness may be subjective or not routinely assessed. Patients with disorders known to cause hypomagnesemia should be taught the possible symptoms of hypomagnesemia, hypocalcemia, and hypokalemia. In addition, such patients should be encouraged to eat foods high in magnesium, such as meat, green vegetables, whole grains, and nuts.

Hypermagnesemia

Hypermagnesemia is an excess of magnesium in the extracellular fluid. In hypermagnesemia, the serum concentration of magnesium is greater than 2.2 mEq/L.[97]

Clinical antecedents

Hypermagnesemia does not occur frequently, because the kidneys are able to excrete excess quantities of magnesium. Therefore, the primary precipitating factor for hypermagnesemia may be decreased excretion of magnesium by the kidneys due to renal dysfunction. Other factors may include adrenal insufficiency, shock, hypothermia, and increased magnesium intake. The increased intake may result from intravenous magnesium solutions, intramuscular injections, or use of magnesium-containing antacids or gels.[98]

Critical referents

Excessive numbers of magnesium ions lead to interference with neuromuscular transmission. Clinical effects follow a typical pattern, beginning with general neuron transmission defects resulting in weakness, fatigue, and warmth or flushing. Skeletal muscles are affected as magnesium levels rise, and involuntary muscles such as the heart and diaphragm are the last to be affected.

Resulting signs and symptoms

Clinical presentation of hypermagnesemia is directly related to the degree of increase of magnesium. A patient with a slightly increased magnesium level may be asymptomatic; a patient with an excessive magnesium level may experience detrimental effects in every system. Signs and symptoms of hypermagnesemia as they relate to level of excess are outlined in Table 5-24.

The most significant laboratory value to assess is the serum magnesium level, which if greater than 2.2 mEq/L indicates a problem.[99]

Nursing standards of care

There are two goals for the nursing and medical interventions with a hypermagnesemic patient.

Table 5-24 Signs and Symptoms of Hypermagnesemia

Serum Magnesium Level (mEq/L)	Body System	Signs and Symptoms
2.2–3.0		None
3.1–5.0	Vascular	Hypotension
	Gastrointestinal	Nausea Vomiting
	Nervous	Depressed deep tendon reflexes
5.1–7.0	Nervous	Drowsiness Depression
7.1–10.0	Nervous	Loss of deep tendon reflexes Seizures
	Muscular	Weakness
	Cardiac	Sinus bradycardia Prolonged P-R interval Prolonged Q-T interval
10.1–15.0	Respiratory	Hypoventilation
	Muscular	Paralysis
	Nervous	Coma
15.1–20.0	Cardiac	Cardiac arrest
	Respiratory	Apnea

Source: Adapted from Kinney, M. R., Packa, D. R., and Dunbar, S. B. (1988). *AACN'S Clinical Reference for Critical Care Nursing.* 2nd edition. New York: McGraw-Hill Book Company.

First, because of the neuromuscular involvement, it is necessary to control the environment, manage outside stimulation, and provide for the patient's safety and comfort. The patellar reflex of patients suspected of having hypermagnesemia should be checked, and emergent interventions to reduce magnesium levels should be instituted if it is diminished or absent. The patient must be assessed frequently for neurological status, muscular involvement, cardiac status, respiratory distress, ECG patterns, other physical findings, and laboratory data.

The second nursing goal is to assist in the determination of the primary cause of the problem and provide supportive treatment measures. The treatment will focus on the cause of the increased magnesium level. If the patient has an increased intake of magnesium, then teaching the patient how to reduce intake will be appropriate. If the patient maintains normal renal function, diuretics and intravenous fluids are appropriate to increase renal excretion of magnesium. If the precipitating factor is renal failure, then dialysis is effective in lowering the magnesium level. In any event, calcium supplement may be considered appropriate therapy to minimize the symptoms of an elevated magnesium level.[100]

Acute Renal Failure

Acute renal failure (ARF) occurs when there is a suddent decline in renal function sufficient to cause solute retention. When this occurs the body's internal homeostasis is lost. Loss of renal function results in a syndrome characterized principally by fluid, electrolyte, and acid-base abnormalities, retention of nitrogenous waste products, poor blood pressure control, and inadequate homeostasis and erythropoiesis. On average, 50% of patients who experience acute renal failure die. The mortality rate for patients with postoperative and trauma-related acute renal failure (60–70%) is higher than that for medical cases (20–50%).[101] The leading cause of death from ARF is infection.

Acute renal failure (ARF) is differentiated from chronic renal failure (CRF) in that the former is usually a reversible process, if the patient survives. Also, the rapid onset of ARF contrasts with the progressive process leading to CRF. ARF patients usually do not experience the profound neurological and musculoskeletal disorders (such as peripheral neuropathies and renal osteodystrophy) that occur with CRF.

Clinical antecedents

Acute renal failure has several causes, many of which can be minimized or eliminated. The general risk factors that predispose a patient to ARF are described in Table 5-25. Prevention of ARF is vital considering the significant mortality rate, and the critical care nurse must be cognizant of these risk factors to prevent it.

It is essential that the practitioner be able to identify specific causes of ARF once it has occurred and, in particular, any reversible component of the process. To facilitate this process, cases of ARF are traditionally divided into three groups based on the mean causative factor: prerenal, intrarenal, and postrenal. Each category includes multiple and varied etiologies.

Prerenal ARF occurs in the setting of decreased renal blood flow. Since renal blood flow is a key determinant of glomerular filtration rate (GFR), a marked reduction of renal blood flow will result in a decreased GFR. This is a functional form of renal failure in which solute retention occurs because of inadequate filtration, but no structural damage occurs.[102] Recovery of kidney function is dependent upon re-establishing adequate blood flow. The conditions that can result in prerenal ARF are listed in Table 5-26.

Intrarenal ARF occurs when there is direct injury to the renal tissue affecting the glomeruli, tubules, or

Table 5-25   Risk Factors That Increase Susceptibility to Acute Renal Failure

Pre-existing renal insufficiency: diabetes, hypertension

Age: very young or elderly

Cardiovascular disorders

Surgery: open heart, abdominal aneurysm repair

Trauma

Exposure to nephrotoxins

Multiple myeloma

Pregnancy

Sources: Compiled with data from Richard, C. J. (1986). Acute renal failure. In C. J. Richard, ed. *Comprehensive Nephrology Nursing.* Boston: Little, Brown & Co., pp. 178–221; Ng, R. C., and Suki, W. N. (1980). Treatment of acute renal failure. In B. M. Brenner and J. H. Stein, eds. *Acute Renal Failure.* New York: Churchill-Livingstone, pp. 229–274.

Table 5-26 Prerenal Causes of Acute
Renal Failure

Hypovolemia:
  Dehydration
  Hemorrhage
  Excessive diuresis
  Third spacing
  Skin losses (diaphoresis, burns)
  Gastrointestinal losses (vomiting, diarrhea, fistulae,
    nasogastric suction)
  Hypoalbuminemia

Reduced Cardiac Output:
  Congestive heart failure
  Pulmonary edema
  Myocardial infarction
  Arrhythmias
  Pericardial tamponade
  Valvular disease

Decreased Peripheral Vascular Resistance:
  Sepsis
  Antihypertensive medications
  Anaphylaxis

Impaired Renovascular Blood Flow:
  Thrombosis
  Embolism
  Dissecting Aneurysm
  Hepatorenal syndrome

Sources: Compiled with data from Corwin, H. L., and Bonventre,
J. V. (1986). Acute renal failure. *Medical Clinics of North
America* 70: 1037–1055; Richard, C. J. (1986). Acute renal
failure. In C. J. Richard, ed. *Comprehensive Nephrology
Nursing.* Boston: Little, Brown & Co., pp. 178–221; Mars, D. R.,
and Treloar, D. (1984). Acute tubular necrosis: Pathophysiology
and treatment. *Heart & Lung* 13: 194–202; Ng, R. C., and Suki,
W. N. (1980). Treatment of acute renal failure. In B. M. Brenner
and J. H. Stein, eds. *Acute Renal Failure.* New York:
Churchill-Livingstone, pp. 229–274; Rudnick, M. R., Bastl, C. P.,
Elfinbein, I. B., and Narins, R. G. (1983). The differential
diagnosis of acute renal failure. In B. M. Brenner and J. M.
Lazarus, eds. *Acute Renal Failure.* Philadelphia: W. B.
Saunders, pp. 176–222.

Table 5-27 Intrarenal Causes of Acute
Renal Failure

Prolonged Prerenal Ischemia

Nephrotoxins:
  Antibiotics (aminoglycosides, cephalosporins, sulfa
    drugs, amphotericin B)
  Drugs (allopurinol, cimetidine, furosemide, heroin,
    thiazides, nonsteroidal anti-inflammatory drugs)
  Contrast media
  Anesthetics
  Heme pigments (myoglobin, hemoglobin)
  Heavy metals (mercury, lead, gold, cis-platinum)
  Organic solvents (ethylene glycol, carbon tetrachloride)

Infectious Processes:
  Glomerulonephritis
  Pyelonephritis

Vascular Disorders:
  Atheroembolic disease
  Vasculitis (systemic lupus erythematosis, polyarteritis
    nodosa)
  Thrombotic states (hemolytic uremic syndrome,
    thrombotic thrombocytopenic purpura, disseminated
    intravascular coagulation)

Trauma

Intrarenal Obstruction:
  Acute urate nephropathy

Transplant Rejection

Sources: Compiled with data from Richard, C. J. (1987). Causes
of renal failure. In L. Lancaster, ed. *Core curriculum for
nephrology nursing.* Anthony J. Janetti, Inc., pp. 55–69; Corwin,
H. L., and Bonventre, J. V. (1986). Acute renal failure. *Medical
Clinics of North America,* 70: 1037–1055; Mars, D. R., and
Treloar, D. (1984). Acute tubular necrosis: Pathophysiology and
treatment. *Heart & Lung,* 13: 194–202; Ng, R. C., and Suki,
W. N. (1980). Treatment of acute renal failure. In B. M. Brenner
& J. H. Stein, eds. *Acute renal failure.* New York: Churchill-
Livingstone, pp. 229–274.

interstitium. The most common type of intrarenal ARF seen in clinical practice is acute tubular necrosis (ATN), major etiologies of which include ischemia, nephrotoxins, and pigment (for example, myoglobin). Causes of intrarenal ARF are listed in Table 5-27. The nurse must pay careful attention to potential nephrotoxins, as many of these drugs are routinely given in the intensive care unit (ICU).

Postrenal ARF occurs when the flow of urine from the renal pelvis through the urinary outflow tract is obstructed. Obstruction of the bladder or urethra by clot or calculus results in bilateral obstruction and renal failure. Bilateral obstruction results in anuria (less than 100 mL of urine excreted in 24 hours). Unilateral obstruction of a single ureter may

be sufficient to induce acute renal failure if the patient has only a single kidney. Alleviation of the obstruction will result in restoration of kidney function. Causes of postrenal ARF are listed in Table 5-28.

In summary, in prerenal and postrenal ARF, the source of the kidney dysfunction is external to the kidney. Prerenal ARF is due to hypoperfusion, and postrenal ARF is due to obstructed urinary outflow. Intrarenal ARF is the only type of ARF caused by direct insult to the renal parenchyma. Prolonged prerenal and postrenal ARF can eventually lead to intrarenal ARF. Regardless of the type of ARF, identification of the cause and its elimination or treatment are essential for re-establishing normal renal function.

Table 5-28 Postrenal Causes of Acute Renal Failure

Urinary Tract Obstruction:
  Calculi
  Blood clots
  Sloughed tissue
  Pus
  Fungi
  Crystals
  Tumor
  Surgical ligation
  Strictures
  Fibrosis
  Congenital abnormalities
  Trauma

Prostatic Hypertrophy

Abdominal/pelvic Tumors

Drugs:
  Antihistamines, ganglionic blocking agents

Sources: Compiled with data from Corwin, H. L., and Bonventre, J. V. (1986). Acute renal failure. *Medical Clinics of North America* 70: 1037–1055; Richard, C. J. (1986). Acute renal failure. In C. J. Richard, ed. *Comprehensive nephrology nursing.* Boston: Little, Brown & Co., pp. 178–221; Mars, D. R., and Treloar, D. (1984). Acute tubular necrosis: Pathophysiology and treatment. *Heart and Lung* 13: 194–202; Freedman, P., and Smith, E. C. (1975). Acute renal failure. *Heart & Lung* 4: 873–878.

Critical referents

The pathophysiology of ARF is varied, depending upon whether the condition is prerenal, intrarenal, or postrenal. In prerenal ARF, where renal blood flow is diminished, the kidney responds to the hypoperfused state by initiating a variety of compensatory and autoregulatory mechanisms. The renin-angiotensin mechanism is stimulated, and the ensuing outpouring of angiotensin serves to maintain renal blood flow by maintaining systemic blood pressure, stimulating aldosterone secretion, and maximizing sodium reabsorption. The tubular network remains functionally intact, as reflected by sodium-free, concentrated urine, indicating maximal reabsorption of water and sodium by the tubules.

The autoregulatory mechanism increases the diameter of the afferent arterioles, thus increasing blood flow into the glomeruli. At the same time, the diameter of the efferent arterioles is decreased, generating a back-pressure that allows for maintenance of the GFR.

These are two potent regulatory mechanisms, but when hypoperfusion is prolonged, their ability to respond is exhausted. Acute renal failure occurs as the blood flow becomes too slow to allow for adequate glomerular filtration.

The pathophysiology of acute tubular necrosis, the most common type of intrarenal ARF, varies depending upon the nature of the original insult. Investigations in this area have incriminated four major potential sources of intrarenal ARF: (1) intrarenal obstruction, (2) back-leak of glomerular filtrate, (3) a reduction of the ultrafiltration coefficient, and (4) a decrease in blood flow. More recent research has focused on subcellular events, in particular, adverse alterations of renal cell calcium regulation. Following ischemic injury, renal vasoconstriction may play a greater role in tubular damage; with nephrotoxic injuries, direct toxicity to the tubular cells resulting in back-leak of filtrate and tubular obstruction may be more prominent. It is likely that each of these potential factors participates to some degree in every type of acute renal failure.

Postrenal ARF evolves when a partial or complete obstruction of the urinary tract results in increased pressure in the collecting system. This increased pressure impedes the outflow of urine from the nephrons into the renal pelvis, resulting in distention of the renal pelvis, a condition known as hydronephrosis. The increased intratubular pressure leads to dilation of the tubules and compression of surrounding structures. Derangement of the prostaglandin balance coupled with these mechanical defects may lead to a resultant decrease in GFR and a decline in renal function. Tubular injury and impairment ultimately result in the abnormal handling of sodium and water and the loss of the kidneys' normal concentrating ability.

Resulting signs and symptoms

The clinical signs and symptoms of prerenal or postrenal ARF will largely depend upon the underlying disease process. The prerenal ARF patient may demonstrate evidence of circulatory inadequacies such as congestive heart failure or pulmonary edema. Patients with postrenal obstruction may present with flank pain or renal colic. The signs and symptoms will disappear quickly with correction of the cause of the prerenal or postrenal ARF.

Urinalysis allows for the differentiation of prerenal, postrenal, and intrarenal ARF; Table 5-29 lists the range of values that indicates each type of ARF. Urine from a prerenal ARF patient reflects intact kidneys in that there are no casts, cells, or debris to indicate kidney damage; the urine is concentrated

Table 5-29 Key Urine and Plasma Values in Differentiating Types of Acute Renal Failure

Value	Prerenal ARF	Intrarenal ARF	Postrenal ARF
Urine sodium (mEq/L)	<10–20	>40	>20
Urine osmolality (mOsm)	>500	<350	<350–400
Urine specific gravity	>1.015	~1.010	~1.010
Urine sediment	No cells, casts, or cellular debris	RBCs, RBC casts WBCs, WBC casts Eosinophils Tubular casts Cellular debris	Possibly RBCs; no other cells, casts, or cellular debris
Plasma urea:creatinine	20:1	10:1	10:1

Sources: Compiled with data from Corwin, H. L., and Bonventre, J. V. (1986). Acute renal failure. *Medical Clinics of North America* 70: 1037–1055; Mars, D. R., and Treloar, D. (1984). Acute tubular necrosis: Pathophysiology and treatment. *Heart & Lung* 13: 194–202; Schrier, R. W. (1981). Acute renal failure: Pathogenesis, diagnosis, and management. *Hospital Practice* 16: 93–112.

and low in sodium, as the tubules are attempting to reabsorb sodium and water to improve perfusion. The plasma urea:creatinine ratio is elevated, as the decreased circulating blood volume falsely elevates the blood urea nitrogen (BUN).

A urine sample from an intrarenal ARF patient may contain red blood cells (RBC), RBC casts, tubular cells, and cellular debris, indicating that direct kidney tissue damage has occurred. White blood cells (WBC) and WBC casts may also be present. As the concentrating ability of the kidney is lost, a dilute urine is produced with an osmolality similar to that of plasma. Urine sodium losses are high because of tubular dysfunction. The urea:creatinine ratio is approximately 10:1.

Urine and plasma values for the postrenal ARF patient are similar to those for the intrarenal ARF patient in terms of urine osmolality, urine specific gravity, and urea:creatinine ratio. However, urine from a postrenal ARF patient has a lower sodium content and lacks cells, casts, and cellular debris. Some RBCs may be present if there is trauma secondary to the migration of renal calculi through the urinary tract.

Being able to differentiate the type of ARF allows the appropriate treatment to be provided. If urinalysis reveals a prerenal or postrenal cause, rapid resolution of the resulting signs and symptoms can be expected once the cause is eliminated. If the etiology is intrarenal in nature, the patient can be expected to progress through the four phases of acute tubular necrosis.

The clinical course of acute tubular necrosis (ATN) traditionally has four phases. Specific signs and symptoms are associated with each phase. The first phase is the initiating phase, during which the

insult is occurring, such as a period of hypotension or exposure to a nephrotoxic antibiotic. It is during this phase that an intensive analysis of the patient's volume status and urine should be undertaken to determine the severity of tubular damage.

The second phase in ATN, the oliguric phase, begins when the patient's urinary output falls below 400 cc in 24 hours. It is important to note that not all patients experience oliguria, but those who do have a higher mortality rate.[103] This phase lasts 5 to 14 days and is considered to be the most dangerous phase.[104] In this stage, the chemical alterations become apparent and manifest themselves in a variety of clinical signs and symptoms and biochemical abnormalities. The name of the syndrome that encompasses these signs and symptoms of renal failure is uremia. The signs and symptoms manifested by the patient in the oliguric phase of ATN are summarized in the nursing care plan at the end of this section.

The cardiovascular system is commonly disturbed in acute renal failure. Since the kidneys' ability to regulate fluid balance is lost in ATN, hypervolemia can easily occur and result in congestive heart failure. Expansion of the extracellular volume will result in hypertension and peripheral edema. Inappropriate triggering of the renin-angiotensin mechanism may contribute to hypertension accompanying ARF. Other disorders affecting the cardiovascular system include hyperkalemia and pericarditis, which may be complicated by cardiac tamponade.

Hyperkalemia is a life-threatening condition, particularly when it evolves rapidly and ECG changes occur. Potassium levels rise in ARF, as the kidneys are unable to excrete this electrolyte. Hyperkalemia increases further in circumstances in which tissue destruction is occurring, such as rhabdomyolysis. Approximately 130–150 mEq/L of intracellular potassium is released into the ECF when tissue destruction occurs. Red blood cells also contain significant quantities of potassium; therefore, internal bleeding or hematoma formation may result in the rapid development of severe hyperkalemia. Hyperkalemia may be aggravated by the inappropriate ingestion of foods or medications containing potassium (for example, potassium penicillin). The significance of hyperkalemia is its cardiotoxicity, which is manifested by conduction defects that can lead to arrhythmias and cardiac arrest. Hyperkalemia may also produce generalized muscle dysfunction evidenced by weakness and, on occasion, flaccid paralysis.

Pericarditis may be seen in rapidly advancing acute renal failure. The most significant complication of pericarditis is the development of pericardial effusion, which, if it occurs rapidly and is large, can result in cardiac tamponade. Pericarditis often presents as pleuropericardial pain but can be clinically silent. The etiology of uremic pericarditis is unclear, but it is thought to be caused by the presence of uremic toxins in the pericardial fluid. It is believed that heparin may also be a factor.

The heart is encased in a thin layer called the visceral pericardium. This layer is separated from the parietal pericardium, which lines the other organs of the chest cavity, by 10–20 mL of fluid. This fluid acts as a lubricant as the heart expands and contracts. Pericarditis begins with an aseptic inflammation in response to the uremic toxins. Fibrin is produced and eventually covers the entire pericardium. Adhesions form, impairing cardiac contraction, and constriction can occur as the inflammatory response increases the fluid volume between the visceral and parietal layers. Heparin may cause blood to move into the pericardial space, further increasing the volume. Characteristically there is a temperature elevation, chest pain, and an audible friction rub to the left of the lower half of the sternum. As fluid continues to exude into the pericardial space, an effusion occurs, which can be diagnosed with an echocardiogram and/or ECG. If untreated, the effusion will progress to tamponade. Tamponade is evidenced by circulatory collapse as the constricted heart can no longer adequately perfuse vital organs or the periphery of the body. Pericarditis should be treated immediately to prevent this potentially fatal event.

Neuromuscular and neurologic disturbances due to the accumulation of uremic toxins are a prominent feature of ARF. As the level of uremia advances, the patient may become fatigued and lethargic, manifest irritability, and have a decreased attention span, which can progress to confusion and ultimately coma. Uremic seizures may occur. The onset of neurologic symptoms is related not only to the degree of uremia but to the rapidity of its development as well.

Respiratory disturbances tend to be related to hypervolemia resulting in pulmonary edema and pleural effusions. A pleural friction rub may be present with the effusion. Pulmonary infections are common in patients with acute uremia and need to be monitored very closely, as infection is the primary cause of death from ARF. This increased susceptibility to infection is due to the altered WBC physiology in uremia and may be intensified if the patient is malnourished. Metabolic acidosis, which often occurs in uremia, may produce tachypnea.

Hematologic disturbances include the development of a qualitative platelet defect leading to a bleeding diathesis,[105] anemia, and increased susceptibility to infection. The alteration in platelet function is somewhat correlated with the evolution of a urea nitrogen level greater than 100 mg/dL. It may be clinically manifested as gastrointestinal hemorrhage, subdural hematoma, pericardial hemorrhage, epistaxis, or ecchymosis. Taking a bleeding time is the easiest way to monitor the platelet defect and the development of a bleeding diathesis.

The anemia of ARF is produced by inadequate erythropoiesis and compounded by the fact that uremia shortens the life span of RBCs. Anemia tends to be most severe during the second week of the course of ARF. Blood losses from phlebotomy and dialysis intensify the anemia. As noted earlier, WBCs are altered in uremia, predisposing ARF patients to all types of local and systemic infections.

Gastrointestinal (GI) symptoms include uremic fetor, which is caused by the degradation of salivary urea to ammonia in the presence of the enzyme urease. The patient may also complain of a metallic taste or lack of taste. Advancing uremia is associated with nausea, vomiting, and mucosal ulceration. The presence of uremic toxins in the GI tract produces these signs and symptoms. Gastrointestinal ulceration is of particular concern because of the increased bleeding tendency. Constipation also tends to occur with advanced uremia.

Integument disturbances are frequently seen in ATN. Many patients complain of itching, which is thought to be caused by calcium phosphate ($CaPO_4$) deposits beneath the skin. If the itching is unrelenting, the patient may excoriate the skin and then become at risk for a local infection. Multiple ecchymotic lesions may develop as a result of the platelet defect of uremia. If the anemia is profound, pallor will be prominent. Uremic frost occurs when uric acid crystals emerge through skin pores and dry, forming a white powdery surface. This sign should never be seen in a well-managed ATN patient.

Biochemical disturbances are a prominent feature of ARF and include calcium-phosphate imbalance, metabolic acidosis, hyponatremia, and hypermagnesemia. In ARF, the ability of the kidneys to excrete phosphate and to activate the vitamin D needed for calcium absorption in the gut is impaired. The serum calcium level falls below 8.5 mg/dL, and the serum phosphate level rises above 4.5 mg/dL. Skeletal disturbances including bone demineralization and metastatic calcifications can result. A low serum calcium level results in parathormone (PTH) secretion. Parathormone stimulates reabsorption of calcium from the bone into the blood. Alkaline phosphatase increases, indicating active bone demineralization. If large quantities of phosphate (5.5 mg/dL or more) are circulating in the blood when endogenous calcium is released from the bone or exogenous supplements are given, the calcium binds with the phosphate, forming insoluble $CaPO_4$ complexes. (In ARF there is often a high phosphate level as the kidney is the primary excretory organ for phosphate.) These complexes can be deposited in the heart valves and muscle, brain, lungs, blood vessels, soft tissue, joints, and skin. The deposits are called metastatic calcifications and are likely to occur when the calcium-phosphate product (the serum calcium level multiplied by the serum phosphate level) is 70 or greater. They can impair the function of the organ or tissue in which they are deposited. Renal osteodystrophy, which occurs with protracted bone demineralization, is usually only seen in chronic renal failure patients.

Hypocalcemia develops in part because of precipitation of calcium with phosphate, particularly where there is damaged tissue, but also because renal failure reduces the kidneys' ability to generate active vitamin D. In cases of severe trauma, marked levels of hypocalcemia may be seen, but despite this, tetany is not commonly encountered.

Metabolic acidosis is a common acid-base disturbance in ARF, with the serum bicarbonate falling on average 1–2 mEq per day. The average noncatabolic adult produces about 1 mEq of acid per kilogram per day. These acid end-products are usually excreted along with hydrogen ions in the urine. In ARF the excretion is impaired, as well as the production of bicarbonate and ammonia, which are needed to correct acidosis. When the renal buffering mechanism fails, the patient becomes tachypneic as the body makes an effort to lower the carbon dioxide (CO_2) level and achieve respiratory alkalosis. If untreated, metabolic acidosis will result in lethargy and stupor.

The final biochemical disturbances are hyponatremia and hypermagnesemia. In ARF hyponatremia is caused by the dilutional effect of hypervolemia as the renal excretory mechanism for water is impaired. The resulting signs and symptoms are neurologic in nature, as the hyponatremia causes cerebral edema. The symptoms can be fairly benign (for example, nausea and malaise) until the sodium level falls below 125 mEq/L. Hypermagnesemia occurs because the kidney is the primary excretory organ for magnesium. A summary of expected biochemical disturbances is provided in Table 5-30.

An additional feature of ARF is the development of nutritional disturbances. The majority of such patients are in a state of catabolism with a negative nitrogen balance. With the significant weight loss that can occur, malnutrition may evolve rapidly in such patients. This is of great concern, as malnutrition interferes with the healing of tissue and reduces the body's ability to fight infection.

Drug metabolism disturbances are a particular problem in the oliguric phase of ARF. A multitude of drugs such as gentamicin, vancomycin, and tobramycin are excreted via the kidneys.[106] Other drugs are metabolized by the liver, and their metabolites must be excreted by the kidneys (for example, Meperidine). When the GFR and urinary output are decreased, these drugs can accumulate rapidly in the serum to toxic levels.

In the face of the life-threatening physical manifestations of ARF, it is essential not to lose sight of the psychologic disturbances that can occur. Patients are anxious and fearful at the loss of a body function often taken for granted. They may actually grieve for this loss of function. Depression is also common, as the patient feels powerless to combat this illness. If the patient has been independent, his or her self-concept may be greatly altered, further increasing the anxiety level.

In summary, the oliguric phase of ATN is a multisystem disease with many serious and debilitating signs and symptoms. Primary causes of death in this phase are infection and gastrointestinal bleeding. Meticulous assessments and early identification of the signs and symptoms are critical to minimize their effects.

The third phase of ARF is the diuretic phase. It begins when renal tubular cell recovery starts and is manifested primarily by a rising urine output. Although urine output may increase, the glomerular filtration rate may not improve for several days; therefore, BUN and creatinine levels may continue to rise. When it occurs, the improvement in GFR is marked by a drop in the BUN and creatinine levels. An osmotic diuresis may occur during this phase if

Table 5-30 Expected Biochemical Disturbances in Oliguric Phase
of ATN

Substance	Normal Value	Expected Value in Oliguric Phase[a]
Blood urea nitrogen	12–25 mg/dL	60–120 mg/dL
Creatinine	0.4–1.5 mg/dL	6–12 mg/dL
Sodium	135–145 mEq/L	N or <135 mEq/L
Potassium	3.5–5.0 mEq/L	N or >5.0 mEq/L
Carbon dioxide	24–30 mEq/L	<24 mEq/L
Calcium	8.5–10.5 mg/dL	N or <8.5 mEq/L
Phosphate	3.0–4.5 mg/dL	N or >4.5 mEq/L
Alkaline phosphatase	0–95 IU/L	N or >95 IU/L
WBC count	4,500–11,000 mm^3	N or >11,000 mm^3
Hematocrit	36–46%	<35%

[a]N = normal; lab value normals are the standard set by the Johns Hopkins Hospital Laboratories.

large amounts of solute have accumulated; if distal tubular function is slow to recover, a nephrogenic form of diabetes insipidus may develop. This phase may last for one to two weeks with a gradually decreasing diuresis as the concentrating mechanism becomes re-established and the accumulated solutes are excreted.

As in the oliguric phase, tendencies for bleeding and infection must be monitored closely. Some GI disturbances such as nausea may continue because it can take several days to lower the BUN and creatinine values. Drug metabolism and excretion will also remain abnormal early in this phase. Many of the psychological problems will continue until renal function is fully re-established.

New disturbances in the diuretic phase are related to fluid and electrolyte imbalances. The nurse's role in management of these problems is addressed in the care plan at the end of this section. A fluid deficit can occur as a result of the diuresis and sodium losses when tubular patency is gradually restored, especially if sodium and water restrictions remain and diuretic use continues.

Hypokalemia is also a problem in this phase, as there are renal losses of potassium. Levels can quickly fall below 3.5 mEq/L. This problem is increased if dietary potassium restrictions continue to be enforced and diuretics are in use. Hypomagnesemia may also be seen.

The diuretic phase heralds the beginning of the re-establishment of normal kidney function, but the patient remains in a precarious state, and close surveillance of fluid and electrolyte balances is required.

The primary causes of death in this phase are infection and GI bleeding.

The fourth and final phase in the clinical course of ARF is termed the recovery phase. Tubular function and the concentrating mechanism are restored. Urine output, BUN, creatinine, electrolyte, hematology, and acid-base results, and blood pressure readings return to normal in most patients. If the basement membrane of the nephron was damaged, nonfunctional scar tissue will fill the area. If a significant number of nephrons have had such damage, recovery may be incomplete. The majority of patients will have perfectly normal renal function, although special testing may identify subtle permanent tubular defects. This phase can take from 1 to 12 months for resolution. Generally, all restrictions imposed during the prior phases are lifted.

Nursing standards of care

The basis of nursing management of ARF patients is the identification and elimination of the cause. When ARF is established, the nurse focuses on minimizing the symptoms and preventing progression of the renal failure.

The oliguric phase The key to correcting fluid balance disturbances that affect the cardiovascular and respiratory systems is to maintain the patient at his or her dry (fluid-free) weight. Judicious administration of fluid is essential; the daily fluid intake should be restricted to 400–600 cc plus the previous day's output.[107] (This level of fluid intake is allowed because approximately 400–600 cc is lost insensibly each day.) In the intensive care setting, this is a difficult restriction to meet, and administration of diuretics, dialysis, or slow continuous ultrafiltration (SCUF) may be necessary to prevent fluid overload. (These modalities will be discussed in a later section of the chapter. See the nursing care plan for the management of hypertension in fluid overload.)

The treatment of hyperkalemia is of paramount importance, given the cardiotoxic potential of the potassium ion. Hyperkalemia is a particular problem with metabolic acidosis. In acidosis, potassium shifts out of the cells into the serum. Administering sodium bicarbonate ($NaHCO_3$) will temporarily shift potassium back into the cells. Note that the effect is only temporary (lasting 2–3 hours) and can result in sodium and water retention.[108]

An infusion of 50% dextrose and insulin is another temporary corrective measure. Insulin is capable of shifting potassium back into the cells, an effect that lasts 4–6 hours.[109] The dextrose is administered simultaneously to counter the potential hypoglycemic effect of the insulin.

When hyperkalemia is severe and arrhythmias are present, calcium chloride or calcium gluconate may be given intravenously to stabilize cell membranes from depolarization, thus decreasing the potential for arrhythmias in the hyperkalemic state. The protective effect lasts about a half-hour.[110] None of the above measures actually removes potassium from the body. To effect permanent potassium removal, other measures must be instituted.

Sodium polystyrene sulfonate (Kayexalate) with sorbitol is another treatment for hyperkalemia. It can be given orally or rectally and leads to the exchange of sodium for potassium in the gut. The bound potassium is then excreted in the bowel movement, which is stimulated by the sorbital. It can take several hours for the desired effect to occur. As with the use of sodium bicarbonate, sodium and water retention can occur, as 1 mEq of sodium is left behind for every potassium ion lost. When all of these measures fail or, if significant ECG changes are present, emergent hemodialysis is performed.

In treating pericarditis, pericardial effusion, and cardiac tamponade, removal of the uremic toxins and reversal of the inflammatory process is essential. Steroids and/or nonsteroidal antiinflammatory medications are often used in conjunction with dialysis to remove the uremic toxins. When the patient is hemodialyzed, the smallest possible dose of heparin is used, since heparin can cause blood to exude into the pericardial space. Failure of these conservative measures may necessitate the creation of a pericardial window or pericardial stripping to relieve the constriction of the heart by the fluid between the pericardial layers. Cardiac tamponade and circulatory collapse necessitate urgent intervention, including pericardiocentesis.

Neuromuscular and neurological disturbances occur in direct response to the level of uremia and the rapidity with which it has developed. It is essential to protect the confused or disoriented patient from injury. Frequent orientation to time, place, and person is important. The patient needs to be reassured that the changes in mental status are due to the underlying renal condition and are reversible. Dialysis is the primary method of treatment, but aggressive dialysis should be avoided, since rapid correction of uremia may actually aggravate the degree of neurological disturbance. This condition is known as dialysis disequilibrium syndrome, and it results from a rapid shift of fluid into the brain when aggressive dialysis produces rapid and marked reductions in serum osmolality below the blood-brain barrier. The high solute concentration in the brain compared to the rest of the body creates an osmotic gradient, and fluid shifts into the brain to decrease the solute concentration. The patient presents with signs of cerebral edema. This can occur during the dialysis treatment or many hours after. Prevention of this syndrome is key, and this is done by providing frequent short dialysis treatments to gradually lower the uremic toxin level.

The management of respiratory disturbances is dependent on preventing fluid overload and the development of infection. It is essential to protect the patient from infection and to treat infections that do occur aggressively. As noted earlier, infection is the primary cause of death in ARF. If antibiotics are ordered, careful attention must be given to the dose and dose interval.

The patient with acute renal failure should be carefully observed for hematologic disturbances and, in particular, signs and symptoms of bleeding. Stool, emesis, and urine should be assessed for the presence of blood. Whereas acute hemorrhage may not result in a decrease in hematocrit, hematocrit tests should be closely monitored to detect repeated or chronic loss of blood. Bleeding time is the best indicator of the likelihood of hemorrhage due to the bleeding diathesis of uremia. With patients with a long bleeding time, extra vigilance is required. A biochemical clue to internal bleeding is an inordinate elevation of serum urea nitrogen, which results from metabolic breakdown of the protein in blood. Detecting and eliminating any source of bleeding is essential. Symptomatic management of bleeding in uremia includes transfusions and dialysis. Transfusions replenish the RBC mass, and dialysis removes the BUN that accumulates. Treatments for the platelet defect of uremia include desmopressin acetate (DDAVP), cryoprecipitate, and estrogens.

Other hematologic disturbances include increased susceptibility to infection and anemia. Limiting invasive procedures and closely observing the patient for signs of infection (such as a temperature or elevated WBC) are vital. When the hematocrit falls and the patient begins to exhibit signs of decreased oxygenation (such as fatigue, shortness of breath, and/or chest pain), transfusions are indicated. If the patient is on dialysis, it is best to give transfusions during dialysis, as the potassium that is released as RBCs are lysed in passing through the IV needle is dialyzed off. Limiting phlebotomy procedures is also important. The nurse must also keep in mind that a small amount of blood is lost with each hemodialysis treatment. Exogenous erythropoietin is not of benefit in acute anemia; it will take 10–14 days for a response to be seen.

Gastrointestinal disturbances are common in acute renal failure. Their management is described in the nursing care plan. Antacids and H_2-receptor blocking agents are commonly used in an attempt to reduce gastric acidity and mucosal ulceration. It is important to note that if antacids are used, they should not contain magnesium (as do Maalox and Mylanta). Patients with acute renal failure cannot excrete magnesium and will develop hypermagnesemia. In addition, cimetidine, a commonly used histamine H_2-receptor antagonist, may accumulate if the dosage is not reduced and can cause cardiac and neurologic depression or platelet activity.

Management of integument disturbances is detailed in the nursing care plan. The biochemical disturbances of acute renal failure require a variety of treatments. The most important biochemical disturbance encountered in acute renal failure is hyperkalemia (discussed earlier). In managing calcium-phosphate imbalances, the primary goal is to lower the serum phosphate level. This is usually done with aluminum-containing antacids (for example, Amphogel or Alternagel), which act as phosphate binders in the gastrointestinal tract. These are most effective if given with meals, as they act to bind phosphate contained in food. The bound phosphate is excreted in the stools. These antacids can cause constipation. In alleviating the constipation, it is necessary to avoid magnesium-containing laxatives such as milk of magnesia and magnesium citrate. Fleet enemas should also be avoided, as they have a significant phosphate content. Reduction of the serum phosphate level should result in an increase in the serum

calcium level. If serum calcium fails to return to normal, the nurse should be cautious about administering exogenous calcium in view of the potential for precipitating metastatic calcifications.

Metabolic acidosis can be treated with sodium bicarbonate infusion, but the infusion of sodium in a person with acute renal failure may result in rapid volume expansion or pulmonary edema. Dialysis is the definitive treatment for metabolic acidosis, as the dialysate contains a buffer. If the metabolic acidosis is mild, more conservative measures may be taken, such as the administration of oral alkalizing agents, for example, sodium citrate with citric acid (Bicitra, Shohl's solution). These agents act to neutralize accumulated body acids. When correcting for metabolic acidosis, it is essential to observe for the development of hypocalcemic tetany, which can occur if the correction is too rapid.

Prevention is the key with regard to hyponatremia and hypermagnesemia. To prevent hyponatremia, free-water intake must be restricted. If severe hyponatremia (serum sodium less than 120 mEq/L) occurs, hypertonic saline infusions or dialysis may be required to prevent the development of cerebral edema. Avoidance of magnesium-containing preparations is the defense against hypermagnesemia. These include magnesium-containing antacids and laxatives.

Nutritional management centers on providing adequate nutrition to prevent catabolism and negative nitrogen balance and restricting the intake of electrolytes, protein, and water that the impaired kidneys are unable to excrete. Specific details of this management are contained in the nursing care plan.

Acute renal failure interferes with the metabolism and excretion of many drugs. The importance of carefully monitoring drug administration to ARF patients cannot be overemphasized. Every oliguric patient's drug regimen must be reviewed. Toxic levels of certain antibiotics can further damage the kidney. Metabolites of meperidine, which is metabolized by the liver, must be excreted by the kidneys. If meperidine is given to the patient in ARF, the metabolites can accumulate, leading to an increased and prolonged drug effect and seizure activity. It is important to consider the decreased excretory capacity of the kidneys when administering any drug to a patient in the oliguric phase.

As with any acute illness, there are multiple psychological disturbances. These disturbances and the recommended management are described in the nursing care plan.

The diuretic phase   Care of hematologic, gastrointestinal, drug metabolism, and psychological disturbances should continue as described above for patients in the oliguric phase. Acid-base and calcium-phosphate imbalances should gradually be resolving, and as they do, certain medications such as oral alkalizing agents and phosphate binders may need to be withdrawn. Fluid and electrolyte disturbances require continued vigilant surveillance in the diuretic phase.

The patient should be assessed for hypovolemia, which can occur as a result of the diuresis. Fluid and sodium restrictions may be eliminated, and oral or IV fluid replacement may be needed to keep up with urinary losses until the diuresis is complete.

Along with hypovolemia, there can be hyponatremia (which enhances fluid loss), hypokalemia, and hypomagnesemia. The patient must be assessed for signs and symptoms of these electrolyte losses. Exogenous supplements may be required. With hypokalemia, it is important to rule out alkalosis as a cause, since alkalosis prompts the loss of potassium ions in exchange for hydrogen ions.

The recovery phase The patient in this phase is usually nearly ready for discharge or is at home. It is important to educate the patient about symptoms that should be reported (such as decreased urine output) and any dietary or fluid restrictions that are to continue after discharge. Finally, follow-up is vital, to ensure that complete or partial function is restored and maintained.

Renal Replacement Therapies

When conservative measures (medications, diet, and fluid restrictions) fail to bring about the desired reversal of fluid and uremic complications, renal replacement therapies (RRT) may be ordered. Such therapies are either intermittent (hemodialysis and peritoneal dialysis) or continuous (slow continuous ultrafiltration, continuous arteriovenous hemofiltration, and continuous arteriovenous hemodialysis). Table 5-31 lists the indications for these modalities. Their basic principles, complications, and nursing management are described below.

Intermittent Renal Replacement Therapies

Hemodialysis Dialysis is a process whereby undesirable solutes (such as urea, creatinine, potassium, and phosphate) and body water are removed via differential diffusion and ultrafiltration, respectively, across a semipermeable membrane. In hemodialysis (HD), blood from the patient passes through channels separated from a special fluid (the dialysate) by a semipermeable membrane. The pores in the membrane are large enough to allow urea, creatinine, and electrolytes to move into the dialysate from the blood (see Figure 5-18). Solute removal occurs via diffusion (molecules move from an area of higher concentration to an area of lower concentration). Because the dialysate contains no urea, creatinine, or phosphate and only a small amount of potassium, these solutes shift readily from the blood into the dialysate down a chemical gradient.

Fluid removal, or ultrafiltration, takes place in response to hydrostatic and osmotic forces. Water is moved through the pores of the semipermeable membrane into the dialysate just by the force of the patient's blood pressure and of the blood pump on the dialysis machine. This pressure can be increased

Table 5-31 Indications for Renal Replacement Therapies

Type of Therapy	Indications
Dialysis	BUN > 60–100 mg/dL Creatinine ≥ 6–10 mg/dL Potassium ≥ 6 mEq/L with ECG changes CO_2 ≤ 15 mEq/L Volume overload: pulmonary edema, congestive heart failure, pericardial effusion, cardiac tamponade Change in mental status not attributable to other causes
Continuous renal replacement therapies:	
SCUF	Volume overload in hemodynamically unstable patients or patients refractory to diuretics (such as patients recovering from myocardial infarction, cardiac surgery, or abdominal aortic aneurysm repair) Oliguric patients requiring large volumes of IV fluids for hyperalimentation or drugs
CAVH/CAVHD	Waste product, acid, electrolyte, and fluid removal in patients who are mildly to moderately catabolic and hemodynamically unstable

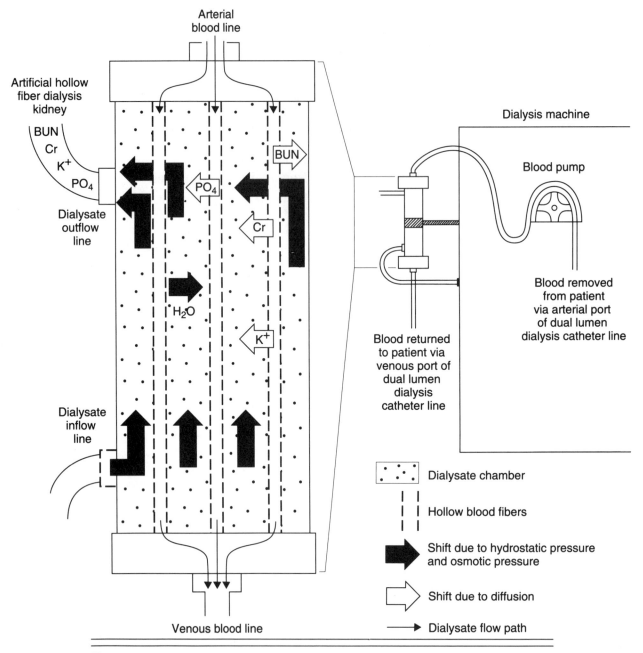

Figure 5-18   Hemodialysis

by creating a vacuum in the dialysate compartment to literally pull body fluid through the pores. The combination of the blood and dialysate pressures is called hydrostatic pressure. Additional fluid removal can be achieved through osmosis (fluids move from an area of low solute concentration to an area of high solute concentration). Glucose is added to the dialysate to achieve this shift. Hydrostatic forces account for most of the ultrafiltration that occurs in HD.

Hemodialysis is the fastest, most efficient means of solute and water removal. It is the treatment of choice when emergent dialysis is needed, as long as the patient is hemodynamically stable.

Hemodialysis requires access to the patient's vascular system. Usually a temporary subclavian, internal jugular, or femoral venous dual-lumen catheter is placed at the bedside. One lumen takes the patient's blood to the HD machine, and the second lumen allows its return. Catheters should be observed for integrity and bleeding after treatments, as they are heparinized. A patient with a femoral line should be on bedrest to prevent any trauma to the femoral vein.

Occasionally a patient may have a surgically placed intravenous access for dialysis, such as an arteriovenous (AV) native fistula, graft, or shunt (see

Table 5-32 and Figure 5-19). It is essential that procedures such as intravenous line placement, blood drawing, or blood pressure *not* be done on a limb with a surgically placed access. Any of these procedures can impair blood flow, which could result in clotting of the access. It is important to note that an AV shunt can be used immediately. In CRF patients who require HD, native and graft fistulas are used to gain access to the circulatory system. Table 5-32 provides descriptions of these devices.

Hemodialysis is performed by a specially trained nurse or technician. An average treatment lasts 2–4 hours. Treatments are usually done every other day, but the frequency depends on the patient's condition. Before beginning the treatment, the intensive care nurse should perform a complete assessment including vital signs, weight, and pulmonary and cardiac auscultation. Certain medications should not be given just prior to dialysis because of their dialyzability. Some common dialyzable and nondialyzable medications are listed in Table 5-33.

Fluid removal during dialysis is based on daily weight, making accuracy critical. During dialysis, the patient should be assessed for headache, nausea, vomiting, chest pain, and restlessness, all of which could indicate hypotension. Hypotension is a potential problem during dialysis because approximately 250 cc of blood is removed from the patient's circulation during the treatment. Cramping due to fluid removal and seizures due to rapid osmolar shifts can also occur. As was mentioned earlier, rapid osmolar shifts result in a syndrome called dialysis disequilibrium. The patient will show signs and symptoms of cerebral edema, including headache, nausea, and confusion, which can progress to seizures, lethargy, and coma. Treatment is directed toward re-establishment of normal osmolality. The patient should also be assessed for bleeding, as heparin is used to keep the blood from clotting when it comes in contact with the foreign surfaces of the tubes and artificial kidney. When the treatment is completed, the patient's previously assessed parameters should be reviewed,

Table 5-32 Types of Vascular Access for Hemodialysis

Type	Description	Nursing Care	Complications
Arteriovenous shunt	Silastic catheter which has two teflon tips. Tips are surgically placed into an artery and a vein. Silastic portion of catheter is brought to outside of body via puncture wounds. Can be placed in legs or arms. Used in acute or chronic HD. Can be used immediately.	Dressing care each day Palpate for thrill (vibration due to rapid blood flow) and auscultate for bruit over venous portion of shunt every 8 hours. If absent, clotting has occurred. Assess for clotting (separation of serum and whole blood in tubing). No procedures on shunt arm (i.e., blood drawing, IVs, or blood pressures).	Infection Clotting Bleeding secondary to dislodgement
Arteriovenous native fistula	Surgical anastomosis of an artery and vein. Completely internal. Vessel accessed using large bore needles. Used in chronic HD. Takes 4–6 weeks to heal.	Palpate for thrill and auscultate for bruit every 8 hours. No procedures on native fistula extremity.	Infection Clotting
Arteriovenous graft fistula	Surgical placement of artificial graft between an artery and vein. Completely internal. Graft accessed using large bore needles. Use for patients with fragile or limited blood vessels. Used in chronic HD. Takes 2–4 weeks to heal.	Palpate for thrill and auscultate for bruit every 8 hours. No procedures on graft extremity.	Infection Clotting

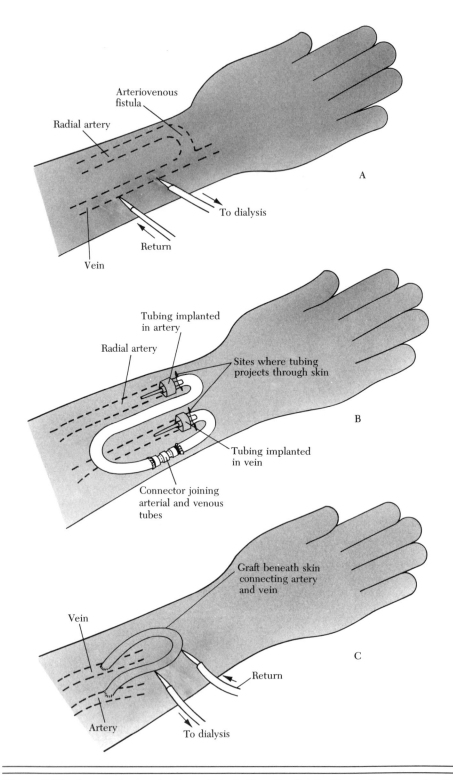

Figure 5-19   Access Devices for Hemodialysis (A, native fistula; B, arteriovenous shunt; C, graft fistula)

Table 5-33 Nondialyzable and Dialyzable Medications (partial listing)

Nondialyzable Medications	Dialyzable Medications
Prazosin	Cimetidine
Furosemide	Multivitamins
Insulin	Aspirin
Haloperidol	Phenobarbitol
Digoxin	Aztreonam
Amphotericin B	Cefoxitin
Phenytoin	Gentamicin
Morphine sulfate	Flucytosine
Propranolol	Neomycin
Clonidine	Tobramycin
Nifedipine	Ticarcillin
Nitroglycerin	Nitroprusside

with careful attention to the blood pressure and fluid status changes.

Peritoneal dialysis If a patient requires dialysis but is hemodynamically unstable and/or has limited cardiac function, peritoneal dialysis (PD) may be considered. It is a slower process, requiring about 24 hours to achieve the result that HD can obtain in 2–4 hours. In PD, the peritoneal membrane acts as the semipermeable membrane. A PD catheter is placed at the bedside or in the operating room to gain access to the peritoneal cavity (see Figure 5-20). Dialysate can be instilled manually or by using a computerized machine (cycling machine).

The PD catheter is used to infuse dialysate into the peritoneal cavity. The fluid dwells in the cavity from 20 minutes to 5 hours, depending on the patient's fluid and electrolyte balance. As with HD, solutes are removed via diffusion. BUN, creatinine, phosphate, and potassium shift from the blood vessels in the peritoneum into the dialysate. Fluid removal is achieved by adding dextrose to the dialysate, which creates an osmotic gradient. The dialysate can contain 1.5%, 2.5%, or 4.25% dextrose. The higher the concentration of dextrose, the greater the fluid removal rate. At the end of the prescribed dwell time, the dialysate, excess body water, and solutes are drained out. A full cycle of PD (fill, dwell, and drain) is termed an exchange. In patients with acute renal failure who undergo PD, an exchange is usually done every hour for 24–48 hours.

As with HD, a preassessment is done before initiating PD treatment. During the treatment, the nurse must assess the volume drained at the end of each exchange. Normally the drained volume should be equal to the volume instilled. If it is less, the catheter may not be draining properly, a higher concentration of glucose may be needed for fluid removal, or the patient may be dehydrated. If dehydration is ruled out, attempts should be made to reposition the patient to enhance outflow. The drained dialysate should be clear yellow in color and slightly frothy (a result of the protein content). Cloudy fluid indicates peritonitis. Brown fluid occurs with bowel perforation. Blood-tinged fluid is not unusual after a new catheter is placed, but the fluid should clear after four or five exchanges unless active bleeding is taking place.

The dressing over the catheter site should be assessed for clear drainage. If the dressing requires frequent changes due to saturation, dialysate is leaking from around the catheter. Decreasing the volume of dialysate may be necessary. A normal fill volume is 1–2 L. Smaller volumes (less than 1.5 L) are used with new catheters to prevent initial leaks. Protein losses and hyperglycemia should also be monitored. Protein loss in PD can be significant, as the peritoneum is very porous to protein. Hyperglycemia can occur if glucose is absorbed from the dialysate during the dwell time. This is particularly a problem if the dwell time lasts several hours.

Peritoneal dialysis is the method of choice for use with the very elderly, the very young, with patients with advanced cardiac disease, and if gradual changes in blood chemistries and fluid status are desirable. It should not be used to treat severely catabolic patients or patients with life-threatening arrhythmias due to hyperkalemia. It is also contraindicated in patients with peritonitis, recent bowel surgery, or respiratory insufficiency, as the fluid in the peritoneum decreases the lung volume.

Continuous Renal Replacement Therapies

A newer group of treatment options for the fluid and blood chemistry abnormalities associated with ARF are the continuous renal replacement therapies (CRRT), including slow continuous ultrafiltration, continuous arteriovenous hemofiltration, and continuous arteriovenous hemodialysis. For these modalities, an arterial and a venous line (7–8 French) are required. The femoral artery and vein are the safest placement sites, but occasionally an arteriovenous shunt is used. A small, highly porous hemofilter is attached between the arterial and venous lines. The hemofilter requires minimal blood volume (approximately 30–80 mL) to prime it compared to an HD

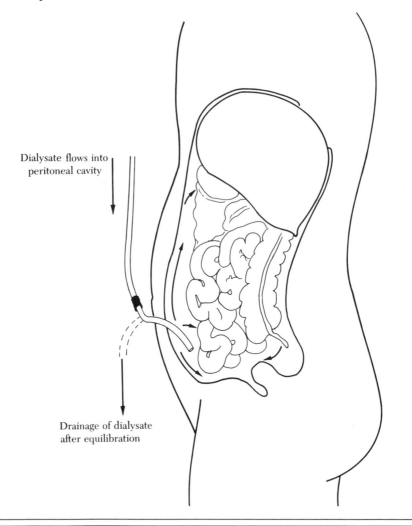

Dialysate flows into
peritoneal cavity

Drainage of dialysate
after equilibration

Figure 5-20 Peritoneal Dialysis Catheter

filter, which requires a much larger volume (approximately 250 mL); the hemofilter thus causes less hemodynamic instability. Blood is circulated through the filter solely by the patient's arterial pressure. A mean arterial pressure of 80 mm Hg is all that is required to achieve adequate flow.[111] Heparin is usually required to prevent clotting as the blood contacts the foreign surfaces of the tubing and hemofilter. Continuous renal replacement therapies can be done continuously for hours, days, or weeks. A benefit of these therapies is that a blood pump and dialysis machine are not needed to propel and monitor the blood flow. Eliminating the blood pump eliminates the need for a dialysis nurse or technician.

Slow continuous ultrafiltration (SCUF) In SCUF, the force of the blood pressure pushes body fluid through the pores of the hollow fibers of the hemofilter. This fluid then drains into a bag (see Figure 5-21). Approximately 100–300 cc can be removed hourly. BUN, creatinine, and other dissolved solutes

are moved through the pores along with the body water. This process is called convection. The primary purpose of SCUF is fluid removal. Changes in the patient's solute concentration due to convection are minimal.

Continuous arteriovenous hemofiltration (CAVH) With CAVH, larger volumes of fluid are removed (600–900 cc). A portion of this fluid (500–800 cc) is then replaced. With this method, 100–300 cc of fluid can be removed hourly. The composition of the replacement fluid is based on the patient's electrolyte needs; this fluid is given not only to replace some of the fluid removed but also to dilute the remaining toxins in the blood plasma and provide needed electrolytes. CAVH therapy removes fluid via hydrostatic pressure and waste products and electrolytes by convection (see Figure 5-22).

Continuous arteriovenous hemodialysis (CAVHD) Continuous arteriovenous hemodialysis (CAVHD) is a process that combines dialysis and CAVH. Dialy-

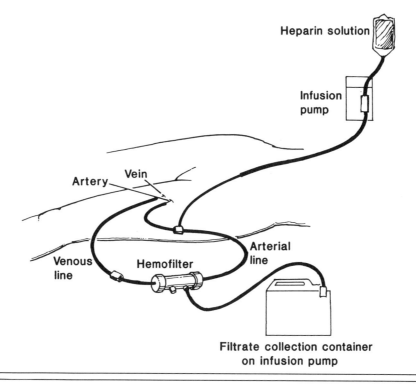

Heparin solution

Infusion pump

Vein

Artery

Arterial line

Venous line

Hemofilter

Filtrate collection container on infusion pump

Figure 5-21   Slow Continuous Ultrafiltration (SCUF)

sate is run through the hemofilter counter to the blood flow. The dialysate bathes the hollow fibers of the filter and causes a shift of BUN, creatinine, potassium, and phosphate via diffusion, and a shift of water via osmosis (in response to a gradient created by glucose). It is the same process as HD, but it operates at a much slower blood flow rate (see Figure 5-23).

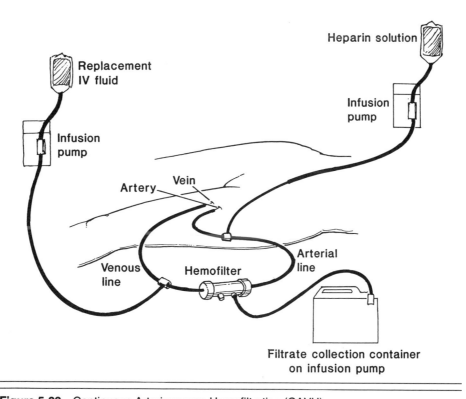

Heparin solution

Replacement IV fluid

Infusion pump

Infusion pump

Artery   Vein

Arterial line

Venous line

Hemofilter

Filtrate collection container on infusion pump

Figure 5-22   Continuous Arteriovenous Hemofiltration (CAVH)

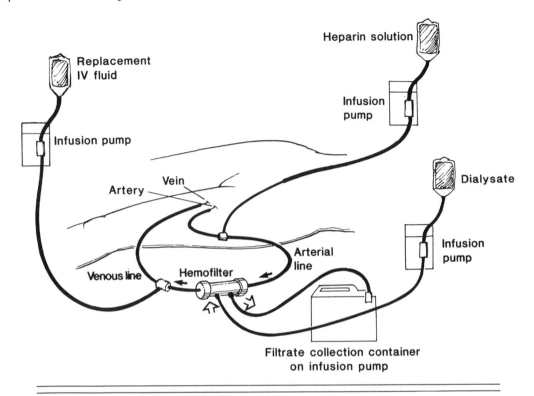

Figure 5-23 Continuous Arteriovenous Hemodialysis (CAVHD)

Prior to initiating any of these therapies, the nurse should conduct a patient assessment similar to that preceding HD. Once the treatment is initiated, heparin infusion, coagulation, and signs of bleeding must be monitored. Regardless of the modality used, the process is safest if net hourly fluid loss does not exceed 300 cc. The extremities where the lines are placed must be assessed every 4 hours for neurovascular changes. Any changes may necessitate removal of the catheter. The hemofilter must be assessed for clotting, which is indicated by decreased hourly fluid removal, streaking of the hemofilter fibers, cold blood tubings, or separation of serum from whole blood in the blood lines. If clotting occurs, all replacement fluid and dialysate infusions should be stopped immediately to prevent fluid overload.

Continuous renal replacement therapies provide a means to remove large quantities of fluid and correct electrolyte and blood chemistry abnormalities via convection and/or diffusion in hemodynamically unstable patients. These therapies should not be used with patients who are severely catabolic or acidotic, because of the gradual nature of the changes they effect.

Continuous Venovenous Therapies (CVVT) A new type of continuous therapy called continuous venovenous therapy (CVVT) is now available. Based on the arteriovenous therapies, CVVT involves placing a single dual-lumen dialysis catheter in a large vein. The hemofilter circuit is placed between the two lumens of the venous catheter. Because there is

no arterial pressure to pump blood through the hemofilter circuit, a small simplified dialysis machine must be used. The machine is equipped with a blood pump, an air detector, and other simple alarm features. Rather than having a dialysis nurse or technician at the bedside, intensive care nurses are taught how to monitor the pump. CVVT provides results similar to the arteriovenous therapies, but avoids the risks associated with the placement of a large arterial catheter. In CVVT, continuous venovenous ultrafiltration (CVVU) is equivalent to SCUF, continuous venovenous hemofiltration (CVVH) to CAVH, and continuous venovenous hemodialysis (CVVHD) to CAVHD.

Acute renal failure is a condition that affects virtually every system in the body. Its etiologies are multiple. Patients in the intensive care setting are exposed to numerous factors that can predispose them to the development of ARF. The intensive care nurse's first responsibility is to prevent ARF by being aware of which patients are at high risk and of the events that can lead to ARF. If renal failure develops despite these efforts, then symptomatic treatment is essential to reduce the severity of the homeostatic disturbance until such time as kidney function is recovered. Above all the nurse must remember that the mortality rate with ARF is 50%.

The following nursing care plan summarizes critical care practices for the management of acute renal failure.

Nursing Care Plan for the Management of the Patient with Acute Renal Failure (Oliguric Phase)

Diagnosis	Signs and symptoms	Intervention	Rationale
Fluid volume excess	Peripheral edema CHF Crackles on lung auscultation Elevated CVP Jugular venous distention S3 gallop Tachycardia Hypertension Weight gain I > 0	Assess weight daily	To reveal total body water
		I & O at least every 2–4 hours	Best assessment of total body water
		Frequent assessment of VS (every 2–4 hours)	To identify tachycardia, hypertension, which indicate CHF
		Fluid restriction (400–600 cc plus previous 24-hour output)	To prevent overload
		Sodium restriction (2 gm)	To reduce fluid retention
		Administer prescribed diuretics	To enhance volume removal
		Dialysis or slow continuous ultrafiltration (SCUF) as needed	Corrective therapy for fluid volume excess (close observation identifies electrolyte disturbances, intolerance of fluid removal with hypotension, and dialysis disequilibrium)
		Assess heart sounds for heart failure every 4–8 hours	To identify early heart failure or pericardial friction rub
		Assess breath sounds every 4–8 hours	To identify pulmonary edema
		Assess CVP at least every 8 hours	To indicate how heart is handling fluid volume excess
Decreased cardiac output related to hypertension	Elevated systolic and diastolic readings High systemic vascular resistance (if Swan-Ganz catheter is inserted) Fullness in head, dizziness, or headache	Sodium and fluid restrictions	To decrease circulating blood volume, which may contribute to hypertension
		Administer antihypertensives as prescribed	Drugs commonly used to reduce hypertension include beta blockers, vasodilators, and angiotensin-converting enzyme inhibitors
		Administer nitrates or vasodilating agents as prescribed	

Nursing Care Plan for the Management of the Patient with Acute Renal Failure (Oliguric Phase)

Diagnosis	Signs and symptoms	Intervention	Rationale
		Dialysis if hypertension is severe and uncontrolled	Assists in correcting severe and life-threatening hypertension
		Neurologic evaluation at least every shift for potential neurologic complications of hypertension	Reduces risk of complications of increased intracranial pressure (stroke, bleeding)
		Symptomatic treatment for headaches or other symptoms	Pain relief may help decrease BP
		Rest and quiet	To reduce workload on heart, oxygen consumption, and possibly BP; rest reduces sympathetic stimulation and may assist in maintaining BP
Decreased cardiac output related to pericarditis, pericardial effusion, or tamponade	Chest discomfort Fever In tamponade: Pericardial friction rub Tachypnea Cyanosis Muffled heart sounds Narrow pulse pressure Absent or diminished point of maximal impulse Absent peripheral pulses Increased JVP Pulsus paradox Equilibration of heart pressures: CVP = PAP = PCWP	Dialysis	Removes toxins that cause effusions
		Limit heparin use	Heparin can cause blood to exude into pericardial space, which can increase effusion
		Administer steroids or nonsteroidal antiinflammatory drugs as ordered	To reduce inflammation and discomfort
		Monitor heart sounds and vital signs at least every 4 hours; print out pulsus paradox on arterial line and report if greater than 10 mm Hg; assess lung sounds, JVP, CVP, PAP, and PMI at least every 4–8 hours	To evaluate symptoms of developing tamponade

Diagnosis	Signs and symptoms	Intervention	Rationale
		Compare peripheral and central pulses for difference at least each shift	Indicative of tamponade
		Review chest x-ray to evaluate cardiac silhouette	An ongoing comparison allows early detection of any cardiac enlargement
		Prepare fluid challenge if tamponade is suspected	First treatment is expansion of vascular volume
		Keep pericardial tap tray available for emergency use	Emergency pericardiocentesis may be necessary
		Monitor for developing cardiac effusion to determine patient's candidacy for pericardial catheter with or without sclerosing or pericardial window	Planned intervention for developing effusion is preferable
Alteration in electrolyte balance related to hyperkalemia	Potassium > 6 mEq/L ECG changes: peaked T waves, prolonged QRS, prolonged P-R, depressed ST segment, and absent or flattened P wave Bradycardia Asystole Muscle weakness Flaccid paralysis Diarrhea Hyperactive bowel sounds	Restrict potassium from oral and parenteral sources (40–60 mEq/day)	To reduce exogenous potassium
		Monitor for ECG changes	Allows early detection of common and life-threatening arrhythmias with hyperkalemia
		Assess patient for extrarenal sources of hyperkalemia (GI bleeding, blood transfusions, muscle or tissue breakdown)	Permits staff to eliminate contributing problems
		Administer prescribed drugs: Sodium bicarbonate: 1–2 ampules (44–88 mEq); observe for sodium and fluid overload with administration	To shift potassium ions into cells

Nursing Care Plan for the Management of the Patient with Acute Renal Failure (Oliguric Phase)

Diagnosis	Signs and symptoms	Intervention	Rationale
		Dextrose 50% and insulin: 50 mL dextrose 50% with 5–10 units regular insulin	Insulin shifts potassium ions into cells; dextrose prevents hypoglycemia
		Sodium polystyrene sulfonate (Kayexalate) with sorbitol: 15–60 g Kayexalate can be given orally, via NGT, or via enema	Kayexalate is an exchange resin which exchanges K^+ for Na^+ in the gut; K^+ is then excreted in bowel movements
		Calcium gluconate (10%): 10–30 mL over at least 5 minutes; monitor ECG, as arrhythmias can occur	Increases threshold for arrhythmias
Alterations in sensory-perceptual activities and alterations in thought processes related to neurological disturbances	Elevated BUN (60–100 mg/dL) Irritability Changes in mental status Confusion Seizure activity Tremors Abnormal muscle movements	Assess patient's mental status and level of consciousness	Provides early evidence of neurological compromise
		Orient patient	Reduces risk of injury
		Provide safety measures	Protects patient from injury in the event of seizure or falls resulting from altered mental state
		Dialysis	Removes wastes and toxins that may contribute to altered mental states
		Reassure patient when anxious	To allay patient's anxiety
		Give information repeatedly	To allay patient's anxiety, increase patient's adherence to care regimen, and compensate for patient's impaired memory

Diagnosis	Signs and symptoms	Intervention	Rationale
Impaired gas exchange related to respiratory disturbances due to pulmonary edema	Rales Rhonchi Dyspnea	Assess daily weights, vital signs, and I&O	Allows for assessment of fluid status
		Fluid restriction (400–600 cc in addition to previous 24-hour output)	Reduces risk of fluid overload
		Sodium restriction	Reduces risk of fluid retention
		Administer prescribed diuretics	Assist in fluid removal
		Dialysis or slow continuous ultrafiltration (SCUF)	To help in fluid removal
		Auscultate breath sounds; monitor pulse oximetry and ABGs PRN	To allow for early diagnosis and treatment of respiratory distress
		Evaluate PAP and PCWP at least every 4 hours	To allow for early detection and treatment of heart failure
Ineffective breathing pattern related to pleural effusion	Pleural friction rub Dyspnea Tachypnea Abnormal ABGs (decreased O_2, increased CO_2) Elevated WBC Elevated temperature Tenacious sputum, productive cough	Maintain sodium and fluid restrictions	Minimizes fluid overload, which exacerbates respiratory distress
		Treat cardiac disorders (congestive failure), as ordered	Congestive failure exacerbates respiratory distress
		Auscultate breath sounds; monitor pulse oximetry and ABGs PRN	Provides information on patient's respiratory status and allows for timely intervention
		Administer oxygen as ordered	To increase oxygenation to tissues and to treat symptoms of respiratory distress
		Assist with pleural tap PRN	To improve breathing capacity
		Encourage coughing and deep breathing	Enhance ventilation
		Elevate head of bed	To provide for symptomatic relief
		Administer antibiotics and/or diuretics as ordered	To treat and/or prevent infectious complications and volume overload, which increase work of breathing

Nursing Care Plan for the Management of the Patient with Acute Renal Failure (Oliguric Phase)

Diagnosis	Signs and symptoms	Intervention	Rationale
Alteration in tissue perfusion and fluid volume deficit, related to bleeding tendency due to hematological disturbances	Elevated BUN Oral or GI bleeding Occult blood in stool Decreased hematocrit	Perform hematology and coagulation studies; assess patient for signs of bleeding	To allow for early detection and treatment of bleeding
	Abnormal coagulation tests (PT, PTT, fibrinogen)	Limit activity if Hct is extremely low (<20–25%)	To minimize hypoxia
		Transfuse patient as ordered (preferably when patient is on dialysis)	Provides immediate increase in Hct; dialysis during transfusion allows for the removal of K^+ released from damaged RBCs
		Minimize invasive procedures (IM, SQ injections, ABG or blood drawing)	Reduce risk of bleeding
		Administer local and systemic agents to enhance clotting	Uremic toxins cause platelet dysfunction
Potential for infection	Elevated WBC Elevated temperature Symptoms of infection	Assess temperature each shift	To detect early symptoms of infection
		Assess patient during each shift for signs of local or systemic infection	
		Limit invasive procedures	To decrease risk of infection
		Strict use of aseptic technique	To minimize patient's exposure to infectious agents
Alteration in tissue perfusion, related to anemia	Decreased Hct (<35%) Pallor Fatigue Dyspnea Chest pain	Administer oxygen as ordered	To facilitate oxygenation of tissues
		Limit activity if Hct is extremely low	To minimize hypoxia, which could lead to injury from fainting, etc., and to protect patient from complications of cardiac ischemia

Diagnosis	Signs and symptoms	Intervention	Rationale
		Administer transfusion as ordered; in chronic patients, administer erythropoietin	To improve oxygen-carrying capacity of blood
Alteration in oral and GI mucosa, related to uremia	Oral bleeding and ulcerations Stomatitis GI bleeding and ulcers Xerostomia	Oral assessment every 4–8 hours	To detect abnormalities requiring intervention
		Provide for oral hygiene (avoid alcohol products)	To protect patient from bleeding and ulcerations and resultant complications
		Rinse mouth with mouthwash or saline	Soothes mucous membranes
		Assess stool and emesis for occult blood	To allow early detection of bleeding due to GI ulcers
		Dialysis	To remove uremic toxins that cause GI irritation
Potential for alteration in nutrition related to GI disturbances	Ammonia odor on breath Metallic taste in mouth Loss of appetite Nausea and vomiting	Administer vitamins as prescribed; provide small frequent meals and divide fluid restriction over 24 hours	To improve nutritional intake and fluid balance and prevent GI disturbances when eating
		Administer antiemetic, antacid, and H_2-antagonist as ordered	To decrease nausea and GI irritation due to secretion of gastric acid and uremic toxins
		Dialysis to remove uremic toxins	To prevent GI complications that stem from uremic toxins
Alterations in skin integrity related to integument disturbances	Pallor Dry, itchy skin Ecchymosis Excoriation/infection Uremic frost Edema	Meticulous skin care with superfatted soaps, bath oils, and lotion	To decrease skin lesions or breakdown
		Frequent repositioning of patient	To improve circulation and prevent pressure spots
		Use of low airflow bed if skin is in poor condition	To prevent pressure spots

Nursing Care Plan for the Management of the Patient with Acute Renal Failure (Oliguric Phase)

Diagnosis	Signs and symptoms	Intervention	Rationale
		Protection from injury	Skin of ARF patient is more likely to be injured and risk of infection is greater if skin integrity is compromised
		Administration of antihistamine	To relieve pruritis
Alteration in electrolyte balance related to hyperphosphatemia or hypocalcemia	Calcium < 8.0 mg/dL Phosphate > 5 mg/dL Product of calcium and phosphate > 70 Increased parathormone (PTH) Increased alkaline phosphatase Bone demineralization Metastatic calcifications Bone pain	Restrict organ meats and green vegetables	Phosphate present in these foods
		Administer Amphogel/Alternagel	Aluminum-based antacids bind phosphate in the gut
		Administer activated vitamin D if phosphate < 5	Facilitates Ca absorption from gut; if PO_4 > 5 do not give vitamin D, as $CaPO_4$ deposits can occur
		Assess patient for constipation and administer non-magnesium stool softeners PRN	Phosphate binders may cause constipation The kidney is the primary excretory organ for Mg; products containing Mg can lead to hypermagnesemia
		Assess patient for bone pain and administer analgesics as ordered	Calcium-phosphate deposits may be very painful
		Dialysis	To remove phosphate
		Assess patient for leg cramps and tetany	Signs of hypocalcemia
		Monitor ECG	To assess for cardiac rhythm changes resulting from hypocalcemia
Alteration in regulation related to metabolic acidosis	pH < 7.35 Venous carbon dioxide ≤20 mEq/L Tachypnea Lethargy Stupor Coma	Administer oral alkalyzing agents as ordered	Correct acidosis
		If serum CO_2 < 15 mEq/L, administer sodium bicarbonate cautiously	Corrects acidosis but can cause retention of sodium and water

Diagnosis	Signs and symptoms	Intervention	Rationale
		Observe for hyperkalemia	Hydrogen ion loss can result in retention of potassium ions to maintain ionic balance
		Dialysis	Dialysate contains buffers that neutralize acids in blood
		Observe for hypocalcemic tetany	May occur if acidosis is corrected too quickly
		Monitor ABGs or venous pH as directed	To allow for early detection of problems and evaluation of treatment
Alteration in electrolyte balance related to hyponatremia	Sodium < 125 mEq/L Nausea Malaise Headache Lethargy Altered mental state Seizures Coma	Fluid restriction	To restore sodium level without causing fluid overload
		Hypertonic saline solutions if patient is symptomatic or if sodium level is below 115 mEq/L	To replace sodium and to prevent further complications
		Dialysis	To remove excess fluid so sodium concentration will increase
		Safety precautions	Seizures may occur with severe hyponatremia
Alteration in electrolyte balance related to hypermagnesemia	Magnesium > 2.0 mEq/L Decreased reflexes Muscle weakness Drowsiness Heart block	Avoid all magnesium-containing preparations	To decrease risk of hypermagnesemia
		If hypermagnesemia is severe, administer calcium chloride as ordered	To oppose the effects of magnesium on cardiac muscle
		Administer diuretics as ordered	To enhance magnesium excretion
Potential for nutritional intake less than body requirements due to catabolism, nausea, vomiting, anorexia, stomatitis, or malabsorption	Elevated BUN Hypoalbuminemia Weight loss Negative nitrogen balance	Administer vitamins as prescribed	To protect patient from vitamin deficiency
		Maintain daily dietary restrictions regardless of oral or parenteral intake: protein (40–60 g), potassium (40–60 mEq), sodium (2 g), and phosphate (500–1000 mg)	Partially or completely damaged kidneys cannot excrete adequate amounts of waste products and excess electrolytes

Nursing Care Plan for the Management of the Patient with Acute Renal Failure (Oliguric Phase)

Diagnosis	Signs and symptoms	Intervention	Rationale
		Dialysis	To remove BUN, creatinine, potassium, sodium, phosphate, and fluids
		Assess weight and general nutritional status daily; if parenteral nutrition is used, be sure renal restrictions of fluid and electrolytes are followed	For adequate nutritional support without causing further complications related to renal compromise
		Antiemetics PRN as ordered	To relieve nausea, vomiting and improve oral intake
Alteration in regulation related to drug metabolism disturbances	Elevated serum levels of drugs and/or metabolites that are normally excreted Prolonged effects of sedatives and paralytics Signs and symptoms of drug toxicities	Monitor antibiotic administration, especially aminoglycosides, cephalosporins, antifungals; measure therapeutic levels as indicated	To minimize additional renal injury from nephrotoxins; to prevent toxic accumulation of drugs that depend on renal excretion
		Decrease dose, increase dosage interval, or eliminate known nephrotoxins	To prevent toxic effects of these drugs
		Monitor antibiotic levels closely	To avoid overdoses
		Avoid the use of meperidine; cautiously administer drugs that depend on renal excretion or nondialyzable substances (e.g., phenothiazines)	Meperidine metabolites are dependent on renal excretion; accumulated metabolites can cause an increased drug effect and lead to seizure activity

Diagnosis	Signs and symptoms	Intervention	Rationale
		Monitor for side effects and toxicities of medications	Medication accumulation enhances toxicities
Potential for anxiety and fear related to ICU admission, physical prognosis, etc.	Anxiety Grief Depression Fear of death Refusal of care Crying	Explain the acute nature of the illness to the patient and family	To facilitate patient's understanding of status and prognosis
		Reassure patient and family that all appropriate measures will be taken	To help allay fears
		Allow patient and family to verbalize concerns and take part in decision-making process; explain all procedures	To facilitate patient's understanding, provide coping strategies, and promote adherence to regimen
		Implement nonpharmacological relaxation techniques	To allow for rest and relaxation that will help patient gather strength to cope
		Refer patient and family to support group	To give patient maximal support
		Explore patient's resources if renal failure becomes chronic and requires dialysis or transplant	To facilitate full use of available resources

Nursing Care Plan for the Management of the Patient with Acute Renal Failure (Diuretic Phase)

Diagnosis	Signs and symptoms	Intervention	Rationale
Alteration in fluid volume: deficit related to fluid balance disturbances (hypovolemia)	Dry mucous membrane Poor skin turgor Weight loss Hypotension Dizziness	Assess weight, vital signs, and I&O daily	To determine fluid status
		Assess need to revise sodium or fluid restrictions or use of diuretics	To maintain adequate fluid volume
		Administer parenteral fluid or oral replacement fluids as ordered to keep up with urine output	To protect patient from further dehydration
		Discourage patient from independent activity until hypotension and/or dizziness resolves	To protect patient from injury
Alteration in electrolyte balance related to hyponatremia	Dry mucous membranes Poor skin turgor Weight loss Hypotension Dizziness Serum sodium < 135 mEq/L Altered mental status Tremors Seizures	Push fluids as ordered; assess need to revise sodium restrictions and use of diuretics	To prevent dehydration and maintain fluid and electrolyte balance
		Assess need for exogenous sodium supplementation	To correct hyponatremia
		Neurological assessment and seizure precautions PRN if sodium is extremely low	To identify neurologic changes and protect patient from seizure-related complications
Alteration in electrolyte balance related to hypokalemia	Serum potassium < 3.5 mEq/L ECG changes: flattened T waves and presence of U waves Constipation Muscle weakness, fatigue	Assess need to eliminate potassium restriction	Intake should not be limited when patient is hypokalemic
		Assess patient for alkalosis	pH increases lead to serum hypokalemia
		Determine if cause of hypokalemia is use of diuretics and if so discuss with MD if diuretics can be eliminated	Diuretics cause excretion of K^+; diuretics can often be discontinued in this phase to allow K^+ to stabilize

Diagnosis	Signs and symptoms	Intervention	Rationale
		Administer exogenous potassium supplements as ordered	To correct hypokalemia
		Assess abdomen and bowel sounds	To allow for early diagnosis and treatment of ileus (frequently seen with hypokalemia)
		Monitor ECG for changes indicative of hypokalemia and administer antiarrhythmics as necessary	To protect patient from complications and life-threatening arrhythmias caused by hypokalemia
Alteration in electrolyte balance related to hypomagnesemia	Hyperirritability Tetany Leg and foot cramps Chvostek's sign Confusion Arrhythmias Seizures	If patient is symptomatic, administer IM or IV magnesium as ordered	To prevent or decrease complications from hypomagnesemia
		Monitor ECG for arrhythmias	To protect patient from complications and life-threatening arrhythmias caused by hypomagnesemia
		Provide supportive care for muscle cramps	To decrease discomfort of cramps
		Provide neurological assessment and seizure precautions	To identify neurologic changes and protect patient from injury in the event of seizure activity caused by hyperirritability related to hypomagnesemia

Medications Commonly Used in the Care of the Patient with Acute Renal Failure

Medication	Effect	Major side effects
Activated vitamin D (Rocaltrol)	Allows for absorption of calcium from gut	Hypercalcemia
Aluminum-based phosphate binders (Amphogel, Alternagel, Basagel, Alucaps)	Bind with phosphate in the GI tract	Constipation Hypophosphatemia
Angiotensin-converting enzyme inhibitors (ACE inhibitors; Captopril)	Reduce BP by blocking conversion of A1–A11 renin-angiotensin vasoconstriction and aldosterone fluid retention	Hypotension Proteinuria Altered taste
Beta blockers	Lower BP by slowing heart rate	Bradycardia CHF symptoms Glucose intolerance Fatigue Impotence
Calcium channel blockers	Vasodilation reduces blood pressure	Orthostasis Heart block
Calcium chloride, carbonate, oracetate	Increase serum calcium	Bradycardia if administered too fast Dysrhythmias Phlebitis Hypercalcemia
DDAVP (Desmopressin)	Enhances platelet aggregation	SIADH
Diuretics (Furosemide, thiazides)	Cause renal excretion of excess Na^+ and H_2O	Hypokalemia Hypocalcemia Transient deafness if given rapidly Transient paresthesias Hypomagnesemia
Erythropoietin (epoetin alfa, recombinant human erythropoietin)	Stimulates bone marrow to produce RBCs	Iron overload Bone pain
Histamine (H2) blocker (Cimetidine, Famotidine)	Reduces secretion of HCl, ulcer preventative	Platelet abnormalities Rash
Hydralazine (Apresoline)	Reduces BP by arteriolar vasodilation	Tachycardia Sodium retention Drug-induced lupus Hypotension
Kayexalate (sodium polystyrene sulfonate) with Sorbitol	Enhance exchange of sodium ions for potassium ions in GI tract	Diarrhea Bowel necrosis
Sodium bicarbonate ($NaHCO_3$)	Binds with hydrogen ions to correct acidosis and hyperkalemia	Sodium and fluid overload

Compiled by B. Shelton, 1991.

Renal Trauma

Trauma care has become a major concern of critical care nurses over the past decade. Approximately 10% of all abdominal trauma injuries result in renal trauma.[112] The mortality rate among victims of renal trauma is 6–12%; early and accurate recognition of renal injury is an important aspect of maintaining this low rate. Those at greatest risk for mortal kidney injury are the elderly, drug or alcohol abusers, and those with pre-existing renal disease.[113] The complications of kidney injury include wound infection, tissue inflammation, hemorrhage, kidney dysfunction, and kidney removal. Therefore, the most immediate concern is to maintain cellular perfusion by establishing a patent airway, maintaining respirations, and promoting an adequate circulating volume. Trauma to the kidney is usually a direct result of some form of injury to the body. The injury may be of a nonpenetrating (blunt) or a penetrating type. Nonpenetrating injuries account for 70–80% of renal trauma; penetrating injuries account for 20–30% of renal trauma.[114] Penetrating and nonpenetrating wounds can also cause associated nonrenal injuries involving organs such as the liver, small intestine, colon, stomach, spleen, pancreas, chest, vena cava, aorta, and ureter.[115] This section will concentrate on kidney injury.

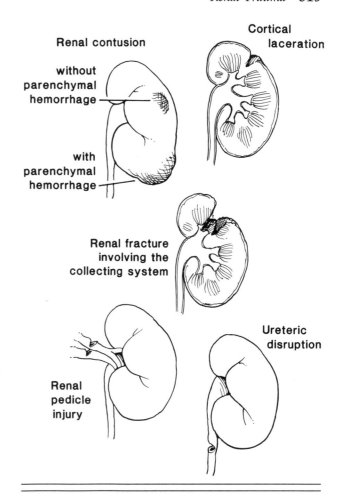

Figure 5-24   Types of Renal Trauma

Clinical antecedents

The most common antecedent to renal trauma is a motor vehicle accident. Blunt injury is the most likely etiology, although acceleration-deceleration injuries are likely to cause tearing of the blood vessels. Other precipitators of renal trauma are gunshot wounds, stab wounds, work-related injuries, wounds from penetrating projectiles, impact with steering wheels, direct blows, falls from heights, sports injuries, and pedestrian injuries.[116] Fractures of ribs number 1 through 12 are often associated with renal lacerations.[117]

Critical referents

Renal trauma may be classified into five major categories of injury (see Figure 5-24). The first type of injury is a contusion, which may cause hematomas, hematuria, or a small renal cortex tear. This type of injury may include hemorrhage, or it may be relatively minor; 60–80% of all renal injuries are of this type.[118] These injuries most often result from compression of the kidney between the lower ribs and the vertebral column, as seen in cases of blunt trauma. The second type of injury is cortical laceration, which involves deep renal tissue tears. The third type of injury is a renal fracture, which involves various tears throughout the renal tissue and the collecting system. The fourth type of injury includes vascular involvement in which the renal artery is disrupted.[119] A fifth type of injury involves ureteric disruption.[120]

Resulting signs and symptoms

One of the most important diagnostic tools in assessing renal trauma is a complete history of the precipitating event. Important data to collect include the time and location of injury, a description of associated pain, the patient's medical history, and the time of the patient's last meal. Motor vehicle accident victims are frequently complex cases that present with many injuries, but information regarding the type of accident, speed of the vehicle, and position of the person in the vehicle may help predict the severity of renal injury. Any history of hypertension should be noted, as severe renal injury can lead to hypertension later.

The clinical presentation of a patient suffering from renal trauma depends upon the type of injury. The nurse should always suspect renal trauma when evaluating a patient who has sustained blunt trauma to the abdomen, back, pelvis, or flank regions. Abdominal assessment is likely to reveal the extent of renal injury. Fifty to sixty percent of blunt injuries to the kidneys and eighty to ninety percent of penetrating renal injuries are accompanied by other system injuries.[121] A finding of ecchymosis over the flank (Grey-Turner's sign) indicates a retroperitoneal hematoma.[122]

If a patient sustains a penetrating injury, the physician or nurse should assess the wound carefully for depth, direction, and amount of damage. Entrance and exit sites should be noted, as they may give clues regarding location and severity of internal injury. This information will help evaluate renal involvement. If the penetrating object is still present within the patient, no attempt to remove it should be made. After the patient is assessed quickly and carefully and attempts to restore cardiovascular and respiratory status are made, the patient is transported to the operating room for removal of the object.

A patient with renal injury will often complain of flank tenderness or upper abdominal and back pain. This pain can also radiate to the groin or shoulder and may be accompanied by nausea.[123]

Physical findings in the event of either penetrating or nonpenetrating injury may include changes in respiratory and cardiovascular status related to a loss of circulating volume. The initial assessment may indicate hypotension, diaphoresis, tachycardia, bleeding (outwardly or internally), Kussmaul's breathing, changes in level of consciousness, and hematuria. There may be severe pain, broken ribs, tenderness, and ecchymosis present.[124]

Complications from renal trauma are extensive. They can include hemorrhage, shock, sepsis, retroperitoneal bleeding, fistulas, abscess formation, ileus, hypertension, chronic pyelonephritis, renal failure, or a nephrectomy.[125] These complications arise from a loss of blood, infection, or renal tissue disruption.

In conjunction with a thorough physical exam of the patient, radiologic tests may provide some key information to determine the extent of the injury.

Kidney-ureter-bladder (KUB) radiography allows visualization of the ribs and vertebrae surrounding the kidney. Assumptions about the kidney involvement may be based on these findings. For example, if fractures of the ribs and vertebrae are noted, there may be possible renal damage. If the kidney outline cannot be detected, then blood or urine seepage may be possible.

The intravenous pyelogram (IVP) is a basic diagnostic test for detection of renal trauma. An intravenous, iodine-based dye makes the structures of the kidneys visible, and renal function can then be evaluated. Nuclear imaging is an alternative diagnostic tool for use with those patients who are allergic to the contrast medium of an IVP; this methodology is limited, however, by its inability to detect lesions smaller than two centimeters and its lack of sensitivity to vascular disorders.[126] Although it offers valuable information about general renal perfusion, it does not offer information about renal injury.

A renal ultrasound test uses high-frequency sound waves to detect renal abnormalities. Although it is painless and noninvasive, it also does not offer conclusive information. A renal angiogram is performed when severe injury is suspected and kidney viability is of concern. A renal computed tomography (CT) scan is not usually used as an initial assessment tool but can provide the most accurate information about renal masses and lesions.

Any renal trauma patient should be monitored carefully by assessing vital signs frequently and taking complete blood counts daily. These tests give a good indication of the integrity of renal vessels to, from, or within the kidneys. Blood urea nitrogen, serum creatinine, creatinine clearance, and hourly intake and output measurements help to assess renal function.[127] The most relevant laboratory study in cases of renal trauma is the gross and microscopic urinalysis. Eighty to ninety percent of all renal trauma patients have hematuria, although severity of hematuria is not necessarily highly correlated with extent of injury. Any hematuria is sufficient cause for a more extensive evaluation.

Nursing standards of care

Initial management of the renal trauma patient centers around stabilization of the victim after the injury. The stabilization phase involves restoring adequate ventilation and circulating volume and determination of the extent of the injury. The maintenance phase for the renal trauma patient focuses on preventing infection, managing pain, and reducing the possibility of decreased circulating volume.

If there is suspicion of internal bleeding or if a flank mass is present, abdominal girths can provide some information about a hematoma. Palpation of the mass might dislodge the clot and cause further bleeding.[128]

Nursing management of patients with more severe renal trauma is more extensive. Vital signs must be monitored more frequently. Laboratory values such as hematocrit, hemoglobin, BUN, creatinine, creatinine clearance, electrolytes, and coagulation profiles are assessed regularly. Hourly intake and output values are closely monitored.[129] Surgical exploration may be necessary to repair any vascular interruptions, to drain hematomas, to repair urine collection systems, or to remove the kidney. Bleeding and urine seepage from the surgical site must be evaluated. In any event, adequate hydration is indicated. Fluid resuscitation with colloids, crystalloids, and blood products may be used.[130] Every patient with severe renal trauma must be monitored for fluid overload. Therefore, a central venous catheter or pulmonary artery catheter may be needed, and skin turgor checks, breath sound assessments, intake and output measurements, and vital sign checks are essential.

The renal trauma patient is a prime candidate for infection. Care should be taken when managing and monitoring drainage lines and any surgical wound. Aseptic technique should be instituted at all times. Antibiotic therapy may be started prophylactically. Laboratory values, vital signs, and temperature must be evaluated. Drainage insertion sites and any surgical wound must be evaluated for redness, swelling, pain, odor, warmth, and drainage.[131]

Minimization of pain is another goal in managing the renal trauma patient. The patient may experience severe flank pain as well as incisional pain. An analgesic is recommended for comfort. The nurse should take care to assess for the complications of urinary retention when using narcotics for pain management. Psychosocial support for the patient and family will depend upon the extent of the injury and the prognosis for the patient.[132]

The most common complication of renal trauma is the destruction of renal tissue with associated renal failure. Patients often require long-term dialysis management or become candidates for renal transplant. The care of these patients is the same as for others in renal failure.

Kidney Transplantation

Kidney transplantation attempts were recorded as early as 1933, but the first successful transplant was accomplished between identical twins in 1954.[133]

United Network for Organ Sharing (UNOS) statistics from 1988 reveal that over 9,000 kidney transplants were performed that year.[134] According to UNOS, the survival rate among patients with cadaveric transplants was 92%, with a graft success of 81%. Recipients of a kidney from a living relative had a 97% survival rate, with a 91% graft success. Due to the success of transplantation, there were almost 18,000 patients waiting for a kidney as of December 1990; 847 of those potential recipients had been added to the waiting list during the month of December alone.[135]

The cost of transplantation is about one-third the cost of dialysis.[136] Federal funding has been available for dialysis and transplantation since 1972, and it was estimated that almost $4 billion would be spent to care for more than 90,000 patients with end-stage renal disease during 1991.[137]

End-stage renal disease (ESRD) is the primary indication of the need for kidney transplantation. There are many conditions that can lead to ESRD; a few are listed below.

Hypertension
Glomerulonephritis
Pyelonephritis
Diabetic nephropathy
Hereditary or congenital conditions
Systemic lupus erythematosus

Contraindications to renal transplantation include the following:

Active malignancy
AIDS
Active tuberculosis
Systemic infection
Active IV drug abuse
Advanced cardiopulmonary disease
Active vasculitis or glomerulonephritis
Inability to maintain medical regimen

Recipient selection criteria vary among transplant centers. Candidates over 60 years of age may now be considered after careful evaluation, and some patients receive transplants before ever receiving dialysis.[138] As of 1988, UNOS policy required that candidates be screened for HIV; however, a positive result on that screening is not a contraindication for kidney transplant unless AIDS is actually present.[139]

Medical and psychological evaluations are performed at the transplant referral center. A complete history and physical is done, with emphasis on the condition causing the renal disease and any other current health problems. Laboratory and diagnostic procedures should include the following:

Complete blood count
Chemistry and coagulation panels
ABO and HLA tissue typing
Viral titers
Chest and abdominal x-rays
Abdominal ultrasound
Voiding cystourethrogram

Evaluation for hepatitis-B antigen is particularly important, because liver disease contributes to the mortality rate of transplant patients, and its presence is complicated by nephrotoxic immunosuppressive agents. Consultations with psychiatric staff and social workers take place, and other specialty consultations are arranged as necessary.

The psychological evaluation is essential to determine the potential candidate's understanding of the process and ability to cope with the life-long medical regimen it imposes.[140] The patient's record of compliance with dialysis routines or medications and any history of substance abuse are carefully evaluated.

The waiting time for a cadaveric kidney may be from a few months to several years, depending upon the amount of preformed cytotoxic antibody present, the candidate's health status, and the availability of allografts.[141]

Potential living related donors are also carefully evaluated both physically and psychologically before being accepted.[142] It is essential that the donor offer a kidney of his or her own free will and fully understand the risks and benefits.

An appropriate donor is both ABO- and HLA-compatible. A six-antigen HLA match has the greatest potential for success but is rarely found in other than an immediate family member. The administration of cyclosporine has greatly improved the success of poorly matched pairs. After a cadaveric kidney is typed, it will first be offered to a six-antigen match on the UNOS list. If there is no six-antigen match, the kidney will remain in the local region for the recipient who is most appropriate according to the predetermined UNOS scoring system.[143]

Allograft retrieval is accomplished through a flank incision from a living related donor. An abdominal incision is used for a cadaveric retrieval, and both kidneys are removed.[144] Improvement of preservation solutions permits the maintenance of kidneys for up to 48 hours before transplantation, but most are transplanted within 24 hours.[145]

The donor allograft is placed extraperitoneal in the iliac fossa, making it convenient to anastomose to the iliac vasculature and the bladder.[146] The native kidneys are usually left intact, as nephrectomy has been associated with increased mortality rates.[147] Nephrectomy is done for recipients with hypertension resulting from the kidney disease, renal tumor, or conditions that cause chronic urinary tract infection that could result in infection of the allograft.[148]

Postoperative medical emphasis is on maintaining renal function and fluid and electrolyte balance and on the prevention and early recognition of complications. Fluid management is evaluated on the basis of urine output and CVP measurements.[149] A massive diuresis may result from filtering BUN (which acts as an osmotic diuretic), intraoperative hydration, or postoperative tubular dysfunction (which decreases the kidneys' normal concentration ability).[150] The diuresis may be seen for several hours or days, gradually decreasing as the BUN and creatinine levels normalize.

Acute tubular necrosis (ATN) can result from ischemic damage due to long preservation time or delayed surgical reconstruction. ATN may last for days or weeks and is treated with diuretics or dialysis.[151] Dialysis is avoided in the early postoperative period if possible because of the bleeding risk associated with the required anticoagulation; it is sometimes performed immediately prior to transplantation to avoid the bleeding risk.[152]

Common electrolyte imbalances include hyperkalemia, hypokalemia, and hyperglycemia.[153] Hyperkalemia may occur with ATN, allograft rejection, or banked blood transfusions. Cyclosporine can also exacerbate the imbalance. Hyperkalemia is treated by dialysis, by Kayexalate and sorbitol, or by administration of dextrose and insulin in acute situations.[154] Hypokalemia results from diuresis, use of diuretics, or gastrointestinal loss. Potassium is replaced as necessary because hypokalemia may contribute to paralytic ileus or dysrhythmias.[155]

Hyperglycemia may be related to use of large volumes of dextrose intravenous fluids during surgery, from a steroid effect, or from the stress response to surgery. Hyperglycemia is of greater concern in the diabetic recipient and must be monitored for closely.

Complications related to the surgical procedure are uncommon.[156] Vascular leak or graft rupture create symptoms similar to those of hemorrhage or shock, accompanied by abdominal swelling or tenderness and bleeding at the suture line. Ureteral obstruction can occur from adhesions or improper placement of the ureter in the bladder. Problems such as ureteral leak and ureteral fistula can result and can be identified by intravenous pyelogram, renal scan, or cystogram.

Infection is the most common cause of mortality in renal transplant recipients.[157] Bacterial, fungal, and viral infections can overwhelm the immunocompromised patient. Pneumocystis carinii and Legionella pneumophila are frequently responsible for pneumonia. Candida may be found in the wound or as a gastrointestinal infection. The most common viral agents include cytomegalovirus, herpes, and Epstein-Barr virus.[158] Cultures may be done when infection is suspected or on a routine basis.

Most transplant recipients will experience at least one episode of rejection. Hyperacute rejection rarely occurs but may be seen, even in HLA-matched individuals, in the presence of preformed antibodies that do not appear in recent screenings.[159] Accelerated rejection may also occur in recipients with high levels of preformed cytotoxic antibodies. This type of rejection may present as disseminated intravascular coagulation (DIC). Rejection is most often identified by rising BUN and creatinine levels and decreased urine output. A biopsy is done if physical and laboratory findings are not conclusive.[160] Rejection is treated with a high-dosage steroid bolus, increased steroid dosage with a taper, or OKT-3. The routine administration of immunosuppressive agents including steroids, azathioprine (Imuran), and/or cyclosporine (Sandimmune) is used to minimize the occurrence of rejection.[161]

Nursing management of the kidney transplant recipient focuses on the maintenance of fluid and electrolyte balance, promotion of comfort and safety, and assessment for complications. The following nursing care plan outlines the standard practices of critical care following kidney transplantation.

Nursing Care Plan for the Management of the Kidney Transplant Patient

Diagnosis	Signs and symptoms	Intervention	Rationale
Potential fluid volume deficit related to diuresis	Hypotension Decreased urine output Decreased CVP Laboratory signs of hemoconcentration	Careful I&O	Assists in recognition of fluid imbalance or altered urine output
		Frequent assessment of blood pressure and CVP	Hypotension exacerbates renal insufficiency and electrolyte imbalances
		Daily weight	Reflects total body fluid
Potential fluid volume excess related to ATN or graft rejection	Hypertension Pulmonary edema Peripheral edema	Careful I&O assessment	Excess fluid volume may indicate renal insufficiency and graft rejection
		Frequent assessment of blood pressure and CVP	Provide valuable hemodynamic information
		Auscultation of breath sounds	Excess fluid may manifest as CHF
		Assessment of response to diuretic therapy or dialysis	Lack of response indicates need for more extreme measures
Alteration in electrolyte balance: hyperkalemia related to ATN, kidney rejection, or blood transfusions	Elevated potassium level Peaked T waves, widening QRS complex, and ST depression Bradycardia Muscle twitching Muscle weakness	Monitor serum potassium as ordered	Hyperkalemia potentiates dysrhythmias
		Observe ECG for indications of potassium increase	ECG changes indicate greatly increased K^+
		Monitor response to administration of Kayexalate or dextrose and insulin	Provides information to guide additional interventions
Alteration in electrolyte balance: hypokalemia related to diuresis, diuretic therapy, or GI loss	Decreased potassium level Flat T waves, U wave, or prolonged Q-T interval	Monitor serum potassium as ordered	Hypokalemia potentiates dysrhythmias and may contribute to paralytic ileus
		Observe ECG for indications of potassium decrease	ECG may reflect moderate decrease in potassium
		Monitor response to replacement therapy	Many clinical factors and medications enhance K^+ loss and contribute to replacement needs

Diagnosis	Signs and symptoms	Intervention	Rationale
Hyperglycemia related to IV dextrose solutions, steroid effect, or response to stress of surgery	Elevated serum glucose level Presence of glucose in urine	Monitor serum and urine glucose frequently	Glucose monitoring is particularly important in diabetic patients
		Administer insulin as ordered and monitor response	Insulin needs will vary with physiologic stress level and medications
Pain related to surgical incision	Complaints of incisional pain Splinting Restricted movement	Place patient in position of comfort	Patient's chance of returning to normal activity is enhanced when pain is well managed
		Medicate as ordered with continuous or intermittent analgesics	
		Monitor response to analgesics	
Potential for injury: graft dysfunction related to rejection	Elevated BUN and creatinine Decreased urine output	Monitor for trends in laboratory values	Rejection must be differentiated from infection to ensure appropriate therapy
		Measure urine output hourly and note any trend	Urine output is a sensitive indicator of graft rejection
		Administer immunosuppressive agents as ordered	These agents are the most important factors influencing graft rejection
Potential for infection related to immunosuppressive therapy	Symptoms of pneumonia Wound or gastrointestinal infection	Observe for symptoms of infection	Immunosuppression allows acquisition of virulent organisms that would not cause infection in a patient with a normal immune system, reactivation of latent organisms, or infection caused by normal body flora
		Obtain surveillance cultures as ordered	To detect early colonization prior to clinical infection
		Monitor culture findings	Positive cultures require immediate antibiotic treatment
		Maintain scrupulous hand washing and basic infection control principles	Nosocomial infections can be prevented with careful technique

CHAPTER 5 POST-TEST

1. Which symptom usually indicates bilateral mechanical obstruction of the renal arteries?
   a. oliguria
   b. anuria
   c. proteinuria
   d. hematuria

2. The single most useful test for the measurement of glomerular filtration is:
   a. urea clearance.
   b. creatinine clearance.
   c. uric acid clearance.
   d. protein clearance.

3. Of the following medications, which will not be removed by hemodialysis?
   a. phenobarbitol
   b. chlorpromazine
   c. procainamide
   d. theophylline

4. Laboratory abnormalities that can be anticipated in the patient experiencing renal failure include:
   a. hypernatremia and hyperkalemia.
   b. hypercalcemia and hypomagnesemia.
   c. hyperphosphatemia and anemia.
   d. azotemia and hypophosphatemia.

5. The most common cause of death in the patient with acute renal failure is:
   a. cardiac tamponade.
   b. hepatorenal syndrome.
   c. neurologic crisis.
   d. infection.

6. The majority of reabsorption of the glomerular filtrate takes place in:
   a. the collecting duct.
   b. Henle's loop.
   c. the proximal tubule.
   d. the distal tubule.

Refer to the following clinical vignette to answer questions 7 through 9.

M. M. is a 34-year-old patient with Crohn's disease admitted for acute abdominal pain, intractable vomiting, and dehydration. In the ED she presents with frequent premature ventricular contractions and a five-beat run of ventricular tachycardia. Her 12-lead ECG shows prominent U waves with sinus bradycardia. She is admitted to the CCU for monitoring and evaluation of her cardiac status. Her chemistry results are as follows:

Na: 148 mEq/L
Cl: 100 mEq/L
K: 3.0 mEq/L
Mg: 0.9 mEq/L
Glucose: 166 mg %
BUN: 28
Phosphate: 4.8 mEq/L
Ca: 8.5 mEq/L

7. The most likely etiology of the patient's ventricular dysrhythmias is:
   a. hypokalemia.
   b. hypermagnesemia.
   c. cardiac ischemia.
   d. Wolff-Parkinson-White syndrome.

8. The physician orders Ringer's lactate at 200 cc/hr, potassium supplementation of 80 mEq over 5 hours, and magnesium sulfate of 1 g over 1 hour. In response to these orders, the nurse should:
   a. refuse to give the potassium supplement at the prescribed rate.
   b. when one line is available, start the magnesium before the potassium.
   c. suggest that a lidocaine drip be added to the medication orders.
   d. question whether the magnesium dose is too high.

9. Nursing care measures that will allow assessment and management of complications in this patient include:
   a. placing the patient on a protocol to rule out MI.
   b. bedrest.
   c. taking seizure precautions.
   d. use of a noninvasive BP cuff for blood pressure readings every 15 minutes during magnesium infusion.

10. Cardiac complications seen in the patient with renal failure may include all of the following *except*:
    a. pericardial tamponade.
    b. cardiomyopathy.
    c. hypertension.
    d. autonomic neuropathy with tachy-brady syndrome.

ENDNOTES

1. Porth, C. M. (1986). *Pathophysiology: Concepts of Altered Health States.* 2nd edition. Philadelphia: J. B. Lippincott.

2. Ibid.

3. Guyton, A. C. (1986). *Textbook of Medical Physiology.* 7th edition. Philadelphia: W. B. Saunders.

4. Lancaster, Larry, ed. (1987). *Core Curriculum for Nephrology Nursing.* Pitman, NJ: Jannetti, Inc.

5. Porth, op. cit.

6. Alspach, J. G., ed. (1991). *Core Curriculum for Critical Care Nursing.* 4th edition. Philadelphia: W. B. Saunders.

7. Guyton, op. cit.

8. Alspach, op. cit.

9. Guyton, op. cit.

10. Ibid.

11. Ibid.

12. Keyes, J. L. (1990). *Fluid, Electrolyte, and Acid-Base Regulation.* Boston: Jones and Bartlett.

13. Ibid.

14. Walpert, N. (1990). Calcium metabolism disorders. *Nursing 90* (7): 60–64.

15. Keyes, op. cit.

16. Alspach, op. cit.; Kinney, M. R., Packa, D. R., and Dunbar, S. B. (1988). *AACN's Clinical Reference for Critical Care Nursing.* 2nd edition. New York: McGraw-Hill Book Company.

17. Richard, C. L. (1987). *Comprehensive Nephrology Nursing.* Boston: Little, Brown & Co.

18. Ibid.

19. Ibid.

20. Ibid.

21. Ibid.

22. Valtin, H. (1979). *Renal Dysfunction: Mechanisms Involved in Fluid and Solute Imbalance.* Boston: Little, Brown & Co.

23. Kinney, Pack, and Dunbar, op. cit.

24. Ibid.

25. Valtin, op. cit.

26. Zaloga, G. P., and Chernow, B. (1987). Life-threatening electrolyte and metabolic abnormalities. In Parillo, J. E., ed., *Current Therapy in Critical Care Medicine.* Toronto: B. C. Decker, pp. 245–257.

27. Ibid.

28. Ibid.

29. Kinney, Packa, and Dunbar, op. cit.

30. Ibid.

31. Emanuelsen, K., and Rosenlicht, J. (1986). *Handbook of Critical Care Nursing.* New York: John Wiley & Sons.

32. Kinney, Packa, and Dunbar, op. cit.

33. Valtin, op. cit.

34. Kinney, Packa, and Dunbar, op. cit.

35. Keyes, op. cit.

36. Rose, B., and Black, R. (1988). *Manual of Clinical Problems in Nephrology.* Boston: Little, Brown & Co.

37. Grauer, K., and Curry, R. W. (1988). *Clinical Electrocardiography.* Oradell, NJ: Medical Economics Books.

38. Innerarity, S. A. (1990). Electrolyte emergency in the critically ill renal patient. *Critical Care Nursing Clinics of North America 2* (1): 89–99.

39. Kinney, Packa, and Dunbar, op. cit.

40. Emanuelsen, op. cit.

41. Ibid.

42. Kinney, Packa, and Dunbar, op. cit.

43. Ibid.; Valtin, op. cit.

44. Zaloga and Chernow, op. cit.

45. Grauer and Curry, op. cit.; Innerarity, op. cit.

46. Kinney, Packa, and Dunbar, op. cit.

47. Gahart, op. cit.

48. Rose and Black, op. cit.

49. Kinney, Packa, and Dunbar, op. cit.

50. Keyes, op. cit.

51. Zaloga and Chernow, op. cit.

52. Keyes, op. cit.

53. Kinney, Packa, and Dunbar, op. cit.

54. Schrier, R. (1986). *Renal and Electrolyte Disorders.* Boston: Little, Brown & Co.

55. Ibid.; Walpert, op. cit.

56. Grauer and Curry, op. cit.

57. Innerarity, op. cit.

58. Guyton, op. cit.; Emanuelsen, op. cit.

59. Kinney, Packa, and Dunbar, op. cit.

60. Ranson, J. H. C. (1985). Risk factors in acute pancreatitis. *Hospital Practice 20* (4): 69–73.

61. Ibid.; Kinney, Packa, and Dunbar, op. cit.; Green, L., and Ringenberg, Q. S. (1988). Current concepts in the management of hypercalcemia of malignancy. *Hospital Formulary 23* (3): 268–287.

62. Keyes, op. cit.

63. Ibid.; Ranson, op. cit.

64. Kinney, Packa, and Dunbar, op. cit.; Johnson, B. L., and Gross, J. (1986). *Handbook of Oncology Nursing.* New York: John Wiley and Sons.

65. Kinney, Packa, and Dunbar, op. cit.

66. Walpert, op. cit.

67. Ranson, op. cit.; Green and Ringenberg, op. cit.

68. Walpert, op. cit.; Kinney, Packa, and Dunbar, op. cit.

69. Kinney, Packa, and Dunbar, op. cit.

70. Ibid.

71. Guyton, op. cit.; Alspach, op. cit.

72. Zaloga and Chernow, op. cit.; Innerarity, op. cit.

73. Kinney, Packa, and Dunbar, op. cit.

74. Alspach, op. cit.; Keyes, op. cit.

75. Kinney, Packa, and Dunbar, op. cit.

76. Gyton, op. cit.; Alspach, op. cit.

77. Kinney, Packa, and Dunbar, op. cit.

78. Keyes, op. cit.

79. Kinney, Packa, and Dunbar, op. cit.

80. Kinney, Packa, and Dunbar, op. cit.; Emanuelsen, op. cit.

81. Guyton, op. cit.; Kinney, Packa, and Dunbar, op. cit.

82. Kinney, Packa, and Dunbar, op. cit.

83. Ibid.; Emanuelsen, op. cit.

84. Kinney, Packa, and Dunbar, op. cit.; Grauer and Curry, op. cit.

85. Ibid.

86. Kinney, Packa, and Dunbar, op. cit.

87. Innerarity, op. cit.

88. Zaloga and Chernow, op. cit.

89. Innerarity, op. cit.

90. Ibid.

91. Gahart, op. cit.

92. Ibid.

93. Innerarity, op. cit.

94. Gahart, op. cit.

95. Ibid.

96. Keyes, op. cit.

97. Kinney, Packa, and Dunbar, op. cit.

98. Ibid.

99. Ibid.

100. Ibid.

101. Schrier, R. W. (1981). Acute renal failure: Pathogenesis, diagnosis, and management. *Hospital Practice 16*, 93–112.

102. Mars, D. R., and Treloar, D. (1984). Acute tubular necrosis—Pathophysiology and treatment. *Heart & Lung, 13*, 194–202.

103. Schrier (1981), op. cit.; Anderson, R. J.; Linas, S. L.; and Berns, A. S. (1977). Nonoliguric acute renal failure. *NEJM 296:* 1134–1138.

104. Coleman, E. A. (1986). When the kidneys fail. *RN 49:* 23–38.

105. Castaldi, P.; Rozenberg, M.; and Stewart, J. (1966). The bleeding disorder of uremia. *Lancet 2:* 66–69.

106. Golper, T. A., and Bennett, W. M. (1984). Drug usage in dialysis therapy. In A. R. Nissenson, R. N. Fine, and D. E. Gentile, eds. *Clinical dialysis.* Norwalk, CT: Appleton-Century-Crofts, pp. 609–624.

107. Schrier (1981), op. cit.; Ng, R. C., and Suki, W. N. (1980). Treatment of acute renal failure. In B. M. Brenner & J. H. Stein, eds. *Acute renal failure.* New York: Churchill Livingstone, pp. 229–274.

108. Lancaster, L. (1987). Manifestations of renal failure. In L. Lancaster, ed. *Core curriculum for nephrology nursing.* Pitman, NJ: Janetti, Inc., pp. 29–42.

109. Carbone, V. & Bonato, J. (1985). Nursing implications in the care of the chronic hemodialysis patient in the critical care setting. *Heart & Lung 14:* 570–578.

110. Coleman, E. A. (1986). When the kidneys fail. *RN 49:* 23–38.

111. Lievaart, A., and Voerman, H. J. (1991). Nursing management of continuous arteriovenous hemodialysis. *Heart & Lung 20* (2): 152–160.

112. Smith, Mary Fallon. (1990). Renal trauma: Adult and pediatric considerations. *Critical Care Nursing Clinics of North America 2* (1): 67–77.

113. Walsh, P., Gittes, R., Perlmutter, A., and Stomey, T. (1986). *Campbell's Urology.* Philadelphia: W. B. Saunders.

114. Alspach, op. cit.

115. Walsh et al., op. cit.

116. Alspach, op. cit.; Walsh et al., op. cit.

117. Walsh et al., op. cit.

118. Ibid.

119. Cook, op. cit.

120. Walsh et al., op. cit.

121. Smith, op. cit.

122. Kidd, op. cit.

123. Dunham, C. M., and Cowley, R. A. (1986). *Shock Trauma/Critical Care Handbook.* Rockville, MD: Aspen Publishers, pp. 253–265.

124. Alspach, op. cit.; Kidd, op. cit.

125. Cook, op. cit.; Dunham and Cowley, op. cit.

126. Walsh et al., op. cit.

127. Kidd, op. cit.

128. Ibid.

129. Alspach, op. cit.; Kidd, op. cit.

130. Ibid.; Cook, op. cit.

131. Alspach, op. cit.; Kidd, op. cit.

132. Ibid.

133. Cunningham, N. (1990). Postoperative care of the renal transplant patient. *Critical Care Nurse 10* (9): 74–80; Palumbi, M. A. (1990). Historical perspective. In K. M. Sigardson-Poor and L. M. Haggerty, eds. *Nursing Care of the Transplant Recipient.* Philadelphia: W. B. Saunders.

134. UNOS. (1991). *UNOS Update 7* (1).

135. Ibid.

136. Perryman, J. P., and Stillerman, P. U. (1990). Kidney transplantation. In S. L. Smith, ed. *Tissue and Organ Transplantation: Implications for Professional Nursing Practice.* St. Louis: Mosby.

137. Smith, S. L. (1990). Historical perspective of transplantation. In S. L. Smith, ed. *Tissue and Organ Transplantation: Implications for Professional Nursing Practice.* St. Louis: Mosby.

138. Perryman and Stillerman, op. cit.

139. Perryman and Stillerman, op. cit.

140. Holechek, M. J., Burrell-Diggs, D., and Navarro, M. O. (1991). Renal transplantation: An option for end-stage renal disease patients. *Critical Care Nursing Quarterly 13* (4): 62–71.

141. Stieber, A., Gordon, R. D., Marsh, J. W., Rosenthal, J. T., and Starzl, T. E. (1989). Critical care in kidney transplantation. In W. C. Shoemaker, S. Ayers, P. R. Holbrook, and W. L. Thompson, eds. *Textbook of Critical Care Medicine.* 2nd edition. Philadelphia: W. B. Saunders.

142. Sigardson-Poor and Haggerty, op. cit.; Holechek, Burrell-Diggs, and Navarro, op. cit.

143. Perryman and Stillerman, op. cit.

144. Haggerty and Sigurdson-Poor, op. cit.

145. Perryman and Stillerman, op. cit.

146. Sigurdson-Poor and Haggerty, op. cit.

147. Perryman and Stillerman, op. cit.

148. Haggerty and Sigurdson-Poor, op. cit.

149. Perryman and Stillerman, op. cit.; Stieber et al., op. cit.

150. Haggerty and Sigurdson-Poor, op. cit.

151. Ibid.

152. Perryman and Stillerman, op. cit.; Stieber et al., op. cit.

153. Haggerty and Sigurdson-Poor, op. cit.; Perryman and Stillerman, op. cit.

154. Cunningham, op. cit.

155. Haggerty and Sigurdson-Poor, op. cit.

156. Ibid.; Stieber et al., op. cit.

157. Stieber et al., op. cit.

158. Stieber et al., op. cit.

159. J. Hart, personal communication, April 1991.

160. Stieber et al., op. cit.

161. Stieber et al., op. cit.

6 The Gastrointestinal System

CHAPTER 6 PRE-TEST

J. M., a 69-year-old man, experienced a sudden agonizing knifelike pain in the epigastrium, radiating to his back. Concerned that he might be having a heart attack, his friends brought him to the emergency department. Physical exam revealed a moderately distressed man with epigastric pain, nausea, and vomiting. No previous medical problems were noted except Type II diabetes, and an attack of cholecystitis one year ago. He smokes a pack of cigarettes per day and drinks between 1 and 6 beers per day.

1. Given the presenting symptoms only, the most likely medical diagnosis is:
   a. gastric or duodenal ulcer.
   b. gangrenous gallbladder.
   c. acute pancreatitis.
   d. dissecting aortic aneurysm.

2. The most helpful diagnostic test for differentiation of this disorder is:
   a. serum amylase level.
   b. serum acid phosphatase.
   c. abdominal flat plate.
   d. abdominal CT.

3. Nursing priorities for care of the patient with acute abdominal perforation include:
   a. abdominal assessment, providing emotional support.
   b. provide comfort, assess for fluid and electrolyte status.
   c. assess oxygenation, assess for acute renal failure.
   d. obtain type and crossmatch for blood, assess for infection.

4. The organ most likely to be injured in blunt abdominal trauma is the:
   a. stomach.
   b. small intestine.
   c. liver.
   d. spleen.

5. Sympathetic stimulation of the mesentery of the GI tract leads to:
   a. diarrhea.
   b. decreased motility.
   c. increased peristalsis.
   d. a vagal response.

T. J. is a 56-year-old male presenting to the medical ICU after being brought to the ED with bizarre behavior and an unsteady gait. His family states that he lives alone, and is visited occasionally by two sisters and a nephew. Upon admission, the nurse notes an

emaciated man with an enlarged and taut abdomen. Multiple bruises are noted on the legs and arms; the patient's gums are bleeding, there is palmar erythema, and intention tremors are present. He denies discomfort and is disoriented to time and place. A serum chemistry shows:

Na 149 mEq/L
Cl 100 mEq/L
K 3.2 mEq/L
BUN 30 mg/dL
Creatinine 1.2
CO_2 22 mEq/L
Ca 8.9 mg/dL
Phos 3.5 mg/dL
Mg 1.7 mEq/L
Cholesterol 220 mg/dL

6. The disorder Mr. J. most likely exhibits is:
   a. acute hepatitis.
   b. cardiac cirrhosis.
   c. alcoholic cirrhosis.
   d. bowel obstruction.

7. A complication the nurse might anticipate in this patient would be:
   a. hypotension.
   b. diverticulosis.
   c. hepatitis B.
   d. esophageal varices.

8. Laboratory values seen with acute viral hepatitis include:
   a. leukocytosis.
   b. extremely high alkaline phosphatase levels.
   c. elevated transaminases.
   d. hyperalbuminemia.

9. The gastrointestinal surgery indicated for a recurrent ulcer in the antrum of the stomach is:
   a. antrectomy and vagotomy.
   b. Bilroth I.
   c. Bilroth II.
   d. portacaval shunt procedure.

10. Postoperative management of the patient who has had the surgery described above will include:
    a. educating the patient regarding fat intolerance.
    b. monitoring for pseudocyst formation.
    c. histamine blockers.
    d. vitamin B_{12} replacement for life.

Gastrointestinal Anatomy and Physiology

The gastrointestinal (GI) system plays a major role in the body's physiological functioning by providing a mechanism for the body to process and distribute nutrients. This system allows the body to ingest nutritional materials and fluids from external sources, digest them into forms that can be used by cells, and absorb these materials into the circulation so that they can be disseminated. The process makes nutrients from a single source of ingestion available throughout the body. The gastrointestinal system is also responsible for concentrating and eliminating the undigestible substances and various waste products that result from metabolism.

The gastrointestinal system is composed of several parts which are divided into two categories: the muscular tube, or canal, and the accessory organs (Figure 6-1). The tube, also known as the gastrointestinal tract (GI tract), or gut, is continuous from mouth to anus and has several divisions. These are the upper (absorptive) and lower (secretory) GI tracts, terms that loosely describe these parts' primary functions of absorption and secretion. In total, these tracts encompass the oral cavity, esophagus, stomach, small intestine, and large intestine. The upper GI tract consists of all parts of the system up to and including the small intestine; the lower GI tract

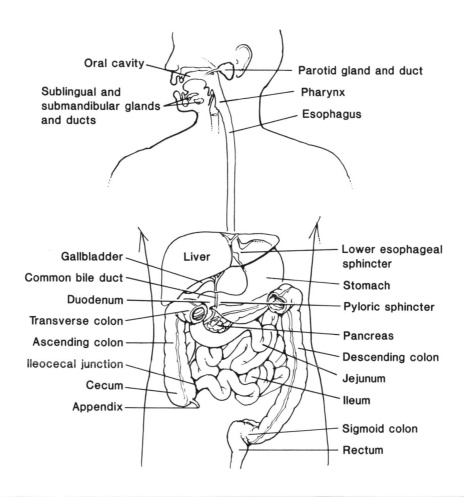

Figure 6-1   Anatomy of the Gastrointestinal System

consists of the large intestine alone. The accessory organs include the pancreas, liver, and gallbladder.

Structure of the Gastrointestinal Walls

The walls of the GI tract have four layers, each of which has a unique structure and function. The outermost of these layers is called the serosa. Although the serosa varies in thickness and composition throughout the GI tract, its function remains the same—protecting and suspending the gastrointestinal structures within the body cavities.

The next layer of the GI tract wall is the muscular layer. This is divided into two distinct layers defined by the direction in which the muscle cells are arranged. Adjacent to the serosa, the muscle cells lie longitudinally along the canals. The innermost muscle layer is circular, with cells lying perpendicular to the longitudinal muscle cells. This distribution of muscle allows for the motility patterns that are characteristic of the gut. The stomach contains an additional oblique layer of muscle that facilitates the churning and mixing of gastric digestion.

With only a few exceptions, the muscle tissue of the GI tract is primarily involuntary—its activity is beyond conscious control. The upper esophagus is an exception; some of the muscle there is striated to allow for voluntary initiation of swallowing. When this muscle is rendered dysfunctional by damage to cranial nerve IX, dysphagia (difficulty in swallowing) results. Striated muscles can also be found in the external anal sphincter, permitting conscious control over defecation.

The submucosa is the third layer from the outside of the wall of the GI tract. This is largely a supportive structure and contains most of the blood and lymphatic vessels. Most of the nerves that service the gut are also found in this layer. Diseases of the internal lumen of the GI tract, such as tumors or inflammatory bowel disease, often involve this layer, leading to possible hemorrhage. The individual with colon cancer is not likely to have symptoms until the submucosa is involved, when localized pain or bleeding becomes apparent. By this time, the disease has frequently already traveled to distant body organs via the lymphatic system.

The innermost layer of the GI tract is the mucosa. This layer comes in contact with all ingested materials and is composed predominantly of epithelial and secretory cells. The nature of the secretions varies greatly from one area of the system to another, depending upon the behavior that is characteristic of that region. Also within this area are lymphoid follicles, called Peyer's patches, that are active in antibody synthesis and assist in the immune response of the body. Extending out from the mucosa of the small intestine are villi, which are fingerlike extensions that serve to increase the surface area and therefore the absorptive capabilities of the intestine.

Since a single epithelial layer may separate the intestinal lumen from the capillaries, the gastrointestinal mucosa is particularly susceptible to bleeding secondary to erosion or mechanical injury. Injured mucosa can also lead to altered permeability of nutrients or an exchange of bacteria between the GI tract and the blood.[1] This makes maintenance of the integrity of GI mucosa of particular concern to critical care nurses.

Gastrointestinal Innervation

Gastrointestinal function is controlled by two major sources of innervation: the intrinsic (or enteric) nervous system and extrinsic nervous influences. Four cranial nerves in the central nervous system also control the initial mastication and deglutition process.

The intrinsic nervous system of the gut is independent of central nervous system control and contains two networks. The first network is called the myenteric (Auerbach's) plexus and lies between the longitudinal and circular muscle layers. The primary influence of the myenteric plexus is on muscle tone and rhythm; thus it influences gastrointestinal motility. The myenteric plexus is also responsible for effective esophagogastric sphincter closure and peristaltic movements of the GI tract.[2] The second network is termed the submucosal (Meissner's) plexus, and it separates the circular muscle and submucosal layers of the wall of the gut. The submucosal plexus primarily influences the secretions of the GI tract. Nerves of the intrinsic nervous system also relay sensory information about distention and pain to the central nervous system.

Extrinsic input is supplied by the central, parasympathetic, and sympathetic nervous systems. The parasympathetic nerves that influence functioning of the GI tract arise from two spinal segments: the medulla and the sacral segment. Stimulation of the parasympathetic system tends to enhance most gastrointestinal functions by causing secretion of acetylcholine and increasing glandular secretions. Parasympathetic stimulation of the GI tract is most likely to increase the tone of gastrointestinal smooth muscles, to stimulate peristaltic activity, and to decrease sphincter tone.

Both motor and sensory sympathetic nerve fibers that influence the organs of the gastrointestinal system arise from the thoracic and lumbar regions of the spinal cord. They are diverted to the appropriate portions of the gut through the sympathetic ganglia. Sympathetic nervous system fibers run alongside the blood vessels of the gut and secrete norepinephrine; this results in an inhibition of gastrointestinal activity.

Four cranial nerves and the "swallowing center" of the brain provide nervous stimulation to assist in the pharyngeal stage of the swallowing reflex. The trigeminal nerve assists in digestion by providing sensory input to the maxillary (lips, cheek, and hard palate) and mandibular (tongue, buccal mucosa, and lower jaw) areas. Motor fibers innervate the muscles necessary for mastication. The glossopharyngeal nerve provides sensory input to the back of the tongue, the pharynx, and the soft palate. Its motor fibers enhance the activity of the vagus nerve. The vagus nerve provides the major stimulus for involuntary swallowing by innervation of the palatal, pharyngeal, and laryngeal muscles. Finally, the hypoglossal nerve is a motor nerve responsible for muscular activity of the tongue.

In order to maximize the digestive and absorptive capabilities of the GI tract, a variety of muscular activities occur. The two basic muscular movements that occur throughout the entire GI tract are mixing and propulsion. Each area utilizes them in a fashion consistent with its function. Mixing movements act to integrate the digestive secretions and the ingested food and fluids, facilitating the breakdown of nutrients into molecules that can be absorbed into the bloodstream. These movements also enhance the process of absorption by constantly shifting the portions of digested materials so that they are exposed to all of the mucosa within the intestines. Propulsive movements serve to move the gastrointestinal contents toward the anus. These movements are called peristalsis and occur most commonly in response to distention of the lumen of the gut.

Other factors that stimulate peristalsis are extrinsic sympathetic nervous signals and irritation of the epithelial layer of the intestinal tract. This is the mechanism of action for some laxatives, such as milk of magnesia. Peristaltic movement occurs because a group of muscles that encircles the lumen of the gut constricts and creates a pocket of digested material. As the muscles below the pocket relax, the longitudinal layers of the gut constrict and push the bolus down the lumen. This process is repeated to propel the contents of the gut forward. The amount of peristalsis that occurs and the distance the bolus travels after peristalsis is initiated depend upon the strength of the initial stimulus, nervous impulses, and hormonal influences. Factors that influence peristaltic action are listed in Table 6-1.

Table 6-1 Factors That Stimulate and Inhibit Peristalsis

Stimulation	Inhibition
Moderate distension of GI wall	Severe GI wall distention
Parasympathetic nervous system stimulation	Sympathetic nervous system stimulation
Acetylcholine	Norepinephrine
GI hormones	Pain
Hunger	Fear
Alcohol	Sadness or depression
Coffee	Shock
Anger and hostility	
Anxiety	

Gastrointestinal Circulation

The organs of the GI system require a continuous large volume of blood flow to support their many functions. Consequently, the GI system receives 25–30% of the cardiac output. This is the largest proportion allocated to any body system. Arterial supply to the GI system arises from four major vessels branching off the abdominal aorta: the celiac artery, the hepatic artery, the superior mesenteric artery, and the inferior mesenteric artery. This arterial system provides large amounts of the metabolic substrates (such as glucose and oxygen) needed for secretion, motility, and absorption.

The large volume of blood flow is also necessary for absorption and transportation of the digested nutrients and fluids. The absorption of nutrients and fluids is facilitated by the dense capillary beds in the submucosal walls of the GI tract. The walls of these capillaries are fenestrated—they contain large openings that encourage rapid transport of molecules. The blood from the capillary beds in the stomach, intestines, and pancreas drains into larger veins arising from each organ, which send it into the portal vein, through the liver, out the hepatic vein, and into the inferior vena cava. This is normally a very low-pressure system, permitting rapid blood flow. Reductions in blood flow and subsequent increased venous pressures lead to portal hypertension.

The design of the GI circulation serves a number of purposes. It allows for independent regulation of blood flow to the organs of the GI tract while maintaining a standard blood flow to the entire portal system. The liver is also exposed to all of the materials absorbed by the circulation of the GI tract, with both metabolic and immunologic benefits.

Endocrinology

There are many intrinsic and extrinsic chemicals that affect the gastrointestinal functions of secretion and motility. The endocrine tissues of the GI tract are unusual, because most are in the form of diffusely scattered cells rather than concentrated glands. The chemicals secreted by these tissues can exert their influence either by being released into the bloodstream and traveling to their target organ or cells (in the case of hormones) or by diffusing across the extracellular spaces to adjacent cells. The chemicals are categorized as hormones, peptides, or enzymes. No matter what the mechanisms of their dispersal is, the changing levels of these chemicals regulate the amount and composition of digestive juices and the rate of peristalsis. The interaction and interdependency of these hormonal substances are demonstrated by the sequence of events that follow the ingestion of a meal. When a meal is ingested, the stomach becomes distended and gastrin is released. This stimulates the secretion in the stomach of acid and pepsinogen, which act to break down the food into usable substrates. When the partially digested acidic contents of the stomach are emptied into the duodenum, secretin, cholecystokinin (CCK), and serotonin are released to inhibit gastric acid secretion and to stimulate secretion of bircarbonate and water by the pancreas. Figure 6-2 diagrams these enzymatic interactions. The digestive hormones influencing both gastric activity and the digestive processes are described in detail in Table 6-2.

Structure and Function of Gastrointestinal Organs

Oral and Pharyngeal Cavities

The oral and pharyngeal cavities provide the main port through which nutrients and fluids enter the body. The pharynx has three distinct divisions: the nasopharynx, the oropharynx, and the laryngeal pharynx. The nasopharynx is composed of the hard

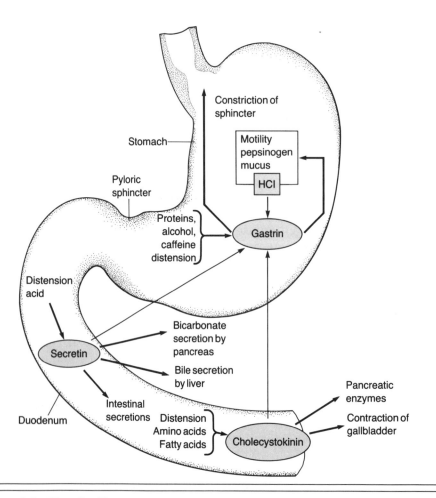

Figure 6-2   Digestive Hormones

Table 6-2 Gastrointestinal Hormones

Hormone	Site of Secretion	Secretion Stimulated By	Secretion Inhibited By	Actions
Gastrin	Antrum of stomach Proximal small intestine	Distention of antrum or fundus of stomach Certain foods (meats, ethanol) Alkaline pH of stomach	Decrease in stomach pH to < 1.5 Hypoglycemia Fat in duodenum Somatostatin release Secretin release	Increase in acid secretion by parietal cells Stimulation of pepsin release Increased gastric blood flow
Secretin	Duodenum Jejunum	Duodenal acidification Ingestion of ethanol	Neutralization of intestinal content	Stimulates secretion of water and bicarbonate by pancreas Decreases gastric acid secretion and gastric emptying Decreases motility of colon
Gastric inhibitory peptide (GIP)	Duodenum Jejunum	Ingestion of carbohydrates and fats		Inhibition of gastric acid secretion Inhibition of gastric motility
Insulin	Pancreatic beta cells	Increase in blood glucose levels Increase in blood amino acid levels Increased levels of gastrin, CCK, secretin, GIP	Decrease in blood glucose levels	Promotes uptake and storage of glucose by liver and muscle cells Promotes synthesis of fatty acids from excess glucose Promotes protein formation
Somatostatin	Throughout gut and pancreas, as well as in nervous system, body fluids, and tissues	Vagal stimulation Ingestion of meal Intestinal intraluminal acid and bile Circulating nutrients Release of CCK, GIP, glucagon, secretion	Decreased vagal tone Release of substance P, serotonin, prostaglandin	Inhibits: Salivary gland secretion Gastric acid, pepsin, and intrinsic factor secretion Gastric motility Pancreatic bicarbonate and enzyme secretion Gallbladder contraction Small intestine motility and carbohydrate absorption Blood flow to gut and liver Release of gastrin, CCK, VIP, GIP, secretin, insulin Increases: Gastric mucus production Levels of glucose and ketones in blood

(continued)

Table 6-2 Gastrointestinal Hormones (*continued*)

Hormone	Site of Secretion	Secretion Stimulated By	Secretion Inhibited By	Actions
Substance P	Throughout the GI tract and in the central nervous system	Food in the gut		Contraction of intestinal smooth muscle and gallbladder Decrease in bile flow Increase in pancreatic juice output
Histamine	Mast cells in gut mucosa (especially the stomach) Circulating basophils	Ingestion of food, especially meat	Gastrin release Blocker stimulation	Stimulation of gastric acid and pepsin secretion Increase in gastric mucosal blood flow Contraction of gallbladder and relaxation of sphincter of Oddi Increase in GI motility
Serotonin	Throughout GI tract	Vagal stimulation Increased intraluminal pressure in gut Acid and fat in duodenum	Somatostatin	Inhibits gastric acid secretion and gastric mucin production Stimulates intestinal secretions Decreases pancreatic secretion of water and bicarbonate while maintaining enzyme secretion
Cholecystokinin (CCK)	Small intestine	Products of fat and protein digestion in intestinal lumen Duodenal acidification	General anesthesia Presence of bile in duodenum	Stimulates contraction of gallbladder Stimulates secretion by pancreas of enzymes and bicarbonate as well as release of insulin Stimulates intestinal motility Inhibits contraction of lower esophageal sphincter and sphincter of Oddi Creates feeling of satiety
Glucagon	Pancreatic alpha cells	Drop in plasma glucose levels Rise in plasma amino acid levels Norepinephrine Acetylcholine	Rise in plasma glucose levels	Increases blood glucose levels by promoting conversion of glycogen and proteins to glucose in the liver and stimulating conversion of fat to glucose

Table 6-2 *(continued)*

Hormone	Site of Secretion	Secretion Stimulated By	Secretion Inhibited By	Actions

Vasoactive intestinal peptide (VIP)	Throughout GI tract, pancreas, salivary glands, other organ systems			Vasodilation in most vascular beds of the body
				Gastrointestinal effects:
				  Inhibits secretion of acid and pepsin
				  Increases cyclic AMP levels
				  Inhibits gastrin release
				  Stimulates pancreatic secretion of bicarbonate, water, and enzymes
				  Stimulates gallbladder secretion
				  Increases release of fatty acids and glucose from adipose tissue and liver

and soft palates and the nasal cavities. This structure assists in swallowing by elevating the soft palate and preventing food reflux into the nasal cavities. The oropharynx consists of the lips, buccal mucosa, teeth, salivary glands, tongue, and uvula. The laryngeal pharynx includes the area between the nasopharynx and esophagus. Its major structure is the epiglottis, which is essential in preventing pulmonary aspiration during deglutition (swallowing). It is the interaction of the divisions of the pharynx that begins the digestive process. These structures work together to break down the food into smaller particles, dilute and lubricate them, and initiate the enzymatic processes of the gut.

Saliva is produced in the oral cavity and serves many functions. Saliva is produced primarily by three pairs of glands: the parotid glands, the submandibular glands, and the sublingual glands (shown in Figure 6-1). Saliva is usually a nonviscous fluid composed of water, mucin, electrolytes, and enzymes (amylase and lingual lipase). The saliva has both a protective and a digestive capacity. Saliva contributes to overall oral health by preventing dental caries and inflammation of the mucosa. It contains bicarbonate and has numerous antimicrobial proper-

ties. The bicarbonate acts to neutralize the acid from ingested materials and from bacterial metabolism. (It also plays a role in the lower esophagus by buffering acid that has refluxed from the stomach.) The naturally alkaline environment of the oral cavity can be maintained in the critically ill patient with saliva substitutes and bicarbonate mouth care regimens.[3] The importance of saliva is evidenced by the increased incidence of dental caries and oral fungal superinfection with thrush in patients with xerostomia, a condition of reduced or absent saliva. Elderly persons, brain-injured patients, and those receiving radiation therapy to the mouth or neck region are especially at risk.

Saliva also aids in the process of digestion. The water and mucin in saliva lubricate the ingested materials and facilitate swallowing. Saliva also contains the digestive enzymes amylase (which begins the degradation of starches into disaccharides) and lingual lipase (which begins the degradation of lipids into fatty acids). Patients with xerostomia do not initiate starch and lipid breakdown in the mouth and may demonstrate altered digestive functions.

Saliva production is stimulated by cues related to eating. Before the actual ingestion of food, the rate of salivation is increased, stimulated by the anticipation of food. Once food is ingested, salivation is further stimulated by the proprioceptive (touch) reflex and the gustatory (taste) reflex. The rate of saliva production is mediated by the autonomic nervous system, with the parasympathetic pathway being the most important regulator. Impulses from both branches of the autonomic nervous system lead to increased salivation. However, the amount and consistency of the secretions vary. With parasympathetic stimulation, the rate of salivary secretion is increased four- to eightfold, creating a watery saliva. Sympathetic stimulation leads to only one-fifth the normal rate of secretion, with the product being more viscous. Factors that can stimulate the sympathetic response and subsequently decrease the rate of saliva secretion include sleep deprivation, fear, anxiety, mental effort, and dehydration.

Esophagus

The esophagus lies behind the trachea and larynx and connects the oral cavity to the stomach (see Figure 6-1). Its primary function is to serve as a passageway for ingested foods and fluids. At the lower end of the esophagus lies a region called the lower esophageal (cardiac) sphincter. This area is capable of increased muscular constriction whose purpose is preventing the reflux of irritating gastric contents into the esophagus. Without this sphincter, reflux would occur, as pressure in the stomach (an intra*abdominal* organ) tends to be higher than pressure in the esophagus (an intra*thoracic* organ). Some factors that tend to lower the effective pressure of the lower esophageal sphincter and thus increase the risk of reflux are listed in Table 6-3.

Hiatal hernia is a physical syndrome consisting of a weakened lower esophageal muscle with possible partial sphincter opening. Patients with hiatal hernias are more likely to experience reflux than patients with normal musculature.

Swallowing, also known as deglutition, occurs in three stages. Each requires coordination of several structures and muscles. The first, the oral phase, is

Table 6-3 Factors That Increase Esophageal Reflux

Hormones: secretin, cholecystokinin, anticholinergic drugs
Cigarettes
Alcohol
Fatty foods
Increased abdominal mass: tumors, pregnancy, obesity, ascitic fluid, splenomegaly

usually initiated voluntarily and involves the pushing of food toward the back of the mouth by the tongue. When the food reaches the back of the mouth, it stimulates the pharyngeal phase, in which voluntary control is lost and reflex activity takes over. The pharyngeal phase involves muscle movements to channel the food into the esophagus while protecting against aspiration. The tongue lifts to block reflux back into the mouth, the soft palate lifts to block entry into the nasopharynx, and the epiglottis closes to prevent movement of material into the trachea and airways. An understanding of these mechanisms makes it clear why infants with cleft palate have nasopharyngeal aspiration and alcohol-induced incompetence of the epiglottis can lead to pulmonary aspiration. As muscle tension pulls the larynx forward during this process, the pharyngeal-esophageal sphincter (or hypopharyngeal sphincter) opens, allowing the food to be propelled into the esophagus.

Once the food enters the esophagus, the final phase of swallowing occurs. In this esophageal phase, the ingested materials are moved toward the stomach by a combination of gravity and peristalsis. The amount of peristalsis required depends upon the position of the body and the consistency of the food. An upright position and more liquid food facilitate swallowing and require less assistance by peristalsis. The clinical application of this fact is the practice of positioning patients at risk for aspiration (such as patients suffering from stroke or recently extubated patients) in a high Fowler's position before giving them fluids to assess their swallowing competence.

Peristalsis in the esophagus occurs secondary to the contraction of the circular muscle in the walls. This activity is termed primary peristalsis if it is a continuation of the swallowing process begun in the mouth. It is termed secondary peristalsis, however, if the muscle contractions are stimulated by local irritation of the mucosa. This occurs most frequently when the ingested food remains in the esophagus after the initial swallowing activity or if gastric contents are refluxed into the base of the esophagus. Completion of the swallowing process requires relaxation of the lower esophageal sphincter (also known as the cardiac sphincter) to allow the food to enter the stomach.

Stomach

The main functions of the stomach are the storage and mechanical breakdown of ingested materials in preparation for the final stages of digestion and absorption as they travel down the GI tract. The stomach is divided into three regions: (1) the fundus (cardiac portion), or upper region; (2) the body, or middle region; and (3) the antrum, which is an elongated, constricted region at the lower end of the stomach that connects to the pyloric sphincter and duodenum (see Figure 6-3). The inner angle of the stomach is termed the lesser curvature, and the outer angle is the greater curvature. The primary function of the upper portion (fundus and body) is to receive the food and secrete digestive enzymes. The lower portion (antrum and pylorus) is responsible for mixing and moving the contents into the duodenum.

The internal anatomy of the stomach includes three smooth muscle layers, a submucosa, and an innermost layer of mucosa with many folds and ridges called rugae. The rugae are located only on the greater curvature of the stomach; they allow for distention of the stomach after a large quantity of food is ingested. The mucosa is a combination of three kinds of cells, each secreting digestive or protective substances. The parietal cells are responsible for secreting hydrochloric acid (HCl), which is important for digesting amino acids. Chief cells secrete pepsinogen, and the mucous cells provide a protective layer of mucus along the mucosal layer.

The stomach is bordered on either end by thickened rings of circular muscle, known as sphincters, which control the rate at which food enters and leaves this organ. Movement of food within the stomach is accomplished by mild mixing waves, which stir the food around and break it down. In order to move contents out of the stomach, peristaltic waves must start in the body of the stomach and move with increasing force toward the pylorus.

Gastric secretion The stomach secretes between 1.5 and 3.0 L of mucus, gastric juice, and digestive enzymes each day, depending upon diet and hormonal and nervous stimuli. Mucus is secreted by the

cardiac cells and forms a continuous layer along the inside of the stomach. The gastric juice contains several components: hydrochloric acid, gastrin, pepsinogen, gastric lipase, and gastric amylase. These and other digestive enzymes secreted to break down food substances into nutrients are listed in Table 6-4.

Mucus is the gel-like substance secreted by the mucous and chief cells located throughout the stomach. Mucus assists digestion by mixing with and lubricating the ingested food mass, but its primary function is to protect the mucosal lining of the stomach from abrasion and degradation by hydrochloric acid and enzymes. Mucus is secreted continually and forms a layer over the epithelial lining of the stomach. This layer is mobile and is replaced immediately if it is disrupted. Any interruption of the mucous layer (such as from alcohol ingestion) will lead to inflammation and ulceration of the mucosal lining as it is exposed to hydrochloric acid and pepsin.

Hydrochloric acid is one of the more important substances secreted by the stomach; it is produced by the parietal (or oxyntic) cells in the body of the stomach. This acid serves many purposes, including the denaturing of proteins, the activation of gastric enzymes, and the limitation of the growth of ingested microorganisms. Hydrochloric acid also functions to lower the stomach pH to a level conducive to gastric activities. Gastric activity is optimized at a pH less than 3.5; gastric functions are inactive at a pH greater than 6.0.

Pepsinogen is another major component of the gastric secretions. Pepsinogen is secreted by the chief cells in the body and antrum of the stomach and is converted to pepsin in the presence of hydrochloric acid. Pepsin is the active form of this proteolytic enzyme, which initiates protein catabolism by breaking certain amino acid bonds. This prepares the

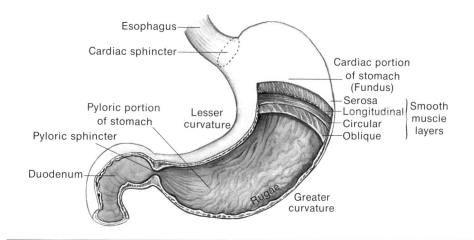

Figure 6-3 The Stomach

Table 6-4 The Digestive Enzymes

Location of Digestive Activity	Digestive Secretion	Source	Enzyme	Enzyme Action
Mouth	Saliva	Salivary glands	Amylase (ptyalin)	Converts starch to maltose
Stomach	Gastric juice	Stomach lining	Pepsin	Converts proteins to proteoses and peptones Converts nucleoproteins to peptones and nucleic acids
Small intestine	Bile	Liver	Rennin —	Converts casein to calcium paracaseinate Emulsifies fats; no enzymatic activity
	Pancreatic juice	Pancreas	Trypsin	Converts peptones to polypeptides
			Pancreatic amylase (amylopsia)	Converts starch and glycogen to maltose
			Pancreatic lipase	Converts fats to fatty acids and glycerol
			Ribonuclease	Converts nucleic acids to nucleotides
	Intestinal juice	Small intestine (crypts of Lieberkühn)	Enterokinase	Converts polypeptides to amino acids
			Sucrase	Converts sucrose to glucose and fructose
			Maltase	Converts maltose to glucose
			Lactase	Converts lactose to glucose and galactose
			Lipase	Converts fats to fatty acids and glycerol
			Nuclease	Converts nucleic acids to nucleotides

Source: Anderson, P. D. (1984). *Human Anatomy and Physiology: Implications for Health Professionals.* Monterey, CA: Wadsworth Publishing Co., p. 484.

ingested proteins for further digestion and absorption in the intestines.

Other substances secreted by the stomach include intrinsic factor, which is necessary for the absorption of vitamin B_{12}, and the weak enzymes gastric lipase and amylase. The lipoprotein substance called intrinsic factor is produced by parietal cells in the antrum, travels to the epithelium of the ileum, and coats the ileal cells to allow absorption of vitamin B_{12}. If either the antrum of the stomach or the ileum is resected, vitamin B_{12} cannot be absorbed, and pernicious anemia results.

Gastric secretion occurs in three phases. The first phase is termed the cephalic, or nervous, stage and is initiated by the sight, smell, or thought of food. When these stimuli occur, the vagus nerve sends impulses to the stomach to secrete hydrochloric acid, pepsinogen, and mucus. This phase can last 30–45 minutes and prepares the stomach for the expected food.

The second phase of gastric secretion is termed the gastric, or hormonal, phase. This phase is initiated when food reaches the antrum of the stomach and stimulates the release of the hormone gastrin. Gastrin then travels to the parietal cells of the stomach and stimulates an increased rate of hydrochloric acid secretion. The release of gastrin continues until the pH of the stomach drops to 1.5 or less. This release of gastrin and subsequent acidification of the stomach are stronger with greater degrees of gastric distention, in the presence of substances such as ethyl alcohol and meats, and with an alkaline gastric pH. This fact provides the rationale for providing small, frequent, nonmeat meals to patients with existing gastric irritation such as gastritis or ulceration. It also reinforces the current practice of administering hydrochloric acid inhibitors without antacids to patients at risk for gastric ulceration.[4]

The third and final phase of gastric secretion is termed the intestinal phase. The small intestine plays a primary role in nutrient absorption. It is in the small intestine that digestion of most nutrients is completed. The digestive process results in absorbable molecules such as glucose, amino acids, fatty acids, and vitamins, which can easily enter the circulatory system. The intestinal phase begins with the entrance of acidic gastric contents into the duodenum. The hormones secretin and cholecystokinin are released and inhibit gastric emptying and secretion of gastric hormones. The release of secretin and cholecystokinin continues whenever certain stimulating criteria are met: (1) when the gastric contents entering the small intestine contain fats, (2) when the small intestine is distended, (3) when the materials entering the duodenum are hypertonic or hypotonic, or (4) when anything is irritating the small bowel. Several substances also stimulate increased gastric secretion whenever they are ingested. These include alcohol, caffeine, fats, carbohydrates, proteins, condiments, and drugs such as cholinergics, reserpine, anticholinergics, and steroids.

Gastric motility The movement of gastric contents toward the pyloric valve is accomplished by waves of constriction that are rather weak in the fundus and become much more intense as they reach the antrum. In fact, by the time the contractions reach the pyloric region, they are intense wringing movements that greatly raise the pressure in the distal portion of the stomach. This process is facilitated by the stomach's fourth muscle layer, the oblique layer. Contraction of this muscle layer creates the wringing motion of gastric propulsion.

When the strength of the wave is stronger than the strength of the pyloric sphincter, the chyme (partially digested food materials) will be squirted into the duodenum. Only small amounts of the chyme will be dumped into the duodenum at any one time. The back-and-forth movement of the mass that occurs as the sphincter is opened and closed aids in the digestive process. The control of the pyloric sphincter is determined by the pH, content, and consistency of the chyme itself. Therefore, just as the cardiac sphincter is in control of influx and reflux of substances into and out of the stomach, the pyloric sphincter controls the rate of efflux of substances from the stomach into the duodenum. The rate at which gastric contents are propelled into the duodenum is regulated by stimuli from the stomach and duodenum. In the stomach, distention caused by ingested materials triggers the release of the hormone gastrin. Gastrin initiates propulsive contractions in the stomach and inhibits constriction of the pyloric valve. In this way, emptying of the gastric contents into the duodenum is facilitated.

When an excess volume of chyme or gastric contents rich in certain materials enters the duodenum, a combination of nervous and hormonal factors inhibits the propulsive contraction of the stomach and increases the tone of the pyloric valve. This inhibition of gastric emptying involves a combination of intrinsic nervous reflexes, extrinsic nervous stimuli, and the hormones cholecystokinin, secretin, and gastric inhibitory peptide. Characteristics of chyme that inhibit gastric emptying include the presence of hydrochloric acid, proteins, fats, solutions that are hypertonic or hypotonic, and any irritating materials. Overall, this inhibition of gastric motility works to allow only as much material to enter the duodenum as can be properly neutralized and digested.

Vomiting, or retrograde peristalsis, occurs when the upper GI tract becomes excessively irritated, distended, or excitable. Nervous impulses are transmitted to the vomiting center in the medulla of the brain, and messages are sent to the muscles of the stomach, small intestines, diaphragm, and abdominal muscles to signal the need for a change in motor activity. These messages lead to a retrograde peristalsis starting at the ileum, which forces the intestinal contents back into the duodenum and stomach. The diaphragm and abdominal muscles contract simultaneously, squeezing the stomach and raising the intragastric pressure. Next, the lower esophageal/cardiac sphincter relaxes, and the gastric contents are expelled. This continues until the irritating materials are expelled or the distention is resolved.

Small Intestine

The small intestine plays a primary role in the digestion and absorption of ingested nutrients and fluids. It is in the small intestine where the process of digestion of most nutrients is completed. The resulting molecules of glucose, amino acids, fatty acids, and vitamins can be easily absorbed into the circulatory system through the walls of the intestine.

The small intestine is approximately 22 feet long and is divided into three segments (refer to Figure 6-1). These segments are the duodenum (10 inches long, connected to the stomach), the jejunum (the middle segment, 8 feet long), and the ileum (averaging 12 feet long and connected to the large intestine). Each end of the small intestine is bordered by a valve, the pyloric valve at the beginning and the ileocecal valve at the end. The ileocecal valve lies at the junction of the small and large intestine and controls the flow of materials into the large intestine while preventing reflux of material back into the ileum.

The mucosa and submucosa of the small intestine are attached to the circular folds surrounding the lumen. These folds greatly increase the surface area available for secretion, digestion, and absorption. These folds are most numerous in the lumen of the duodenum and gradually decrease in number through the jejunum and ileum. The surface area of the small intestine is further increased by the presence of millions of villi, or fingerlike projections that line the lumen of the small intestine. Each villus contains capillaries and lacteals (lymphatic vessels). The structures of these villi aid in the mixing of intestinal contents and facilitate digestion and absorption.

Secretion in the small intestine Lining the lumen are two types of glands. Brunner's glands are found in the duodenum, and they manufacture mucus, which protects the duodenal mucosa and neutralizes the hydrochloric acid in the chyme entering from the stomach. Secretion of mucus by Brunner's glands is stimulated by the hormones secretin and glucagon. The other type of gland is in the form of indentations in the mucosa at the base of each villi; each indentation is lined with secretory cells. These intestinal glands, or crypts of Lieberkühn, secrete a clear yellow fluid called succus entericus. The succus entericus is rich in enzymes, including enterokinase,

which converts the trypsinogen secreted by the pancreas into trypsin for protein digestion.

The nutrients absorbed in the small intestine include water, electrolytes, iron, fats, proteins, and carbohydrates. Carbohydrates, proteins, and fats provide glucose and essential substrates for cellular metabolism. Recognition of the physiology of their absorption will assist the critical care nurse in anticipating nutritional deficits and their clinical consequences. Absorption of nutritional factors by the small intestine is summarized in Table 6-5.

In addition to the substrates required for metabolism, the body needs a readily available supply of vitamins and minerals. The small and large intestine assist in the absorption of these substances from ingested foods and fluids. The significance of vitamins and minerals to homeostasis is evidenced by the array of diseases or physical symptoms that occur when the diet is deficient in these substances. Summaries of these essential substances and their impact on body processes are provided in Tables 6-6 and 6-7.

Motility in the small intestine Movement of materials within and through the small intestine is facilitated by several processes. The movements of the villi help to keep the intestinal contents and digestive secretions well mixed while providing more contact between the digested nutrients and the lumen of the bowel. Rhythmic segmentations are circular contractions at intervals along the small intestine, which give it the appearance of a chain of sausage links. The main purpose of these contractions is to mix intesti-

Table 6-5 Intestinal Nutrient Absorption

Substance	Mechanism	Area of Absorption	Comments
Water	Active transport into portal circulation	Jejunum, primarily the large intestine	Exchange 8–9 L/day
Electrolytes	Passive and active transport into portal circulation	Especially in proximal small intestine	Na^+, Cl^-, K^+ nitrate, and HCO_3 readily absorbed
Carbohydrates	Active transport into portal circulation	Duodenum	Sodium enhances active transport of glucose
Protein	Active transport into portal circulation	Primarily in jejunum and ileum	Requires several enzymes to break down
Fats	Active transport to lymphatics	Jejunum	Must be broken down into fatty acid aggregates called micelles for absorption
Iron	Active transport after binding to albumin	All areas of small intestine	Requires ascorbic acid for absorption
Calcium	Active transport into portal circulation	Duodenum	Requires vitamin D; activated in kidney
Vitamins	Passive diffusion	All parts of small and large intestine	Fat-soluble vitamins (A,D,E,K) require bile salts

Table 6-6 Major Minerals

Mineral	Sources	Contribution	Daily Requirement	Effects of Excess	Effects of Deficiency
Calcium	Dairy products, eggs, fish, soybeans	Bone structure, blood clotting, muscle contraction, excitability, synapses	About 1 g	None	Tetany of muscles, loss of bone minerals
Chlorine	All foods, table salt	Acid-base balance, osmotic equilibria	2–3 g	Edema	Alkalosis, muscle cramps
Cobalt	Meats	Necessary for hemoglobin formation	Not known	None	Pernicious anemia
Copper	Liver, meats	Necessary for hemoglobin formation	2 mg in adults	None	Anemia (insufficient hemoglobin in red cells)
Fluorine	Fluoridated water, dentifrices, milk	Hardens bones and teeth, suppresses bacterial action in mouth	0.7 ppm in water is optimal	Mottling of teeth	Tendency to dental caries
Iodine	Iodized table salt, fish	Synthesis of thyroid hormone	0.1–0.2 mg in adults	None	Goiter, cretinism
Iron	Liver, eggs, red meat, beans, nuts, raisins	Oxygen and electron transport	16 mg in adults	May be toxic	Anemia
Magnesium	Green vegetables, milk, meat	Bone structure, cofactor with enzymes, regulation of nerve and muscle action	About 13 mg	None	Tetany
Manganese	Bananas, bran, beans, leafy vegetables, whole grains	Formation of hemoglobin, activation of enzymes	Not known	Muscular weakness, nervous system disturbance	Subnormal tissue respiration
Phosphorus	Dairy products, meat, beans, grains	Bone structure, intermediary metabolism, buffers, membranes, phosphate bonds, essential for energy (ATP)	About 1.5 g	None	Unknown; related to rickets; loss of bone mineral
Potassium	All foods, especially meats, vegetables, milk	Buffering, muscle and nerve action	1–2 g	Heart block	Changes in ECG, alteration in muscle contraction
Sodium	Most foods, table salt	Ionic equilibrium, osmotic gradients, excitability in all cells	About 6 g for adults	Edema, hypertension	Dehydration, muscle cramps, kidney shutdown

(continued)

Table 6-6   Major Minerals (*continued*)

Mineral	Sources	Contribution	Daily Requirement	Effects of Excess	Effects of Deficiency
Sulfur	All protein-containing foods	Structural, as amino acids are made into proteins	Not known	Unknown	Unknown
Zinc	Meat, eggs, legumes, milk, green vegetables	Part of some enzymes	Not known	Unknown	Unknown

Source: Adapted from James E. Crouch and J. Robert McClintic, *Human Anatomy and Physiology*, 2nd edition. New York: John Wiley & Sons.

nal contents and digestive secretions and to enhance absorption of nutrients by assuring that all portions of intestinal contents have contact with the intestinal walls. Rhythmic segmentations also have the effect of "milking" the small blood and lymphatic vessels of the intestine, facilitating rapid turnover of blood supply in the region. Peristaltic waves occurring in response to stretching of the intestinal mucosa facilitate the movement of intestinal contents forward through the small intestine. The distention also stimulates the release of serotonin, which increases the sensitivity of the intestinal musculature to nervous excitation and contraction.

Large Intestine

The large intestine plays a significant role in the reabsorption of water, electrolytes, and vitamins as well as in the storage and elimination of the waste products of digestion. The large intestine stretches from the ileocecal valve to the anus and is 5–6 feet long (refer to Figure 6-1). The first segment of the large intestine, immediately following the ileum, is the cecum. The cecum is only 2–3 inches long; it begins at the ileocecal junction and ends in a blind pouch attached to the veriform appendix. The next 4 to 4½ feet of the large intestine is divided into four segments, which are anatomically similar. Adjacent to the cecum is the ascending colon, which extends up the right side of the abdomen to the level of the liver, where it bends to the left (hepatic flexure). The next segment, the transverse colon, lies across the upper edge of the abdominal cavity between the liver and the spleen; at the spleen it bends downward (splenic flexure). The descending colon extends down the left side of the abdomen to the level of the left iliac crest. The sigmoid colon is the last of these

segments, and is characterized by the S shape that it forms as it turns to join the rectum. The rectum comprises the last 7 inches of the gastrointestinal tract, and it ends with the anal canal.

The muscular layer of the large intestine contains three heavy bands of longitudinal muscle called the tenaie coli. The tenaie coli are significantly shorter than the large intestine itself. They work by pulling one end of the intestine toward the other, causing it to pucker, forming small sacs called haustra. The purpose of these haustra is twofold: they increase the surface area available for absorption, and they allow for better movement of the solid contents of the large intestine.

Secretion in the large intestine   The large intestine is not responsible for secretion of digestive enzymes but does contain epithelial cells, which secrete mucus to lubricate the thickening mass of waste products from digestion. The large intestine is the primary location for the absorption of water and also participates in electrolyte absorption.

The mucosal cells of the large intestine are also partly responsible for the breakdown of urea into ammonia. In normal circumstances, this activity serves to conserve nitrogen, but when there is excessive urea, the reabsorption of it by the large intestine exceeds the liver's capacity to convert it into a usable nitrogen source, and excessive BUN results.

Derivation of certain vitamins from the breakdown of cellulose occurs in the large intestine. This process requires the presence of intestinal bacteria generally referred to as the "normal flora of the GI tract." The most common of these bacteria are the aerobic Escherichia coli and the anaerobic Bacterio-

Table 6-7 Principal Vitamins

Vitamin	Sources	Contribution	Daily Requirements	Effects of Deficiency
Fat-soluble Vitamins				
Vitamin A (precursor: carotene)	Animal fat, milk, fish liver oils	Vision (rhodopsin)	5000 IU	Skin disorders, night blindness, bone and nerve disorders
Vitamin D (calciferol)	Fish liver oils, milk, eggs	Calcium and phosphorus regulation	400 IU	Rickets, osteomalacia
Vitamin E	Rice oils, wheat germ	Reproduction (in experimental animals)	Not known	Sterility
Vitamin K	Green vegetables	Blood clotting	Not known	Coagulopathies
Water-soluble Vitamins				
Thiamine (B_1)	Peas, yeast, beans, nuts	Metabolism of energy-rich carbohydrate molecules	1.5 mg	Beriberi, neuritis
Riboflavin (B_2)	Liver, milk, meat, eggs	Oxidation	1.5–2.0 mg	Skin lesions
Nicotinic acid (niacin)	Meat, fish	Cellular oxidation	17–20 mg	Pellagra, skin lesions, dementia
Folic acid	Liver, cereals, green vegetables	Red cell maturation	1–2 mg	Anemia
Pyridoxine (B_6)			Unknown	
Vitamin B_{12}			2–5 mg	
Vitamin C (ascorbic acid)	Citrus fruits, tomatoes	Capillary function	75 mg	Scurvy

Source: Adapted from Anderson, P. D. (1984). *Human Anatomy and Physiology: Implications for Health Professionals.* Monterey: Wadsworth Publishing Company, p. 474.

ides fragilis. Vitamins synthesized in this manner are folic acid, vitamin K, riboflavin, and nicotinic acid.

Motility in the large intestine Several forms of motility are evident in the large intestine. A receptive relaxation of the cecum allows the contents of the ileum to enter the large intestine. Further along the large intestine, pendulum movements occur. These consist of continuous forward and backward shiftings of the intestinal contents between the haustra. Pendulum movements facilitate absorption by mixing and exposing all portions of the materials to the walls of the large intestine. Intestinal contents are moved forward by these pendulum movements, but at a slow rate. In the more terminal segments of the large intestine, particularly the colon, an adaptive relaxation creates storage space for feces that have yet to be eliminated. When the elimination reflex is stimulated, mass peristaltic movements begin. These are slow, irregular, yet forceful waves of contractions that move the contents of the large intestine forward for elimination.

Elimination Elimination occurs when the defecation reflex is stimulated by intestinal contents entering the rectum. Distention of the rectal wall stimulates relaxation of the internal anal sphincter and temporary constriction of the voluntary external anal sphincter. When a conscious decision is made to defecate, the external anal sphincter is relaxed, allowing the feces to be eliminated. This process can be enhanced by extrinsic influences such as parasympathetic stimulation (causing contractions of the muscles of the ascending and sigmoid colons) and voluntary muscle contractions of the thoracic, abdominal, and diaphragmatic muscles. All of these additional forces work to increase intraabdominal pressure and facilitate evacuation.

Feces are water (75%) mixed with solid waste products. Waste products include bacteria (30%), fat (10–20%), protein (2–3%), undigested roughage (30%), inorganic matter (10–20%), and dead epithelial cells.[5] The brown color of feces is caused by a bilirubin derivative called stercobilinogen.

When defecation is difficult, straining may occur. During straining, the voluntary contractions of the thoracic, abdominal, and diaphragmatic muscles can be assisted by Valsalva's maneuver. Valsalva's maneuver is a forced expiration against a closed glottis. It creates a rapid increase in intraabdominal pressure and facilitates defecation. This straining process stimulates the parasympathetic vagus nerve and can produce heart rate changes (an initial bradycardia followed by tachycardia and then a return to bradycardia). Also, increases in the thoracic and abdominal pressures will cause a pooling of blood in the extremities, decreasing cardiac preload and output. All of these changes can be potentially dangerous in an already compromised individual.

Pancreas

The pancreas (Figure 6-4) is a soft, lobulated organ located in the epigastrium and left upper quadrant of the abdomen. The pancreas is divided into three major segments: the head, nestled under the curve of the duodenum; the body (central portion), which extends horizontally across the top of the abdomen and behind the stomach; and the tail, which extends almost to the spleen on the left side of the abdomen.

The basic functional units of the pancreas are the acini, which are alveolar structures lined with secretory cells. Each acinus contains a duct through which the digestive secretions drain. Several acini combine to form a lobule; lobules are joined by connective tissue to form lobes. These lobes together form the pancreatic gland.

The secretions from the acini drain into progressively larger ducts, which eventually drain into the main duct, called the duct of Wirsung. The duct of Wirsung extends the length of the pancreas and may either join with the accessory pancreatic duct of Santorini or enter the duodenum separately at a point above the common bile duct. The pancreatic duct (duct of Wirsung) eventually joins with a short segment of the common bile duct just above the ampulla of Vater, where both then empty into the duodenum. The sphincter of Oddi protects the duodenal junction of the pancreas from autodigestion by preventing reflux of chyme and pancreatic enzymes up through the duct and into the pancreas. Spasm of this sphincter, resulting in acute abdominal pain, may occur with ingestion of large amounts of fats or with administration of certain narcotics.

The pancreas performs both exocrine and endocrine functions. There are two major exocrine functions: first, the pancreas secretes a variety of enzymes for digestion as listed in Table 6-4. The main enzymes are trypsinogen, amylase, lipase, and ribonuclease. (The pancreas also secretes maltase, lactase, and sucrase, which convert disaccharides to simple sugars, and nuclease, which converts proteins to amino acids.) The acini are primarily involved in the production of very alkaline digestive juices, secreting between 1500 and 2000 cc each day.[6]

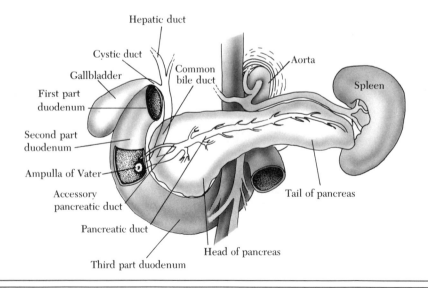

Figure 6-4 The Pancreas

This production is continuous, but secretion increases with ingestion of food substances. Second, the pancreas secretes large amounts of water and bicarbonate. These alkaline secretions work to neutralize the acidic chyme ejected from the stomach into the duodenum and create an environment in which the digestive enzymes can work efficiently. They also dilute the intestinal contents so as to protect the mucosa.

Secretion by the pancreas is regulated in part by the gastrointestinal hormones. Secretin is released from the duodenum in response to stimulation by food and acid in the lumen. Secretin then stimulates the pancreas to produce a watery secretion rich in bicarbonate and low in enzymes.

Cholecystokinin is also secreted by the duodenum and upper jejunum in response to food substances, particularly proteins and fats. Cholecystokinin stimulates the production of a pancreatic secretion rich in enzymes and bicarbonate to facilitate the completion of digestion of all food substances. Other hormones that affect pancreatic secretion are listed in Table 6-2.

Endocrine function of the pancreas involves the release into the circulation of three hormones that affect the uptake and utilization of nutrients by the body. These hormones are secreted by three types of islet cells embedded in the lobules of acinar tissue.

The alpha cells produce glucagon, which primarily serves to prevent hypoglycemia by blocking insulin's action when normoglycemia is reached. The beta cells secrete insulin, which is necessary for the cellular use of ingested or stored glucose. Finally, the delta cells produce somatostatin, whose principal role is to slow the assimilation of food from the gut, thus preventing the rapid exhaustion of nutrients absorbed.[7] (See Table 6-2 and the chapter on the endocrine system for further details.)

Liver

The liver is the largest organ in the body, weighing between three and four pounds. It is located in the right upper quadrant of the abdomen immediately below the diaphragm (see Figure 6-5). The liver is surrounded by a protective layer of connective tissue, Glisson's capsule, which envelops the blood vessels and bile ducts as they enter and leave the liver. This entire structure is covered by the peritoneal membrane, which folds back upon itself to form ligaments that help to suspend the liver in the abdominal cavity. One of these, the falciform ligament, also serves to divide the liver into the right and left lobes. The right lobe is the larger of the two and is subdivided into the right lobe proper, the quadrate lobe, and the caudate lobe.

The functional unit of the liver is the lobule; the

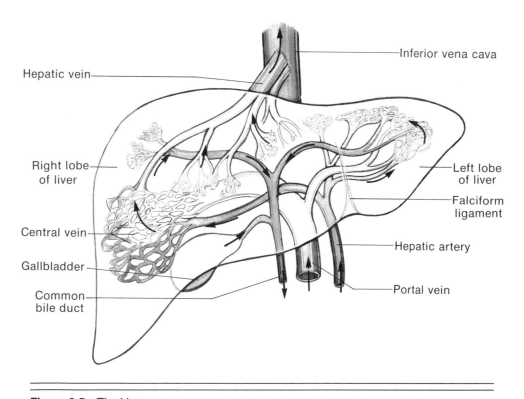

Inferior vena cava
Hepatic vein
Right lobe of liver
Central vein
Gallbladder
Common bile duct
Left lobe of liver
Falciform ligament
Hepatic artery
Portal vein

Figure 6-5 The Liver

liver contains from 50,000 to 100,000 lobules. Each lobule is composed of plates of hepatic cells (hepatocytes), which are responsible for many of the liver's functions. Each lobule has its own branch of the hepatic artery, the portal vein, and the bile duct.

The lobules receive both arterial and venous blood. Arterial blood, carrying oxygen needed for basic metabolic functions, is delivered to the hepatocytes via the hepatic artery. Venous drainage from the GI tract is carried into the liver by the portal system, which has collected blood from the inferior and superior mesenteric veins and the splenic vein. This arrangement allows the hepatocytes to be continuously exposed to venous blood rich in nutrients and fluids. All of this blood passes through the sinusoids, which are the conduits between the portal triad and the central vein. The blood then drains out of the central vein into the hepatic vein, which ultimately connects to the inferior vena cava. Normally there is little or no resistance to blood flow into, through, or out of the liver. If obstruction occurs, portal circulation is compromised and complications ensue. (Portal hypertension is discussed in more detail later in this chapter.)

The plates of hepatic cells radiate around a central vein and are surrounded by narrow spaces. These spaces, called the spaces of Disse, are similar to the interstitial spaces between cells and allow for rapid diffusion of nutrients and fluids between the hepatocytes and the blood. Lining the endothelial walls that separate the sinusoids from the spaces of Disse are the Kupffer cells. These cells perform an immunologic function of phagocytosis and destruc-

tion of old or defective red blood cells and any foreign materials absorbed through the gut. Blood flow through the plates starts at the periphery in the portal venules and travels through the hepatic sinusoids to the central vein (see Figure 6-6).[8]

Other structures also drain the lobules. Lymphatic vessels carry away excess fluid and protein that accumulates between the hepatocytes. The bile canaliculi begin between the hepatocytes and drain the bile produced and excreted by the hepatic cells. The bile drains into the right and left hepatic ducts, which join together to form the main hepatic duct. This in turn drains into the cystic and common bile ducts.

Hepatic functions   The liver performs a wide variety of functions related to metabolism, coagulation, blood storage, and detoxification. The liver is involved in the metabolism of all nutritional substances. Carbohydrate metabolism begins with the absorption of glucose, fructose, and galactose from the gut. These simple sugars are then converted to glycogen and deposited in the liver for storage. When blood glucose levels drop, this glycogen is degraded into glucose in the liver by the process of glycogenolysis. Glucose and glycogen can also be synthesized from fats and proteins via the process of gluconeogenesis. In this case, the catabolism of muscle protein provides the liver with amino acids, which it can use to form glycogen. These processes play an extremely important role in the maintenance of constant blood glucose levels.

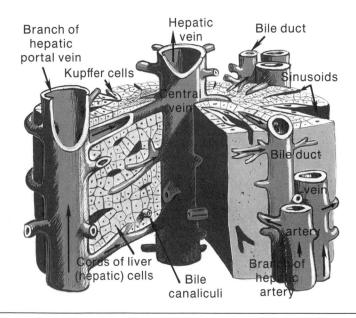

Figure 6-6   Microanatomy of the Liver

The liver is involved in protein metabolism through the synthesis and conversion of amino acids absorbed from the gut and formed from fats and carbohydrates during the process of amination. Plasma proteins produced as part of this synthesis process include albumin for the maintenance of blood oncotic pressure and most of the coagulation proteins necessary to form a fibrin clot.

Deamination of amino acids to carbohydrates or fats also occurs in the liver, either to meet immediate energy demands or for storage purposes. This process of deamination results in the formation of ammonia, which is then converted to urea for excretion. Urea is excreted for the most part by the kidneys. If the liver is dysfunctional, the synthesis of urea is compromised, and an excessive amount of ammonia (NH_3) remains in the body. A patient found to have an increasing amount of ammonia in the face of a decreasing BUN is showing signs of an ominous liver process; the cause of the problem may be difficult to determine if concommitant renal failure is present. (The discussion of hepatic encephalopathy later in this chapter provides more details on ammonia production and side effects.)

Fat metabolism begins with the breakdown of ingested fats into glycerol and fatty acids, which are absorbed through the intestines and transported to the liver. In the liver, the fatty acids are split into acetylcoenzyme A (acetyl CoA), which enters the Krebs cycle in the hepatic mitochondria, resulting in the release of large amounts of energy. Excess acetyl CoA is converted to ketone bodies, which are transported to other body tissues and then converted back to acetyl CoA to supply local cellular energy needs.

The liver is also involved in the formation of cholesterol from fat metabolism. Much of the cholesterol is converted to cholic acid, a basic component of bile salts that promotes the digestion and absorption of fats. Finally, the liver extracts excess carbohydrates from the bloodstream and converts them to triglycerides, which are transported to the adipose tissue for storage.

The liver also plays a role in vitamin storage, especially of the fat-soluble vitamins. Large quantities of vitamins A, D, B_{12}, and K and the mineral iron are stored in the hepatic parenchyma, sometimes in amounts sufficient to prevent deficiencies for months to years.

Production of bile is another metabolic function of the liver. Although bile is primarily an excretory product of the liver, it is essential for the absorption of fats and fat-soluble vitamins from the gut. Bile salts are the end-products of cholesterol metabolism and the most abundant component of bile. The high cholesterol levels commonly found in patients with obstruction high in the biliary tree demonstrate the importance of bile salts. Bile salts aid in the hydrolysis and absorption of fat-soluble vitamins by forming complexes with the lipid molecules (micelles) that are highly water-soluble and easily transported across the intestinal lumen. Cholecystitis, a disorder involving blockage of bile drainage, typically presents with light, fatty stools (steatorrhea). It reflects the lack of bile pigment that gives feces their typical brown color, as well as an inability to absorb fats.

Bile pigments, including the major pigment, bilirubin, are also found in bile. Bilirubin is formed in bone marrow, in the spleen, and elsewhere during the breakdown of damaged red blood cells. When first formed, bilirubin is in its unconjugated form and is not water-soluble. When this unconjugated (or indirect) bilirubin reaches the liver, it is combined with glucuronic acid and is converted into the conjugated (direct) form, which is water-soluble and can be excreted in the bile. When the conjugated bilirubin reaches the intestine, it is converted by bacteria into urobilinogen compounds. When found in the stool, these compounds are called stercobilinogen. Some bilirubin is recirculated to the bone marrow; most is excreted in the urine (urobilinogen). In times of high bilirubin load or hepatic failure, urine urobilinogen levels will increase until a threshold is reached; then bilirubin will remain unconjugated and produce clinical jaundice. Other components of bile include unconverted cholesterol, phospholipids, potassium, sodium, chloride, and water.

The liver performs a variety of coagulation functions, beginning with the absorption and storage of vitamin K. Vitamin K is essential for the formation of many coagulation factors within the liver. In particular, the liver is involved in the formation and release of clotting factors V, VII, VIII, IX, and X, as well as prothrombin and fibrinogen. At the same time, the liver produces an endogenous form of heparin that helps to maintain the flow of blood throughout the tissues.

The liver is important for the maintenance of a normovolemic state through its ability to store excess blood volume. The hepatic sinusoids are very distensible and can enlarge to accommodate up to 400 cc of blood. This blood can then be shunted into the circulation if hypovolemia occurs.

The liver is responsible for a number of detoxification functions. First, the phagocytic, or Kupffer, cells that line the hepatic sinusoids remove more than 99% of the abnormal cells, foreign proteins, and bacteria that enter the bloodstream from the intestines. Next, the liver is responsible for the detoxification and conversion of ammonia to urea so that it can be eliminated in the urine. Ammonia is a normal by-product of metabolism, but it is also toxic to tissues. Finally, the liver is involved in the detoxification of many drugs, hormones, and foreign substances by converting them to a water-soluble form so that they can be excreted in the bile or urine. Substances detoxified by the liver include drugs such as narcotics, penicillins, sulfonamides, benzodiazepines, and hormones (such as the sex hormones estrogen and testosterone, the corticosteroid cortisol, and the mineralocorticoid aldosterone).[9]

Hepatocellular enzymes When evaluating the liver, it is common to review the level of hepatocellular enzymes that are found in the circulating blood volume. They are often used as indicators of hepatocellular damage. Four enzymes are commonly measured: aspartate aminotransferase (AST/SGOT), alanine aminotransferase (ALT/SGPT), alkaline phosphatase (Alphos), and GGT. These are summarized in Table 6-8.

AST is a transaminase found also in the heart, kidney, skeletal muscle, and brain; therefore, it is not specific for liver disease. The ALT enzyme, however, is found primarily in the liver and is therefore more specific for liver evaluation. Both AST and ALT are released in the event of hepatocellular compromise or destruction. The clinician must evaluate the levels in relation to the clinical presentation and use assessment skills to differentiate hepatic from nonhepatic disease.

Alkaline phosphatase is an enzyme found to be active in the bone, intestine, liver, and placenta. If the patient is not pregnant or suffering from bone disease, elevations of this enzyme may occur from an increase in its synthesis by the hepatocytes or biliary tract. Such an elevation is an indication of decreased functioning within the biliary tract.[10]

Table 6-8 Indicators of Hepatic Dysfunction

Item Measured	Indicative Of
Transaminases: SGOT/AST SGPT/ALT GGT	Hepatocellular injury or biliary tract obstruction/dysfunction
5' nucleotide	Differentiates source: bone vs. liver alkaline phosphatase
Proteins: Albumin Globulin Clotting factors: I, II, V, VII, IX, X	Liver protein synthesis
Ammonia	Alterations in urea synthesis

The enzyme GGT is found in the hepatic and biliary system but also within other tissues. Its usefulness is in its correlation with alkaline phosphatase for the assessment of biliary tract disease. If both are elevated, it is likely that the patient is suffering from biliary disease. Unfortunately, GGT may also be elevated in pancreatic, cardiac, renal, and pulmonary disease and is therefore not specific.

Assessment of the Gastrointestinal System

With gastrointestinal disorders, as with any other disease state, a thorough assessment of the patient, including personal and family history, physical findings, subjective complaints, and diagnostic test data will provide the clinician with the best possible information with which to make judgments and decisions. Some organs in the gastrointestinal system are similar to one another in structure and function and work together; others function independently. For this reason, assessment parameters are often divided to cover the gastrointestinal tract, the pancreas, the liver, and the spleen. Key assessment criteria and their potential implications are addressed in the following discussion.

History

The patient's personal and family history is an essential component of the nursing assessment process. Whenever possible the personal history should include information regarding the areas listed in Table 6-9.

The patient's and family's past medical history can often provide the nurse with clues regarding the current complaint. Pertinent information to obtain may fall under any of the areas listed in Table 6-10.

Physical Assessment

Physical assessment of the gastrointestinal system includes an oral exam, abdominal assessment, gastrointestinal drainage assessment, and nutritional assessment.

The oral exam of the critically ill should include evaluation of each of the following: voice, ability to swallow, lips, tongue, saliva, mucous membranes, gingiva, and teeth or dentures. The oral cavity often reflects other health problems of the patient and should be assessed at least daily. A tool for evaluating this area of the gastrointestinal system is shown in Table 6-11; an algorithm for management of problems in the oral mucosa is sketched in Figure 6-7.

Table 6-9 Pertinent Elements of Current Medical History for GI Assessment

General Category of Information	Specific Data
State of nourishment	Weight gain or weight loss over specific time frame (more than 20% weight loss over 2 months*) Recent changes in hair, skin, or mucous membranes Usual diet, recent diet Routine daily caffeine consumption (include colas, chocolate)
Changes in appetite	Increased or decreased; food intolerances and time frames Relationship of changes to life stresses, other symptoms Altered taste sensations
Changes in bowel habits*	Stool color and consistency (relate changes to time, food, caffeine) Recent diarrhea; type, amount, frequency of agents to treat; length of time; accompanying symptoms such as blood, mucus, fevers Recent constipation; amount, color, shape, accompanying pain
Difficulty swallowing*	As related to type, amount, consistency, or temperature of food Related to recent fevers Personal history of tobacco use (especially chewing tobacco, pipe, cigar) pack-years = # packs/day × # years smoked
Heartburn, indigestion	Relationship to meals, certain foods, amount eaten Concomitant history or risk factors for heart disease
Alcohol intake	Type of liquor usually consumed (brand names may be helpful to determine alcohol proof) Average daily amount (experts say that if patient reports over 2–3 drinks/day, actual consumption is potentially three times greater than patient admits)
Easy bruising or bleeding	Related to injury, dependent, or spontaneous Associated with telangiectasis

*Warning signal of cancer

Table 6-10 Pertinent Elements of Patient and Family History for GI Assessment

Disease	Implications
Oral ulcers	Potential malnutrition, immunodeficiency, oral disease, food or drug intolerances
Gastritis or gastric/ duodenal ulcers	Recurring ulcer or extension of gastric irritation, vomiting blood Potential perforation
Lower GI irritation	Potential for ulcerative colitis or Crohn's disease (pain, bleeding, diarrhea) Diverticulitis, internal and external hemorrhoids Some etiologies can produce bowel obstruction or perforation
Exposure to dysentery or known GI contagions	Differentiate infectious and noninfectious diarrhea
Hepatitis, cirrhosis	Previous disease increases risk of hepatic failure with additional insult Increased risk of hepatic tumor Rule out hepatic causes of biliary obstruction
Cholecystitis	Identify potential etiology of GI distress, rule out as a cause of biliary obstruction
Pancreatitis	High risk of recurrence, associated hepatic/biliary complications common May help identify etiology of GI distress, glucose intolerance, or electrolyte abnormalities
Previous surgeries	Various organs' proximity to surgery site may predispose them to complications Can rule out some etiologies of GI distress
Medication history	Many drugs interfere with GI function, irritate GI tract Medications to particularly note include steroids, salicylate derivatives, nonsteroidal antiinflammatory agents, antibiotics
History of diabetes	Predisposes individual to cholecystitis and more severe gall bladder disease, pancreatitis
Occupational history	Some GI disorders may be stress-induced or related to sitting, standing, etc.

Table 6-11 Oral Assessment Scale

Parameter	Level 1	Level 2	Level 3	Level 4	Score
Lips	Smooth, soft, pink, moist	Wrinkled, dry, spots of redness	Rough, dry, swollen	Dry, cracked bleeding	_____
Tongue	Firm, pink, without fisures	Dry, pink with reddened areas	Dry, swollen, reddened	Coated, tip red, sides ulcerated	_____
Mucous Membranes	Moist	Slightly dry	Dry, inflamed, may have white coating	Very red with pinpoint brown spots or ulcerations	_____
Gingiva	Moist	Slightly dry	Reddened with ulcerations	Very red, shiny, with ulcerations	_____
Teeth	Without debris	Debris present	Debris clinging to half the enamel	Enamel surface covered with debris	_____
Saliva	Thin, watery	Increased in amount and viscosity	Scanty, mouth dry	Thick and ropey, viscid and mucid	_____
Ability to Swallow	Without difficulty	Discomfort present	Diminished gag reflex and/or pain on swallowing	Absent gag reflex and/or inability to swallow	_____
				TOTAL SCORE	_____

INSTRUCTIONS: Assign a point-value equivalent to the level observed for each parameter. Add all points and use scale below to determine appropriate management strategy, as outlined in Figure 6–7.

SCALE
  < 8   Level 1
  8–12   Level 2
  13–18 Level 3
  >18   Level 4

Source: Adapted from Shelton, B., and Weikel, D. (1990). Alterations in the oral mucosa: Assessment to intervention. *AACN's Proceedings 1990 National Teaching Institute.* Newport Beach, CA, p. 154.

The physical exam of the abdomen and GI system is performed in a slightly different manner than are other system assessments. It is important for the nurse to conduct an abdominal assessment in the following order: inspection, auscultation, percussion, and palpation. Auscultation is performed prior to percussion and palpation so that normal gastrointestinal processes are not accentuated by the exam. The exam should be performed with the patient in a completely supine position whenever possible, although raising the knees does help the patient relax for the palpation phase.

In inspection, the nurse should locate the abdominal landmarks noted in Figure 6-8, then mentally divide the abdomen into assessment regions. Regional assessment may follow either the nine-region method or the four-quadrant method. The division of the abdomen into four quadrants using the umbilicus as a central point is most common. The quadrants and regions and their abdominal contents are shown in Figure 6-9. Important aspects of abdominal inspection include observing for skin changes, scars or wounds, rashes, vascular nevi, distended veins, pulsations, and masses or protrusions. In emaciated patients, aortic pulsations and peristaltic activity may be seen during the abdominal exam.

The next step in the abdominal assessment is auscultation. Each quadrant of the abdomen should be listened to for several minutes with the bell of a stethoscope. The normal bowel sounds are caused by the movement of both air and water through the lumen of the intestine. These sounds vary from barely distinguishable low reverberations to louder, high-pitched noises. Bowel sounds may be normoactive, hyperactive (frequent or continuous and high-pitched), or hypoactive (fewer than 10–15 gurgling noises in a 2–3-minute period of time). Bowel sounds are not really "absent" unless no peristaltic noises are heard for a full 5 minutes. It may be helpful to listen to the abdomen again after percussion and palpa-

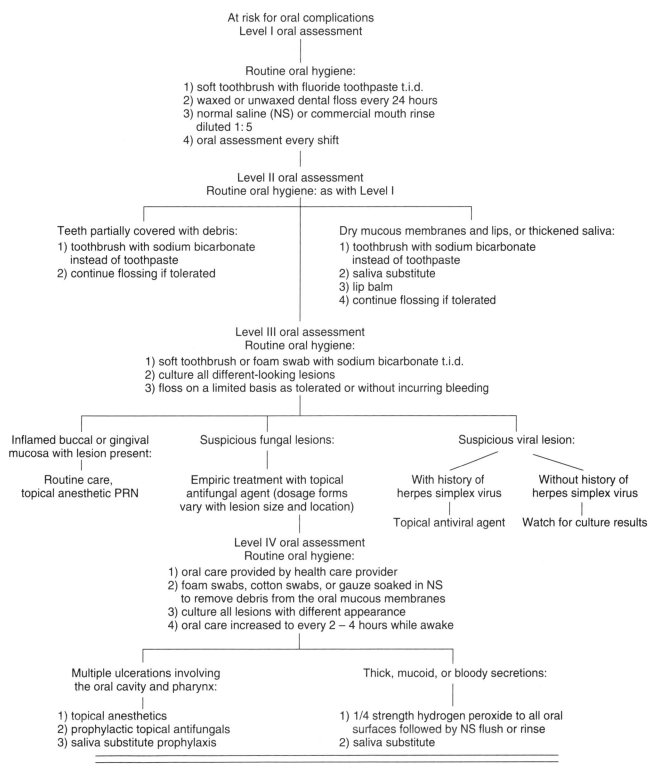

At risk for oral complications
Level I oral assessment

Routine oral hygiene:

1) soft toothbrush with fluoride toothpaste t.i.d.
2) waxed or unwaxed dental floss every 24 hours
3) normal saline (NS) or commercial mouth rinse
   diluted 1:5
4) oral assessment every shift

Level II oral assessment
Routine oral hygiene: as with Level I

Teeth partially covered with debris:

1) toothbrush with sodium bicarbonate
   instead of toothpaste
2) continue flossing if tolerated

Dry mucous membranes and lips, or thickened saliva:

1) toothbrush with sodium bicarbonate
   instead of toothpaste
2) saliva substitute
3) lip balm
4) continue flossing if tolerated

Level III oral assessment
Routine oral hygiene:

1) soft toothbrush or foam swab with sodium bicarbonate t.i.d.
2) culture all different-looking lesions
3) floss on a limited basis as tolerated or without incurring bleeding

Inflamed buccal or gingival
mucosa with lesion present:

Routine care,
topical anesthetic PRN

Suspicious fungal lesions:

Empiric treatment with topical
antifungal agent (dosage forms
vary with lesion size and location)

Suspicious viral lesion:

With history of
herpes simplex virus

Topical antiviral agent

Without history of
herpes simplex virus

Watch for culture results

Level IV oral assessment
Routine oral hygiene:

1) oral care provided by health care provider
2) foam swabs, cotton swabs, or gauze soaked in NS
   to remove debris from the oral mucous membranes
3) culture all lesions with different appearance
4) oral care increased to every 2 – 4 hours while awake

Multiple ulcerations involving
the oral cavity and pharynx:

1) topical anesthetics
2) prophylactic topical antifungals
3) saliva substitute prophylaxis

Thick, mucoid, or bloody secretions:

1) 1/4 strength hydrogen peroxide to all oral
   surfaces followed by NS flush or rinse
2) saliva substitute

Figure 6-7 Algorithm for Management of Alterations in the Oral Mucosa

tion, as bowel sounds may be stimulated during these procedures. Common GI disorders and the resulting bowel sound changes are noted in Table 6-12. Other sounds that may be heard in the abdomen include a venous hum, a peritoneal friction rub, and bruits. A venous hum is an infrequent finding but may occur in the cirrhotic patient with extensive portal hypertension. It is audible as a sustained pulsing sound in the epigastric region. Peritoneal friction rubs, also rare, are associated with irritation

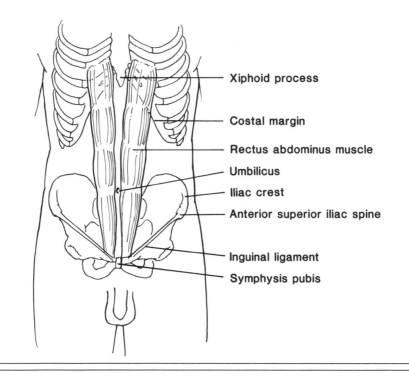

Figure 6-8 Identifying Surface Landmarks

of the contact area between the peritoneum and the abdominal organs. Such a rub is most likely to be heard in the splenic or hepatic region. It usually indicates an inflammatory process or an enlarged organ and thus is often associated with malignant processes. Bruits may be heard over any of the major abdominal arteries if there is turbulent flow due to partial obstruction.

Percussion of the abdomen is used to determine the size and location of some of the abdominal organs

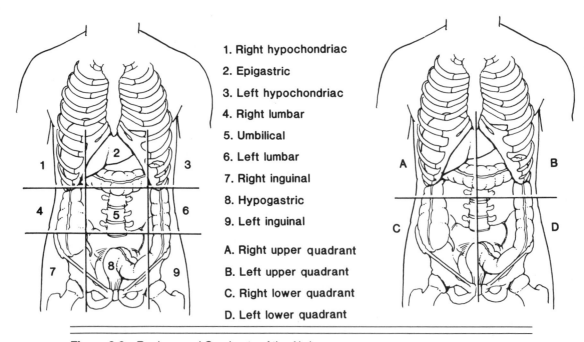

1. Right hypochondriac
2. Epigastric
3. Left hypochondriac
4. Right lumbar
5. Umbilical
6. Left lumbar
7. Right inguinal
8. Hypogastric
9. Left inguinal

A. Right upper quadrant
B. Left upper quadrant
C. Right lower quadrant
D. Left lower quadrant

Figure 6-9 Regions and Quadrants of the Abdomen

Table 6-12 Conditions That Affect Bowel Sounds

Condition	Type of Sound
Peritonitis	Hypoactive or absent
Paralytic ileus	Hypoactive
Inflammation	Hypoactive
Intraabdominal bleeding	Hypoactive
Pneumonia	Hypoactive
Hypokalemia	Hypoactive
Gastric bleeding	Hypoactive
Hyperkalemia	Hyperactive
Gastroenteritis	Hyperactive
Diarrhea	Hyperactive
Esophageal bleeding	Hyperactive
Mechanical obstruction	Hypoactive or absent (lower quadrants); hyperactive (epigastrium)

and the presence and location of fluid and air in the cavity. When percussing, the nurse moves the hands clockwise, starting in the left or right upper quadrants, unless the patient complains of pain in a specific location. Painful abdominal areas should be percussed last. Normal abdominal percussion findings are hollow tympanic sounds over the abdomen, except for the dullness that is usually found over the liver and spleen. Liver percussion should include assessment of the midclavicular costal margin (the right lobe of the liver) and the midsternal area (the left lobe of the liver). Different conditions (pleural effusions or abdominal masses) may interfere with dullness in the abdominal cavity; thus, findings of dull percussion sounds should not be used for diagnosis without other supportive assessment findings. The stomach when empty is tympanic and can be percussed along the lower left costal margin. If the tympanic area is larger, gastric dilation may be suspected. Splenic dullness should be noted posterior to the midaxillary line at the level of the tenth rib.

Palpation is the last and probably most important step in evaluating the abdomen. Deep palpation is performed to assess for organ size and position, and light palpation to assess discomfort or minor alterations. The positioning of the patient is the same for this phase; having the patient empty the bladder and raise the knees to relax the abdominal muscles will enhance the accuracy of findings. Palpation of the liver edge is accomplished by placing one hand under the patient at the level of the eleventh rib and

pressing upward. The other hand is placed on the right side of the abdomen below the area of liver dullness and with the fingers pointing upward. When the patient takes a deep breath, the examiner should push the fingertips upward and in to palpate the liver's border. This edge is usually palpable, firm and smooth. If the liver is enlarged, of a nodular texture, or irregularly shaped, this should be noted. Enlarged, smooth, nontender livers are most indicative of early cirrhosis; irregularly shaped livers often contain malignant tumors. A tender, slightly enlarged or normal-sized liver is characteristic of hepatitis. The spleen is palpated by approaching from the right side and reaching across the patient's body with the left hand. This hand supports the ribcage as the right fingertips palpate under the costal margin during exhalation. The spleen is normally not palpable, and even when enlarged it often takes deep palpation to feel it.

Palpation is also useful for differentiating the location and character of abdominal pain. The abdominal organs are visceral organs, containing few pain receptors; therefore, organ pain is characteristically dull, diffuse, and generalized, and not associated with muscular rigidity. Peptic ulcers, intestinal obstructions, and splenomegaly are examples of conditions that cause visceral pain. Liver pain is caused by swelling of or injury to the liver capsule, as there are no sensory nerves within the liver itself. Somatic pain is elicited if the skin, fascia, or other abdominal surfaces are inflamed. An excellent example of somatic pain is the discomfort associated with cholecystitis or appendicitis. When either of these inflammations includes the internal peritoneal lining, the pain becomes the characteristic rebound tenderness. Rebound tenderness is elicited when the inflamed peritoneum is pressed against organs. Upon palpation, there is no pain, but when the fingers release the abdomen, the return of the abdomen to a resting state produces a sharp and severe localized pain. In addition to cholecystitis and appendicitis, common causes of rebound tenderness include severe, life-threatening GI disorders such as bowel strangulation or perforation, bowel infarction with necrosis, acute pancreatitis, intraabdominal abscesses or infections, and peritonitis (as is seen with abdominal surgery or peritoneal dialysis). Somatic pain is also more localized than organ pain and is usually accompanied by involuntary rigidity (guarding) of the abdominal muscles.

The presence of abdominal pain should be thoroughly investigated in all circumstances. A careful medical and family history can often assist the clinician in developing a list of potential etiologies. Information that should be elicited from the patient re-

Table 6-13 Characteristics of Pain in GI Assessment

Pain Characteristic	Implications of Finding
Onset of pain: time, relationship to exercise, rest, position	Helps diagnose upper and lower GI and eating disorders; useful for hiatal hernia, ulcers, cholecystitis
Nature of pain: visceral or somatic, dull, aching, sharp, rebound	Helps narrow the range of suspected intra-abdominal problems, provides information for choosing other diagnostic tests
Referral of pain to other locations	Determines involvement of other organs; certain pains are classic indicators of certain disorders

garding pain falls into the broad categories listed in Table 6-13.

The need to assess drainage or excretion will vary, depending upon the patient's specific problems and severity of illness. Healthy individuals with intact GI tracts will not drain gastrointestinal secretions externally and thus are not at risk for complications related to loss of such secretions. Artificial drainage tubes may be placed temporarily or perma-nently in any organ of the GI tract; ostomies may be created surgically. The ostomy or tube is named after the site it is draining; for example, an ileostomy is a loop of bowel brought to the skin surface to drain the ileum, and a biliary stent is a tube placed in the common bile duct to drain bile. Nurses should be familiar with the specific care of each of these drain-age devices and aware of the potential physiologic problems the patient is at risk to develop. Because

Table 6-14 Imbalances that May Occur with Abnormal Avenues of Output

Fluid	pH	Content (mEq/L)	Likely Imbalances with Significant Losses
Gastric juice (fasting, NG suction)	1–3	Na^+ 60 K^+ 10 Cl^- 85 HCO_3^- 0–15	Metabolic alkalosis Potassium deficit Sodium deficit Fluid volume deficit
Small intestine (suction) Jejunum	7–8	Na^+ 111 K^+ 4.6 Cl^- 104 HCO_3^- 31	 Metabolic acidosis Potassium deficit Sodium deficit
Ileum		Na^+ 117 K^+ 5.0 Cl^- 105	Fluid volume deficit
New ileostomy		Na^+ 129 K^+ 11 Cl^- 116	Potassium deficit Sodium deficit Fluid volume deficit Metabolic acidosis
Biliary tract fistula	7.8	Na^+ 148 K^+ 5.0 Cl^- 101 HCO_3^- 40	Metabolic acidosis Sodium deficit Fluid volume deficit
Pancreatic fistula	8.0–8.3	Na^+ 141 K^+ 4.6 Cl^- 76 HCO_3^- 121	Metabolic acidosis Sodium deficit Fluid volume deficit

Sources: Bland, J. (1963). *Clinical Metabolism of Body Water and Electrolytes.* Philadelphia: W. B. Saunders Company; Guyton, A. C. (1976). *Textbook of Medical Physiology.* 5th edition. Philadelphia: W. B. Saunders Company.

Table 6-15 Measurements for Nutritional Assessment

Measurement	Purpose	Process
Weight	Represents total of all body constituents; indicates changing nutritional reserves; basis for other anthropometric measures	Use same scale, clothing, time of day; measure—do not accept patient's report
% usual body weight (UBW)	Reflects weight change	$\% \text{ UBW} = \dfrac{\text{Current wt}}{\text{Usual wt}} \times 100$
% weight change	Identifies risk factor of weight loss and is considered for given time period	$\dfrac{\text{Usual wt} - \text{actual wt}}{\text{Usual wt}} \times 100$
Midarm circumference (MAC)	Reflects muscle and fat	Using metal tape measure, measure circumference of arm at midpoint between acromial process of scapula and olecranon process of ulna
Triceps skin-fold thickness (TSF)	Estimates subcutaneous fat stores and energy reserves (not degree of malnutrition); <40% standard indicates severe depletion	Caliper measurement of nondominant arm at midpoint; measure and add to subscapular skin-fold thicknesses; use usual weight percentile to determine expected TSF percentile; normal: male, 11 mm; female, 19 mm
Midarm muscle circumference (MAMC)	Reflects skeletal muscle protein mass; <80% standard indicates severe depletion	Indirectly estimated from midarm circumference: MAMC = MAC − (0.314 × TSF mm); use usual weight percentile to determine expected MAMC percentile; normal: male, 27.0 cm; female, 21.3 cm
Subscapular skin-fold thickness (SST)	Estimates subcutaneous fat	Caliper measurement 1 cm below tip of right scapula; use usual body weight percentile to determine SST percentile.
Creatinine/height index (CHI)	Comparison of actual urinary creatinine to the theoretical ideal urinary creatinine can estimate the percentage of lean muscle mass	$\text{CHI} = \dfrac{\text{actual urinary creatinine}}{\text{ideal urinary creatinine}} \times 100$
Albumin levels	Low levels reflect loss of visceral process needed to maintain tissue synthesis; decreased albumin indicates poor nutrition or excessive catabolism for 10 days or more	Laboratory test
Serum transferrin	Transferrin is responsible for iron transport; high levels occur when the serum contains insufficient oxygen to bind with iron; decreased levels occur with protein malnutrition. (Alternate test is total iron binding capacity, TIBC.)	Laboratory test
Total lymphocyte count	Malnutrition is associated with depressed immune competence and decreased lymphocyte count	$\dfrac{\% \text{ lymphocytes} \times \text{WBC}}{100}$
Cell-mediated immunity	Skin tests for mumps or candida and PPD tests are negative in the patient with malnutrition and impaired cell-mediated immunity	Intradermal skin tests of substances administered; wheal is read 24–48 hours later; collect 24-hour urine for nitrogen and obtain serum BUN and creatinine at end of 24 hours

Table 6-16 Blood Test Abnormalities
in GI Disorders

Test	Abnormalities
Hematology	Anemia from folic acid, B_{12}, iron deficiency; elevated WBCs from GI infections and peritonitis
Coagulation	PT prolongation with gut malabsorption and liver disease; fibrinogen level increased in early cirrhosis and decreased in hepatic coma
Electrolytes	Ca, Cl, Mg, Ph, K, Na absorbed by small intestine
Enzymes	SGPT levels elevated with liver disease; amylase synthesized by salivary glands and pancreas, increased with pancreatic disease, narcotic use, mumps; lipase elevated with pancreatic disease; alkaline phosphatase elevated with biliary obstruction, hyperparathyroidism, bone tumors and diseases, cirrhosis
Hormones	Insulin reduced with diabetes mellitus; serum gastrin elevated with gastric tumors
Proteins	Albumin greatly decreased and alpha globulin increased with Laennec's cirrhosis, hepatitis; serum haptoglobin and transferrin decreased with hepatocellular disease

the tubes or ostomies drain gastrointestinal secretions, and it is important for nursing staff to recognize the possible electrolyte and acid-base imbal-

ances that may result from excessive drainage from any of these sites. A summary of common imbalances is given in Table 6-14 (page 856). The skin integrity surrounding all of these drainage areas should be meticulously maintained, as the acidic or alkaline nature of the drainage predisposes patients to skin breakdown.

Poor nutritional status is common among critically ill patients. The nurse's ability to assess baseline information and changes in nutritional status can affect the outcome of many critical illnesses. Many physiological disorders place patients at risk for nutritional deficiencies. The goal of nutritional assessment should be to predict requirements, not to diagnose malnutrition. A complete nutritional assessment should include (1) nutritional history, (2) anthropometric measurements, (3) assessment of somatic protein mass, (4) assessment of visceral protein mass, and (5) assessment of immunocompetence.[11] A summary of techniques to assess patients' nutritional status and the purpose of each assessment is given in Table 6-15 (page 857).

Diagnostic Tests

A wide variety of laboratory studies and diagnostic tests are used in diagnosing gastrointestinal disorders, and these can often be tailored to provide conclusive diagnostic evidence. There are no generalized gastrointestinal laboratory profiles but rather many tests, which may be significant in particular disorders. Some of the more common blood test findings that can facilitate differential diagnosis and therapeutic monitoring in gastrointestinal disorders

Table 6-17 Diagnostic Studies for Gastrointestinal Disorders

Type of Procedure	Clinical Indications	Examples
X-rays	Organ size, position and intactness, relationships among organs	Abdominal flat plate Barium swallow or enema
CT scans	Vascular problems, abscesses, pancreatitis	Abdominal CT
Nuclear medicine studies	Organ enlargement, character of masses, hematomas, presence of foreign body or substance	Venogram
Ultrasonography	Define etiology of masses (cysts, abscesses, neoplasms); differentiate foreign bodies (for example, gallstones)	Abdominal ultrasound Liver ultrasound Pelvic ultrasound
Scopic procedures	Visualization of internal diameter of GI tract	Esophagogastroduodenoscopy Colonoscopy Endoscopic retrograde cholangiopancreatoscopy (ERCP)
Biopsies	Cytopathic diagnosis of known abnormality	Liver biopsy Paracentesis

are outlined in Table 6-16. Specific nursing implications of laboratory tests are discussed with individual disorders.

There are basically four types of diagnostic studies: (1) radiology and CT scanning, (2) nuclear medicine studies, (3) invasive scopic (viewing) or sampling (paracentesis) procedures, and (4) sonography. Indications for the use of each of these general categories are listed in Table 6-17.

A clear understanding of normal gastrointestinal anatomy and physiology provides the critical care nurse with the knowledge base essential to the provision of wholistic patient care. Even if the patient does not have a primary gastrointestinal disorder, it is likely that either the ongoing disease process or the treatment regimen will have some effect on gastrointestinal function. Physiological mechanisms are always interrelated; differential diagnosis in patients with gastrointestinal complaints is a challenge. Good assessment skills focused upon pertinent history, specific symptoms, and therapeutic interventions are essential to good patient management. Thorough assessment of the patient with gastrointestinal symptoms often uncovers multisystem problems. The critical care nurse can actively participate in early recognition and differential diagnosis of the common gastrointestinal disorders described in the following sections.

Intestinal Infarction

Intestinal infarction is a significant reduction of blood flow to the gut that produces ischemic and necrotic tissue damage to the intestinal mesentery. Infarction of the intestines may be due to external factors related to inadequate cardiac output and its perfusing ability or may be related to localized lack of blood flow to the intestine. Infarction can occur anywhere in the gastrointestinal system; in this section infarction is discussed only in relation to the small or large intestine.

Clinical antecedents

Under normal circumstances, the bowel receives approximately 25–30% of the cardiac output. With low cardiac output, this is reduced and may be insufficient for tissue survival. Such a problem is enhanced when hypotension from low blood volume or flow stimulates the stress response of the sympathetic nervous system, causing shunting of blood

away from the gut and to the brain and heart. Conditions that cause bowel infarction are categorized according to the etiology of the perfusion deficit: low cardiac output, hypovolemia, or sympathetic nervous system stimulation. These antecedents are summarized in Table 6-18.

Low cardiac output can result from heart failure from coronary artery disease, acute myocardial infarction, or dysrhythmias. Direct myocardial depression can result from medications, hypoxia, acidosis, or sepsis.

Hypovolemia occurs as a result of dehydration, exsanguination, surgery, or capillary leak syndrome. At least 20% of the circulating volume must be lost before orthostatic changes occur.[12] It is estimated that greater than 30% of the total blood volume must be lost before the onset of frank hypotension and subsequent disruption of blood flow to the organs.[13] Unfortunately, the gut may be more sensitive to injury from flow reductions in malnourished patients and patients with liver or portal system disease or intraperitoneal irritation and edema. The nurse should be aware that for critically ill patients, a mild blood flow reduction is likely to have a greater than normal effect on mesenteric blood flow and may result in bowel ischemia or infarction.

Another reason blood may not flow freely through the GI circulation is occlusion or constriction of any of the mesenteric vessels. Reduced mesenteric circulation can occur from thromboses, clotting disorders (for example, DIC), or strangulation of the bowel. Ischemic bowel disease of a nonacute nature is likely to be a manifestation of atherosclerotic disease. This type of ischemia typically affects the left colon and resolves without infarction in 90% of all cases.[14] Severe vasoconstriction, as with vasopressor

Table 6-18 Clinical Antecedents of Intestinal Infarction

General Category	Specific Antecedents
Low cardiac output states	Angina Myocardial infarction Myocarditis/cardiomyopathy Pericarditis/effusion/tamponade Dysrhythmias
Hypovolemia	Dehydration Hemorrhage Capillary leak
Sympathetic nervous system stimulation	Hypertension Renin-angiotensin stimulation Adrenergic stimulants (epinephrine, norepinephrine)

or vasopressin (Pitressin) use, may also precipitate bowel ischemia from low blood flow.

Critical referents

The consequence of low blood flow to any region of the body is ultimately tissue injury and death (see Figure 6-10). The severity and duration of the flow reduction will greatly affect the organ's ability to recover. Arterial blood flow is necessary to carry oxygen and other essential nutrients to the tissues. When this flow is compromised, the body compensates by converting to anaerobic metabolism, which does not require oxygen. Anaerobic metabolism can produce glucose for the body's homeostatic functions but does not feed oxygen to surrounding tissues for their cellular respiration process. In addition, anaerobic metabolism results in production of the cellular metabolite lactic acid. Localized hypoxia and lactic acid production lead to tissue ischemia and necrosis.

Necrosis of the bowel, more commonly known as bowel infarction, can be pathophysiologically likened to a myocardial infarction. If the surrounding blood vessels are able to provide a collateral network of blood supply to the affected area of the bowel, tissue damage can be limited, and recovery will be complete. If circulation is not restored by either collateral supply or return of the normal blood flow, larger areas of bowel become necrotic, and the characteristic symptoms of bowel infarction become evident. Bowel infarctions have a much broader impact than necrosis of other organs. Necrosis of bowel tissue is particularly likely to be a problem because the normal bacteria that reside in the GI tract may cross into the bloodstream and cause septicemia or may be released into the peritoneum and cause peritonitis. In addition, the GI tract depends upon all related organs for the processing and excretion of food products. When bowel ischemia or inflammatory edema occurs, functional performance is compromised, and bowel obstructions can occur.

Resulting signs and symptoms

Signs and symptoms of an intestinal infarction in an alert patient are usually readily recognized. Ischemic injury to visceral organs produces a dull

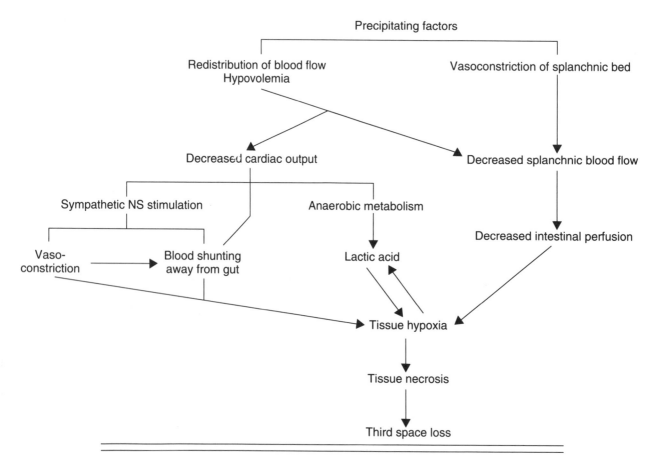

Figure 6-10   Pathophysiology of Intestinal Infarction

somatic pain in the region of the injury. Consequently, the critical care nurse should anticipate finding localized and dull but persistent discomfort of the abdomen. The location of the pain will assist in predicting the organ involved (the duodenum, other parts of the small intestine, or the distal large intestine). Rebound tenderness indicates peritoneal irritation from gastrointestinal rupture, which may occur as a complication of ischemia and infarction.

Systemic symptoms of a necrotic or infectious process will usually be present and may include fever, malaise, chills, and hypovolemia. The immune system's response to infection often leads to vascular volume depletion with ascites, or distended abdomen. Signs that frequently accompany these symptoms include leukocytosis, elevated erythrocyte sedimentation rate, amylasemia, or air in the bowel loops (evident on x-ray).

Patients often complain of nausea and may present with vomiting. These symptoms are indicative of the mechanical obstruction caused by edematous bowel segments or dysfunctional portions of the bowel. These symptoms may be significant enough to require vigorous fluid repletion, and patients should be assessed every shift for signs and symptoms of dehydration: orthostasis, hypotension, low CVP readings, poor skin turgor, fever, hypernatremia, high serum osmolality, and oliguria.

Chronic intestinal ischemia can occur in conjunction with extensive atherosclerosis. Chronic ischemia presents with more nonspecific symptoms such as crampy postprandial periumbilical abdominal discomfort.[15] Other associated symptoms may include steatorrhea, diarrhea, constipation, abdominal bloating, or abdominal bruit.[16]

The most dangerous symptoms of bowel infarction are those that result from an intraabdominal sepsis. Intraabdominal sepsis occurs from translocation of bacteria from the gut to the peritoneum. This is facilitated by the capillary permeability that occurs as part of the inflammatory response in the area of necrosis. Intraabdominal sepsis symptoms include high fevers, altered mental status, respiratory distress, sudden hypovolemia with evidence of abdominal fluid accumulation, hypotension, and rebound tenderness.

Laboratory tests that may provide useful information regarding the patient's condition include serum chemistries, serum osmolarity, CBC with differential, amylase levels, and lactic acid levels. Each test contributes information regarding the possibility of infarction but cannot be used for diagnosis without other tests.

All patients with suspected bowel infarction should have abdominal flat-plate and upright x-rays. These assist the clinician in identifying free air or abnormal fluid levels in the abdomen, an indication of perforation. Differentiating between perforation and infarction may be clinically impossible until symptoms of intraabdominal sepsis indicate that a perforation has occurred.

Nursing standards of care

When bowel ischemia or infarction is suspected, the patient should be evaluated immediately for potential surgical risk. Although infarctions may be managed medically, many symptomatic infarctions proceed to disruption of the bowel or septicemia and require surgical resection.[17]

Methods of increasing perfusion to the gut have been used with high-risk patients or those with early and vague symptoms. Medications commonly used to increase mesenteric circulation include renal-dose dopamine and nitroglycerin. Both agents increase renal blood flow, but through different mechanisms. Dopamine in doses between 1 and 4 μcg/kg/min has been shown to proportionately increase the blood through the splanchnic capillary bed. This may facilitate circulation to the tissues with reduced ischemic injury. In large thromboses or late infarction, this therapy will be of little help in reversing the process. Nitroglycerin (usually given intravenously) causes selective venodilation and dilates the coronary and splanchnic arteries. This vasodilation has been shown to reduce the abdominal pain associated with intestinal infarction.[18]

Surgical interventions for the patient with life-threatening bowel infarction will vary according to the location and extent of injury. The goal is always to preserve as much bowel as possible, so resections with end-to-end anastamoses are preferred. This surgery should not greatly interrupt the digestive processes unless the duodenum or jejunum is resected. (Surgeries on specific areas of the intestines are discussed later in this chapter.) When a resection with end-to-end anastomosis is not possible, then a partial resection with either a temporary or a permanent colostomy is performed. (Specific nursing care of the patient with a colostomy is described in the nursing care plan for GI surgery.)

Nursing care of the patient with a bowel infarction primarily involves assessment and evaluation. Early recognition of intestinal ischemia can significantly limit tissue damage and the incidence of septicemia. The top-priority goals of nursing care are (1) interventions for patient comfort, (2) maintenance of nutrition, and (3) recognition of obstruction and perforation.

Intestinal Obstruction and Perforation

Intestinal obstruction occurs when there is a blockage of the small or large intestine that retards the natural progression of digestive processing. The obstructing mechanism may be mechanical or paralytic (functional) in nature. Mechanical obstructions may be further classified according to acute or chronic presentation, partial or complete obstruction, and involvement of the small or large intestine. Intestinal pseudo-obstruction is a term used to describe a condition in which symptoms of intestinal obstruction are evident, but no actual obstruction can be confirmed by routine diagnostic procedures. All of these syndromes are common in the critically ill patient as a result of electrolyte disorders and complex intraabdominal processes.

An obstruction becomes a bowel perforation when the intraluminal pressure exceeds the bowel's resistive capacity and a rupture of the bowel membrane occurs. With perforation, the bowel contents at that area are released into the peritoneum, producing irritation and potential infection. This clinical complication is life-threatening and demands immediate surgical intervention.

In the early twentieth century, mortality from bowel obstruction exceeded 50%, but now the mortality rate is only approximately 10%.[19] This reduction in mortality can be attributed to advances in antibiotic therapy, decompression techniques, and fluid and electrolyte replacement.

Clinical antecedents

Intraabdominal pathology is the most common cause of all bowel obstructions. Small bowel obstructions are more common, and abdominal adhesions are the leading etiology of such obstructions.[20] Obstructions of this area are considered to be less life-threatening if they rupture, as the small intestine does not contain microorganisms that may cause sepsis. The large intestine is most likely to be obstructed as a result of malignant tumor.[21]

Bowel obstructions are classified according to the mechanism of blockage: (1) intraluminal obstruction is a mass in the internal lumen of the bowel; (2) mural obstructions arise from lesions of the bowel wall; (3) extramural obstruction is compression of the bowel by external structures; and (4) digestive obstruction is caused by a lack of propulsion of digestive contents through the bowel. Examples of the common etiologies are given in Table 6-19.

When the lumen is obstructed but the blood flow to the mesentery remains intact, the obstruction is a simple obstruction. When the blood flow to the obstructed area is also compromised, the obstruction is termed a strangulated obstruction. Closed-loop obstruction occurs when a bowel is looped over itself and blocked on both ends, resisting both regurgitation and normal progression of the intestinal contents.[22] The condition is known as volvulus, or strangulated hernia.

Approximately 20% of "acute abdomen" admissions in surgery departments are cases of intestinal obstruction.[23] Hernias had been the most common cause of obstruction until ten years ago, but early medical management of herniation has improved. Abdominal adhesions are now the most common etiology of bowel obstruction.[24] Etiologies will vary with age groups; hernias remain the most common in childhood, but tumors and diverticulitis are most common in patients over 65 years of age.

Critical referents

The three types of intestinal obstruction produce variations of the same clinical syndrome—blockage

Table 6-19 Classifications of Intestinal Obstruction

Mechanical	Functional
Intraluminal obstruction	Neuromuscular defects
Gallstones	Megacolon
Fecal impactions	Mesenteric vascular
Intussusception	occlusion
Polypoid tumors	Paralytic ileus (electrolyte
Foreign bodies	peritonitis, sepsis)
Lesions of the bowel	Vascular occlusion
Tumor	
Congenital disorders:	
Meckel's diverticulum,	
imperforate anus, atresia	
Inflammatory disease:	
diverticulitis, Crohn's	
disease, ulcerative colitis	
Strictures: inflammatory	
bowel, radiation,	
endometriosis, Kaposi's	
sarcoma	
External lesions	
compressing bowel	
Tumor	
Anomolous vessels	
Abscesses and	
hematomas	
Volvulus	
Adhesions	
Hernia	

of flow of the digestive contents. The clinical consequences will vary with the level of intraluminal pressure; rupture (perforation) can result when the pressure becomes too high.

Paralytic obstructions are those resulting from reduced peristalsis at any area along the GI tract. Paralytic obstruction of the small intestine, particularly the ileus, is a common complication of critical illness. It is associated with electrolyte disturbances (hypokalemia, hypocalcemia, or hypomagnesemia), surgical or traumatic manipulation of the bowel, peritonitis, and gram-negative sepsis. Medications known to reduce gastric motility (including the phenothiazines, Lomotil, and probanthine) are also possible precipitators of paralytic ileus. The precise mechanism that produces paralytic ileus is unknown, but several plausible theories have been postulated. One proposes that the etiologic factors may be similar to the normal physiologic suppression of GI motility. Consequently, any disorders that create excess catecholamines or contribute to autonomic smooth muscle inhibition of peristalsis can lead to paralytic ileus. Some mechanisms that may be encountered in the ICU setting include vasopressor therapy; use of benzodiazepines, narcotics, or histamine blockers; hormonal stress response; fear; and bowel ischemia. Another theory focuses upon the adrenal axis of the stress response. According to this theory, stress triggers the release of pituitary hormones, which act upon target organs that produce epinephrine, stimulating the release of adrenocorticotropic hormones. These steroids then inhibit gastric motility and may lead to paralytic ileus.[25]

Strangulated bowel is an intestine that has been twisted so severely at one spot that there is no lumen left through which products can pass. In intussusceptive obstructions, the bowel has turned in upon itself. One portion of the bowel is enveloped by the next, leading to functional impairment. This twisting also blocks all blood flow to the strangulated area and leads to bowel ischemia and cessation of peristalsis. No bowel contents can move beyond the point of blockage. In adults the most common cause of intussusception is an abnormality of the bowel wall, such as polyps, diverticulae, or tumors.

Intraluminal obstructions do not allow sufficient space inside the lumen of the bowel for normal digestion and propulsion to take place. The digestive contents back up and adhere together, forming an obstructive mass. Fluid and gas accumulate proximal to the obstruction. The location of the obstruction in part predicts the nature of the gas that accumulates and is transported into the bloodstream. In the small intestine, carbon dioxide (CO_2) and nitrogen accumulate from normal processes and cannot be excreted. The breakdown of fatty acids in the region also causes increased levels of carbon dioxide and produces a more severe metabolic acidosis in this type of obstruction. Colonic obstruction, which occurs where normal GI flora produce methane, leads to increased abdominal gas, distention, and increased serum ammonia levels. Prolonged partial obstruction may occur in the case of strictures or inflammation; patients suffering partial obstructions should be observed carefully for signs and symptoms of complete obstruction.

One of the most important events occurring during simple obstruction is the loss of fluid and electrolytes. As the intestine distends, the intraluminal pressure exceeds the surrounding abdominal pressure. The net result is that fluid is trapped in the obstructed area and then leaks from the intestine into the peritoneum. Proximal bowel obstruction will lead to emesis rather than the severe fluid depletion seen with distal small intestine obstruction. The nature and severity of electrolyte disturbances will vary with the location of the obstruction.

Extrinsic lesions compressing an area of the bowel may also cause occlusion of normal digestive processes. Adhesions, the most common etiology of simple obstruction, form fibrous bands connecting areas of the bowel together. These bands compress, or kink, areas of the bowel and lead to backup of fluid and gas.

Intestinal perforation may be the ultimate complication of either an obstruction (which causes high intraluminal pressures with bowel rupture) or erosion of the intestinal wall by lesions such as tumors or ulcerations. Perforation of the small intestine leads to the release of intestinal fluid rich in enzymes but deficient in bacteria. (This type of fluid differs from colonic fluids, which are rich in bacteria but lack enzymes.) The release of intestinal fluid results in a chemical peritonitis, but not necessarily sepsis. A colonic perforation is more likely to cause septicemia.

Resulting signs and symptoms

The signs and symptoms of bowel obstruction can be divided into primary effects (those directly related to the obstruction) and secondary effects (the consequences of the obstructive process). In 1978, Stewardson reviewed the symptomatology of 238 patients with bowel obstruction. He found the most common presenting symptoms to be leukocytosis, fever, tachycardia, and localized abdominal pain. In 90% of the patients exhibiting at least two of these signs, gangrenous bowel was found upon surgery.[26]

The primary effects include abdominal discomfort, distention, and bowel sound changes. The pain associated with obstruction is moderate to severe, crampy, with a crescendo-decrescendo pattern and rebound tenderness signifying the progression to perforation. Abdominal pain due to an obstruction often occurs after eating and is separated by times of no pain. The frequency of discomfort in small intestine obstruction has been shown to be greater than that in large intestine obstruction. Severe pain without periods of remission is characteristic of strangulation and should be investigated promptly. Some reports note that the pain lessens in intensity as abdominal distention becomes more prominent.[27]

Abdominal distention occurs with both mechanical and paralytic ileus and is difficult to differentiate on routine abdominal films, which show evidence of gas in both disorders. Bowel sounds are hyperactive proximal to the site of obstruction and hypoactive, quiet, or absent distal to the obstruction.

The fluid drained during management of obstructions may be green, bilious (golden), bloody, or frankly fecal. Drainage from the small intestine develops an overgrowth of bacteria while stagnant in the intestine. It is important for critical care nurses to know that prolonged intestinal ischemia during this process can lead to high levels of bacterial growth and the production of a fecal-appearing and odorous small intestine drainage.

Obstructions found high in the GI tract lead to backup of gastric contents with vomiting, possibly without abdominal distention. With obstructions occurring in the lower GI tract, stools are likely to be absent or thin and ribbonlike, and the abdomen will be distended.

After an evaluation of the physical status of patients with potential obstruction or perforation, laboratory and radiologic studies are necessary to confirm the likely location and etiology. Serum laboratory studies that are routinely ordered for patients with potential obstruction and perforation of the intestine include hematocrit, sodium, potassium, magnesium, calcium, BUN, amylase, and osmolality. Leukocytosis may be used to evaluate different types of obstruction. Simple obstruction will cause mild elevations in the WBC count ($10.0–15.0/mm^3$), strangulation will probably cause moderate elevations ($15.0–25.0/mm^3$), and mesenteric occlusion or perforation will produce high WBC counts ($25.0/mm^3$).[28] The laboratory tests will provide information regarding intravascular fluid shifts and possible malabsorption of essential electrolytes. Nurses should be aware that other nutrients not commonly measured will also be deficient in cases of lower small bowel obstruction. These may include zinc, copper, iron, vitamin K, and folic acid. Loss of these minerals and vitamins can cause poor wound healing, coagulopathies, and various types of anemia.

Despite a large quantity of physical and laboratory indicators of intestinal obstruction, definitive diagnosis of strangulation is possible in only three-quarters of cases. A summary of significant signs and symptoms of different types of obstructions is given in Table 6-20. Radiologic exam of the abdomen is considered the primary source of confirmation of a diagnosis of bowel obstruction. Three-position abdominal x-rays should be taken to evaluate all possible etiologies of obstruction. The patient is instructed to sit upright, to lie flat, and to lie on his or her side. The side selected will vary with the location of abdominal discomfort. Paralytic and mechanical ob-

Table 6-20 Clinical Presentations of Bowel Obstruction

Parameter	High Small Bowel	Low Small Bowel	Large Bowel
Onset	Acute	Short-term but less acute	Insidious
Emesis	Prominent symptom, often feculent	Vomiting present on occasion, but not feculent	Absent or occurs very late
Pain	Frequent crampy, crescendo-decrescendo pain, every 4 to 5 minutes	Crampy intermittent pain; less frequent (every 15 to 20 minutes)	Crampy, less severe pain; not associated with eating
Abdominal distension	Minimal or absent	Noticeable	Pronounced
Bowel habits	Watery fluid from rectum	Obstipation once distal tract emptied	Diarrhea, ribbon-like stools, and eventually obstipation
Dehydration	Early, life-threatening	Moderate, may be life-threatening	Late
Electrolyte and acid-base imbalances	Common, but not severe	Common, severe	Rare

structions of the small bowel often look similar on x-ray, but key differences do exist. Paralytic ileus is most likely to show copious gas throughout the intestine and colon, high fluid levels in the intestine, and a severely elevated diaphragm. Simple mechanical obstructions present with low gas levels in the colon, moderate fluid levels in the intestine, and a mildly elevated diaphragm.[29]

When a colonic obstruction is confirmed by x-ray, a barium study is usually indicated to identify the precise type of obstruction (paralytic, simple mechanical, or strangulated). However, the risks of complete obstruction or perforation associated with this procedure may outweigh its benefits in some clinical situations.

After thorough physical, laboratory, and radiologic assessment have indicated that an obstruction exists, a treatment paln geared to the patient's specific etiology and clinical condition must be formulated.

Nursing standards of care

Conservative management of intestinal obstruction is preferred whenever there is little risk of perforation or sepsis. Conservative management consists of (1) giving the patient nothing by mouth, (2) providing gastroduodenal decompression, and (3) correcting the underlying etiology. When the patient has an intestinal obstruction of whatever origin, the digestive and absorptive functions of the GI tract are incompetent and must be addressed through external means.

It is important to eliminate all ingested food and water until the disorder is resolved. Stimulation of the intestine during this time will only serve to increase the abdominal pain and intraluminal pressure, as well as cause reverse peristalsis. Even ice or sips of fluid can be dangerous as precipitators of these problems. If food and fluid cannot be provided intravenously, supplementation of both should be considered. Patients cannot tolerate the withholding of fluid for more than 8–12 hours, and food abstinence exceeding 3 days may lead to nutritional deficiencies. Many patients will be supplemented with peripheral or parenteral hyperalimentation.

Decompression of excess fluid and air above the obstruction and removal of the normal digestive secretions, which cannot be processed, is accomplished via nasogastric suction. A Levin or sump tube is placed in the stomach or high duodenum to drain secretions produced in this area, thoroughly rest the obstructed gut, and reduce the risk of pulmo-

nary aspiration. High small bowel obstructions, particularly those of a mechanical nature, may be treated with a Cantor or Miller-Abbott intestinal tube. This is a mercury-tipped tube that is passed into the stomach; changes in the patient's position and normal peristaltic waves facilitate its progression into the distal small bowel. This treatment is indicated in partial and complete lower small intestine obstructions. The tube may be able to pass through partial obstructions and drain the small bowel from the distal side, or may lessen the acute symptoms by forging a pathway through the bowel lumen. This is considered a short-term measure and may not be sufficient with severe obstructions.

When conservative measures for relief of obstruction fail, endoscopic or surgical intervention may be indicated. Bowel obstructions requiring surgical intervention are usually not paralytic and rarely involve the distal colon. Some advocate early surgery to provide the patient with the best opportunity for an uncomplicated recovery. Surgery should be performed before extreme abdominal distention and dehydration occur. Four situations call for the use of surgery as an emergent procedure: strangulation, early mechanical obstruction, colonic obstruction, and closed-loop obstruction. Surgical procedures for relief of intestinal obstruction vary according to the location and etiology of the obstruction. Common surgical procedures may include excision of external factors compressing the bowel, enterotomy and removal of the obstruction, resection with an end-to-end anastomosis, and formation of a cutaneous ostomy. The goal of all surgical procedures is to remove all ischemic or necrotic tissue to prevent sepsis and gangrene.

Pre- and postoperative vascular volume assessment through a central venous catheter is essential, as is accurate intake and output assessment using a Foley catheter. Volume replacement with electrolyte-rich fluids (Ringer's solution or Ringer's lactate) and antibiotics is used with all patients. Postoperative care is the same as with all abdominal surgeries. Fluid sequestration in the abdomen and the resultant hypovolemia are more prevalent in this type of patient than in those who have undergone other stomach, esophageal, or colorectal procedures.

The nursing care of the patient with obstruction or perforation of the intestine is highly variable, because of the various types of obstruction and the many functional areas of the GI tract. Nurses caring for these patients are challenged to provide concise and complete descriptions of all symptoms to assist in locating the obstruction. Frequent laboratory monitoring and careful fluid balance assessment are essential for regulation of the treatment plan. The major objectives of a nurse caring for a patient with potential obstruction or perforation should be (1) to assist in the maintenance of fluid, electrolyte, and nutritional balance through assessment and medical or surgical intervention; (2) to provide for patient comfort by decreasing abdominal pain and distention and maintain the decompression tubes used in treatment; (3) to observe the patient for acute life-threatening complications such as strangulation, perforation, septicemia, or adult respiratory distress syndrome.

Nursing Care Plan for the Management of the Patient with Intestional Infarction, Obstruction, or Perforation

Diagnosis	Signs and symptoms	Intervention	Rationale
Fluid volume deficit due to fluid shifts	Decreased CVP Orthostasis or frank hypotension Increased weight Increased abdominal girth	Monitoring vital signs often, including temperature, respiration, BP, and CVP	Hypotension from fluid shifts is common in perforation; increased temperature is indicative of dehydration or septicemia
	Excessive output from NG tubes or drains	Administer fluids or colloids PRN (Ringer's lactate, Ringer's solution, blood products, albumin)	High-solute fluids may be less likely to leak from vascular space
		Weigh patient every day	Weight is a good indication of fluids in body (but not in vascular space)
		Keep meticulous I&O records	
		Monitor electrolytes twice daily	Electrolyte abnormalities (decreased calcium, magnesium, and potassium) are common with obstructions
		Monitor and note any diarrhea or emesis	Diarrhea and emesis exacerbate electrolyte abnormalities
		Measure abdominal girth every shift	Increasing abdominal girth results from fluid shifts in abdomen (common with perforation and lower bowel obstruction)
		Measure GI drainage at least every 8 hrs; replace output as often hourly as indicated	Massive GI losses must be replaced hourly to minimize fluid volume deficit

Nursing Care Plan for the Management of the Patient with Intestinal Infarction, Obstruction, or Perforation

Diagnosis	Signs and symptoms	Intervention	Rationale
Potential for infection	Fever Leukocytosis Diagnostic evidence of abscess or infection Feculent NG drainage	Culture blood and all excretions whenever there is a change in appearance or a change in patient's condition	New infections may be evident in cultures at any time, purulent drainage is not always evident with infection
		Monitor CBC differential at least every 3 days (possibly every day)	Elevated granulocytes (neutrophils, basophils, and eosinophils) indicate a bacterial infection (left shift)
		Monitor temperature every 2–4 hours Administer antibiotics as ordered and monitor antibiotic levels; stat antibiotics (within 1 hour) of suspected perforation	Fever is often an early sign of infection, although subnormal temperatures are also potentially dangerous
		Monitor characteristics of NG drainage	Feculent NG drainage is present with high bacteria and stagnant secretions
Altered nutrition: intake insufficient for body requirements	Weight loss greater than or equal to 10% of baseline Hypoalbuminemia Anergy to skin tests Elevated BUN or nitrogenous wastes in urine	Assess etiologies of reduced nutrition (catabolism, disrupted GI tract, vomiting, diarrhea)	Various etiologies of malnutrition need to be corrected in different fashions
		Obtain consult with nutritionist	Nutritionist will perform anthropometric tests and other assessments of nutritional demands
	Negative nitrogen balance identified through 24-hour urine and nitrogen intake tests	Administer nutritional supplements (PPN, TPN) as ordered	Most patients will require nutritional support until GI tract function returns

Diagnosis	Signs and symptoms	Intervention	Rationale
	Muscle wasting	Maintain NPO status with obstruction or perforation	To avoid contamination of gut with flora
	Oral lesions		
	Poor condition of skin, hair, nails	Accurate I&O measurements	To avoid dehydration
	Anemia	Provide skin care precautions to prevent breakdown	Malnourished patients have less integumentary reserve and are likely to experience skin breakdown
	Vomiting with decreased K, Ca$^+$, Mg$^+$, Cl$^-$		
Pain	Patient complains of discomfort	Assess pain location, precipitators, and alleviators	Abdominal pain may be characteristic of specific etiology
	Abdominal muscle rigidity	Pain medication as ordered for postoperative care or acute management; evaluate pain on scale of 1 to 10 (or other appropriate scale) before and after administration of medication	All patients should be relieved of discomfort, but caution should be exercised to avoid masking differential pain, which may be diagnostic
	Abdominal guarding		
	Nonverbal cues of abdominal discomfort (such as clutching, positioning, restlessness, or tachypnea)		
	Rebound tenderness		
		Provide nonpharmacological interventions for pain relief and diversional activities	Nonpharmacological pain management may enhance efficacy of other pain management strategies
		Administer stool softeners while patient is on medication	To avoid complication of constipation, which contributes to ileus
		Provide pillow for splinting abdomen for coughing and deep breathing postoperatively	Enhances effectiveness of coughing
		Place patient in position of comfort	Patients with ascites are more comfortable in low Fowler's; patients with rebound tenderness are more comfortable with knees flexed

Nursing Care Plan for the Management of the Patient with Intestional Infarction, Obstruction, or Perforation

Diagnosis	Signs and symptoms	Intervention	Rationale
Altered tissue perfusion in brain, lungs, heart, kidneys	Confusion Hypoxemia Hypotension Oliguria Cyanosis	Provide vigorous volume expansion with some obstructions and all perforations	Fluid can shift into peritoneum and cause severe hypovolemia
		Assess weight every day, abdominal girth every shift, CVPs every 4 hours, and vital signs every 2 hours	To evaluate both intravascular and extravascular volume
		Neurological assessment or mini mental exam at least every shift	Neurological changes may reflect changes in tissue perfusion
		Respiratory status with pulse oximetry and ABGs after potential perforation	Patients with perforation are extremely prone to ARDS
		Urine output measurement every 1–2 hours after suspected perforation	Provides a good measurement of vascular volume
Potential for ineffective gas exchange	Signs and symptoms of respiratory distress: hypoxemia, peripheral cyanosis, and/or air hunger	Coughing, deep breathing, and incentive spirometry every 4 hours; perform FVC or FEV when tachypnea, dyspnea, or hypoxemia indicates possible ARDS	Patients are at high risk for development of ARDS after perforation
		Perform ABGs as ordered to evaluate respiratory distress or monitor oxygen therapy	ABGs are the best indicator of respiratory failure, which is one of the most common complications of perforation
		When possible, use prophylactic pulse oximetry for perforations	Oximeter approximates O_2 saturation and will show occurrence of hypoxemia

Diagnosis	Signs and symptoms	Intervention	Rationale
Potential for injury related to mechanical devices used to decompress intestine	Heme positive gastric secretions Gastric secretion pH < 3 Nare erosion	Maintain NG tube per hospital policy; check NG/intestinal tube placement and patency every 4 hours	Aspiration is potential complication of misplaced NG tube
		Monitor gastric drainage tube output; perform heme test; plan for fluid and electrolyte replacement	Excessive gastrointestinal drainage may cause dehydration
		Administer antacids, sucralfate, or histamine blockers as ordered;	Ulcer prevention regimens are usually implemented when patients have NG or intestinal tubes
		If intestinal tube is used: do not tape to nose; document markings on daily flow sheet; have patient rotate positions every 2 hours for up to 2 days while passing tube	Tube relieves obstruction by moving through intestinal tract via peristaltic waves and positioning. Monitoring progression of tube ensures efficacy of treatment
Alteration in elimination	Obstipation Abdominal distention	Evaluate abdominal girth and evidence of distention	
	Thin, ribbon-like stools	Monitor stool output and describe appearance and heme test	Watery stools indicate small bowel obstruction; thin, ribbon-like stools indicate large bowel obstruction

Medications Commonly Used in the Care of the Patient with Intestinal Infarction, Obstruction, or Perforation

Medication	Effect	Major side effects

Antibiotics (coverage for gram-negative anaerobes):
  Aminoglycoside
  Penicillin
  Beta lactam
  Clindamycin
	Reduce bacterial contamination of peritoneum, prevent sepsis	Hypersensitivity reactions
		Renal dysfunction
		Ototoxicity
		Diarrhea, GI distress
		Other drug-specific effects
		Risk of superinfection with fungus

Dopamine (1–4 mcg/kg/min)	Stimulates dopaminergic receptors to cause renal and splanchnic vasodilation	Tachycardia, dysrhythmias Peripheral constriction Hypertension Tissue necrosis with extravasation
Nitroglycerin	Venodilation and vasodilation to increase blood flow to mesentery	Hypotension Headache
Neostigmine	Parasympathomimetic agent that inhibits cholinesterase and enhances cholinergic activity such as GI motility. Used in ileus, but should be avoided in patient with obstruction.	Tremors, muscle fasiculations Weakness Bradycardia Hypotension

Gastrointestinal Bleeding

Gastrointestinal bleeding is identified when frank or old blood is lost through a gastrointestinal orifice. (Oral or gum bleeding is not usually included within this definition.) The gastrointestinal tract is particularly prone to bleeding because of the extensive vasculature that lies close to the mucosal surface. People normally lose small amounts of blood daily via the GI tract from normal red cell hemolysis and minor abrasions of the mucosa; however, acute gastrointestinal bleeding is abnormal and is a common reason for admission to the ICU as well as a complication encountered by ICU patients. Statistics show that 70% of patients with gastrointestinal disease will present with gastrointestinal bleeding,[30] but in as many as 80% of these cases, the bleeding stops spontaneously without treatment.[31] Hemorrhage (loss of more than 1000 cc of blood) is more significant in patients with hematemesis (vomiting of blood) than in those with hematochezia (bright red blood from the rectum) or melana (black, tarry stools). The mortality rate of these patients is also 50% higher.[32] Despite technological advances in intensive care, acute GI hemorrhage still results in a 10% mortality rate.[33] Etiologies and specific therapies for gastrointestinal bleeding from various sites will differ, but general assessment and management is the same in all cases.

Clinical antecedents

Gastrointestinal bleeding can range from occult (heme test positive without visible blood) to frankly hemorrhagic. Gastrointestinal bleeding is classified as upper or lower GI bleeding based upon the location of bloody drainage. Melana usually indicates bleeding in the esophagus, stomach, or duodenum, but slow bleeds occurring lower in the GI tract may also present as melana. Examples of different types of upper and lower GI bleeding are listed in Table 6-21. Rarely does bleeding occur from the middle of the intestine (jejunum or ileum). The most common causes of upper GI bleeding are (1) peptic ulcers, (2) erosive gastritis, (3) esophageal varices, and (4) esophageal tears.[34] There are numerous other causes of GI bleeding, and for all of these there are classic populations at risk and presenting symptoms. Recognition of specific risk factors such as age, concurrent medical conditions, and medication profiles may assist in the identification of etiology. For example, lower GI bleeding in the older patient is likely to result from tumors, diverticulitis, or ischemic colitis, none of which are common in young adults. Many nongastrointestinal medical conditions predispose patients to GI bleeding. The most common are uremia, hepatic failure, trauma, burns, and alcoholism. Medications most often associated with a predisposition for GI bleeding are listed in Table 6-22.

The first goal of caregivers of patients with acute gastrointestinal hemorrhage is the isolation of the bleeding site and institution of the specific measures that will alleviate the bleeding. Thus, differentiation of the etiology is essential.

Critical referents

Whatever its etiology, gastrointestinal bleeding causes loss of vascular blood components and accumulation of blood in the GI tract. The major physiologic effect is profound hypovolemia. Significant blood loss from either the upper or lower GI tract can lead to life-threatening perfusion deficits and coagulopathies. Pathophysiological effects are primarily the same as those of hemorrhagic shock. Blood lost from the vasculature stimulates the sympathetic nervous system (SNS) and baroreceptors within the carotid vessels. Sympathetic stimulation causes peripheral vasoconstriction, increased heart rate, increased inotropic force of the heart, central shunting of blood, and fluid conservation. Both SNS and baroreceptor stimulation cause the release of ADH and potentiate sodium and water retention.

Pathophysiology of specific GI bleeding varies according to the site involved. The most common causes of GI bleeding in the ICU are esophageal varices, peptic ulcers (gastric and duodenal), abdominal trauma, and inflammatory or ischemic bowel disease. To understand these specific presentations and pathophysiology, it is essential to be familiar with the normal blood supply of the GI tract. The arterial blood supply is so extensive that erosions into the walls of any GI structure are likely to produce arterial bleeding. A knowledge of the GI vessel network and the anatomic area each vessel supplies allows the nurse to predict that a doudenal ulcer may produce bleeding from the gastroduodenal artery, for example, or that a colorectal bleed involves the inferior mesenteric artery.

Venous circulation of the GI tract was outlined earlier in the section on gastrointestinal anatomy and physiology. Venous systems are generally low-pressure systems, but pressure may be increased with high volumes of blood flow or reduced liver capacity. This high pressure and congestion of blood within

Table 6-21 Common Types of Gastrointestinal Bleeding

Location	Disorder	Population at Risk	Level of Risk	Signs and Symptoms
Upper GI Tract Esophagus	Esophagitis	Immunosuppressed Those with infections of oral cavity or esophagus Recipients of chemotherapy Recipients of head and neck radiation therapy	Moderate	Dysphagia Hematemesis
	Mallory-Weiss tears at gastroesophageal junction	Any age, though often older adults During vomiting, coughing	Severe	Sudden, severe blood loss (hematemesis) after coughing or retching
	Esophageal varices	Cirrhosis Portal hypertension Alcohol abuse	Severe	Sudden severe blood loss (hematemesis) Sense of impending doom Maroon stool
	Also: Esophageal ulcer, cancer, or rupture			
Stomach or large bowel	Peptic ulcer (gastric or duodenal)	Hypersecretion of HCl Stress (physical or emotional) Alcohol abuse	Severe	Gastric/abdominal pain relieved by eating Duodenal/abdominal pain that increases after eating Melana Hematemesis
	Erosive gastritis	Adults, usually over 25 years old	Moderate	Abdominal pain not relieved by eating Melana Hematemesis
	Crohn's disease, ileitis	Young adults	Moderate	Abdominal cramping after eating Melana Fever Moderate diarrhea
Lower GI Tract Large bowel	Meckel's diverticulum	Children and young adults Familial tendency	Mild	Moderate bleeding, red or maroon in color
	Ulcerative colitis	Those receiving antibiotics or radiation to abdomen Familial tendency	Moderate	Crampy pain prior to or during defecation Frankly bloody stools Diarrhea
	Diverticulosis	Likelihood increases progressively with age after 40	Mild	Crampy abdominal pain during defecation Bloody diarrhea
	Polyps	All ages Familial tendency	Mild	Occult blood in stool Blood mixed with stool Usually painless bleeding from rectum Usually mild blood loss
	Colorectal carcinoma	Familial tendency High-fat, low-fiber diet Refractory, untreated ulcerative colitis	Mild	Painless, occult or obvious blood in stool Thin, ribbon-like stools Low back pain
Rectum/anus	Hemorrhoids	Obese persons Those who sit much of the time	Mild	Blood with stool or directly from rectum
	Anorectal fissure	Any age Constipation and passage of hard stools Anorectal sex	Mild	Blood with stool or directly from rectum
	Also: Ischemic, antibiotic, or radiation- or chemotherapy-induced colitis Amyloidosis Aortic-intestinal fistula			

Table 6-22 Medications Predisposing Patients to GI Bleeding

Class of Medication	Examples
Salicylates and derivatives	Aspirin Bufferin Alka-Seltzer Cold formulas
Antiinflammatory agents	Indomethacin Phenylbutazone Naprosyn Corticosteroids
Antibiotics	Tetracycline Erythromycin Flucytosine Rifampicin
Anticoagulants/ antiplatelets	Warfarin Heparin Streptokinase Urokinase Activase Dipyrimadole
General	Oral potassium chloride Cancer chemotherapy agents Alcohol

the gastrointestinal venous system, known as portal hypertension, leads to distention and inappropriate stretching of the veins. Weakened areas in the venous walls are called varicosities, or varices. Although varicosities may occur in any vein, their occurrence within the gastrointestinal vessels heralds a potential risk of rupture and bleeding. Clinically significant, bleeding varicosities are most likely to be present in the esophagus, duodenum, or rectum. Esophageal varices cause the most acute and life-threatening of all GI bleeding. Patients with esophageal varices are usually cirrhotic and suffering from high portal pressures. This increases the risk of hemorrhage with rupture of the varicosity. The mortality rate among patients who begin bleeding from esophageal varices is 65%, and bleeding recurs in 65% of those who do survive the first hemorrhagic event.[35] Only 25% of patients with esophageal varices survive longer than 2 years.[36]

Direct erosion or damage to a section of the GI system will also lead to gastrointestinal bleeding. Upper GI bleeding is a result of erosions (ulcers) of the esophagus, stomach, and duodenum; erosions comprise 50–70% of all upper GI bleeds.[37] These ulcers are all termed peptic ulcers, but each has specific defining characteristics, as outlined in Table 6-23.

A Mallory-Weiss syndrome is a tear of the mucosa near the gastroesophageal junction. The patient presents with severe vomiting or recent trauma and has sudden, severe, gastrointestinal hemorrhage with hematemesis. Although uncommon, it is a well-described syndrome and should be considered in the differential diagnosis of severe acute upper GI bleeding.

Lower GI bleeding has been associated with a variety of etiologies ranging from hemorrhoids to transmural intestinal erosion resulting from tumors or inflammatory bowel disease. Bleeding risks ranging from mild to moderate or severe have been associated with these various etiologies. The clinical signs of various degrees of blood loss are listed in Table 6-24.

Resulting signs and symptoms

It is important for the nurse to make astute observations regarding the nature, color, severity, and resolution of any GI bleeding. Occult blood in the stool is usually indicative of loss of less than 15–20 mL of blood per day.[38] Black, tarry stools (melana) will occur when the loss has been at least 60 mL of blood per day or when blood has remained in the gut for 6–8 hours.[39] Blood loss of greater than 60 cc but less than 500 cc for up to three days will produce melana.[40] Patients with losses greater than 500 cc are likely to be hemodynamically unstable.[41] Minor blood loss may produce hemodynamic changes in elderly or anemic patients, as their reserve blood supply is smaller than that of the younger, normovolemic patient. Brisker rates of bleeding produce characteristic symptoms such as hematemesis or hematochezia. As many as 50% of patients with hematemesis also present with melana, but the reverse is not true.[42] On occasion, blood remains in the GI tract for a time and may range from dark red to maroon when expelled by vomiting or from the rectum. Blood that has come in contact with gastric acid becomes dark and looks like coffee grounds. In assessment it is important to document the relationship of the bleeding to past medical history (bleeding occurring in same or different location), emotional distress, medications, drainage tube manipulation, and specific laboratory values (for example, platelet count).

The major signs of gastrointestinal bleeding are hypovolemia and acute compromise in tissue perfusion. Common symptoms of hypovolemia may include tachycardia, orthostasis or hypotension, syncope, light-headedness, nausea, sweating, thirst, anxiety, hypothermia, oliguria, and low central venous pressure. The degree of hypotension and

Table 6-23   Classification of Peptic Ulcers*

Type	Risk Factors	Pathophysiology	Frequency	Likelihood of Developing into Malignancy	Hemorrhagic Tendency
Esophageal erosions	Candida esophagitis Caustic ingestion Existing varices Mucosites from cancer chemotherapy	Toxic ingestion or high portal pressures produce tissue injury and partial thickness erosion	Unusual	Unlikely	Severe
Gastric erosions	Aspirin Alcohol Caustic ingestion	Exposure of gastric mucosa to toxic substances with partial thickness erosion	Very common in ICU or with NG suction	Mild	Mild to severe
Gastric ulcer	Previous gastric surgery Hyperacidity	Break in mucosal barrier allowing backwash of HCl; most common in pylorus	20% of all peptic ulcers	Severe	Severe
Duodenal ulcer	Corticosteroids Hyperacidity	Increased amounts of HCl in duodenum	80% of all peptic ulcers	Unlikely	Moderate
Stress ulcer	Sepsis Trauma Shock Burns (Curling's ulcer) Head injury (Cushing's ulcer)	Ischemic damage to gastric mucosa causing ulceration of stomach, esophagus, or duodenum	Occurs in approximately 40% of risk groups	Mild (depends upon site)	Mild to moderate

*Peptic ulcers can be esophageal ulcers, gastric ulcers, or duodenal ulcers (including stress ulcers)

tachycardia at presentation and prior to fluid administration approximately reflects the amount of blood lost. In severe hypovolemia, all organs are affected by the compromised cardiac output and many show signs or symptoms of dysfunction or failure. Ischemic complications such as myocardial infarction or acute renal failure are not uncommon. Table 6-25 summarizes the clinical signs and symptoms seen in the patient suffering GI bleeding.

When bleeding in the GI tract occurs, a large amount of blood remains in the GI canal and participates in exchange through the mucosal wall. The heavy blood (protein) load within the GI tract leads to increased BUN, increased total bilirubin, possible elevated hepatic transaminases, low transferrin and ferritin levels, elevated reticulocyte levels, and hyperphosphatemia. These laboratory tests are not always abnormal and may be dependent upon the amount of blood lost, how quickly it was lost, and the patient's specific organ function. It is important to realize that the hematocrit is not always an accurate reflection of the severity of GI bleeding because of the consequences of hemoconcentration. Hemoglobin levels, RBC indices, and red cell morphology may be more helpful in determining amount of blood lost.

Table 6-24   Clinical Presentation in Acute Gastrointestinal Hemorrhage

Blood Loss	Clinical Presentation
Less than 500 cc	Patient is usually asymptomatic
Less than 20% blood volume (approximately 1000 cc)	Orthostasis
Approximately 40% or more of blood volume loss (approximately 2000 cc)	Shock

Table 6-25 Signs and Symptoms of GI Bleeding

Cause	Symptoms
Blood loss	Melana
	Hematemesis
	Hematochezia
	Coffee-ground emesis
	Bloody drainage
	Cyanosis
	Low Hct/Hgb/RBC
	Elevated reticulocytes
	Decreased platelets
	Abnormal coagulation profile
	Elevated BUN
Hypovolemia	Anxiety, confusion
	Tachypnea, dyspnea, hypoxemia, cyanosis
	Tachycardia, dysrhythmias, systolic murmur
	Hypotension, orthostasis, CVP < 1 mm Hg
	Oliguria/anuria, high urine specific gravity
	Thirst
	Poor skin turgor
	Elevated BUN and creatinine
	Hypernatremia
	Hyperosmolarity
Blood replacement	Hypothermia
	Coagulopathy
	Hypocalcemia
	Hyperkalemia
	Metabolic acidosis

For example, microcytic anemia (small RBCs) is a signal of chronic blood loss, and a decreased MCH (mean corpuscular hemoglobin) indicates that hemoglobin saturation is decreased, reflecting RBCs lost. Blood remains in the GI tract for up to 7–12 days after a hemorrhage has occurred.[43] The patient with GI bleeding may require massive blood transfusions, which cause additional lab abnormalities (see Table 6-16).

Diagnostic evaluation of GI bleeding can be divided into procedures used for suspected upper GI bleeds and those for lower GI bleeds. With any patient presumed to have significant lower GI bleeding, a nasogastric tube should be passed to rule out the possibility of a rapid upper GI bleed. Radiologic and endoscopic procedures are the preferred method of determining the source of bleeding. An overview of nonlaboratory diagnostic procedures is given in Table 6-26. Radiologic procedures such as upper or lower GI series can be combined with special examination of the suspected area of bleeding. Unfortunately, these procedures are of limited use during active bleeding. Scopic procedures (endoscopy, sigmoidoscopy, and proctoscopy) allow direct visualization of the GI tract and potential access for surgical interventions such as cautery or laser surgery. They are the preferred methods of confirming GI bleeding. When scopic procedures do not reveal a bleeding site and the patient continues to suffer from life-threatening bleeding, arteriography is employed. It is recommended that arteriography be employed when (1) bleeding persists long enough to cause hemodynamic instability; (2) active bleeding persists despite a known source; and (3) patient shows evidence of significant "coffee ground" material but bleeding is not brisk enough to be noted on endoscopic exam.[44] Cannulation of the descending aorta and any of the gastrointestinal branches (gastroduodenal, superior mesenteric, or inferior mesenteric) may provide information regarding arterial bleeding not visible through endoscopy. Surgical correction may be performed but is often not possible because the bleeding is beyond the reach of the catheter. When arteriography fails to identify the site of bleeding, an unusual test called a bleeding scan may be performed. Bleeding scans are most useful in the diagnosis of intermittent bleeding, provided it occurs within 24 hours of injecting technetium-99.[45] Surgical exploration may be required in a small number of patients, but it is a last resort because it carries with it a high morbidity and mortality.

Nursing standards of care

Conservative medical management of GI bleeding is preferred and attempted in all patients with bleeding of unknown origin. The conservative approach includes the use of nasogastric tubes with lavage, gut rest, and blood volume and product replacement. During this therapy, patient risk factors as well as the nature, location, and severity of the bleeding will indicate which diagnostic procedures should be emphasized. If bleeding is not severe, the patient will be stabilized, and radiologic procedures will be performed after the resolution of bleeding. Specific risk factors such as alcoholism or existing coagulopathies may dictate a more aggressive and immediate diagnostic evaluation.

Vascular volume replacement is essential for tissue survival and reduction of multisystem side effects. Vascular volume should be replaced with normal saline, lactated Ringer's solution, and albumin until blood products are available.[46] Intravenous fluid should be run "wide open" until the blood pressure stabilizes and then should be adjusted to match the volume lost until vital signs stabilize. As

Table 6-26   Diagnostic Tests for Determining Site of GI Bleeding

Test	Area	Indications
Endoscopy		
Esophagogastroduodenoscopy	Esophagus, stomach, duodenum	Hematemesis
Endoscopic retrograde cholangiopancreatography (ERCP)	Ampulla of Vater for pancreas Cystic duct	Suspected pancreatitis or cholangitis with bleeding
Colonoscopy	Descending colon up to flexure of transverse colon	Hematochezia (blood may be darker, indicating higher lesion) Inconclusive sigmoidoscopy
Sigmoidoscopy	Sigmoid colon up to curve of descending colon	Hematochezia (rapid, bright red blood loss) Inconclusive proctoscopy
Proctoscopy	Rectum and beginning of sigmoid colon	Hematochezia Pre-existing hemorrhoids Screening for colorectal cancer
Radiography		
Barium swallow	Entire upper GI tract	Melana Intermittent heme-positive NG drainage or hematemesis
Barium enema	Lower GI tract	Melana after barium swallow that is inconclusive Intermittent, not severe hematochezia
Angiography		
Arteriogram	Any GI artery branch of the aorta can be visualized	Refractory bleeding with inconclusive barium studies or scopic procedures Rapid, life-threatening blood loss of unknown origin

blood products become available, red blood cells will be administered as the first priority unless the cause of bleeding is a coagulopathy (such as thrombocytopenia), indicating the need for specific component replacement first. A maximum of 3 points rise in the hematocrit with each unit of blood can be expected if the patient is no longer bleeding.[47] Because the lost blood also contained coagulation proteins, care must be taken to replace these with platelets, fresh frozen plasma, and possibly cryoprecipitate as well. (Additional information regarding massive transfusions and their side effects can be found in the chapter on Hematology.)

A nasogastric tube is inserted in all patients with upper GI bleeding. After tube placement is confirmed by withdrawal of identifiable stomach contents or by air injection, the tube is flushed with tepid normal saline until the returns are clear. It is recommended that flush solutions be allowed to drain freely or with minimal suction to prevent injury to the stomach mucosa.[48] The amount of flush required to eliminate bleeding should be documented. Some ICUs set up a continuous three-way flush system; others perform this procedure manually. Several methodologies that were used in the past are now

believed to contribute to gastric mucosal ischemia and possible bleeding. For example, it is no longer considered appropriate to lavage with iced fluid or diluted vasopressor substances (norepinephrine).[49]

If the bleeding is difficult to resolve, some practitioners advocate sending a sample of the gastric aspirate for hematocrit and hemoglobin evaluation. This will demonstrate how much blood is actually being lost, unlike the measurement of diluted bloody fluid. Gastric heme testing should be performed routinely throughout the recovery period. Much controversy has surrounded the use of antacids to increase gastric pH to reduce GI bleeding. Current thinking is that the alkaline pH levels of gastric secretions stimulate the constant secretion of HCl, potentially leading to ulceration[50] and aspiration pneumonia. Current recommendations support the use of histamine blockers (ranitidine, cimetidine, Famotidine) to block HCl secretions and prevent ulcers, with the addition of sucralfate (Carafate) and possibly antacids if ulcers do form.[51]

In severe upper GI bleeding that occurs above the level of the stomach (gastroesophageal junction, esophagus), a balloon tamponading tube (either a Sengstaken-Blakemore or a Minnesota tube) may be

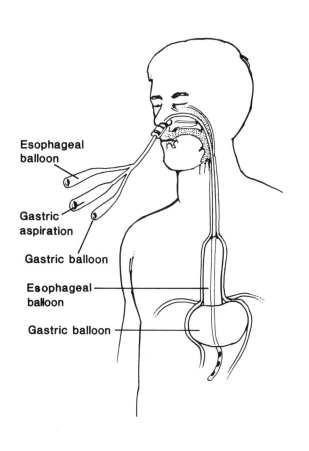

Esophageal
balloon

Gastric
aspiration

Gastric balloon

Esophageal
balloon

Gastric balloon

Figure 6-11   Sengstaken-Blakemore Tube

inserted. This therapy is at least temporarily effective in 40–85% of patients.[52] A diagram of the Sengstaken-Blakemore tube is shown in Figure 6-11. The Minnesota tube is similar, except that it also has an esophageal aspiration port that is designed to prevent the aspiration of fluids that accumulate above the esophageal balloon. The tube is inserted into the stomach, and the stomach balloon is inflated and pulled up against the esophageal-cardiac junction. If bleeding is from above this point, the tube is held in traction while the esophageal balloon is also inflated. These two balloons alleviate hemorrhage by applying direct pressure to the bleeding site. In either case, the tube is pulled into a traction position to maintain pressure. Stabilization of the traction position externally is essential; in some cases this is accomplished by use of a special traction block or by taping the tube to a hat worn by the patient. This therapy should be reserved for extreme and unresponsive bleeding, as it has been proven only temporarily successful and may cause local tissue necrosis. Most centers now

attempt both arteriography and vasopressin administration prior to using this measure.

Arteriography with cautery has become the state-of-the-art management approach for both upper and lower GI bleeds.[53] Cautery or laser-beam therapy causes tissue necrosis and coagulation of the bleeding site. Specific ulcerations may be responsive to these therapies. However, friable mucosa with diffuse bleeding is unlikely to respond as markedly. If the site of bleeding cannot be isolated or specifically treated during arteriography, infusion of vasopressin into the splanchnic bed (intraarterially, or intravenously) may be attempted. Vasopressin (Desmopressin) causes specific mesenteric and coronary vasoconstriction, and can reduce bleeding through a reduction of blood flow to the area and decreased portal vein pressure. The normal dosage is usually 0.1–0.9 unit/min, although some literature will suggest doses up to 1.5 unit/min.[54] This therapy is recommended for short-term use only and if continued for more than 72 hours may increase the risk of ischemic events. Some clinicians now advocate the use of intravenous nitroglycerin in conjunction with vasopressin in order to reduce the latter's cardiovascular side effects.[55] There are also anecdotal reports of the effectiveness of high-dose estrogen therapy and somatostatin infusion in the management of GI bleeding.

Management of the patient with gastrointestinal bleeding requires extensive analytical and decision-making skills. Clinicians are often confused by differences between upper and lower GI bleeding and the various treatment options. Several algorithms to assist in this decision-making process are shown in Figure 6-12.

Vigilant monitoring of the complete blood count, reticulocyte count (a count of young RBCs released from the bone marrow during anemic stress), coagulation studies, and calcium levels will assist clinicians in assessing the patient's response to therapy. Other laboratory studies that may complement this focused view of the patient include renal function tests, hepatic function tests, and BUN levels.

Surgical intervention for GI bleeding is reserved for the patient with refractory bleeding caused by identified, surgically correctable problems such as trauma to the GI tract, peptic ulcers, inflammatory bowel disease, or ischemic colitis. Other disorders such as esophageal varices may require surgical intervention once bleeding has resolved. Common surgeries for GI bleeding and the post-operative management of these patients are described in the following section on GI surgery. Surgery usually involves removal of the severely ulcerated area and reanastomosis between the stomach, duodenum,

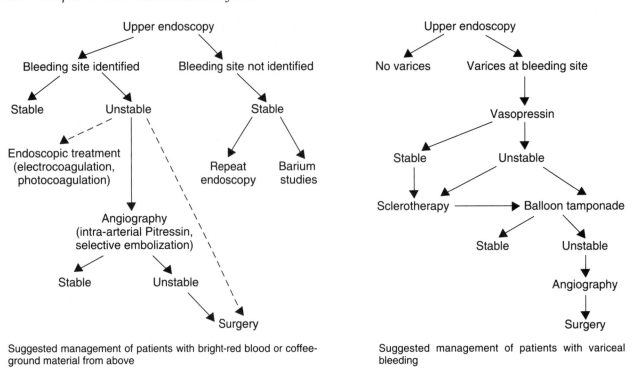

Suggested management of patients with bright-red blood or coffee-ground material from above

Suggested management of patients with variceal bleeding

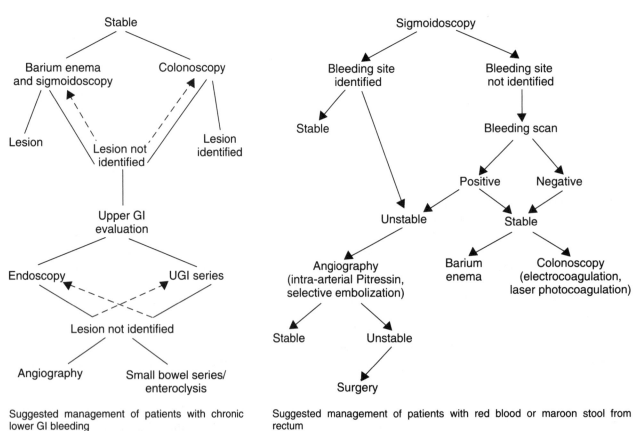

Suggested management of patients with chronic lower GI bleeding

Suggested management of patients with red blood or maroon stool from rectum

Figure 6-12   Algorithms for Management of Various Types of Bleeding

and/or jejunum. Severing of the vagus nerve (vagotomy) may also be performed in certain circumstances. Removal of certain parts of the stomach may lead to deficiency of intrinsic factor and pernicious anemia.

The role of the nurse in management of GI bleeding focuses upon risk assessment, emergency management, and evaluation of responses to therapy. Care of GI bleeding patients is labor-intensive and requires rapid decision making. Nurses must be proficient in managing NG or Sengstaken-Blakemore tubes, volume expansion and transfusion therapy, and vasopressin administration. Goals of nursing care include (1) assessment of risk for bleeding and/or risk of tissue perfusion deficits from existing bleeding; (2) control and assessment of severity of GI bleeding through noninvasive techniques (NG tube flush, administration of medication, intake and output measurements, hemodynamic monitoring); (3) maintenance of the comfort and stability of the patient during therapy for GI bleeding; and (4) assessment and planning for vascular volume or blood product replacement.

Nursing Care Plan for the Management of the Patient with Gastrointestinal Bleeding

Diagnosis	Signs and symptoms	Intervention	Rationale
Impaired tissue integrity near the site of GI bleeding	Active or occult bleeding (heme positive, hematemesis, hematochezia) Decreased Hct, Hgb, or RBC count Ulceration evident during scopic procedure	Insert NG tube as appropriate and maintain according to institutional protocol; check patency with gentle aspiration to avoid mucosal injury; maintain with straight drainage or low intermittent suction (less than 120 mm Hg)	Removal of blood is necessary to prevent nausea, vomiting, and elevated BUN levels; suction greater than 100–120 mm Hg can cause gastric irritation, which increases risk of bleeding
		Administer GI mucosal coating agents as ordered (sucralfate)	To prevent injury by HCl and promote healing of tissue
		Administer antacids as ordered	To increase pH of stomach/duodenal secretions, reducing risk of ulceration (note that alkaline pH increases gastric acid secretion, causing constant secretion of acid unless patient is given histamine blockers concomitantly)
		Administer histamine blockers as ordered (monitor for thrombocytopenia and side effects)	To decrease acid secretion, which reduces risk of ulceration (but thrombocytopenia may increase risks of bleeding from existing injured areas)
		Record blood loss accurately; measure all outputs (including phlebotomy); weigh dressings as indicated	To estimate replenishment needs (phlebotomy is a common source of obscure blood losses)
		Perform Hct, Hgb on bloody secretions to ascertain amount of blood (should be less than 18 mg %)	Hct or Hgb reflects amount of blood (as opposed to other components) in secretions

Diagnosis	Signs and symptoms	Intervention	Rationale
		When using Sengstaken-Blakemore tube: during insertion, inject air slowly and observe for signs and symptoms of esophageal rupture or respiratory distress; maintain traction on tube; gastroenterologist to deflate balloon periodically; check and record balloon pressures every 8 hours (maximum 35–40 mm Hg)	Slow inflation is necessary to evaluate the effect of balloon inflation on airway patency; excessive quantity of air or rapid inflation may rupture the esophagus
Altered tissue perfusion	Anxiety, confusion, restlessness Oliguria Decreased cardiac output Metabolic acidosis Hypotension Dyspnea, hypoxemia Angina Abdominal pain	Assess fluid volume status every hour via vital signs, CVP, and cardiac indices as appropriate	Tissue perfusion may be reflected in vital signs
		Do orthostatic checks when patient is not frankly hypotensive	Orthostasis is an early indication of vascular volume depletion
		Administer crystalloids as ordered; follow patient's weight and I&O with hemodynamics	Crystalloids replace vascular volume but may hemodilute the patient
		Administer colloids as ordered, and observe for allergic reactions	Colloids may help pull additional fluid into vascular space
		Administer renal-dose dopamine as ordered and monitor urine output (minimum 30 cc/hr)	Increasing renal perfusion may decrease risk of ARF
		Administer inotropic agents as ordered	Increasing cardiac output may compensate for decreasing circulating blood volume

Nursing Care Plan for the Management of the Patient with Gastrointestinal Bleeding

Diagnosis	Signs and symptoms	Intervention	Rationale
		Perform blood chemistries 3–5 times/week and hepatic profiles 3 times/week	To monitor for signs of organ failure related to poor perfusion
		Check oxygen saturation and ABGs for signs and symptoms of respiratory distress; administer oxygen as ordered	Hypoxemia indicates inadequate circulating hemoglobin
		Perform 12-lead ECG with chest discomfort and with initiation of vasopressin therapy	Cardiac ischemia and infarction may occur as a result of decreased oxygen carrying capacity or with coronary constriction with vasopressin
		Perform ECG monitoring	To note dysrhythmias or ischemia
		Administer vasopressin 0.2–1.2 I.U. as ordered; monitor ECG, chest discomfort, abdominal discomfort, urine output	Diminished coronary and splanchnic circulation are anticipated, but may produce deleterious complications such as MI or bowel infarction
		Administer nitrate with vasopressin as ordered	Counteracts coronary vasoconstriction of medication
Impaired gas exchange related to decreased oxygen-carrying capacity	Hypoxemia Dyspnea Cyanosis Anemia	Give supplemental oxygen as ordered and as indicated by patient's complaints of respiratory distress	To increase patient's comfort
		Monitor using periodic pulse oximetry, if possible, continuously during massive hemorrhage and/or replacement of blood products	Massive hemorrhage leads to decreased oxygen carrying capacity as well as blood loss

Diagnosis	Signs and symptoms	Intervention	Rationale
		Plan care to provide frequent rest periods	Activity increases oxygen demand and consumption
		Monitor oxygen extraction data (SVO$_2$)	Determines tissue utilization of oxygen
		Plan care to provide frequent rest periods	Activity increases oxygen demand and consumption
Potential decrease in body temperature related to blood loss and/or massive transfusions	Temperature less than 36°C Cool skin Coagulopathies	Use blood warmer to administer packed RBCs and IV fluids when patient is hypothermic	To reduce hypothermia
		Assess for coagulopathies related to administration of cold blood	Coagulopathies occur with hypothermia
		Keep patient covered with blankets or warming blanket; cover patient's head to decrease heat loss	To maximize patient warming (but do not warm faster than 1°C/hr)
Alteration in fluid volume (deficit) related to blood loss	Anxiety, restlessness Orthostasis or hypotension Tachycardia CVP less than 1 mm Hg Decreased Hgb, Hct, and RBC count	Administer hypertonic crystalloids or colloids as ordered	To maintain circulating volume and thus tissue perfusion
		Monitor volume intake and output with weight and CVP	To assess for vascular volume status and gain information regarding total body volume
		Use MAST trousers temporarily in acute situation until operating room is available or volume replacement is successful	To shunt blood flow centrally to perfuse major organs
Pain related to ulcerations	Subjective cues of discomfort Nonverbal cues of discomfort	Pain assessment at least every shift	Level of pain gives clues to disease process and guides intervention
		Administer analgesia as ordered	Pain increases sympathetic nervous system stimulation and worsens vasoconstriction

Medications Commonly Used in the Care of the Patient with Gastrointestinal Bleeding

Medication	Effect	Major side effects

Antacids:
  Mylanta
  Maalox
	Alkalinize the pH of gastric secretions to reduce risk of erosion by HCl	Diarrhea (certain products cause constipation)
		
		Altered taste sensations

Colloidal fluids (albumin, plasma protein fraction)	Increase oncotic pressure to expand vascular volume	Allergic or anaphylactic reaction Volume overload
Dopamine	Low dosage (1–4 mcg/kg/min) for renal perfusion; higher dosage is inotropic	Tachycardia, dysrhythmias Hypertension, peripheral vasoconstriction Extravasation, possibly leading to tissue necrosis

Histamine blockers:
  Famotidine
  Ranitidine
  cimetidine
	Block secretion of HCl in the stomach to decrease risk of ulceration and aid in ulcer healing	Confusion, somnolence
		Thrombocytopenia
		Dizziness, headache
		Constipation
		Neutropenia
		GI distress

Sucralfate	Direct coating of ulcerated areas of the stomach or small intestine	Constipation Rash
Vasopressin: Desmopressin	Mesenteric and coronary vasoconstriction, reduces blood flow to gut	Angina Myocardial infarction Bowel infarction SIADH Sweating Tremors Abdominal cramps, nausea, diarrhea Rhinitis (with nasal formulation)

Abdominal Trauma

Abdominal trauma is any injury resulting from penetrating or blunt injury to the body anywhere from the nipple line to mid-thigh.[56] Abdominal trauma may injure the internal organs through rotational, crushing, shearing, deceleration, burst, or penetrating injury. Blunt trauma to the abdomen is less common in motor vehicle accidents than head or musculoskeletal injury and is thus more likely to elude diagnosis. The spleen, liver, kidneys, and small bowel are the most frequently injured abdominal organs, although other injuries may occur.[57]

Clinical antecedents

All abdominal injury is classified as either blunt or penetrating trauma. Blunt trauma to the abdomen can be incurred from crush injuries, falls, sports injuries, or motor vehicle accidents (MVAs), which are the most common cause. Individuals most likely to suffer blunt abdominal injury in an MVA are those not using seat belts, drivers injured by steering wheel impact, passengers or pedestrians suffering acceleration-deceleration injuries, and individuals thrown from the motor vehicle.

Penetrating injury may result from stab or gunshot wounds. Penetrating stab wounds may be a result of any sharp object impaling the abdomen, including knives, ice picks, sharpened wood objects, or metal rods. Victims of domestic disputes, robbery and rape victims, and adolescents or young adults who have been in fights are likely to present with stab wounds of the abdomen. As few as 30–40% of victims of abdominal stab wounds sustain actual visceral injury, whereas more than 90% of victims of abdominal gunshot wounds sustain visceral damage.[58] Edwards and Gaspard reported that 14% of 35 patients with abdominal gunshot wounds that did *not* penetrate the abdomen still had visceral injury.[59] This is most likely due to the blast effect of the gunshot wound—damage from bullets does not necessarily follow the pathway between the entrance and exit sites. Instead, the injury will be dependent upon the trajectory of the bullet, its speed, and any deflection off of bony structures.[60] In addition, 25% of lower chest wounds produce intraabdominal visceral injury.[61]

Critical referents

Victims of abdominal injury from traumatic causes are likely to present with any of three types of injury: gastrointestinal vessel injury, laceration of abdominal organs, or crush injury with tissue damage and hemorrhage. The nature and severity of symptoms will vary with the type of injury and the area of the abdomen affected. Lacerations are more common in penetrating trauma; all types of injury occur in blunt trauma.

The gastrointestinal system is a highly vascular area of high blood flow. Most abdominal injuries result in some vascular injury with significant hemorrhage. Major life-threatening bleeding can occur from any of the arteries in the abdomen, the portal vein, or the inferior vena cava. Damage to the descending aorta is relatively rare in the trauma survivor but, if present, is accompanied by shock. Emergency management may require a thoracic approach to ligate the thoracic aorta until emergency surgery can be performed. A significant number of these patients do not survive. If this emergency measure is required, the kidneys are greatly compromised, and renal failure is a likely outcome.

Hemorrhage of the abdominal arteries from blunt injury will usually occur at juncture points, frequently from ragged tears within the intima of the abdominal vessels. These vessels bleed intraperitoneally, and the injury may present as retroperitoneal hematomas. Centrally located retroperitoneal hematomas above the pelvis usually herald multiorgan injury.[62] Eighty percent of blunt abdominal trauma includes the pelvis. For this reason, evaluation of retroperitoneal hematomas should include assessment for pelvic injury. Hepatic bleeding occurs most often within the organ and will frequently (50% of the time) stop spontaneously due to tamponade by the limiting hepatic capsule.[63] Since each hepatic sinusoid contains an artery and a vein, the liver is highly susceptible to bleeding.

Portal vein bleeding occurs with penetrating trauma 90% of the time.[64] Such trauma are frequently associated with concomitant visceral injuries of the inferior vena cava, pancreas, stomach, or liver. Bleeding occurs rapidly and may not be distinguished from arterial hemorrhage. Exploration and surgical ligation is the only treatment strategy acceptable for patients experiencing portal vein bleeding.

Injury to the inferior vena cava is a life-threatening event occurring in 1 in 50 gunshot wounds to the abdomen.[65] One-third of such patients die of exsanguination before reaching the hospital, and another third die during hospitalization. A single puncture of the vena cava with the impaling weapon left in place is less likely to produce hemorrhage and shock, as the blood loss is kept to a minimum by the weapon. Gunshots or blunt trauma are more likely to be associated with gaping holes or ragged tears of the vena cava, which are fatal. The infrarenal area of the inferior vena cava is most susceptible to penetrating injury, although hepatic injury is also prevalent.

Laceration of a specific abdominal organ is almost always a result of penetrating trauma other than gunshot wounds. The small bowel is least likely to be injured in a stab wound, and it is hypothesized that its relative mobility and slippery exterior allow it to move away from the impaling object. Injuries to the stomach are also relatively uncommon because of its floating and protected position. The terminal large intestine also resides in a protected position and escapes injury. Eighty percent of bowel injuries occur between the duodenojejunal junction and the terminal ileum, 10% in the duodenum, and 10% in the large intestine. The liver is the second most injured organ in penetrating trauma. As gunshot wounds increasingly outnumber stab wounds among ER patients, the incidence of liver injury increases as well.[66] A list of the potential injury sites with pertinent clinical information is presented in Table 6-27.

The usual mechanism of intestinal injury induced by blunt trauma is crushing of the small bowel against the vertebral column. Rupture of the small bowel may also occur from shearing forces upon the abdomen, which cause increased intraluminal pressures and explosive rupture from the high pressure. Exploration often shows multiple transections, particularly with blunt trauma. Tearing of the mesentery from the bowel without luminal injury deprives the bowel of necessary blood supply and may result in bowel infarction and necrosis if it is not noted upon initial exploration. When evaluating for potential structural damage in abdominal injury, the clinician must consider the type of injury, the vascularity of the area, and the probable internal contents of the digestive tract at the area of injury. For example, injury to the duodenum results in pancreatic enzyme release with peritonitis, and injury to the colon causes bacterial contamination of the peritoneum with intraabdominal sepsis.

Resulting signs and symptoms

As noted, the signs and symptoms associated with abdominal trauma will vary with etiology (blunt or penetrating injuries) and the organs affected (see Table 6-27). Symptoms of acute blood loss should be routinely assessed in patients with abdominal injury, as many of them will have significant bleeding. Clues of abdominal bleeding include abdominal pain, increased abdominal girth, Grey-Turner's sign (flank bruising), Cullen's sign (periumbilical bruising), Bal-

lance's sign (dullness of the flank areas upon auscultation, with the right flank dullness disappearing with position changes), Kehr's sign, Coppernail sign (bruising of the scrotum or labia), and hypotension. Symptoms of peritonitis indicate perforation of abdominal organs and may include rebound tenderness, fever and leukocytosis, absent bowel sounds, and acute hypovolemia with hypotension. Ruptured organs may present with hemorrhagic signs and symptoms, friction rubs if the injury involves the liver or spleen, or signs associated with perforation, such as hyperresonance, abdominal distention, or air under the diaphragm on abdominal films. In patients with pancreatic injury, electrolyte disturbances such as hyperglycemia and hypokalemia may also occur. A serum amylase analysis should be obtained for all patients with potential abdominal injury; if elevated, amylase level is a relatively reliable indicator of intraabdominal injury. Amylase levels may rise as early as 2 hours after injury, but, unfortunately, an increase in amylase does not indicate the nature of the injury or provide an indication for surgical intervention.[67]

The pregnant patient with abdominal trauma presents a unique challenge for assessment of injury. Pregnancy naturally lifts the bladder out of the pelvic region and into the abdomen, predisposing the pregnant woman to bladder and ureter injury. Vaginal bleeding is more likely to occur and signals possible fetal distress that requires immediate follow-up. Pelvis vasculature increases during pregnancy, and this fact places the mother at high risk for retroperitoneal bleeding if a pelvic fracture occurs. Other normal physiological changes related to pregnancy that may alter the clinical presentation of such a patient are vascular volume overload, respiratory alkalosis, ST changes on ECG, abdominal rigidity, and decreased bowel sounds.[68]

All blunt abdominal trauma patients should have a nasogastric (NG) tube inserted to assess for upper GI bleeding. This also provides a means of decompressing the bowel for life-saving procedures or abdominal paracentesis. The presence of a NG tube also permits the administration of contrast material for various radiologic and CT studies.

In multiple trauma, the abdominal injury may be missed in the initial assessment due to the more life-threatening symptoms of head and chest injury or more obvious orthopedic trauma. This fact necessitates a protocolized plan for assessment of abdominal organ damage. When traditional abdominal assessment with palpation does not elicit a pain response, a needle paracentesis is indicated. Bloody drainage (a positive finding) has been determined to be 95% accurate for diagnosis of intraabdominal

Table 6-27 Types of Abdominal Trauma

Anatomic Area	Etiology	Clinical Presentation	Diagnosis	Treatment	Complications
Stomach	Penetrating trauma of upper left abdomen	Hematemesis Signs and symptoms of hemorrhage Signs and symptoms of peritoneal bleeding	Bloody aspirate via Levin tube Celiotomy	Double sutured surgery followed by peritoneal lavage; subcutaneous tissue may be left open	Hemorrhage Leakage from suture line with subhepatic or subphrenic abscess
Duodenum	10% of penetrating/blunt abdominal trauma Patients received blow to lower chest or upper abdomen Blunt trauma to abdomen (e.g., in child abuse) with submucosal hematoma, which causes intestinal obstruction	Injury may be retroperitoneal so abdominal symptoms are not present (late duodenum or early jejunum) May cause rapid peritoneal irritation Likely retroperitoneal hematoma Crepitation or bile-stained fluid in the lateral region may be noted on peritoneal lavage Bile-stained fluid from abdominal wounds	Needle paracentesis of RUQ of abdomen Abdominal x-rays may show air around right kidney Exploratory celiotomy	Suture closure if possible Resection with end-to-end anastomosis Y loop of the proximal jejunum over the damaged duodenum Reimplantation of the common bile duct may be necessary Pancreatico-duodenectomy for severe trauma including ampulla of Vater (especially if pancreas is hemorrhaging) Duodenal diverticulization: removal of gastric antrum, closure of duodenal stump and Billroth II procedure Gastrojejunostomy with vagotomy; duodenum is cannulated with a rubber tube and bile is diverted via T-tube Gastrotomy with pyloric exclusion; side-to-side gastrojejunostomy with duodenal repair and pyloric closure Submucosal hematomas may be treated with hematoma evacuation, duodenal resection, or nonsurgical gut rest	Dumping syndrome Poor fat absorption Pancreatic cysts or fistulae Duodenal and pancreatic fistulae Fluid and electrolyte disturbances Duodenal fistulae Fluid and electrolyte disturbances Malnutrition

(continued)

Table 6-27 Types of Abdominal Trauma (*continued*)

Anatomic Area	Etiology	Clinical Presentation	Diagnosis	Treatment	Complications
Small bowel (other than duodenum)	80% of all abdominal trauma between duodenojejunal junction and terminal ileum Crushing small bowel against vertebrae causes tears Shearing and tearing forces in acceleration-deceleration injury May tear mesentery from bowel Most common injury in cases of abdominal penetrating trauma	Acute abdominal pain and fluid imbalances Signs and symptoms of obstruction and or perforation Bowel contusions often more serious than first appears; necrosis may occur later after injury	Abdominal flat, upright, and side-lying x-rays for air Peritoneal lavage	Closure of each tear or group of tears is usual surgery Surgical debridement may be necessary with extensive tissue injury Surgical resection with end-to-end anastomosis may be performed if other repairs not possible	Late bowel infarction Sepsis Malabsorption syndrome
Colon/rectum	Penetrating wounds often result from industrial accidents involving blasts or flying objects Explosives, compressed air, or gunshot wounds common etiology Instrumentation injury during sigmoidoscopy or injury during sexual acts Accidental colonic or rectal perforation during pelvic surgery	Acute abdominal pain Signs and symptoms of sepsis Rectal hemorrhage Fecal material from lower abdominal wounds	Proctoscopy Sigmoidoscopy Abdominal flat, upright, and side-lying x-rays for air Gastrografin may be used if dye study is essential	Aggressive fluid management Broad spectrum antibiotics (gram-positive and gram-negative coverage) ASAP Surgical closure should be performed only if tissue destruction is minimal Significant injury (especially with fecal contamination) should have colon exteriorized temporarily Proximal colostomy with closure of distal colon (loop for less severe injury and double-barrel for more severe injury) Bowel resection with ileotransverse colostomy if injury to ileocecal area Use of surgical drains for all post-op patients	Hemorrhagic or septic shock Wound dehiscence and evisceration Malabsorption

Table 6-27 *(continued)*

Anatomic Area	Etiology	Clinical Presentation	Diagnosis	Treatment	Complications
Liver	Second most commonly injured organ in both penetrating and blunt trauma 80% of liver trauma is from penetrating trauma 20% of liver trauma is from blunt injury	Symptoms of acute hemorrhage and hypovolemic shock Increased abdominal girth RUQ pain	Depends on location and details of injury Signs and symptoms of hemorrhage Peritoneal lavage with bloody returns	Immediate surgical exploration to arrest bleeding sites Surgical maneuvers may block blood flow into liver for short periods Drainage of hematomas to external drain, especially in perihepatic areas Removal of lateral half to two-thirds of right twelfth rib facilitates drainage Not necessary to surgically correct nonbleeding injuries Suture of bleeding vessels with supplemental Surgicel or Avitene A vascular section of omentum may be used to compress liver to control bleeding Resectional debridement or limited wedge resection Severe and extensive liver injury especially involving major vessels may require hepatic lobectomy	Subhepatic and subphrenic abscesses Hemorrhage

Reduced hepatic ability to clear toxic substances |
| | Hepatobilia, upper or lower GI hemorrhage, obstructing jaundice, colicky abdominal pain | | CT scan useful in determination of subcapsular hematoma Hepatic arteriography | Vascular isolation with a venocaval shunt used especially if the vena cava injured Subcapsular hematoma may be monitored for continued bleeding and surgically evacuated only with serious bleeding | Renal failure Peripheral ischemia

Hepatobilia (blood in bile) |

hemorrhage.[69] Needle paracentesis is performed bilaterally on the anterior abdomen, on either side of the rectus abdominus. Paracentesis of all four quadrants used to be recommended, but recently this has been shown to be unnecessary.[70] Unfortunately, a negative finding may be inconclusive, and a repeat needle paracentesis with peritoneal lavage is required. A trocar or dialysis catheter is inserted into

Table 6-28 Diagnostic Procedures for Abdominal Trauma

Test	Indications	Clinical Significance
Laboratory tests		
Complete blood count	All trauma	Detection of hemorrhage; caution should be used at trusting this test alone
Serum electrolytes	All trauma	Possible hyperglycemia and hypokalemia. These are indicative of small bowel or pancreatic injury. Transient glucose elevations are to be expected and need only be monitored.
Serum creatinine	All trauma	Provides a baseline for assessment of renal insufficiency
Serum amylase	All trauma	Reliable indicator of intraabdominal injury (pancreas, duodenum, upper small intestine); isoenzyme amylase may be more specific for pancreatic injury
Urinary sediment, blood	All trauma	Hematuria or sediment may indicate renal injury
Arterial blood gases	All trauma	Hypoxemia, acid-base balance
Radiology		
Chest and abdomen upright films	Stable trauma victims	Diagnose presence of pneumoperitoneum
Abdominal flat plate films	Stable trauma victims	Changes in size, shape or position of viscera may provide indirect evidence of solid viscera rupture; hemorrhage into the organ shows as increased density or displacement of nearby organs
Upper GI	Stable patients with negative mini-lap	May reveal intramural hematomas of the small bowel
Intravenous pyelogram	Blunt trauma or suspected renal injury	Detects breaks in integrity of GU system
Computerized tomography		
CT of abdomen	Suspected liver/spleen injury; suspected retroperitoneal injuries	Diagnosis of hematomas within visceral organs in the peritoneal cavity
Arteriography		
Abdominal arteriogram	Blunt abdominal trauma	Helpful for diagnosing vessel abnormalities by allowing selective catheterization of the celiac, mesenteric, or renal vessels
Paracentesis		
Peritoneal lavage	Abdominal injury with negative peritoneal tap; inconclusive abdominal findings; patients with altered consciousness	More accurate diagnosis of intraabdominal hemorrhage or bowel perforation than with peritoneal tap; assesses presence of RBCs, WBCs, amylase; *not* recommended for patients with gunshot wounds to chest or abdomen, or with stab wounds to back; patients with previous abdominal procedures; patients in late pregnancy or with dilated bowels
Culdocentesis	Females with blunt abdominal trauma	Diagnostic for retroperitoneal bleeds/hematomas

the mid-abdomen above the symphysis pubis. The lower peritoneal cavity is aspirated and assessed for nonclotting blood (evidence of peritoneal fluid rather than vessel aspirate). The yield of positive aspirate is higher with this procedure. However, a negative aspirate is followed by an infusion of 1000 cc of normal saline or Ringer's lactate and position changes prior to vacuum removal of the fluid. The

Table 6-29 GI Surgeries

Surgery	Description	Indications	Special Nursing
Esophagus			
Esophageal resection	Resection of a portion of the esophagus with an end-to-end anastomosis	Small esophageal tumor, especially in middle portion	Airway protection Supplemental feeding No manipulation of NG tube
Blunt esophagectomy	Removal of the lower portion of the esophagus with close-over of the esophageal stump; a gastrostomy or jejunostomy is created for feeding	Tumor in lower third of esophagus Caustic ingestions	Airway protection Gastrostomy care NPO forever
Colon interposition	A section of the esophagus is removed and replaced with a portion of the colon in order to preserve the alimentary canal	Caustic ingestions Small esophageal tumors Young patients	Supplemental feeding Relearn swallowing No manipulation of NG tube
Esophagogastrectomy	Portion of the esophagus and stomach removed with anastomosis to jejunum; involves thoracic approach	Tumor at lower end esophagus and involving stomach	No manipulation of NG tube Pernicious anemia Electrolyte imbalances Malabsorption; weight loss
Partial esophagectomy	The proximal portion of the esophagus is removed with gastric pull-up (the remainder of the esophagus and stomach are pulled up and connected to short end of the proximal esophagus)	Tumors in lower two-thirds of esophagus	Tendency for reflux Small frequent feeding No manipulation of NG tube
Fundoplication or Nissan procedure	Gastric wrap around lower esophagus to tighten the sphincter area	Zenker's diverticulum	Airway protection No manipulation of NG tube Elevation of head of bed

(continued)

fluid is quantitatively analysed for RBCs, WBCs (>500/mm^3), bacteria, food, and amylase. The number of RBCs that is significant remains controversial, ranging from 500/mm^3 to 100,000/mm^3.[71] The limitations of this diagnostic tool are its inability to detect retroperitoneal, diaphragmatic, or pancreatic injuries.

When the patient is stable, a variety of radiologic or noninvasive scanning studies may be performed. These are summarized in Table 6-28.

Nursing standards of care

Techniques for management of patients with abdominal trauma are prioritized according to the need for stabilization and the potential threat to life. Not all abdominal injuries require surgical exploration or repair. Maintaining a decompressed, quiet abdomen will provide the basis for accurate assessment. This requires the insertion of both an NG tube and a Foley catheter. Diagnostic studies are fairly accurate for determining acute life-threatening events but may miss the more covert injuries. Injuries likely to elude diagnosis include pancreatic in-

jury, slow hepatic or splenic bleeding, and bleeding from mesenteric vessels. In many patients, the only therapy required may be an NG tube, ongoing laboratory studies (CBC, chemistry, amylase), and frequent abdominal assessment. With all patients, assessment for bleeding or rupture of abdominal organs should be performed throughout the recovery period.

The usual medical protocol after diagnosis of acute intraabdominal injury with organ rupture or bleeding is exploratory surgery. Exploratory surgery is done through a celiotomy, which requires a long mid-line incision to provide access to all areas of the abdomen. Intraoperative arteriography may also be performed to ensure that all blood vessels are intact. A summary of possible gastrointestinal surgeries for specific injuries or conditions is given in Table 6-29.

Initial nursing care will be directed toward the top-priority life-saving measures during stabilization and diagnosis of the extent of injury. Important nursing outcomes include the stabilization of vascular volume, establishment of effective breathing patterns with adequate ventilation, and normalization of body fluids and electrolytes. Significant nursing goals for the patient who has sustained traumatic abdominal injury include (1) maintenance of comfort

Table 6-29 GI Surgeries (*continued*)

Surgery	Description	Indications	Special Nursing
Stomach			
Vagotomy	Division of the vagus branches to prevent impulse from reaching the stomach	Chronic gastritis Ulcers	Provide comfort measures if patient complains of fullness Decreased gastric secretion Decreased gastric motility
Pyloroplasty	Enlarging of the pyloric sphincter to establish an enlarged outlet	Patients with vagotomy	Dumping syndrome
Antrectomy	Removal of the antrum of the stomach; remaining stomach is anastomosed to the duodenum; usually performed with a vagotomy	Gastric and pyloric ulcers	No manipulation of NG tube Possible pernicious anemia Dumping syndrome
Gastroenterostomy	Creation of an anastomosis between the posterior wall of the stomach near the antrum and the jejunum	Duodenal trauma Ulcers	Electrolyte disturbances Poor fat metabolism No manipulation of NG tube
Gastrostomy tube placement	Incision into the antrum of the stomach for the purpose of placing a permanent feeding tube	Comatose patients requiring long-term feeding or frequent esophageal surgeries	Check feeding residuals Elevate head of bed
Gastric resections: Total gastrectomy	Stomach removed, with anastomosis of the esophagus to jejunum using thoraco-abdominal incision	Trauma Severe multiple gastric ulcers	Poor nutrient absorption, weight loss No manipulation of NG tube Care of thoraco-abdominal incision
Bilroth I	Removal of part of the distal portion of the stomach with an anastomosis to duodenum (pylorus and antrum removed)	Ulcers of the pylorus	Pernicious anemia Dumping syndrome No manipulation of NG tube
Bilroth II	Partial removal of the stomach (pylorus and antrum); removal of lower portion of the stomach and anastomosis to jejunum	Ulcers of distal stomach and duodenum	Dumping syndrome Poor fat absorption Electrolyte abnormalities
Pyloric exclusion surgery	Gastrostomy on greater curvature of antrum; pylorus is closed and a side-to-side gastrojejunostomy is done	Trauma to distal stomach and duodenum	Pernicious anemia Dumping syndrome No manipulation of NG tube
Small intestine			
Ileostomy	Opening of the ileum to the surface of the abdomen	Crohn's disease Traumatic injury to colon	Unformed stools Electrolyte disturbances
Small bowel resection	Resection of a portion of small bowel with end-to-end anastomosis	Crohn's disease Ulcerative colitis Trauma Tumor	Altered water reabsorption Possible colostomy Altered vitamin absorption
Large intestine			
Colectomy (subtotal or total)	Resection of portion or entire colon, with end-to-end anastomosis or colostomy	Tumors Crohn's disease Ulcerative colitis Trauma to portion of colon	Altered water absorption Possible temporary colostomy Possible vitamin malabsorption
Colostomy	Portion of the colon brought through the abdominal wall, creating a temporary or permanent opening; stool is semi-formed, nonirritating; temporary colostomies usually located in mid-left or transverse colons	Colectomy Gut rest	Colostomy care and patient education Note whether colostomy is temporary or permanent Skin care Colostomy drainage assessment
Abdominal-perineal resection	Radical, traumatic procedure including an abdominal procedure with colostomy and transected rectum without anal closure	Tumors of sigmoid or rectum	Perineal drains No rectal procedures or suppositories; high risk of infection in rectal incision
Proctosigmoidectomy	Perineal resection of part of the rectum with the large intestine pulled downward and anastomosed; external sphincter preserved	Rectal trauma or tumors	Temporary colostomy common No rectal procedures Less pre-defecation urge

Table 6-29 *(continued)*

Surgery	Description	Indications	Special Nursing
Pancreas			
Distal pancreatectomy	Removal of the tail of the pancreas, with pancreatic head and end of the duct of Wirsung oversewn	Isolated pancreatic tumor or trauma	Decreased fat absorption Possible pancreatic abscesses Possible glucose or electrolyte problems
Pancreatico-duodenectomy (Whipple procedure)	Removal of the head of the pancreas, the entire duodenum, a portion of the jejunum, the distal third of the stomach, the lower half of the common bile duct, and a portion of the pancreatic duct with re-establishment of the continuity of the biliary, pancreatic, and GI systems	Pancreatic cancer or extensive trauma	Pancreatic pseudocysts common Pancreatic-intestinal fistulae Altered fat absorption
Pancreaticojejunostomy (Roux en Y procedure)	Jejunum sectioned, with duodenum partially removed and jejunal anastomosis to the body of the pancreas; the other end of the jejunum is translocated later into the small intestine	Pancreatic cancer or trauma of pancreas and duodenum	Altered fat absorption Electrolyte disorders Possible pernicious anemia
Liver			
Subsegmental (wedge) resection	The removal of an area of the liver that is less than a segment and not along an anatomic dissection plane	Small localized benign tumors	Possible hemorrhage Vascular volume deficit
Left lateral segmentectomy (lobectomy)	Excision of a liver mass to the left of the left segmental fissure along an anatomic plane	Extensive trauma to the segment or tumors and cysts confined to the segment	Hypertension Vascular volume deficit
Left medial segmentectomy	Resection between the main interlobar fissure and the left segmental fissure	Benign tumors of this area	Vascular volume deficit
Left lobectomy	Excision of all hepatic tissue to the left of the main lobar fissure	Tumors of the left medial or lateral segments	Hemorrhage Hypoalbuminemia Vascular volume deficit
Right lobectomy	The removal of the liver to the right of the main lobar fissure	Tumors involving only the right lobes	Vascular volume deficit Hypertension Hypoalbuminemia
Extended right lobectomy	Excision of the entire right lobe plus the medial segment of the left lobe	Tumors extending from right lobe into medial segment	Hemorrhage Vascular volume deficit Hypoalbuminemia Signs of reduced liver capabilities
Infusaid pump placement	Pump implanted into a surgically constructed subcutaneous pocket in the abdominal wall; catheters are threaded into the right, left, or both hepatic arteries	Primary or metastatic tumors of the liver	Chemotherapy follow-up Limits on air travel
Hepatic artery dearterialization or embolization	Intentional embolization or detachment and ligation of one of the hepatic arteries	Tumors in one lobe or another	Symptoms of liver dysfunction
Splenectomy	Left lateral incision	Splenic infarctions, trauma	High risk of bleeding High risk of infection

and relief of pain, (2) prevention of infection, (3) maintenance of fluid balance and nutrition, (4) helping the patient and family to cope with the situation.

Gastrointestinal Surgery

Surgical intervention is a common therapeutic approach to gastrointestinal problems. Surgical procedures vary extensively and may involve access to the thoracic, abdominal, and pelvic cavities. Both emergent and elective surgical interventions are employed for GI disorders, and both involve a broad spectrum of anesthetic techniques and invasive monitoring. Many patients who have undergone complex or extensive gastrointestinal surgery require critical care intervention for a period of time. Such surgery affects the interaction of many physiologic functions and is often the etiology of multisystem organ failure. Surgeries requiring critical-care management strategies will be emphasized within this section.

Clinical antecedents

Gastrointestinal surgery is performed for injuries or diseases of the GI tract that involve hemorrhage or disruption of the digestion of nutrients. Abdominal surgery is performed to treat vascular, gastrointestinal, urologic, and pelvic disorders. Refer to Table 6-29 for descriptions of surgical procedures and the common disorders treated with surgeries of the abdomen.

Critical referents

The pathophysiology of specific gastrointestinal disorders and their associated surgical intervention are addressed throughout this chapter; this section provides a general overview of commonalities in GI surgery.

All abdominal surgeries involve resection of the abdomen for surgical manipulation of the abdominal organs. This necessitates resection of the three layers of abdominal muscles, which produces significant postoperative abdominal pain and difficulty with the deep breathing and coughing needed to prevent atelectasis and postoperative pulmonary infections. Weakened abdominal muscles are prone to atrophy;

wound dehiscence is also common in the case of poor nutrition or abnormal wound healing.

Abdominal surgery for any reason results in manipulation of the bowel with at least short-term suppression of peristalsis. In addition, there is a risk that injury to the GI tract will cause enzyme or bacterial release into the peritoneum. Chemical or mechanical peritonitis are common complications of surgery, although intraabdominal sepsis only occurs when the bowel contents contaminate the abdomen.

The location and aggressiveness of the surgery will directly dictate the type of nursing care required and suggest possible complications to be anticipated. The degree to which and length of time during which digestive functions will be interrupted vary depending on the surgery but are often correlated with the amount of bowel manipulation or anesthesia. After surgery, peristaltic and motility functions cease for a time, necessitating bowel rest until their return.

Trauma and surgery as well as anesthesia stimulate the patient's stress response. This surge of sympathetic hormones may have immediate or later effects upon the recovering patient. The immediate effect of the release of epinephrine is the stimulation of antidiuretic hormone (ADH). ADH causes renal conservation of fluid and sodium, resulting in fluid overload, hemodilution, and oliguria. Later effects involve the adrenal axis of the stress response. Approximately 7–14 days after the initial stressor, cortisol elevations lead to hyperglycemia, fluid retention, mood swings, and decreased resistance to infection. Although not always seen in the ICU setting, the impact of the stress response upon patient recovery should be considered.

Resulting signs and symptoms

The postoperative abdominal surgery patient usually shows the anticipated late effects of anesthesia and evidence of altered digestive functions. Anesthetic effects will vary, depending on the individual patient, the agent used, and the length of surgery.

After abdominal surgery, there is significant discomfort requiring continual assessment and analgesia. Pain is a result of muscular, soft tissue, and visceral injury and will subside within approximately 3–5 days of surgery. Abdominal pain is often continuous, nonlocalized, and radiating into the back or legs. As the patient heals and becomes more mobile, surgical discomfort subsides but may be replaced with pain from gas accumulation in the GI tract. Walking and the return of peristaltic activity generally alleviate this discomfort.

Abdominal surgery often compromises the patient's pulmonary capacity from both anesthetic effects and hypoventilation related to abdominal discomfort. An early postoperative fever is common and is usually related to hypoventilation and retained pulmonary secretions. Other symptoms the patient may present with are dyspnea, tachypnea, diminished breath sounds, coarse crackles or gurgles on auscultation, and a productive cough. Diagnostic signs evidencing these pulmonary problems may include hypoxemia in blood gases, inadequate FVC (forced vital capacity) and NIF (negative inspiratory force), or hypoventilation on chest x-ray.

Altered digestive function is common in all patients who have had gastrointestinal surgery. Dysfunction may be short- or long-term, temporary or permanent. For the first several days, most surgery patients requiring intensive care will have an NG tube in place. This tube should drain yellow (stomach), golden (duodenum), or dark green (high jejunum) secretions. If secretions are light green, tube placement may be too far into the jejunum. In patients who have had surgeries involving the esophagus, stomach, or small intestine, the NG tube should not be manipulated by nursing staff. Drainage of secretions occurs until bowel sounds return, flatus is passed through the rectum, and fluids are tolerated. These are the criteria that indicate that the GI tract is functional and intact. Complications that may arise include paralytic ileus or poor nutrient absorption related to surgical removal or displacement of the stomach or intestine. Some manifestations of these complications are dumping syndrome, persistent abdominal distention, or diarrhea.

Postoperatively, wounds may be closed or open; closure may involve sutures, retention sutures, or staples. Wounds are closed in uncomplicated and clean abdominal surgeries. Either sutures or staples are acceptable; use of one or the other depends on the preference of the surgeon. Retention sutures are used to supplement routine closure in the obese patient. They are placed at regular intervals (every few inches) along the suture line.

With open wounds, the subcutaneous tissue is left open and the viscera are closed with sutures. Open wounds are reserved for the contaminated injury (trauma, perforation) and allow periodic cleansing and/or antibiotic flushes of the area. It is believed that closing contaminated wounds may increase the risk of infection and/or wound dehiscence and evisceration. With potentially infectious wounds, drains may be placed into the surgical site to facilitate drainage and prevent intraabdominal sepsis. The drains may be flexible Penrose drains or reservoir drains such as the Jackson-Pratt drain.

Drainage will vary according to specific circumstances of the patient, but it should be clear, serous, or serosanguinous. Purulent or excessively bloody drainage is an abnormal finding.

Ostomies are closed- or open-loop externalizations of the bowel. A closed-loop ostomy will be opened several days after surgery. Ostomies are covered with drainage bags that provide an external exit for wastes of digestion. The location of the ostomy will predict the consistency of the contents. Ileostomies produce continuous watery yellow diarrhea and cause severe and persistent electrolyte disturbances. Colostomies drain only the colon or sigmoid area and emit intermittent fecal material that may not even require a drainage bag.

Other clinical findings that may occur in some patients include hypotension, tachycardia, hypovolemia, oliguria, edema, and lethargy. Essential laboratory values that should be monitored postoperatively for all patients include CBC and chemistry. Other studies ordered routinely for some patients are liver function tests and coagulation tests. Chest x-rays are routinely obtained to evaluate the patient's ventilatory capacity; abdominal x-rays or CT scans are used to assess for postoperative complications such as fistulae or abscesses.

Nursing standards of care

Routine medical follow-up for abdominal surgery patients will include brisk intravenous fluid replacement, antibiotic administration, intake and output measurement, wound care, and pulmonary hygiene measures. The nurse will also ensure that the patient remains comfortable and free of acute post-op complications. Common postoperative complications and key nursing implications are noted in Table 6-30.

Fluid management postoperatively will involve administering a mildly hypertonic electrolyte solution (such as normal saline with potassium chloride or D5 normal saline, Ringer's, or Ringer's lactate) at 100–250 cc/hr. The patient will be observed for cardiac tolerance (heart rate and BP), volume depletion or overload (CVP), and urinary output. Serum electrolytes will be monitored to ensure replacement of gastrointestinal losses without overload.

Pain management may consist of intermittent intravenous or intramuscular injections of pain medication or, more commonly now, a continuous intravenous medication via patient-controlled pump (patient-controlled analgesia, or PCA). Frequent and sufficient pain relief permits the patient to practice

Table 6-30 Postoperative Complications of Abdominal Surgery

Complication	Signs and Symptoms/Intervention
Paralytic ileus	Keep patient NPO; consider supplementation NG tube for decompression Bowel sounds, abdominal girth
Mechanical obstruction	Cantor tube, NG tube Reoperation Vomiting Hyperactive or quiet bowel sounds Abdominal pain Electrolyte monitoring
Infections	Bowel decompression Peritoneal lavage, drainage from surgical drains or open wounds Antibiotics Drainage observations, cultures Vital signs
Abscess formation	Surgical drainage, drains Antibiotics Localized pain, pocket of drainage
Wound infections, dehiscence, evisceration	Wound packing (iodophor gauze, wet to dry, Dumborrow's solution) Antibiotics Nutritional support Reoperation
Fistulas	Bowel decompression and rest Replace fluid and electrolytes Drains Nutritional support
Respiratory compromise	Cough, deep breathe, ambulate Pain medication Early fevers

deep breathing and coughing to reduce atelectasis and facilitates the increasing activity that improves lung status.

Some patients require nasogastric or intestinal suction until peristaltic activity resumes. Management of the drainage tube involves routine assessment for position, patency, and nature of drainage. Many patients will receive histamine-blocking agents to reduce hydrochloric acid production and potential stress ulceration. However, recent literature does not support the use of routine intermittent antacids as a preventive measure.[72]

Wound care varies drastically from one patient to another. Among the options are dry sterile dressings, wet to dry dressing, antibiotic-soaked gauze, electrolyte-soaked gauze, and vaseline dressing. Most closed wounds are covered for 3 days to a week, with daily soap and water or iodine cleansing until sutures are removed. Surgical drains are covered with sterile dressings until removed. Routine culture of drainage should be performed when drains are left in for more than a week or when the nature of the drainage appears unusual. Open wounds require wet or wet to dry dressings several times a day until closure begins. Ostomy care varies with location of the externalization but includes skin care, replacement of fluid and electrolyte losses, and odor management.

All postoperative patients receive antibiotics. Prophylactic antibiotics given prior to gastrointestinal surgery include agents effective against common gram-negative anaerobes. These include cephalosporins and clindamycin.[73] Bacteria most likely to produce polymicrobial postoperative infections in gastrointestinal surgical patients are Escherichia coli, enterococci, pseudomonas, klebsiella, and proteus. A beta-lactam antibiotic such as Ceftazidime or Cefotaxime may be used alone. However, patients at risk for the occasional pathogen streptococcus may receive a combination antibiotic regimen of an aminoglycoside (Gentamycin, Amikacin, Tobramycin) and a penicillin derivative (Ticarcillin, Ampicillin, Pipercillin).[74]

The nurse's role in managing the postoperative gastrointestinal surgical patient involves complex assessment of various body systems and prevention of complications. The major nursing goals are to make the patient comfortable via pain relief, to maintain gastric decompression, to care for the wound, and to encourage activity. The nurse is also responsible for recognition of early sepsis and fluid or electrolyte imbalances. The major responsibilities in nursing management of postoperative patients are outlined in the care plan that follows.

Nursing Care Plan for the Management of the Patient with Gastrointestinal Trauma and Surgery

Diagnosis	Signs and symptoms	Intervention	Rationale
Lack of knowledge of surgical procedure and outcomes	Questions by patient and family Anxious behavior Inability of patient to describe surgery and possible postoperative problems	Ascertain patient's level of knowledge about procedures	To establish baseline
		Provide preoperative teaching prior to hospital admission when possible	Studies show retention is less than optimal if info is provided after admission; pre-op teaching has been shown to decrease postop complication rates
		Describe anticipated surgery and time frames	Anxiety may be alleviated by increased knowledge of what to expect; definition of time frames reinforces goal-oriented recovery
		Reassure patient about availability of analgesia	Many patients fear pain and the inability to control it
		Demonstrate and have patient perform deep breathing and coughing	Preoperative competence and understanding of coughing and deep breathing enhances patient's performance postoperatively
Pain related to tissue injury or operative procedure	Complaints of abdominal, back, or leg discomfort Abdominal muscle rigidity Inability to cough or ambulate Nonverbal cues of discomfort	Assume pain is present in first 24 hours, and administer medication as ordered	Postoperative pain may be severe in the first 24 hours, and inadequate relief leads to decreased mobility and/or ventilation
		Provide consistent pain relief as patient requests; reassess patient's pain frequently to determine need for dose adjustment	Pain relief may improve patient's compliance with activity and breathing exercises; medication may not be adequate so adjustments may be indicated

Diagnosis	Signs and symptoms	Intervention	Rationale
		Consider PCA pump as appropriate; if using pump, document hourly and supplemental doses taken, as well as patient's attempts at administration, and evaluate need for increased hourly dose	To provide rapid pain relief and control for the patient; PCA pump has been shown to be more effective than analgesics administered exclusively by nurse
		Provide care to the patient with epidural analgesia according to hospital protocol; check catheter site every 4 hours for potential dislodgement; check vital signs every hour for 4 hours; do not flush catheter	Epidural analgesia is more potent and effective; however, may have potentially more serious systemic side effects
		Identify all locations and severity of pain	Pain may be deferred; 10–40% of all patients with abdominal surgery have back pain; severity of pain may indicate need for increased medication
		Use a scale for assessing level of pain (1–10 scale or smiling/frowning faces) Check admission trauma or operative report for extent of injury or surgery	Simple pain scales that do not require reading are easiest to use and analyze when frequent adjustment of analgesics is necessary
Fluid volume deficit related to fluid shifts or losses through surgery or inflammatory response to trauma	Anxiety, restlessness Tachycardia Orthostasis or hypotension CVP < 1 mm Hg PCWP < 8 mm Hg ST depression on ECG	Administer hyperosmolar crystalloids (D_5NS, Ringer's, RL) or colloidal fluids to replenish vascular volume; document estimated blood loss (EBL) on chart postoperatively	Blood lost during surgery must be replaced with both crystalloids and colloids to maintain blood pressure, electrolytes, oxygen-carrying capacity, and normal coagulation

Diagnosis	Signs and symptoms	Intervention	Rationale
	Tachypnea, dyspnea, and hypoxemia Oliguria, high urine specific gravity Hyperosmolarity	Weigh patient every day; assess I&O every 1–2 hours	To determine total body fluid and assist in assessing vascular volume
		Replace drainage from tubes if excessive	To prevent dehydration
		Assess hemodynamic parameters every hour until patient is stable, then when changes in vital signs or hemodynamic readings occur	Changes may reflect additional bleeding
		Evaluate signs and symptoms of organ perfusion deficits (mental status changes, oliguria, chest pain, dyspnea) and initiate renal dopamine, nitroglycerin, or supplemental oxygen PRN	Perfusion deficits may indicate need to increase vascular volume, cardiac output, or manipulation of preload and afterload
		Replace blood components as ordered	To restore vascular volume
Alteration in nutrition (intake less than body requirements) related to trauma, surgical procedure, or prolonged gastrointestinal rest	Weight loss > 10% of IBW Hypoalbuminemia Anemia, leukopenia, or thrombocytopenia Ketonuria or ketoacidosis Proteinuria Intake less than 1000 cal/day Continuous NG tube suction Absent bowel sounds	Obtain nutritional consultation early in postop or posttrauma period	To assist in the assessment of the patient's nutritional and metabolic needs and determine the anticipated length of time for deficits
		Obtain (via nutritionist) diagnostic studies for nutritional assessment (anthropometric measurements, total protein levels, urine protein levels)	Full nutritional profile facilitates determination of appropriate nutritional supplement
		Develop nutritional supplementation plan based on patient's requirements and physical limitations (enteral, peripheral, parenteral)	Calorie requirements and fluid volume tolerance will vary with patient

Nursing Care Plan for the Management of the Patient with Gastrointestinal Trauma and Surgery

Diagnosis	Signs and symptoms	Intervention	Rationale
		Maintain NG tube per hospital protocol	With some surgeries NG tube should *not* be manipulated
		Assess bowel sounds and abdominal distention at least every shift	Return of bowel sounds may indicate discontinuance of NG tube
Potential for trauma related to necessary diagnostic procedures (peritoneal lavage)	Hypotension Hypoxemia or signs of respiratory failure Signs and symptoms of hypovolemia Fever	Prepare abdomen for needle aspiration of both sides	To establish a sterile area of skin
		Decompress abdomen with NG tube prior to procedure	To prevent potential bowel perforation
		Prepare specimen tubes for collection of hematology, amylase, and culture specimens	Diagnostic tests will determine perforation or peritonitis
Potential for ineffective airway clearance and impaired gas exchange	Fever Tachycardia Decreased oxygen saturation Hypoxemia Diminished breath sounds or crackles, especially in lung bases	Have patient perform coughing and deep breathing when possible; for patient on ventilator, deep breathe and suction at least every 4 hours	To prevent pneumonia
		Encourage patient to change position every 2 hours	To prevent pneumonia
		Encourage patient to get out of bed by second postoperative day, and ambulate as ordered	Enhances ventilation and reduces risk of postoperative pneumonia; enhances return of musculoskeletal strength; promotes circulation and healing
		Productive cough or significant sputum should be sent for culture	Positive sputum cultures indicate the need for antibiotic administration or change

Diagnosis	Signs and symptoms	Intervention	Rationale
		Obtain sputum culture and chest x-ray with every fever spike (>101°F)	Fever may be an early symptom of pneumonia
		Observe for signs and symptoms of ARDS	ARDS is a common complication of massive tissue injury and surgery
Impaired physical mobility	Musculoskeletal injuries	Passive ROM exercises every 8 hours	To prevent contractures
	Lethargy, coma, heavily sedated state	Turn and reposition patient every 2–4 hours	To prevent contractures and improve circulation and ventilation
	Paralyzed through injury or for therapeutic reasons	Skin care every 8 hours: massage with lotion; check for breaks in integrity	Immobile patients are prone to skin breakdown
		Use special low-airloss bed when skin is fragile or becomes reddened	To decrease pressure points and reduce risk of skin breakdown
		Consult with rehab or PT as appropriate	To develop a body maintenance program specific to the patient's deficits and needs
Potential for infection related to intraabdominal sepsis	Fever	Take patient's temperature at least every 4 hours; report temperatures greater than 101°F or less than 96°F	Often the first sign of infection is fever, but body temperature less than normal may also indicate sepsis
	Leukocytosis		
	Purulent or cloudy drainage from wounds or drains		
	Poor wound healing	Evaluate each episode of hypotension or respiratory distress for potential sepsis	Unexplained hypotension or drop in CVP and Swan-Ganz values may indicate sepsis
	Abdominal pain, distention, or tautness		
	Wound dehiscence or evisceration	Culture suspicious wounds or drainage every 3 days after a positive culture	Antibiotics may need to be added or changed based on culture results
		Monitor CBC daily	To assess for leukocytosis and whether there is a left shift (bacterial, fungal infections) or a right shift (viral infections)

Nursing Care Plan for the Management of the Patient with Gastrointestinal Trauma and Surgery

Diagnosis	Signs and symptoms	Intervention	Rationale
		Administer postoperative antibiotics as ordered; obtain peak and trough levels as ordered	Antibiotic levels reflect whether quantity of antibiotic being used is sufficient for bactericidal activity
		Recognize abnormal culture and antibiotic reports	To help identify when organisms become resistant and antibiotics need to be changed
		Assess abdomen and wounds for abnormal pain, discharge, and increased girth	Localized abdominal symptoms may indicate intraabdominal sepsis

Acute Pancreatitis

Acute pancreatitis is an inflammatory process that presents with a variety of clinical symptoms and degrees of severity. As many as 15–30% of patients with pancreatitis develop critical complications requiring aggressive management.[75] As yet the medical community has been unable to identify specific factors that predict which patients will be prone to these complications.

Pancreatitis is classified according to the acuteness of the disease and by the underlying pathophysiologic process. Acute pancreatitis is usually edematous or hemorrhagic in form; chronic pancreatitis may present as acute, relapsing, or hemorrhagic (and thus is also addressed in this section).

Clinical antecedents

The precise etiology of acute pancreatitis is unknown, although the major risk factors comprising 65–90% of all cases are alcohol-related or associated with biliary tract disease.[76] Idiopathic pancreatitis, or pancreatitis of unknown etiology, comprises 10–20% of all cases.[77] Alcohol consumption has classically been associated with the more indolent and insidious chronic pancreatitis, although not in all cases. Pancreatitis in the young is almost always associated with blunt abdominal trauma or surgical manipulation during bowel or hepatic surgeries. Trauma is more commonly associated with hemorrhagic pancreatitis, and surgical manipulation usually results in the edematous form. Furthermore, a number of medications, infectious diseases, and miscellaneous precursors have also been implicated in the development of pancreatitis; these are listed in Table 6-31.

Critical referents

Since the precise etiology of acute pancreatitis is only postulated, pathophysiologic mechanisms precipitating pancreatic episodes are equally puzzling. Some theories label alcohol as a direct toxin to the pancreas; others merely suggest that it triggers excess pancreatic secretions. What is clear is that clinical studies have indicated increased pancreatic secretions and spasm of the sphincter of Oddi after alcohol consumption. Another theory proposes that there is damage to the pancreatic outflow tract from alcohol consumption, stones, or other toxins. Because of the ensuing pancreatic incompetency, bile and duodenal juices may be splashing into the duct of Wirsung. Enterokinase, an enzyme known to liberate pancreatic enzymes, is contained in duodenal juice, and thus a reiterative cycle is created.

Although specific mechanisms are not known, all theories propose excessive activation of pancreatic

Table 6-31 Precipitators of Acute Pancreatitis

Pharmacologic Agents	Infectious Disease Factors	Miscellaneous
Antihypertensive drugs such as methyldopa	Mumps	Scorpion bites
Antimicrobials 　Nitrofurantoin 　Sulfonamides 　Tetracycline	Coxsackie virus (simular to poliomyelitis) Mononucleosis Viral hepatitis	Exposure to organophosphorus insecticides Hypercalcemia
Chemotherapeutic agents 　L-Asparaginase		Hyperlipidemia Hyperparathyroidism
Diuretics 　Ethacrynic acid 　Furosemide 　Thiazide diuretics		Inflammatory diseases 　Systemic lupus erythematosus 　Crohn's disease 　Thrombotic thrombocytopenia purpura
Immunosuppressives 　Azathioprine 　Cyclosporine		Pregnancy Ulcer disease
Miscellaneous drugs 　Amphetamines 　Corticosteroids		

enzymes with or without obstruction of the pancreatic duct. It is known that excess pancreatic enzymes accumulate within the pancreas, causing a variety of reactions, all culminating in edema of acinar cells and autodigestion of the pancreas. The process unfolds as follows: a blockage of the flow of pancreatic enzymes (kallikrein, elastase, phospholipase A, and chymotrypsin) causes those enzymes to back up and stagnate in the ducts and acini of the pancreas. Kallikrein causes vasodilation and increased vascular permeability. Phospholipase A activates substances that are toxic to red blood cells. Elastase and chymotrypsin have been shown to cause damage to the blood vessels. This damage includes rupture of local vessels, leading to minimal to quite severe hemorrhage within the pancreas. Furthermore, the accumulation of trypsinogen becomes so great that it negates the action of trypsin inhibitor, so trypsin becomes activated. Trypsin activation spreads rapidly and activates most of the proteolytic enzymes. The activated enzymes begin digesting the pancreas itself, as well as the fat in and around the organ.

Resulting signs and symptoms

Clinical presentations of pancreatitis may vary greatly. The physical symptom most often noted is epigastric pain. The onset of pain is usually sudden but occurs within a few hours of the beginning of the inflammation. Most patients experiencing pancreatitis describe the pain as constant, boring, or aching, and at least half of them describe it as radiating to the back. Pain may also be intense in the left subcostal or retrosternal areas level with the second lumbar vertebra. Anecdotal reports note that pain seems to be more severe when the patient experiences the hemorrhagic form of pancreatitis and that it becomes more diffuse as the attack progresses.[78] In an attempt to alleviate discomfort, some patients assume a sitting or knee-to-chest position, which does not always prove helpful; but lying flat or eating and drinking seem to increase discomfort. Pain that radiates to the left shoulder, although uncommon, can be seen when the tail of the pancreas is involved and diaphragmatic irritation results.

Other gastrointestinal symptoms may include nausea, vomiting, loose and foul-smelling stools, and abdominal distention. The abdominal distention has been noted to be a result of a paralytic ileus (in 40% of all patients).[79] It may also be a result of flatus, although release of pancreatic enzymes may cause increased peritoneal fluid secretion and ascites. Nursing assessment of the abdomen should include

measures to differentiate guarding or diffuse tenderness from rebound tenderness, which indicates either peritoneal irritation due to enzyme release or the presence of pancreatic hemorrhage. Rigidity is not usually noted. Percussion, abdominal girth, and weight changes may provide additional information regarding the presence of ascites. Diarrhea, melana, hematemesis, and jaundice occur in a small percentage of patients (the latter possibly being a result of biliary tree obstruction, obstruction of the head of the pancreas, or pseudocyst formation).

One of the most acute and common manifestations of acute pancreatitis is vascular volume depletion, secondary to 20–30% of the vascular volume being released for third-space fluid accumulation. Symptoms of volume depletion may present as acute hypotension or be as subtle as orthostatic pulse or blood pressure changes and weight gain. Patients presenting with these signs and symptoms should be assessed for other antecedents to acute pancreatitis to ensure prompt intervention. Hypoalbuminemia is frequently present and may increase the incidence of shock in these patients. Resulting intravascular volume depletion also may contribute to the incidence of renal failure. Hypotension sufficient to cause oliguria is of particular concern, because oliguria will further exacerbate tendencies toward renal failure. Specific assessment parameters that may reflect vascular volume include orthostatic vital signs, central venous pressures, urinary output, urine specific gravity, electrolyte and CBC values, and skin conditions such as edema or poor turgor.

Low-grade fever (99–102°F or 38–39°C) is another common presentation in early acute pancreatitis but usually does not persist. The fever may be related to pancreatic inflammation or peritoneal irritation. When fevers are elevated for prolonged periods (longer than 10 days) and accompany other unresolving pancreatic symptoms, formation of a pancreatic abscess should be suspected. Pancreatic abscesses are notoriously difficult to treat and aways require surgical intervention.

Respiratory distress may occur in severe cases of acute pancreatitis and is often considered a poor prognostic sign. One-third to one-half of all patients with acute pancreatitis have some symptoms of respiratory dysfunction.[80] Thirty percent of mortalities in cases of pancreatitis are actually caused by respiratory failure.[81] The most critical time to assess for this complication is within the first 48 hours. It is believed that it is a direct result of pancreatic enzyme damage to lung tissue. The pancreatic enzyme lipase has been documented to cause fat necrosis in the alveoli, with resultant fat embolization. Clinical presentation of enzymatic destruction of lung tissue mimics the symptoms of adult respiratory distress syndrome (ARDS) with acute hypoxemia and fluid accumulation. Furthermore, elevation of the diaphragm due to abdominal distention may be a factor contributing to some patients' distress symptoms. Chest radiologic exam may reflect diffuse white infiltrates as seen with adult respiratory distress syndrome or acute pulmonary edema. Pancreatic enzyme seepage into the pleural space results in the production of excessive pleural fluid and development of pleural effusions in approximately 5–15% of all pancreatitis patients.[82] This accumulation more often occurs in the left lung and causes symptoms of diminished breath sounds, dyspnea, and cough.[83]

In patients with hemorrhagic pancreatitis, abdominal skin discoloration of the periumbilical area, known as Cullen's sign, reflects severe hemorrhagic disease. The discoloration is usually bluish-purple or dusky and increases as the disease progresses. Turner's sign is an identical skin discoloration in the flank region that is also indicative of hemorrhagic pancreatitis.

The above physical assessment findings, considered in conjunction with etiologic suspicions and laboratory analysis, can reflect the type of pancreatic disease and the prognosis, as well as pinpoint actual and potential nursing problems. Laboratory studies and radiologic procedures may be used to more clearly confirm the diagnosis of acute pancreatitis. The test most often used is the serum amylase level. One of the most sensitive indicators, the serum amylase level begins to elevate within 3–6 hours of the onset of the disease. A value of greater than 500 Somogyi units is considered diagnostic of acute pancreatitis. Unfortunately, this exam is not specific, and values may be elevated by many gastrointestinal diseases as well as by opiate use, burns, cerebral trauma, ectopic pregnancy, and renal failure. Additionally, the serum amylase level returns to normal within 2–3 days of the incident and is thus not useful in evaluating patients long after the onset of symptoms. Urine amylase levels or serum lipase levels have been shown to be more reflective of pancreatic secretion levels; these values stay elevated for five to seven days and thus are more useful diagnostically. The amylase:creatinine ratio, although used extensively in past years, has not proven an effective diagnostic tool because it often yields false positive or negative results and because of variability in test performance among laboratories.[84] A recently developed test used in the diagnosis of pancreatitis is the radioimmunoassay of serum elastase. Elastase is responsible for the degradation of a collagen, elastin. Large amounts of elastin are found in the pancreas and destroyed in pancreatitis.[85] A new laboratory test of pancreatic isoamylase levels is currently being investigated and shows some promise as a more specific indicator of pancreatitis.[86]

Consequential laboratory findings that are a result of the enzyme leakage associated with pancreatitis include leukocytosis, hypoalbuminemia, hypocalcemia, hyperglycemia, hypertriglyceridemia, and elevated LDH and SGOT enzymes. These tests cannot be considered diagnostic, but they have been shown to provide potentially useful prognostic information and are used extensively to guide treatment decisions. Systemic symptoms may reflect the commonly found laboratory abnormalities listed above. Hypocalcemia may result in signs of tetany: muscle tremors, muscle cramps, or positive Trousseau's sign. Hyperglycemia and glycosuria may lead to symptoms of dehydration, extreme thirst, polyuria, confusion, or hypotension. Hyperkalemia may cause cardiac arrhythmias or muscle flaccidity. An increased level of lipase (one of the major pancreatic enzymes) causes fat necrosis in many areas of the body, with resulting fat nodules on the liver, in the lungs, and subcutaneously. Fat necrosis also causes serum hyperlipidemia.

Abdominal ultrasound is used for detection of structural abnormalities in the pancreas. If ultrasound is inconclusive, an abdominal CT scan may be performed, although as many as 14–21% of patients with acute pancreatitis have normal CT scans.[87] If the etiology remains mysterious, it may be helpful to obtain endoscopic information via endoscopic retrograde cholangiopancreatography (ERCP). This test may reveal a hitherto undiscovered but treatable biliary tract disease, although it presents some risk of worsening the pancreatitis, as it has been implicated as the cause of pancreatitis in a small percentage (less than 1%) of patients.[88]

The above diagnostic procedures have proven accurate in confirming the diagnosis of pancreatitis in all acute and most chronic cases, although timing is essential with all procedures.

Nursing standards of care

Medical intervention is usually aimed at resting the pancreas while seeking the cause of the problem and preventing life-threatening complications. Pancreatic rest is achieved by nasogastric intubation and maintaining the patient on NPO status. Use of pancreatic-enzyme inhibitors has been investigated and has shown some promise, although conservative management is still preferred. Surgery may be indicated if the cause of the pancreatitis is thought to be biliary tract disease, but it is considered to be risky if performed during acute pancreatitis or in cases of hemorrhagic disease. Surgery may be the treatment of choice with prolonged symptoms indicative of pseudocyst formation. Finally, peritoneal lavage has been used to provide symptomatic relief in the face of severe disease, but although symptoms are improved, outcomes and underlying disease processes remain unchanged.

Nursing management of patients with pancreatitis should center on actual and potential problems identified through assessment and documentation of risk and precipitating factors. Problems should be prioritized to allow individualization of care and achieve the nursing goals of (1) promoting the comfort of the patient, (2) decreasing pancreatic stimulation, and (3) preventing life-threatening complications. The following nursing care plan describes standard critical care practices used in cases of pancreatitis.

Nursing Care Plan for the Management of the Patient with Acute Pancreatitis

Diagnosis	Signs and symptoms	Intervention	Rationale
Alteration in comfort due to tissue injury, diaphragmatic irritation, and destruction and interruption of blood supply	Epigastric, back, or left shoulder pain Edema Nausea and vomiting Cullen's sign Turner's sign	Decrease physical activity and provide bedrest	Decreased physical activity reduces pancreatic secretion
		Place patient in position of comfort, possibly upright or in knee-chest position	To alleviate discomfort
		Provide Demerol as ordered	Opiates increase spasm of sphincter of Oddi
		Administer papaverine or anticholinergics as ordered	To reduce pancreatic secretions
		Administer anxiolytics PRN	Anxiety increases pancreatic secretions
Alteration in fluid volume (deficit) from fluid shifts, NG suction, and vomiting	Fluid shifts Nausea and vomiting Hemorrhage CVP < 1 mm Hg Orthostasis Hypotension Pleural effusion	Maintain careful I&O records	To assess insensible losses; capillary leak syndrome leads to hypovolemia
		Ascertain urine specific gravity, urine osmolarity, electrolytes, albumin, and hemoconcentrated lab values	Hypovolemic changes should be reversed as early as possible
		Monitor abdominal girth, systemic and peripheral edema, weight gain	To assess for fluid shifts
		Observe for tachycardia, weak and thready pulses, low CVP, orthostatic changes, and changes in neurological status	Signs of fluid volume deficit

Nursing Care Plan for the Management of the Patient with Acute Pancreatitis

Diagnosis	Signs and symptoms	Intervention	Rationale
		Observe for hypocalcemia, tetany, Trousseau's sign, Chevostek's sign, and arhythmias	Pancreatic secretions bind with free serum calcium, producing varying levels of hypocalcemia, which may become life-threatening
Alteration in nutrition (intake less than body requirements) due to nausea and vomiting, increased pancreatic enzyme function, and abnormal fat metabolism	Hyperglycemia	Frequent oral care	NPO status and poor nutrition contribute to oral pathologies
	High-fat stools		
	Gycosuria	Observe characteristics of NG tube drainage	Acute disease states inhibit ability to absorb and use nutrients
	Increased BMR		
	Malnutrition	Progress diet to low-fat foods as soon as ileus resolves (as evidenced by flatus or stool)	Diseased pancreas is unable to tolerate high-fat foods
	Abnormal liver enzymes		
	Hyperlipidemia		
	Nausea and vomiting	Monitor glucose levels and check for glycosuria	Impaired insulin secretion leads to hyperglycemia
		Avoid caffeine, alcohol, and nicotine	Increase pancreatic secretions
		Observe for hepatocellular dysfunction, jaundice, and hyperbilirubinemia	Hepatic failure leads to decreased fat metabolism and exacerbates malnutrition
		Assess gastrointestinal motility	Risks of impaired motility and absorption increase with pancreatic complications
		Administer peripheral or total parenteral nutrition as ordered	Patients are NPO for extended periods and frequently require nutritional supplementation
		Administer anti-emetics as ordered	Caution must be taken to alleviate discomfort of nausea and vomiting without adversely decreasing GI motility

Diagnosis	Signs and symptoms	Intervention	Rationale
Potential for infection and injury related to necrosing pancreatic secretions, pancreatic abscess, pseudocysts, and fistulas	Diminished breath sounds Hypoxemia, dyspnea, or tachypnea Cyanosis Mental confusion Leukocytosis, pus formation Hyperthermia	Observe for crackles, gurgles, diminished breath sounds, and ABG changes Monitor for fever and institute measures to decrease body temperature (antipyretics, tepid baths) Observe for signs of abdominal complications such as discomfort, distention, or palpable masses In the event of fistula, provide diet high in protein and calories Provide meticulous skin care	Respiratory compromise is secondary to immobility and disease processes Low-grade changes in temperature may be early signs of infection; fever states increase metabolic rate and catabolic states Risk of pancreatic abscesses and fistulae is high To fortify body to fight infection To reduce risks and exacerbation of infection
Potential for alteration in oxygenation due to rise in diaphragm caused by ascites, pleural effusions, and ARDS	Diminished breath sounds Hypoxemia, dyspnea, or tachypnea Central cyanosis Mental confusion	Careful assessment of breath sounds and breathing patterns Monitor ABGs as ordered Assess for fluid shifts to abdomen Assess pulmonary compliance via pulmonary function tests or changes in peak airway pressures Maintain deep breathing, coughing, and turning routines	Early detection of respiratory compromise facilitates early intervention Early changes in ABGs indicate metabolic and respiratory alkalosis, which can quickly develop into metabolic acidosis Ascites leads to respiratory compromise Early detection of pulmonary fluid leak or ARDS facilitates timely restoration To decrease risk of atelectasis and accumulation of pulmonary secretions

Nursing Care Plan for the Management of the Patient with Acute Pancreatitis

Diagnosis	Signs and symptoms	Intervention	Rationale
Patient lacks knowledge of disease, possible complications, and treatments	Verbalization of lack of knowledge Behavior that exhibits lack of insight into disease or risk factors	Review probable etiology and precursors of pancreatitis	Solid understanding of causes helps patient adhere to interventions
		Explore rehabilitation programs if indicated	Timely intervention for alcohol abuse facilitates restoration function
		Reinforce the importance of prompt reporting of signs and symptoms indicating further pancreatic problems	Early detection of complications facilitates timely and appropriate interventions
		Provide advice about low-fat diets and stress importance of avoiding alcohol	Maintaining the appropriate diet reduces recurrences of pancreatic disease

Medications Commonly Used in the Care of the Patient with Acute Pancreatitis

Medication	Effect	Major side effects
Histamine blockers	Block production of HCl by the stomach and decrease ulcer formation; decreased HCl reduces pancreatic secretion as well	Thrombocytopenia Neutropenia Confusion Somnolence Dizziness, headache Constipation GI distress
Meperidine: Demerol	Relief of abdominal pain	Hypotension Constipation Sensory changes
Neostigmine	Parasympathetic antagonist; decreases HCl secretion and peristalsis	Ileus
Anticholinergics (Donnatol, belladonna, Pro-Banthine)	Relieve pain by inhibiting motility and gastric secretion	Dry mouth Tachycardia Constipation Urinary retention

Hepatic Disorders: Overview

Patients in critical care areas frequently develop hepatic dysfunction, although only occasionally is it the primary reason for ICU admission. The various hepatic disorders have differing etiologies, presentations, and prognoses. The sections that follow describe physiologic conditions and pertinent nursing implications of acute and chronic hepatitis, cirrhosis, portal hypertension, and hepatic encephalopathy. Table 6-32 provides an overview and comparison of laboratory findings in some of these disorders.

Acute Hepatitis

Hepatitis is defined as an inflammation of the liver that causes hepatocyte injury and may lead to func-tional impairment. The cause can be viral, alcoholic, or toxin- or drug-related. This section will focus on the clinical findings, ramifications, and treatment of acute hepatitis. The mechanism of transmission and injury will be investigated. This discussion will serve as a foundation for later discussions of chronic hepatitis, fulminant hepatitis, cirrhosis, and portal system disease processes.

Clinical antecedents

Viral hepatitis   Viral hepatitis is the result of exposure to a viral pathogen that infects and potentially compromises the liver. The most common forms of the inflammation are hepatitis A, hepatitis B, non-A, non-B hepatitis, hepatitis C, hepatitis D, and hepati-

Table 6-32   Common Laboratory Findings with Hepatic Disease

Type of Disease	SGOT/AST SGPT/ALT	Alkaline Phosphatase	Bilirubin	Albumin	Prothrombin Time	Other
Fulminant (acute) hepatic failure	Increased 10–20 times normal; fall with progression of disease	No increase unless cholestatic process is also present	Normal at onset; rises progressively; may be 15–20 mg/100 mL	Normal initially; falls with disease process	Prolonged *early;* may be 8–10 times normal value	Transaminases will decrease with progression; indicates greater than 80% loss of liver
Acute hepatitis	Elevated at least 10 times normal limit	Less than twice normal unless patient is jaundiced or cholestatic process is present	Direct/indirect increased in icteric phase	Normal initially; decreases as damage progresses	Normal initially; prolonged *later*	If transaminases are greater than 5000 IU/L, condition is probably drug related; if rash, eosinophilia; if fever, rule out hypersensitivity
Alcoholic hepatitis	SGOT/AST up to two times SGPT/ALT	Two to three times normal	Ranges from normal to 20 mg/100 mL	Decreases if cirrhosis is developing	Three to four times longer	If condition is progressing toward cirrhosis, patient may be unresponsive to vitamin K therapy
Chronic hepatitis	Elevated for more than 6 months	One to two times normal	2–10 mg/100 mL	Decreases; reflects degree of cirrhosis	Prolonged; reflects degree of cirrhosis	Increased SGOT/SGPT and alkaline phosphatase may last for months to years; if active phase of CAH, levels may approach those found with disease
Cirrhosis	Elevated moderately; varies; depends upon degree of active inflammation	Elevated three to ten times normal with obstructive disease or cholestasis	Slightly elevated direct/indirect	Decreased slightly	Prolonged	Elevated globulin; hyperglobulinemia

Table 6-33 Comparisons of Type A, Type B, and Non-A, Non-B Hepatitis

Feature	Hepatitis A	Hepatitis B[b]	Non-A, Non-B Hepatitis Bloodborne (Hepatitis C)	Non-A, Non-B Hepatitis Enteric (Hepatitis E)
Incubation	15–45 days (mean 30)	30–180 days (mean 60–90)	15–160 days (mean 50)	14–60 days (mean 40)
Onset	Acute	Often insidious	Insidious	Acute
Age preference	Children, young adults	Any age	Any age, but more common in adults	Young adults (20–40 years old)
Transmission route:				
Fecal-oral	+++[a]	–	Unknown	+++
Other nonpercutaneous[c]	+/–	++	++	+/–
Percutaneous	Unusual	+++	+++	–
Severity	Mild	Often severe	Moderate	Mild
Prognosis	Generally good	Worse with age, debility	Moderate	Good
Progression to chronicity	None	Occasional (5–10% of cases)	Occasional (10–50% of cases)	None
Prophylaxis	IG	Standard IG (not documented) HBIG, hepatitis B vaccine	?	?
Carrier	None	0.1–30%[d]	Approximately 1%	None

[a]Pluses and minuses indicate the likelihood that a given type of hepatitis will be transmitted in a certain way.
[b]Concomitant delta hepatitis is similar in these features to hepatitis B, but outcomes are more severe.
[c]For example, sexual or maternal-neonatal contact
[d]Varies considerably throughout the world; see text
Source: Dienstag, Wands, and Isselbacher, Acute hepatitis. In *Harrison's Principles of Internal Medicine*, pp. 1327.

tis E. They are distinguishable by their mode of transmission and potential for progressive disease; their clinical presentations, however, are almost identical. The general characteristics of each type are summarized and compared in Table 6-33. There are other viral entities that will produce a hepatitis phenomenon with similar symptoms; they are listed in Table 6-34.

Hepatitis A virus (HAV) is transmitted primarily by the fecal-oral route and in very rare cases by

Table 6-34 Various Viral Causes of Hepatitis

Coxsackie virus
Cytomegalovirus
Epstein-Barr
Herpes simplex
Infectious mononucleosis
Rubella
Yellow fever

parenteral mechanisms. It has been found in the liver, bile, stools, and blood of infected individuals. It is prevalent in areas of poor sanitation and/or overcrowding. Contaminated shellfish, food, milk, or water may spread the disease; transferral between family members and within hospitals is also common.[89] The potential rate of infection is very high in those practicing oral-anal sex.[90] The course of the disease is diagrammed in Figure 6-13.

Hepatitis B virus (HBV) is transmitted primarily by contact with body fluids, especially blood. In the past, exposure was commonly associated with transfusions, but recent education has focused more on the potential of exposure from dental instruments, tattooing, sexual acts, autolancet platforms, and the sharing of needles—or any other means by which blood may be exchanged. The virus has also been found in semen and saliva, but not in stools. The likelihood of developing hepatitis after a transfusion is related to the category of transfusion and the treatment that the blood product has received prior to administration. If the product has been heated to 60°C or super-cooled (for example, albumin or im-

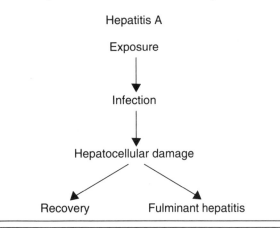

Figure 6-13   Progression of Hepatitis A

mune globulin), the risk of viral transmission is negligible. The greatest risk involves receiving factors concentrated from multiple pooled donors; whole blood, single-donor platelets, and plasma transfusions present only an average risk.[91] The likelihood of acquiring hepatitis B from a blood transfusion has also dropped significantly with the advent of blood bank screening programs that are specific for the virus; hepatitis B now accounts for only 5–10% of posttransfusion hepatitis.[92] The course of the disease is diagrammed in Figure 6-14.

Like hepatitis B, non-A, non-B hepatitis is also transmitted primarily by contact with body fluids. Since the screening for hepatitis B has eliminated it as the primary source of posttransfusion hepatitis, it is

apparent that some other pathogen is responsible for this process. Researchers have isolated a virus called hepatitis C. However, there are still cases of posttransfusion hepatitis that occur in the absence of either hepatitis B or hepatitis C serology, implicating at least one other virus in the presentations; thus, the classification of non-A, non-B continues to be used. The course of the disease is diagrammed in Figure 6-15.

With the increased study of hepatitis has come the recognition of two new viral pathogens: hepatitis D (delta hepatitis) and hepatitis E. Hepatitis D is found only in individuals who are hepatitis B–positive, because it is somewhat parasitic. That is, the delta virus is an incomplete virus that requires the specific double-shelled structure of the hepatitis B virus for replication and expression.[93] As soon as the underlying hepatitis B infection is completed and the virion is extinct, delta hepatitis is also necessarily extinct. The hepatitis D infection either can be initiated with the hepatitis B infection (coinfection) or can superimpose itself on a patient who is acutely or chronically infected with hepatitis B (superinfection). The mode of transmission varies depending on the geographic area in which the infection is acquired. In certain Mediterranean countries, for example, hepatitis D is endemic to the hepatitis B population and is transmitted mainly by sexual or maternal-neonatal contact.[94] In areas without this endemic population, the disease is primarily confined to those who have frequent contact with blood and blood products. This accounts for the increased

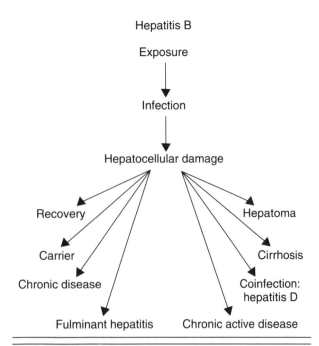

Figure 6-14   Progression of Hepatitis B

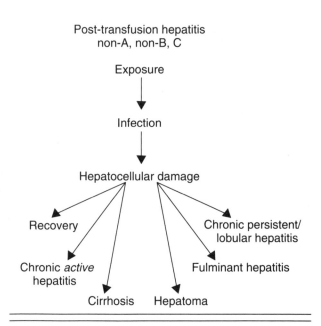

Figure 6-15   Progression of Post-Transfusion Hepatitis Non-A, Non-B, C

level of the disease among drug addicts and hemophiliacs. Recent studies have shown a fatality rate as high as 5% in drug addicts with simultaneous acute infection of hepatitis B and D.[95] Figure 6-16 diagrams the course of the disease.

Hepatitis E is an enterically transmitted pathogen that has been discovered in populations who were resistant to hepatitis A and did not have bloodborne risk factors. It has been identified in India, Asia, Africa, and Central America, and has arisen following monsoons, earthquakes, and natural disasters that result in crowded and unsafe sanitary conditions. It seems to favor young adults and is extremely pathogenic in pregnant women. The overall fatality rate is 1–2% in the general population, but among pregnant women it may be as high as 10%.[96]

Alcoholic hepatitis Alcoholic hepatitis is a result of chronic alcohol ingestion. The disorder is often accompanied by, but is not dependent upon, malnutrition. A nutritional deficit may, however, potentiate the disease process. Hepatitis usually follows the development of alcoholic fatty liver, a condition in which the hepatocytes are distended and distorted by fatty deposits within the cells and surrounding tissues. If the process is severe, the in-house mortality rate may exceed 50%.[97] If alcohol ingestion is discontinued while symptoms are still mild, clinical recovery may be complete. Unfortunately, many alcoholics experience multiple bouts of hepatic inflammation and compromise and develop irreversible liver damage.[98]

Toxic or drug-induced hepatitis Hepatocellular damage follows the exposure to or ingestion of toxic substances or pharmacologic agents. Toxic substances can generally be categorized by their presentation: they cause either direct toxicity or idiosyncratic reaction. Direct toxicity is often a predictable event; that is, the damage that occurs is dose-related and is seen in enough patients that the clinician can expect a specific form and degree of liver compromise with a given type and dose of drug. The reaction usually occurs within the first several hours of ingestion. These findings are also reproducible. Either the agent is a poison in its ingested form, or the liver metabolizes it into a toxic element which is damaging to the hepatic cells. Examples of such agents are acetaminophen, carbon tetrachloride, and the deadly mushroom *Amanita phalloides*.[99]

Idiosyncratic reactions occur unpredictably and vary in strength and prognosis among individuals. Their occurrence is not related to dosing and may develop any time within the treatment regimen. The classic examples of idiosyncratic reactions occur as a result of halothane anesthesia, isoniazid therapy, or use of phenytoin.

It should be noted that there are hepatotoxic drug reactions that do not present the hepatocellular damage that is seen with acute or chronic hepatitis. The drugs involved may diminish hepatic function without evidence of the destruction at the cellular level that occurs with toxic or idiosyncratic reactions. Those affected present instead with cholestatis, as determined by the presence of increased alkaline phosphatase and/or bilirubin.[100] Oral contraceptives and haloperidol often contribute to this sort of symptomatology.

Critical referents

Viral hepatitis Very little is known about the specific mechanisms of injury from hepatitis A, non-A, non-B hepatitis, and delta hepatitis. Evidence regarding the pathogenicity of hepatitis B, however, has led investigators to believe that the presentation and outcome of infection with the hepatitis B virus are related to the immunologic response of the host. This theory is supported by the fact that patients who are carriers of the hepatitis B virus do not always show histologic changes upon biopsy, which implies that the virus itself is not the injurious agent.[101] Theoretically, as the virus becomes incorporated into the hepatocyte cell wall, the change in cell structure triggers the immune system to respond as if the cell were diseased.[102] It is thought that the incorporation of minute amounts of the core antigen in the surface of the cell membrane may be the triggering factor for T-lymphocytes. This immune response is also considered the mediator of the extrahepatic findings of hepatitis B; immune complexes are deposited on

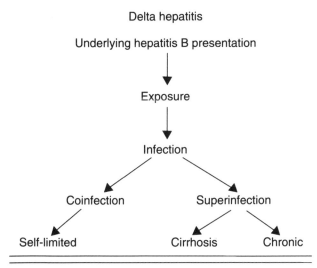

Figure 6-16 Progression of Delta Hepatitis

tissue blood vessel walls and stimulate the complement system, resulting in a syndrome resembling a serum sickness.[103]

The specific histological changes that occur within the liver are relatively similar with all of the different viral etiologies. These changes are detailed in Table 6-35. The basic presentation is compromised cellular integrity and structure, ranging from inflammation and infiltration to necrosis and collapse. These make the liver incapable of carrying out the basic functions that are required of it on a daily basis: synthesis of coagulation factors and plasma proteins, detoxification of exogenous and endogenous toxins and foreign products, and maintenance of energy supplies (gluconeogenesis, glucogenesis, and glucogenolysis).

Some patients present with a more severe process than those described in Table 6-35. In these patients, large numbers of collapsed cells and destruction of the reticulin framework within lobules leads to a development of a "bridgework" of cellular debris between different vascular areas of the lobules. This hepatocellular derangement, known as bridging necrosis, is often found in the patient who progresses to cirrhosis, but no specific and reproducible prognostic value has been identified with its presentation.[104]

Alcoholic hepatitis The mechanism of injury in alcoholic hepatitis is the alcohol itself; the liver metabolizes the alcohol instead of nutrients such as carbohydrates and glucose. The long-term result of this is the deposition of fats within the liver cells and subsequent destruction of the hepatocytes. The destructive process is not a simple one; the alcohol is oxidized to form acetaldehyde and a compound called NADH. The formation of excess amounts of this compound results in the altering of normal metabolic pathways and an increased utilization of oxygen. The preferential use of alcohol over fats results in a decreased utilization of fatty acids for nutrition and increased production of triglycerides.[105] The process of gluconeogenesis is impaired, and therefore glucose supplies within the liver are reduced. If the alcohol consumption continues for a prolonged period of time, the hepatocellular destruction will begin to resemble that seen with viral hepatitis. There will be ballooning of cells, degeneration and necrosis, and infiltration of the liver by leukocytes and lymphocytes. Mallory bodies, severely damaged hepatocytes that are surrounded by polymorphonuclear leukocytes, are a classic finding in alcoholic hepatitis.

Toxic or drug-induced hepatitis The mechanism behind toxic and drug-induced hepatitis depends upon whether it is a direct injury or idiosyncratic process. Some ingested agents cause a specific and direct injury to the hepatocytes. In the case of idiosyncratic reactions, the theory is that hepatocellular damage is the result of an immune-mediated hypersensitivity response and/or a reaction to the metabolites of the ingested agent.

Each individual toxin will produce its own form of hepatocellular and lobular damage; if it is a direct process, the structural changes are relatively consistent and identifiable. For example, acetaminophen toxicity creates a centrilobular necrosis, whereas the

Table 6-35 Histological Findings in Acute Hepatitis

Hepatitis A,B,D, and non-A, non-B	Hepatitis C	Hepatitis E
Panlobular infiltration with mononuclear cells: small lymphocytes, occasional plasma cells and eosinophils	Relatively little inflammation	Marked cholestasis
Hepatic cell necrosis: cell degeneration and necrosis, ballooning of cells, acidophilic body formation, cell dropout	Substantial increase in activation of sinusoidal lining cells	Degenerative and necroinflammatory changes in the parenchyma
Hyperplasia of Kupffer cells	Fat deposits	Coagulative liver-cell necrosis
Variable degrees of cholestasis	Occasional bile duct lesions with biliary epithelial cells stacked without disturbance of basement membrane	
Hepatocellular regeneration		
Retention of reticulin framework		
Portal tract inflammation and constriction		

Source: Adapted from Magun, Acute and chronic hepatitis, in Bongiovanni, *Essentials of Clinical Gastroenterology;* and Dienstag, Wands, and Isselbacher, Acute hepatitis, in *Harrison's Principles of Internal Medicine.*

mushroom *Amanita phalloides* produces massive hepatic necrosis.[106] If the damage is idiosyncratic in nature, the changes may look like those found with viral hepatitis (as in halothane reactions), or they may mimic cholestatic disease (as in anabolic steroid toxicity); one agent may cause different presentations in different patients.[107] In the case of drugs such as oral contraceptives or Haloperidol, the cholestatic picture is probably related to a change in the liver's ability to exchange metabolites through to the bile.[108]

Resulting signs and symptoms

Viral hepatitis The early signs of acute viral hepatitis are insidious and often mistaken for a flu-like illness. The patient experiences fatigue, anorexia, nausea, and tiredness that is relieved by a rest or a night's sleep; persistent activity results in extreme fatigue by the end of the day. There may also be abdominal pain and vomiting. These symptoms usually abate with the onset of jaundice. The prodromal period, which varies according to the type of hepatitis, may last anywhere from 7 days to 10 weeks.[109] The icteric phase, when the patient notices darkened urine, lightened feces, and/or frank jaundice, often brings the patient to a physician for evaluation. Some patients will have jaundice so mild as to go unnoticed; they are asymptomatic and diagnosis will only take place during routine examination or after laboratory tests are conducted because the patient learns that he or she has been exposed. On evaluation, it is common to find the patient has a smooth, tender and palpable liver. Splenomegaly is present in approximately 20% of patients;[110] occasionally generalized lymphoadenopathy is also present.[111] The recovery phase is marked by the absence of the symptomology but continued hepatic enlargement and biochemical abnormality.

The most frequent measurement made in suspected or confirmed cases of hepatitis is of the serum transaminases (ALT and AST). These are commonly found to be at least ten times greater than normal; they may reach peak levels ranging from 400 to 4000 IU or more and will decrease as the patient enters the recovery phase. Serum bilirubin of 5–20 mg/dL, divided equally between conjugated and unconjugated forms, is frequently found as the jaundice becomes apparent. If the level is consistently above 20 mg/dL, the disease is likely to be very severe.[112] Alkaline phosphatase will be normal or only mildly elevated. The serum albumin in early disease will be normal to slightly low, and the prothrombin time

(PT) will be anywhere from normal to one to two times normal. If the PT is greatly prolonged, evaluation for severe hepatic necrosis should be initiated; it indicates a poor prognosis. There is frequently evidence of leukopenia, lymphopenia, and neutropenia in the pre-icteric phase.[113]

There are some signs that are specific to each viral etiology. Hepatitis A virus may be accompanied by a low-grade fever (38–39°C); the onset of symptoms is usually more abrupt in hepatitis A than in hepatitis B.[114] The patient who presents with the usual hepatitis findings but also with arthralgia, high fever, and urticarial rash is displaying signs of hepatitis B.[115] The patient who has been stable in his or her presentation of chronic hepatitis B but suddenly experiences a worsening of symptoms (including a sudden increase in transaminase levels) should be evaluated for superinfection with hepatitis D.[116]

Truly definitive diagnosis of any of these diseases is based on the serological marker. Each disease, except non-A, non-B hepatitis, has its own diagnostic marker. With hepatitis A, the antibody to HAV (anti-HAV) of the IgM class of immunoglobulins starts to show up in the serum early in the disease; its appearance there coincides with the disappearance of HAV in the stool. After approximately 4–6 weeks, the antibody is transformed into an antibody of a different class, which appears to confer life-long immunity to hepatitis A.[117]

The serology of hepatitis B is somewhat more complicated; this virus is a double-shelled DNA virus made up of an inner core that contains the hepatitis B core antigen and an outer envelope that contains the hepatitis B surface antigen. A third antigen, the hepatitis B "e" antigen, is also found in the serum of patients with hepatitis B; its exact placement in the virion is not clear.[118] These markers are good indicators of the disease process and progress; the sequence of their appearance is summarized in Table 6-36. The first diagnostic marker measurable is the hepatitis B surface antigen (HBsAg), which usually appears 1–2 months after exposure and approximately 1 month before clinical jaundice is seen. Approximately 1–2 months after the disappearance of the hepatitis B surface antigen, the hepatitis B surface antibody (HBsAb) is present in the serum. This indicates that the patient is nearing the end of the acute phase of the illness. In between the disappearance of the HBsAg and the development of the HBsAb, the hepatitis B core antibody (HBcAb) is detectable. This core antibody confirms the viral etiology even when the surface antigen or antibody is not detectable. If the antibody is of the IgM class of immunoglobulins, it is indicative of an acute infection. If it is of the IgG class, it is indicative of remote

Table 6-36   Example of Possible Serology Time Sequence in Hepatitis B Patient

Time Frame	Event
Week 0	Exposure to hepatitis B
Week eight	Hepatitis B surface antigen detectable in serum
Week ten	Hepatitis B "e" antigen and core antibody detectable in serum
Week twelve	Jaundice detectable
Week fourteen	Hepatitis B "e" antigen disappears
Week sixteen	Hepatitis B surface antigen disappears
	Hepatitis B core antibody detectable
Week twenty	Hepatitis B surface antibody detectable

exposure. Since the core antigen is deep within the virion, it is not routinely detectable except by direct examination of the infected liver cells (that is, a liver biopsy); it is the antibody to the core antigen that is detectable in the serum. The hepatitis B "e" antigen (HBeAg) is present in all acute infections and is thought to be a measurement of high viral replication and infectivity; it usually disappears a few weeks before the HBsAg disappears. The hepatitis B "e" antibody (HBeAb) is thought to be associated with decreased infectivity and replication.[119] It is important to know that the indicator of the level of immunity garnered from the hepatitis vaccine is the development of the hepatitis B surface antibody, *not* the hepatitis B core antibody. Those individuals who have actually had the hepatitis B infection and developed their own immunity will have both the hepatitis B surface antibody and the hepatitis B core antibody.[120]

The advent of a test for hepatitis C has assisted in the diagnosis of this pathogen and the ruling out of non-A, non-B hepatitis, but only to a small extent. There may be delays of 3 months to 1 year between exposure to the disease and the development of detectable serum levels of the hepatitis C antibody (HCAb).[121]

Serological measurement of hepatitis D is usually based on the presence of the anti–hepatitis D virus antibody. The diagnosis can be established by the detection of the antidelta antibodies either in the serum or in the liver via biopsy. If the delta infection is self-limited, then there will be a slow depletion of the antidelta antibody following clinical recovery.[122]

Alcoholic hepatitis   The patient presenting with alcoholic hepatitis usually comes in for evaluation because of the pain, fevers, anorexia, and vomiting associated with the disease, as opposed to the jaundice that brings in viral patients. Fever is usually less than 39.4°C in such patients, and vomiting may be uncontrollable. Right upper quadrant abdominal pain signals an enlarged and tender liver, and splenomegaly may be present. If the patient has already progressed to cirrhosis, then the liver may be shrunken and difficult to palpate. Spider angiomas may be visible. The classic signs of chronic liver disease, such as ecchymosis, fluid retention, and jaundice, may also be present. Parotid enlargement, vitamin deficiencies, and palmar erythema are common.[123]

Laboratory values will differ from those seen with viral hepatitis. There is a mild increase in the transaminases; the SGOT/AST is usually greater than the SGPT/ALT. If the transaminase levels are greater than 300 units, other etiologies or complications of liver disease should be investigated.[124] (If the bilirubin and alkaline phosphatase levels are both increased, this may be indicative of the cholestatic complications that are sometimes seen with alcoholic liver disease.) Anemia and leukocytosis may be present. The prothrombin time (PT) may be prolonged in the patient with hepatitis and may be uncorrectable even with vitamin K and/or fresh frozen plasma. As the liver may be incapable of the usual glucose metabolism, measurements of serum glucose upon admission and throughout the clinical course are recommended.

Toxic or drug-induced hepatitis   There are no standard presentations among patients with drug-induced hepatitis; the patient may have symptoms that range from a slight increase in hepatic enzymes to complete liver failure. If the transaminase elevation is greater than 5000 IU/L, there is a high probability that the injury is drug-related.[125] If the presenting symptom is a hypersensitivity reaction, then fever, rash, arthralgia, and eosinophilia will frequently be present. The presentation is usually abrupt and may start as long as 2 weeks to 2 months after the exposure to the offending drug.[126] There are a few medications whose specific side effects have been well documented and are treatable; unfortunately, that is the exception rather than the rule. Acetaminophen is one of those; it is possible to measure the serum level and determine whether it is over the threshold beyond which hepatitis will consistently occur. The serum level can also act as a predictor of the extent of hepatic disease that the patient will experience. Appropriate, immediate, and intensive treatment of drug-induced hepatitis is essential.[127] Ethical guidelines (and common sense) prevent the reintroduction of a known idiosyncratic reactive drug to a patient who has shown previous compromise with its use; severe complications may ensue.

Nursing standards of care

Viral hepatitis The management of acute hepatitis usually requires little action from health care professionals. Supportive measures and recognition of the signs and symptoms of progression toward chronic or fulminant hepatitis or cirrhosis are the standards of care. The patient is encouraged to rest in hope of alleviating the exhaustion that often accompanies the disease. Medications are held to a minimum in order to decrease the amount of work required of the liver. Alcohol is generally prohibited, and the patient is advised to limit the amount of fat in the diet; this advice is not usually necessary, as the patient's nausea increases with the ingestion of fat. If the patient is unable to maintain adequate hydration and nutrition (1000 kcal/day), he or she may well require hospitalization.[128] If the patient is elderly, has developed compromising ascites, is encephalopathic, or has an elevated prothrombin time, hospitalization is usually required until his or her condition can be brought under control. Recovery may take several weeks to months and is complete when the patient has normal liver function tests, is asymptomatic and jaundice-free, and has a non-tender liver.[129] Patients with hepatitis A or E can expect a complete recovery within 1–2 months. Three-quarters of patients with uncomplicated hepatitis B or C recover within 3–4 months.[130]

Unfortunately, there are patients who do not return to their previous level of health following infection with viral hepatitis. The least pathologic of these is the patient who shows basic "post-hepatic syndrome," a generally less severe version of the presenting symptoms of anxiety, fatigue, failure to thrive, and some right upper quadrant pain. This syndrome is basically a prolonged recovery period from the initial insult.[131]

There are some more severe complications that result from the viral infiltration of the liver. The least pathological of the viral forms of the disease is hepatitis A. It is generally less severe than hepatitis B and does not develop into a chronic hepatitis, although some patients do develop a cholestatic hepatitis that may last up to 3 months.[132] A very small group of those infected with hepatitis A go on to develop fulminant hepatitis, but this is uncommon. Patients most prone to the development of this complication are those over the age of 60.[133]

Although 90% of patients with hepatitis B recover without further problems, hepatitis B is more likely to cause complications such as chronic hepatitis and fulminant hepatic failure.[134] Five to ten percent of patients with hepatitis B continue to have signs of hepatitis after 6 months. Those who maintain a consistent circulating level of the surface antigen without the development of the surface antibody have not been able to neutralize the hepatitis B virus and are chronic carriers. They are infectious if they also have circulating hepatitis B "e" antigen. The carrier state may last for months or years or may decline and disappear at any time.[135] The second and more severe complication is a state of chronic active hepatitis, found in about 10% of the patients who suffer from acute hepatitis B infections.[136] Fulminant hepatitis can also result from hepatitis B infection, especially in the presence of hepatitis D; it can be extremely devastating. There is a risk of hepatoma associated with consistent hepatitis B infection, whether in the carrier or the chronic state.

Chronic hepatitis is a common complication of non-A, non-B hepatitis. Studies have shown that at least 50% of the patients who are infected with non-A, non-B hepatitis develop a chronic hepatitis, which causes fluctuating or persistent mild elevation of serum transaminases.[137] Liver biopsies often show chronic active hepatitis with potential to progress to cirrhosis, as well as some evidence that perhaps chronic non-A, non-B hepatitis is involved in the development of hepatomas.[138] Awareness of these potential problems will assist the clinician in providing the best possible support and preventive medicine.

Although the clinical presentation of hepatitis D is similar to those of other viral forms of hepatitis, the resulting infection is more severe and carries a higher mortality rate. The acute coinfection is usually self-limited and results in a basically unchanged course of the hepatitis B disease. The acute superinfection, however, often results in a chronic hepatitis that may develop into cirrhosis.[139] The patient who was stable during the course of the chronic hepatitis is often left with worsened baseline illness and symptomatology.[140] The best therapy available is to prevent the disease by ridding the patient of the hepatitis B virus.

Prophylaxis against viral hepatitis is recommended whenever possible. Anyone who is at risk for exposure to hepatitis B can receive repeated injections of a hepatitis B vaccine that is designed to confer surface antibody immunity. If an unvaccinated individual has already been exposed to the hepatitis B virus, combination therapy involving the hepatitis B vaccine and hepatitis B immune globulin is recommended. The appropriate dose will depend upon the type of exposure (needle stick, perinatal exposure, or sexual contact) and the age and immunosuppressive history of the individual.[141]

Immune globulin contains hepatitis A antibodies and is recommended either before exposure or early in the incubation period of hepatitis A infection. The prophylactic use of immune globulin is recommended when there is intrafamilial risk of exposure and in day-care centers (or similar settings) for staff or children in contact with the contaminated individual. It is commonly recommended for travelers to foreign countries where the disease is endemic.

There is no specific vaccine for hepatitis D; rather, immunity is conferred by vaccinating populations at risk for hepatitis B. Since the delta virus cannot survive without the use of the hepatitis B shell, this approach should prevent infection with hepatitis D.

Similarly, there is no specific prophylactic measure against non-A, non-B hepatitis. Postexposure efficacy of a single dose of immune globulin has not been established. The best measure available now is the ability to screen out hepatitis C from blood donations, thereby reducing the risk of transfusion-related contamination.

Alcoholic hepatitis As for viral hepatitis, the basic nursing role with a patient with alcoholic hepatitis is supportive. Patients with severe fever, jaundice, or prolonged PT will need to be hospitalized. The goals are to assist the patient in withdrawal from alcohol, to maintain fluid and electrolyte balances, and to evaluate the potential for a secondary infection. While hospitalized, the patient can be evaluated for diseases that result from excessive alcohol ingestion, such as pancreatitis, diabetes, and ulcerations. Recognition of the special needs that this patient may have while recovering from alcohol abuse may prompt the use of thiamine to prevent Wernicke's encephalopathy, vitamin K for prolonged PT, and fluids to replete a hypermetabolic and consistently febrile state.[142] Special measures for management of delirium tremens and the associated complications should be instituted as necessary. The ultimate goal is to prevent further ingestion of alcohol and the progression of hepatocellular disease.

Toxic or drug-induced hepatitis In the case of toxic or drug-induced hepatitis, the first priority is to remove the offending agent whenever possible. Watching the liver functions until such time as the levels return to normal is recommended; if at the end of 6 months the levels have not returned to baseline, a liver biopsy to look for chronic hepatitis or cirrhosis may be indicated. (A liver biopsy to look for specific pathology may be performed earlier in the course of

the disease if a specific drug cannot be implicated as the cause.) The biopsy allows the clinician to look for a recognizable pattern, which may suggest a specific kind of drug reaction.

Care of the patient with hepatitis encompasses many areas of nursing practice. The nursing care plan at the end of this section suggests nursing diagnoses and interventions appropriate for patients with various forms of hepatitis.

Fulminant Hepatitis

Fulminant hepatitis is a clinical disorder defined as hepatocellular necrosis and hepatic encephalopathy following the onset of a clinical illness. This rare but extremely dangerous complication of viral illness has a mortality rate of more than 50%.[143] Drug overdose and exposure to toxins may also precipitate the disease.

Clinical antecedents

Any agent that causes injury to the liver can be the precipitating factor for fulminant hepatic failure. It is commonly associated with viral hepatitis, especially hepatitis B. Those hepatitis B patients who are also coinfected or superinfected with hepatitis D have been proven to be at a greatly increased risk for the development of fulminant hepatic failure.[144] Hepatitis A and non-A, non-B hepatitis are also precipitating disease states, but consistent data as to their frequency is not available. Other viral infections (herpes simplex, cytomegalovirus, adenovirus, and Reye's syndrome) are precipitators, as is Wilson's disease, an inherited disorder characterized by abnormal copper levels and depositions within the body. Drug overdosing, exposure to poisons such as the *Amanita* mushroom, or idiosyncratic responses to halogenated anesthetics have also been identified as causative agents. Pregnant women who are near term and present with pre-eclampsia or fatty livers have developed this deadly disease as well.[145]

Critical referents

The pathogenesis of fulminant hepatitis is related more to the complications of the liver failure than to the actual liver destruction itself. These effects are listed in Table 6-37 and diagrammed in

Table 6-37 Effects of Hepatic Failure

Decreased phagocytic activity

Decreased manufacturing of bile salts

Inability to recycle bile salts

Decreased conjugation of bilirubin

Decreased bile flow

Decreased carbohydrate metabolism

Increased serum cholesterol

Decreased protein synthesis

Decreased conversion of urea

Decreased mineral storage

Decreased vitamin storage

Decreased detoxification abilities

Figure 6-17. The effect of liver failure on organs cannot be overstated. The patient with fulminant hepatic failure is without a functioning liver. The liver shrinks in size and functional ability as the disease progresses, with massive liver cell necrosis occurring faster than any regenerative process can counteract it. The remaining hepatocytes are not enough to sustain basic homeostatic functions. The ramifications of the loss of hepatocellular function are listed in Table 6-38.

Table 6-38 Clinical Consequences of Pathogenic Changes in Fulminant Hepatitis

Alkalosis

Cerebral edema

Renal failure

Ventilatory disturbances

Electrolyte disturbances

Neurological deterioration, coma, death

Hypoglycemia

Sepsis

Nutritional deficit

Pancreatitis

Acute hepatic encephalopathy is the hallmark of fulminant hepatitis and is often the first symptom detected. The most common mechanism of this deterioration is cerebral edema, which is found in up to 80% of the patients in severe coma.[146] Intracranial hemorrhage and edema are structural causes of hepatic encephalopathy; metabolic causes include hypoglycemia, electrolyte imbalances, and medications. Increased intracranial pressure (ICP) is not uncommon.

Coagulopathies result from the loss of the clotting factors that the liver normally produces. With-

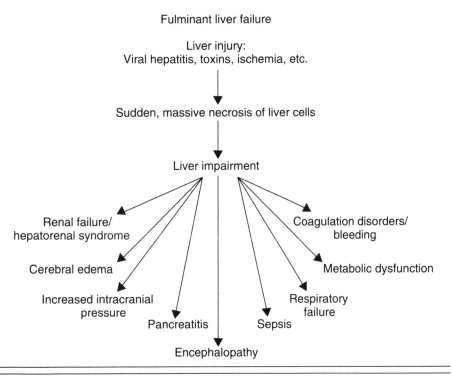

Figure 6-17 Progression of Fulminant Liver Failure

out these factors, bleeding may result and can range from minimal to massive amounts. Gastrointestinal hemorrhage is very common and is promoted by the increased acidity of the gastric fluid. Fluctuating or nonexistent vitamin K levels will potentiate or allow bleeding that would not otherwise be an issue.

Renal failure may result from acute tubular necrosis (ATN), glomerulonephritis, or hepatorenal syndrome. Whereas the first two are not limited to hepatic disease, hepatorenal syndrome is an unusual process that is directly related to liver disease. This renal failure is not the result of renal tissue malfunction; in fact, the kidneys of victims of hepatorenal syndrome have been used successfully as donor organs. The problem in this case is related to altered blood flow into the cortex of the kidney. It is postulated that the fluid shifting that occurs with rapid diuresis and/or ascites production or removal may potentiate this process by diminishing renal perfusion. Hepatorenal syndrome is a diagnosis made after all other renal etiologies are ruled out.

Electrolyte and glucose abnormalities are also common in fulminant hepatitis. Hyponatremia is related to the overall fluid volume overload that occurs with liver failure; the total body sodium may actually be close to normal.[147] If the patient is too vigorously repleted or if the fluid balance shifts, hypernatremia will result. Hypokalemia is usually the result of renal wasting, vigorous diuretic therapy, nasogastric suctioning, or vomiting. Hypoglycemia results from the loss of the liver's gluconeogenic and glycolytic abilities. It may also relate to a deterioration of the liver's ability to break down endogenous insulin.[148] Hypocalcemia and hypomagnesemia may also occur, and monitoring for these conditions is recommended.

Alkalosis is a common finding in patients with fulminant hepatitis. A number of factors may contribute to the alkalosis: hypokalemia, hydrogen ion exchange in and out of the cells, the loss of carbon dioxide with hyperventilation, renal dysfunction, urea accumulation, gastric aspiration, or vomiting. Metabolic acidosis is a rare finding and should trigger an investigation into possible lactic acid accumulation.

The nutritional status of the patient with fulminant hepatitis is not easily maintained. Altered mental status and liver function decrease both the quantity of nutrients the patient ingests and the ability of the liver to remove and distribute the essential nutrients. Carbohydrate, protein, and glucose metabolism is markedly diminished, and protein challenges can precipitate or worsen hepatic encephalopathy.

Sepsis is, unfortunately, a disastrous complication of fulminant hepatitis. Immune system mediators (e.g., leukocytes, complement) are either destroyed or inactivated by the liver failure and associated organ failure. Gram-negative, gram-positive, and fungal infections may develop. Standard use of H_2 antagonists that lower the pH of the stomach by blocking Hcl production, use of broad-spectrum antibiotics that potentiate superinfections, and increased use of invasive procedures as the disease progresses are all potential causes of infection.

Pancreatitis is a side effect of fulminant hepatitis and should be suspected in the patient experiencing a sudden hypotensive and hypovolemic episode. Abdominal pain and increased amylase levels can also be present even when pancreatitis is not found during detailed examination.[149]

Resulting signs and symptoms

Neurological manifestations of the disease can range from slight confusion to nonresponsive hepatoencephalopathic coma. The cerebral edema will result in increased intracranial pressure and its associated symptoms. Unfortunately, it is often difficult to differentiate the patient *with* cerebral edema from the patient who has these symptoms *without* cerebral edema. As the cerebral edema and ensuing coma are classic differentiators of fulminant hepatic failure, it is important to attempt a delineation. Neurological deficits may show as unequal pupil size (anisocoria), decerebrate posturing, myoclonus, and abnormal oculovestibular and oculocephalic reflexes. Hyperventilation will occur early in the process, slowing to abnormal rates and rhythms and eventual apnea as the coma progresses. Increased intracranial pressure always demands immediate and aggressive evaluation for intervention.

Coagulation defects are noted in the laboratory by increased prothrombin time and elevated levels of fibrinolysis products. Evaluation for signs and symptoms of internal and external bleeding should be done daily, if not hourly; the disease process and the patient's response will dictate the frequency required. Prophylactic treatment for coagulation defects is not usually recommended, as the patient frequently cannot tolerate the fluid load that accompanies blood product repletion. If, however, active bleeding is occurring, repletion of coagulation factors may be required, and careful monitoring is necessary.[150]

Blood urea nitrogen is not a sensitive indicator of renal function in the patient with liver failure. Urea is made by the liver, and as the liver fails, urea production will be impaired. Levels can therefore be misleading. Creatinine, although a better measure, may be dumped in the urine more easily if the patient has extensive renal tubular damage and thus may not be a reliable measure either.[151] Urine output and characteristics (electrolytes, creatinine, specific gravity, etc.) are probably the best indicators of renal function.

Electrolyte and glucose abnormalities are measured in the serum. Specific monitoring of sodium, potassium, calcium, and magnesium is recommended. All will be decreased in the patient with liver failure, as will glucose concentration. Concurrent sampling of the urine may help identify the role of the kidneys in the imbalances.

The signs and symptoms of sepsis are the same as those expected in any patient: hypotension, tachycardia, respiratory distress, fever, and vasodilation/constriction. Evaluation should therefore follow the same protocol that would be used for any other patient in sepsis. The only inhibitory factor should be consideration of the special bleeding and immune problems that patients with liver disease experience. The real challenge for the clinician is in singling out the signs of sepsis from the signs associated with overall hepatic failure and the multisystem response that results.

Weight loss, protein intolerance, and a decreased appetite are important evidence of fulminant hepatitis that can be noted during nutritional evaluation. The provision of adequate nutrition in the face of diminished metabolic capabilities is a constant challenge.

Pancreatic evaluation includes measurement of amylase and evaluation of insulin/glucose requirements and a subjective review and assessment. The latter will prove difficult if the patient is in the late stages of encephalopathy.

Nursing standards of care

Mortality rates of patients with fulminant hepatitis approaches 60–90%, irrespective of the causative agent.[152] Death is usually a result of the irreversible complications that result from loss of liver function. Identifying the etiology of the disease may help somewhat; if the toxin is acetaminophen overdose and the appropriate antidote is given quickly enough, supportive care may lead to a full recovery. Wilson's disease, on the other hand, requires liver transplantation if the patient is to survive, as all other therapies are ineffective. Similarly, if the process is the result of overwhelming viral injury, death will occur unless liver transplantation is possible.

Medical and nursing care should be directed toward the prevention or management of the multi-

ple complications of disease. Basic concepts such as protection from injury and minimal administration of drugs that may interfere with examinations are important.

Neurological complications require both basic and advanced technical and clinical management. Management of cerebral edema and increased intracranial pressure is of paramount importance. All possible measures should be taken to prevent increases of the intracranial pressure or to decrease ICP when it does rise: elevation of the head of bed, establishment of a quiet environment, cautious diuretic therapy, minimal stress from medical/nursing procedures, and mechanical hyperventilation are all possible interventions. Mannitol is an osmotic diuretic frequently used for diuresis, but its use is not recommended in patients with renal failure or those who have an osmolality of greater than 315 mOsm with a cerebral perfusion pressure of less than 60 mm Hg.[153] The goal is to remove free water to promote decreased cerebral edema. The goal of hyperventilation is to establish a pCO_2 of 28–32 mm Hg; this will promote cerebral vasoconstriction. EEGs to monitor progression or lessening of symptoms are helpful but do not replace thorough physical and neurological examinations by both medical and nursing staff. Coordination of staff when conducting these examinations will decrease the overall stimulation of the patient. Measurement of intracranial pressure is of the utmost importance if the patient is a transplant candidate; sustained ICP above 30 mm Hg has been associated with neurological deficits that do not resolve even after successful transplants and thus may affect the decision of the transplant team regarding candidacy.[154] Administration of lactulose or neomycin to either remove or decrease production of contributing nitrogenous bodies may be initiated but will not resolve the underlying liver disease.

Bleeding is best managed by prevention. Safety precautions to prevent falls, needle sticks, self-induced injuries, and tissue injuries should be initiated. Physiological factors such as decreased vitamin K availability or utilization, decreased clotting factors, and cascade disruption can be addressed by repletion of the appropriate factor or compound. Repletion must be done carefully, as the patient is at risk for development of DIC as a result of decreased clearance of products of fibrinolysis. Prophylactic antacid or H_2 antagonist therapy is standard but must proceed carefully; decreased mental ability leaves the patient at risk for aspiration of gastric contents, and accompanying renal failure prolongs the serum concentrations of any drugs given.

Renal failure is difficult to reverse and this may be impossible if it is the result of hepatorenal syndrome (renal failure resulting from hepatic failure).

Hemodialysis and/or continuous arteriovenous hemofiltration is an option and is normally used for hyperkalemia and fluid overload. Ultrafiltration for fluid only is an option for the patient who needs only fluid removed. Any approach that results in fluid shifting must be undertaken very carefully, as this process has been implicated in the development of hepatorenal syndrome. The decreased serum sodium may also be corrected with dialysis or ultrafiltration as total body fluid volume is decreased. Repletion of sodium is best done cautiously, as rapid change (a serum increase of greater than 20 mEq in 24 hours) is associated with central pontine damage.[155] If dialysis is required and the patient is a candidate for transplant, avoid the use of the left femoral vein if at all possible so that it may be used for the venovenous bypass necessary during the transplant procedure. Repletion of low potassium must be undertaken very carefully, especially if the patient is going to be receiving a transplant; large releases of potassium occur with graft reperfusion.

Respiratory complications frequently result from the decreased cough reflex ineffective and respiratory patterns that accompany hepatic coma and cerebral edema. Intubation allows for good pulmonary toilet and protects the airway. The use of an endotracheal tube (7.5–8.0 French) allows easy access should bronchoscopy be required.

Alkalosis can sometimes be prevented by careful use of an NG tube. Aggressive gastric suctioning or use of alkalyzing agents often causes alkalosis. Alkalosis resulting from hypokalemia, impaired renal function, and altered central respiratory drive are harder to avoid.

Immune system deficits are also difficult to overcome. Prophylactic administration of broad-spectrum antibiotics is not recommended, because of the potential for superinfection and nephrotoxicity. Conventional therapy involves frequent blood culturing for bacteria and viruses, with antibiotic therapy only if an organism is identified or sepsis occurs.

Nutritional approaches depend on the individual patient's clinical conditions. A low-sodium, low-potassium, and low-protein regimen is recommended. Amino acid formulas have been developed for severely compromised patients, but these must be accompanied by some protein for proper dietary maintenance.

Chronic Hepatitis

Chronic hepatitis is a term that refers to a group of disorders characterized by hepatic inflammation or necrosis and elevated transaminases that continue for a period of 6 months or more. Chronic hepatitis is categorized on the basis of the different architectural changes that occur within the liver as a result of the disease process. The types include chronic persistent hepatitis, chronic lobular hepatitis, and chronic active hepatitis. It is important for the clinician to identify a patient's specific clinical syndrome so that proper treatment regimens may be instituted.

Clinical antecedents

Chronic hepatitis may result from many different insults to the liver. These are listed in Table 6-39. The most common insult is viral, such as hepatitis B, non-A, non-B hepatitis, hepatitis C, and hepatitis D.[156] Although data is inconclusive, it appears unlikely that hepatitis E is a cause of chronic hepatitis, as the disease is often relatively mild and of short duration. Hepatitis A is the only viral hepatitis that doesn't cause chronic disease. Chronic hepatitis may also be caused by medications, metabolic disorders, and autoimmune diseases. In some patients, however, the causative agent may never be identified; such patients are said to be suffering from idiopathic hepatitis.

Chronic persistent and chronic lobular hepatitis are the result of hepatitis B or non-A, non-B infection. No other etiologies are identified at present.

Chronic active hepatitis (CAH) can be caused by chemical insults, hepatitis B, or non-A, non-B hepatitis. Drug therapy, such as the use of methyldopa, oxyphenisatin, or isoniazid, has been shown to cause the development of CAH. Approximately one-third of the cases start suddenly after acute viral hepatic illness.[157] Hepatitis B surface antigen has been found in 20–30% of the patients with CAH, indicating that persistent active hepatitis B infection may be a predisposing factor.[158] Those with positive hepatitis B "e" antigen and hepatitis B DNA serology upon diagnosis of CAH are in a stage of active viral repli-

Table 6-39 Precipitators of Chronic Hepatitis

Type of Chronic Hepatitis	Precipitator
Persistent Hepatitis/Lobular Hepatitis	Hepatitis B Non-A, non-B hepatitis
Active Hepatitis	Chemical insults Hepatitis B Non-A, non-B hepatitis Drug therapy Acute viral infection Idiopathic hepatitis

cation and infectivity and are therefore continuously exposing the liver to viral injury. Not only is the hepatitis B patient who becomes superinfected with hepatitis D at a much greater risk of developing chronic active hepatitis, but the clinical course of the disease (if it does develop) is usually much more severe.

Critical referents

Chronic persistent and chronic lobular hepatitis are generally not life-threatening disorders. It is important to differentiate the presentations by histological evidence. Liver biopsies of the patient with chronic persistent hepatitis are defined by an infiltration into the portal area of the liver by mononuclear cells; this infiltration does not extend into the lobule, and there is no necrosis at the periphery of the lobule. Chronic lobular hepatitis is similar but *does* involve lobular inflammation and focal hepatocellular necrosis, especially during the active phase.[159] It is characterized by cycles of remissions and active phases. Despite the damage to the liver that occurs with these changes, it is rare for either chronic persistent or chronic lobular hepatitis to progress to hepatic failure and/or cirrhosis, and the architecture of the liver remains intact.

Chronic active hepatitis (CAH), on the other hand, has extremely pathogenic effects. It is recognized by its active inflammation, functional deterioration, necrosis, and fibrosis. Eventually, it may lead to liver failure and death. Infiltration of plasma and mononuclear cells into the portal zone extends into the liver lobules, with hepatocyte destruction occurring at the periphery of the lobule.[160] This is called piecemeal necrosis. This necrosis extends into the periportal area and leads to areas of focal necrosis. If severe, the necrosis will "bridge" between adjacent portal tracts or between portal tracts and portal veins. This results in the formation of tissue necrosis and fibrotic areas. The process will occur at different rates and locations throughout the liver. The patient may have some areas of patchy involvement surrounded by either areas that have not been injured or areas that were previously injured but are now regenerating. The end result is a liver with areas of viable tissue, areas of necrotic tissue, and fibrous connective bands between them.

Recent literature has identified the increasing role of the immune system in the development of CAH.[161] It is believed that the immune system is conditioned or controlled by genetic factors. Evidence of interaction of T-lymphocytes and plasma cells in hepatocellular destruction and fibrotic development, as well as the presence of circulating "autoantibodies," lends credence to this theory. For example, lupoid hepatitis is characteristically found in women who are negative for the hepatitis B surface antigen.[162] Other autoimmune diseases such as thyroiditis, ulcerative colitis, and glomerulonephritis may also be associated with CAH. The immune reaction may be at the cellular level, with lymphocytes becoming sensitized to antigens on the hepatocyte cell membrane, or at a humoral level, as supported by the development of extrahepatic features such as arthralgias, arthritis, rashes, glomerulonephritis, and a decreased complement level.[163]

Death from chronic active hepatitis within the first 2 years is usually from liver failure and coma. If death occurs after this period, it is usually a complication of the compromised liver, such as variceal bleeding, infection, or other systemic side effects. It is unusual for patients testing negative for hepatitis B surface antigen to develop primary hepatocellular carcinoma after CAH, in contrast with the high rate found among hepatitis B carriers with CAH/cirrhosis.[164]

Idiopathic chronic hepatitis results from a source that is never clinically or histologically identified. The clinical course is not significantly different from that of viral hepatitis, except that it is more severe initially; therefore, these patients may come in for evaluation earlier than patients with viral disease.

The prognosis for patients with chronic hepatitis is entirely dependent upon the form of the disease from which they suffer. Chronic persistent hepatitis is extremely unlikely to progress to cirrhosis or chronic active hepatitis. If, however, the patient suffers from chronic active hepatitis, the causative agent will determine the prognosis. Eighty percent of patients with CAH that arises from hepatitis B will survive 5 years; if cirrhosis is present in addition to CAH, the survival rate drops to 55%. The prognosis is less hopeful for patients with chronic hepatitis arising from non-A, non-B hepatitis. Autoimmune hepatitis patients who have SGOT levels greater than five times the normal *and* hypergammaglobulinemia will die within 3 years if no treatment is undertaken. Those who have SGOT levels greater than ten times normal, regardless of gammaglobulin levels, are also found to have a survival rate of only 3 years.[165]

Resulting signs and symptoms

The patient with chronic persistent or chronic lobular hepatitis is usually asymptomatic, although some report anorexia, fatigue, and occasional nausea and vomiting. The liver is slightly enlarged and tender to palpation. Mild increases in aminotransferase and alkaline phosphatase may last for months to years. If chronic lobular hepatitis moves into an active phase, the aminotransferase levels may approach those found with acute viral hepatitis.

The clinical course of chronic active hepatitis may begin asymptomatically and end in death. The majority of patients are unable to tell when the disease started, as the onset is insidious and occurs over a period of weeks to months. Other patients experience a sudden onset similar to that of acute hepatitis, but the specific histopathologic events within the liver occur over the next 12–24 months.[166]

The specific signs and symptoms of CAH are those found in the majority of patients with liver disease. Malaise, anorexia, low-grade fever, and fatigue are common. Persistent and/or recurrent jaundice is a sign of severe liver disease. Hepatomegaly, splenomegaly, and right upper quadrant pain may also be present, along with the signs and symptoms of portal hypertension. Serological testing may show development of various antibodies, including antibodies to smooth muscle, mitochondria, and systemic lupus. Extrahepatic disturbances may also be present; they are more common in women than men and in patients who exhibit no history of hepatitis B.[167] Some typical extrahepatic signs are listed in Table 6-40.

With the progression of the hepatic disease, complications of long-term liver disease such as coagulopathies, variceal bleeding, hypersplenism, and encephalopathy become a part of the clinical picture. The presence of circulating autoantibodies against DNA, IgG, and smooth muscle is indicative of an immunologic disorder. The signs and symptoms are similar to those of chronic viral hepatitis. In severe cases, fever and extrahepatic manifestations are common. If the patient is symptomatic, physical examination will show hepatosplenomegaly, palmar erythema, and spider angiomata.[168]

Finally, although they don't correlate to either severity of disease or prognosis, lab values can assist in monitoring progression or recovery. SGOT and SGPT may range between 100 and 1000 units. The serum bilirubin ranges anywhere from 2 to 10 mg/dL and, with a decreasing albumin, indicates the presence of active disease and/or cirrhosis. Hypergammaglobulinemia is present if there has been extensive plasma cell infiltration. The prothrombin time is frequently prolonged, especially late in the disease process or with an active phase.

Nursing standards of care

The only way to know the proper treatment and prognosis for the patient with chronic hepatitis is by histological identification of the specific form of the disease. This can only be accomplished through liver biopsy. Despite the depth of medical knowledge regarding the complexities of chronic hepatitis, there are still very few treatment modalities.

The patient with the best chance of remission without deterioration is the one with chronic persistent or chronic lobular hepatitis; it is rare for either of these to progress to hepatic failure or cirrhosis. Clinicians should be aware that patients in remission from chronic active hepatitis will have symptoms similar to those with chronic persistent or chronic lobular hepatitis. Chronic active hepatitis should be suspected if there is a sudden change or progression in the disease process. If the patient is found to suffer from either chronic persistent or chronic lobular hepatitis, medical treatment involves only a follow-up every 6 to 12 months to watch for the rare progression to chronic active hepatitis.

If the diagnosis is chronic active hepatitis, specific therapies should be initiated, depending upon the origin of the disease. If the hepatitis is the result of a drug reaction, removal of the causative agent is the immediate action to be taken and will result in improvement of histopathological, clinical, and chemical measures. If the CAH is not associated with hepatitis B or non-A, non-B hepatitis, glucocorticoids may be beneficial, as the process may be immune-mediated. There is evidence to suggest that this therapy may prolong survival through the difficult first year. Protocols for length of administration and

Table 6-40 Extrahepatic Signs and Symptoms in CAH

Amenorrhea

Anemia

Arthralgia

Arthritis

Bloody diarrhea (from associated ulcerative colitis)

Dermatologic eruptions (macular, papular, acne)

Pericarditis

Pleurisy

Scleral icterus

Sicca syndrome

Source: Wands and Isselbacher, Chronic hepatitis. In *Harrison's Principles of Internal Medicine*, p. 1339.

doses vary, but all regimens begin with high-dose prednisone or prednisilone that is decreased gradually. A positive result (evidenced by clinical, biochemical, and histologic remission) has been found in more than 60% of the cases treated this way.[169] These responses may take weeks to months to become apparent, and future liver biopsies may give evidence of chronic persistent hepatitis. The use of Azathioprine and concomitant lower-dose steroid therapy has been attempted in patients who could not otherwise tolerate the high dose of glucocorticoids. Again, dosages and regimens vary, but the therapy has met with some success in slowing the progression to cirrhosis.[170] Unfortunately, relapse with this disease is common, and a cure is not available at this time.

If the patient is a carrier of hepatitis B surface antigen but is asymptomatic, no treatment is required. If the patient is positive for hepatitis B surface antigen *and* is symptomatic, glucocorticoid therapy will not help and may in fact cause harm. Alpha-interferon is the most promising therapy presently under investigation. It has shown some ability to reduce or eliminate viral replication. Other therapies that have been attempted are listed in Table 6-41; their effectiveness is still under study.

Nursing responsibilities for the management of chronic hepatitis are focused on prevention of further injury, implementation of the treatment regimen, and management of symptoms and side effects. This is a chronic illness and therefore requires continuous and consistent monitoring not only for medical but also for psychological ramifications.

Cirrhosis

Cirrhosis is the result of massive liver tissue injury from a variety of etiologies. The damage that is sustained by the liver is irreversible and pathological. Lobular distortion resulting from fibrotic tissue development is a characteristic finding on biopsy. There are many different mechanisms of injury, the most common of which is alcohol toxicity.

Clinical antecedents

There are four general categories of cirrhosis, delineated by their method of presentation and causative agents: alcoholic, postnecrotic, biliary, and cardiac cirrhosis. Alcoholic cirrhosis is probably the most familiar to both health professionals and the general public, and it is among the most preventable. Postnecrotic cirrhosis follows hepatitis B infection, especially if this has been complicated by hepatitis D. Non-A, non-B hepatitis and immune disorders are also catalysts of cirrhosis. Biliary cirrhosis is defined by the site of biliary obstruction that has caused the injury to the liver hepatocytes. Primary biliary cirrhosis is the result of an autoimmune disorder that has caused damage to the intrahepatic bile ducts. Sec-

Table 6-41 Potential Therapies for CAH

Acyclovir
Adenine arabinoside
Adenine arabinoside monophosphate
Azathioprine
Cyclophosphamide
D-penicillamine
Interleukin 2

Source: Wands and Isselbacher, Chronic hepatitis. In *Harrison's Principles of Internal Medicine*, p. 1340.

Table 6-42 Etiologies of Cirrhosis

Etiology	Examples
Infectious diseases	Viral hepatitis
	Toxoplasmosis
	Schistosomiasis
	Brucellosis
Inherited and metabolic disorders	Hemochromatosis
	Wilson's disease
	Glycogen storage disease
	Hereditary fructose intolerance
	Fanconi's syndrome
Drugs and toxins	Methyldopa
	Methotrexate
	Isoniazid
	Oxyphenisatin
	Arsenicals
	Pyrrolidizine alkaloids (used in the treatment of veno-occlusive disease)
	Oral contraceptives (Budd-Chiari disease)
Other or unproven causes	Sarcoidosis
	Graft-versus-host disease
	Chronic inflammatory bowel disease
	Cystic fibrosis
	Jejunoileal bypass
	Diabetes mellitus

Table 6-43   Cirrhosis

	Alcoholic	Postnecrotic	Primary Biliary	Secondary Biliary	Cardiac
Also known as	Portal, Laennec's nutritional or fatty cirrhosis	Toxic, nodular, posthepatic, postviral, or multilobular cirrhosis	Cholangitic, obstructive, or biliary cirrhosis	Biliary cirrhosis	
Cause	Fatty deposition within liver parenchyma; decreased nutritional status	Follows severe hepatitis B, hepatitis D, non-A, non-B hepatitis, chronic active hepatitis; autoimmune disease, Wilson's disease, hemochromatosis	Unknown primary cause; associated with autoimmune diseases: calcinosis, Raynaud's disease, sclerodactyly, telangiectasia, sicca syndrome, autoimmune thyroiditis, renal tubular acidosis	Longstanding total or partial obstruction of larger extrahepatic ducts: post-op strictures, gallstones, chronic pancreatitis, sclerosing cholangitis	Right-sided heart failure
Structural changes	Cell necrosis and collapse, fine scarring, fibrotic connective tissue bands; small regular nodular development	Cell necrosis and collapse; irregular patterns of nodular regeneration, hepatocyte collapse; connection of triads by bands of connective tissue; fibrosis and lobular collapse	Chronic inflammation, edema and necrosis of portal triads; fibrous obliteration of bile ducts	Biliary stasis with dilation of portal tracts, edema, and fibrous development; possible sites of biliary rupture	Dilation of hepatic sinusoids; necrosis, and development of fibrotic bands
Physical findings	Liver initially large, shrinks with disease process	Liver shrunken and distorted	Liver shrunken and distorted	Liver shrunken and distorted	Tense, swollen liver capsule

ondary biliary cirrhosis is the result of extrahepatic blockage of the bile ducts and may be associated with biliary stricture or sclerosing cholangitis. Cardiac cirrhosis occurs in the presence of severe right-sided heart disease that causes right ventricular failure.[171] Cirrhosis can also result from a variety of infections, medications, metabolic, and hereditary factors that are listed in Table 6-42 (page 929).

Critical referents

Cirrhosis is the end result of prolonged pathological processes occurring within the liver. As healthy cells are exposed to various pathogenic agents, they and their support structures are destroyed. The natural response of the liver to this injury is to attempt to regenerate the injured area. Unfortunately, the body's defense response is to deposit collagen in the injured area. These deposits become organized into bands of fibrotic tissue. The fibrotic bands of tissue may grow separately or together; if they connect, a reorganization of the liver's basic structure occurs. If the reorganization is extreme, the outcome will be an irregular nodular organ with pathological twisting, disorganization, and constriction of hepatic cells and plates. The vascular structure, which normally offers little resistance to flow and easy access to all lobes and structures, becomes very difficult to perfuse. If vascular flow is not regained or maintained, the result is necrosis and/or atrophy. The overwhelming extent of injury and compromise is fatal. Each type of cirrhosis causes this process in its own individual way; Table 6-43 gives comparisons of the types of cirrhosis, which are discussed below.

Alcoholic cirrhosis is the result of hepatocellular damage that occurs with long-term alcohol abuse. The altered metabolic pathways within the liver lead to fat deposition within the cellular framework with resulting hepatocyte compromise. Over a period of time, the injury and fibrosis that are the hallmarks of cirrhosis develop and destroy the liver.

Postnecrotic cirrhosis is the result of necrosis, collapse, and fibrosis from a source of inflammation within the liver. In this disorder, the bands of connective tissue join together and connect many portal triads, which causes total disorganization of both structure and function within the liver.

Primary biliary cirrhosis also results in fibrous restructuring of the liver, but the mechanism of injury here is an infiltration of inflammatory cells. These cells infiltrate tissue of the bile ducts and destroy them, decreasing the number available between the lobes. There is hepatocyte necrosis and growth of a network of fibrotic tissue that spans the liver. This process can take months or years to reach completion.

Secondary biliary cirrhosis results from consistent partial or complete obstruction of the common bile duct or its branches. This causes bile to be trapped within the liver. As this continues, there is dilation of the bile ducts and potential for cholangitis as the infiltrates around the ducts increase. Eventually the ducts become swollen and fibrotic and may rupture, causing areas of necrosis. As expected, the injured areas between the fibrotic tissue attempt to regenerate themselves, and a finely nodular cirrhosis results.

Cardiac cirrhosis is the result of right-sided heart failure. The inability of the heart to completely empty

Table 6-44 Alteration of Glucose Metabolism in Cirrhosis

Type of Alteration	Contributing Factors

Hyperglycemia	Decreased hepatic glucose uptake
	Decreased hepatic glycogen synthesis
	Hepatic resistance to insulin
	Portal-systemic glucose shunting
	Peripheral insulin resistance
	Hormonal abnormalities (serum)
	  Increased glucagon
	  Decreased cortisol
	  Increased insulin (decreased in hemochromatosis)

Hypoglycemia	Decreased gluconeogenesis Decreased hepatic glycogen content Hepatic resistance to glucagon Poor oral intake Hyperinsulinemia secondary to portal-systemic shunting

Source: Podolsky, Derangements of hepatic metabolism. In *Harrison's Principles of Internal Medicine*, p. 1312.

the ventricle impedes the flow of blood from the liver to the heart. This results in a pooling of blood and engorgement of the hepatic sinusoids, ischemia, necrosis, and fibrosis.[172]

Resulting signs and symptoms

The cirrhotic patient exhibits the expected complications of liver failure. Complications such as with coagulation deficits, metabolic and nutritional compromise, ascites, peripheral venocongestion, portal hypertension, hepatic encephalopathy, electrolyte imbalances, and alterations of glucose metabolism are common to all patients. Table 6-44 lists the factors that contribute to altered glucose metabolism in cirrhosis. Symptoms specific to each form of cirrhosis and their causes are listed in Table 6-45.

The only way to identify a specific type of cirrhosis is to examine the liver tissue itself. Both percutaneous and transvenous liver biopsy allow the clinician to take a tissue sample from within the liver. Percutaneous liver biopsy requires the investigator to pierce the liver from the exterior. The technique is illustrated in Figure 6-18. Since the procedure necessitates piercing of the diaphragm and pleura, it can lead to complications such as pneumothorax and bleeding. In the case of transvenous biopsy, bleeding

Table 6-45 Signs and Symptoms of Cirrhosis

Type	Symptom	Cause
Alcoholic cirrhosis	Azotemia	Prerenal kidney failure
	Bruising	Loss of coagulation factors
	Clubbing of fingers	Circulatory compromise
	Decreased body hair (men)	Disturbance of hormone metabolism
	Glucose intolerance	Endogenous insulin release
	Gynecomastia (men)	Disturbance of hormone metabolism
	Hemolytic anemia	Hypercholesterolemia
	Hypokalemia	Hyperaldosteronism (exchange with K^+)
	Hypomagnesemia	Urinary losses/dietary deficiency
	Jaundice	Impaired bilirubin metabolism
	Menstrual irregularities	Disturbance of hormone metabolism
	Palmar erythema	Disturbance of hormone metabolism
	Respiratory alkalosis	Central hyperventilation
	Spider angiomas	Disturbance of hormone metabolism
	Testicular atrophy	Disturbance of hormone metabolism or ingestion of toxic ETOH
	Virilization (women)	Disturbance of hormone metabolism
	Weakness/fatigue	Loss of energy stores
	Weight loss/loss of muscle	Anorexia/malnutrition
Postnecrotic cirrhosis	Azotemia	Prerenal kidney failure
	Glucose intolerance	Endogenous insulin release
	Hemolytic anemia	Hypercholesterolemia
	Hypokalemia	Hyperaldosteronism (exchange with K^+)
	Hypomagnesemia	Urinary losses/dietary deficiency
	Respiratory alkalosis	Central hyperventilation
Primary biliary cirrhosis	Bone pain/osteomalacia	Impaired vitamin D uptake
	Bruising	Impaired vitamin K uptake
	Dermatitis	Impaired vitamin E uptake/EFA deficiency
	Night blindness	Impaired vitamin A uptake
	Pruritus/jaundice/dark skin	Bilirubin deposition and accumulation
	Steatorrhea	Impaired bile excretion
	Xanthelasmas/xanthomas	Prolonged elevation of serum lipids
Secondary biliary cirrhosis	Bone pain/osteomalacia	Impaired vitamin D uptake
	Bruising	Impaired vitamin K uptake
	Dermatitis	Impaired vitamin E uptake/EFA deficiency
	Fever/RUQ pain	Cholangitis/biliary colic
	Night blindness	Impaired vitamin A uptake
	Pruritus/jaundice/dark skin	Bilirubin deposition and accumulation
	Steatorrhea	Impaired bile excretion
	Xanthelasmas/xanthomas	Prolonged elevation of serum lipids
Cardiac cirrhosis	Pulsatile liver (early)	Tricuspid regurgitation
	Severe RUQ pain	Stretching of Glisson's capsule

from the site *within* the liver will be recirculated; bleeding from percutaneous biopsy tends to accumulate in the abdomen and will not be recirculated. If the patient is thrombocytopenic or has coagulation disorders, severe ascites, or infection of the proposed biopsy area or surrounding tissue, percutaneous biopsy may be contraindicated. If extrahepatic biliary obstruction is suspected, the risk of possible biliary peritonitis from increased intrahepatic biliary pressure must be weighed against the benefits of the examination.[173] The histopathological findings ex-

pected with different disease processes were listed earlier in Table 6-43.

If biopsy is not feasible, noninvasive techniques may be utilized. Liver-spleen scans measure the uptake of radioisotopes by the liver and spleen and allow the investigator to measure the size of those organs and detect possible portal hypertension. Other techniques include ultrasound and CT scanning, which, although they may not be diagnostic for cirrhosis specifically, will aid in the evaluation of size and form of the liver and associated organs.

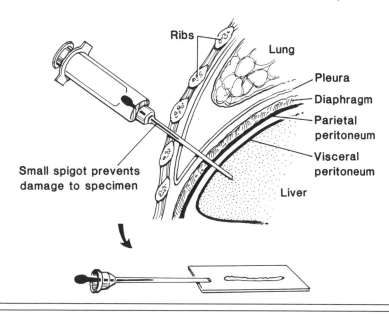

Figure 6-18 Percutaneous Liver Biopsy

Labels in figure: Ribs, Lung, Pleura, Diaphragm, Parietal peritoneum, Visceral peritoneum, Liver, Small spigot prevents damage to specimen

Nursing standards of care

Treatment of the cirrhotic patient focuses upon the removal of predisposing factors: elimination of alcohol intake, treatment of chronic/acute inflammation, removal of biliary obstruction, or correction of right-sided heart failure. Basic to the care of all cirrhotic patients is the recognition of the common side effects of liver failure (ascites, portal hypertension/encephalopathy, variceal hemorrhage, etc.). Nurses are responsible for the prevention of side effects and/or their management if they are present. Limitation of known stressing agents (alcohol, drugs metabolized by the liver, etc.) is fundamental. The patient's medication and social profile should be evaluated, and all potentially hepatotoxic factors eliminated.

Avoidance of alcohol by a patient with alcoholic cirrhosis may limit disease progression. Only 5% of those who continue to drink despite major complications live as long as 5 years.[174] Care of such patients is mostly supportive, with any treatments geared toward managing the complications. Colchine, a drug commonly used for gout, may slow the progression of the disease and increase life expectancy by inhibiting collagen formation within the diseased liver.[175] If the patient is not showing signs and symptoms of hepatic coma, a diet with a protein requirement of 1 g/kg and 2000–3000 kcal/day with vitamin and thiamine supplements is appropriate. This diet *must*

be discontinued if signs or symptoms of hepatic coma develop. The importance of total abstinence from alcohol cannot be overemphasized with this patient population. Assisting patients to find an alcohol abuse treatment program and supporting them and their family members may be the most important intervention that health care personnel can implement.

The only treatment option available with postnecrotic cirrhotic patients is supportive care; in 75% of cases the disease is progressive despite such care and the patient dies within 1–5 years. Death usually occurs from the complications of liver compromise rather than from the primary injury.

There is no treatment regimen for primary biliary cirrhosis at this time, although some delay of symptoms may result from use of colchine, as mentioned above. The goal of treatment is to keep the patient as comfortable as possible by diminishing or alleviating the symptoms. Cholestyramine, a drug that binds with excess bile salt and promotes its excretion in the feces, may be used to help decrease pruritus and lower hypercholesterolemia. Dietary manipulation to minimize fat intake helps decrease the incidence of steatorrhea, and vitamin D repletion will help prevent the pain associated with osteomalacia. Liver failure and death resulting from primary biliary cirrhosis will usually occur within 5–10 years after initial diagnosis. Death is frequently the result of variceal hemorrhage and/or infection.[176]

Secondary biliary cirrhosis is treated by surgical or endoscopic removal of the obstruction. If this isn't possible, as in the case of sclerosing cholangitis, antibiotics may help control superinfection and are sometimes used to suppress its recurrence. If the underlying process can be either reversed or halted, the prognosis for symptom reduction and survival is much improved. If this is not possible, there is a steady progression to terminal cirrhosis. Similarly, cardiac cirrhosis is cured only by removal of the underlying cardiac problem. If that is not possible, treatment options are nonexistent, and care must be supportive in nature.

Nursing Care Plan for the Management of the Patient with Hepatic Disorders

Diagnosis	Signs and symptoms	Intervention	Rationale
Altered elimination: diarrhea or oliguria related to disease process	Steatorrhea Diarrhea Decreased urinary output Light-colored feces Increased BUN and creatinine Increased urine specific gravity	Decrease fatty intake (diet should include minimal animal products); do not administer fat emulsions unless patient is evaluated for tolerance	The patient's body is unable to provide the bile salts necessary for the metabolism of fats
		Administer fluids cautiously, using colloids if patient is also hypoalbuminemic	Liquid stools deplete the body of circulating volume required for tissue perfusion
		Administer GI antimotility agents (Lomotil, tincture of opium); monitor for constipation	Slowing the peristaltic activity will increase absorption rates and decrease fluid loss
		Protect rectal area from breakdown: encourage frequent cleaning; offer sitz baths; educate the patient on importance of keeping the area clean; utilize protective creams if area becomes raw	The patient is at increased risk for infection and perianal breakdown
		Monitor intake and output carefully and document CVP and weight when giving fluid replenishment or diuretic	Fluid balance is precarious due to predisposing factors for both overhydration and dehydration
		Check urine specific gravity every shift	To obtain information regarding kidneys' ability to concentrate and potential need for volume replacement
		Evaluate urine electrolytes and creatinine as appropriate	To monitor for acute renal failure related to hepatorenal syndrome

Nursing Care Plan for the Management of the Patient with Hepatic Disorders

Diagnosis	Signs and symptoms	Intervention	Rationale
Potential for altered nutrition: intake greater than body requirements	Increasing BUN Increasing serum ammonia Liver progressively larger and firmer Steatorrhea Xanthelasmas/xanthomas Hypoalbuminemia	Limit amount of protein in diet (meat, eggs, beans) based on patient presentation and laboratory values	The patient will not be able to process all the protein that is provided by the normal diet
		Avoid blood in GI tract; use NG tube with lavage as indicated	Blood breaks down into protein and increases ammonia
		Low sodium and potassium diet	To help prevent fluid overload, hyperkalemia, and hypernatremia
		Palpate liver every shift	Baseline and follow-up assessment of liver size and consistency will allow for recognition of rapidly deteriorating liver function and increasing distention
		Monitor BUN, ammonia, electrolytes, and osmolarity	To evaluate liver function, volume regulation, systemic ramifications of disease, and response to therapy
		Note characteristics of stool (color, consistency, and frequency)	The patient is unable to provide the bile salts necessary for the metabolism of fats and is prone to fatty and frequent stools
Potential for altered nutrition: intake less than body requirements	Weight loss Nausea and vomiting Dehydration Lack of appetite Osteomalacia	Encourage small, frequent meals	Smaller, more frequent meals are more easily digested
		Have patient avoid fatty foods and meals late in the day	The patient will have little tolerance for fatty foods and digests slowly

Diagnosis	Signs and symptoms	Intervention	Rationale
	Dermatitis Glucose and electrolyte abnormalities	Monitor electrolytes and glucose levels; replete vitamins as required; educate the patient about the need for adequate nutrition to facilitate recovery	The patient is unlikely to be taking in enough sustenance to maintain adequate levels of vitamins, electrolytes, protein, or fluids
		Record daily weights as needed	To provide both information to clinicians and support for the patient who is trying to maintain or gain weight
		Administer insulin as ordered	Decreased liver function may lead to decreased glucose storage and increased circulating glucose
		Administer thiamine to patient with alcoholic hepatitis before glucose administration	Administration of thiamine will help prevent Wernicke's encephalopathy in the alcoholic patient receiving glucose
		Administer vitamin K as needed for coagulation abnormalities	GI absorption of vitamin K may be irregular and liver synthesis of coagulation proteins is disrupted
Potential fluid deficit related to nausea and vomiting or fluid shifts	Poor skin turgor Increased specific gravity Increased BUN Increased serum osmolality and Hct Poor oral intake CVP < 1 mm Hg Orthostasis Nausea, vomiting	Encourage small, frequent amounts of food and drink	Patients are often able to tolerate small amounts taken more frequently more easily than large amounts taken at a single sitting
		Provide IV hydration if required, possibly including electrolyte and vitamin repletion; tailor fluid administration to sodium and glucose levels of each individual; administer colloids, albumin, and blood products as indicated	Electrolyte, glucose, coagulation factors, albumin, and RBC transfusions will correct underlying abnormalities while providing necessary fluid and osmotic agents

Diagnosis	Signs and symptoms	Intervention	Rationale
		Administer antiemetics as ordered	To decrease the incidence of nausea and vomiting, which may be decreasing the patient's interest in food and worsening fluid balance
		Restrict free water and sodium intake	If the sequestration of fluid is related to the pathological accumulation of ascites or third spacing, restriction of free water and excess sodium is indicated
		Utilize large molecular repletion factors	Repletion of fluid should be done with agents that can pull fluid back into the circulation from extracellular spaces
		Administer potassium-sparing diuretics as ordered (e.g., Spironolactone)	These diuretics spare potassium, decreasing incidence of hypokalemia and its associated alkalosis, which worsens ammonia accumulation
Self-care deficit related to immobility and discomfort	Inability to carry out normal activities of daily living or to maintain baseline activity Increased pain and decreased tolerance of pain	Splint patient's right side as required	To help the patient support tender areas, which may be inhibiting movement
		Explain to patient that this present level of extreme fatigue is unlikely to be a permanent condition (in cases of acute/chronic hepatitis)	As the patient begins systemic recovery from the disease, energy levels start returning; the fatigue and inability to perform normal activities can be psychologically frightening and troublesome for the patient

Diagnosis	Signs and symptoms	Intervention	Rationale
		Promote rest and relaxation, with limited activity and body stress	The patient will be able to sustain activities if they are performed a little bit at a time; rest promotes healing of the stressed system
		Allow change of position and use of occupational and physical therapy as recovery progresses	Occupational and physical therapy will assist the patient in recognizing limitations of strength and provide mental stimulation
Potential for health risk to others	Family members or friends sharing food, water, or bathing	Educate the family and significant others and health-care personnel regarding the modes of transmission and methods to prevent transmission of the various viral hepatitis diseases	The protection of all those in contact with the patient will prevent further spread of infection
	Family members or friends demonstrating signs and symptoms of hepatitis	Follow serology data and inform patient of infectious status	Patients' awareness of infectious capacity will assist in protecting those around them
		Consider immunoglobulin or hepatitis vaccination for others at risk of contracting hepatitis	Prophylaxis against disease acquisition (not available for all types of hepatitis and may need sequential administration for effectiveness)
		Use enteric feeding while patient is hospitalized	To protect patient and health-care workers against contracting and spreading disease
		Institute universal precautions in caring for patients	Reduces risk for health care providers of acquiring hepatitis
Potential for pain related to disease process (swelling of the liver)	Complaints of right upper quadrant pain	Position patient on left side	Pain is the result of stretching of the capsule surrounding the liver
	Guarding of side when moving or during physical examination	Teach patient splinting techniques to be used during movements	Splinting helps prevent jarring and painful movements
	Inability to take deep breath without discomfort		

Nursing Care Plan for the Management of the Patient with Hepatic Disorders

Diagnosis	Signs and symptoms	Intervention	Rationale
	Nonverbal cues of discomfort	Consider use of narcotic analgesics for pain relief, but administer cautiously to avoid toxicity; utilize narcotics that are responsive to reversal agent whenever possible	Narcotics and sedatives may relieve pain and encourage good breathing and ambulation as needed; patients with liver disease may have difficulty clearing substances from the serum and thus narcotics and sedatives may have a longer than normal half-life
		Encourage nonpharmacological methods of relieving discomfort (relaxation, meditation, diversion)	Nonpharmacological methodologies may enhance medication effects and reduce need
		Have patient rate pain on a scale (1–10 or least to worst) before and after interventions	To evaluate effectiveness of medication regimen
Potential noncompliance in abstaining from alcohol	Continued deterioration of liver function tests	Enroll patient in alcohol withdrawal program	Support groups are often very helpful to patients trying to abstain from alcohol
	Lateness or missing of appointments with health-care team	Educate patient regarding morbidity and mortality from alcoholic hepatitis	Knowledge of the prognosis with continued ingestion of alcohol may help patient abstain
	Progression to cirrhosis or findings of pancreatitis or ketoacidosis	Involve family and significant others in treatment plan or in support groups	Family and significant others can support the patient as he or she tries to withdraw from alcohol; support groups can help family members affected by the disease process and behavior of the alcoholic patient
	Development of ineffective coping mechanisms		

Diagnosis	Signs and symptoms	Intervention	Rationale
Potential impaired tissue integrity related to decreased clotting factors, vitamin K deficiency, and decreased fibrinogen production	Bruising Ecchymosis Bleeding Heme positive stool or urine Decreased Hct or Hgb Prolonged bleeding time and PT/PTT time	Provide coagulation factors and vitamin K repletion as necessary	The compromised liver is unable to provide the coagulation factors required for clotting and maintenance of hemostasis; repletion of vitamin K is appropriate with progressive disease
		Prevent injury by limiting invasive procedures	Maintenance of skin and structural integrity will limit the potential sites of bleeding
		Educate patient regarding potential for bleeding due to disease process	Patient recognition of bleeding and tissue compromise will assist the caregiver in recognizing potential health problems; involving the patient in his or her own care provides him or her with an amount of control
		Monitor stool and urine for evidence of bleeding	To aid in recognition of early bleeding
		Provide GI prophylaxis as ordered, including antacids, coating agents, and avoidance of acidic substances	Increased acidity potentiates bleeding in the gastric system
		Use topical hemostatics as appropriate	Local measures may assist in halting bleeding without increasing protein load as blood products do
		Administer blood components required for hemorrhage	Acute hemorrhage can occur and must be treated supportively with blood products to prevent hemodynamic compromise

Nursing Care Plan for the Management of the Patient with Hepatic Disorders

Diagnosis	Signs and symptoms	Intervention	Rationale
Potential or actual alteration in skin integrity related to rash, pruritis, edema	Uncontrollable itching Swelling/tearing of skin Erythematous rash Jaundice	Administer antipruritic drugs as ordered (Benadryl, Atarax)	Allergic reactions to drugs frequently cause pruritic reactions, which respond to antihistamine therapy; jaundice causes itching
		Use cooling baths and soaks; use cooling (mentholated) lotions	Cooling baths and lotions help block the painful itching sensation
		Use agents that bind with bile salts	To remove the offending agents from the circulation and keep them from being deposited and causing irritation of the skin
		Provide diversional activities as appropriate	To divert patient from focusing on itching
		Binding/wrapping of hands as needed; clip nails	To prevent the patient from injuring fragile skin
		Provide means of communicating with staff by leaving call light within reach and assure patient that staff will be in every 15 minutes to check on him/her while he/she is without the use of his/her hands	Patients must be assured of safety and companionship
Potential for body image disturbance and situational low self-esteem	Depressed mood Feelings of defeatism Loneliness Reluctance to have visitors Jaundice Ascites and edema	Provide emotional support; refer patient to mental health worker or social worker as needed	Mental health workers and staff can provide support to the patient and family members in difficult times
		Assist patient to develop morale booster plan	The patient may be able to identify ways to maintain morale; use of these by staff members will build a strong and trusting relationship

Diagnosis	Signs and symptoms	Intervention	Rationale
		Provide diversional activities	To take patient's mind off the problem
		Enhance patient's appearance with robes, scarves, etc.	Encourage normal activities to enhance appearance and boost self-esteem
Potential for fluid volume deficit secondary to paracentesis, third-spacing, and dehydration	Hypotension Tachycardia Poor skin turgor Decreased urinary output Orthostasis Peripheral edema Ascites Increased specific gravity	Monitor CVP every shift and blood pressure at least every 4 hours; monitor PCWP every 4 hours or as ordered; assess urinary volume and quality as ordered; weigh patient every day or more frequently as ordered	Monitoring of intravascular fluid volume and comparison with weights, vital signs, intake, and output assists the clinician in determining appropriate methods of volume repletion and manipulation
		Measure abdominal girth every day or more frequently as ordered	Third spacing depletes intravascular volume
		Use colloids, albumin, and blood products as ordered for repletion of fluid volume in hypotensive crisis	Use of volume expanders assists in the correction of hypotension
Potential for infection secondary to immunosuppressive therapy, cirrhosis, or autoimmune hepatitis	Hypotension Tachycardia Fever Elevated WBC count Decreased WBC count Hyper/hypothermia	Minimize invasive procedures and exposure of the patient to infectious agents; no contact with oral polio vaccines or live virus vaccines; minimize exposure to childhood disorders such as chicken pox	Limiting exposure to these pathogens decreases the risk of compromising disease states
		Monitor temperature and vital signs as ordered	Vital signs reflect ongoing or potential sepsis, especially as the steroids may suppress fever
		Administer antibiotics as ordered	Antibiotics will supplement the compromised immune system and treat ongoing infections

Nursing Care Plan for the Management of the Patient with Hepatic Disorders

Diagnosis	Signs and symptoms	Intervention	Rationale
		Monitor CBC for decreased absolute neutrophil count	Neutropenia may occur with hepatic disease
		Culture all drainage with fever work-up or routinely as ordered	Surveillance cultures and cultures at the time of fever may reveal new sites or pathogens causing infection
		Initiate care plans for treating septic patients	Sepsis is a common complication of hepatic failure
Lack of knowledge regarding esophageal varices and medical management of cirrhosis or hepatitis	Questions from patient and family regarding bleeding, discomfort, and complications related to disease process Inappropriate questions to or expectations of health care practitioners	Explain disease process and interventions as they occur	Patients and families will be less fearful of the ramifications of the disease process if they are kept up to date on the content and goal of care being given
		Reinforce any information that is given to the patient and family by repetition; use pictures and diagrams whenever possible	Repeating information and using audiovisual aids help patient retain information
		Involve social work staff and clergy as available and desired by patient	Nonmedical personnel are sometimes much less threatening and more approachable by family members; many patients use religious faith as a coping mechanism
Potential for tissue injury related to liver biopsy	Increasing abdominal girth Decreased blood pressure Decreased Hct or Hgb	Measure abdominal girth before and 1–2 hours after procedure until other bleeding monitoring is discontinued	Baseline and followup measurements allow evaluation for distention due to potential bleeding

Diagnosis	Signs and symptoms	Intervention	Rationale
	Decreased level of mentation Decreased oxygen saturation Tachycardia Dyspnea Complaints of right upper quadrant pain	Monitor bleeding indicators before and after biopsy at least every shift and per physician's orders (PT/PTT); monitor CBC every 8 hours for 32 hours or more often if ordered Have blood components (PRBC/FFP/platelets/ cryoprecipitate) available before procedure is initiated	The patient undergoing evaluation for hepatitis will usually have a preexisting coagulopathy; proper evaluation of bleeding time, repletion factors that may be required, and the overall patient condition will facilitate recovery from the procedure
		Check vital signs every 15 minutes for first hour, then every 30 minutes for 2 hours, and then every hour until patient is stabilized	A percutaneous biopsy will cause bleeding into the abdominal cavity; the patient who hemorrhages following a transvenous biopsy will most likely bleed into the hepatic circulation, decreasing the risk of hypovolemia; evaluate for bleeding within the capsule, as it may cause rupture or tamponade the circulation
		Monitor oxygen saturations during procedure and hourly for 4 hours afterward and ABGs as indicated	Respiratory distress and hypoxemia may be indicative of hypovolemia and/or impending rupture of hepatic capsule
		Position patient per institutional protocol following procedure: right side down for capsular tamponade may be indicated	Positioning the patient on the right side following biopsy compresses the puncture site
		Bed rest for 24 hours following procedure	Bed rest is recommended to protect the area of injury
		If appropriate, decompress bowel with NGT prior to tap	Reduces risk of bowel perforation

Nursing Care Plan for the Management of the Patient with Hepatic Disorders

Diagnosis	Signs and symptoms	Intervention	Rationale
Potential for injury related to paracentesis	Hypotension Tachycardia Fever Abdominal pain Bleeding Increased abdominal girth Intravascular volume depletion	Measure baseline abdominal girth before procedure; monitor every 1–2 hours for 8 hours, then every shift for three shifts or until patient shows no signs of bleeding internally	To indicate potential hemorrhage into abdominal cavity and to allow for comparison of distention before and after fluid removal
		Monitor coagulation factors and obtain CBC before procedure and every 8 hours for 24 hours or until patient shows no signs of bleeding; maintain platelet level and Hct/Hgb/PT/PTT per physician's orders; monitor for signs and symptoms of transfusion reactions with administration of blood products and signs and symptoms of fluid overload associated with fluid administration	Paracentesis is an invasive procedure that requires careful monitoring of the patient's ability to clot at potential sites of bleeding
		Culture ascitic fluid for microorganisms (fungal, bacterial, and viral pathogens)	Ascites may become infected and compromise the patient
		Observe for air returns in paracentesis needle; monitor bowel sounds, abdominal tenderness, and vital signs after procedure in suspected bowel perforation	Signs of bowel perforation

Diagnosis	Signs and symptoms	Intervention	Rationale
		Obtain syringe full of ascitic fluid from person performing paracentesis early in the procedure and set it aside where it will not be disturbed: if the solution does not clot, then it is peritoneal in origin; if the solution does clot, then it is likely to be vascular in origin	If the fluid is not from the peritoneum, measures to compress the site of bleeding and address potential compromise to the patient must be investigated
		Sedate and medicate the patient prior to and following the procedure	Patients need to be cooperative and calm for the procedure and may experience pain as a result of the fluid removal
		Obtain post-tap abdominal x-ray	To note perforation
		Administer IV fluids as required	To maintain intravascular volume; third-space shifts from intravascular to interstitial areas are uncommon but possible

Portal Hypertension

The portal veins collect blood from the abdominal viscera and mesentery and feed it through the liver and the hepatic vein into the inferior vena cava. The portal circulation is normally characterized by low vascular resistance. A blockage of blood flow into or through the liver leads to increased venous pressures and is referred to as portal hypertension. Although a simple disease by definition, the systemic ramifications of portal hypertension are complex. The consequences of portal hypertension are splenomegaly, ascites, variceal bleeding, and hepatic encephalopathy. If recognition of these signs and symptoms is delayed or ignored, the clinical course can be fatal.

Clinical antecedents

The causes of portal hypertension can be broken down into four categories: three defined by the location of the blockage of the flow within the liver (presinusoidal, sinusoidal, or postsinusoidal), and one related to the amount of blood that flows to the liver. Presinusoidal resistance results from a blockage proximal to the hepatic sinusoids, such as that found with portal vein thrombosis. It is the second most common cause of portal hypertension. Significant portal vein obstruction may result from cirrhosis, infection, pancreatitis, or abdominal trauma, or it can be without a specific precipitating event. Schistosomiasis, an unusual presinusoidal disorder, is a parasitic disease that takes place within the liver but before the actual sinusoids. In this case, the compromise of blood flow is within the liver itself, but the disease is presinusoidal.

Sinusoidal resistance is obstruction that occurs because of a compression or blockage within the sinusoids themselves, and is frequently the result of a cirrhotic liver process. In fact, the most common cause of portal hypertension in the United States is cirrhosis; more than 60% of patients with cirrhosis exhibit clinically significant portal hypertension.[177]

Postsinusoidal processes result from blockage of the inferior vena cava or the hepatic vein, such as is seen with Budd-Chiari syndrome. These blockages prevent the emptying of the blood from the sinusoids. Veno-occlusive disease, with the associated injury to the hepatic venules, is also classified as a postsinusoidal injury. Veno-occlusive disease may arise from the use of chemotherapeutic agents, such as Busulfan or Cyclophosohamide.[178] Constrictive pericarditis or severe right-sided heart disease may

also lead to post-sinusoidal disease. Budd-Chiari and veno-occlusive diseases are not common primary causes of portal hypertension.

Portal hypertension that occurs not from blockage within the hepatic system but from an increased flow into the liver is less common, but possible. Splenomegaly or arteriovenous fistulas have been found to cause such a condition. Basically, any disease process that inhibits blood flow *through* the liver or causes an exceptional increase of blood supply *to* the liver can result in portal hypertension. Although these delineations are helpful in identifying the site of blockage, it is important to recognize that blockages may occur simultaneously at more than one location.

Critical referents

The pathophysiology of portal hypertension is best understood by an appreciation of the initial pathophysiological changes associated with the hypertension: splenomegaly, ascites, varix development, and encephalopathy.

The portal circulation normally exhibits very low vascular resistance. There are no valves within the hepatic circulation, and the sinusoids themselves offer little resistance to flow. The blood pressure within a healthy portal system normally measures between 10 and 15 cm water, or 7–10 mm Hg.[179] Consequently, the vasculature within the liver is designed to work best under conditions of little resistance to high flow. If something either causes a break in the flow itself or makes it more difficult for blood to flow into the liver, the vasculature must adjust to the new flow. If the aberrant situation cannot be rectified, blood pressure within the portal system increases. Portal hypertension exists when that pressure is greater than 30 cm H_2O or 20 mm Hg.[180] If the hypertension persists, collateral flow from the high-pressure portal venous circulation to the lower-pressure systemic venous circulation may be established in order to accommodate the flow change.

The resistance to blood flow into the liver affects the ease with which blood flows *out* of the spleen. The congestion within the liver causes a pressure buildup against the flow from the spleen into the portal vein, which leads to a corresponding congestion within the spleen. This congestion is termed congestive splenomegaly. It is most often seen in the patient with severe hepatic disease and secondary portal hypertension, which causes splenomegaly. Primary splenomegaly that causes a secondary portal hypertension is rare, but not unheard of.[181] The danger for the patient with splenomegaly arises from the risk of destruction or consumption of the spleen. The degree of thrombocytopenia, anemia, and leukopenia that may occur can vary greatly.

Ascites is the accumulation of fluid within the peritoneal cavity and is one of the most common side effects of portal hypertension. It may occur from various mechanisms related to hydrostatic pressure changes or lymphatic obstruction, as follows:

1. As pressure within the portal system rises, the hydrostatic gradients within the circulation alter, favoring a shift of fluid from the intravascular space to the peritoneal cavity.
2. The liver disease that usually accompanies portal hypertension causes decreased albumin production. This alters the colloidal pressures found within the vascular space and predisposes the patient to a shift of fluid into the peritoneal cavity, especially in the presence of increased portal pressure.
3. The liver has a decreased ability to manage the amount of lymphatic circulation presented to it. A deterioration of the sinusoids and lymphatics leads to a weeping of lymphatic fluid into the peritoneal cavity.

Aside from the mechanical aspects of ascites development, some theories say that supplemental factors predispose a patient to the development of ascites. These theories focus on the fluid and sodium imbalance that is present in the patient with ascites. One theory argues that as blood backs up and pools within the splanchnic bed, the body senses intravascular volume depletion. This imbalance is recognized by the kidneys, which activate aldosterone and renin and cause sodium and water retention. The second theory argues that there is *no* primary fluid deficit, but rather an inappropriate retention of fluid and sodium by the renal system, which causes a fluid-sodium imbalance.[182] Whatever the cause, once ascites has developed, the patient is in the unfortunate position of being in a state of total body fluid excess with intravascular volume depletion because the fluid is sequestered in the abdominal cavity.

The collateral channels, or varices, that the body creates to help relieve the build-up of pressure can be fatal. Although these collaterals work to decrease portal pressure, they are not strong vessels. They become engorged and develop into tortuous varices that are fragile and bleed easily as they become distended. These channels are most commonly found around the rectum (hemorrhoids), the cardioesophageal junction (esophagogastric varices), the retroperitoneal space, and the falciform ligament of the liver (periumbilical or abdominal wall collaterals). Figure 6-19 illustrates some types of collateral channels.

The most common site of variceal bleeding is from the gastroesophageal junction.[183] The degree of portal hypertension and the size of the varices are thought to influence the likelihood and significance of bleeding. Massive variceal bleeding is a life-threatening event that requires immediate and aggressive intervention to prevent hemodynamic compromise. The first priority of critical care management is to respond to the life-threatening vascular volume depletion. Once the patient is sufficiently stabilized, an investigation of the exact source of bleeding can be conducted, and appropriate treatment options can be organized. Forty to seventy percent of the patients who hemorrhage from such varices die from the initial episode.[184]

Resulting signs and symptoms

The presentation of portal hypertension will vary among patients, depending upon their state of health, the degree of hypertension, and the precipitating factors. The major manifestations and the resulting signs and symptoms of the disease all relate to the obstruction of normal blood flow and the development of collateral circulation. Most patients who are being evaluated for portal hypertension have already been diagnosed with some type of liver disease. Portal hypertension should be suspected in the presence of splenomegaly, ascites, varices, or peripheral venocongestion, as exhibited by pitting edema. If these symptoms are found in a patient without a previous history of liver disease, an evaluation of potential causes of hepatic congestion is indicated.

Splenomegaly is found on abdominal palpation of the patient with portal hypertension, although the size of the spleen does not always correlate with the severity of the hypertension. Enlarged spleens may present as generalized abdominal discomfort or fullness and are painful to palpation. A nontender, enlarged spleen demonstrates advanced hepatosplenic disease. Laboratory findings of thrombocytopenia, leukopenia, and anemia will assist the practitioner in identifying splenic overactivity, although these findings are also present in other disease processes and therefore must be viewed appropriately.

The accumulation of fluids associated with ascites is usually not detected by the patient or clinician until increasing abdominal girth causes discomfort. The portal pressure that helps to push fluid out of the

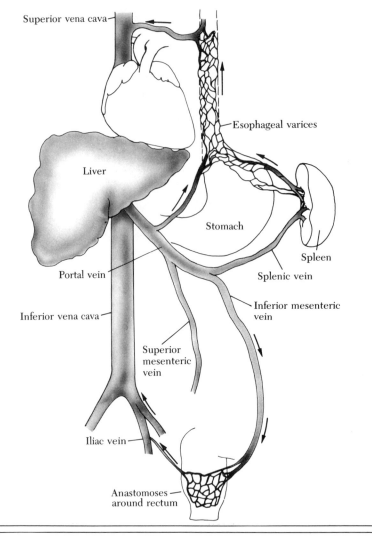

Figure 6-19 Collateral Venous Channels

hepatic circulation also opposes the reabsorption of fluid from the peritoneal cavity back into the circulation. As the amount of fluid within the abdomen increases (usually to levels greater than 500 cc), physical examination will confirm a fluid wave and a shifting dullness to percussion. The patient may complain of difficulty in taking a full breath, a feeling of fullness after small meals, and an increased frequency of gastric reflux. Further physical examination may reveal a raising of the lower lung borders upon percussion and/or auscultation, as well as a displacement of the cardiac point of maximal impulse. The elevation of the diaphragm that accompanies the fluid accumulation interferes with both the quality and comfort of breathing and will increase the risk of pulmonary compromise. Extremely severe ascites causes engorgement of the abdominal vessels as well. Severe ascites is illustrated in Figure 6-20.

Ultrasound and computerized tomography are successful in detecting even very small amounts of ascitic fluid within the abdomen and may guide clinicians in determining appropriate therapy. The shifting of fluids and solute concentration leaves the patient with continuously changing blood chemistry and composition. Some common abnormalities include hypoalbuminemia, hypernatremia, elevated blood urea nitrogen, and increased ammonia levels.

The classic findings in the patient with compensatory channel development are easily recognized: hemorrhoids and abdominal varices. Caput medusae are abdominal varices that radiate from the umbilicus toward the xiphoid and rib areas and are easily visualized on physical examination. Endoscopic examination allows the visualization of varices of the stomach and esophagus; cannulation of the

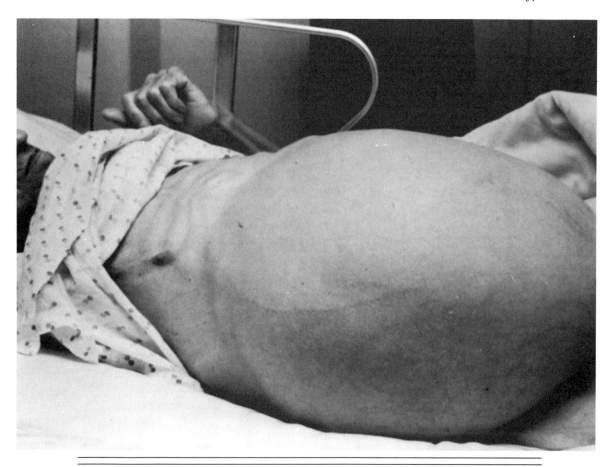

Figure 6-20 Severe Ascites

portal venous system allows direct measurement of pressures for definitive diagnosis or in preparation for surgical intervention. Angiography may also help in diagnosis or in the location of a bleeding varix. Varices present few primary symptoms leading to health evaluation unless tissue injury and bleeding have occurred. Bleeding is most likely to occur and may present as either a slow oozing bleed or a sudden massive hemorrhage. The clinical presentation is the best indicator of the severity of bleeding from this site. The recognition of black, tarry, or melanotic stools may be the first clue that bleeding is occurring. These symptoms are often mistakenly diagnosed as lower GI bleeding, particularly if few risk factors for portal hypertension exist. Variceal bleeding can also be massive and without warning. The most likely source for massive hemorrhage is where the vena cava and azygous veins join with the smaller vessels of the esophagus.[185] The cause of bleeding can be anything that causes an increase in abdominal pressure and is commonly as negligible as a sudden sneeze, vomiting, or coughing. Hematemesis can result in a loss of a very large amount of

blood. The patient with sudden bleeding of esophagogastric varices often complains of sudden and overwhelming nausea and a sense of impending doom. Variceal bleeding is bright red in color and may be pulsatile if hepatic pressures are extremely high. Secondary symptoms may range from mild tachycardia and orthostasis to a shock state requiring intensive support. Rapid evaluation of the source of hematemesis may be attempted through endoscopic procedures, although the large amount of visible blood may obscure diagnosis. Severe bleeding warrants angiography or emergency exploratory surgery.

The collateral channels that are developed in portal hypertension divert blood containing nutrients and cellular waste products away from the liver, and subsequently liver function is both compromised and bypassed. The resulting build-up of both endogenous and exogenous toxins leaves the patient compromised at best and a classic candidate for hepatic encephalopathy. The signs can range from a mild personality change to total and irreversible coma. Figure 6-21 diagrams the course of the disease.

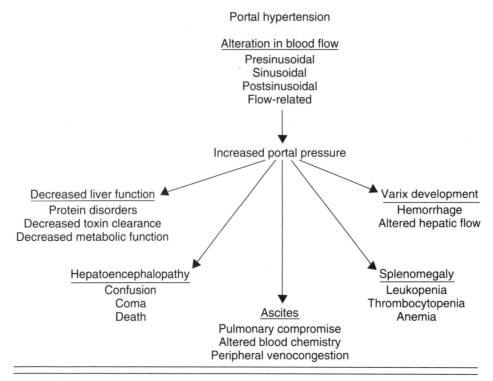

Portal hypertension

Alteration in blood flow
Presinusoidal
Sinusoidal
Postsinusoidal
Flow-related

Increased portal pressure

Decreased liver function
Protein disorders
Decreased toxin clearance
Decreased metabolic function

Varix development
Hemorrhage
Altered hepatic flow

Hepatoencephalopathy
Confusion
Coma
Death

Ascites
Pulmonary compromise
Altered blood chemistry
Peripheral venocongestion

Splenomegaly
Leukopenia
Thrombocytopenia
Anemia

Figure 6-21   Progression of Portal Hypertension

Nursing standards of care

Treatment of the patient with portal hypertension is typically aimed at alleviating the specific side effects and symptoms that are associated with the disease, although elimination of the cause of the hypertension (for example, cure of the patient with alcoholic hepatitis or other liver disease) may result in some decrease of portal pressure. The primary cause of portal hypertension, however, is cirrhosis, which remains virtually irreversible in today's treatment realm.

Some surgical and endoscopic techniques are designed to reduce the hypertension itself. Surgical techniques permanently direct flow around the blockage and provide a route of flow that connects the portal and systemic blood flow via vessels that can accommodate the pressure gradient. Two examples of new flow routes created surgically are illustrated in Figure 6-22. In 95% of the emergency cases, the surgical shunt will stop variceal bleeding.[186] The shunts are delineated by the amount of flow that continues to feed the liver. Nonselective shunts decompress the entire portal system; examples of this are the portacaval and the proximal splenorenal shunts shown in Figure 6-22. In the portacaval shunt, the portal vein is anastomosed to the inferior vena

cava; if this technique is used, the only flow into the liver is via the hepatic artery. With the use of the proximal splenorenal shunt, the spleen is removed, and the splenic vein is connected to the renal vein. This allows for continuation of flow via the hepatic vein and artery, while allowing for the decompression of the portal system and associated varices. Of the two techniques, the portacaval shunt is faster and requires less operative time and is therefore often the choice for use in emergency situations. Unfortunately, such shunts are associated with an increased hepatic encephalopathy and failure. Selective shunting, such as that seen with the distal splenorenal shunt, is designed to bypass specific varices while maintaining some flow through to the liver. There is usually a less immediate decrease in the portal pressure, and therefore it may not be the procedure of choice in an emergency. The retention of both arterial and venous hepatic flow is responsible for the decreased incidence of hepatic encephalopathy in these patients. Unfortunately, there is no evidence to support the use of these shunts to prevent the development of varices; there is less development of variceal bleeding, but there is increased hepatic encephalopathy.[187] Even in those patients who received shunts following variceal bleeding, there was not a significant increase in survival rate, and the development of hepatic encephalopathy was the same for both

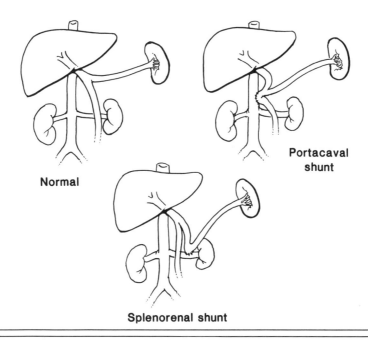

Normal

Portacaval shunt

Splenorenal shunt

Figure 6-22 Portalsystemic Anastomoses

groups. Those with shunts developed encephalopathy as a result of hepatic failure; those without shunts developed it following hemorrhage.[188]

Splenomegaly does not usually require intervention. Symptomatic splenomegaly that accompanies portal hypertension may necessitate splenectomy if the compromise is severe, especially if the patient is a candidate for shunt surgery. If the splenomegaly is the cause rather than the side effect of the portal hypertension, removal of the spleen may be indicated.

Sclerosis is the process of thrombosing the varix and thus reducing the risk of bleeding. Agents used to sclerose esophageal varices include sodium tetradecy sulfate, morrhuate sodium, and thrombin in dextrose.[187] This procedure requires use of an endoscopic apparatus that allows visualization of the varices. The sclerosing agent is then injected either directly into the varix or into the tissue surrounding the varix by a needle-tipped catheter that can be passed via the endoscope. If possible, the process of sclerosing should continue until the suspected varices are completely destroyed; this often requires serial endoscopic procedures and injections. The success rate of sclerotherapy after single variceal bleeding approaches 90%, but the procedure is not indicated as a prophylactic among patients at risk for bleeding.[190]

Temporary reduction of portal pressure and portal bleeding can be achieved by the use of intravenous or intraarterial vasopressin infusions. Vasopressin (Pitressin, antidiuretic hormone) is a selective vasoconstricting agent that causes splanchnic vasoconstriction and decreases portal blood flow. Infusion can be either intraarterial or systemic; there seems to be little difference in effectiveness. Bleeding is controlled in up to 80% of the cases; rebleeding occurs in more than half of the cases after the vasopressin is tapered off or stopped.[191] Vasopressin also selectively vasoconstricts the coronary arteries and can lead to life-threatening cardiac ischemia or infarction if not used judiciously. Some clinicians advocate the use of concomitant topical or intravenous nitroglycerin to prevent these complications in high-risk patients.[192] Other side effects include intravascular volume overload, hyponatremia, intestinal ischemia or infarction, and renal compromise.

Some investigators have proposed the use of beta-adrenergic receptor blockers such as propranolol to decrease portal venous pressure by decreasing the heart rate. Venodilating agents such as nitrates may also be used to reduce pressure. Investigations of the efficacy of such therapy continue.[193]

Despite many creative medical and surgical therapies, portal hypertension is generally unresponsive to attempts at primary management. As a result, treatment interventions are usually directed toward alleviating the symptoms or decreasing the pathology associated with the complications of portal hypertension.

Initial treatment for ascites is the removal of the predisposing factor, liver disease. Unfortunately, this is often an impossible task. Given this, the goal shifts to the relief of discomfort and stress associated with the ascites and prevention of further accumulation of fluid. First, restriction of sodium and fluid intake is recommended, with bedrest to assist in renal clearance. Therapies to reduce or remove the ascites must be instituted carefully. If the fluid is to be removed via diuretic therapy, care must be taken to ensure that the patient does not become hypovolemic as intravascular volume is removed before the ascitic fluid is reabsorbed. Removal that is too rapid can leave the patient with fluid and electrolyte imbalances, decreased circulating volume, and associated renal perfusion deficits, which potentially lead to hepatorenal syndrome and encephalopathy.

Diuretics such as Aldactone (spironolactone) and Triamterene are preferred because they are potassium-sparing. They work by counteracting salt retention and potassium excretion by the distal tubule that is the hallmark of hyperaldosteronism. Effective blocking of the aldosterone mechanism can be documented by monitoring diuresis and urinary lab values. An increase in sodium excretion and a decrease in potassium excretion will indicate successful therapy. If diuresis is not achieved with first-line medications, thiazide diuretics, which act upon the proximal tubules, may be added. Again, the interventions must be monitored carefully for potential side effects. Recent recommendations suggest that the goal for weight loss should be less than 1.0 kg daily if the patient has ascites *and* peripheral edema. If only ascites is present, then weight loss should not exceed 0.5 kg per day.[194]

If fluid removal is to be by direct aspiration of the ascitic fluid (paracentesis), many of the same concerns are raised. Removal of the fluid from one compartment may encourage the body to attempt equalization from another compartment, namely the intravascular space. Frank hypotension or orthostasis may occur if fluid removal is too rapid. Reaccumulation is a frequent problem. If paracentesis is combined with carefully monitored intravenous albumin repletion, larger amounts of fluid may be removed safely. The ascitic solution should be examined carefully: cloudy fluid is associated with infection; bloody fluid with malignancies, tuberculosis, or a traumatic procedure; and milky fluid is indicative of lymphatic obstruction such as that seen with lymphomas.[195]

Surgical implantation of a peritovenous shunt between the peritoneal cavity and the superior vena cava allows for drainage of the ascitic fluid from the peritoneal cavity (see Figure 6-23). Such shunts are placed within the abdominal cavity; one-way valves allow fluid to exit the peritoneal cavity when the intraperitoneal pressure exceeds the venous pressure by more than 3–5 cm H_2O.[196] One such shunt, called the Denver shunt, also has a manual pump

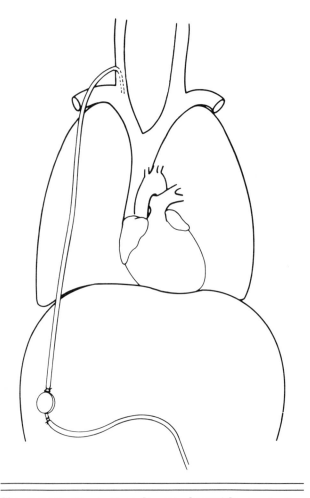

Figure 6-23 The LeVeen Shunt to Control Severe Ascites

that allows the doctor or nurse to force fluid out of the abdominal cavity and into the venous circulation. The rest are dependent upon pressure gradients for fluid shifting. The return of ascitic fluid to the general circulation allows for the correction of side effects associated with the development of ascites, such as plasma volume depletion, hormonal imbalances, and increased portal pressures.[197] Unfortunately, there are multiple problems associated with the use of peritovenous shunts. The shunts themselves are prone to obstruction, and the patient may experience bacterial infection, coagulopathies, pulmonary edema, and/or GI bleeding.[198]

For some patients, ascites does not reduce with standard therapy. If the patient is severely deficient in albumin, combining salt-poor albumin to pull in fluid from the abdominal cavity and careful diuresis to remove it from the circulation may be effective.

The patient with severe variceal bleeding requires immediate expert medical attention. Vigorous replacement of circulating volume, including the use of colloids, packed cells, and coagulation factors, is essential. Yet health care personnel must be aware that overrepletion might actually cause an increase in portal pressure. Intensive monitoring will include hemodynamic monitoring of blood pressure and central venous and pulmonary pressures, multiple large-bore IV accesses, and consistent expert evaluative skills. Approximately half of all hemorrhages are stopped without medical intervention.[199] Unfortunately, there is no way to know which patient will rebleed. For patients whose bleeding does not stop spontaneously, balloon tamponade or use of vasopressin can be implemented.

Balloon therapy involves the passage of a triple-lumen (Sengstaken-Blákemore) or four-lumen (Minnesota) tube into the stomach. The Minnesota tube has an additional feature, an esophageal aspiration port to drain blood from the esophageal area. The gastric balloon of the tube is inflated first, and then the apparatus is pulled back to compress the cardiac portion of the stomach. If that is insufficient to stop the bleeding, the esophageal balloon is also inflated, compressing the bleeding vessels within the esophagus. Balloon therapy is considered a short-term solution, and balloon pressures are monitored carefully. Potential complications of this therapy include esophageal erosion or rupture, aspiration, airway compromise and a high level of patient discomfort. (Refer to the earlier section on gastrointestinal bleeding for more information on this therapy.)

Nursing care of the patient with portal hypertension requires a high level of assessment and interpretive skills on the part of the nurse. Evaluation of physical and laboratory findings on a daily basis determines which therapies are effective and which are not. Care of the patient with portal hypertension focuses upon: (1) recognition of patients at risk for portal hypertension and teaching preventive strategies; (2) the prevention, recognition, and treatment of bleeding; (3) prevention, recognition, and treatment of ascites; (4) prevention, recognition, and treatment of splenomegaly and encephalopathy; (5) promotion of patient involvement in the management/treatment plan.

Hepatic Encephalopathy

When the liver is first compromised, clinical management strategies focus upon the recognition and treatment of the immediate ramifications of the disease. These include life-threatening coagulation disorders, impaired detoxification, and synthetic processing. In prolonged or extreme disease, however, the clinician must include yet another problem among the patient care issues—deteriorating neurological function, known as hepatic encephalopathy.

Clinical antecedents

Unfortunately, the exact cause of hepatic encephalopathy remains somewhat of a mystery. It is associated with both acute and chronic liver failure. The encephalopathy itself may be acute and reversible or chronic and progressive.[200] Three consistent precipitating factors have been identified: gastrointestinal bleeding, increased dietary protein, and electrolyte disturbances. In almost all cases of hepatic encephalopathy, a thorough examination and history will lead to the identification of one of these as a direct precipitator of the development of encephalopathy. Other potential contributors to hepatic encephalopathy are superimposed acute viral hepatitis, extrahepatic bile duct obstruction, or surgery in a patient with cirrhosis.

Critical referents

Cellular level The pathophysiology of hepatic encephalopathy is based upon an excess of nitrogenous wastes within the body and the inability of the liver to clear these and other waste products. These products have a direct and deleterious effect that leads to the development of hepatic encephalopathy.

Nitrogenous wastes from within the body are primarily the result of protein degradation. Small amounts of ammonia, a nitrogenous product, are produced normally by the liver and kidneys. The primary sources of ammonia, however, are protein digestion within the small intestine and metabolism of urea in the colon. Bacteria within the intestine facilitate the deamination of amino acids and proteins, releasing ammonia. Any increased intake of protein (including increases resulting from enteral or parenteral high-protein nutritional support) will result in a correlative increase in nitrogen production.

The liver is responsible for the conversion of ammonia into excretable urea. A problem arises when the increased protein uptake and/or ammonia production is greater than the liver can tolerate. The nitrogenous wastes are not detoxified by the liver and therefore accumulate in the circulation, where they cross into and become toxic to the nervous system. In the case of a shunt, either physiological or surgical, the liver never has the opportunity to pro-

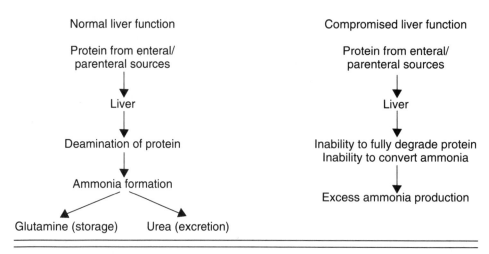

Figure 6-24   Liver Function

cess the nitrogenous wastes in the blood. Figure 6-24 illustrates both normal and abnormal liver function.

Multiple toxins are cleared from the blood by the liver on a daily basis; ammonia is only one of them. The fact that the liver is compromised or bypassed means that any circulating toxin can accumulate and be a potential cause of deteriorating mental status. The discussion that follows will focus on ammonia production and accumulation, as it is the primary agent implicated in hepatic encephalopathy.

Hypokalemia is another potential cause of increased ammonia production. With hypokalemia, potassium is drawn out of the cell and into the intravascular fluid as the body attempts to normalize the potassium ions of the intravascular fluid. In exchange, sodium and hydrogen move into the cell, creating an acidotic environment within the cell, but a systemic alkalosis. The hydrogen that moves into the cell may be the result of the conversion of ammonium (NH_4^+) to ammonia (NH_3). This increases the total amount of serum ammonia. Figure 6-25 illustrates the process.

Systemic alkalosis of any origin will increase the ratio of nonionic/uncharged ammonia (NH_3) to ionic/charged ammonium (NH_4^+); the movement of hydrogen into the cell reduces the serum hydrogen available for the conversion of ammonia to ammonium. The alkalosis will also stimulate increased renal production of ammonia. It is only the uncharged ammonia that is gaseous and therefore able to cross the blood-brain barrier. The ammonia will move preferentially toward an acidotic environment. If the acidotic environment is within the central nervous system, the ammonia will cross the blood-brain barrier. Once in the brain, ammonia is metabolized into glutamine, which is an inactive substance but a precursor for several neurotransmitters. It is

theorized that glutamine either competes for neurotransmitter receptors or increases development of inhibitory neurotransmitters, which leads to diminished mentation.[201] Figure 6-26 illustrates the process.

Almost all patients with hepatic encephalopathy have increased serum ammonia levels, and recovery from hepatic encephalopathy is accompanied by a decreasing serum level. The correlation, however, is not exact; the degree of encephalopathy is not always proportional to the degree of ammonia intoxication. There is, however, a good correlation between the amount of glutamine found in the cerebrospinal fluid and the degree of encephalopathy.[202]

No one knows what the exact mechanism of injury is once the ammonia has crossed into the

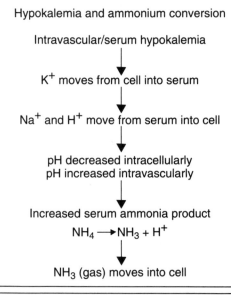

Figure 6-25   Hypokalemia and Ammonium Conversion

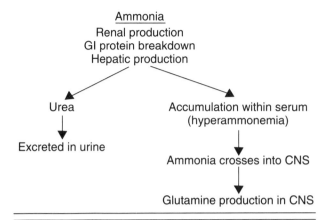

Figure 6-26 Movement of Ammonia in Systemic Alkalosis

brain; several theories exist, but none is definitive. These theories focus not only on the substitution of ammonia into neural pathways but also on possible physiological changes of the brain cells into which ammonia enters. Other metabolites and compounds are thought to produce hepatic encephalopathy, either independently or in combination with ammonia. Some of these are listed in Table 6-46. It is most likely that no single substance is totally responsible for the development of encephalopathy; rather, the condition is a result of the combination of agents. The exact mechanism of their pathogenesis is uncertain at this time.

Research into the role of gamma-aminobutyric acid (GABA) has led to a belief that it is important in the development of hepatic encephalopathy.[203] Increased concentrations of GABA result in reduced levels of consciousness. GABA is responsible for the inhibitory action of benzodiazepines such as Valium; if there is no GABA, benzodiazepines do not have any effect upon the brain.[204] An increased level of GABA in the CNS may be the result of the liver's

inability to clear out the amino acids that are the precursors of this neurotransmitter or perhaps the result of an increased permeability of the blood-brain barrier to those same amino acids. GABA and other amino-acid derivatives are thought to disturb the balance of inhibitory and excitatory neurotransmitters in the brain, and some may actually act as false neurotransmitters. Regardless of specific action, the end result is hepatic encephalopathy.

Gross Pathogenesis The patient who comes in with large-scale GI bleeding in the presence of liver disease is at risk of developing hepatic encephalopathy. Blood within the GI tract is protein-laden, and the natural digestive process will convert that protein to ammonia. Electrolyte and acid-base disturbances may also precipitate encephalopathy by creating an alkalotic environment. The most common causes of imbalances that create an alkalotic environment are the injudicious use of diuretics, vigorous paracentesis, and/or vomiting. Use of central nervous system depressants such as benzodiazepines and barbiturates or hypoxia may either cause or obscure the actual etiology of hepatic encephalopathy. Acute infections have also been identified as possible causative agents because the increased catabolic activity may result in protein breakdown and ammonia production.

The decisive factors in the development of hepatic encephalopathy are the degree of hepatic compromise, the amount of nitrogenous substances circulating, and the shunting of blood past the liver. Disease processes such as hepatitis, cirrhosis, and hepatoma cause destruction within the liver, leaving it unable to perform the detoxification that the body requires on a daily basis. The shunting of blood flow can be caused by disease processes, collateral circulation, or surgical procedures.

Table 6-46 Potential Agents of Hepatic Encephalopathy

Short-chain fatty acids
Ketones
Mercaptans
Phenol
False neurotransmitters
Ammonia
Bile salts
Gamma-aminobutyric acid

Source: Rothstein and Herlong, Neurologic manifestations of hepatic disease, *Neurologic Clinics*, 7(3):563–574.

Resulting signs and symptoms

Cerebral edema is a common finding in the patient with hepatic encephalopathy. Clinically, any neurological derangements may be encountered; however, there are some classic signs of the disease that aid in its recognition and diagnosis. The most unique is asterixis, which when found in conjuction with liver disease, is known as "liver flap." Asterixis is abnormal muscle tremors that create haphazard and involuntary jerking movements, especially of the hands. The best means of measuring this is by having the patient hold his or her arms out with hands dorsiflexed. If asterixis is present, the patient will be unable to hold the hands in this position, and they will flap up and down rapidly. In order to test this, the patient must be awake and strong enough to follow commands and maintain voluntary muscle control. Fetor hepaticus is the name given to the unusual musty odor of the breath and urine of the patient with hepatic encephalopathy. An EEG will show symmetric, high-voltage, slow wave patterns in advanced encephalopathy, but few if any changes early in the disease.[205]

Frequently, family members are the first to recognize the subtle and insidious changes that accompany hepatic encephalopathy in the patient with chronic liver failure. These same changes are much easier to recognize in the patient with acute liver failure (such as fulminant liver failure), as they occur rapidly and are more dramatic and the patient is often undergoing intensive observation. The early changes range from mild personality changes, mood disturbances, and confusion to deterioration in motor skills and job performance and reversal of sleep patterns. Research findings have shown that patients often show the deterioration in manual skills before they show signs of intellectual deterioration; this reinforces the importance of measuring both parameters in the evaluation of hepatic encephalopathy.[206]

Clinical signs and symptoms are commonly grouped into the following four stages.

Stage I: The first stage of hepatic encephalopathy is not usually recognized except in hindsight, when the history of the patient is reviewed with family and friends. There is a slight change in personality and behavior, and there may be evidence of either euphoria or depression. Mentation is compromised, as exhibited by slower and slightly slurred speech and a change in the sleep-wake pattern. Asterixis may or may not be present, and the EEG is usually normal.

Stage II: This stage is more clinically pronounced than the first and is characterized by a further decrease in the cerebral functioning; the patient is lethargic and disoriented regarding time, place, and person. Fine-muscle coordination begins to deteriorate, and there is difficulty in adding, subtracting, and drawing. Asterixis and EEG changes are noted.

Stage III: At this stage, the patient is extremely confused, and speech is often incoherent. The majority of the time is spent sleeping: when the patient is awakened, his or her behavior is often disruptive and beligerent. Asterixis (if elicited) and EEG changes continue to be evident.

Stage IV: In this stage, the patient is comatose. Initially, there may be response to painful stimuli, but none later. EEG presentations are always abnormal. There will be no asterixis.

Figure 6-27 demonstrates the deterioration of writing and apraxia that occurs with hepatic encephalopathy.

Unfortunately, there is no specific test designed to definitively diagnose hepatic encephalopathy. The best indicator is a measurement of serum ammonia concentration; normal serum ammonia is less than 50 μmol/L. It is important to measure the ammonia in a consistent manner, as values will differ between arterial and venous samples; small amounts of ammonia will be taken up by the muscles, and a small amount will be excreted by the lungs. CSF is normal upon exam, although increased glutamine levels may be measurable and may correlate with degrees of hepatic encephalopathy. Computerized tomography of the brain will not reveal any abnor-

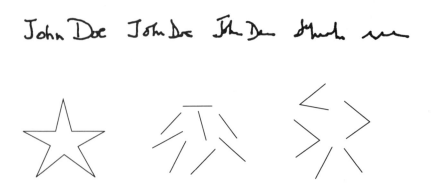

Figure 6-27 Deterioration of Handwriting and Constructional Apraxia with Progressive Portal Systemic Encephalopathy

malities. Unfortunately, many other diseases mimic hepatic encephalopathy, making diagnosis difficult. These are detailed in Table 6-47.

Given the confusion that can arise in trying to diagnose hepatic encephalopathy, the following summary may be helpful as a guideline. If the following major factors are present, then hepatic encephalopathy should be ruled out:

1. Acute or chronic hepatocellular disease and/or extensive portal-systemic shunts
2. Disturbances of mentation and awareness, which may vary in severity and frequency
3. Shifting combinations of neurologic symptoms, including asterixis, rigidity, hyper-reflexia, and occasionally seizures
4. Nonspecific symmetric, high-voltage, slow wave EEG findings[207]

Nursing standards of care

The first step in caring for the patient with hepatic encephalopathy is the identification of the precipitating event. If it is identifiable, specific mea-

Table 6-47 Differential Diagnoses for Hepatic Encephalopathy

Type of Disease	Example
Cerebral disease	Head injury; bilateral hematoma
	Chronic meningitis (tuberculous)
	Encephalitis
	Polioclastic
	Demyelinating
	Wernicke's encephalopathy
	Delirium tremens
Metabolic disorders	Uremia
	Diabetic ketoacidosis
	Hypoglycemia
	Hypothermia
	Hyperammonemia (other than hepatic)
	Hypercapnia (respiratory failure)
	Anoxia
	Korsakoff's syndrome
	Wilson's disease
	Alcohol intoxication
Endocrine disorders	Hypopituitarism
	Hypothyroidism
	Adrenal failure
Drug use	Narcotics and sedatives

sures may be available to correct it and prevent potentially fatal complications. Supportive strategies that allow the liver to rest and perhaps regenerate may be the only other alternative.

If the patient's ammonia is increased, measures must be initiated immediately to lower it. If the increased ammonia is from protein breakdown resulting from gastrointestinal bleeding, the intestine must be cleaned of any blood. The same is true if the protein deposits in the bowel are the result of constipation, ileus, or any other process that slows the passage of bowel contents. Aggressive feedings above the requirements for an individual patient will cause a protein imbalance. The alcoholic/cirrhotic patient, when presented with a normal protein load, may well not have the liver reserve required to process it, and restriction or elimination of dietary protein may be required. Finally, the patient who is in a catabolic state from infection will require aggressive therapy in order to rid the body of yet another source of ammonia.

Regardless of the source of the encephalopathy, the clinician does have several drugs that can help to stop or slow protein breakdown. The first is neomycin, a broad-spectrum antibiotic that destroys the normal bacterial flora of the bowel responsible for the breakdown of protein into ammonia. Neomycin is poorly absorbed through the bowel, but still must be given carefully (especially to the renally impaired), as it is excreted renally and is nephrotoxic. Use of this drug requires judicious monitoring of the blood urea nitrogen and creatinine. Side effects of neomycin include ototoxicity, yeast superinfection, and lethargy.

Lactulose is another drug used to reduce ammonia levels. This synthetic disaccharide is converted in the colon to lactic and acetic acids, which decrease the pH of the bowel. Ammonia in the blood is attracted to an acidic environment and is therefore pulled out of the blood and into the colon. Once in the colon, ammonia is not reabsorbed and will become part of the stool. The second action of lactulose is as an osmotic cathartic, which facilitates excretion of the ammonia-laden stool. Lactulose can be given orally or by enema. Oral doses are frequently made more tolerable by mixing them with fruit juices. The therapeutic goal is two to three soft, acidic stools per day. Unfortunately, side effects of lactulose include abdominal cramping, bloating, diarrhea, nausea and vomiting, and electrolyte imbalances.

With recent findings concerning the role of GABA in hepatic encephalopathy, research has focused upon the use of benzodiazepine-receptor antagonists in the patient with hepatic encephalopathy. Findings on one such product, Flumazenil, suggest that elimination of relapsing encephalopathy is feasible.[208] This drug has recently been made available in the United States. It has not been studied extensively, but investigations are under way.[209]

If hypokalemic alkalosis is a precipitating factor, careful repletion of potassium is required. Normalization of potassium may restore intracellular and extracellular balances of ammonia. Repletion to the point of hyperkalemia may result in acidosis with exacerbation of hepatic encephalopathy.

Injudicious use of narcotics and other hepatic-excreted or hepatotoxic drugs is one of the most avoidable precipitators of hepatic encepalopathy. Early recognition of hepatic compromise and dose adjustment and/or restriction can prevent further damage.

Acid-base balance can be partially restored by ventilatory manipulation; the patient on a ventilator can be made hypercapnic. Hypercapnia theoretically assists in two ways: it causes a shift in the acid-base balance of the serum, and it stimulates the utilization of carbon dioxide to facilitate ammonium production.[210] This effect is reflected in the following equation:

$$NH_3 + CO_2 + H_2O \longrightarrow H_2CO_3 + NH_3 \longrightarrow$$

Ammonia   Carbonic acid

$$HCO_3^- + NH_4^+$$

Ammonium

If these mechanisms are not successful, hemodialysis may be tried in an attempt to reduce the ammonia load. This therapy is not widely successful, and the patient who does not respond to the above therapies is not likely to survive.

Nursing responsibilities focus on recognition of the disease process, prevention of complications, facilitation of removal of ammonia, and protection of the compromised patient. As treatment is primarily oriented toward symptomatic support, the nurse plays an essential role in administering medication, monitoring dietary and fluid restrictions, and evaluating the patient. Appropriate monitoring of blood concentrations of encephalopathic markers, blood chemistries, and initiated therapies is of paramount importance.

Nursing Care Plan for the Management of the Patient with Portal Hypertension or Hepatic Encephalopathy

Diagnosis	Signs and symptoms	Intervention	Rationale
Potential alteration in vascular volume: excess portal pressure	Splenomegaly Ascites Peripheral venocongestion (edema) Abdominal distention Leukopenia, anemia, thrombocytopenia	Administer diuretics (Aldactone, thiazide, and loop diuretics); monitor for side effects of excessive diuresis, such as hypotension, tachycardia, orthostasis	Decreased circulating volume should help decrease portal blood flow and pressure gradient (Aldactone is potassium-sparing; other diuretics should be used as needed and for those refractory to Aldactone therapy)
		Avoid splenic palpation	Palpation may cause spleen to rupture
		Administer pain medications carefully for discomfort related to splenic enlargement or distention	To help increase tolerance to activity and promote increased lung expansion
		Raise head of bed to 30 degrees	Increasing the angle of recline may help increase lung expansion and decrease pain
		Prepare and care for the patient receiving a surgical shunt for redirection of portal blood flow; for the patient receiving a peritovenous shunt, NPO before surgery and until bowel sounds return following surgery	For aspiration precautions and to allow the bowel to rest after surgical manipulation
		Monitor abdominal girths for signs and symptoms of leakage at the anastomosis; evaluate the patient for decreasing ascites, variceal pressure, and increased or decreased liver function	Increasing girth and worsening liver function tests may indicate hemorrhage or a blocked catheter; decreasing girth and improving liver function tests may indicate appropriate response to the surgical procedure

Nursing Care Plan for the Management of the Patient with Portal Hypertension or Hepatic Encephalopathy

Diagnosis	Signs and symptoms	Intervention	Rationale
		Monitor weight every day and intake and output every 8 hours; monitor Hct, temperature, and dressing site for signs and symptoms of infection	Shifts of fluid from the peritoneum may cause fluid and electrolyte instability as ascites is reabsorbed
		Monitor electrolytes every day and potassium every 6–8 hours until patient is stabilized	Potassium levels often fall following diuresis
		Patient may wear abdominal binder after wound is healed to increase abdominal pressure	Increased abdominal pressure will favor fluid passing out of the abdomen and into the venous circulation via the peritovenous shunt
Potential for injury related to venous congestion of the portal circulation	Variceal development: esophageal, rectal, periumbilical, or esophagogastric Decreased protein production (coagulopathies, hypoalbuminemia, edema, ascites) Diminished toxin clearance	Have patient avoid sitting on hemorrhoids, avoid vascular volume overload, abstain from activities that increase intraabdominal pressure (lifting, tight belting, abdominal restraints or compressors)	Elimination of excess fluid from the abdomen and avoidance of activities that increase intraabdominal pressure will decrease venous pressure and the potential for exacerbation of bleeding
		Utilize diuretic therapy or needle removal of fluid in abdomen	Ultrafiltration and associated mechanisms of fluid clearance will aid in fluid removal
		Limit sodium and fluid intake	Restriction of fluid and sodium will decrease the potential for fluid accumulation

		Assess patient for development of bleeding from varices or as a result of diminished coagulation factor availability: heme test all stool and emesis; monitor PT/PTT, Hgb, Hct, bleeding times, and CBCs	Portal hypertension results in dilated varices, which are prone to bleeding; diminished production of coagulation factors leaves the patient more susceptible to bleeding; CBCs will indicate the degree to which splenic sequestration is occurring
		Monitor liver and chemistry panels for albumin, sodium, potassium, serum osmolarity, ammonia, SGOT/SGPT, total/direct bilirubin, urea, creatinine, ammonia, and CBCs	To determine liver function or dysfunction
		Replete albumin and coagulation factors as ordered	To assist in maintaining fluid balance and coagulation
		Assess patient for signs and symptoms of hepatic encephalopathy: test for cognitive and synthetic thought processing and ability of patient to perform multiple integrated tasks; use in conjunction with thorough neurological examination	Multilevel testing is a better indicator of loss of higher-level integrative thought processing; use in conjunction with thorough and consistent neuro examinations will assist the clinician to recognize subtle changes
		Adjust medication dosages to reflect diminished hepatic clearing of narcotics, antibiotics, and endogenous toxins	Adjustments must be made for the decreased clearance and degradation of medications to preclude overdosing

Nursing Care Plan for the Management of the Patient with Portal Hypertension or Hepatic Encephalopathy

Diagnosis	Signs and symptoms	Intervention	Rationale
Potential alteration in vascular volume (deficit) related to variceal bleeding and ascites	Hypotension Orthostasis Tachycardia CVP < 1, PCWP < 8 Lightheadedness, nausea, vomiting Increased or decreased weight Output greater than intake	Fluid repletion with colloidal and/or hyperosmolar substances, coagulation factors (maintain type and cross match throughout hospital stay); observe for signs and symptoms of transfusion reaction; monitor carefully for overrepletion of lost fluid volume	Rapid and safe repletion of vascular volume is imperative
	Hypoalbuminemia Increased fibrin split products Mild or massive hemorrhage (bright red blood from rectum, black tarry stool, heme-positive stool or emesis, hematemesis)	Monitor vital signs and utilize invasive measures (Swan-Ganz, arterial lines, CVP); watch for signs and symptoms of hypovolemic shock	Careful and consistent measurement of circulating volume is imperative
		Utilize Sengstaken-Blakemore tube for tamponading of esophageal bleed	Balloons of tube apply direct pressure on area of bleeding; care of the patient with Sengstaken-Blakemore tubes is important to reduce the risks associated with placement and use
		Monitor stomach and esophageal balloon pressures every 4–8 hrs.; report pressures > 30 mm Hg to MD	Excessive balloon pressures lead to tissue necrosis
		Monitor drainage from stomach lumen continuously; also from esophageal lumen if Minnesota tube is used	Returns will determine efficacy of therapy and blood product replacement
		Monitor continuously for signs of respiratory distress; anchor end of tube to an external foam block or helmet-type device	Bleeding above the esophageal balloon can compromise the airway, as can balloons that pull upward out of place

Diagnosis	Signs and symptoms	Intervention	Rationale
		Prepare patient for endoscopy for evaluation and potential sclerosing of esophageal bleed: NPO; sedation as tolerated and ordered; obtain consents from patient or surrogate	Maintaining NPO status decreases the potential for aspiration; sedation helps to calm the patient; and consents are necessary for any invasive procedure
		Monitor patient receiving vasopressin therapy to decrease GI bleeding: cardiac monitoring for changes in ST segment; intake and output every 8 hours; administer vasopressin via central line or intraarterially	Vasopressin can cause constriction of cardiac and splanchnic arteries with ischemia requiring concomitant administration of nitroglycerin to alleviate it
		Following paracentesis, check vital signs every 15 minutes for first hour, then every 30 minutes for 2 hours, then every hour until patient is stable	Vital signs will indicate continued loss of systemic vascular volume from shifting of fluids or perforation of a vessel
		Send sample of fluid for culture to evaluate for infection; monitor dressing site every shift	Peritonitis may result from introduction of infected materials into ascitic fluid or the bloodstream following paracentesis
		Measure abdominal girth every shift and have patient report discomfort PRN	To allow for recognition of internal hemorrhage
		Following portal system bypass: monitor dressing for bleeding from surgery; monitor vital signs per recovery room and OR protocol; monitor bleeding time and CBC, assess for hepatic encephalopathy; assess liver enzymes and electrolyte panels daily; monitor abdominal girth for signs and	If blood flow bypasses the liver, there is potential for increased hepatic encephalopathy from the increase in circulating toxins; a history of portal hypertension means the patient has had an alteration in vascularity of the surrounding area and is at increased risk for bleeding

965

Nursing Care Plan for the Management of the Patient with Portal Hypertension or Hepatic Encephalopathy

Diagnosis	Signs and symptoms	Intervention	Rationale
		symptoms of leakage at the anastomosis; evaluate the patient for decreasing ascites, variceal pressure, and increased or decreased liver functions; monitor weight and intake and output daily	
Potential alteration in thought process related to decreased clearance of toxins	Decreased level of consciousness Confusion Disturbance of sleep/wake cycle Shortened attention span Lethargy Coma Increased serum ammonia Increased glutamine in CSF Asterixis Increased BUN Hepatorenal syndrome	Rule out other potential causes of decreased thought process (cerebral bleed, overdose, etc.) Monitor ammonia (serum) every day and glutamine (CSF) and electrolytes with each liver panel Assess both memory and integrative thought processes (use of constructional testing and repetitive scales/association formats) Institute precautions against falls and protective restraints PRN; institute aspiration precautions Avoid hepatotoxic drugs and monitor levels of drugs that are excreted via the liver; if narcotics or benzodiazepine are to be used, be cognizant of route of excretion and the ability to reverse the agent	Hepatic encephalopathy mimics other cerebral disorders that cause changes in mentation Ammonia and glutamine are recognized indices of hepatic encephalopathy; electrolytes indicate other potentiating factors Testing should reflect both basic and higher-level thought processes Patient safety must be maintained at all times Decreased hepatoclearance may lead to overdosing and subsequent complications

Diagnosis	Signs and symptoms	Intervention	Rationale
		Observe for signs of central brain failure (hypoventilation, apneustic respirations, hypoxemia/hypercarbia, no response to stimuli, posturing, and comatose state)	Early recognition of impending problems can assist the clinician in identifying treatment options and in working with patient and family to determine goals for long-term therapy
Potential for ineffective breathing pattern related to encephalopathy	Dyspnea Apneustic respirations Hypercapnia Hypoxemia Copious oral/airway secretions	Elevate head of bed 30° or place patient in side-lying position	Reduces risk of aspiration
		Assess airway competence, cough, and gag reflex at least every 8 hrs.	Provides predictive information on airway competence
		Assess pulse oximetry and ABGs PRN and as ordered	Identifies oxygenation or ventilation difficulties
		Monitor for airway competence in patients with esophageal bleed and potential aspiration and in those with increased diaphragm level (and decreased pulmonary excursion) found with ascites accumulation; encourage coughing and deep breathing exercises	Massive esophageal bleeding leaves the patient at risk for aspiration; elevated diaphragm makes it difficult to maintain good pulmonary toilet
Potential alteration in nutrition related to inability of liver to utilize nutrients	Hyperglycemia Hypoglycemia Lipidemia Muscle wasting Vitamin deficiency Ketones in urine Hypercholesterolemia Hyperammonemia Elevated BUN	Assess patient's nutritional status with nutritionist and determine most appropriate means of providing nutrition to patient and most appropriate concentration/constitution	Patients with long-term/severe liver disease are unable to break down and utilize nutrients necessary for maintenance of body processes
		If patient is hyperglycemic, administer insulin as ordered, and limit amount of exogenous glucose intake; monitor for signs and symptoms of insulin reaction following	Patient is unable to degrade and store glucose secondary to loss of hepatocellular function and processing; insulin receptors may respond sporadically to insulin therapy

Diagnosis	Signs and symptoms	Intervention	Rationale
		administration of ordered doses; monitor glucose levels at least every 4 hours until patient is stabilized	
		If patient is hypoglycemic, administer glucose solutions as ordered, and monitor serum glucose for signs and symptoms of hyperglycemia	The patient has not been able to store glucose for future use
		Provide exogenous vitamin K weekly for the depleted patient, or more frequently if patient is bleeding; provide vitamin D and vitamin B as ordered	Vitamin K is necessary for coagulation; decreased levels of vitamin D can lead to demineralization of bone and potential osteomalacia and fractures; decreased levels of vitamin B lead to potential neurologic problems, including palsy
		Eliminate alcohol intake	Preferential use of alcohol over other energy substrates potentiates liver disease

Medications Commonly Used in the Care of the Patient with Hepatic Disorders, Portal Hypertension, or Hepatic Encephalopathy

Medication	Effect	Major side effects
Azathiaprine	Purine antagonist and antimetabolite; exact mechanism of immunosuppression unknown (may inhibit RNA/DNA synthesis or may be incorporated into nucleic acids, causing cell malfunction)	Bone marrow depression Nausea and vomiting Anorexia Diarrhea Increased serum alkaline phosphatase and bilirubin May cause veno-occlusive disease and progressive liver disease with chronic use Rash Drug fever Serum sickness Arthralgia Raynaud's disease Pulmonary edema
Cholestyramine	Absorbs bile acids in the intestine and forms nonsoluble absorbable complex that is excreted in the feces	Constipation, impaction, hemorrhoids Abdominal pain, distention, bloating Nausea and vomiting Anorexia Biliary colic Hyperchloremic acidosis and increased urinary calcium excretion Rash and irritation of the skin, tongue, and perianal area
Colchine	Weak antiinflammatory action, appears to reduce the inflammatory response to the deposition of monosodium urate crystals in joint tissues	Nausea and vomiting Abdominal discomfort Diarrhea Thrombophlebitis at injection site Bone marrow depression Bladder spasm Paralytic ileus Hypothyroidism

Medications Commonly Used in the Care of the Patient with Hepatic Disorders, Portal Hypertension, or Hepatic Encephalopathy

Medication	Effect	Major side effects
Immune Globulin IV	Provides passive immunity by increasing antibody titer and antigen-antibody reaction potential	Occasional hypotension and clinical manifestations of anaphylaxis Mild chest, hip, joint, or back pain Myalgia Nausea, vomiting Chills, fever Headache Urticaria Flushing Dyspnea Wheezing and cyanosis
Lactulose	Metabolism of sugar in the lower intestinal tract; acidifies the contents of the colon; cathartic action; increases water content in stool	Gaseous distension, belching, flatulence Borborygmi Fluid loss Hypokalemia and hypernatremia Nausea and vomiting
Neomycin	Aminoglycoside; antibiotic; bacteriocide	Diarrhea

Liver Transplantation

Liver transplantation in a human was first attempted by Starzl in 1963, and he accomplished the first successful liver transplant in 1967.[211] Since that time thousands of liver transplants have been accomplished throughout the United States and Europe. Liver transplantation is a viable alternative for persons suffering from irreversible end-stage liver disease, which leads to life-threatening complications from loss of the myriad of normal liver functions. The one-year survival rate for patients with liver transplants in 1988 was 76%.[212]

Clinical antecedents

There are many conditions that can lead to the need for transplantation: advanced liver disease, malignancy, fulminant hepatic failure, and metabolic dysfunction, as outlined in Table 6-48. The metabolic diseases are seen most frequently in pediatric patients.

The criteria for recipient selection vary at each transplantation center. As more knowledge is gained and transplantation techniques improve, the number of recipients has increased and the contraindica-

Table 6-48 Antecedents of Liver Transplantation

Antecedent	Examples
Advanced liver disease	Chronic active hepatitis Primary biliary cirrhosis Sclerosing cholangitis Alcoholic cirrhosis Budd-Chiari syndrome Biliary atresia
Malignancy	Hepatocellular Cholangiocarcinoma
Metabolic disorder	Wilson's disease Alpha 1-antitrypsin deficiency Protoporphyrin excess Crigler-Najjar syndrome Glycogen storage disease Tyrosinemia

Fulminant hepatic failure	Acute viral hepatitis:
	  Hepatitis B
	  Non-A, non-B hepatitis
	  Chronic active hepatitis
	  Epstein-Barr
	Drug-induced hepatitis
	Toxic-induced hepatitis

Table 6-49 Contraindications for Liver Transplantation

Absolute Contraindications	Relative Contraindications
Active alcohol or drug abuse	Active sepsis outside the liver
Extrahepatobiliary malignancy	Patient over 60 years of age
Advanced cardiopulmonary disease	Positive hepatitis B antigen
Patient's inability to comprehend the nature and costs of procedure	Advanced chronic renal disease not associated with liver disease
	Prior complex liver or biliary surgery
	Positive HIV status
	Portal-vein thrombosis

tions have become less absolute. Table 6-49 lists absolute and relative contraindications for liver transplantation.

After a potential recipient is referred to a transplantation center, physical, psychological, and financial evaluations must be completed before the person can be accepted as a transplant candidate.[213] Laboratory studies, including viral titers and cultures, blood typing, chemistries, and hematology, are evaluated for transplant information and general physical status. Ultrasound, computerized tomography, magnetic resonance imaging, and duplex scans may be done to evaluate the anatomy of the liver and the surrounding area. An evaluation of other chronic diseases is also conducted.

The psychological evaluation is performed to determine the patient's understanding of the illness; the frequency of substance abuse (if any) and its contribution to the patient's condition; the patient's expectations of the transplant; the patient's coping ability and support system; and the presence of any psychiatric illness. The candidate must understand the enormity of the liver transplantation process and be willing to commit to lifelong follow-up and immunosuppressive therapy in order to maintain the health of the graft. The family must also be able to support the undertaking.[214] The financial burden of transplantation may be met through insurance, cash, or fundraising. The costs of ongoing medical care and immunosuppressive therapy must also be considered. In 1983, the cost of liver transplantation was estimated to be $238,000 for the first year.[215]

Critical referents

An appropriate donor is identified by matching the ABO blood type and approximate physical size of the recipient. It is essential that the donor liver and cardiovascular system be supported to preserve normal function. Vasopressors are used sparingly when necessary to maintain adequate hemodynamic stability. The retrieval of the graft takes from 3 to 4 hours.[216] The liver is cooled and infused with a high-potassium solution to maximize preservation. Solutions that are currently used allow the liver to be maintained for 20–24 hours and still function normally.[217]

The surgery may require 8–12 hours and be complicated by portal hypertension and coagulopathies that are commonly found with end-stage liver disease. A venovenous bypass between the femoral and axillary veins is used to prevent additional venous hypertension secondary to cross-clamping the portal blood system.[218] The vascular anastomoses are completed first, followed by the biliary reconstruction. Three drains are placed above and below the graft, and a T-tube or stent is placed to facilitate bile drainage during healing.

Resulting signs and symptoms

The postoperative medical emphasis is on maintaining appropriate fluid status, electrolyte balance, coagulation, and liver, kidney, and cardiopulmonary function.[219] The abdominal drains may produce a large volume with the reaccumulation of ascites, especially if preoperative ascites was present. Liver function can be observed from inspection of the T-tube. Normal bile will be dark golden in color, later turning slightly green. Ischemia or necrosis of the graft may be evidenced very dark and muddy bile.

Most patients will have some coagulopathy. The previously disturbed coagulation status is complicated by an average replacement of 8–15 units of packed red blood cells intraoperatively. The prothrombin time should gradually return to normal as liver function improves.

Routine chest x-rays are done to assess for pleural effusions, which commonly occur on the right side and are related to subdiaphragmatic manipulation during surgery. Major pulmonary problems are not usually associated with the effusion.

Good graft function will contribute to hemodynamic stability. Initial cardiac output is frequently elevated. Metabolic alkalosis indicates appropriate liver function as the citrate from blood replacement is broken down into bicarbonate. Mechanical ventilation is maintained until the alkalosis is controlled in order to prevent the compensatory hypoventilation that would occur. A hydrochloric acid infusion may be necessary to correct the imbalance. Elevated serum glucose levels are common with normal graft function and may require insulin. A very low blood sugar may indicate poor liver function.

Sudden elevation in serum transaminases or bilirubin may indicate hepatic artery thrombosis, sepsis, or rejection. If the hepatic vessels are shown to be patent, a biopsy is done to differentiate infection from rejection. The correct diagnosis is essential, because if immunosuppression therapy is increased to treat rejection, the patient will be at even greater risk for infection.

Drug therapy includes antibiotic coverage and immunosuppression.[220] Antibiotics for common biliary pathogens (e.g., aminoglycosides, cephalosporins) are administered preoperatively and continued for two days following surgery. Immunosuppression is provided by steroid therapy, azathioprine, cyclosporine, or OKT3. Steroids are initiated preoperatively, and the patient is weaned daily until a maintenance dose is attained.

Azathioprine (Imuran) is an antimetabolite that interferes with antibody production; it may be used either as primary therapy or for rejection. Bone marrow suppression is the primary side effect of the drug, and the patient's white blood count must be followed closely. Cyclosporine (Sandimmune) was credited with significantly improving transplantation when it was introduced in 1972.[221] The drug inhibits the specific T cells that respond to transplant antigens, but it does not interfere as much as other immunosuppressants with the normal ability of the body to prevent bacterial infection. The primary side effect of the drug is nephrotoxicity, which tends to be dose-related. OKT3 is a monoclonal antibody that also responds to specific T cells. OKT3 is generally used to treat rejection or when cyclosporine cannot be used because of renal impairment. FK-506 is a new fungal metabolite that is being studied at transplant centers in comparison with cyclosporine. It has shown great initial promise, and it is anticipated that it will prove to be very successful for primary therapy and the treatment of rejection.

Nursing standards of care

Nursing management of the liver transplant recipient focuses on maintenance of the cardiovascular system, assessment for complications, and promotion of comfort and safety. Cardiovascular alterations may be related to fluid volume. Fluid volume excess can result from aggressive fluid resuscitation, stress response, and renal failure, which occurs in approximately 20% of transplant patients.[222] A fluid volume deficit can be related to hemorrhage or third-space loss. Hypovolemia is a concern because it contributes to acute tubular necrosis, especially in the presence of cyclosporine.[223]

Electrolyte and acid-base imbalances occur frequently.[224] Hypokalemia often results from the large intraoperative losses of ascitic fluid and the vascular shifts that occur after the donor liver is flushed of the high-potassium preservation solution. Hypomagnesemia is related to preoperative malnutrition, use of diuretics and cyclosporine, and the hypocalcemia that may occur with massive blood transfusions. Hyperglycemia is a positive indicator of liver function and may also be related to stress and steroid therapy. Metabolic alkalosis is secondary to the large citrate volume in the transfused blood. The citrate is metabolized to bicarbonate by a functioning liver.

Infection and rejection are the most serious complications postoperatively.[225] Vascular complications include thrombosis at the cannula sites of the venovenous bypass and hepatic artery or portal vein thrombosis.[226] Primary graft dysfunction may be related to inadequate preservation, ischemia during donor death, or unknown reasons.[227] Retransplantation is often required for primary graft dysfunction. Impaired gas exchange may be related to pleural effusion, prolonged anesthesia, immobility, or ventilatory impairment from diaphragm manipulation.[228]

Patient comfort is affected by the extensive abdominal incision that parallels the diaphragm. Pain management may be difficult, depending on the ability of the new graft to adequately metabolize the analgesics.[229] Promotion of the safety of the transplant patient focuses on infection control practices and prevention and recognition of complications.

The following nursing care plan gives a general outline of the care required following liver transplantation.

Nursing Care Plan for the Management of the Patient with a Liver Transplant

Diagnosis	Signs and symptoms	Intervention	Rationale
Potential fluid volume excess related to stress response, fluid resuscitation, or renal insufficiency	Hypertension Pulmonary edema Peripheral edema	Careful I&O records; frequent assessment of blood pressure, CVP, and PAP; auscultation of breath sounds; evaluation of response to diuretic therapy	Excess fluid volume must be recognized and treated as quickly as possible
Potential fluid volume deficit related to third-space shift or hemorrhage	Hypotension Decreased urine output Decreased CVP or PAP	Careful I&O records, including assessment of abdominal drains; frequent assessment of blood pressure, CVP, and PAP	Hypotension exacerbates renal insufficiency; hemorrhage must be recognized and treated promptly
Alteration in electrolyte balance: hypokalemia related to fluid losses and potassium shifts	Decreased potassium level ECG changes	Monitor serum potassium as ordered; observe ECG for flat T wave, U wave, or prolonged Q-T interval; evaluate response to replacement therapy	Hypokalemia potentiates dysrhythmias
Hypomagnesemia related to preoperative malnutrition, diuretic therapy, and cyclosporine	Decreased magnesium level Tetany, jerking, seizures Irritability, confusion	Monitor serum magnesium as ordered; evaluate response to replacement therapy	Magnesium contributes to central nervous system, neuromuscular, and cardiac function
Hyperglycemia related to return of liver function, stress response, or steroids	Elevated serum glucose level Presence of glucose in urine	Monitor serum and urine glucose frequently; administer insulin as ordered and monitor response	Hyperglycemia is a positive sign if it indicates a functioning liver; but severe hypoglycemia may indicate graft failure
Alteration in acid-base balance: metabolic alkalosis related to citrate metabolism	Irritability, disorientation Dysrhythmias Decreased ventilation	Monitor ABGs; administer HCl infusion as ordered; monitor respiratory rate	May prevent weaning from ventilator due to compensatory decreased respiratory drive

Diagnosis	Signs and symptoms	Intervention	Rationale
Impaired gas exchange related to pleural effusion or impaired diaphragm function	Decreased pO_2 or O_2 saturation Increased pCO_2 Decreased ventilation	Monitor ABGs or pulse oximeter; monitor respiratory effort; suction patient at least every 2–4 hours; reposition patient at least every 2 hours	Aggressive respiratory management is essential to minimize and prevent respiratory complications
Pain related to surgical incision	Complaints of incisional pain Splinting Restricted movement	Place patient in position of comfort Medicate as ordered with continuous or intermittent narcotic; monitor response to narcotic administration, including pain relief and level of consciousness	To help to alleviate pain Narcotics are metabolized in the liver and must be administered very carefully in order to assess for changes in level of consciousness that can reflect liver function
Potential for bleeding related to venovenous bypass and graft anastomoses	Bleeding at axillary and femoral venovenous bypass sites Continued bloody drainage from abdominal drains Decreased Hct or Hgb Hypotension	Monitor venovenous bypass sites for bleeding; measure output from abdominal drains hourly, noting amount, character, and trends of drainage; monitor Hct and Hgb as ordered; monitor for signs of hypotension and shock	Venovenous sites and anastomoses are at risk of bleeding, especially in the presence of coagulopathy
Potential for graft dysfunction related to ischemia, rejection, or idiopathic causes	Elevated transaminase levels and bilirubin Decreased bile production Decreased urine output Prolonged coagulation time Depressed neurological function Metabolic alkalosis Hypoglycemia	Monitor for trends in laboratory values; measure bile drainage and urine output hourly, noting trend Administer prostaglandin as ordered and monitor response of bile output	Primary graft failure must be differentiated from infection and rejection in order to treat appropriately Prostaglandin may be administered in an attempt to cause vasodilation and improve blood flow

Nursing Care Plan for the Management of the Patient with a Liver Transplant

Diagnosis	Signs and symptoms	Intervention	Rationale
Potential for infection related to immunosupppressive therapy	Symptoms of pneumonia, peritonitis, septicemia, endocarditis, urinary tract infection, or hepatitis Presence of organisms on routine cultures Presence of opportunistic pathogens (CMV, candida, pneumocystis carinii, herpes)	Observe for symptoms of infection; obtain surveillance cultures as ordered; monitor culture findings and relate to system pathology; maintain scrupulous handwashing and basic infection-control principles	Immunosuppression allows acquisition of virulent organisms that do not cause infection when system is normal, reactivation of latent organisms, or infection by normal body flora
Potential for rejection related to incompatible donor and recipient tissues	Elevated bilirubin with or without elevated transaminase levels Decreased bile drainage Change in color of bile drainage, from golden to colorless Rejection noted upon biopsy	Administer immunosuppressive agents as ordered (steroids, cyclosporine, azathioprine, OKT3); monitor bilirubin and transaminase levels and amount and appearance of bile; monitor biopsy reports	Most transplant recipients experience some degree of rejection; immunosuppressive therapy is given to prevent rejection, and additional steroid therapy or other immunosuppressive agents are administered to treat rejection
Lack of knowledge on the part of recipient and family regarding recovery, complications, and ongoing health maintenance	Verbalization of lack of knowledge about prognosis or fear of complications and death	Explain postoperative routine to family and recipient; provide realistic information regarding infection and rejection Describe ongoing administration of immunosuppressive therapy; initiate consultation for financial support if needed	Thorough understanding by recipient and family members assists in recovery and compliance Lifelong immunosuppressive therapy is costly and costs must be considered before discharge

Nutritional Disorders in the Critically Ill

Technological advances have given many critically ill patients increased chances of survival, though they require extensive periods of recovery. Throughout critical illness and recovery, maintaining adequate nutrition is a continual challenge to clinicians. As many as 50% of all hospitalized patients suffer from protein-calorie malnutrition.[230] Many critically ill patients require supplemental nutritional support during their illness. Research studies in this field have shown overwhelming evidence of the importance of nutritional status to the eventual recovery of these patients.[231] As a result, aggressive nutritional support has become commonplace in ICUs today. Nutritional support is defined as a balance of nutrient substrates (carbohydrates, fats, proteins) given to patients with normal metabolic demand and oxygen transport to replenish both calories and nutrients.[232] Few critically ill patients have normal metabolism and oxygen utilization. The new concept of metabolic support focuses on nutrients and calories needed to prevent organ failure. This section will address the differences between these patient groups and implications for critical care management.

Clinical antecedents

Patients are identified as nutritionally deficient when their nutrient intake is not equivalent to their energy requirements. Most institutional policies identify groups of patients who meet these criteria and qualify for supplementation. An example of a general policy is to consider nutritional supplementation for all patients whose enteric intake has been or will be withheld for at least 7–10 days.[233] In simple terms, this includes any patients who (1) cannot eat, (2) will not eat, (3) cannot eat enough, or (4) should not eat. A summary of patient groups likely to meet these criteria is given in Table 6-50.

Recognition of patients at risk for nutritional deficit promotes early assessment and intervention in the critical care setting. Patients at risk should have a nutrition consult and complete physiological and laboratory nutritional assessment. Nutritional assessment parameters gathered by various methods

Table 6-50 Patient Groups Likely to Require Nutritional Support

Patient Behavior	Precipitating Conditions
Cannot eat	Laryngectomy
	Coma
	Burns
	Trauma
Will not eat	Depression
	Neurological impairment
Cannot eat enough	Cancer chemotherapy
	Cancer radiation therapy
	Sepsis
	Hyperthyroidism
Should not eat	GI surgery
	Acute pancreatitis
	Crohn's disease in exacerbation
	Acute GI bleed
	Abdominal trauma
	Intestinal obstruction
	Intestinal fistulae

Table 6-51 Nutritional versus Metabolic Support

	Nutritional Support	Metabolic Support
Setting failure	Malnutrition	Hypermetabolism/organ
Basis	Starvation	Metabolic stress
Focus	Restoration of organ function; emphasis on visceral proteins and lean body mass	Preservation of structures and function; no substrate limitation; support of metabolism
Fuel	Glucose	Mixed
Nonprotein cal/g nitrogen	$\geq$150/L	$\leq$100/L
Protein (g/kg · day)	1.15	2.0–3.0
Percentage of nonprotein calories as fat	0–80	30–40

Source: Cerra, F. B. (1987). Hypermetabolism, organ failure and metabolic support. *Surgery 101*(1).

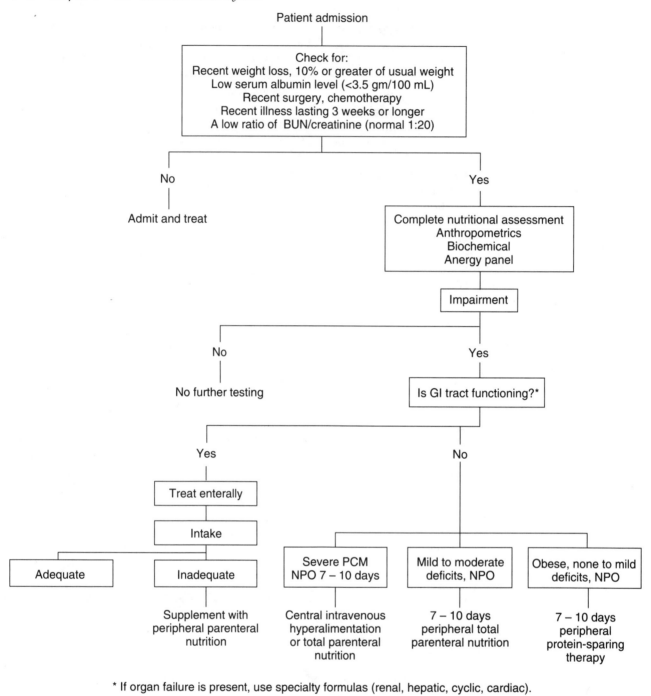

Figure 6-28 Decision Process for Nutritional Support

reveal nutrition history, information about somatic protein mass, visceral protein mass, catabolic rate, and fat stores. These assessments allow the nurse to draw conclusions about the caloric needs of the patient based on currently available substrate and predicted needs. Newer approaches to nutritional assessment advocate a more thorough review of the patient's energy expenditures, to permit a decision between nutritional supplementation or metabolic

support. These two types of parenteral feeding have similar components in different concentrations. The key differences between nutritional supplementation and metabolic support are outlined in Table 6-51.

The decision to provide supplementation is based on the clinical and biochemical findings from assessment. Clinicians must then determine the type of nutrition indicated in each patient's case. The three major types of alimentation are peripheral (by

Table 6-52 Nutrition and Disease

Disease	Dietary Considerations
Cardiac	Ethanol has minor effect on plasma triglycerides Coffee: no confirmed studies of effect on heart If carbohydrate is main source of energy, patient is less prone to myocardial infarction. Link between obesity and low levels of HDL cholesterol: obese patients are prone to hypertension and hyperglycemia Salt: the amount that may have an effect is dependent on individual susceptibility; for example, blacks and whites have same dietary intake, but blacks have higher incidence of hypertension

Cardiac cachexia
  Longstanding CHF (related to decreased CO and impaired delivery of nutrients and malabsorption in GI tract)
  Perioperative cardiothoracic
	Potassium supplements (diuretics)
	Sodium restriction
	Increased carbohydrates
	Replace Na^+ and fluid
	Protein intake 1 g/kg
	Carbohydrates for energy stores

COPD
  Dyspnea interferes with eating
  Diaphragmatic restrictions imposed by full stomach
  Loss of palate secondary to chronic production of sputum
  Gastric irritation associated with bronchodilators
	Need to increase calories above RDA because of the increased work of breathing
	Remember when weaning ventilator patients that high amounts of glucose cause glucose induced CO_2 production and can induce respiratory failure, making weaning unsuccessful.

Cancer
Main problem is weight loss due to:
  Chemotherapy
  Aversion to food
  Depression and loss of appetite secondary to diagnosis
  Self-induced "food fad cures"
  Changes in carbohydrate and fat metabolism
	Patient may need supplemental/enteral feedings
	Drugs to decrease nausea and increase appetite

Renal disease Retention of nitrogenous wastes, fluid, Na^+ and K^+	Need diet low in proteins and high in carbohydrates Decrease fluids according to % of renal function

Liver disease
  Interferes with production of glucose or utilization of glucose
  There is hepatic accumulation of triglycerides
  Protein deamination of plasma protein
	Need to give diet of vegetables/dairy products, which decreases aromatic amino acids
	Give medication that decrease production or retention of ammonia

GI disease
  Gastrectomy
 	
  Inflammatory bowel disease (ulcerative colitis; Crohn's disease)
  Bowel resection
 	
  Internal fistula
	Six small meals daily; eliminate liquids with meals to prevent dumping
	Rest bowel
	TPN
	Rest bowel
	Prolonged TPN until healing occurs
	Replace fluids and electrolytes
	TPN

vein), enteral (orally or into the GI tract), and parenteral (into a central venous access). Determination of the best mode or combination is based upon the patient's clinical disorder and metabolic needs. A sample algorithm for this decision-making process is outlined in Figure 6-28.

The next step in this process is to determine whether enteral or parenteral feeding is most appro-

Table 6-53 Types of Nutritional Supplementation

Type	Indications	Advantages	Disadvantages	Complications
Peripheral	Minor nutritional deficits Inadequate fat stores for daily requirements Good peripheral veins Good hepatic and respiratory function Minimal or no fluid restrictions Anticipated supplementation not greater than 7–10 days Sensory/perceptual changes (i.e., absent gag reflex) *Contraindications:* Patient to be without nutrition for more than 7 days Patient critically ill or catabolic	Inexpensive Easy to use Maintains nutrition	Limited ability to supplement calories Access to veins Potential impaired tissue integrity Potential for infection	Phlebitis Fluid over-load Electrolyte disturbances (hyperchloremic acidosis) and deficiencies
Enteral	Ability to tolerate GI feeding Patient comatose or neurologically impaired Disease involves esophagus Impaired ability to swallow Excessive refractory diarrhea *Contraindications:* Nausea and vomiting Upper GI tract disorder involving bleeding or malabsorption	Preserves normal GI flora and integrity Mimics normal eating Moderately inexpensive	Malabsorption problems Potential for aspiration	Diarrhea Patient does not absorb supplement Aspiration
Parenteral	Debilitating illness lasting more than 2 weeks Loss of at least 10% of pre-illness weight GI disorders preventing absorption Chronic vomiting and diarrhea Poor tolerance for long-term enteral feeding Limited or no oral intake for over 7 days Serum albumin less than 3.5 gm/dL Sensory/perceptual changes (i.e., absent gag reflex) *Contraindications:* Short-term need for nutrition Inadequate central venous access	Easy to use Provides complete nutrition and high calories needed by catabolic patients	Expensive Limits patient activity Potential for infection	Hyperglycemia Hyperosmolar nonketotic syndrome Electrolyte disorders (hypokalemia hypocalcemia, hypomagnesemia, hypophosphatemia) Metabolic acidosis Hepatic dysfunction Air embolism Hypervolemia

priate. It is universally agreed that enteral nutrition should be attempted whenever possible.[234] It is inexpensive, allows for more normal nutrient utilization, maintains the integrity of the GI tract, and may prevent translocation of bacteria from the GI tract to the bloodstream.[235]

Parenteral nutrition may be given either peripherally or by central vein (total parenteral nutrition). Peripheral nutrition can provide approximately 1500–2500 calories per day and is usually used as a short-term measure with critically ill patients with a planned short-term illness (such as surgery), as an adjunct to enteral nutrition, or when central venous access is temporarily not possible or is not desired. Total parenteral nutrition alone can deliver 5000–8000 calories per day and all necessary protein, vitamins, and minerals.

Critical referents

Essential nutrients found in food provide the substrate needed to perform body functions such as maintenance of tissues, enhancement of growth, promotion of enzyme production and activity, maintenance of normal cellular activities, and development of energy stores. When a person does not consume adequate quantities of carbohydrates, fats, and proteins, body maintenance is hindered. An average adult requires 2000–3000 calories per day (30–40 kcal/kg). Critical illness alters metabolism and energy expenditure in many ways. It is estimated that burn and trauma victims require up to 10,000 calories per day.[236] When the body has insufficient quantities of nutritional factors or is utilizing more energy than usual for body maintenance, it converts its tissue reserves to energy. The most common type of nutritional deficiency is protein-calorie malnutrition.

In the normal adult, carbohydrates are the preferred energy source, but in high metabolic states protein synthesis is impaired and there is a shift in the body's fuel sources away from glucose and toward amino acids. To meet metabolic demands the body first converts all available complex sugars to simple sugars, then manufactures glucose from readily available or ingested lipids (broken into free fatty acids) and proteins (broken into amino acids). During starvation, the body converts glycogen (stored as carbohydrates in the liver) into energy (a process called glycogenolysis); the end result of the process is the production of glucose. Unfortunately, the body's total supply of glycogen is likely to be used within 24 hours when extreme physical stress occurs. Fat stores are then broken down into free fatty acids and glycerol to be used for energy. When fatty acids are used for energy, the metabolic end products are glycerol (used to make triglycerides) and ketones. When these are in excess, the end result will be ketosis and acidosis. Amino acids are needed for synthesis of the body's proteins, which may be used for energy in extreme circumstances. Since amino acids (the usable metabolites of protein breakdown) cannot be stored, the use of protein for energy requires breakdown of body proteins. Most nutritional supplementation plans are designed to correct nutritional deficiencies and maintain protein synthesis, positive nitrogen balance, visceral tissue function, and body mass. These goals are inadequate to meet the needs of hypercatabolic patients; thus, the new concept of metabolic support has emerged. Metabolic support provides partial calorie replacement and emphasizes specialized nutrients to sustain vital organ structure and limit use of body protein stores.

Resulting signs and symptoms

Nutritional deficiencies seen in the critical care setting primarily originate from protein-calorie malnutrition, although specific vitamin deficiencies may also be seen. The signs or symptoms of nutritional deficiencies are widely variable, depending on disorder and individual patients. The critical care nurse can anticipate finding weight loss, muscle atrophy, poor skin and hair quality, lack of concentration, and immunoincompetence (seen as infections) in the population of patients who become severely protein-calorie malnourished. Nutritional assessments should readily reveal these deficits. Anorexic patients who eat but do not consume a sufficient quantity of food are likely to have more insidious symptoms and show evidence of protein-calorie malnutrition early, in the form of certain vitamin deficiencies.

Nursing standards of care

Certain physiologic disorders predispose patients to particular nutritional deficits and supplemental needs. Commonly encountered diseases with related dietary limitations include diabetes, congestive heart failure, and renal failure. These patients should receive diets or supplements specially formulated for their clinical disorders. A list of commonly encountered disorders and their specific dietary considerations is given in Table 6-52 (page 979).

Once an actual or potential nutritional deficiency has been identified, critical care clinicians should promptly evaluate the patient for the most appropriate supplementation plan. Ideally, patients who are able to eat should continue eating regardless of the supplement plan. In fact, some patients are able to maintain their nutritional status through high calorie/high protein supplements. (Milkshakes with eggs added may be enough to meet these patients' needs; many commercial products are also available.)

Table 6-54 Techniques and Rationales in Passive Replacement Nutrition

Type of Nutrition	Specific Nursing Care	Rationale
Peripheral nutrition: Amino acids 3–4.25% (1–2 L/day) with electrolytes combined with dextrose 5–10% (3–4 L/day) and 10–20% fat emulsion (500 cc/day) Total calorie capacity: 1400–2000 cal/day	Insert at least #20 or larger intravenous catheter for peripheral nutrition; assess every shift for phlebitis	Large-bore catheter needed for viscous fluid and large hourly volume
	Maintain aseptic technique and use a dedicated intravenous line	Glucose solution predisposes patient to infection
	Monitor glucose levels via Dextrostix every 6 hours until patient is stable	Urine glucose is not considered an accurate reflection of blood glucose; high-glucose solution predisposes patient to hyperglycemia
	Check hepatic enzymes every other day; do not give fat emulsion of transaminases or bilirubin in amounts greater than hospital standard or physician's orders	Fat emulsions tax the liver's ability to break down and utilize nutrition
	Administer trace vitamins and minerals daily	To meet daily requirements
	Monitor laboratory tests for efficacy and side effects of therapy (serum chemistries, protein levels, and transaminases)	Altered nutritional product formulation or calorie levels may be indicated; some side effects of alimentation may require treatment
Enteral nutrition: Premixed commercial nutritional supplements can be given in concentrated or diluted form Total calorie capacity: 1800–2800 cal/day	Provide NG tube care per institutional policy	Proper tube position and patency are essential for an enteral nutritional plan
	Consult with nutritionist for best enteral formula: oligomeric formulas are hyperosmolar and easily digested but expensive; polymeric are semi-isotonic or hypertonic solutions with high carbohydrate/fat ratio, intact protein, and low residue; modular or special sectional formulas are customized for specific patient needs	Patient tolerances of whole protein, lactose, and other nutrients are variable, necessitating individualized plan for nutrition; type and location of feeding tube or patient's condition may also influence this decision
	Start nutrition slowly to assess tolerance	Change may be necessary if patient is intolerant
	If supplement is given continuously, check for residual volume every 2–4 hours (when approximately 300 cc have been given); if no residual volume remains after three checks, checks may be done less frequently	Residual volumes greater than the previous hour's intake indicate reduced absorption of feeding
	Glucose test aspirate from ET tube every day if patient is ventilated	To check for silent aspiration; aspiration of enteral feeding will cause positive glucose checks
	Maintain elevation of head of bed at approximately 30 degrees or position patient on side	To prevent aspiration
	Check medications for agents that are poorly absorbed with food or milk items; stop feedings prior to administration	Medications given per NG tube may not be absorbed because of incompatibility with certain enteral feeding formulas

Table 6-54 *(continued)*

Type of Nutrition	Specific Nursing Care	Rationale
	Check glucose levels at least twice daily for hypo/hyperglycemia	High glucose content may lead to hyperglycemia
	Monitor patient for diarrhea; administer antidiarrheals or bulking agents as needed	Diarrhea is a common side effect that reduces absorption and decreases the benefit of nutrition
	Weigh patient every day	To evaluate maintenance or improvement of nutritional status
	Check nutritional parameters every week (protein levels, iron/transferrin levels)	To assess patient's response to nutrition and whether it should be maintained
Total parenteral nutrition (TPN) Complete alimentation formula (CAF) Dextrose 20–25%; amino acids 3–4.25%; electrolytes, minerals, vitamins, 10–20%; fat emulsion (250–500 cc/day) Total calorie capacity: 2000–4000 cal/day	Assist in insertion of TPN line using sterile technique; maintain sterility and closed system for TPN infusion; use a dedicated line for TPN infusion whenever possible	To avoid infection
	Monitor catheter site for infection with each dressing change	To note phlebitis or infection early
	Culture blood from TPN lumen with fever spikes	To identify whether the catheter is the source of septicemia
	Assess glucose every 6 hours for 2 days; if no problem is evident, assess every day from then on	Hyperglycemia is a common complication, but need not always be present
	Use a filter on tubing to reduce administration of microaggregates to patient	To reduce contaminants
	Monitor vascular volume for overload (BP, CVP, weight)	Large volume of solution may lead to hypervolemia and congestive heart failure
	Check all TPN solutions against original orders and daily chemistry to determine that electrolyte additives are appropriate; report need for changes	Orders frequently change daily; electrolytes become imbalanced due to fluid shifts or medications
	Examine the solution for cloudiness; return to pharmacy if it is cloudy	Cloudiness indicates contamination
	Administer concomitant histamine blockers	To block HCl secretions since patient is NPO and is at risk for ulcers
	Encourage food supplementation if this is safe for the patient	To increase calories, provide sense of well-being, maintain integrity and flora of GI tract
	Be certain that vitamin K is replenished weekly while patient is on TPN	Vitamin K needs to be replaced in NPO patient but does not require daily supplementation
	Record I&O every 8 hours and obtain weight every day	To assess fluid balance and whether nutrition should be maintained at steady state

As previously mentioned, there are three choices for passive replacement nutrition: enteral, peripheral, and parenteral. Peripheral nutrition is seldom used alone in the critical care setting but may be used in conjunction with enteral feedings. A comparison of indications for the different methods of nutritional supplementation, advantages and disadvantages of each method, and criteria for choosing one supplementation plan over another are given in Table 6-53 (page 980). Techniques and rationales for each nutritional option are given in Table 6-54 (pages 982–983).

Enteral nutrition should be used whenever possible because it is relatively noninvasive and inexpensive, limits the patient less, and preserves GI integrity. Enteral feedings are usually delivered through special nasogastric feeding tubes or via tubes placed surgically into the esophagus, stomach (g-tube), or jejunum (j-tube). The physician's choice of feeding tube may be determined by the patient's unique GI condition, personal preferences, ability to participate, or anticipated length of need. Enteral feedings are either elemental or defined (lactose-free, clear liquid).

Parenteral nutrition is the most common form of supplement used in the critical care area. Parenteral nutrition provides the highest amount of protein and calories of any supplement option, as well as flexibility for electrolyte and mineral replacement. Even though its use is prevalent, it is not without extreme cost, technological demands, and complications.

Although they provide symptomatic and short-term relief for nutritional deficiencies, these options are not usually implemented as long-term life-saving measures unless they enable the patient to have a better quality of life and participate more fully in his or her own care. It has long been controversial whether to nutritionally support patients who are unable to participate in their care in any other way. Health care professionals are frequently called upon to determine whether nutritional supplements are adjunctive, helpful interventions for patients who are unable to eat or life-support for the individual who cannot participate in other aspects of daily living. This ethical dilemma will not be easily resolved, but it is the role of all caregivers to determine the patient's wishes regarding the institution, maintenance, or discontinuation of nutrition when changes in the clinical condition occur. This should continue to be part of providing nutritional support to the critically ill.

CHAPTER 6 POST-TEST

1. Chronic hepatitis is most likely to be the consequence of:
   a. Hepatitis A.
   b. Hepatitis B.
   c. fulminant hepatitis.
   d. alcoholic cirrhosis.

2. The neurologic manifestations of hepatic encephalopathy are most likely the result of:
   a. hyperammonemia.
   b. hyperbilirubinemia.
   c. cerebral edema.
   d. hyperosmolarity.

Ms. S. K. is a 64-year-old COPD patient admitted two weeks ago for respiratory failure. On admission pneumonia was diagnosed, but Ms. S. K. is currently afebrile and has limited sputum production. The physicians are concerned that her intolerance of weaning attempts is the result of inadequate nutrition and respiratory muscle weakness. Supplemental nutrition is required. Answer the following questions regarding nutritional support of this patient.

3. Tests that may be performed to assess Ms. S. K.'s nutritional status include:
   a. triceps skin-fold, tissue HLA tests.
   b. 24-hour-urine creatinine clearance, ideal body weight.
   c. serum immunoglobulin levels, triglyceride levels.
   d. serum transferrin levels, total lymphocyte count.

4. The nutritional supplementation most appropriate for this patient is:
   a. peripheral nutrition.
   b. enteral nutrition.
   c. parenteral nutrition.
   d. high-glucose, low-fat parenteral regimen.

5. An encouraging postoperative finding in liver transplantation is:
   a. dark brown bile drainage from the T-tube.
   b. hypertension.
   c. hyperglycemia.

   d. metabolic acidosis.

6. The primary digestive role of the small intestine is:
   a. secretion of enzymes.
   b. resorption of water.
   c. transport of vitamin K.
   d. absorption of nutrients.

Mr. J. S., 44 years old, is brought to the ED with complaints of dull, aching, left upper quadrant abdominal pain partially relieved by eating, and hemepositive stools. The nurse determines a history of ulcerative colitis and vomiting of dark brown material one time in the past week. Immediately after admission, Mr. S. complains of acute nausea and has a 200 cc maroon stool. Answer the following questions regarding Mr. S.:

7. The most likely etiology of Mr. S.'s bleeding is:
   a. gastric ulcer.
   b. Crohn's disease.
   c. diverticulitis.
   d. hemorrhoids.

8. The current symptoms indicate that:
   a. the bleeding has probably increased from the original bleeding site.
   b. the bleeding is coming from a new site.
   c. Mr. S. has a perforated ulcer.
   d. blood loss is sufficient to cause hypotension.

9. The most common etiology of bowel obstruction is:
   a. inflammation.
   b. paralytic ileus.
   c. adhesions.
   d. hernias.

10. The order in which abdominal assessment should be conducted is:
    a. percussion, auscultation, palpation.
    b. palpation, percussion, auscultation.
    c. palpation, auscultation, percussion.
    d. auscultation, palpation, percussion.

ENDNOTES

1. Carrico, C. J.; Meakins, J. L.; Marshall, J. C.; Fry, D.; and Maier, R. V. (1986). Multiple-Organ-Failure syndrome—The gastrointestinal tract: the "motor" of MOF. *Archives of Surgery* 121(2): 197–200.

2. Alspach, J. G., ed. (1991). *Core Curriculum for Critical Care Nursing.* 4th edition. Philadelphia: W. B. Saunders, Inc.

3. Russell, M. T.; and McElwee, M. R. (1988). Compensating for xerostomia in the critically ill patient. *Critical Care Nurse* 7(3): 98–103.

4. Lacroix, J.; Infante-Rivard, C.; Jenicek, M.; and Gauthier, M. (1989). Prophylaxis of upper gastrointestinal bleeding in intensive care units: a meta analysis. *Critical Care Medicine* 17(9): 862–869.

5. Alspach, op. cit.

6. Ibid.

7. Guyton, A. C. (1986). *Textbook of Medical Physiology*. 7th edition. Philadelphia: W. B. Saunders Company.

8. Isselbacher, K. J.; and Podolsky, D. K. (1991). Biologic and clinical approaches to liver disease. In Jean D. Wilson, ed. *Harrison's Principles of Internal Medicine*. 12th edition. New York: McGraw-Hill, Inc., pp. 1301–1303.

9. Podolsky, D. K.; and Isselbacher, K. J. (1991). Derangements of Hepatic Metabolism. In Jean D. Wilson, ed. *Harrison's Principles of Internal Medicine*. 12th edition. New York: McGraw-Hill, Inc., pp. 1311–1317.

10. Podolsky, D. K.; and Isselbacher, K. J. (1991). Diagnostic Tests in Liver Disease. In Jean D. Wilson, ed. *Harrison's Principles of Internal Medicine*. 12th edition. New York: McGraw-Hill, Inc., pp. 1308–1311.

11. Alspach, op. cit.

12. Bongiovanni, G. L. (1988). Gastrointestinal bleeding. In Gail L. Bongiovanni, ed. *Essentials of Clinical Gastroenterology*. New York: McGraw-Hill.

13. Ibid.

14. Eastwood, G. L. (1985). Approach to gastrointestinal bleeding. In J. M. Rippe; R. S. Irwin; J. S. Alpert; and J. E. Dalen, eds. *Intensive Care Medicine*. Boston: Little, Brown & Co.

15. Kaldor, P. K. (1988). Gastrointestinal Patient Care Problems. In M. R. Kinney; D. R. Packa; and S. B. Dunbar, eds. *AACN's Clinical Reference for Critical Care Nursing*. 2nd edition. New York: McGraw-Hill Book Company.

16. Ibid.

17. Ibid.

18. Boley, S. J. (1988). Collateral blood flow in segmental intestinal ischemia: Effects of vasoactive agents. *Surgery* 104(3): 583–584.

19. Guyton, op. cit.

20. Ibid.

21. Ibid.

22. Schwartz, S. T.; Shires, G. T.; and Spencer, F. C., eds. (1989). *Principles of Surgery*. 5th edition. New York: McGraw-Hill Book Company.

23. Ibid.

24. Ibid.

25. James, R. S. (1985). Intestinal obstruction, pseudo-obstruction, and ileus. In M. H. Sleisenger; and J. S. Fordtran, eds. *Gastrointestinal Disease*. 4th edition. Philadelphia: W. B. Saunders Company.

26. Stewardson, R. H.; Bombeck, T.; and Nyhus, L. (1978). Critical operative management of small bowel obstruction. *Annals of Surgery* 187: 189–192.

27. James, op. cit.

28. Schwartz, op. cit.

29. Ibid.

30. Peterson, W. L. (1985). Gastrointestinal bleeding. In M. H. Sleisenger; and J. S. Fordtran, eds. *Gastrointestinal Disease*. 4th edition. Philadelphia: W. B. Saunders Company.

31. Schaffner, J. (1991). Upper and lower gastrointestinal bleeding. *Proceedings Critical Care Medicine 91*. Rockville, Md.: CCM.

32. Richter, J. M.; and Isselbacher, K. J. (1991). Gastrointestinal bleeding. In J. D. Wilson, ed. *Harrison's Principles of Internal Medicine*. 12th edition. New York: McGraw-Hill, Inc.

33. Schaffner, op. cit.; Katschinski, B. D.; Logan, R. F.; Davies, J.; and Langman, M. J. (1989). Audit of mortality in upper gastrointestinal bleeding. *Postgraduate Medical Journal* 65(770): 913–917.

34. Richter and Isselbacher, op. cit.

35. Kaldor, op. cit.

36. Pierce, J. D.; Wilkerson, E.; and Griffiths, S. A. (1990). Acute esophageal bleeding and endoscopic injection sclerotherapy. *Critical Care Nurse* 10(9): 67–72.

37. Ibid.

38. Eastwood, op. cit.

39. Ibid.; Richter and Isselbacher, op. cit.

40. Richter and Isselbacher, op. cit.

41. Ibid.; Bongiovanni, Gastrointestinal bleeding.

42. Richter and Isselbacher, op. cit.

43. Ibid.; Bongiovanni, Gastrointestinal bleeding.

44. Bongiovanni, Gastrointestinal bleeding.

45. Ibid.

46. Ibid.

47. Ibid.

48. Marshall, J. B. (1990). Acute gastrointestinal bleeding: A Logical Approach to Management. *Postgraduate Medicine* 87(4): 63–70.

49. Kaldor, op. cit.

50. LaCroix et al., op. cit.

51. Ibid.

52. Pierce, Wikerson, and Griffiths, op. cit.

53. Sugawa, C. (1989). *Surgical Clinics of North America*. 69(6):1167–1183.

54. Vallerand, A. H.; and Deglin, J. H. (1991). *Drug Guide for Critical Care and Emergency Nursing*. Philadelphia: F. A. Davis Company; Burns, S. M.; and Martin, M. J. (1990). VP/NTG therapy in the patient with variceal bleeding. *Critical Care Nurse* 10(9): 42–49.

55. Burns and Martin, op. cit.

56. Alspach, op. cit.

57. Thal, E. R.; McClelland, R. N.; Jones, R. C.; Perry, M. O.; and Shires, T. (1989). Abdominal Trauma. In S. I. Schwartz; G. T. Shires; and F. C. Spencer, eds. *Principles of Surgery*. New York: McGraw-Hill Book Co.

58. Thal et al., op. cit.; Bastnagel, P. J. (1989). Abdominal Trauma. In V. D. Cardona; P. D. Jurn; P. J. Bastnagel-Mason; A. M. Scanlon-Schilip; and S. W. Veisse-Berry, eds. *Trauma Nursing: From Resuscitation through Rehabilitation*. Philadelphia: W. B. Saunders Company.

59. Edwards, J.; and Gaspard, D. J. (1974). Visceral injury due to extraperitoneal gunshot wounds. *Archives of Surgery* 108: 865.

60. White, K. M. (1989). Injuring mechanism of gunshot wounds. *Critical Care Nursing Clinics of North America* 1(1): 97–103.

61. Dunn, P. A. (1990). Assessing a pregnant woman after trauma. *Nursing 90* 20(12): 53–57.

62. Thal et al., op. cit.

63. Ibid.

64. Ibid.; Bastnagel, op. cit.

65. Bastnagel, op. cit.

66. White, op. cit.

67. Thal et al., op. cit.

68. Dunn, op. cit.

69. Thal et al., op. cit.

70. Ibid.; Bastnagel, op. cit.

71. Thal et al., op. cit.

72. Schaffner, op. cit.

73. Bartlett, J. (1990). *1989–90 Pocketbook of Infectious Disease Therapy*. Baltimore: Williams and Wilkins.

74. Ibid.

75. McPhee, M. (1985). Treatment of acute pancreatitis. *Hosptial Practice* 20(6): 83–88.

76. Brown, A. (1991). Acute pancreatitis: pathophysiology, nursing diagnosis and collaborative problems. *Focus on Critical Care* 18(2): 121–131.

77. Brown, op. cit.

78. Ranson, J. H. C. (1985). Risk factors in acute pancreatitis. 20(4): 69–73.

79. Brown, op. cit.

80. Brown, op. cit.; Ricketson, C. A. (1983). Acute pancreatitis. *Critical Care Update*: 40–49; Jeffries, C. (1989). Complications of acute pancreatitis. *Critical Care Nurse* 9: 38–48.

81. Brown, op. cit.

82. McPhee, op. cit. Jeffries, op. cit.

83. Toskes, P. P. (1985). Recurrent acute pancreatitis. *Hospital Practice* 20(7): 85–92.

84. Ricketson, op. cit.; Toskes, op. cit.

85. Brown, op. cit.

86. Nasrallah, S. M. (1985). The management of acute pancreatitis. *Critical Care Quarterly* 82: 15–19.

87. Brown, op. cit.

88. Toskes, op. cit.

89. Dienstag, J. L.; Wands, J. R.; and Isselbacher, K. J. (1991). Acute Hepatitis. In Jean D. Wilson, ed. *Harrison's Principles of Internal Medicine*. 12th edition. New York: McGraw-Hill, Inc., pp. 1322–1337.

90. Keith, J. S. (1985). Hepatic Failure: Etiologies, Manifestations, and Management. *Critical Care Nurse* 5(1): 60–86.

91. Dienstag, Wands, and Isselbacher, op. cit.

92. Ibid.

93. Hoofnagle, J. H. (1989). Type D (Delta) Hepatitis. *Journal of the American Medical Association* 261(9): 1332–1335.

94. Hoofnagle, op. cit.

95. Dienstag, Wands, and Isselbacher, op. cit.

96. Ibid.

97. Podolsky, D. K.; and Isselbacher, K. J. Cirrhosis of the Liver. In Jean D. Wilson, ed. *Harrison's Principles of Internal Medicine*. 12th edition. New York: McGraw-HIll, Inc.

98. Podolsky and Isselbacher, Cirrhosis of the liver.

99. Dienstag, Wands, and Isselbacher, op. cit.

100. Ibid.

101. Ibid.

102. Magun, A. M. (1988). Acute and chronic hepatitis. In Gail L. Bongiovanni, ed. *Essentials of Clinical Gastroenterology*. New York: McGraw-Hill, Inc.

103. Dienstag, Wands, and Isselbacher, op. cit.

104. Ibid.

105. Magun, op. cit.

106. Dienstag, Wands, and Isselbacher, op. cit.

107. Ibid.; Magun, op. cit.

108. Dienstag, Wands, and Isselbacher, op. cit.

109. Magun, op. cit.; Alspach, op. cit.

110. Dienstag, Wands, and Isselbacher, op. cit.

111. Iber, F. L.; and Baum, R. A. (1987). *Gastroenterology*. New York: Elsevier Science Publishing Co. Inc.

112. Dienstag, Wands, and Isselbacher, op. cit.

113. Alspach, op. cit.; Iber and Baum, op. cit.

114. Keith, op. cit.

115. Iber and Baum, op. cit.

116. Magun, op. cit.

117. Keith, op. cit.; Magun, op. cit.; Alspach, op. cit.

118. Keith, op. cit.; Magun, op. cit.

119. Magun, op. cit.; Alspach, op. cit.; Iber and Baum, op. cit.

120. Iber and Baum, op. cit.

121. Dienstag, Wands, and Isselbacher, op. cit.

122. Aach, R. D. (1987). Primary Hepatic Viruses: Hepatitis A, Hepatitis B, Delta hepatitis and Non-A, Non-B Hepatitis. *Transfusion Transmitted Viruses: Epidemiology and Pathology*. American Association of Blood Banks.

123. Magun, op. cit; Iber and Baum, op. cit.

124. Podolsky and Isselbacher, Cirrhosis of the liver.

125. Magun, op. cit.

126. Ibid.

127. Ibid.; Iber and Baum, op. cit.

128. Magun, op. cit.

129. Ibid.; Keith, op. cit.; Iber and Baum, op. cit.

130. Dienstag, Wands, and Isselbacher, op. cit.

131. Alspach, op. cit.

132. Magun, op. cit.

133. Ibid.

134. Dienstag, Wands, and Isselbacher, op. cit.

135. Keith, op. cit.; Magun, op. cit.; Jones, P. F.; Brunt, P. W.; Mowat, N.; and Ashley, G., eds. (1985). *Gastroenterology*. Chicago: Yearbook Medical Publishers, Inc.

136. Magun, op. cit.

137. Ibid.

138. Aach, op. cit.

139. Hoofnagle, op. cit.

140. Magun, op. cit.

141. Dienstag, Wands, and Isselbacher, op. cit.

142. Ibid.

143. Fagan, E. A.; and Williams, R. (1990). Fulminant Viral Hepatitis. *British Medical Bulletin* 46(2): 462–480.

144. Ibid.; Hoofnagle, op. cit.

145. Dienstag, Wands, and Isselbacher, op. cit.

146. Fagan and Williams, op. cit.

147. Shearman, D. J.; Finlayson, N. D. C.; and Carter, D. C. (1989). Fulminant (acute) hepatic failure. In *Diseases of the Gastrointestinal Tract and Liver*. Edinburgh: Churchill Livingstone.

148. Ibid.

149. Ibid.

150. Schafer, D. F.; and Donovan, J. P. (1990). Fulminant Hepatic Failure. In Theodore M. Bayless, ed. *Current Therapies in Gastroenterolgy and Liver Disease*. 3rd edition. Toronto: B. D. Decker, Inc.

151. Ibid.

152. Magun, op. cit.

153. Schafer and Donovan, op. cit.

154. Ibid.

155. Levinsky, N. G. (1991). Fluid and Electrolytes. In Jean D. Wilson, ed. *Harrison's Principles of Internal Medicine*. 12th edition. New York: McGraw-Hill, Inc.

156. McIntyre, N. (1990). Clinical presentation of acute viral hepatitis. *British Medical Bulletin* 46(2): 533–547.

157. Wands, J. R.; and Isselbacher, K. J. (1991). Chronic Hepatitis. In Jean D. Wilson, ed. *Harrison's Principles of Internal Medicine*. 12th edition. New York: McGraw-Hill, Inc.

158. Ibid.

159. Magun, op. cit.

160. Ibid.; Wands and Isselbacher, op. cit.

161. Wands and Isselbacher, op. cit.

162. Magun, op. cit.

163. Wands and Isselbacher, op. cit.

164. Skinner, C. A. (1988). Neoplasms of the Gastrointestinal Tract. In Gail L. Bongiovanni, ed. *Essentials of Clinical Gastroenterology*. New York: McGraw-Hill.

165. Magun, op. cit.

166. Wands and Isselbacher, op. cit.

167. Ibid.

168. Regenstein, F.; and Perrillo, R. P. (1990). Chronic Hepatitis. In Theodore M. Bayless, ed. *Current Therapies in Gastroenterology and Liver Disease*. 3rd edition. Toronto: B. C. Decker, Inc.

169. Wands and Isselbacher, op. cit.

170. Ibid.

171. Podolsky and Isselbacher, Cirrhosis of the liver.

172. Ibid.

173. Bongiovanni, G. L. (1988). Hepatic Cirrhosis. In Gail L. Bongiovanni, ed. *Essentials of Clinical Gastroenterology*. New York: McGraw-Hill.

174. Podolsky and Isselbacher, Cirrhosis of the liver.

175. Jarmilla, J. P. (1991). Colchine for liver cirrhosis. *Hospital Pharmacy* 26: 251–271.

176. Podolsky and Isselbacher, Cirrhosis of the liver.

177. Ibid.

178. Grandt, N. C. (1989). Hepatic veno-occlusive disease following bone marrow transplantation. *Oncology Nursing Forum* 16(6): 813–817.

179. Podolsky and Isselbacher, Cirrhosis of the liver.

180. Ibid.; Given, B. A.; and Simmons, S. J. (1984). Hepatic Disorders. In *Gastroenterology in Clinical Nursing*. St. Louis: C. V. Mosby.

181. Podolsky and Isselbacher, Cirrhosis of the liver.

182. Ibid.

183. Ibid.

184. Given and Simmons, op. cit.

185. Podolsky and Isselbacher, Cirrhosis of the liver.

186. Bongiovanni, G. L. (1988). Variceal Bleeding and Portal-Systemic Shunts. In Gail L. Bongiovanni, ed. *Essentials of Clinical Gastroenterology*. New York: McGraw-Hill.

187. Ibid.

188. Ibid.

189. Kalloo, A. N. (1990). Sclerotherapy of Esophageal Varices. In Theodore M. Bayless, ed. *Current Therapies in Gastroenterology and Liver Disease*. 3rd edition. Toronto: B. C. Decker, Inc.

190. Podolsky and Isselbacher, Cirrhosis of the liver.

191. Ibid.

192. Burns and Martin, op. cit.

193. Podolsky and Isselbacher, Cirrhosis of the liver.

194. Ibid.

195. Weesner, R. E. (1988). Complications of Cirrhosis. In Gail L. Bongiovanni, ed. *Essentials of Clinical Gastroenterology*. New York: McGraw-Hill.

196. Bongiovanni, Variceal bleeding.

197. Ibid.

198. La Villa, G.; Gines, P.; and Arroyo, V. (1990). Hepatorenal Syndrome and Ascites. In Theodore M. Bayless, ed. *Current Therapies in Gastroenterology and Liver Disease*. 3rd edition. Toronto: B. C. Decker, Inc.

199. Podolsky and Isselbacher, Cirrhosis of the liver.

200. Ibid.

201. Rothstein, J. D.; and Herlong, H. F. (1989). Neurologic Manifestations of Hepatic Disease. *Neurologic Clinics* 7(3): 563–574.

202. Ibid.

203. Shearman, D. J.; Finlayson, N. D. C.; and Carter, D. C. (1989). Hepatic encephalopathy. *Diseases of the Gastrointestinal Tract and Liver*. Edinburgh: Churchill Livingstone.

204. Rothstein and Herlong, op. cit.

205. Podolsky and Isselbacher, Cirrhosis of the liver.

206. Shearman, Finlayson, and Carter, Hepatic encephalopathy.

207. Podolsky and Isselbacher, Cirrhosis of the liver.

208. Rothstein and Herlong, op. cit.

209. Ibid.

210. Mitchell, R. B.; Wagner, J. E.; Karp, J. E.; et al. (1988). Syndrome of Idiopathic Hyperammonemia after High-Dose Chemotherapy: Review of Nine Cases. *The American Journal of Medicine* 85: 662–667.

211. Smith, S. L. (1990). Historical Perspective of Transplantation. In S. L. Smith, ed. *Tissue and Organ Transplantation: Implications for Professional Nursing Practice*. St. Louis: C. V. Mosby.

212. UNOS. (1991). *UNOS update* 7(1).

213. Bass, P. S.; Bindon-Perler, P. A.; and Lewis, R. L. (1991). Liver Transplantation: The Recovery Phase. *Critical Care Nursing Quarterly* 13(4): 51–61.

214. Maddrey, W. C.; Friedman, L. S.; Munoz, S. J.; and Hahn, E. G. (1988). Selection of the Patient for Liver Transplantation and Timing of Surgery. In W. C. Maddrey, ed. *Transplantation of the Liver*. New York: Elsevier.

215. Starzl, T. E.; Demetris, A. J.; and Van Thiel, D. (1989). Liver Transplantation. *The New England Journal of Medicine* 321(16): 1092–1099.

216. Miller, H. D. (1989). Liver Transplantation: Postoperative ICU Care. *Critical Care Nurse* 8(6): 19–31.

217. Meyers, W. C.; and Jones, R. S. (1990). *Textbook of Liver and Biliary Surgery*. New York: Lippincott; Shaw, Jr, B. W.; and Wood, R. P. (1988). The Operative Procedures. In W. C. Maddrey, ed. *Transplantation of the Liver*. New York: Elsevier; Starzl, Demetris, and Van Thiel, op. cit.

218. Meyers and Jones, op. cit.; Gordon, R. D.; Makowka, L.; Bronsther, O. L.; Lerut, J. P.; Esquivel, C. O.; Iwatsuki, S.; and Starzl, T. E. (1987). Complications of Liver Transplantation. In L. H. Toledo-Pereyra, ed. *Complications of Organ Transplantation*. New York: Marcel Dekker; Maletic-Staschak, S. (1984). Orthotopic Liver Transplantation: The Surgical Procedure. *AORN Journal* 39(1); 35–39.

219. Klein, A. (1990). Postoperative Care of the Liver Transplant Patient. Unpublished manuscript.

220. Klein, op. cit.; Marsh, J. W.; Gordon, R. D.; Stieber, A.; Esquivel, C. O.; and Starzl, T. E. (1989). Critical Care of the Liver Transplant Patient. In W. C. Shoemaker et al., eds. *Textbook of Critical Care Medicine*. 2nd edition. Philadelphia: W. B. Saunders.

221. Vargo, R. L.; and Rudy, E. B. (1989). Infection as a Complication of Liver Transplant. *Critical Care Nurse* 9(4): 52–62.

222. McMaster, P.; Kirby, R. M.; and Gunson, B. K. (1987). Liver Transplantation. In G. R. D. Catto, ed. *Clinical Transplantation: Current Practice and Future Prospects*. Boston: MTP Press.

223. Marsh et al., op. cit.

224. Gruppi, L. A.; Killen, A. R.; and Rodriguez, W. (1990). Liver Transplantation: Key Nursing Diagnoses. *Dimensions of Critical Care Nursing* 9(5): 272–279; Smith, S. L.; and Ciferni, M. (1990). Liver Transplantation. In S. L. Smith, ed. *Tissue and Organ Transplantation: Implications for Professional Nursing Practice*. St. Louis: C. V. Mosby; and Staschak, S.; Zamberlan, K. (1990). Liver Transplantation: Nursing Diagnoses and Management. In K. M. Sigardson-Poor and L. M. Haggerty, eds. *Nursing Care of the Transplant Recipient*. Philadelphia: W. B. Saunders.

225. Marsh et al., op. cit.; Smith and Ciferni, op. cit.; Carithers, Jr., R. L.; Fairman, R. P.; Mendez-Picon, G.; Posner, M. P.; Mills, A. S.; and Friedenberg, K. T. (1988). Postoperative Care. In W. C. Maddrey, ed. *Transplantation of the Liver*. New York: Elsevier; Ciferni, M.; and Kelly, A. (1990). Cytomegalovirus Infection in the Liver Transplant Patient: A Case Study. *Critical Care Nurse* 10(5): 10–21.

226. Miller, op. cit.; Starzl, Demetris, and Van Thiel, op. cit.; Gordon et al., op. cit.; Gruppi, Killen, and Rodriguez, op. cit.

227. Starzl, Demetris, and Van Thiel, op. cit.; Gordon et al., op. cit.; Marsh et al., op. cit.; Gruppi, Killen, and Rodriguez, op. cit.

228. Starzl, Demetris, and Van Thiel, op. cit.; Miller, op. cit.; Gruppi, Killen, and Rodriguez, op. cit.; Smith and Ciferni, op. cit.

229. Gruppi, Killen and Rodriguez, op. cit.; Grenvik, A.; and Gordon, R. (1987). Postoperative Care and Problems in Liver Transplantation. *Transplantation Proceedings* 19(4): 26–33.

230. Minnick, L. (1984). Nutrition in the Critically Ill. *University of Maryland Basic Intensive Care Course.*

231. Apelgren, K. N.; Rombeau, J. L.; Twonsey, P. L.; and Miller, R. A. (1982). Comparison of nutritional indices and outcome in critically ill patients. *Critical Care Medicine* 10: 305–307.

232. Cerra, F. B. (1987). Hypermetabolism, organ failure, and metabolic support. *Surgery* 101(1): 1–14.

233. Naccarto, D. V. (1987). *Guide to Parenteral Nutritional Therapy.* Baltimore: University of Maryland Medical Systems.

234. Kaldor, op. cit.; Naccarto, op. cit.; Berger R.; and Adams, L. (1989). Nutritional support in the critical care setting (part 2). *Chest* 96(2): 372–380.

235. Carrico et al., op. cit.

236. Springhouse Corporation. (1991). *Clinical Skill-builders—IV Therapy.* Springhouse, Pa.: Springhouse Corporation.

7 The Endocrine System

CHAPTER 7 PRE-TEST

1. The alpha cells of the pancreas secrete:
   a. glucagon.
   b. epinephrine.
   c. catecholamines.
   d. insulin.

2. The hypothalamus controls the release of pituitary hormones by:
   a. positive feedback—the appropriate level of hormone acts as a stimulus to release the releasing factors.
   b. negative feedback—the appropriate level of hormone shuts off the release of releasing factors.
   c. osmotic feedback—the appropriate level of hormone causes osmotic diffusion into the hypothalamus and shuts off the release of releasing factors.
   d. antibody feedback—antibodies formed by hormones block the release of releasing factors.

3. In DKA the serum potassium is:
   a. low until hyperglycemia is corrected.
   b. elevated for several hours after the glucose returns to normal.
   c. normal but becomes elevated after the hyperglycemia is corrected.
   d. elevated but falls rapidly after the hyperglycemia is corrected.

4. Nursing care of the patient receiving a continuous insulin drip should include:
   a. urine dipstick for glucose every 6 hours.
   b. nothing by mouth.
   c. serum glucose levels every hour for 2 hours, then every 2 hours.
   d. use of plastic bags and buretrols.

Refer to the following clinical vignette to answer questions 5 and 6.

K. J., a 44-year-old firefighter, was thrown from a moving fire engine and incurred a frontal head injury. He has received treatment for acute cerebral edema and has an intraventricular catheter installed in the lateral ventricle. Other injuries are limb fractures and a splenic rupture, requiring splenectomy. The nurse caring for K. J. notes increasing difficulty arousing him, hyperventilation, hypothermia, ICP of 19 mm Hg, and increased urine output.

5. These symptoms are the hallmark of:
   a. syndrome of inappropriate ADH.
   b. diabetes insipidus.
   c. HHNK.
   d. primary pituitary ischemia or necrosis.

6. The first intervention for this patient will probably be:
   a. to increase intravenous fluids.
   b. to obtain a repeat CT scan.
   c. drainage of CSF.
   d. to change antibiotics.

Overview of the Endocrine System

Unlike other organ systems that are anatomically continuous and sequential in function, the endocrine system and its suborgans have discrete physical structures and physiologic functions. The endocrine organs are called glands because their secretions—hormones—have a regulatory effect on a variety of metabolic functions. Endocrine organs are so named because hormones are secreted internally, rather than externally like the gastrointestinal system's digestive secretions. They also do not have ducts regulating their release of secretions as exocrine glands do. Many of the endocrine organs do stimulate one another's action, but each is a separate entity and will be addressed separately with respect to anatomy, physiology, and pathophysiologic disorders.

The body's endocrine organs include hypothalamus, pituitary, parathyroids, thyroid, adrenals, pancreas, ovaries, and testes. These are shown with their anatomical locations in Figure 7-1. The critical care nurse should be familiar with physiologic principles and pathophysiologic disorders of the pituitary, thyroid, adrenal, and pancreas glands even though the critical care certification exam tests only pituitary and pancreatic disorders.

Two differences exist between the endocrine system and other body systems. The first is the speed at which it functions. Endocrine function is the

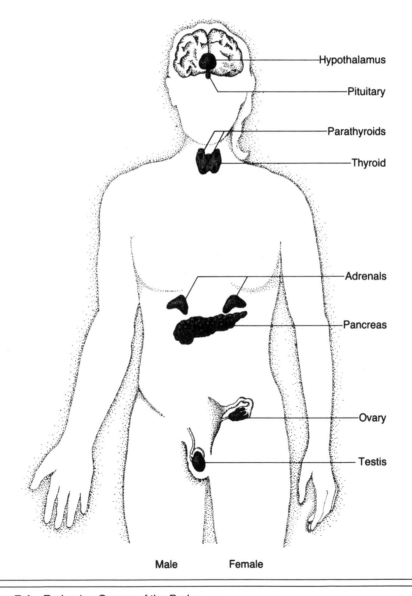

Male   Female

Figure 7-1   Endocrine Organs of the Body

slowest of all body functions, because its role is maintaining a homeostatic balance of biochemical reactions, which requires several feedback and integrated activities. Another important difference is the nature of the organs' activities. Endocrine glands do not initiate an activity, such as muscle contraction or digestion, but instead regulate various existing activities of other organs.

Endocrine system function is controlled by the nervous system. Occasionally, direct control is exerted, as in the direct stimulation of the adrenal gland by sympathetic hormones. More often, however, indirect control is achieved through hypothalamic regulation. The general mechanism by which endocrine glands function is feedback loops. These control systems ensure that secretions are produced at the proper times and in the appropriate amounts; that is, feedback loops initiate and cessate the hormonal responses. They do this by providing messages regarding the need for more or less hormone to continue a body function. Within the feedback loop is the ability to turn on or turn off specific hormone production. The hormone released by the target endocrine gland provides feedback that influences release of either the releasing or inhibiting substance of the hypothalamus or the pituitary hormone. If the effect is to inhibit the overall response of the system, it is termed negative feedback. If the effect is to stimulate further hormone release, it is termed positive feedback. The director of feedback mechanisms in the endocrine system is the nervous system organ, the hypothalamus. It performs this role by responding to feedback from target tissues or processes. When the pituitary gland directly influences the hypothalamus's secretion of regulating substances, the process is termed the short feedback loop. When the target organ signals the hypothalamus via intermediate messages to the pituitary gland, the process is termed the long feedback loop. Many glands have both mechanisms for regulating release of their hormones. This is exemplified by the diagram of feedback loops for thyroid hormones in Figure 7-2.

Hormones produced by the endocrine glands are of two major types: protein-derived (amino acids), such as hormones of the pituitary, thyroid, and pancreas, and lipids, such as the hormones produced by the adrenal cortex and the gonads. The two types of hormones differ in their ability to enter the cells of their target organ: protein-based hormones achieve their purpose by binding on receptor sites, and lipid hormones enter the cell and act directly on it. Cell-penetrating hormones (lipid-based) have a more rapid action and are less easily blocked. Protein-based hormones requiring receptor sites also require cyclic AMP (energy) to pass into the target

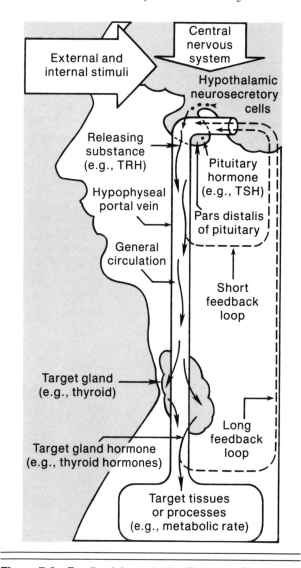

Figure 7-2 Feedback Loops in the Endocrine System

cell. This requirement is significant in states of altered glucose availability, such as sepsis. Prostaglandins are a group of recently identified hormone-like compounds found throughout the body. It is believed that they are the second messenger in the active transport of protein-based hormones and can accelerate many reactions through facilitation of hormone transport into cells. Prostaglandins or prostaglandin inhibitors are now being used in various settings by clinicians who are attempting to alter the natural history of a body process. For instance, prostaglandins are used in obstetrics to assist in the induction of labor.[1] Also, some researchers are using them investigationally for treatment of adult respiratory distress syndrome (ARDS) and sepsis.[2]

Disorders of the endocrine glands involve either hypersecretion or hyposecretion, and severity is determined by the degree of dysfunction. A broad range of these disturbances from barely detectable to life-threatening can be seen. Hypersecretion and hyposecretion are often clinical opposites and will present in a contrasting manner. Individual variations in response to hormonal dysfunctions will be related to the patient's age, gender, and state of physical health. The critically ill patient is at particular risk for endocrine disturbances because of multisystem injury and health compromise.

The Pituitary Gland

The pituitary gland, also known as the hypophysis, is a small gland the size of a lima bean located at the base of the brain beneath the third ventricle and attached to the hypothalamus by a stalk-like structure. The pituitary gland is divided into two independent lobes with very different functions. The anterior portion of the pituitary gland is termed the adenohy-

pophysis and is composed of glandular epithelial tissue. The anterior lobe is connected to the hypothalamus by a network of capillaries called the portal system. Release of hormones stored within the anterior pituitary is regulated by releasing hormones synthesized in the hypothalamus. The posterior portion of the pituitary gland is derived from the brain and is directly connected to the hypothalamus; it is termed the neurohypophysis. Hormones from the hypothalamus are stored in the neurohypophysis and are released in response to neural stimulation. The two lobes of the pituitary are so different in both composition and stimulation that they are usually referred to as two separate glands—the anterior pituitary and the posterior pituitary. Figure 7-3 is a diagram of the pituitary gland showing the location of important anatomical structures and the approximate areas of release for pituitary hormones.

The anterior pituitary gland is often described as

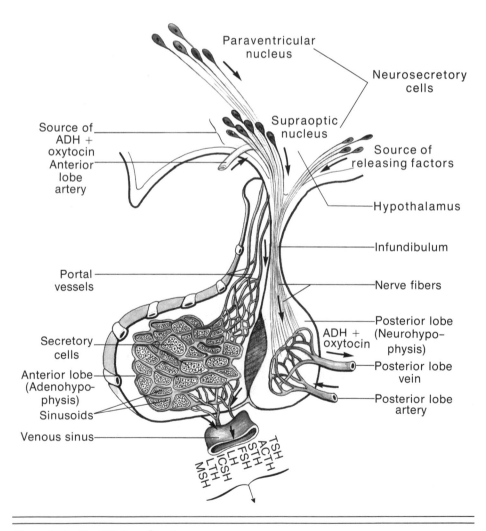

Figure 7-3 The Pituitary Gland

the "master gland of the endocrine system" because of its important influence on regulation of the other endocrine glands. Six hormones, called trophic hormones, are produced in the adenohypophysis; all of these are responsible for growth or for stimulation of other hormones. The names and effects of these are noted in Table 7-1. The level of each of these various trophic hormones from the adenohypophysis is regulated by the level of circulating hormone that exists. When the level reaches a threshold low, the hypothalamus generates a releasing hormone, which travels down the portal system to the anterior pituitary and stimulates the release of more trophic hormone, which acts directly on the target gland. When a specific target gland's hormone level rises, the rise serves to turn off the release of trophic hormone. This complex communication system regulates hormone levels within a narrow range, creating a steady state, without large deviations in hormones at any given time. This relationship between pituitary trophic hormones, target organs, and target organ hormones is depicted in Figure 7-4. Prolactin is the only anterior pituitary hormone regulated by inhibition from the hypothalamus.

Disorders of the pituitary involve undersecretion (hyposecretion) or oversecretion (hypersecretion) of one or multiple pituitary hormones. Disorders involving the growth hormone include dwarfism (decreased growth hormone) and gigantism or acromegaly (increased growth hormone). The neurohypophysis is the storage area and point of release for the hypothalamic hormones antidiuretic hormone (ADH) and oxytocin. External stimulants, such as plasma osmolality for ADH and infant suckling for oxytocin, cause the release of these hormones. Disorders of hyposecretion or hypersecretion of the neurohypophysis are most often neurological in origin.

Evaluation of pituitary function is usually hormone-specific. Based on presenting symptoms, tests of availability of and responsiveness to feedback loops assist clinicians in determining the etiology of

Table 7-1 Hormones of the Anterior Pituitary

Hormone	Effects/Functions	Selected Disorders
Adrenocorticotropic hormone (corticotropin, ACTH)	Stimulates production of glucocorticoids by adrenal cortex	Undersecretion may lead to symptoms of Addison's disease. Oversecretion may lead to symptoms of Cushing's syndrome.
Melanocyte-stimulating hormone (MSH)	Stimulates pigment production in skin	
Growth hormone (somatotropin, GH)	Promotes growth of body tissues	Undersecretion may produce pituitary dwarfs. Oversecretion may cause gigantism or, in adults, acromegaly.
Thyroid-stimulating hormone (thyrotropin, TSH)	Stimulates production and release of thyroid hormones	Undersecretion may lead to symptoms of hypothyroidism. Oversecretion may lead to symptoms of hyperthyroidism.
Follicle-stimulating hormone (FSH)	Initiates maturation of ovarian follicles or stimulates spermatogenesis	Undersecretion may cause hypogonadotropic eunuchoidism in males and amenorrhea in females.
Luteinizing hormone (LH)	Causes ovulation and stimulates ovary to produce estrogen and progesterone	Infertility
Interstitial cell-stimulating hormone (ICSH)	Stimulates androgen production by interstitial cells of testis	
Prolactin (LTH)	Stimulates secretion of breast milk	Undersecretion may cause failure to lactate after giving birth. Oversecretion may lead to lactation without recently having given birth.

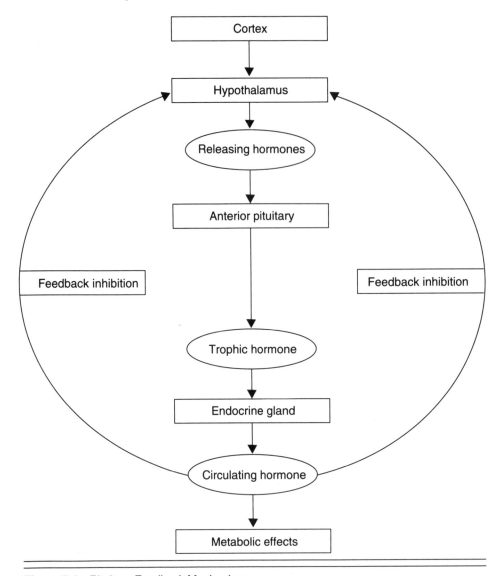

Figure 7-4   Pituitary Feedback Mechanisms

pituitary disorders. Most patients will also undergo a brain scan or magnetic resonance imaging (MRI) of the brain to rule out tumors or compression disorders. The specific pituitary disorders important for critical care nurses to recognize and manage are those involving faulty ADH release: secretion of inappropriate ADH (hypersecretion of ADH) and diabetes insipidus (hyposecretion of ADH).

Antidiuretic Hormone (ADH)

Antidiuretic hormone (vasopressin) is a peptide hormone produced by nuclei in the hypothalamus, primarily the supraoptic nuclei. Packaged in neurosecretory granules, it travels down axons to the posterior pituitary. It is released into the bloodstream by the posterior pituitary in response to changes in osmolality and volume of extracellular fluids. ADH level is thought to be regulated by three major physiological processes: osmoreceptors, baroreceptors, and the juxtaglomerular apparatus of the kidney. These processes are all thought to be involved in sensing volume (pressure) and osmolality changes. A summary of these complex interrelated factors is presented in Table 7-2.

The osmoreceptors found in the hypothalamus are sensitive to both sodium concentration and osmolality in the cerebrospinal fluid (CSF) and respond to minute increases of 1–2% by stimulating ADH release. If osmolality continues to increase, the sensation of thirst is also triggered.

Systemically, ADH release is triggered by the baroreceptors present in the carotid arteries, left atrium, aortic arch, and pulmonary veins in response

Table 7-2 Mechanisms Affecting Release of ADH

Origin	Mechanism
Hypothalamus	Heightened osmolarity triggers the osmoreceptors to increase ADH production and to signal the pituitary gland.
Pituitary gland	Increased ADH is secreted and transmitted through the blood to the kidneys.
Kidneys	Increased ADH causes more fluids to be reabsorbed into the circulatory system.
Circulatory system	Pressure receptors in the heart vessels and carotids sense the increased fluid volume and transmit this message to the brain.
Brain	Osmoreceptors and the pituitary gland are sent the signal to decrease ADH production and secretion.

to decreases in circulating volume of 5–10%, including decreases in cardiac output and blood pressure. Hypovolemia can trigger the release of angiotensin, which enhances the release of ADH from the posterior pituitary. The combined effect of systemic hypovolemia (decreased effective circulating volume) and increased osmolality is an extremely potent stimulus for ADH secretion. Table 7-3 lists the most important factors regulating ADH release from the posterior pituitary.

The Thyroid Gland

The thyroid gland is a bilobular gland located in the anterior neck, on either side and below the larynx.

Table 7-3 Factors Affecting Release of ADH

Stimulating Factors	Suppressing Factors
Increased osmolality	Decreased osmolality
Decreased volume	Increased volume
Decreased pressure	Increased pressure
Increased sodium in CSF	Ethanol
Positive pressure breathing	Corticosteroids
Angiotensin	Anticholinergics
Stress, pain	Phenytoin
Increased temperature	Decreased temperature

The right and left lobes are connected by a narrow isthmus that overlaps the trachea. The four parathyroid glands are located on the posterior surface of the thyroid gland (Figure 7-5). Internally, the gland consists of cuboidal vesicles called thyroid follicles, separated by specialized cells known as parafollicular cells. In the center of each follicle, the primary thyroid hormones, triiodothyronine (T_3) and thyroxine (T_4), are synthesized. These hormones exert their influence on many metabolic functions of the body, especially growth. The term *thyroid hormone* refers to both of these substances. Most thyroid hormone in the systemic circulation is inactive and bound to a protein called thyroid-binding globulin (TBG). The small amount of unbound hormone in circulation is the active form. Another hormone, calcitonin, is generated in the parafollicular cells. Calcitonin is able to lower calcium but is not the major regulator of calcium levels.

Thyroid hormone has diverse physiologic effects, but the primary one is the enhancement of the basal metabolic rate. Increased thyroid hormone is present in hypermetabolic states. Growth and tissue synthesis (especially related to protein), stimulated by thyroid hormone, increase metabolic rate, energy utilization, and oxygen consumption. Thyroid hormone is also responsible for some aspects of absorption and metabolism of carbohydrates, conversion of lipids to glucose (glycogenolysis), desaturation of fats, and lowering of serum cholesterol levels. Although the precise mechanism is unknown, thyroid hormone is known to have a synergistic relationship to catecholamines. This synergy promotes additive sympathetic metabolic effects and enhances neurotransmission and reflex activity. Less is known about the activity of calcitonin (thyrocalcitonin). It is unaffected by thyroid-stimulating hormone (TSH). Increased serum levels of ionized calcium stimulate the release of thyrocalcitonin, which monitors the serum levels and governs serum adjustments by exerting an influence on the rate of bone resorption (breakdown). Specific up-regulation of serum calcium levels occurs in response to parathormone, a parathyroid hormone.

Thyroid hormone levels are regulated by the hypothalamus, the pituitary gland, iodine transport capabilities, and calcium levels. All the hormones involved in this regulation process are outlined in Table 7-4, and the feedback loops were described earlier, in Figure 7-2. The thyroid hormone called thyroxine is released and regulates thyroid function by three mechanisms within the long and short feedback loops (Figure 7-6). In the long feedback loop, a high level of thyroxine inhibits the release of thyrotropin-releasing hormone (TRH) from the hy-

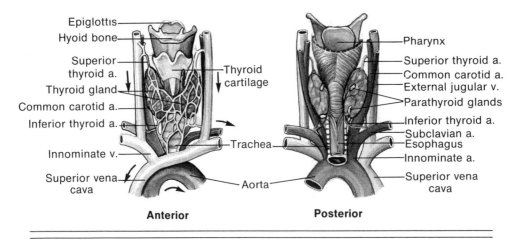

Figure 7-5 The Thyroid Gland

pothalamus, which instructs the anterior pituitary to stop releasing thyroid-stimulating hormone (TSH). The second mechanism in the long feedback loop involves the manner in which thyroxine inhibits the release of TSH by direct messages to the anterior pituitary. In the short feedback loop, the stimulated pituitary gland signals the hypothalamus that sufficient thyroxine is in the system. Stimulation of the thyroid gland by TSH causes T_3 and T_4 to be separated from thyroglobulin and become activated.

Eighty percent of activated thyroid hormone is T_4 (80–100 mcg daily), and 20 percent is T_3 (30 mcg daily). Once liberated from the follicular cells, these thyroid hormones bind with thyroid-binding globulin (TBG) and thyroid-binding prealbumin (TBPA). The T_4 hormone is inactive but is readily activated when transformed into T_3 by an enzyme that removes the iodine from the molecule. This enzyme, 5'-deiodinase, is reduced in the critically ill patient who is suffering caloric deprivation or receiving amiodarone, iodine contrast, propranolol, glucocorticoids, or PTU (propylthiouricil).

Thyroid hormone levels can also vary because of alterations in iodine consumption. The most common source of iodine for thyroid function is dietary intake from iodized salt or fluorinated water. Iodine is essential for the binding of thyroid hormone to TBG in the follicular cells. Without this iodine link, hormones cannot adequately react to TSH levels.

Overfunctioning (hyperthyroidism) or underfunctioning (hypothyroidism) of the thyroid gland will produce inappropriate quantities of thyroid hormone and generally affect the rate of metabolism and growth. Disorders of the thyroid gland are most likely to reflect alterations in T_3 and T_4 levels; they do not seem to reflect alterations in calcitonin levels. Hyperthyroidism and hypothyroidism may result in clinical crises requiring critical care intervention, but they can also be precipitated by critical illness itself. The primary presentation of thyroid disorders in the critical care unit is through the multisystem symptoms they generate. These disorders and their pertinence to critical care practice will be addressed later in this chapter.

Table 7-4 The Thyroid Hormones

Factors Regulating Thyroid Functions	Feedback Loops
Triiodothyronine (T_3)	Increased $T_4 \rightarrow$ decreased TRH $\rightarrow$ decreased TSH $\rightarrow$ decreased T_3 and T_4
Thyroxine (T_4)	
Thyrotropin-releasing hormone (TRH)	Increased $T_4 \rightarrow$ decreased TSH
Thyroid-stimulating hormone (TSH)	
Thyrocalcitonin	
Thyroxine-binding globulin (TBG)	
Thyroxine-binding prealbumin (TBPA)	
5'-deiodinase	

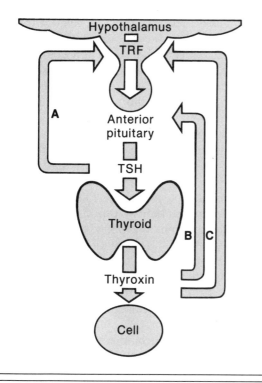

Figure 7-6 Feedback Mechanisms for Thyroid Hormones

The Adrenal Glands

The adrenals are a pair of glands that lie at the apices of each kidney (Figure 7-7). Despite their small size, they exert important physiologic effects on the entire body. Each adrenal gland is composed of two separate sections, the adrenal cortex and the adrenal medulla, which produce distinct hormones.[3]

The outer portion of the gland, the adrenal cortex, secretes three types of hormones. The cortex can be further divided into three regions, or zones, where these hormones are secreted. Directly beneath the capsular cover is the outermost region, the zona glomerulosa, where the mineralocorticoids are secreted. The middle zone, or zona fasciculata, and the innermost zone, or zona reticularis, are responsible for glucocorticoid and sex hormone secretion respectively.[4]

The inner portion of the gland, the adrenal medulla, is related functionally to sympathetic neurons. It secretes the catecholamines, epinephrine and norepinephrine, in response to sympathetic stimulation.[5]

The hormones of the adrenal cortex are synthesized from the steroid cholesterol and thus are termed corticosteroids. They are divided into three classes as previously described: the glucocorticoids, the mineralocorticoids, and the androgens (or sex hormones). Since androgens are not of great significance in critical care, they will not be discussed in this text.[6]

Cortisol is the principal glucocorticoid in the body and is responsible for at least 95% of adrenocortical secretory activity. Glucocorticoids are secreted by the zona fasciculata and zona reticularis regions of the adrenal cortex in response to serious infection, trauma, stress, or debilitation. They are essential for survival under emotional, physical, or chemical stress.[7]

A patient with a normally functioning adrenal cortex will respond to major stresses by increasing the amount of adrenocorticotropic hormone (ACTH)

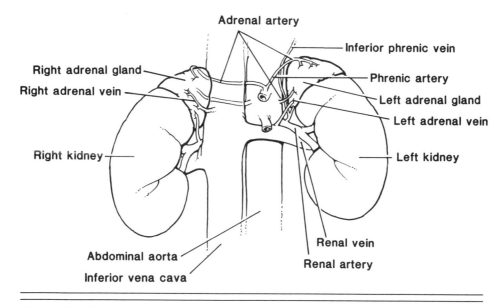

Figure 7-7 The Adrenal Glands

released and the activity of the adrenal cortex. Release of glucocorticoids from the adrenal cortex depends upon the release of ACTH from the anterior lobe of the pituitary gland. The stimulus for release of ACTH is the presence of corticotropin-releasing factor (CRF) secreted by the hypothalamus. CRF is carried to the anterior pituitary where it stimulates ACTH secretion. The stress response begins with release of CRF and then ACTH, followed by glucocorticoid secretion from the adrenal cortex (Figure 7-8).[8]

The release of glucocortoids is affected not only by stress, but also by diurnal sleep-activity cycles (activity in the early morning hours and inactivity in late evening) and by serum concentrations of cortisol. The negative feedback effect of cortisol in the blood will lead to decreased formation of CRF in the hypothalamus and of ACTH in the anterior pituitary. Plasma cortisol levels are therefore regulated by this negative feedback loop. This mechanism is not dependent upon the source of glucocorticoids. In situations in which exogenous glucocorticoids are responsible for plasma level elevation, CRF and ACTH are still decreased.[9]

The anterior pituitary also plays a role in maintaining the structural integrity of the adrenal cortex. In conditions in which ACTH is inhibited or absent, the adrenal cortex will atrophy and become incapable of synthesis and secretion of glucocorticoids and mineralocorticoids. The cortex may also become less responsive to the stress stimulation by ACTH. This can occur in the patient with prior or ongoing exogenous glucocorticoid administration.[10]

The glucocorticoids affect all cells of the body, especially the liver. Liver gluconeogenesis is stimulated concurrently with a reduction in glucose utilization by the cells, leading to elevations in blood glucose concentration. Protein metabolism is also affected: as storage is diminished in all cells except the liver, protein synthesis is decreased and protein catabolism is increased, except in the liver. Fat metabolism is influenced by glucocorticoids: as fatty acids are mobilized from adipose tissue, glucose conversion to fat is stimulated, and the use of fatty acids for energy is promoted. Glucocorticoids also exert an antiinflammatory response, which may interfere with a patient's response to infection as well as suppress delayed sensitivity reactions. In addition, glucocorticoids have an immunosuppressive action related to their lympholytic abilities. An excess of glucocorticoids leads to Cushing's syndrome; a deficiency leads to Addison's disease and, potentially, adrenal crisis.[11]

The mineralocorticoids are so called because of their effect on electrolytes of the extracellular fluid, mainly sodium and potassium. Aldosterone is the principal mineralocorticoid and is secreted in the zona glomerulosa. It is responsible for regulation of sodium and potassium movement through the renal tubules. Specifically, it increases sodium reabsorption and therefore indirectly increases extracellular fluid volume and enhances potassium excretion.[12] Aldosterone release is stimulated when the serum level of potassium or the ratio of serum potassium to serum sodium increases. In addition, the renin-angiotensin mechanism and the presence of ACTH

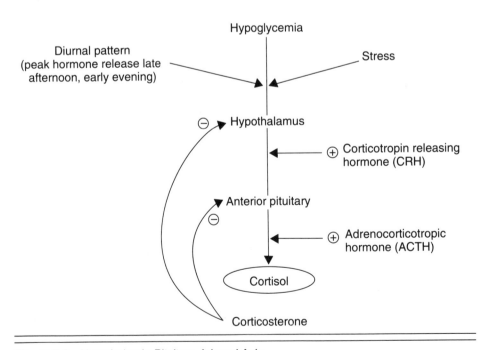

Figure 7-8 Hypothalamic-Pituitary-Adrenal Axis

regulate aldosterone secretion. An excess of aldosterone leads to hyperaldosteronism with resultant hypokalemia, muscle weakness, and, possibly, paralysis. Hypertension may also occur from the increase in extracellular fluid volume. A deficiency of aldosterone is termed Addison's disease, which may progress to adrenal crisis.[13]

The adrenal medulla is responsible for synthesizing and secreting epinephrine and norepinephrine, the hormones known as the catecholamines. The catecholamines serve as the body's first line of defense against stress, and their secretion is a reaction to, for example, fear, anxiety, pain, trauma, strenuous exercise, fluid loss, and hypoxia. Catecholamines are also synthesized in sympathetic nerve fiber endings, the brain, and some peripheral tissues.[14]

Epinephrine comprises 80% of the adrenal medulla's secretions of catecholamines. Its major action is the "fight-or-flight" response, and it affects both alpha- and beta-adrenergic sites but predominantly the latter. Essentially, alpha-adrenergic effects include peripheral vasoconstriction, mydriasis, and increased sweating. Beta-adrenergic effects are vasodilation, inotropic and chronotropic cardiac stimulation, bronchodilation, and diminished gastrointestinal motility (see Table 7-5). Epinephrine causes selective vasodilation in heart and skeletal muscle. Its release is governed by sympathetic nervous system stimulation as well as by substances such as insulin and histamine.[15]

Norepinephrine affects predominantly alpha-adrenergic sites. It has a more intense effect on skeletal muscle vasculature than epinephrine does,

and it produces increased peripheral vascular resistance. Norepinephrine, however, has less intense effects on cardiac and metabolic function than epinephrine does. It is important to note that without adequate levels of cortisol, the norepinephrine-mediated vasoconstriction and epinephrine-mediated metabolic responses do not occur.[16]

The Endocrine Pancreas

The endocrine functions of the pancreas are contained within the main pancreas and performed by specialized cells. The pancreas's major anatomical structures are referred to as the head (which lies posterior and connected to the duodenum), the neck (joining the major areas), the body, and the tail (which lies on the inferior surface of the spleen). The location of the pancreas and its relationship to various gastrointestinal structures facilitate its exocrine functions of supporting the breakdown of lipid food substances. A main pancreatic duct, the duct of Wirsung, runs the length of the organ and provides the vesicle for the transportation of pancreatic enzymes to the GI tract. The exocrine hormones most often associated with the pancreas are somatostatin, gastrin, amylase, and lipase. The pancreas is composed of a combination of cells with exocrine functions and those with endocrine functions. The microanatomy of the pancreas is depicted in Figure 7-9. Pyramidal structures, each with its own secretory tract, are lined with cuboidal secreting cells that form canals, referred to as acini. The randomly situated pyramids and secretory cells are termed the islets of Langerhans and are responsible for the endocrine hormones that are secreted by the pancreas. Acini are most commonly located in the tail of the pancreas and are functionally separated into the central area (called the cortex) and the distal canal (called the medulla). The secretions of the endocrine pancreatic cells are transferred directly into the circulation within the pancreas.

The cells of the islets of Langerhans are identified by the Greek letters alpha, beta, and delta. The centrally located alpha cells secrete glucagon in response to decreasing serum glucose levels, whereas the peripheral (medulla) beta cells secrete insulin when serum glucose levels are high. The delta or D cells located within the islets (cortex) are thought to release gastrin (also known as pancreatic polypeptide) and somatostatin, which inhibit the secretory activity of alpha and beta cells.[17] Because of the proximity of the delta cells to the alpha cells, the impact on the level of glucagon (secreted by alpha cells) is thought to be stronger than that on the level of insulin (secreted by beta cells). Somatostatin's

Table 7-5 Adrenergic Receptors and Their Functions

Alpha Receptors	Beta Receptors
Vasoconstriction	Vasodilation (B₂)
Iris dilation	Cardioacceleration (B₁)
Intestinal relaxation	Increased myocardial strength (B₁)
Intestinal sphincter contraction	Intestinal relaxation (B₂)
Pilomotor contraction	Uterus relaxation (B₂)
Bladder sphincter contraction	Bronchodilation (B₂)
	Calorigenesis (B₂)
	Glycogenolysis (B₂)
	Lipolysis (B₁)
	Bladder relaxation (B₂)

Source: Langfitt, D. (1984). *Critical Care Certification Preparation and Review.* Bowie, MD: Robert J. Brady.

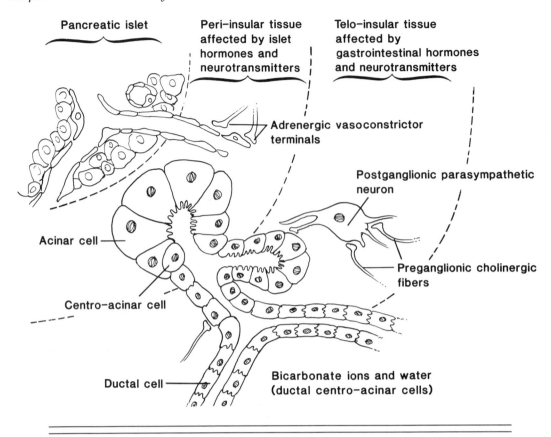

Figure 7-9   Microanatomy of the Pancreas

precise mechanisms are unknown, but it is believed that they involve neurohormonal pathways and transmitter substances such as acetylcholine.

The regulation of insulin and glucagon is controlled by a negative feedback mechanism involving blood glucose levels. Figure 7-10 is a schematic diagram of this feedback loop. The functioning of this loop is best tested by the glucose tolerance test (GTT), which involves administration of a concentrated glucose solution after a period of 3–4 hours of fasting. Serial blood glucose levels then demonstrate the body's ability to recognize the glucose load and secrete insulin appropriately—not deficiently, not excessively. When disorders of insulin or glucagon secretion exist, symptoms of hypoglycemia or hyperglycemia will occur.

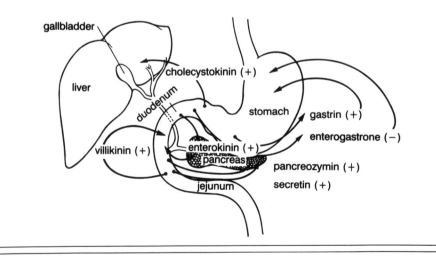

Figure 7-10   Glucose Feedback Loop

Secretion of Inappropriate ADH

The clinical syndrome of secretion of inappropriate antidiuretic hormone (SIADH) is generally seen in association with other disease states. Its incidence in critically ill patients is unknown. Mild cases may often go unrecognized but can complicate the care of patients with other, coexistent disease states. SIADH may also present as a medical emergency and, if inadequately treated, may be fatal or have permanent neurological sequelae.

In SIADH, multiple factors (often disease states) act to disrupt the feedback mechanism that normally controls the volume of body water and the dilution of sodium. Some of these factors act centrally on the pituitary itself; others act directly on the distal tubules and collecting ducts of the nephron. Disease-related causes of SIADH tend to fall into three categories: malignancy, CNS disease, and pulmonary disease.

The most common reason for SIADH is ectopic production of an ADH-like compound by tumors, particularly small cell (oat cell) carcinoma of the lung. Research has shown that the ADH synthesized by, stored in, and released from these malignant cells is identical to the ADH produced in the pituitary gland.

Central nervous system disorders may also increase ADH production. The disorders may be the result of generalized edema or may be localized in the hypothalamic and pituitary region.

It is believed that normal pulmonary tissue has the capacity to produce and secrete ADH but does not usually do so unless damaged. Pulmonary diseases or barotrauma causing injury to the pulmonary tissue will result in secretion of inappropriate ADH. Common etiologies of pulmonary-induced ADH include bacterial or viral pneumonias, tuberculosis, and certain fungal pneumonias such as aspergillus. Many mechanically ventilated patients or those with pulmonary contusion develop ADH from barotrauma. Use of higher levels of PEEP or patient asynchrony with the ventilator increases this risk.

Many medications, acting either centrally or on the nephron, have been implicated in the etiology of SIADH. Finally, factors such as nausea, stress, pain, and trauma may cause SIADH, presumably by central action. The risk factors for the development of SIADH are outlined in Table 7-6.

Critical referents

ADH exerts its antidiuretic effect on the distal tubules and collecting ducts of the kidney, increasing their permeability to water. This is accomplished by the binding of ADH to specific receptor sites on cell membranes, which triggers changes in enzyme activity and subsequent changes in the cell membranes' permeability to water. As a result, free water is conserved by the body, diluting solutes and lowering plasma osmolality. Normally, when fluid and solute homeostasis is restored, ADH secretion is inhibited. (Figure 7-11 illustrates the feedback control of ADH release.) In SIADH, this negative feedback is disrupted; excess free water is conserved by the body, both increasing fluid volume and decreasing osmolality.

When ADH is secreted in excessive amounts, it inhibits aldosterone, which is the hormone primarily responsible for the conservation of sodium in the body. Aldosterone, secreted by the adrenal cortex, acts directly on the kidney to promote potassium loss and sodium retention, in response to feedback control involving the afferent arterioles and juxtaglomerular apparatus.

Sodium, the most abundant and most important cation in the body, is usually maintained within a narrow range of concentration by the direct action of aldosterone and the indirect action of ADH. Sodium is responsible for maintaining the osmotic pressure of extracellular fluid (ECF), participates in most biochemical reactions in cells, is involved in nerve and muscle action potentials, and, as sodium bicarbonate, is the most important buffer in extracellular fluid. Its importance is illustrated by the fact that the ratio of minimum to maximum tolerated concentrations of sodium is less than 1:2; for hydrogen and potassium the ratio is about 1:10. The primary function of sodium is the osmotic role it plays in maintaining extracellular fluid volume in the human body, which is 60% water. "Volume consists primarily of water, and sodium is the 'sponge' that holds the water upon which ECF volume so heavily depends."[18] SIADH, by disrupting this delicate balance of volume and sodium, thus affects numerous systems of the body. The specific pathophysiologic consequences of reduced sodium (hyponatremia), as found in SIADH, are addressed in the chapter on the renal system.

Resulting signs and symptoms

The clinical signs and symptoms of SIADH vary with the severity of the syndrome. Mild cases may

Table 7-6 Clinical Antecedents of SIADH

Ectopic Production	CNS Disorders	Pulmonary Disorders	Medications	Disruptions of Homeostasis
Lung cancers	Trauma	Lung trauma	Morphine	Nausea
Carcinoma of pancreas	Tumor	Bacterial pneumonia	Barbiturates	Vomiting
Carcinoma of duodenum	Subarachnoid hemorrhage	Viral pneumonia	Vincristine (Oncovin)	Stress
Carcinoma of bladder and prostate	Cerebral atrophy	Pulmonary tuberculosis	Cyclophosphamide (Cytoxan)	Trauma
Lymphosarcoma	Cerebrovascular accident	Aspergillus pneumonia	Cisplatin	Pain
Thymoma	Encephalitis	Mechanical ventilation (especially when PEEP is employed or patient is asynchronous with the ventilator)	Chlorothiazide (Diuril)	Surgery
Reticulum cell sarcoma	Meningitis		Tricyclic antidepressants	Hemorrhage
Ewing's sarcoma	Guillain-Barré syndrome		Fluphenazine (Prolixin)	
Hodgkin's disease	Lupus erythematosus	Empyema	Carbamazipine (Tegretol)	
Malignant histiocytosis		Pneumocele	Acetaminophen	
Tuberculosis		Chronic obstructive lung disease	General anesthetics	
Lung abscess			Nicotine	
Pneumonia			Chlorpropamide (Diabinese)	
Chronic lung infection			Tolbutamide (Orinase)	
Status asthmaticus			Phenformin (DBI, Meltrol)	
Aspergillosis			Isoproterenol (Isuprel)	
Hypothyroidism				
Hypopituitarism				
Addison's disease				
Porphyria				

mimic other diseases and go unrecognized. Initially water retention is the primary feature of SIADH; as the syndrome progresses, serum sodium levels decrease, and water intoxication occurs. It is helpful to know the signs and symptoms of falling sodium levels, as summarized in Table 7-7.

Mild SIADH, with near normal serum sodium levels of 125–134 mEq/L, usually presents as weight gain without edema and mild mental status changes. These changes may include vague complaints, such as headache, weakness, and sleepiness, and some confusion or disorientation. The gastrointestinal system is also affected by water retention, anorexia being the chief complaint. Muscle cramps may also occur.

If SIADH progresses, serum sodium levels will continue to fall. At levels of 115–124 mEq/L, more marked changes in mental status are seen, including personality changes, irritability, lethargy, and sluggish deep tendon reflexes. Weakness is a major

complaint. The patient is nauseated and may have abdominal cramping, vomiting, and diarrhea. Water continues to be retained, and oliguria is usually seen at this stage.

Severe SIADH is characterized by serum sodium levels below 115 mEq/L in an adult. Children are less able to tolerate low sodium levels and may have life-threatening symptoms with serum sodium levels below 128 mEq/L. Seizure activity and coma will progress to death if severe SIADH is not treated.

Physical assessment of the patient with SIADH reveals clinical signs and symptoms associated with water retention and low sodium levels. Laboratory tests are necessary in order to diagnose SIADH and differentiate it from other possible causes of sodium depletion and fluid overload. A list of both primary (related to sodium and water levels) and secondary (resulting from volume changes) laboratory values seen with SIADH is presented in Table 7-8. Serum sodium levels and serum osmolality are checked and

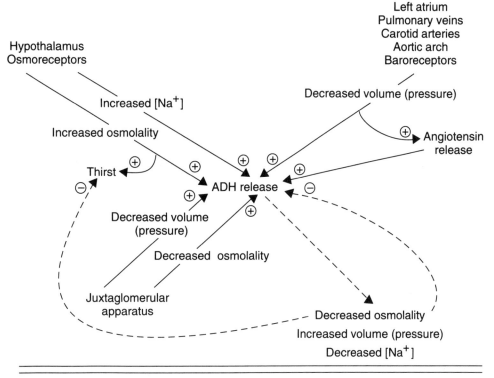

Figure 7-11 Feedback Control of ADH

are below normal ranges (135–145 mEq/L for sodium, 275–295 mOsm/kg for serum osmolality) in SIADH. It is helpful to analyze urine sodium and osmolality concurrently. In SIADH, the kidneys are unable to diurese water or conserve sodium in spite of the serum values. Thus, urine osmolality is greater than plasma osmolality and, in fact, is usually greater than 1200 mOsm/kg. Urine sodium is usually normal or higher than normal, with the kidneys spilling more than 220 mEq of sodium in 24 hours.

Other, more definitive tests may be needed to differentiate SIADH from other possible causes of dilutional hyponatremia. The differential diagnosis includes evaluation for congestive heart failure, cirrhosis, hypervolemia, hypothyroidism, Addison's disease, and Rocky Mountain spotted fever. Plasma and urine ADH levels can be measured by a radioimmunoassay. A water load test can be given. The patient drinks 25 cc/kg of water every 4 hours. Urine output and urine and serum osmolalities are serially measured. In a normal individual, about 80% of the ingested water will be excreted in 4 hours. During

Table 7-7 Relation of Clinical Symptoms to Severity of Hyponatremia

Classification	Serum Na$^+$ (mEq/L)	Symptoms
Mild	125–135	Asymptomatic; confusion, fatigue
Moderate	118–124	Weakness, short-term memory loss, inappropriate behavior, lethargy
Severe	112–117	Coma, seizures

Table 7-8 Results of Laboratory Studies Suggestive of SIADH

Increased urinary osmolality*

Increased urinary sodium*

Decreased urinary aldosterone

Decreased serum osmolality*

Hyponatremia*

Dilutional hypokalemia

Dilutional hypocalcemia

Normal BUN

Normal creatinine

Normal thyroid hormones

Normal adrenal cortical hormones

*Classic lab values

this time, urine osmolality will fall while plasma osmolality will be maintained within normal limits. In SIADH, less than 40% of the water may get excreted, and urine osmolality remains normal or high. Other tests that may be done to diagnose SIADH include cortisol levels, T_3 and T_4 levels, and serum electrolyte levels. Changes in mental status may require further investigation to ensure that there are not other causes—for example, brain metastases in a patient with lung cancer.

Nursing standards of care

Medical intervention includes eliminating the cause of SIADH as well as correcting hyponatremia and hypervolemia. Underlying causes, such as malignancies or drugs, are investigated. Treatment of the causative disease or discontinuation of the implicated drug usually stops the inappropriate secretion of ADH. Correction of the fluid and sodium status is also required.

Treatment of SIADH varies, based on the severity of the accompanying hyponatremia. The patient's clinical status also determines treatment, because different individuals may exhibit different symptoms with the same serum sodium level.

Mild SIADH is treated with fluid restriction to 800–1000 mL/day. This prevents further fluid overload and sodium dilution. The patient's fluid and electrolyte status will equilibrate over time. More rapid correction of sodium levels is hazardous and may precipitate seizures and other central nervous system symptoms caused by sudden fluid and electrolyte shifts.

More severe SIADH is generally treated with hypertonic saline (3% NaCl) and forced diuresis with a loop diuretic agent. Hypertonic saline is given intravenously, generally as 250–500 mL over several hours, followed by an intravenous diuretic (such as furosemide). This procedure allows a more rapid correction of low serum sodium and elimination of free water. Hypertonic saline infused alone is not effective, as most of the administered sodium is excreted in the urine. Fluid restriction continues, with the patient allowed as little as 500 mL/day.

There are also medications that may be tried, particularly for chronic SIADH. Few patients can tolerate prolonged fluid restriction, and there are many situations (for example, a patient with lung cancer) where it may be impossible to remove the cause of SIADH. Demeclocycline (Declomycin) is an oral tetracycline derivative that acts by blocking the effect of ADH on the kidneys. Its usual dosage is 600–1200 mg daily (in children, 6–12 mg/kg/day given in divided doses). Side effects include photosensitivity, hematologic changes, skin rashes, azotemia, and superinfection. In the patient with concurrent liver failure, demeclocycline may precipitate acute renal failure. Antacids, food, and dairy products may interfere with demeclocycline's absorption, so the patient should be instructed to take it on an empty stomach. It may also decrease the effectiveness of oral contraceptives. Because it is a tetracycline, demeclocycline is contraindicated during pregnancy and lactation, and, like antibiotics in general, its administration may interfere with the diagnosis of infections.

Lithium carbonate is sometimes used, and it also acts by blocking the renal effect of ADH. It has several toxic side effects, including gastrointestinal irritation, tremors, weakness, and cardiac irritability. Phenytoin (Dilantin) is occasionally used to manage SIADH. It acts by centrally inhibiting ADH release.

Nursing management of the patient with SIADH includes management of the signs and symptoms of fluid overload and hyponatremia. Since this may be a progressive, life-threatening syndrome, anticipation of its potential complications and understanding of its pathophysiology are essential. Actual problems are identified based on physical assessment, history from the patient and family, and interpretation of laboratory and diagnostic data. Education of the patient and family can enhance adherence to fluid restrictions as well as lessen anxiety. Prioritization of problems should be individualized, based on the patient's need for safety, comfort, and prevention of life-threatening complications. The following care plan delineates the nursing management of the patient with diagnosed SIADH. This plan of care may also be adapted to any patient with hyponatremia and hypervolemia.

Diagnosis	Signs and symptoms	Intervention	Rationale
Alteration in fluid volume: fluid excess related to decreased output due to inappropriate ADH secretion	Increased weight Intake greater than output Oliguria Normal or high specific gravity of urine Jugular vein pulsations Positive hepatojugular reflex Crackles (rales), gurgles (rhonchi), cough Weakness, fatigue Blood pressure changes Third heart sound Edema	Keep careful I&O records; calculate fluid balance every 8 and 24 hours; weigh patient daily or twice a day and compare with admission and normal weight	Output should equal or exceed intake to correct hypervolemia
		Auscultate breath sounds in all lung fields every 8 hours; check temperature every 4 hours	Early detection of pulmonary complication facilitates treatment
		Auscultate heart sounds for S_3	Early detection of cardiac failure facilitates treatment
		Maintain fluid restriction as ordered, spreading intake throughout day in conjunction with patient preferences; avoid administration of free water in any form (enema, NG tube flush, or mixed with tube feedings); encourage intake of fluids with high sodium content (bouillon, tomato juice, milk, orange juice)	Patient is already hypervolemic, and fluid restriction will enhance development of hyperosmolarity with subsequent turn-off of SIADH
		Plan active or passive range-of-motion exercises every 4 hours and change of position every 2 hours if patient is not ambulatory	Movement and position changes prevent venous pooling and decrease incidence of complications related to immobility

Nursing Care Plan for the Management of the Patient with Secretion of Inappropriate ADH

Diagnosis	Signs and symptoms	Intervention	Rationale
Alterations in thought processes related to increased extracellular fluid volume and decreased sodium levels in central nervous system	Confusion, disorientation Anxiety, restlessness, altered attention span Combativeness Lethargy, weakness Decreasing level of consciousness Decreased deep tendon reflexes, seizure activity, impaired cranial nerve function	Neurological assessment hourly to every 8 hours (dependent on degree of deficit)	To reveal small changes in central nervous system function that will necessitate more aggressive treatment of SIADH
		Reorient confused patient to place, person, and time with each interaction	Constant reinforcement assists in maintaining safety of patient with poor memory
		Protect patient from injury with padded side rails, close observation, use of physical restraints	Patient may not recognize own limitations and may injure self
		Seizure precautions	Seizures due to hyponatremia are possible
		Maintain elevation of head and minimize activities that increase intracranial pressure (suctioning, Valsalva maneuver, vomiting)	SIADH causes cerebral edema, which increases intracranial pressure and affects central nervous system function, conditions that may progress to brainstem herniation and death
		Encourage family and significant others to participate in reorienting patient and provide contact with normal events (news, information about home and family)	Familiar persons are often most successful in reorienting the confused patient
		Respect individuality and privacy of patient as much as possible	It can be easy to forget issues of privacy when patient is not conversing normally and participating in care

Diagnosis	Signs and symptoms	Intervention	Rationale
Anxiety related to perceived threat to biological integrity or possibly to altered central nervous system function	Expressed feelings of apprehension, nervousness, helplessness, fear, tension, loss of control Irritability, anger, agitation, combativeness Inability to rest or sleep Crying, withdrawal, forgetfulness, inability to concentrate Increased heart rate Increased BP Insomnia Tremors Weakness Diaphoresis	Promote a therapeutic relationship with patient by acknowledging anxiety, communicating empathy, and accepting patient's individuality Provide reassurance by staying with patient, speaking slowly and calmly, allowing patient to use appropriate coping mechanisms (verbalizing anxiety, crying, walking, diversional activity) Decrease sensory stimulation by providing quiet environment; promote normal sleep by darkening room at night and minimizing interruptions Provide explanations of disease process, treatments, drugs, routines, and procedures at level appropriate to patient's comprehension and level of anxiety	Anxiety may interfere with healing and adherence to care regimen Measures promoting empathic awareness between nurse and patient decrease anxiety Rest and sleep promote healing and decrease anxiety Understanding of what is happening increases the patient's sense of self-control thereby decreasing anxiety
Alteration in nutrition: intake less than body requirements related to anorexia due to excess fluid volume	Disinterest in food, history of decreasing dietary intake Decreased muscle mass (mid-arm circumference) Brittle hair and nails History of abdominal cramping, constipation, diarrhea, or vomiting	Auscultate bowel sounds Offer frequent small meals or snacks throughout day; maintain calorie count; encourage foods with high caloric content if tolerated	Poor absorption and edema of bowel may occur and will be evidenced by diminished bowel sounds Good nutrition will promote healing and decrease the incidence of complications from immobility

Diagnosis	Signs and symptoms	Intervention	Rationale
		Encourage foods with high sodium content; provide mouth care before and after meals and PRN	Fluid restriction and anorexia both decrease saliva production and increase the risk of oral complications such as ulcers, dry mouth, and tooth decay
		Provide frequent oral care; use saliva substitutes or hard candies	Fluid restrictions cause extreme thirst and anorexia
Potential for injury related to sensory or motor deficits due to hyponatremia or cerebral edema	Impaired ability to communicate needs, decreased level of activity, and/or impaired ability to care for self

Impaired sight or hearing

Seizure activity | Reorient confused patient to place, person, and time with each interaction; supervise activities and provide assistance as necessary; maintain uncluttered environment; keep bed at lowest feasible position, with padded side rails in place when patient is unattended | Disoriented patient is at high risk for self-injury while hospitalized; promoting a safe environment minimizes the risk of injury |
| | | If restraints are required to protect an agitated patient from self-injury, they should be used for the minimum time possible and should be removed every 4 hours to check underlying skin for injury | Physical restraints may be required, but should be used cautiously |
| | | Check patient's medications and history for possible psychotropic agents, including antiemetics, analgesics, and/or tranquilizers or indications of alcohol and/or drug abuse | The patient with SIADH who is agitated and confused should not be sedated as this may mask further deterioration in mental status |

Diagnosis	Signs and symptoms	Intervention	Rationale
Lack of knowledge about SIADH	Misconceptions Requests for information Nonadherence with treatment plan	Determine patient's knowledge and ability to learn; identify learning objectives and determine methods of learning that patient finds most useful (visual or audio aids, demonstration, booklets, discussion); develop teaching plan for patient and family using varied methods	Learning needs and abilities vary with age, education, illness, and culture
Nonadherence with fluid restriction related to negative side effects (thirst, discomfort)	Nonadherence or discrepancy between history given and physical exam (weight, lab values, etc.)	Assess for level of understanding of disease process and treatment plan; correct knowledge deficit; assess patient and family's attitudes toward illness and possible need for psychological support	The ability to tolerate discomfort depends partly on understanding and acceptance of the reason for discomfort
		Encourage patient's participation in care (allow patient to make own choices about types of fluids taken and distribution of fluids throughout day); Develop contract with younger patient	Patient participation in self-care promotes independence, wellness, and self-esteem
		Provide alternatives to fluids (mouth care, gum, hard candies)	Comfort measures may make fluid restriction more tolerable
		Establish goals that will allow modification of fluid restriction (for example, when weight decreases 1 kg, fluid intake may be increased by 250 cc/day)	Flexibility in therapeutic plan allows patient to make choices and allows fluid leeway for the nonadhering patient

Medications Commonly Used in the Care of the Patient with Secretion of Inappropriate ADH

Medication	Effect	Major side effects
Demeclocycline, Demecycline	Blocks effects of ADH on the kidneys	Photosensitivity Skin rashes Azotemia Superinfection Bone marrow suppression
Diuretics (furosemide, bumetamide)	Excretion of excess vascular water	Hypokalemia Hypocalcemia Hypomagnesemia Transient deafness
Hypertonic NS (3% or 5%)	Increases sodium content and osmolarity Assists in hemoconcentration	Vascular volume overload Hypernatremia
Lithium carbonate	Blocks effects of ADH at the cellular level	GI distress Tremors Weakness Cardiac irritability
Phenytoin	Blocks ADH release by the brain	Gum hyperplasia Rashes Altered coagulation

Diabetes Insipidus

Diabetes insipidus (DI) is a disease state characterized by thirst and frequent urination. These symptoms, also found in diabetes mellitus, arise in DI from a completely different cause. Diabetes insipidus is the deficiency of antidiuretic hormone (ADH, or vasopressin). ADH is the hormone responsible for regulating the volume and concentration of body water.

Clinical antecedents

Diabetes insipidus can be the result of a defect in the synthesis of ADH, a defect in the mechanism of release of ADH, or, rarely, a primary renal defect in which the renal tubular cells are unable to respond to the hormone. It may be a transient syndrome associated with other illness or trauma, or it may be a permanent disease state.

Central (neurogenic) causes of DI include diseases and homeostatic changes that disrupt the production or release of ADH. Trauma, cerebral edema, tumors of the hypothalamus or pituitary, and some drugs are common causes of DI. When a cause of DI cannot be determined, it is called primary, or idiopathic, DI. Idiopathic DI is believed to comprise 30–50% of all cases.[19]

Renal (nephrogenic) causes of DI include renal failure, some medications, pregnancy, and inherited defects in the ability of renal tubular cells to respond to ADH. Nephrogenic DI is usually less severe than central DI. The risk factors and causes of DI are outlined in Table 7-9.

Critical referents

The decreased activity of ADH in diabetes insipidus results in the loss of free water from the body. This loss may be due to insufficient amounts of ADH being synthesized and released or to its effect on the distal tubules and collecting ducts of the kidney being blocked. Destruction of the supraoptic nuclei in the hypothalamus or of the axon tracts connecting the nuclei with the posterior pituitary results in a complete loss of ADH and a permanent DI state. Disruption or compression of the pituitary stalk (during surgery or as a result of trauma or tumor) usually causes transient DI. Nephrogenic DI involves the reabsorption function of the renal tubules—there is reduced tubular response to vasopressin with subsequent diuresis.

Resulting signs and symptoms

The patient with DI presents with extreme polyuria, nocturia, and polydipsia. If the thirst center is intact and the patient with DI is alert and able to drink, the body fluids lost through the kidneys will

Table 7-9 Antecedents of Diabetes Insipidus

	Physical Antecedents	Medications
Central (neurogenic)	Head injury Neurosurgery Craniopharyngioma Glioma Astrocytoma Brain metastases (especially from leukemia, breast cancer) Meningitis Encephalitis Aneurysm Idiopathic Inherited defect	Ethanol Reserpine Morphine Chlorpromazine Phenytoin
Renal (nephrogenic)	Polycystic kidney disease Pyelonephritis Pregnancy Idiopathic Inherited trait	Lithium carbonate Demeclocycline Methoxyflurane

be replaced by drinking. The patient with DI who is unable to sense thirst or unable to drink is at great risk for overwhelming dehydration and will have a more obvious clinical presentation. The urine is dilute, with a low specific gravity and osmolality. Urine output is greater than 250 mL/hr. In severe cases, 10–15 L of urine a day may be excreted. This occurs in spite of a hyperosmolar serum and extracellular fluid and triggers extreme thirst. Concentration of body fluids also results in a relative hypernatremia. Alcohol's suppression of ADH release results in a mild transient DI, familiar to some as the classic hangover: "the morning after" is characterized by thirst and a headache, which result from fluid and electrolyte shifts in the central nervous system; dehydration, which results from the inappropriate loss of body fluid via the kidneys; and adversely affected energy level and ability to concentrate. Diabetes insipidus, whatever the cause, is characterized by dehydration, thirst, and, sometimes, mental status changes, all of which are related to the shifts of fluids and electrolytes that may be occurring. The signs and symptoms of DI (inadequate ADH) and SIADH (excessive ADH) are compared in Table 7-10.

The degree of dehydration is assessed by physical examination as well as laboratory data. Mild dehydration includes dry mucous membranes, tachycardia, and possibly weight loss. Moderate dehydration progresses to include poor skin turgor, dry skin, postural hypotension, and complaints of weakness and thirst. In cases of severe dehydration, tachycardia is accompanied by decreased pulse volume and pulse pressure, hypotension, and decreased central venous pressure. Body temperature is often increased. The patient is unable to sweat and has a dry mouth with no saliva production.

Mental status changes seen with DI include lethargy, irritability, combativeness, and delirium. Such changes are due to rapid shifts of fluid and electrolytes in the central nervous system. These may result from too rapid correction of fluid and electrolyte deficits as well as from the physiological changes associated with DI. In some circumstances, DI has been noted to be triphasic; that is, a transient occurrence lasting 2–3 days is followed by resolution and then recurrence after an additional 2–3 days.[20] This occurs most commonly after trauma or surgery. The critical care nurse should observe the patient for this phenomenon by monitoring fluids, electrolytes, and clinical symptoms throughout the high-risk period.

Laboratory tests are also done to differentiate DI from other possible causes of hypovolemia and hypernatremia; excessive water intake and excessive administration of parenteral fluids must be ruled out. Results of serum studies that indicate DI include (refer to Table 7-10) an elevated osmolality (greater than 295 mOsm/kg), normal glucose, and hypernatremia (greater than 150 mEq/L). Urine osmolality is inappropriately low (less than 200 mOsm/kg; specific gravity 1.002 to 1.006). Following a head injury or neurosurgery, these laboratory findings are generally sufficient to diagnose DI in the presence of extreme polyuria.

Another test to diagnose DI, particularly in the absence of strong etiology, is the dehydration test, or water deprivation test. The patient is deprived of fluid for 6–8 hours, and serial urine specimens are collected until the urine osmolality has stabilized (variation of less than 30 mOsm/kg between three consecutive specimens). The patient is then given 5–10 units of aqueous ADH subcutaneously, and urine osmolality is measured 1 hour later. The patient who does not have DI is able to concentrate urine during dehydration, so urine osmolalities are higher than serum osmolalities. Because the urine is already maximally concentrated, when ADH is given,

Table 7-10 Comparison of Signs and Symptoms of SIADH and Diabetes Insipidus

Parameter	SIADH	Diabetes Insipidus
Urinary output	Moderately high	Extremely high
Vascular volume (CVP)	Extremely high	Extremely low
Altered mental status	Severe	Mild
Thirst	—	Moderate
Skin	Edema, dry, temperature normal	Poor turgor, dry, warm
Serum osmolality	<280 mOsm	>295 mOsm
Serum sodium	<130 mEq/L	>150 mEq/L
Urine osmolality	High	Low

osmolality does not increase further. The patient with DI, on the other hand, is unable to concentrate urine during dehydration, so urine osmolalities remain lower than serum osmolalities. In neurogenic DI, urine osmolality increases significantly in response to ADH injection; in nephrogenic DI, urine osmolality remains low. These findings are summarized on Table 7-11. During this test the patient is hospitalized and must be carefully monitored for symptoms of dehydration and hypovolemic shock. Weights and vital signs should be recorded. Blood and urine specimens are collected frequently during the test, and the nurse enforces complete fluid restriction.

Occasionally a hypertonic saline infusion test is used to diagnose DI. In this test, saline is infused intravenously, and serial blood and urine specimens are collected for determination of sodium and osmolality. The patient with DI will continue to exhibit a free water diuresis during this test, with low urine sodium and osmolality. Consequently, serum sodium and osmolality will continue to rise. The patient must be closely monitored for symptoms of water overload and hypernatremia. This test, as well as the dehydration test, may need to be discontinued if the patient is unable to tolerate the volume and electrolyte shifts that occur.

Other diagnostic tests ordered may include x-rays and visual field testing. Head x-rays, computerized axial tomography, and magnetic resonance imaging disclose hypothalamus or pituitary lesions and defects. Lesions in this area can compress the optic chiasm, resulting in bitemporal visual field loss.

Nursing standards of care

Patients with partial DI may tolerate their disease without treatment, provided that they have an intact thirst mechanism and the ability to take fluids at will.

Medical intervention in complete DI is based on the augmentation or replacement of active ADH. Mild neurogenic DI is treated with medications that enhance the action of ADH. Most frequently chlorpropamide (Diabinese), an oral hypoglycemic, is given in doses ranging from 200 to 500 mg per day. It stimulates the release of ADH from the pituitary as well as enhances its effect on the kidney; hypoglycemia may result. Chlorpropamide's action is nullified by alcohol. Other medications sometimes used to treat mild DI include carbamazepine (Tegretol) and clofibrate. Carbamazepine is an anticonvulsant with some liver, bone marrow, and central nervous system toxicities. Doses of 400–600 mg per day are used for DI. Clofibrate is a hypolipidemic agent that may cause muscle aches. Doses of 2000 mg per day are used to treat DI. Both of these drugs act by enhancing the activity of ADH. In more severe DI, ADH is given intranasally, intravenously, intramuscularly, or subcutaneously. Mammalian ADH and synthetic ADH are both available for use. Vasopressin (Pitressin) and the longer-acting vasopressin tannate are forms of mammalian ADH. Vasopressin is given at 5–10 units 2 to 4 times a day to an adult. Vasopressin tannate may be given at 1.5–5 units every 2 to 3 days if DI persists. Both drugs are contraindicated in the first stage of labor and in coronary artery disease and should be used cautiously with pregnancy, epilepsy, migraine, asthma, hypersensitivity, and renal disease and with elderly persons and children. The vasopressin compounds interact with many substances. These interactions are summarized in Table 7-12.

Desmopressin (DDAVP, or 1-desamino-8-D-arginine vasopressin) is a synthetic ADH that may be administered intravenously (1–2 units) in transient DI or intranasally (5–20 units per day) in permanent DI. Desmopressin may cause headaches, nausea, nasal congestion and rhinitis (when administered intranasally), abdominal cramps, flushing of the skin, and increased blood pressure. Its use is con-

Table 7-11 Results of Water Deprivation Test

Diagnosis	Maximum Urine Osmolality (mOsm/L)	Urine to Serum Osmolality Ratio after Vasopressin	Urine to Serum Osmolality Ratio
Normal	800–1200	>1	>1
Partial DI (pituitary)	100–200	Unchanged	<1
Complete DI (neurogenic)	100–200	<1	<1
Nephrogenic DI	<150	Unchanged	<1

Table 7-12 Vasopressin (Pitressin) Interactions

Effects	Causative Substances
Increased pressor effects	Ganglionic blockers
Increased antidiuretic effects	Chlorpropamide Fluorocortisone Carbamazepine Acetaminophen Urea Cyclopropamide Clofibrate Tricyclic antidepressants
Decreased antidiuretic effects	Lithium Heparin Alcohol Demeclocycline Epinephrine Colchicine

traindicated in the patient with hypertension or hypersensitivity and during pregnancy and lactation. It should be used cautiously in the patient with coronary artery disease.

Nephrogenic DI does not respond to the administration of ADH, because it results from a defect in the ability of the renal tubular cells to respond to the hormone. Medical management consists of administering a thiazide diuretic—usually hydrochlorothiazide—in doses of 50–100 mg/day, combined with a sodium-restricted diet. This combination usually reduces urine output significantly.

Nursing management of the patient with DI includes management of the symptoms of fluid deficit and hypernatremia. Severe DI may result in hypovolemic shock. Excessive volumes of urine may cause dilation of the bladder and ureters. Assessment of problems is based on physical examination, history from the patient and family, and interpretation of laboratory and diagnostic data. Prioritization of problems is individualized, based on the patient's needs for safety, comfort, and prevention of life-threatening complications such as dehydration. The following care plan delineates the nursing management of the patient with DI. It can also be adapted to many patients with hypovolemia and hypernatremia.

Nursing Care Plan for the Management of the Patient with Diabetes Insipidus

Diagnosis	Signs and symptoms	Intervention	Rationale
Alteration in fluid volume (deficit) related to increased output (polyuria) due to decreased ADH secretion or activity	Weakness Thirst Fatigue Sudden weight loss Dilute urine, increased urine output Decreased venous filling (low CVP) Decreased skin turgor Dry mucous membranes and/or skin Hypernatremia Hemoconcentration Increased pulse rate and decreased pulse volume and pressure Hypotension Increased temperature	Carefully record intake and output; calculate fluid balance every 8 hours; weigh patient daily or twice a day and compare with admission and normal weight; monitor urine output and specific gravity	Excessive urine output leads to hypovolemia; signs and symptoms of hypovolemia should be closely monitored and corrected as soon as possible; comparison of daily weight with admission weight better reflects total body fluids; specific gravity and urine output indicate effectiveness of therapy; low specific gravity and high output not desirable
		Monitor vital signs, orthostatic vital signs, and other hemodynamic parameters, as indicated	Provide a complete picture of fluid balance
		Maintain skin integrity and prevent excessive dryness	Fluid losses enhance risk of dryness and poor skin turgor, increasing risk of altered skin integrity
		Provide frequent oral and eye care	To prevent injury due to dryness
		Assist body cooling, as appropriate (cool environment, reduced bedding and clothes, tepid sponge bath, hypothermia blanket)	Excessive dehydration will lead to hyperthermia with subsequent increased metabolic demands
		Replace fluids as ordered	To ensure restoration of fluid balance while underlying problem is being addressed

Nursing Care Plan for the Management of the Patient with Diabetes Insipidus

Diagnosis	Signs and symptoms	Intervention	Rationale
Alterations in thought processes related to decreased extracellular fluid volume and increased sodium levels in central nervous system	Confusion, disorientation Anxiety, restlessness, altered attention span Combativeness Lethargy, weakness, decreasing level of consciousness Decreased deep tendon reflexes Seizure activity Impaired cranial nerve function	Conduct neurological assessment every hour to every 8 hours (dependent on degree of deficit); reorient confused patient to place, person, and time with each interaction	Neurological assessment may reveal small changes in central nervous system function that necessitate more aggressive treatment of DI
		Protect patient from injury (padded side rails, close observation, and/or physical restraints)	Patient is at risk for injury due to confusion
		Seizure precautions	Seizures due to hyper-natremia are possible
		Maintain elevation of head and minimize procedures that increase intracranial pressure (suctioning, Valsalva maneuver, vomiting)	Increasing the ICP may increase cerebral edema, worsening altered thought processes
		Encourage family or significant other to participate in reorienting patient and to provide contact with normal events (news, information about home and family)	Familiar persons are often most successful at reorienting the confused patient
		Respect individuality and privacy of patient as much as possible	It can be easy to forget issues of privacy when patient is not convers-ing normally and participating in care
Anxiety related to perceived threat to biological integrity or possibly to altered central nervous system function	Expressed feelings of apprehension, nervousness, helplessness, fear, tension, loss of control Irritability, anger, agitation, combativeness	Promote a therapeutic relationship with patient by acknowledg-ing anxiety, communi-cating empathy, and accepting patient's individuality	Anxiety may interfere with healing and adherence to care regimen

Diagnosis	Signs and symptoms	Intervention	Rationale
	Inability to rest or sleep	Provide reassurance by staying with patient, speaking slowly and calmly, allowing patient to use appropriate coping mechanisms (verbalizing anxiety, crying, walking, diversional activity)	Measures promoting empathic awareness between nurse and patient decrease anxiety
	Crying, withdrawal, forgetfulness, inability to concentrate		
	Increased heart rate		
	Increased BP		
	Insomnia	Decrease sensory stimulation by providing quiet environment; promote normal sleep by darkening room at night and minimizing interruptions	Rest and sleep promote healing and decrease anxiety
	Tremors		
	Weakness		
	Diaphoresis		
		Provide explanations of disease process, treatments, drugs, routines, and procedures at level appropriate to patient's comprehension and level of anxiety	Understanding of what is happening increases the patient's sense of self-control thereby decreasing anxiety
Lack of knowledge of DI	Requests for information	Determine patient's level of knowledge and ability to learn	Education regarding recognition of symptoms and risk of occurrence is essential, but may need to be directed to family if patient is incompetent
	Verbalization of misconceptions		
	Inability to follow instructions correctly		
		Work with patient to identify objectives	Mutually agreed-on objectives are an essential element of informed care
		Determine methods of learning that patient finds most useful— e.g., visual or audio aids, demonstration, booklets, discussion; develop teaching plan for patient and family using varied methods and opportunities for feedback and reinforcement	Appropriate methods of teaching enhance retention of important concepts; feedback allows evaluation of whether patient is learning and applying information
		Ascertain patient's and family's understanding of chronicity of disorder	Level of understanding may influence teaching priorities

Medications Commonly Used in the Care of the Patient with Diabetes Insipidus

Medication	Effect	Major side effects
Carbamazepine (Tegretol)	Enhances activity of ADH	Hepatotoxicity Bone marrow suppression Drowsiness
Chlorpropamide (Diabenese)	Stimulates release of ADH from pituitary and enhances ADH's activity on the kidneys	Hypoglycemia
Clofibrate	Enhances activity of ADH	Muscle aches
Vasopressin (regular or tannate)	Synthetic or semisynthetic substitute for ADH	SIADH Coronary ischemia Headache Allergic reaction Hypertension
Desmopressin (DDAVP)	Synthetic form of ADH	Headache Nausea Nasal congestion, rhinitis Abdominal cramps Flushed skin Hypertension Angina, cardiac ischemia

Hyperthyroidism and Thyrotoxic Crisis

Hyperthyroidism (thyrotoxicosis) occurs when an excessive quantity of thyroid hormone is secreted from the thyroid gland or when thyroid hormone remains unbound to thyroid-binding globulin (TBG). The clinical effects of this excess hormone may be readily obvious or subtle. An exaggerated form of this disorder, precipitating life-threatening hypermetabolism, is called thyroid storm or thyrotoxic crisis.

even cause hyperthyroidism. Intrinsic thyroid disease is the most common cause of acute hyperthyroidism. Often hyperthyroidism is not clinically apparent prior to illness, when it is exacerbated by increased demands on the diseased thyroid. Any enlargement of the thyroid gland is termed a goiter. If uniformly enlarged, it is called a diffuse goiter; it may be called a nodular goiter if multiple nodules are present on the thyroid. Thyroid cancer usually presents as a single nodule on the organ. It is important to note that not all etiologies of hyperthyroidism are pathologic; any induced state of hypermetabolism will stimulate the release of thyroid hormones to maintain this state.

Clinical antecedents

Hyperthyroidism may have an intrinsic (within the thyroid) or extrinsic (outside the thyroid) etiology. A list of possible disorders causing hyperthyroidism, according to their stimulating factor, is given in Table 7-13. Understanding the roles of TRH and TSH in the regulation of thyroid hormone makes it easy to see that disorders of the hypothalamus or the anterior pituitary may have an effect on the level of thyroid hormone. Furthermore, it is known that there is a promotional link between catecholamines and thyroid hormones, which may exacerbate or

Critical referents

Pathophysiological changes in hyperthyroidism are dependent upon the specific etiology of the disorder. Pituitary disorders, hypothalamic injury, or other intracranial disorders may have a direct effect on one of the thyroid-stimulating hormones (TRH or TSH), with subsequent increased function. Goiters (thyroid enlargement) are a direct response to reduced hormone stimulation or available substrate (iodine). After gland hypertrophy, thyroid hormone output is increased but does not exceed the

Table 7-13 Clinical Antecedents of Hyperthyroidism and Hypothyroidism

Stimulating Factor	Etiology	
	Hyperthyroid	Hypothyroid
Hypothalamus (TRH)	Injury or stimulus	Injury or stimulus
Anterior pituitary (TSH)	Pituitary adenoma	Pituitary tumor Postpartum pituitary necrosis
Abnormal production of TSH-like substances	Grave's disease	—
Intrinsic thyroid disease	Toxic multinodular goiter Thyroid adenoma Thyroid cancer	Toxic multinodular goiter Thyroid adenoma Thyroid cancer Hashimoto's disease Cretinism Thyroidectomy Radiation exposure
Extrinsic thyroid effects	Surgical injury Sepsis, infection Toxemia of pregnancy Iodine overdose Catecholamines Adolescence	Stressed thyroid

body's metabolic requirements unless other factors interfere. A gland with goiter is termed a nontoxic goiter unless it is stimulating excessive quantities of hormones; then it is referred to as toxic. A toxic goiter is not as likely as a nontoxic one to cause a disproportionately large thyroid, although some enlargement is present in most cases. The development of toxic goiter is the consequence of antithyroid autoantibody production by the patient's lymphocytes.[21] The autoantibody mimics TSH's effects on the thyroid gland but is not regulated by the normal mechanisms. It is a misnomer to use hyperthyroidism to label hypermetabolic states producing increased thyroid hormone. The elevated hormone level is actually a normal physiologic response to increase demand, even though the side effects of excess thyroid hormone present as pathological symptoms and may be detrimental to health.

The critically ill patient may have several causes contributing to a thyroid crisis. For instance, an elderly borderline hyperthyroid patient may present with cardiac abnormalities and, consequently, receive iodine-based dye and/or the antidysrhythmic amiodarone. These precipitators may enhance thyroid output, but, because of the thyroid hormone's long half-life, clinical hyperthyroidism may not occur until 3 weeks later. The symptoms may be mistaken for refractory heart failure, and thus management of the patient becomes confusing.

Resulting signs and symptoms

The clinical presentation of a patient in thyroid crisis is a reflection of the degree of thyroid hormone stimulation. The primary profile is one of hypermetabolism with particular effects on nutrient utilization, cardiovascular response, and neuromuscular activity. Given the primary functions of thyroid hormones, it is not surprising to find such symptoms. A comparison of the major clinical effects of hyperthyroidism and hypothyroidism is provided in Table 7-14.

Clinical laboratory test findings may include leukocytosis, polycythemia, thrombocytosis, hypernatremia, hyperkalemia, and elevated transaminases. The calcium may be normal or mildly elevated, but an elevated level is not related to the thyroid hormone calcitonin. (In fact, calcitonin levels are unaffected in hyperthyroidism.) True calcium regulation is controlled by the parathyroid glands, which are

Table 7-14   Signs and Symptoms of Hyperthyroidism and Hypothyroidism

	Hyperthyroid	Hypothyroid
Cardiovascular effects	Tachycardia, atrial fibrillation Hypertension Increased cardiac output Cardiomyopathy	Bradycardia, lengthened Q-T interval Hypotension Pericardial effusion Cardiac failure
Neurological effects	Impaired concentration Agitation Emotional lability Insomnia Hyperreflexia Muscle weakness Tremors	Apathy, depression Obtundation Hyporeflexia Muscle weakness Seizures
Gastrointestinal effects	Diarrhea Hyperactive bowel sounds Increased appetite	Constipation Adynamic ileus Anorexia
General	Dermopathy (thick skin) Warm, diaphoretic skin Thin, fine hair Exophthalmus Hypocapnia Hyperthermia Weight loss	Cool, dry skin Coarse dry hair Edema Hypercapnia Hypothermia Weight gain
Laboratory	Hyperglycemia Polycythemia	Hypoglycemia Anemia

not necessarily dysfunctional in hyperthyroidism. A notable finding is the high percentage of these patients (10–14% prior to the sixth decade and 40% by the eighth decade) who present with atrial fibrillation.[22] This and other dysrhythmias tend to be refractory to the usual antidysrhythmics and inotropic agents, requiring as much as twice the usual dose for therapeutic effects.[23]

Other clinical symptoms that may be present are heat intolerance, dyspnea or respiratory difficulty, and difficulty swallowing (related to thyroid enlargement). Physical exam changes that may be detectable include eyelid retraction or ptosis, skin hyperpigmentation, thyroid enlargement or bruit, impaired renal concentrating ability, hoarseness, gynecomastia, and amenorrhea.[24] It is important to realize when assessing the hyperthyroid patient that initial signs and symptoms of hypermetabolism lead to organ exhaustion and symptoms similar to those of hypothyroidism—for example, heart failure, respiratory failure, and hypoglycemia. Although clinical presentation is often classic, several diagnostic tests must be performed in order to confirm hyperthyroidism.

A small subset of patients present with what is termed "silent hyperthyroidism." In these patients, the classically noticeable symptoms are not present, but they have atrial fibrillation, heart failure, or even chest pain without cardiac signs.[25] These symptoms are most common in the elderly and in men.

Hyperthyroidism, thyrotoxicosis, and end-stage severe hyperthyroidism may be difficult to differentiate. Thyrotoxic crisis may be the terminal event in a chronic severe hyperthyroid patient or may be a result of an undiagnosed or physically stressed hyperthyroid patient. The classic features of thyrotoxic crisis are those of acute heart failure and severe neuromuscular irritability. The patient may present in a manic state, acutely paranoid, having seizures, in pulmonary edema, demonstrating hypertensive crisis, or in multiorgan failure. The patient may have at least one life-threatening symptom.

The most common diagnostic tests are laboratory evaluations of the level of thyroid-stimulating hormone (TSH) and serum levels of T_3 and T_4. An elevated result for the T_3 resin uptake test indicates increased hormone binding. An elevation of serum T_4 is diagnostic in 90% of all suspected cases of hyperthyroidism.[26] The common diagnostic tests used in diagnosis of thyroid disorders are listed in Table 7-15. Protein-calorie malnutrition, as seen in many critically ill patients, can alter the TSH response to TRH, indicating a hyperthyroidism that does not exist. A TSH stimulation test is likely to be performed to ascertain whether the hyperthyroidism is intrinsic (normal TSH stimulation) or hypothalamic-pituitary in origin (elevated TSH stimulation). Thyroid-binding globulin (TBG) tests are sometimes performed as well, but caution should be taken with their interpretation. This binding protein is decreased with increased serum thyroid hormones but may also be decreased by common medications such as opiates, estrogens, clofibrate, and 5-fluorouracil. A radioactive iodine (I^{131}) uptake scan is utilized when nodules are present to determine their nature. So-called cold nodules (those that do not pick up dye) are indicative of carcinoma; hot nodules (those that pick up dye) are nearly always benign.

Table 7-15 Diagnostic Tests for Thyroid Disorders*

Test	Results Indicating Hyperthyroidism	Results Indicating Hypothyroidism
Serum T_4	Increased	Decreased
Serum T_3	Increased	Decreased
T_3 resin uptake	Increased	Decreased
Serum TSH	Decreased (primary and secondary)	Increased (primary)
T_3	Increased	—
TSH stimulation	Decreased (primary) Decreased with treated Graves or multinodular goiter	Decreased (secondary)
TBG	Decreased	Increased
Cholesterol	Decreased (primary) Normal (secondary)	Increased (primary) Normal (secondary)

*Primary disorders are those originating in the thyroid gland; secondary disorders are those originating in the pituitary gland or the hypothalamus.

Nursing standards of care

The first priority in managing the hyperthyroid patient is to address the hypermetabolic rate. Because there are few therapeutic options to address this condition outside of treatment of the primary thyroid disorder, immediate management of the high levels of thyroid hormones is necessary. Other measures supporting this goal may involve supportive care or blocking of the conversion of T_4 to T_3. Thyroid hormones may be blocked medically with antithyroid medications or by destruction of thyroid tissue with radioactive iodine or surgery. Antithyroid medications are usually attempted prior to the more aggressive interventions.

Because of their swift effects, medications blocking the conversion of T_4 to T_3 may be given immediately. Among these are propylthiouracil (PTU), glucocorticoids, propranolol, or Ipodate. During treatment with these medications, aspirin products should be avoided, as they increase this conversion of T_4 to active thyroid hormone. When PTU and glucocorticoids are used concomitantly, hyperthyroid symptoms usually begin to abate within 24 hours.

Treatment of acute hyperthyroidism almost always includes a thionamide agent such as PTU or methimazole (Tapazole). The remission rate on this therapy ranges from 10% to 50%, but 30 days to several months are required for the full physiological effects to be appreciated. Patients given these medications should remain on them for 6–18 months and should have them withdrawn slowly to prevent thyrotoxicosis. In conjunction with thionamides, inorganic iodide is given to prevent thyroid hormone release. This is usually given approximately 1 hour after the thionamides to prevent the accumulation of the iodide. The iodide does not produce antithyroid effects for 7–14 days. Lithium carbonate, which also inhibits thyroid hormone production and release, may be used instead of inorganic iodide.

Most clinicians currently recommend the use of radioactive iodine as a second-line measure. Because of its long-term effects on growth and fertility, it is seldom used in children, adolescents, and pregnant women. Its advantages are its efficacy (80% response), ease of use, noninvasiveness, and limited side effects. When radioactive iodine is used as a single therapeutic measure, there is some risk of a rebound thyroid storm 10–14 days after treatment.[27] The radioactive iodine immediately suppresses T_3 and T_4 activity, but large quantities of the hormones may be released after the iodine's effects have abated. To prevent this complication, the patient is often treated concomitantly with PTU. The greatest risk of radioactive iodine therapy is that of posttreatment hypothyroidism. The incidence of this side effect is 10% the first year, with an increase of 5% yearly thereafter, and experts predict that all recipients will eventually develop hypothyroidism if they live long enough after therapy.[28] Dosage is based on the size of the gland and its radioactive iodine uptake over a 24-hour period. On occasion, inaccurate assessment of need occurs, and a second dose must be given.

Before radioactive iodine therapy was determined to be safe, surgical removal of the thyroid gland was considered the conventional therapy. This procedure is now reserved for the patient refractory to other measures. A subtotal thyroidectomy is performed, preserving a portion of the thyroid to maintain normal function. Preoperative medical therapy is aimed at inducing a temporary euthyroid state and decreasing vascularity. This therapy includes treatment with a thionamide, iodide preparations, and beta blockers. The iodides are started 7–10 days before the surgery and are given to decrease the vascularity of the organ, making surgery safer. Beta blockers, started 5–7 days prior to surgery, slow the heart rate to reduce cardiovascular risks. Propranolol has been the preferred beta blocker because it also serves to block the conversion of T_4 to T_3.[29] A new approach is to use the ultra-short-acting beta blocker Esmolol to control the heart rate and blood pressure. In addition, reserpine or guanethidine may be used adjunctively to block the catecholamine effects. The potential postoperative complications of a subtotal thyroidectomy are hemorrhage, airway obstruction, infection, hypothyroidism, hypoparathyroidism, and laryngeal nerve injury.

The nursing care of the patient in thyrotoxicosis involves monitoring for heart failure and life-threatening neurological symptoms while providing a supportive and comfortable environment. The variety of possible metabolic derangements requires constant surveillance and laboratory monitoring. The nurse's goals include the following: (1) to provide a safe, comfortable environment conducive to rest and reduction of agitation, (2) to recognize early signs and symptoms of organ exhaustion, malnutrition, and dehydration, and (3) to educate the patient regarding the chronicity of the disease and the planned therapeutic regimen. A complete overview of the nurse's responsibilities in the care of this patient is provided by the care plan that follows.

Nursing Care Plan for the Management of the Patient with Hyperthyroidism

Diagnosis	Signs and symptoms	Intervention	Rationale
Fluid volume deficit: intake less than requirements	Thirst Tachycardia Full, bounding pulses Dry skin, poor turgor CVP < 1 mm Hg	Evaluate fluid volume status by recording vital signs, cardiac pressures, subjective symptoms, I&O	Important to ascertain fluid balance in attempt to maintain tissue perfusion
		Replenish fluid volume, usually with crystalloids, as needed and ordered	Fluid replenishment is usually needed to maintain cardiac output and tissue perfusion
		Provide mouth and skin care	To prevent dry and cracking areas or skin breakdown
		Assess patient for signs and symptoms of high output heart failure (crackles, murmurs or gallops, chest pain, ischemic ECG changes)	Heart failure is usually long-term complication, along with volume deficit and hypermetabolism
		Provide comfort measures for headache, thirst, and dry skin	To minimize patient's discomfort
		Monitor electrolytes for hemoconcentration and subsequent abnormalities related to deviation (hypernatremia, hyperkalemia, hyperosmolarity, hypercalcemia)	All intravascular solutes may be elevated in acute dehydrated period, with clinical manifestations present
		Observe thrombosis precautions	Patient is at high risk for thrombosis or thrombocytosis due to increased blood viscosity
Ineffective breathing pattern or hyperventilation	Hyperventilation (RR > 24/min), shallow breaths Dyspnea Decreased oxygen saturation Numbness and tingling of fingertips	Assess respiratory rate and depth and subjective sensations of dyspnea every 4–8 hours; increase frequency if altered sensorium or low oxygen saturation present	To collect information regarding respiratory compensation for disease process

Nursing Care Plan for the Management of the Patient with Hyperthyroidism

Diagnosis	Signs and symptoms	Intervention	Rationale
		Assess patient for symptoms of hypocarbia (numbness and tingling fingertips); if present, consider using narcotic to slow respiratory rate	Excessive carbon dioxide exhalation occurs
		Provide supplemental oxygen as needed	May be symptomatically helpful
		Monitor for hoarseness, stridor, dysphagia, or pooling respiratory secretions	Postoperative partial thyroidectomy patient is at risk for respiratory compromise due to edema or rupture of suture line
		Keep head of bed elevated postoperatively after partial thyroidectomy	To protect against aspiration
Hyperthermia	Body temperature > 38.5°C Sensations of warmth Flushing Diaphoresis	Administer acetaminophen PRN for elevated temperature	Exogenous means to decrease temperature are often necessary; ASA enhances conversion of T_3, worsening hyperthyroidism
		Cool or tepid baths and showers	Cool or tepid water decreases body temp without inducing shivering
		Use fans and open areas	To decrease sensation of warmth
		Evaluate for concomitant infections	Critically ill hyperthyroid patients may also be hyperthermic with infection

Diagnosis	Signs and symptoms	Intervention	Rationale
Altered nutrition: intake less than body requirements	Weight loss Anorexia Food intake less than normal Altered nutritional assessment parameters (albumin, nitrogen balance, creatinine height index, etc.)	Maintain calorie count Record daily weight Provide small, frequent, high-calorie feedings Arrange for consultation with nutritionist to evaluate need for supplemental nutrition either enterally or parenterally if oral intake is inadequate	To assess intake and pinpoint deficits early Weight is a good indicator of fluid balance, metabolic demands, and insensible loss To help patient ingest sufficient quantities of food Preventative and rehabilitative measure in high-risk patient
Diarrhea	More than 6 loose stools per day Defecation urgency	Give antimotility agents, as ordered (Kaopectate or tincture of opium preferred over anticholinergics, which may increase heart rate Measure I&O Protective cream for perirectal irritation Assess electrolytes daily for losses due to diarrhea; replenish as ordered	To control diarrhea To ensure that dehydration does not occur To aid in prevention of breakdown To allow for early intervention
Sleep pattern disturbances	Insomnia or only short periods of sleep Fatigue, exhaustion Irritability	Provide dark room and uninterrupted periods for rest; administer sedatives as ordered Limit interruptions to allow patient to rest Document sleep patterns	To enhance sleep Short activity periods should be followed by uninterrupted rest periods To provide continuing assessment of problem

Nursing Care Plan for the Management of the Patient with Hyperthyroidism

Diagnosis	Signs and symptoms	Intervention	Rationale
		Assess for neurological changes due to lack of sleep	Common complication of sleep disturbances
		Enlist assistance of family members to plan methods of inducing sleep	Family members know patient's likes and dislikes
Impaired social interaction	Nervousness Inability to concentrate Inability to complete sentences Irritability	Speak in calm tone of voice	To help induce calmness
		Repeat instructions; provide written ones as necessary	To reinforce information
		Involve family in care	Assists patient in following instructions; helps family feel needed
		Assess patient's anxiety level	Anxiety may be secondary or outcome of disorder
		Administer anxiolytics or sedatives, as ordered; evaluate response	Medications may reduce symptoms
Alteration in comfort: fevers, nausea, diarrhea, headache	Verbalization of discomfort Nonverbal cues indicating discomfort	Provide empathy and support for patient and family	To reduce anxiety
		Explain the length of time required for total resolution (4–8 weeks) with medications	Thyroid treatment is a very slow process
		Prepare for possible thyroidectomy	Subtotal thyroidectomy may need to be done to relieve symptoms
		Provide quiet, undemanding environment	To help patient control anxiety, nervousness, and emotional lability

Hypothyroidism and Myxedema Coma

Hypothyroidism is a deficiency in the production of the thyroid hormones T_3 and T_4 either because of primary dysfunction of the thyroid gland or because of inadequate stimulating hormone from the pituitary and hypothalamus. Hypothyroidism is characterized by a slowing of all metabolic processes. When hypothyroidism is present in neonates, it is termed cretinism. In adults, hypothyroidism in its most severe form is called myxedema coma. Currently myxedema coma leading to neurological suppression and death is relatively rare, but it still carries a mortality rate as high as 50%.[30]

Clinical antecedents

Hypothyroidism at birth, or cretinism, may be due to failure of the thyroid gland to develop or to genetic deficiencies of the enzymes necessary for hormone synthesis. Manifestations of cretinism may not be readily apparent at birth but become apparent within the first 2 months of life. This condition is generally considered completely reversible in most cases if diagnosed and treated early.

Hypothyroidism in adults has many of the same etiologic factors as hyperthyroidism but the opposite hormonal problem and clinical features. Hypothyroidism is present in as much as 5% of the population, with clinical presentation peaking between 40 and 60 years of age.[31] Hypothyroid crisis is most often precipitated by a physical or emotional stressor such as severe illness, injury, infection, exposure to cold, or the administration of sedative agents. Sedative agents—such as narcotics, phenothiazines, benzodiazepines, and barbiturates—further depress the central nervous system in a patient with existing CNS suppression caused by lack of thyroid hormones. The most common causes of hypothyroidism are autoimmune responses (Hashimoto's thyroiditis), thyroidectomy, radioactive iodine therapy or radiation to the thyroid area, antithyroid medications such as those used to treat hyperthyroidism, thyroid tumors, and pituitary disease (postpartum necrosis, pituitary tumor).

The critically ill patient may undergo many of the above-mentioned stressors within the context of the present illness and is susceptible to a syndrome of hypothyroidism with a normal thyroid gland. Although this usually resolves without treatment, some clinicians advocate replacement therapy.

Critical referents

The specific pathophysiology of hypothyroidism is the predictable direct reflection of the lack of thyroid hormone. When thyroid hormone is not present to participate in basic metabolic functions, homeostatic activities are considerably slowed. Inadequate thyroid hormone will result in decreased protein, carbohydrate, and lipid metabolism, which often manifests as interstitial accumulations of mucotaneous protein-polysaccharides—thus the name myxedema. Cholesterol level increases as the absence of thyroid hormone prevents its clearance. A common physiological effect is the accumulation of body fluids as the normal mechanisms to eliminate them are altered. This may present as anasarca, cerebral edema, pleural effusions, pericardial effusions, or ascites. The hypothyroid patient has a depressed respiratory center, which leads to a defective hypercapnia respiratory drive. Insufficient substrate available for cardiac function and slowed metabolism present as heart failure.

Resulting signs and symptoms

The common hypothyroid symptoms of fatigue, anorexia, cold intolerance, weight gain, and dry skin become more pronounced as the patient proceeds toward myxedema. In Table 7-14 common symptoms of hypothyroidism are compared to those of hyperthyroidism. In the more severe clinical situation, the patient will be lethargic or obtunded and will present with bradycardia or severe hypoventilation. It is important to note that this is one of the rare circumstances when bradycardia may be accompanied by hypertension because of the high peripheral vascular resistance.[32] Hypoventilation may be characterized by hypoxemia and hypercarbia, but more often the patient has sleep apnea, thought to be centrally regulated.[33] In the extreme case the patient develops the classic facial appearance of periorbital edema, dull expression, and sparse hair. The cardiac failure of hypothyroidism is commonly unresponsive to catecholamines, and since the patient's vascular fluid volume may be in excess, emergency management of complications can be difficult. ECG changes that have been noted are low voltage of the R wave and a prolonged Q-T interval. Serum cardiac enzymes may be altered, since hypothyroidism can cause increased CPK levels without myocardial injury.

Electrolyte abnormalities such as hyponatremia, hypoglycemia, hyperkalemia, and respiratory and metabolic acidosis are common. These abnormal values may represent primary hypothyroidism or acute adrenal insufficiency, which is often present in conjunction with hypothyroidism. Acute adrenal insufficiency may be caused by pituitary hypertrophy or autoimmune adrenal insufficiency.[34] Consequently, the patient with possible myxedema coma should also be treated with corticosteroids for adrenal insufficiency. The diagnosis of hypothyroidism is made by analyzing clinical symptoms and thyroid hormone levels, as with hyperthyroidism (refer back to Table 7-15). The serum T_3 and T_4 levels are reduced, the TSH levels are increased, and the T_3 resin-uptake levels are low in primary hypothyroidism. As in hyperthyroidism, disorders that are hypothalamic-pituitary in origin are best determined by the TSH level and TSH stimulation test. Adrenal insufficiency is often present with symptomatic hypothyroidism, so the patient must be assessed for that as well. While evaluating the patient for thyroid illness, it is important for the ICU clinician to keep in mind that the critically ill may have abnormal thyroid function test results because of the body's response to physiological stress. In such a patient, reductions of T_3 and T_4, as well as mildly reduced or elevated TSH levels, are common. Unless the clinical symptoms are life-threatening, endocrinologists recommend that several thyroid function studies be performed on the patient prior to treatment.

Nursing standards of care

The treatment of hypothyroidism is first and foremost thyroid hormone replacement. Both synthetic agents and natural extracts are available. Commonly used synthetic hormones can be given as T_3 alone (liothyronine, or Cytomel), T_4 alone (levothyroxine, or Levothyroid or Synthroid), or T_3-T_4 combinations (liotrix, or Euthroid or Thyrolar). Thyroid extract, USP, is a naturally occurring thyroid hormone extracted from animals. The most common therapy is the use of levothyroxine, as it provides available hormone without the side effects of administering active hormone.[35] Ascertaining the appropriate dose is at times difficult, because there is no safe measure of the degree of deficit and replacing the hormone too rapidly may lead to heart failure or increased ischemic changes. Based on the hormone's half-life of 7 days and peak effects at 3 weeks, daily doses are given, with dosage adjustments every 3–4 weeks. Clinical improvement is not always a true reflection of the degree of disease resolution and

should be viewed only as a helpful adjunct to thyroid hormone levels. Rapid correction of myxedema can be achieved through the administration of T_3, the active form of thyroid hormone. The patient with longstanding hypothyroidism develops hypertrophy of the pituitary gland and altered output of TSH and ACTH (adrenocorticotrophic hormone). When thyroid hormones are replaced rapidly, the thyroid stimulation is resolved, but a subsequent ACTH deficiency and symptoms of adrenal insufficiency may ensue. Adrenal insufficiency often accompanies hypothyroidism, requiring low-dose hydrocortisone treatment concomitant with thyroid replacement hormone. It is important to administer low levels of glucocorticoid so as not to suppress the thyroid further. Even with effective therapy, however, the patient may not return to baseline physiologic status and may be plagued with complications of a decreased metabolic rate, such as chronic heart failure, angina, or psychiatric disorders.[36]

Supportive management of the hypothyroidism patient's physiological responses is necessary in order to prevent potentially dangerous cardiopulmonary and neurologic consequences. Hypotension in this patient is best managed by conservative fluid administration, despite volume problems, because cardiac dysrhythmias are prevalent when vasopressor substances are used. The hypothermic hypothyroid patient must be returned to a baseline temperature slowly, as rapid rewarming may cause profound hypotension. When the patient presents with respiratory acidosis and hypoventilation, endotracheal intubation and mechanical ventilation are necessary to support gas exchange while the disorder is being corrected. Hypoglycemia can be significant and can enhance the neurologic symptoms related to lower basal metabolism. Treatment with glucose solutions is common, although the patient must be closely monitored for overreplacement. Since infection is a common precipitator of myxedema, assessment and treatment of any existing infectious processes are essential to eventual recovery.

In a few small clinical studies of critically ill hypothyroid patients, thyroid hormone replacement was attempted to reverse the symptoms of hypotension, hypothermia, and bradycardia. There was not a statistically significant patient response to the hormone administration, although it may be argued that the cardiac or neurological patient may benefit from such treatment more than the average patient.[37]

The nursing care of hypothyroid and myxedematous patients requires close observation of central brain function and the patient's ability to protect the airway and maintain normal blood pressure, respiration, and body temperature. Nurses are called upon to monitor for life-threatening organ failure as thyroid replacement therapies are rapidly administered. Primary nursing goals include the following: (1) to prevent life-threatening organ failure from a decreased metabolic rate (seizures, heart failure, respiratory failure, and hypoglycemia), (2) to provide supportive care to alleviate the discomforting symptoms of hypothyroidism, and (3) to assist in planning the regulation of hormone replacement. A complete nursing care plan follows.

Nursing Care Plan for the Management of the Patient with Hypothyroidism

Diagnosis	Signs and symptoms	Intervention	Rationale
Decreased cardiac tissue perfusion	Hypotension Bradycardia Ischemic ECG changes Chest pain Dysrhythmias Pericardial effusions Decreased CO or CI	Monitor patient closely if severe myxedema is present or there is evidence of cardiac dysrhythmias, pericardial effusion, or heart failure	Symptoms of possible but not usual life-threatening cardiac complications
		Do heart sound assessment every 4–8 hours	To note signs of above complications
		Document and report pulsus paradox, diminished peripheral pulses, right heart failure symptoms, pericardial friction rub, or pulse deficit	Signs of pericardial effusion leading to tamponade
		Perform 12-lead ECGs periodically, particularly if condition is complicated by electrolyte disturbances or dysrhythmias	To discover any new ischemic changes or silent MI
		Check echocardiogram, muga, or thallium scan results, as available	Will reflect progressive signs of heart failure
		Monitor electrolytes at least daily	Imbalance can exacerbate cardiac problems
		Implement hypotension precautions	Patient may fall when hypotensive
		Administer vasopressors cautiously	Patients are more prone to dysrhythmias
		Provide rest	Decreases workload on heart
Ineffective gas exchange and breathing pattern related to hypoventilation	Respiratory rate less than 12/min Shallow respirations Sleep apnea (common) Hypercarbia Lethargy	Respiratory assessment every 2–4 hours, particularly when asleep; report rate < 12/min, oxygen desaturation, decreased breath sounds, dull percussion sounds	Symptoms of respiratory failure or developing pleural effusions

Diagnosis	Signs and symptoms	Intervention	Rationale
	Decreased oxygen saturation	Monitor oxygenation if patient is unstable or sat < 95%	Patients are at risk for hypoventilation and hypoxemia
	Hypoxemia	Note presence of dyspnea	Dyspnea is symptom of hypoxemia
	Pleural effusions	Administer supplemental oxygen, as ordered, and for symptomatic relief of dyspnea	Relieve distress, improve oxygenation
		Position patient in semi- or high Fowler's position	To best allow for breathing
		Do incentive spirometry every 4–8 hours	To prevent atelectasis and possible pneumonia
		Monitor patient for increasing lethargy	Symptom of hypercarbia
		Obtain ABGs as ordered to assess ventilation and oxygenation	These patients may experience respiratory compromise
		Avoid medications that are respiratory depressants (e.g., narcotics, benzodiazepines)	May worsen gas exchange problem
Altered thought processes	Confusion, disorientation	Perform neurological assessment every shift, unless changes indicate it should be done more often	To evaluate for ongoing changes or significant symptoms of cerebral edema
	Lethargy		
	Obtundation		
	Coma	Implement seizure precautions	Patient may be prone to seizures because of sodium, hypoxemia
	Inappropriate comments or behaviors		
	Seizures	Evaluate patient's cognitive function, decision-making ability, and memory every shift	These may be early neurologic changes preceding disorientation
		Implement fall precautions	Disoriented patient is prone to falls
		Position to protect airway, if indicated; insert artificial airway PRN; nasotracheally suction PRN	Lethargy may be significant, leaving patient unable to protect airway

Nursing Care Plan for the Management of the Patient with Hypothyroidism

Diagnosis	Signs and symptoms	Intervention	Rationale
		Frequently monitor oxygenation	Neurological changes may be due to many etiologies (such as hypoxemia)
		Monitor electrolytes	To ensure changes are not significant enough to be causing symptoms (hyponatremia, hypocalcemia, hypokalemia, hypomagnesemia)
Alteration in fluid balance: excess	Edema	Record I&O	To assess fluid balance and need for diuresis
	Increased CVP, PA pressures	Weigh patient daily	To evaluate total fluid
	Crackles in lungs	Administer diuretics as ordered	To reduce vascular volume
	Decreased osmolality	Replenish electrolytes with high-concentration electrolyte solutions (Ringer's, RL) after diuresis	To restore depleted electrolytes
	Hyponatremia		
	Cerebral edema		
		Measure CVP and PA pressures at least once per shift and with interventions	To assess vascular volume
		Monitor patient for fluid excess in the lungs—noncardiogenic pulmonary edema	Patient will be prone to oncotic shifts
		Assess patient for signs and symptoms of increased intracranial pressure (weakness, change in mental status, widened pulse pressure, bradydysrhythmias)	Will be present with cerebral edema

Diagnosis	Signs and symptoms	Intervention	Rationale
		Assess for edema	Edematous skin is prone to breakdown
		Provide special skin care or low air-loss bed	To decrease risk of skin breakdown
Hypothermia	Body temperature less than 35°C	Assess body temperature every 4 hours	Hypothermia affects homeostasis, coagulation, and immune responses
	Cool skin	Use blankets, increased room temperature, or warming blanket	To warm patient
		Warm blood, if given	Unwarmed blood enhances hypothermia
Alteration in elimination, constipation	Absent stool for more than 48 hours	Fluid reinforcement, as tolerated without fluid overload problem	To increase water content of stool
	Hard stool	Give stool softener daily	To reduce difficulty of defecating
	Difficulty defecating	Give mild bulking laxative (Metamucil) daily	To increase propulsion through GI tract
		Attempt to get patient to use bedside commode	Enhances ability to defecate for most patients
		Encourage mobility	Enhances peristalsis
		Identify other medications/treatments that may worsen constipation (e.g., narcotics, anticholinergics, beta blockers)	Many health care interventions worsen constipation
Altered health maintenance	Lethargy	Provide physical care during acute disease stages	Patient may be unable to perform care
	Neglect of self-care	Plan self-care in short sessions	To conserve energy
	Poor hygiene	Provide for rest periods	To conserve energy
	Fatigue	Discuss clinical disorder and slow progression back to normal with patient and family	To help patient and family to adapt

Medications Commonly Used in the Care of the Patient with Thyroid Disorders

Medication	Effect	Major side effects
Propylthiouricil (PTU) (Tapazole)	Thionamide agent, used to block conversion of T_4 to active hormone	Iodine accumulation
Supersaturated iodide solution (SSKI)	Suppresses thyroid function and release of hormones	Iodine accumulation
Glucocorticoids	Block release of thyroid hormones	Weight gain Fluid retention Hyperglycemia
Radioactive iodine I^{131}	Immediate suppression of thyroid hormone	Secondary cancer Fertility problems Hypothyroidism
Propranolol Esmolol	Beta blockers; counteract cardiac effects of hyperthyroidism, slow heart rate, decrease blood pressure	Fatigue CHF
Reserpine	Controls catecholamine effects of hormones	Parasympathetic stimulation: bradycardia, GI upset, hyperacidity
Liothyronine (Cytomel)	Replenishes active thyroid hormone	Hyperthyroidism
Levothyroxine (Levothyroid, Synthroid)	Provides thyroid hormone in inactive form to be converted to T_3 as needed	Hyperthyroidism Inadequate hormone
Liotrix (Euthroid, Thyrolar)	Mixed T_3 and T_4, to provide active hormone with reserve to convert as needed for metabolism	Hyperthyroidism Hypothyroidism
Thyroid extract, USP	Naturally occurring thyroid hormone from animals	Allergic reactions

Pheochromocytoma

Pheochromocytoma is a rare catecholamine-secreting tumor of chromaffin tissue. Chromaffin tissue cells are derived from neuroectodermal tissue and are widespread in utero, but most degenerate and disappear after birth. What cells remain are found mainly in the adrenal medulla, with about 5% found elsewhere in the abdomen and pelvis.[38] Despite the rarity, the diagnosis of pheochromocytoma is important because delay in treatment can result in serious morbidity or death. The diagnosis is especially crucial for pregnant women during delivery or for the patient about to undergo surgery for other diseases.[39]

Clinical antecedents

A family history of pheochromocytoma has been identified as a risk factor. Tumor formation has also been linked with other neuroectodermal disease processes.[40]

Critical referents

The catecholamines epinephrine and norepinephrine are normally secreted from the adrenal medulla as a result of sympathetic stimulation. In the case of pheochromocytoma, however, the catecholamines are secreted autonomously as well.[41]

Resulting signs and symptoms

The signs and symptoms of pheochromocytoma are related to the nature of catecholamine secretion. Either of the catecholamines may dominate, but generally the effects of both epinephrine and norepinephrine are visible.[42] Hypertension and symptoms resulting from hypertension, such as headaches, are the most common patient complaints.[43]

Most patients with pheochromocytoma have symptoms that vary in intensity and may be episodic or paroxysmal. Paroxysmal attacks can be precipitated by a number of activities that tend to compress the tumor. These include position changes, exercise, and coughing.[44] Symptoms during an attack classically involve sweating, headache, and palpitations and reflect both vasodilation and vasoconstriction.

Also experienced may be tremors, fatigue, anorexia, nausea, weight loss, hyperglycemia, and visual disturbances. The gastrointestinal disturbances occur in response to sympathetic stimulation and are reflective of a hypermetabolic state. Possible complications of the hypertension include myocardial infarction, cerebral vascular accidents, dissecting aneurysms, or congestive heart failure. Cardiomyopathy may also occur as a result of the effect of catecholamines on the heart.[45]

The symptoms are believed to be caused by bursts of epinephrine from the tumor. The effect of a decreased peripheral vascular resistance along with hypovolemia causes hypotension and subsequent sympathetic stimulation. This stimulation causes the release of norepinephrine from vascular adrenergic nerve endings, which in turn causes vasoconstriction and hypertension. It is believed that the initial burst of epinephrine temporarily depletes the tumor's epinephrine and allows norepinephrine-induced vasoconstriction to dominate, despite sympathetic stimulation of the adrenal medulla and the tumor.[46]

Pheochromocytoma may be difficult to diagnose, and many symptoms may be attributed to anxiety or nervousness. Diagnosis requires an awareness of the peculiar clinical presentation and atypical symptoms. Diagnostic testing begins with 24-hour urine collections to assay for vanillylmandelic acid (VMA), metanephrine, and normetanephrine, which are end-metabolites of the catecholamines. Measurements of plasma epinephrine and norepinephrine are also possible.[47]

After it has been confirmed by biological assay, the tumor needs to be localized by way of a computerized tomography scan, nephrotomography, ultrasonography, or arteriography. Recently, noninvasive techniques for tumor localization have been utilized more frequently because invasive tests can carry significant risk. Invasive tests have been shown to stimulate pheochromocytomas and produce paroxysmal attacks. Patients, therefore, must be prepared for invasive tests in much the same way that they are prepared for surgical removal of the tumor.[48]

Nursing standards of care

Treatment of pheochromocytomas involves excision of the tumor, but presurgical treatment needs to be commenced at least 2 weeks prior to surgical removal.[49] Adrenergic blockers should be administered as soon as the diagnosis is confirmed and before conducting an invasive localization test, in order to reduce or eliminate hypertension and associated symptoms. Adrenergic blockade serves to prevent the crisis brought on by the burst of catecholamine secretion from the tumor that occurs under anesthesia or with tumor manipulation. It also reduces the persistent vasoconstriction and allows for gradual correction of extracellular fluid volume. Treatment of paroxysmal attacks may require a fast-acting antihypertensive agent such as sodium nitroprusside.[50]

The usual technique for adrenergic blockade is to begin with an alpha blocker prior to surgery or invasive testing. Beta blockers are not administered initially, as they may lead to heart failure or pulmonary edema. (Alpha responses are enhanced and the resultant vasoconstriction is not compensated for by vasodilation. Therefore, beta blockers should never precede alpha blockers because of adrenergic stimulation of both alpha and beta receptors in pheochromocytomas.[51]) The drug of choice for selective alpha blockade is phenoxybenzamine (Dibezylene). The usual dose is 10 mg orally, given every 12 hours initially. The dose is increased by 10 mg/day every 2 days thereafter, to a maximum of 200 mg/day. The desired results include disappearance of the tachycardia, control of hypertension, and absence of paroxysmal attacks. Nasal stuffiness and/or pos-

tural hypotension may also occur as blockade is achieved.[52]

Beta blockers may be indicated later in addition to alpha blockers if tachydysrhythmias exist or if the patient is not responsive to alpha blockers alone.[53] The usual drug of choice is propranolol (Inderal), which is given in increasing doses, beginning with 20 mg twice daily, until the arrhythmias disappear.[54]

Postoperatively, the patient may exhibit transient hypoglycemia and hypertension or hypotension, depending upon the extracellular fluid volume of the patient relative to the changed vascular capacity. Persistent hypertension may be indicative of additional tumor.[55] Similar effects may occur during chemotherapy for this disease.

Nursing management requires prompt recognition of hemodynamic changes and appropriate monitoring, including central venous pressure, arterial pressure, and ECG. The patient needs to be frequently monitored during an attack as well as assessed for risks of MI or cerebral vascular attack. The patient should be questioned about the factors that precipitate an attack, and a plan of care should be created that incorporates the alleviation of these factors.[56] A sample care plan for a patient with pheochromocytoma follows.

Nursing Care Plan for the Management of the Patient with Pheochromocytoma

Diagnosis	Signs and symptoms	Intervention	Rationale
Altered level of comfort, related to secretion of catecholamines by tumor	Diaphoresis Restlessness, trembling, insomnia Fear, panic, anxiety Headaches Palpitations, fatigue	Assess factors that are contributing to paroxysmal attacks Plan care to include frequent rest periods Minimize stimuli in patient's environment Administer stool softeners and fluids as ordered Maintain a calm, confident manner Administer analgesics as ordered Safety precautions Provide comfort measures such as assistance with hygiene and a comfortable room temperature	Care should be planned to avoid these factors To minimize fatigue Stimuli such as sudden position changes and straining with bowel movements may cause autonomous secretion of catecholamines Rest and relief of discomfort reduces autonomic secretion of catecholamines Headache and vision disturbances may occur secondary to hypertension Diaphoresis can occur with hypertensive attacks
Altered tissue perfusion, related to catecholamine secretion and subsequent vasoconstriction and vasodilation	Hypertension, orthostatic hypotension Tachycardia, arrhythmias, diminished peripheral pulses Restlessness Crackles (rales) Changes in mentation/motor function Oliguria or anuria Cyanosis or pallor	Perform continual hemodynamic monitoring of cardiovascular status, including assessment of BP, cardiac rhythm and rate Monitor patient for chest pain/angina, dyspnea, JVP Auscultate lung fields for adventitious sounds	Effects of vasoconstriction and/or vasodilation may be seen Arrhythmias can occur from excessive myocardial stimulation Catecholamine-induced myopathy may lead to a diminished cardiac output Potential complications of hypertension include MI, congestive heart failure, and cerebral vascular accident

Nursing Care Plan for the Management of the Patient with Pheochromocytoma

Diagnosis	Signs and symptoms	Intervention	Rationale
		Assess orientation, level of consciousness, reflexes, and motor function	May reveal signs and symptoms of CVA or CHF
		Monitor weight daily; keep I&O records	Assessment for hyperdynamic circulatory function with volume overload
		Administer oxygen as indicated	To increase oxygen availability to tissues
		Administer alpha and beta adrenergic blockers and monitor their effectiveness	Adrenergic blockade will prevent catecholamine secretion from the tumor
Altered nutrition: intake less than body requirements, related to increased metabolic rate	Abdominal pain Lack of interest in food or aversion to eating Weight loss Nausea and vomiting Hypoglycemia	Monitor weight daily; keep I&O records	Excessive catecholamine secretion results in a catabolic state
		Evaluate patient (or obtain nutrition consult) to determine degree of nutritional deficit	Gastrointestinal blood flow decreases in response to catecholamine secretion and leads to nutritional disturbances
		Provide supplemental fluids, usually containing glucose, and modify diet, as indicated	Adequate caloric intake must be assured
		Monitor glucose levels	Glucose levels may be high prior to surgical removal of tumor from glycogenolysis; they may be low following surgical removal from the decrease in circulating catecholamines

Diagnosis	Signs and symptoms	Intervention	Rationale
		Review laboratory data, including albumin, transferrin, amino acid profile, blood urea nitrogen, nitrogen balance, liver function tests, and electrolytes	Provides data on nutritional status
Lack of knowledge of disease, possible complications, and treatments	Verbalization of lack of knowledge Development of preventable complications	Determine patient's level of knowledge and ability to learn	To establish baseline
		Identify support staff requiring information and involve them in learning process	Support staff needs to be aware of signs and symptoms of paroxysmal attacks
		Review etiology of disease and importance of avoiding factors that precipitate paroxysmal attacks	Patient needs to incorporate alleviation of these factors into life-style

Acute Adrenal Insufficiency

Acute adrenal insufficiency (sometimes referred to as acute adrenal crisis) is a medical emergency that may result in fatal cardiac arrhythmias or vascular collapse and shock. The critical care team can reverse a potentially catastrophic sequence of events if the signs and symptoms of acute adrenal insufficiency are recognized promptly and specific life-saving treatment is instituted.[57] The clinical manifestations occur when the function of the adrenal cortex is impaired and there is insufficient production of glucocorticoids and mineralocorticoids or of glucocorticoids alone. This insuffiency leads to fluid and electrolyte disturbances, alterations in fat, carbohydrate, and protein metabolism, and an inability to tolerate stress.[58]

Clinical antecedents

Acute adrenal insufficiency can be a consequence of destruction or dysfunction of the adrenal cortex, referred to as primary adrenocortical insufficiency. Clinical symptoms are not evident until at least 90% of the glandular function is lost.[59] Thus, significant injury must occur before symptoms are present. The most common etiology of primary hypoadrenalism is an autoimmune disorder called Addison's disease. Hypoadrenalism can also occur as a consequence of deficit pituitary ACTH secretion; in that case it is referred to as secondary adrenocortical insufficiency. This problem is more common in the ICU than most clinicians recognize: in a prospective study of 300 consecutive ICU admissions, 92 of the patients were taking therapeutic steroids or had conditions requiring steroid treatment.[60] Common precipitating factors of secondary adrenal insufficiency include stress, rapid withdrawal of steroids, chemotherapy, and diseases of the pituitary gland.

Critical referents

The term Addison's disease is generally used to describe a chronic dysfunction of the adrenal glands. Acute adrenal insufficiency occurs as the disease of chronic insufficiency progresses. This transition from chronic to acute may be demonstrated in patients with Addison's disease who are exposed to a stressor such as infection, trauma, or surgery. When these patients are subjected to such a stressor, they develop an acute need for an increased level of glucocorticoids. If the adrenal cortex is unable to respond by increasing its secretion of glucocorticoids, acute adrenal insufficiency may result.[61]

Most cases of Addison's disease can be attributed to autoimmune destruction of the adrenal cortex, which occurs in approximately 85% of cases. Another 10% arise as complications from tuberculosis, and the remaining 5% from causes such as fungal infections, metastatic cancer, amyloidosis, collagen vascular diseases, or hemorrhagic destruction from anticoagulants, trauma, or infection.[62] Insufficiency related to hemorrhagic destruction may be seen in the Waterhouse-Friderichsen syndrome, usually attributed to meningococcemia.[63] It may also be seen in approximately 15% of septic shock patients.[64]

Secondary adrenocortical insufficiency is caused by disorders of the hypothalamic-pituitary-adrenal (HPA) axis and is most commonly attributed to exogenous glucocorticoid therapy or to primary pituitary or hypothalamic disorders resulting from tumor, infarction, surgery, or radiation. Adrenal insufficiency due to exogenous glucocorticoids—particularly dexamethasone and longer-acting glucocorticoids that block the nocturnal ACTH surge—may result because the high circulating levels of glucocorticoids suppress pituitary release of ACTH. Prolonged administration of exogenous glucocorticoids will produce subnormal ACTH and cortisol responses to stress because the cortisol, acting on the pituitary through the negative feedback mechanism, will inhibit ACTH production. The loss of basal ACTH secretion will eventually result in atrophy of the adrenal cortex and decreased basal secretion of cortisol. The result is not only a decreased ACTH responsiveness to stress but also a diminished adrenal responsiveness to acute stimulation with exogenous ACTH.[65]

Secondary adrenocortical insufficiency may also be exhibited with conditions such as rheumatoid arthritis, chronic pulmonary diseases, and metastatic diseases for which ongoing steroids are included in therapy. When these patients are placed in stressful situations and are not supplied with increases in steroid dosages, the adrenals are not able to respond appropriately, and circulatory collapse may occur. Sudden withdrawal of steroids in these patients may also precipitate an acute adrenal crisis.[66]

Resulting signs and symptoms

Deficiencies in glucocorticoids, or cortisol, will bring about symptoms of hypoglycemia and impaired response to stress. The hypoglycemia is related to impaired gluconeogenesis and fat utilization, caused by the lack of the hormones necessary to aid in the conversion of protein into glucose. The patient exhibits weakness and fatigue, weight loss, anorexia, nausea and vomiting, and diarrhea or constipation. The GI disturbances are a result of the decreased secretion of gastrointestinal digestive enzymes, which in turn is a result of diminished levels of cortisol.[67] Diminished cortisol levels will also stimulate the anterior pituitary to release melanocyte-secreting hormone along with additional ACTH. This will produce the classic physical finding of hyperpigmentation in Addison's disease.[68] A deficiency in glucocorticoids also results in an inability to respond to norepinephrine, which leads to the potential for decreased peripheral vascular resistance and circulatory collapse in the presence of hypovolemia.[69]

Mineralocorticoid deficiency produces fluid and electrolyte disturbances. Specifically, there is renal sodium wasting (and, therefore, water and chloride loss) along with potassium retention. This situation may give rise to hyponatremia, hyperkalemia, hypovolemia, hypotension, and decreased cardiac output (with resultant small heart from a diminished workload). The symptoms include weight loss, dehydration, possible weakness or paralysis from hyperkalemia, and shock.[70]

The patient with chronic adrenocortical insufficiency, therefore, will present with chief symptoms of hyperpigmentation, weakness and fatigue, fever or hypothermia, weight loss, anorexia, and GI disturbances. Exposing the patient to stress can precipitate an adrenal crisis, and acute decompensation can

occur. Symptoms may then expand to include hypotension and cardiovascular collapse, along with changes in mentation and hypoglycemia.[71]

The symptoms of adrenal insufficiency seen in the Waterhouse-Friderichsen syndrome include nausea and vomiting, abdominal pain, headache, and petechiae that may progress to purpura. Fever may be present, and the patient may progress to shock and death within 48 hours of evidence of purpura.[72]

When the adrenal insufficiency is a complication of a disorder of the HPA axis, hyperpigmentation is not present, because pituitary secretion of ACTH and melanocyte-secreting hormone is deficient. Since mineralocorticoid secretion is usually preserved, the manifestations of volume depletion, dehydration, and electrolyte disturbances are also absent. Acute decompensation with hypotension and shock can occur, along with weakness, lethargy, anorexia, nausea and vomiting, and hypoglycemia.[73]

Diagnostic laboratory tests reveal hyponatremia, related to the lack of aldosterone-induced kidney conservation and impaired free water clearance; hyperkalemia, related to aldosterone deficiency and decreased renal perfusion; increased blood urea nitrogen, a consequence of diminished glomerular filtration from hypotension; hypoglycemia, related to impaired gluconeogenesis and lipolysis; frequently acidemia with low plasma bicarbonate, from the loss of aldosterone-promoted hydrogen ion excretion; hypercalcemia or hyperuricemia, a result of volume depletion; and lymphocytosis and eosinophilia.[74] In addition, as Table 7-16 indicates, hormonal assays will demonstrate depressed plasma

Table 7-16 Diagnosis of Adrenal Disorders

Test	Cushing's Syndrome	Addison's Disease
Plasma cortisol	Increased	Increased
Plasma ACTH	Increased (feedback)	Increased (primary)
Serum aldosterone	—	Increased
Urinary hydroxysteroid and 17-ketosteroids and ketogenic steroids	Increased (primary and secondary)	Increased (primary and secondary)
ACTH stimulation	Normal	Increased (secondary)
Metyrapone suppression	Increased	—
Plasma catecholamine (for Pheochromocytoma)		
Urinary vanillylmandelic acid (for Pheochromocytoma)		

cortisol levels as well as depressed or absent urinary hydroxycorticoid and 17-ketosteroid in a 24-hour urine sample.[75] Assessment of possible adrenal insufficiency also includes a rapid ACTH stimulation test. This involves measurement of baseline plasma cortisol levels followed by administration of a synthetic ACTH (such as corsyntropin) and then measurement of plasma cortisol levels 60 minutes after the injection. A decreased adrenal reserve is demonstrated if there is failure of the plasma cortisol level to respond to exogenous administration of ACTH.[76]

Past or present tuberculosis may be revealed on a chest x-ray, or adrenal calcification may be evident on abdominal films, although these conditions are pathognomic of adrenal insufficiency. Chest x-rays may also demonstrate a small cardiac silhouette reflective of hypovolemia.[77]

Nursing standards of care

Adrenal insufficiency in the critically ill patient is a medical emergency requiring immediate fluid and corticosteroid administration. Treatment of acute adrenal insufficiency is specific and is directed at restoration of fluid and electrolyte balances, replacement of hormones, and treatment of the underlying cause. Rapid administration of intravenous fluids, usually normal saline or glucose and normal saline, is needed to correct volume depletion and hypoglycemia. Plasma expanders may be necessary if shock occurs. Vasopressor support may be indicated but requires glucocorticoid replacement in order to be effective.[78] Hyperkalemia is usually responsive to fluid and adrenocorticosteroid replacement and will not require further intervention.[79] Adrenocortical hormone replacement is necessary (options are listed in Table 7-17), usually requiring hydrocortisone

(which has some mineralocorticoid activity of its own) and dexamethasone (which can be used to provide coverage during the ACTH stimulation test since it does not interfere significantly with plasma cortisol levels). Hydrocortisone replacement is given at 30 mg/day (or its equivalent), usually divided to mimic the diurnal pattern of two-thirds of the daily dose in the morning and one-third of the dose in the evening.[80] Severe adrenal insufficiency may require mineralocorticoid replacement with fluorocortisone acetate at 0.05–2.0 mg/day.[81] Antibiotic therapy may be indicated if the crisis was precipitated by an infectious process. Oxygen therapy as well as hemodynamic monitoring with a Swan-Ganz catheter may be necessary if shock ensues. Diet therapy will include foods high in protein and moderate in carbohydrates to manage the hypoglycemia and weakness of acute adrenal insufficiency. The patient with primary adrenal hypofunction may also require mineralocorticoid therapy utilizing fluorocortisone.[82]

When treating acute episodes, the critical care team should remember that any stress sufficient to warrant a patient's receiving intensive care requires an increase in corticosteroid dosage for the patient with adrenal hypofunction. In acute situations, it is better to err on the side of overtreatment than to inadequately dose the patient experiencing fever, infection, sepsis, surgery, or trauma.[83]

Nursing management includes being aware of the patient at risk for adrenal insufficiency, including the patient with Addison's disease who is undergoing a stressful experience or the patient with a history of ongoing glucocorticoid therapy. A critical illness may even trigger a crisis in a patient not known to have a prior history of adrenal insufficiency.[84]

Nursing interventions include administering intravenous fluids, observing for fluid and electrolyte disturbances, monitoring vital signs including heart rate and rhythm, assessing central and peripheral

Table 7-17 Steroid Replacement in Adrenal Insufficiency

Drug	Relative Potency	Average Replacement Dose	Half-life
Cortisol (Solu-cortef hydrocortisone)	1.0	20 mg morning, 10 mg evening	Short
Prednisone	35–40 (night)	5–7.5 mg/day	Long
Prednisolone	4–5	5–6 mg/day	Long
Dexamethasone	30	1.0 mg/day	Long
Betamethasone	30	1.0 mg/day	Very long

perfusion, and monitoring intake and output as well as daily weights for an indication of hydration status. Since this type of patient is sensitive to stressful situations, the nurse must take measures to minimize any stress by providing for periods of rest, carefully explaining all procedures, and furnishing emotional support. The nurse's role in prevention of acute adrenal insufficiency includes educating the patient about the need to increase glucocorticoid therapy during periods of acute illness.[85] A nursing care plan for the patient experiencing acute adrenal insufficiency follows.

Nursing Care Plan for the Management of the Patient with Acute Adrenal Insufficiency

Diagnosis	Signs and symptoms	Intervention	Rationale
Fluid volume deficit related to insufficient secretion of mineralocorticoids and glucocorticoids	Weakness, thirst Decreased venous filling (CVP ≤ 1 cm H_2O) Decreased skin turgor, dry mucous membranes Edema Orthostasis hypotension Tachycardia Decreased urine output and/or concentrated urine Hemoconcentration	Monitor weight daily; keep I&O records; evaluate mucous membranes, skin turgor, and peripheral pulses for hydration status	Excessive sodium excretion and extracellular fluid volume deficiency occur with mineralocorticoid deficiency
		Conduct hemodynamic monitoring and prepare for potential Swan-Ganz monitoring of cardiac output, CVP, and systemic vascular resistance	Hyperkalemia and hyponatremia may contribute to impaired heart function and dysrhythmias; cardiac output, CVP, and systemic vascular resistance are all diminished in acute adrenal insufficiency
		Administer glucocorticoid replacements	Glucocorticoid insufficiency can lead to a diminished vascular tone
		Administer volume and electrolytes replacements	Shock may occur from profound volume deficits
		Monitor patient's response to glucocorticoid and volume replacements	Evaluates effectiveness of therapy
		Administer oxygen as indicated	Provides symptomatic relief of dyspnea related to hypovolemia
		Review laboratory data, including hemoglobin and hematocrit, electrolytes, total protein, and albumin	To monitor for hyponatremia, hyperkalemia, azotemia, hypercalcemia, hyperuricemia, and hypoglycemia

Diagnosis	Signs and symptoms	Intervention	Rationale
		Plan for rest periods as indicated	Weakness may occur from hyponatremia, hyperkalemia, and loss of diurnal activity of glucocorticoids
		Recognize risk to patient by noting precipitating factors	
Sensory-perceptual alteration, related to glucocorticoid deficit	Irritability, restlessness Apprehension, fear Lack of concentration	Reduce patient's exposure to stress and extraneous stimuli	Glucocorticoid deficiency results in an impaired response to stress
	Increased sensitivity to olfactory and gustatory stimuli	Avoid using items (lotions, oils) whose odors may prove irritating to patient	Patient will have increased sensitivity to olfactory and gustatory stimuli
		Reorient patient to time, place, and events as necessary; provide explanations and plan care with patient	Mental and visual acuity is affected by the loss of diurnal peaks of glucocorticoids
		Provide undisturbed rest periods	Allows patient to conserve energy
		Offer reassurance and support	Confused, hypersensitive patient will relax better with supportive caregivers
Altered nutritional status: intake less than body requirements, related to decreased secretion of digestive enzymes	Weight loss Nausea and vomiting Anorexia Abdominal cramps Diarrhea	Monitor weight daily; keep I&O records; evaluate degree of patient's nutritional deficit; provide regular meals in a comfortable environment; determine which foods are best tolerated	Glucocorticoid deficiency leads to decreased secretion of gastrointestinal digestive enzymes, resulting in nutritional imbalances Enhances nutritional maintenance
		Supplement patient's diet with IV fluids containing glucose or enteral feeds, as indicated; observe for signs of hypoglycemia	Glucocorticoid deficiency leads to diminished ability to maintain glucose levels

Nursing Care Plan for the Management of the Patient with Acute Adrenal Insufficiency

Diagnosis	Signs and symptoms	Intervention	Rationale
Lack of knowledge about disease, possible complications, and treatments	Verbalization of knowledge deficit Development of preventable complications	Determine patient's level of knowledge and ability to learn	Self-care education is necessary to avoid potential acute adrenal insufficiency
		Identify support staff requiring information and involve them in learning process	Support staff need to be aware of signs and symptoms of acute adrenal insufficiency
		Review etiology of acute adrenal insufficiency and importance of increasing glucocorticoid therapy during periods of acute illness	Patient needs to recognize symptoms of insufficient glucocorticoid replacement dosages
		Emphasize need for long-term medical follow-up	Patient needs to realize necessity for lifelong therapy

Diabetes Mellitus

Diabetes mellitus is a condition characterized by abnormal utilization of glucose caused by decreased insulin secretion, ineffective glucagon regulatory mechanisms, or peripheral resistance to insulin. Diabetes is not a single disorder but a group of clinical syndromes reflecting glucose intolerance. Table 7-18 presents a summary of the American Diabetes Association's classification of glucose disorders. Table 7-19 summarizes the limits for various laboratory results used in diagnosing diabetes mellitus.

Diabetes mellitus affects 5–7% of the U.S. population.[86] It is one of the leading causes of death in the United States today.[87] Most of the deaths are associated with multisystem complications of the disease—atherosclerotic heart disease, infection, or renal failure. The primary manifestations are those of a chronic disease producing progressive organ failure from inappropriate glucose utilization. There are, however, several acute complications requiring critical care management. Acute hyperglycemia may present as diabetic ketoacidosis or as hyperglycemic, hyperosmolar nonketotic crisis. It is important that critical care nurses recognize these crises and provide immediate intervention as well as constantly monitor for multisystem complications.

The general effects of diabetes produce many nonacute physiological problems that are encountered in the critically ill patient. The chronic state of poor glucose utilization leads to cellular starvation, even in the face of hyperglycemia. Catabolic hormones, such as epinephrine, are secreted in an attempt to meet cellular needs for energy. The systemic effects of prolonged periods of hyperglycemia include profound damage to many cells of the body. Some physiological complications of hyperglycemia and their pathophysiological etiologies are listed in Table 7-20.

The treatment of diabetes involves dietary adjustments, weight loss, and insulin replacement or oral antidiabetic agents. A major part of the nursing care of the stable diabetic may be dietary maneuvers, weight loss programs, and teaching about oral diabetic agents. Critical care nurses are more often involved in the management of acute hyperglycemia or hypoglycemia. The use of insulin in the care of the critically ill requires a knowledge of the onset of action, peak effects, and duration of effects. The critical care nurse must incorporate this information into the patient's routine for activities and meals or enteral feedings. Times of physiological and emotional stress, such as critical illness, will alter the diabetic's insulin needs, necessitating careful monitoring by the critical care nurse.

Monitoring glucose levels has historically involved obtaining intermittent urine or blood specimens, which are tested for glucose. Urine testing for glucose level has been determined to be inaccurate, possibly reflecting a normal level even when blood glucose levels are as high as 300 mg/dL.[88] Variables that may cause increased urine glucose without concomitant serum increases include advanced age, heart failure, renal failure, and many medications. Thus, urine glucose testing should be utilized only when accurate and timely blood glucose testing is unavailable. Blood glucose testing machines that quickly provide results are generally available on most nursing units. The hospitalized diabetic patient should have blood glucose monitored 2–4 times daily. Anxiety, fevers, pain, intravenous administration of fluids, infection, and operative procedures are only a few of the stressors that may contribute to increased insulin needs of the patient. Many clinical conditions and medications have also been associated with altered glucose tolerance or clinical diabetes; these are listed in Table 7-21.

Pancreatic transplant is a strategy aimed at permanent correction of diabetes. Statistics for procedures performed between 1983 and 1986 show that overall 1-year survival of a functional transplanted kidney is 42% and patient survival is 79%.[89] The primary purpose of pancreatic transplant is to restore endocrine function in a difficult to control diabetic with complications such as visual disorders, hypertension, and/or renal failure. Candidates for transplant must be highly motivated and compliant with therapy and cannot have active peptic ulcer disease, malignancy, CAD, or infection. The risks of diabetic complications to those patients should be higher than those associated with the administration of the immunosuppressives necessary to fight rejection.

The procedure involves the transplantation of all or part of a donor pancreas, while leaving the patient's pancreas intact. Many receive a pancreas transplant in conjunction with a kidney transplant. Newer techniques involve implantation of only the islet cells, enclosed within a capsule such as a portal vein or the terminal venules of the liver.[90] The patient's pancreatic exocrine enzymes continue to be released into the GI tract. The donor pancreatic secretions may be diverted into the patient's duct of Wirsung, GI tract, or bladder.[91] Hourly postoperative monitoring of glucose levels is essential to control hyperglycemia with insulin until pancreatic cells are functional. Hyperglycemia will destroy the newly implanted islet cells.[92]

The most feared postoperative complication is rejection. In order to prevent rejection, any of several

Table 7-18 American Diabetes Association's Classification of Glucose Disorders

Statistical Risk Classes*	Distinguishing Characteristics	Clinical Classes	Distinguishing Characteristics
Previous abnormality of glucose tolerance (PrevAGT)	Persons in this category have normal glucose tolerance and a history of transient diabetes mellitus or impaired glucose tolerance.	Diabetes mellitus (DM) Type I Insulin–dependent diabetes mellitus (IDDM)	Patients may be of any age, are usually thin, and usually have abrupt onset of signs and symptoms with insulinopenia before age 40. These patients often have strongly positive urine glucose and ketone tests and are dependent upon insulin to prevent ketoacidosis and to sustain life.
Potential abnormality of glucose tolerance (PotAGT)	Persons in this category have never experienced abnormal glucose tolerance but have a greater than normal risk of developing diabetes mellitus or impaired glucose tolerance.	Type II Non-insulin–dependent diabetes mellitus (NIDDM) (obese or nonobese)	Patients are usually older than 40 years at diagnosis, obese, and have relatively few classic symptoms. They are not prone to ketoacidosis except during periods of stress. Although not dependent upon exogenous insulin for survival, they may require it for stress-induced hyperglycemia and hyperglycemia that persists in spite of other therapy.
		Other types of diabetes mellitus	Patients with other types of diabetes mellitus have certain associated conditions or syndromes.
		Impaired glucose tolerance (IGT) (obese or nonobese)	Patients with impaired glucose tolerance have plasma glucose levels that are higher than normal but not diagnostic for diabetes mellitus.
		Other types of impaired glucose tolerance	Patients with other types of impaired glucose tolerance have certain associated conditions or syndromes.
		Gestational diabetes mellitus (GDM)	Patients with gestational diabetes mellitus have onset or discovery of glucose intolerance *during* pregnancy.

*Used for epidemiologic and research purposes.
Source: American Diabetes Association (1988), p. 4; Adapted from classification developed by an international workgroup sponsored by the National Diabetes Data Group, National Institutes of Health. National Diabetes Data Group: Classification and diagnosis of diabetes mellitus and other categories of glucose intolerance. *Diabetes* 1979 (28):1039–1057.

Table 7-19 Top Limits of Laboratory Tests for the Diagnosis of Diabetes Mellitus*

Biochemical Index	Normal	Acceptable	Fair	Poor
Fasting plasma glucose	115 mg/dL	140 mg/dL	200 mg/dL	>200 mg/dL
Postprandial plasma glucose	140 mg/dL	175 mg/dL	235 mg/dL	>235 mg/dL
Glycosylated hemoglobin	6%	8%	10%	>10%
Fasting plasma cholesterol	200 mg/dL	225 mg/dL	250 mg/dL	>250 mg/dL
Fasting plasma triglyceride	150 mg/dL	175 mg/dL	200 mg/dL	>200 mg/dL

*Adjust for normal values of laboratory, and increase limits for elderly patients.
Source: American Diabetes Association (1988). *The Physician's Guide to Type II Diabetes (NIDDM) Diagnosis and Treatment*, p. 25

immunosuppressive agents may be used: azothioprine, corticosteroids, cyclosporine, or muromonab-CD3. (Refer to the chapter on hematology for more information.) The latest promising agent for preventing rejection of transplanted islet cells is FK 506.[93] Symptoms of rejection include fever, returning hyperglycemia, or hyperamylasemia. Rejection may occur immediately postop or up to months later. Immunosuppressive agents are used for at least a year after surgery; then dosages may be tapered, provided that rejection symptoms are not present. Patients must continue to perform blood glucose tests postoperatively to monitor for late rejection. Rejection unresponsive to immunosuppressives requires removal of the transplanted organ.

Infections are a particularly common postoperative problem and are partly associated with immunosuppressive therapy. Acute cytomegalovirus (CMV) sometimes occurs in patients who did not have the virus prior to transplant. Most adults have had this virus and are not susceptible, but those who are CMV antibody-negative preoperatively may contract CMV from the transplanted organ. Other complications may include pancreatic pseudocysts, peripancreatic seromas, pancreatitis, or poor wound healing. Patients are continuously monitored for fever, abdominal pain, changes in wound drainage, and signs of rejection.

Diabetes has many clinical ramifications for the critical care nurse. It is important that nurses be knowledgeable regarding the assessment and management of these complications. The common glucose disorders are addressed in the following pages.

Diabetic Ketoacidosis

Diabetic ketoacidosis (DKA) is a life-threatening clinical condition with greatly varying presentations. It is the most common endocrine emergency. DKA is characterized by a complete lack of or marked reduction in insulin available within the systemic circulation and severe disturbances in protein, fat, and carbohydrate metabolism.

Clinical antecedents

The etiology of DKA is a lack of insulin. This absence of adequate insulin may be due to undiagnosed diabetes (Type I) or uncontrolled previously diagnosed diabetes. The new diabetic usually presents with DKA that is the result of physiological decompensation brought on by progressive insulin insufficiency. This increasing insufficiency is fueled by the liberation of greater than normal quantities of glucose in response to an acute stressful event. About 25% of patients with insulin-dependent diabetes mellitus (IDDM) are diagnosed after an acute DKA episode.[94]

In the patient with previously diagnosed diabetes, there may be a failure to increase insulin doses despite elevated blood glucose readings and/or increased insulin requirements. Additionally, in the presence of nausea and vomiting, the individual with known diabetes may fail to take the required insulin because of reduced food intake and may present with DKA. Some other causes include insulin resistance, pancreatitis, and conditions requiring an increased insulin supply—for example, severe stress, surgery, trauma, pregnancy, puberty, or infection. Of these, rapid growth (puberty) and infection may be the major precipitating factors of DKA.[95] Meningitis, influenza, and gastroenteritis have caused DKA, but more frequently it is a consequence of respiratory, urinary tract, or skin infection.

Table 7-20 Physiological Effects of Hyperglycemia

Clinical Disorder	Pathophysiology

Atherosclerosis
  Coronary arteries: CAD
  Systemic circulation: hypertension, cardiomyopathy
  Cerebral vessels: increased risk of CVA
  Peripheral vessels: PVD
	Elevated glucose and lipid levels promote the development of atherosclerosis. Further, the renin stimulation occurring with renal involvement causes hypertension, increasing the workload of the heart; decreased oxygenation of myocardial tissue causes compensating ventricular hypertrophy and dilation. Atherosclerosis of cerebral or peripheral vessels leads to failure to perfuse the tissues and a resultant organ failure.

Diabetic retinopathy
  Background diabetic neuropathy (BDR)
  Preproliferative diabetic retinopathy (PPDR)
  Proliferative diabetic retinopathy (PDR)
	Retinopathy seems to be related to uncontrolled glucose levels and degrees of hypertension. It may be a generally benign disorder, called BDR or PPDR, or severe PDR. Clinical findings with BDR include microaneurysms and "dot and blot" hemorrhages of the retina. Complications producing some visual disturbances are macular edema and hard exudates at or near the macula. The proliferative disorder is manifested by cotton-wool spots (soft exudates), which are ischemic infarcts in the inner retinal layer; "beading" of the retinal veins; or intraretinal microvascular abnormalities.

Diabetic renal disease	A number of conditions either precipitate or exacerbate renal dysfunction. They are hypertension, neurogenic bladder, repetitive urethral instrumentation, infection, urinary obstruction, decreased renal blood flow, and nephrotoxic drugs. Diabetic renal disease is hallmarked by nodular and particularly diffuse intercapillary glomerulosclerosis, leading to chronic renal failure.
Diabetic foot problems	Foot lesions in diabetics are the result of peripheral neuropathy, peripheral vascular disease, superimposed infection, or a combination of these effects. Because of peripheral sensory nerve damage caused by the high glucose levels, foot lesions are insensitive, deformed, ischemic, and prone to infection. Hyperglycemia also causes decreased sweating, leading to thickened skin that cracks easily.
Peripheral neuropathies	Hyperglycemia interferes with nerve conduction and leads to chronic and permanent alterations in the sensory components of these peripheral nerves. At times, vibratory sense may be lost and ankle jerk reflexes become absent. The insensitivity and neuropathy may lead to contractures and a deformed foot. Neuropathies are more common bilaterally in the feet than in the upper extremities.

Visceral (autonomic) neuropathies	Visceral neuropathies usually occur in conjunction with peripheral neuropathies, but the two are not necessarily equal in severity.
	  Gastroparesis: delayed emptying or retention of gastric contents causes nausea, vomiting, and abdominal discomfort.
	  Diabetic diarrhea: frequent loose stools, particularly after meals or at night.
	  Neurogenic bladder: decreased sphincter tone leads to urinary retention leading to UTI and possible hydronephrosis.
	  Cardiovascular neuropathy: orthostatic BP or tachydysrhythmias indicate neuropathy of the cardiovascular reflexes.

Impotence	Neuropathies affect nerves responsible for erection. Functional impotence (inability to sustain erection) presents without altered libido or ejaculatory function.

Table 7-21 Clinical Conditions and Medications Causing Glucose Intolerance or Diabetes

Diseases	Medications
Alcoholism	Diuretics
Cerebrovascular accident	Butedimide (Bumex)
Dialysis—hemodialysis, peritoneal dialysis, CAVH dialysis	Chlorthalidone (Hygroton, Combipres, Regroton)
Extensive burns	Clonidine (Catapres, Combipres)
GI hemorrhage	Ethacrynic acid (Edecrin)
Heart disease—hypertension, MI	Furosemide (Lasix)
Hyperlipidemia	Thiazides (Diuril, Hydrodiuril)
Infection	Hormones
Muscular dystrophy	ACTH
Huntington's chorea	Catecholamines (epinephrine, norepinephrine, isoproterenol, levodopa, amphetamines, ephedrine, phenylephrine)
Pancreatitis	Dexatrothyroxine
Renal disease	Estrogens (oral contraceptives)
	Glucocorticoids (cortisone and derivatives)
	Thyroxine and triiodothyronine (toxic levels)
	Psychoactive agents
	Chlorprothixene (Taractan)
	Haloperidol (Haldol)
	Lithium (Lithane, Eskalith)
	Phenothiazines (Thorazine, Trilafon, Etrafon, Triavil, chlorpromazine, Metaclopromide)
	Tricyclic antidepressants: amyltriptyline (Elavil, Endep, Triavil), desipramine (Norpramin, Pertofrane), doxepin (Adapin, Sinequan), imipramine (Presamine, Tofranil), nortriptyline (Aventyl)
	Immunosuppressive agents
	Miscellaneous
	Antineoplastic agents (L-aspariginase)
	Streptozotocin
	Beta-adrenergic blocking agents (propranolol, nadolol, timolol, pindolol, metoprolol, atenolol)*
	Dicumarol derivatives*
	Diphenylhydantoin (Dilantin)
	Indomethacin
	Isoniazid
	Nicotinic acid
	Phenylbutazone*
	Salicylates*
	Sulfonamides*
	Alimentation regimens—peripheral, central, enteral

*Causes hypoglycemia.

Critical referents

DKA results from insulin deficiency and leads to four life-threatening complications: hyperosmolarity, metabolic acidosis, extracellular volume depletion, and electrolyte abnormalities (see Table 7-22).

The initial stage of decompensated diabetes is a period of prolonged hyperglycemia. In normal circumstances, insulin acts as the key that admits glucose into the cells of muscle and adipose tissue.

Table 7-22 Four Pathophysiological Consequences of DKA

Pathology	Etiology
Metabolic acidosis	Ketoacid accumulation
Hyperosmolarity	Hyperglycemia, fluid losses
Hypovolemia	Osmotic diuresis from hyperglycemia
Electrolyte disturbances	Osmotic diuresis, dehydration

Hypoinsulinemia results in the failure of glucose transport into the cells, leading to elevated serum glucose levels (hyperglycemia) and diminished intracellular glucose. The cellular glucose deficiency and the products of cellular metabolic activity stimulate glycogenolysis (breakdown of glycogen in the liver); but while glycogenolysis is activated, glucose synthesis is inhibited and glucose diffuses readily into the blood. New glucose is synthesized by the liver when amino acids are released from protein and glycerol (from fat stores).

If insulin is significantly less than required and carbohydrates cannot be used for energy, the body tries to compensate by burning fats for fuel. When immediate fat stores are depleted, protein stores are converted for energy. In DKA, circulating insulin concentrations are inadequate to inhibit the release of free fatty acids (FFAs) from adipose tissue, and ketosis and acidosis result. As protein and fat stores are utilized, FFAs enter the hepatic circulation. FFAs in the liver cause an accelerated synthesis of acetyl coenzyme A (Co-A). Acetyl Co-A metabolism produces acetoacetic acid (ketoacid), beta-hydroxybutyric acid, and acetone. These three acids—called the ketone bodies—build up in the blood more quickly than they can be metabolized, a condition called ketosis. They then dissociate into ketoanions and hydrogen ions, causing metabolic acidosis. (The complex clinical outcomes of this process are shown schematically in Figure 7-12.) Acetoacetic acid and beta-hydroxybutyric acid are oxidized to acetone and excreted via the lungs. However, poor tissue perfusion escalates the acidosis.

In the nondiabetic individual, glucagon, a hormone secreted by the alpha cells of the pancreas, as discussed earlier, functions in several ways that are in direct opposition to the action of insulin. The most important of these functions is the elevation of blood glucose levels in the presence of too much insulin, preventing hypoglycemia. However, in the diabetic individual with impaired beta cells, glucagon secretion does not appear to be inhibited by elevated blood glucose concentrations and, in fact, has been reported to increase relative to those concentrations, which may further contribute to existing hyperglycemia. The target organ of glucagon is the liver, where it has two major effects on the metabolism of glucose: glycogenolysis and increased gluconeogenesis. These two processes greatly increase the availability of glucose in the body, exacerbating ketosis.

Another counterregulatory hormone that contributes to the progression of ketosis toward acidosis is epinephrine. In DKA, large amounts of stress hormone are present, markedly affecting carbohydrate, protein, and fat metabolism. Epinephrine is important because it not only affects plasma glucose

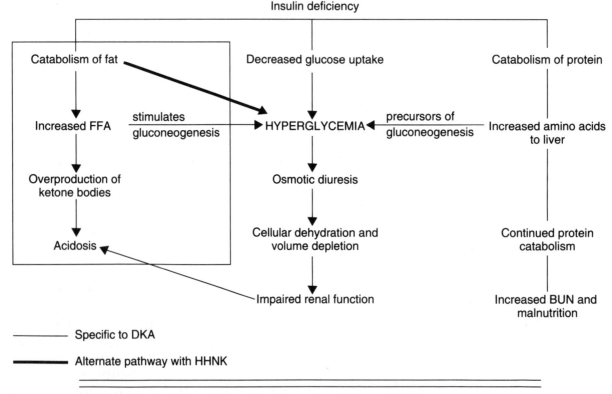

Figure 7-12 Pathophysiology of Hypoglycemia in DKA and HHNK

concentrations, but also simultaneously increases plasma fatty acid concentration and ketosis via the mechanism of hepatic degradation of FFA.

Resulting signs and symptoms

The patient with marked hyperglycemia and hyperketonemic metabolic acidosis may walk into an emergency room unassisted and give a lucid history. The hallmarks of presenting symptoms are hyperglycemia, osmotic diuresis, and metabolic acidosis. Presenting symptoms may include polydipsia, polyuria, and visual disturbances. Other signs and symptoms of DKA include tachycardia, hypotension, warm/dry skin, hyperventilation, weight loss, and dehydration. Dehydration and volume depletion are the result of osmotic diuresis caused by the hyperglycemia and ketonemia.

Nonspecific GI complaints ultimately develop in the majority of patients. These include anorexia, vomiting, and abdominal pain. Abdominal pain may be severe enough, along with leukocytosis, to mimic a surgical abdomen, that is, appendicitis or acute biliary disease. The theoretical etiologies of this abdominal pain include loss of sodium and fluids, ileus, and the high fat content of blood vessels in the intestinal tract.[96] The absence of this symptom in hyperglycemic, hyperosmolar nonketotic coma (HHNK) refutes these explanations, however. The abdominal pain often subsides after fluid replenishment.[97] Unexplained abdominal pain seems to be more prevalent in DKA when the patient is less than 40 years of age and is severely acidotic (serum bicarbonate less than 10 mEq).[98] The hyperlipemia common to DKA is thought to precipitate acute pancreatitis in some individuals.[99]

Infections may be present without fever and are obscured by the leukocytosis (more than 20,000 WBC/mm^3), which may accompany DKA even in the absence of infection. At the time of presentation, the serum potassium may be high, low, or normal. Serum potassium levels are usually normal to high because of the extracellular fluid shifts caused by acidosis. When serum potassium levels are low at presentation, total body deficit of potassium is probable, and the patient requires replenishment.[100] Serum potassium may be truly low (loss of about 6 mEq/kg) or only low in relation to the hyperglycemia. The osmotic diuresis of DKA will also often cause moderate to severe serum hyponatremia, hypophosphatemia, hypomagnesemia, and azotemia. Specific measures aimed at correcting these electrolyte disturbances may be necessary.

Drowsiness related to hyperglycemia can be present for several days prior to the development of ketoacidosis and may signal the possible onset of impaired consciousness in the patient who progresses to a coma. Twenty percent of patients with DKA present with neurological changes, and 10% have actual coma; both conditions are believed to be related to the hyperosmolarity rather than the hyperglycemia itself.[101] Clinical presentation may vary from a mildly decreased level of consciousness to obtundation. The development of changes in level of consciousness, however, is not necessarily always present.

Rapid respirations, known as Kussmaul breathing, are the classic sign of DKA. This type of respiration is a compensatory mechanism for the developing acidosis and serves to reduce acidosis by lowering the arterial PaCO$_2$. The respirations are rapid and shallow, but with increasing acidosis they become slower and deeper. The ability of the nurse to detect acetone (a fruity odor) on the patient's breath seems to be restricted to a fraction of the patients admitted with DKA. Evidence of dehydration is usually present. A comparison of the clinical presentations of DKA and HHNK is presented in Table 7-23.

The metabolic and electrolyte complications of DKA can be as dangerous as the DKA itself and require frequent monitoring. Serum electrolytes are drawn every 1–4 hours.[102] Neurological assessments are performed at least hourly during the initial few hours of treatment, and frequent respiratory assessments for pulmonary edema are performed. Rare complications of DKA include cerebral edema from fluid shifts or acidosis.[103] Vascular thrombosis from hyperviscosity is another rare complication.

Even though the symptoms are classic, DKA can be confused with other acute medical crises. Renal glycosuria of HHNK will produce hyperglycemia, but without associated ketonemia. Salicylate poisoning may cause Kussmaul respirations, glycosuria, and ketonuria, but hyperglycemia is not present. Lead poisoning is known to produce acute changes in level of consciousness, but glucose and ketone levels are only mildly elevated and not in proportion to the mental status changes. Another confusing clinical presentation is that of primary lactic acidosis. The precipitating factors for lactic acidosis do not usually include diabetes, however, and ketonemia is usually not present.

Nursing standards of care

A lack of insulin is the underlying cause of DKA, so the primary objective of therapy is insulin replace-

Table 7-23 Clinical Presentation of DKA versus HHNK

	DKA	HHNK
Age group	Young	Often elderly
Type of DM	I	II
Blood sugar	400–800 mg/dL	>800 mg/dL
Ketosis	+	−
Serum K$^+$	Normal or increased	Normal or decreased
Serum osmolality	<300 mOsm/kg	>300 mOsm/kg
Respirations	Kussmaul	Normal
Temperature	Hypothermic	Hyperthermic
Prodromal period	About one day	Several days

ment to normalize blood glucose. The goal of this replacement therapy is to return the patient's metabolism to a state of carbohydrate utilization. Secondary objectives include restoration of normal circulating blood volume, correction of fluid and electrolyte imbalances, and remediation of the factors that precipitated the development of DKA. Specific measures for management of acute DKA are shown in the following table.

Glucose level	Initial infusion of 10–20 units (0.15 U/kg) regular insulin by bolus IV followed by 5–10 units/hr (0.1 U/kg/hr). This rate may be increased by 50% every 2 hours until the glucose begins to fall.
Fluids	0.9% saline solution at 1 L/hr for 2 hours, then 500 cc/hr until rehydration is established. If rehydration is established and the osmolality remains higher than 295 mOsm/kg, fluids may be changed to 0.45% normal saline.
Acidosis	45 mEq of bicarbonate (one ampule) per liter of fluid may be added to the IV fluid if the arterial pH is less than 7.10. Give 1–2 ampules bolus IV if the pH is less than 7.0 or if cardiorespiratory arrest occurs.
Serum potassium	Add potassium phosphate or chloride to IV fluids.

The aggressiveness of the therapy is determined by the severity of the signs and symptoms.

To return the glucose level to normal, administer 10–20 units (0.15 U/kg) of regular insulin by bolus IV followed by a continuous infusion of insulin at 5–10 units/hr (0.1 U/kg/hr) in IV fluids.[104] The intravenous fluid of choice initially is isotonic (0.9%) normal saline (NS). This provides sodium replenishment and permits a slower return of osmolarity to normal, with reduced risk of cerebral edema.[105] To prevent

loss of insulin due to adherence to the IV tubing, the nurse may flush the tubing with concentrated insulin before filling the tubing with the standard infusion solution. Because of the accompanying dehydration, fluids are administered at 1000 cc/hr for 2 hours (approximately 15 mL/kg/hr), then 500 cc/hr until rehydration is established.[106] Some practitioners continue fluids at 1000 cc/hr until the blood pressure is stable and the urine output is at least 60 cc/hr.[107] After the intravascular volume is replenished, some clinicians recommend changing the IV solution to 0.45% NS. The rationale for this change is that sodium loss is not as great as water loss during diuresis, and 0.45% NS helps prevent hypochloremic metabolic acidosis.[108] Half-normal saline is indicated when the serum osmolarity is elevated.[109]

The treatment of acid-base and electrolyte imbalances may be necessary in the early management of DKA. When acidosis is severe (pH < 7.10), sodium bicarbonate may be added to the intravenous fluid, although in some cases it has been found that there are no alterations in outcome or recovery with the administration of bicarbonate.[110] An additional problem with the correction of acidosis is that it shifts the oxyhemoglobin curve and may enhance hypoxia.[111] Potassium levels are variable; both rehydration and insulin administration may enhance the return of potassium levels to normal.[112] Consequently, replenishment should be performed with caution. If the serum potassium is dangerously low upon admission, potassium chloride or potassium phosphate may be added to the intravenous fluids, usually 20–40 mEq/L, unless the potassium continues to fall.[113] Potassium phosphate has the additional benefit of correcting the hypophosphatemia that often accompanies DKA. Phosphate replacement should be performed extremely cautiously if renal failure exists, as hyperphosphatemia may easily develop.[114] If rehydration causes hypomagnesemia, tetany and seizures are more likely, and magnesium replacement may be indicated for their prevention.

Hourly insulin administration should be continued until blood chemistries have returned to normal for at least 6 hours. Intermediate-acting insulin is usually started at this time, or within 24–48 hours of admission, to fulfill the need for regular insulin. The blood glucose level will be corrected more rapidly than the acidosis; therefore, when glucose becomes less than 250 mg/dL, 5% or 10% IV glucose solutions are given instead of normal saline.[115] DKA may worsen or persist as a result of premature discontinuation of exogenous insulin, and hypoglycemia may occur if the insulin infusion is not supplemented with glucose solutions at that time. It is especially important that the critical care nurse realize that the patient may pass from hyperglycemia to hypoglycemia without ever regaining consciousness; careful evaluation of all diagnostic parameters and blood glucose levels is a necessity.[116]

The nurse's role in the correction of DKA involves vigilant monitoring of serum chemistries and life-threatening symptoms of fluid, electrolyte, and acid-base imbalances. The goal of nursing management is supportive as well as preventive and should include educating the patient so that recurrences of life-threatening DKA can be avoided. The following care plan outlines standard critical care practices.

Nursing Care Plan for the Management of the Patient with Diabetic Ketoacidosis

Diagnosis	Signs and symptoms	Intervention	Rationale
Ineffective breathing pattern	Hyperventilation (marked overbreathing or air hunger)	Establish and maintain a patent airway	To support ventilation and maintain oxygenation
	Kussmaul breathing (rapid/deep)		The comatose patient may require intubation
	Sweet, fruity, sickly smell of ketosis; acetone odor of breath (may be difficult to detect)	Correct pH level	Increased amount of carbonic acid in the blood is a result of decreased pH
	Metabolic acidosis	Monitor ABGs	Indicates resolution of acidosis
Alteration in cardiac output	Tachycardia	Monitor vital signs frequently until the patient is conscious and reasonably alert	Provide assessment of heart's ability to compensate and maintain adequate cardiac output
	Hypotension		
		ECG monitoring	Volume and electrolyte abnormalities may lead to dysrhythmias; CAD is present in most diabetics and may be exacerbated in crisis
		Assess volume status	Volume depletion may lead to shock
Fluid volume deficit	Dehydration	Maintain NPO status	To control glucose and fluid status and protect against aspiration
	Dry, warm skin and mucous membranes		
	Decreased skin turgor	Initiate IV hydration with isotonic or hypotonic saline	Hypovolemic changes should be reversed as early as possible, but at a pace slow enough to avoid cerebral edema
	Orthostatic dizziness		
	Thirst	Start 1–2 large-bore peripheral IVs; infuse NS 100–200 mL at rapid infusion, then 200–500 mL/hr	
	Tachycardia		
	CVP < 1 mm Hg		
	Fever		
		Start CVP line	To determine volume status (hypotension, cardiac or renal impairment)
		Monitor VS every 15 minutes, until stable	For early assessment of changes

Diagnosis	Signs and symptoms	Intervention	Rationale
		Accurate I&O every 2–8 hrs.	Determine intake and output balance
		Check serum osmolarity every 8 hrs.	To evaluate the patient's return to normal osmolarity
Alteration in nutrition	Normal to elevated serum potassium level	Maintain NPO status	Allows IV replenishment without oral interference
	Ketones		
	Polyuria	Start NG tube, PRN	To restore normal carbohydrate, fat, and protein metabolism; to prevent aspiration by nauseated patient with altered mental status
	Polydipsia		
	Weakness and/or anorexia		
	Vomiting	Start IV—continuous infusion insulin 5–10 U/hr; regular insulin bolus dose 0.15 U/kg (before connecting infusion tubing)	To reverse the metabolic abnormalities caused by insufficient insulin
	Diarrhea		
	Gastric distress (abdominal pain)		
	Weight loss		
	Hypokalemia	Run 30 mL insulin solution through tubing	To saturate tubing absorption sites
		Establish urine output goal (based on renal status)	To restore water and electrolyte balance
		Conduct ECG	To estimate the presence of hypokalemia (low T waves with U waves) or hyperkalemia (high, peaked T waves)
		Begin potassium replacement; order lab assessment of serum potassium and alter potassium replacement PRN	To eliminate the catabolic state (potassium wasting in the urine secondary to polyuria, the inability of the kidney to conserve potassium) and the effects of vomiting and/or diarrhea
		5–10% glucose in half normal saline should be added to IV infusion when plasma glucose falls to 250 mg/dL	To prevent hypoglycemia and hypokalemia

Nursing Care Plan for the Management of the Patient with Diabetic Ketoacidosis

Diagnosis	Signs and symptoms	Intervention	Rationale
		Monitor electrolytes during rehydration and insulin administration	Hypomagnesemia and hypophosphatemia can occur
		Provide supportive care for abdominal discomfort (hot pads, pillows, etc.)	Rehydration usually resolves discomfort
		Administer bicarbonate as needed for persistent acidosis (pH < 7.0)	Acidosis should be treated cautiously; pH shifts alter oxygen availability and potassium levels
Impaired gas exchange	Kussmaul breathing	Treat for hyperglycemia	Is underlying cause of acidosis
	Fruity, acetone odor of breath (may be difficult to detect)	Administer sodium bicarbonate (1–2 mEq/kg of body weight as infusion over 2-hour period; amount of bicarb should not exceed 3 mEq/kg over 12 hours)	To correct acidosis
Potential for alteration in consciousness	Altered mental status (drowsiness, lethargy, stupor, coma)	Institute seizure precautions	To protect patient from injury
	Visual disturbances	NPO status	Protection of airway
	Hyperosmolarity	Administer 0.45 NS if osmolarity still > 300 after 4 hours of rehydration	Hypotonic solution reduces risk of worsening osmolarity
		Monitor glucose levels every hour during hydration and insulin administration	Many patients pass from hyperglycemia to hypoglycemia without regaining consciousness
		Neurologic testing with Glasgow coma scale until patient is fully conscious, then add cognitive function tests	DKA may produce long-term neurologic deficits

Diagnosis	Signs and symptoms	Intervention	Rationale
Lack of knowledge of disease, possible complications, and treatments	Nonadherence (fasting) Blood sugars persistently elevated Failure to contact physician when ill Failure to take prescribed insulin Failure to recognize the need for increased insulin with infection, stress, surgery, trauma, or pregnancy	Review basic principles of good diabetic management of medication (changes for sick days), diet, and exercise; stress management Assist the patient in accepting the diagnosis of diabetes Stress the life-threatening nature of DKA Define important diabetes-related concepts for patient: hypoglycemic unawareness, Somogyi effect, diabetic ketoacidosis	Patient needs solid understanding of causes of DKA in order to avoid precipitating crisis, when possible Patient in denial phase will not adhere to care regimen Patient needs to understand that only timely intervention will facilitate reversal Patients are at risk for serious complications related to glucose intolerance

Hyperglycemic Hyperosmolar Nonketotic Coma (HHNK)

Hyperglycemic hyperosmolar nonketotic coma (HHNK), or hyperglycemic dehydration syndrome, is an inherent risk for diabetics who are not ketosis-prone. These patients present with extreme hypertonic dehydration due to severe, uncontrolled blood glucose values, but with no ketosis. This abnormal carbohydrate metabolism is a result of the kidney's inability to excrete sufficient glucose, overproduction of glucose by the liver, and underutilization of glucose by the peripheral tissues.

Clinical antecedents

HHNK occurs most often in persons with mild or undiagnosed diabetes who have some endogenous insulin but not enough to combat hyperglycemia. The syndrome is caused by decreased insulin levels and untreated hyperglycemia. It is most often seen in individuals between the ages of 50 and 70 years, with Type II NIDDM. HHNK occurs with equal frequency in men and women. The typical patient may have NIDDM that is of recent onset or a result of neglect of glucose management. Even individuals who have been well controlled by diet or oral hypoglycemic agents may incur a stressor, such as infection, that alters either glucose mobilization from the liver or insulin requirements.

There are similarities in the precipitating factors for DKA and HHNK. Although HHNK may take a few days to develop, symptoms can appear in a few hours if the patient has experienced infection (particularly pneumonia), major surgery, trauma, severe stress, or any procedure where solutions containing large amounts of glucose are used, such as hyperalimentation or dialysis. Preceding HHNK, the patient may be under medical care for some significant illness—for example, MI, cerebral vascular accident, GI bleeding, or pancreatitis—and drugs used to treat that condition may predispose the patient to HHNK. Other medications that predispose the patient to HHNK are those that impair carbohydrate tolerance or cause the dehydration associated with the onset of HHNK. These medications (listed in Table 7-21) are glucocorticoids, diuretics (particularly thiazides), chlorthalidone, propranolol, immunosuppressive agents, diphenylhydantoin (Dilantin), diazoxide, and infused hypertonic solutions such as Mannitol or Dextran.

Generally, the HHNK patient has a longer history of physical complaints preceding the acute hyperglycemic event than does the DKA patient. The patient with underlying chronic illness is also more likely to develop HHNK because of a reduced tolerance of hyperglycemia and relative lack of support and compensatory mechanisms. Chronic illnesses preceding HHNK are likely to include renal, vascular, and cerebral diseases. (Refer back to Table 7-23 for a comparison of the presentations of the two hyperglycemic disorders DKA and HHNK.)

Critical referents

HHNK is caused by a relative rather than an absolute lack of insulin. This circulating insulin is adequate to prevent the breakdown of fats but inadequate to facilitate carbohydrate metabolism. The sufficient circulating insulin to inhibit lipolysis and its resultant ketone bodies is a primary difference between DKA and HHNK. Normally, ketones produced by the liver are in proportion to the circulating levels of FFAs. However, it seems that the levels of FFAs in HHNK are either normal or lower than those found in DKA. The result of the interaction between the relatively low level of insulin and the excess of antiinsulin hormones—growth hormone, cortisol, and glucagon—leads to an overproduction and underutilization of glucose, causing extreme hyperglycemia. Hyperglycemia is further accelerated by decreased renal excretion.

The characteristic high blood sugars, in the absence of ketoacidosis, cause profound hyperosmolarity, which can lead to dehydration, serious volume depletion, and shock. The osmotic diuresis seen in the patient depletes the total body water by an average of 24% with a loss of approximately 50 mEq/L of both sodium and potassium.[117] Although hypernatremia may be seen, there is a total body depletion of sodium and potassium similar to that of DKA, necessitating replacement via intravenous fluids. The persistent hyperglycemia (glucose levels often over 1000 mg/dL) coupled with the dehydration results in life-threatening hyperosmolarity.[118] This causes a high osmotic gradient to occur at the blood-brain barrier, resulting in cerebral dehydration and the appearance of central nervous system symptoms. If shock is profound or prolonged, a patient in HHNK may develop metabolic acidosis (although the cause for the metabolic acidosis is unknown in the majority of cases), as defined by a serum $PaPCO_2$ level less than 21 mEq/L or an arterial pH of 7.35 or less. This will be lactic acidosis, however, not ketoacidosis. Without early treatment, mortality is significantly higher (40–70%) than with DKA, even in patients of comparable age.[119]

The presence of severe hyperglycemia in the patient with HHNK may be due to factors other than a relative lack of insulin. Approximately 85% of the population will have preexisting renal disease.[120] Normally, the kidneys adjust for hyperglycemia by excreting large amounts of glucose (up to 20 g/hr) in the urine. In a patient with already compromised kidney function, the glomerular filtration rate is reduced, allowing less glucose to escape and increasing the plasma glucose level.

Resulting signs and symptoms

Because of a lack of adequate insulin, the patient with HHNK frequently presents with signs and symptoms similar to those of DKA. Approximately one-third of the patients with HHNK present in coma, and half with impaired consciousness.[121] In some patients, impaired consciousness follows the onset of vomiting. A positive Babinski sign may be present as well, causing the patient to be misdiagnosed with a CVA. Neurological examinations are always abnormal and may include hemisensory defects, transient hemiparesis, aphasia, and hyperreflexia. Seizures related to hyperosmolarity may accompany HHNK, although the electroencephalogram (EEG) is usually normal. Anticonvulsant medications are ineffective in HHNK and decrease the ability of the pancreas to secrete insulin, thereby enhancing hyperglycemia and exacerbating the metabolic acidosis. Neurological reassessment should be done after 48 hours to allow time for resolution of the symptoms. Alterations in consciousness may include drowsiness, disorientation, stupor, or coma. All patients with decreased sensorium should be screened for hyperglycemia so that prompt and appropriate management for HHNK can be started.

Physical examination will reveal severe dehydration but no Kussmaul breathing or acetone breath. Blood pressure may initially be maintained, even with accompanying dehydration, as the extracellular fluid is augmented by the fluid from the intracellular spaces and the catecholamines produce vasocon-

striction. Once the patient is treated with insulin, the glucose moves back into the cells, taking with it the fluid and potassium. After the initial treatment with insulin, this fluid shift accentuates hypotension and may cause shock, which is seen in 30% of the patients presenting with HHNK.[122]

Characteristically, the HHNK patient develops the classic symptoms of polyuria and polydipsia. These symptoms may persist for several days to several weeks, with an average duration of 12 days.[123] They may not be taken seriously until neurological changes occur. Other symptoms include dehydration, dry mucous membranes, poor skin turgor, tachycardia, oliguria, nausea, vomiting, and weight loss. Sodium depletion is generally present but may be an unreliable indicator because the ages and renal capabilities of patients vary.

Laboratory values for the patient with HHNK reflect dehydration and hyperglycemia, without ketone bodies or acidosis in most cases.

Nursing standards of care

A relative rather than an absolute lack of insulin is the underlying cause of HHNK. This insulin deficiency is almost always induced by other precipitating illnesses. It is necessary to detect and correct the underlying cause quickly and at the same time to initiate appropriate and aggressive treatment for correction of this life-threatening condition. Initially, fluid replacement is the most important objective, to correct the severe dehydration and hyperosmolarity. Sodium replacement is another objective, since the patient with HHNK presents with marked symptoms of sodium depletion. Insulin is administered to correct hyperglycemia, and potassium should be used judiciously to correct electrolyte imbalances. Early potassium replacement may be contraindicated by ECG evidence of hyperkalemia, known hyperkalemia, or oliguria.

The goal of nursing management, regardless of the treatment chosen, is to carefully monitor changes in the patient's condition so that fluid and electrolyte requirements can be adjusted to avoid iatrogenic complications such as cerebral edema or hypoglycemia. A nursing care plan for the HHNK patient follows.

Nursing Care Plan for the Management of the Patient with Hyperglycemic Hyperosmolar Nonketotic Coma

Diagnosis	Signs and symptoms	Intervention	Rationale
Alteration in cardiac output	Tachycardia Hypotension Hypovolemia CVP < 1 mm Hg Cool extremities Cyanosis Capillary cell refill < 3 sec	Monitor vital signs frequently until patient is conscious and reasonably alert Assess volume status with orthostasis checks, CVP monitoring, etc. Continuous ECG monitoring Assess 12-lead ECG daily	Vital sign changes such as tachycardia and hypotension may indicate decreased cardiac output To restore the body's normal circulating blood volume; volume depletion may lead to shock Diabetics are already at risk for CAD and stress of crisis may increase risk; altered electrolytes also predispose patient to dysrhythmias
Fluid volume deficit	Dehydration Dry, warm skin and mucous membranes Decreased skin turgor (unreliable, secondary to age) Orthostatic dizziness Hypotension Thirst (unreliable due to possible decrease in mental status; also varies with patient's age) Tachycardia Polyuria	Maintain NPO status Initiate IV hydration with normal saline (5 L during first 12 hours to adequately restore circulation) or half NS (recommended only when there is relative or absolute hypernatremia or if hyperosmolarity continues after rehydration) Start 1–2 large-bore peripheral IVs Start CVP line Monitor VS every 15 minutes, until patient is stable Monitor all intake and output every 2–8 hours	Reduce variables affecting fluid and electrolyte status and protect patient from aspiration Hypovolemic changes should be reversed as early as possible To prevent hypoglycemia, hypokalemia, and cerebral edema To determine volume status (hypotension, cardiac or renal impairment) For early assessment of changes To determine intake and output balance

Diagnosis	Signs and symptoms	Intervention	Rationale
Alteration in nutrition	Normal to elevated serum potassium level; total body potassium depleted	Maintain NPO status	Reduces interference with normalization of glucose and electrolytes; protects patient from aspiration
	Elevated serum glucose (>1000 mg/100 mL)	Correct insulin levels using loading IV dose and subsequent IV infusions of 2–5 U/hr	To reverse the metabolic abnormalities caused by insufficient insulin
		Determine renal status	To restore water and electrolyte balance and guide rehydration plan
		Monitor ECG for potassium changes (hypokalemia: low T waves with U waves; hyperkalemia: high peaked T waves)	Serum potassium levels vary widely and may change with treatment of hyperglycemia
		Monitor serum electrolytes	
		Begin potassium replacement, once urinary output is present (200–400 mEq may be needed in the first 48 hours)	To eliminate the catabolic state (potassium wasting in the urine secondary to polyuria, inability of kidneys to conserve potassium) and the effects of vomiting
		Order lab assessment of serum potassium; alter potassium replacement PRN	
		Test serum glucose levels every 1–4 hours	To assess return to normal and prevent overcorrection
Potential for alteration in consciousness	Altered mental status (drowsiness, lethargy, stupor, coma)	Observe patient for improving sensorium and increasing diuresis	These are signs of improvement
	Positive Babinski's	Maintain NPO status	Protects patient from aspiration
	Transient hemiparesis		
	Aphasia	Initiate seizure precautions	To protect patient from injury
	Hyperflexia	Monitor for neurological deficits	Increasing neurologic deficits are signs of worsening hyperosmolarity or too rapid correction of glucose disorder
	Seizures		
		Assess serum sodium levels	Hyponatremia is common in HHNK and may contribute to altered level of consciousness or seizures

Hypoglycemia

Hypoglycemia is a pathophysiological state in which the glucose requirements of the body outstrip glucose production. It is defined as a blood glucose level less than 50–60 mg/dL and is a frequent complication of the treatment of IDDM and NIDDM.[124] It accounts for approximately 4% of mortality in patients with IDDM.[125] In individuals with diabetes, hypoglycemia is almost always due to too much exogenous insulin or oral hypoglycemic agents, taken either deliberately or accidentally. Occurrences of hypoglycemia are generally characterized as mild to moderate if they can be managed by the patient or severe if assistance from others is needed. Severe prolonged or repeated episodes of hypoglycemia may cause substantial morbidity and/or mortality and can result in permanent brain damage if the patient survives.

Hypoglycemia can be categorized as postprandial, induced, or fasting. These classifications cover a broad range of patients exhibiting hypoglycemic symptoms, not just diabetics.

Clinical antecedents

Hypoglycemia is the most common acute complication of both Type I and Type II diabetes. Common risk factors for the development of hypoglycemia include the use of oral hypoglycemic agents, intensive insulin therapy, and nonadherence or lack of knowledge on the part of the patient. Defective glucose counterregulation, especially when combined with intensive insulin therapy, is another risk factor. After several years of diabetes, the diabetic's counterregulatory response to hypoglycemia is diminished, and the patient loses the ability to recognize symptoms as they develop. The patient is at increased risk for reactions because appropriate action is not taken quickly enough. This lack of timely response is termed hypoglycemic unawareness, and the neuroglycopenic manifestations may be the first symptoms to alert others that the patient is progressing to a severe reaction.[126] In addition, overcorrection of diabetic ketoacidosis can bring on a hypoglycemic crisis.

Hypoglycemic episodes can be precipitated in several ways. Insulin errors, both inadvertent and deliberate, are the most common cause of hypoglycemia. Reversal of morning and evening doses or of fast- and long-acting insulins are examples of these errors. Additionally, improper timing of or changes in the timing of insulin injections in relation to food intake can give rise to hypoglycemia, as can exercise and hot weather.

Changes in the rate at which insulin is absorbed constitute another factor that can induce hypoglycemia. Exercising the extremities can cause more rapid absorption, and a hypertrophied injection site can cause an erratic and unpredictable absorption rate. Switching to more purified insulins or human insulin can speed the rate of absorption.

Alterations in diet, either omitting food or consuming inadequate amounts, can precipitate a hypoglycemic episode. Problems with hypoglycemia can also develop from changing the timing of food intake—for example, delaying meals or snacks—or from prolonged and intense exercise.

Postprandial hypoglycemia occurs in the postoperative GI surgical patient or the child with inherited fructose intolerance. Any time a high-sugar substance is ingested, peristalsis is increased and the small intestine's contents are propelled more rapidly. When this action combines with the secretion of insulin, the individual develops hypoglycemia.[127]

Alcohol, marijuana, and other drugs can prevent awareness of hypoglycemia until it has progressed to a severe stage. The use of alcohol and/or drugs combined with physical activity at social gatherings can obscure the problem and thus preclude initiation of corrective measures, with a resultant sudden onset of severe hypoglycemia. Alcohol ingestion also impairs the body's ability to restore blood glucose levels to normal by inhibiting hepatic gluconeogenesis.

Critical referents

The prompt treatment and prevention of hypoglycemia is crucial because glucose is essential to normal brain metabolism. When glucose is unavailable, intracellular metabolites are used by brain cells for energy, causing changes to occur in membrane transport function, lipid and protein biosynthesis, concentrations of phosphate compounds, and secretion of neurotransmitters. Since it can neither synthesize nor store more than a few minutes' worth of glucose, the brain is dependent on a continuous supply of it and is insulin-insensitive.

Glucose homeostasis is regulated by insulin, glucagon, cortisol, epinephrine, and the growth hormone. The body responds to the hypoglycemic state by suppressing insulin production and increasing secretion of the other hormones. Various physiological conditions could reflect a hypoglycemic state. However, all hypoglycemia is a result of a level of circulating glucose lower than needed to meet requirements. Hypoglycemia develops when the amount of glucose entering the circulation is low compared to the amount of glucose leaving the circulation through glucose utilization—by the insulin-insensitive brain and insulin-sensitive muscle tissue. The primary problem originates from a defect in either glyconeogenesis, glycogenolysis, or carbohydrate absorption, although it may also occur after glucose is removed in large amounts through the adipose tissue, muscle, or liver.

Hypoglycemia is divided into three categories, according to physiological defects: induced hypoglycemia, fasting hypoglycemia, and postprandial hypoglycemia. Induced hypoglycemia is caused by overmedication with insulin or drugs that interfere with glucose metabolism in the liver (such as sulfonylureas, beta blockers, and salicylates) or ingestion of alcohol. Overmedication with insulin is, however, the most common cause. Fasting hypoglycemia occurs when there is a deficit in the nighttime surge of glucose released as a result of the drop in glucose levels during sleep. This occurs in the individual who reduces food intake in the evening hours and thus has insufficient glucose to meet the body's needs during the early morning. Postprandial hypoglycemia is the result of rapid passage of food through the small intestine, which is sufficient to stimulate the release of insulin but not adequate to allow for glucose absorption.

Another type of nighttime hypoglycemia is called the Somogyi effect, or sometimes the rebound effect. An excessive dosing of insulin causes hypoglycemia followed by glucose release and hyperglycemia.[128] Evidence that this condition exists is a wide disparity between the patient's early morning and postprandial glucose levels. The condition may remain undiagnosed for some time because the hypoglycemic period occurs while the patient is sleeping and does not present symptomatically. Treatment of this type of hypoglycemia consists simply of reducing the administration of insulin or oral hypoglycemic agent.

Resulting signs and symptoms

The clinical signs and symptoms of hypoglycemia are similar, regardless of the underlying cause. It is the degree and rate of decline of blood glucose level that result in variable symptoms. A rapid decrease in glucose levels activates the autonomic nervous system, and epinephrine is subsequently released. As the blood glucose level falls into the range 50–70 mg/dL, the central nervous system is stimulated, and the patient may experience sweating, nervousness, trembling, nausea, vomiting, hunger, fatigue, weakness, anxiety, piloerection, tachycardia, and palpitations.[129] When there is a gradually decreased utilization of oxygen by the brain and/or hypoglycemia is severe or prolonged, hypoglycemic symptoms occur more gradually and may include headache, lightheadedness, faintness, visual changes, lethargy, somnolence, and yawning. Additionally, the patient may demonstrate restlessness, agitation, mental confusion, temper outbursts, slurred or thick speech, and strange or bizarre behavior. When the blood glucose level falls below 40 mg/dL, clonic convulsions may develop. This level of dysfunction is usually termed insulin shock.[130] As the blood glucose level continues to decline, the convulsions cease, and the patient proceeds into coma. Glucose levels controlled by insulin tend to fall faster than those controlled by oral hypoglycemics, making the individual with IDDM at higher risk for hypoglycemic shock than the one with NIDDM. The individual without diabetes can also develop diabetic shock if hypoglycemia is significant. The causes of hypoglycemia in this patient include hypopituitarism, hypoadrenalism, renal disease, hepatic disease, and septic shock. Reactive hypoglycemia following high glucose ingestion presents as hypoglycemic symptoms 4–5 hours later.

Chronic alcohol abuse can also cause hypoglycemia by inhibiting glycogen breakdown. The signs and symptoms of alcohol-induced hypoglycemia are primarily neurological in nature: trismus, positive Babinski, hypothermia, extensor rigidity of extremities, and conjugate deviation of the eyes.[131]

Hypoglycemic unawareness, as noted earlier, is a phenomenon that prevents self-recognition of hypoglycemia, which in turn can prevent self-correction as well as timely intervention by the health professional. The patient with hypoglycemic unawareness does not experience early-warning signs such as mood swings or weakness. The patient may be perfectly coherent on admission or may be unusually slow to react, with impaired memory and judgment and can deteriorate directly into an unconscious state. Frequent and prolonged episodes of hypoglycemia can result in extensive and permanent mental or neurological damage.

Nursing standards of care

The distressing symptoms experienced by the patient with episodes of hypoglycemia may range in severity from short-term, subtle behavioral changes to coma or, sometimes, death. It is essential to detect and correct falling blood glucose levels in order to prevent the development of severe hypoglycemia and its attendant neuroglycopenia. The IDDM patient will experience a hypoglycemic episode at some time, and the treatment given depends upon whether the reaction is mild or severe. It should be noted that episodes of hypoglycemia are usually the reason for admission to the critical care area only when they are at their most severe. Significant hypoglycemia may occur in the critically ill patient because of catecholamines, reduced food intake, or physiologic and emotional stress.

Effective prevention and management can be realized only if the patient is performing glucose self-monitoring. In this way, the patient is able to make adjustments in therapy based on test results. Monitoring blood sugar is an essential tool for the patient experiencing hypoglycemic unawareness. The patient should be instructed to immediately treat all blood glucose levels deemed to be in the hypoglycemic range. The challenge of insulin therapy is to achieve euglycemia without producing hypoglycemia. Nevertheless, for the patient, learning to recognize and to treat hypoglycemic symptoms when they do occur are essential survival skills. The objective of treatment is to correct the underlying cause, which generally involves decreasing circulating insulin as well as stimulating the glucose counterregulatory systems.

To prevent progression of symptoms, all episodes of hypoglycemia should be treated promptly. For mild reactions, about 10–15 g of simple sugars will restore blood glucose levels and alleviate symptoms. Fruit juice (unsweetened), hard candy, honey, syrup, and granulated sugar or sugar cubes are all examples of simple sugars that will quickly raise the blood glucose level and stop a reaction. Premeasured glucose tablets are commercially available and have the benefit of helping to avoid overtreatment. Hypoglycemic reactions that occur at night should be treated with a portion of simple sugar followed by a longer-acting mix of carbohydrate and protein such as milk and crackers to prevent further nocturnal episodes.

Moderate hypoglycemic reactions may be treated in the same manner as milder episodes; however, restoration of normal blood glucose may require more time and repeated treatment with substances such as Monogel or icing. If the patient cannot be persuaded to ingest the necessary carbohydrate, glucose may be placed directly on the buccal mucosa or 1 mg of parenteral glucagon may be administered.

The patient experiencing severe hypoglycemia may have impaired consciousness and be unable to swallow oral carbohydrate. The individual should be given either IV glucose or glucagon, if available, immediately. Glucose is administered as 50% dextrose over 1–3 minutes. After this bolus, 5–10% glucose should be administered intravenously until the patient can resume eating. Improvement should be seen within 1–5 minutes after IV glucose and within 15 minutes after the administration of glucagon. Normal mental functioning may not return for several hours following an especially severe or prolonged hypoglycemic episode. If the patient experiences convulsions, headache, lethargy, amnesia, vomiting, and/or decreased muscle control during the episode, further medical attention may be required.

The following nursing care plan addresses the more severe symptoms of hypoglycemia in the critically ill patient.

Nursing Care Plan for the Management of the Patient with Hypoglycemia

Diagnosis	Signs and symptoms	Intervention	Rationale
Alteration in cardiac output	Tachycardia Hypotension Hypothermia Diaphoresis	Monitor vital signs frequently until patient is conscious and reasonably alert	To detect changes in status
Alteration in nutrition	Decreased plasma glucose, < 60 mg/dL Weakness Hunger	Maintain NPO status (depending on state of consciousness)	To protect patient from aspiration
		IV bolus 50% dextrose over 1–3 minutes; IV glucose 5–10 G/hr administered after bolus, until patient can resume PO intake	To reverse the metabolic abnormalities caused by insufficient glucose
		Order lab assessment of plasma glucose	Reflects glucose available for metabolic function and body growth and maintenance; reveals patient trends and response to treatment
Potential for alteration in consciousness	Altered mental status (headache, lightheadedness, drowsiness, lethargy, stupor, coma)	Exercise seizure precautions	To protect patient from injury and aspiration
		Keep flow sheet at bedside	To assess trends
	Visual changes	Assess relationship of changes to insulin administration	Hypoglycemic unawareness and Somogyi effect make hypoglycemia more difficult to predict and manage
Lack of knowledge of disease, possible complications, and treatments	Nonadherence (fasting) Blood glucose persistently low Failure to contact physician	Review basic principles of good diabetic management: medication (changes for sick days), diet, exercise, stress management	Solid understanding of causes of hypoglycemia
	Failure to recognize the need to increase carbohydrate intake	Instruct patient in blood glucose monitoring	Facilitates timely intervention and reversal of hypoglycemia
		Instruct patient to keep glucose supply on person at all times	So patient can take glucose when a rapid hypoglycemic attack occurs

CHAPTER 7 POST-TEST

Refer to the following clinical vignette to answer questions 1 and 2.

P. S. is a 56-year-old ventilator-dependent COPD patient in the MICU. Today you notice that he is more difficult to arouse than usual, and he has gained 2 kg in the past day. Lab results from this morning are as follows:

Na: 122 mEq/L

Cl: 96 mEq/L

K: 3.1 mEq/L

Ca: 8.8 mEq/L

Cr: 1.4 mg %

BUN: 40 mg %

Hct: 24 mg %

Hgb: 8.9 mg %

WBC: 4.9/mm³

Platelets: 166,000/mm³

1. The most likely disturbance represented by this clinical picture is:
   a. acute renal failure.
   b. diabetes exacerbation.
   c. syndrome of inappropriate ADH.
   d. hypocalcemia.

2. The first therapeutic measure to be implemented will probably be:
   a. diuresis.
   b. hypertonic saline infusion.
   c. insertion of an oral airway.
   d. potassium replenishment.

3. ADH is:
   a. produced by the pituitary and stored in the hypothalamus.
   b. responsible for water diuresis and sodium retention.
   c. responsible for water retention and sodium diuresis.
   d. produced in excess quantities in diabetes insipidus.

4. The most common acute crisis of diabetes is:
   a. diabetic ketoacidosis.
   b. hyperglycemic, hyperosmolar nonketotic coma.
   c. hypoglycemia.
   d. myocardial infarction.

5. The major difference between DKA and HHNK are:
   a. the presence of acidosis and the type of diabetes.
   b. the neurological symptoms and the level of glucose.
   c. the presence of ketones and polyuria.
   d. the age of the patient and the type of fluid and insulin treatment.

6. Other complications of diabetes include:
   a. bladder incontinence from neuropathy.
   b. retinal detachment.
   c. constipation.
   d. hypersensitive peripheral skin.

ENDNOTES

1. Farish, D. J. (1993). *Human Biology*. Boston: Jones and Bartlett.

2. Bersten, A., and Sibbald, W. J. (1989). Acute lung injury in septic shock. *Critical Care Clinics* 5(1): 49–79.

3. Sanford, S. J. (1980). Dysfunction of the adrenal gland: Physiologic considerations and nursing problems. *Nursing Clinics of North America* 15: 481–498.

4. Sanford, S. J. (1988). Endocrine crises and patient care. In M. R. Kinney, D. R. Packa, and S. B. Dunbar (Eds.), *AACN's Clinical Reference for Critical Care Nursing*. 2nd edition (pp. 1088–1110). New York: McGraw-Hill; Zaloga, G. P., and Smallridge, R. C. (1985). Thyroidal alterations in acute illness. *Seminars in Respiratory Medicine* 7: 95–99.

5. Zaloga and Smallridge, op. cit.; Sanford (1980), op. cit.

6. Grekin, R. (1986). The adrenal gland. In E. L. Mazzaferri (Ed.), *Textbook of Endocrinology*. 3rd edition (pp. 351–364). Medical Examination Publishing; Ahrens, T.,

and Langfitt, D. (1991). *Critical Care Certification Preparation and Review*. Norwalk, CT: Appleton-Lange.

7. Grekin, op. cit.; Ahrens and Langfitt, op. cit.

8. Sanford (1980), op. cit.; Grekin, op. cit.; Ahrens and Langfitt, op. cit.; Passmore, J. M. (1985). Adrenal cortex. In G. W. Geelhoed and B. Chernow (Eds.), *Endocrine Aspects of Acute Illness* (pp. 97–134). New York: Churchill Livingstone.

9. Sanford (1980), op. cit.; Grekin, op. cit.

10. Sanford (1980), op. cit.

11. Ahrens and Langfitt, op. cit.; Passmore, op. cit.

12. Grekin, op. cit.; Ahrens and Langfitt, op. cit.

13. Gotch, P. M. (1991). The endocrine system. In J. G. Alspach and S. M. Williams (Eds.), *Core Curriculum for Critical Care Nursing*. 3rd edition (pp. 452–494). Philadelphia: W. B. Saunders.

14. Ahrens and Langfitt, op. cit.

15. Grekin, op. cit.; Ahrens and Langfitt, op. cit.; Sanford (1988), op. cit.

16. Sanford (1980), op. cit.; Grekin, op. cit.

17. Williams, P. L.; Warwick, R.; Dyson, M.; and Bannister, L. H. (1989). *Gray's Anatomy*. 37th edition. London: Churchill Livingstone.

18. Methany, N. M., and Snively, W. D. (1983). *Nurses Handbook of Fluid Balance* (p. 38). Philadelphia: Lippincott.

19. Chernow, B., Wiley, S. C., and Zaloga, G. P. (1987). Critical care endocrinology. In J. E. Parillo (Ed.), *Current Treatment in Critical Care Medicine*. Toronto: B. C. Decker, Inc.

20. Ibid.

21. Crowley, L. V. (1992). *Introduction to Human Disease*. 3rd ed. Boston: Jones and Bartlett.

22. Newmark, S. R. (1977). Axioms on hyperthyroidism. *Hospital Medicine* 13(11): 6–17.

23. Braverman, L. E., and Chiovato, L. (1985). Thyroid storm. In J. M. Rippe et al. (Eds.), *Intensive Care Medicine* (pp. 798–801). Boston: Little, Brown.

24. Chernow et al., op. cit.

25. Ibid.

26. Ibid.

27. Braverman and Chiovato, op. cit.

28. Chernow et al., op. cit.

29. Isley, W. L. (1990). Thyroid disorders. *Critical Care Nursing Quarterly* 13(3): 39–49.

30. Chernow et al., op. cit.

31. McMillan, J. Y. (1988). Preventing myxedema coma in the hypothyroid patient. *Dimensions of Critical Care Nursing* 7(3): 136–144.

32. Isley, op. cit.

33. Ibid.

34. Ibid.

35. Sanford (1988), op. cit.

36. Chernow et al., op. cit.

37. Zaloga and Smallridge, op. cit.

38. Weigle, C. G. M. (1987). Metabolic and endocrine disease in pediatric intensive care. In M. C. Rogers (Ed.), *Textbook of Pediatric Intensive Care* (pp. 1057–1109). Baltimore: Williams and Wilkins.

39. Grekin, op. cit.; Goldfein, A. (1983). The adrenal medulla. In F. S. Greenspan and P. H. Forsham (Eds.), *Basic and Clinical Endocrinology* (pp. 311–329). Los Altos, CA: Lange Medical.

40. Ayala, L. A. (1985). Pheochromocytoma. In G. W. Geelhoed and B. Chernow, (Eds.), *Endocrine Aspects of Acute Illness* (pp. 239–256). New York: Churchill Livingstone.

41. Grekin, op. cit.; Sanford (1988), op. cit.

42. Grekin, op. cit.

43. Ayala, op. cit.

44. Ibid.

45. Goldfein, op. cit.

46. Sanford (1980), op. cit.; Sanford (1988), op. cit.

47. Grekin, op. cit.; Weigle, op. cit.; Ayala, op. cit.

48. Ayala, op. cit.

49. Chernow et al., op. cit.

50. Sanford (1988), op. cit.; Weigle, op. cit.; Goldfein, op. cit.; Ayala, op. cit.

51. Grekin, op. cit.; Ayala, op. cit.

52. Goldfein, op. cit.; Ayala, op. cit.

53. Liddle, G. W. (1981). The adrenal. In R. H. Williams (Ed.), *Textbook of Endocrinology*. 6th edition (pp. 249–292). Philadelphia: W. B. Saunders.

54. Ayala, op. cit.

55. Weigle, op. cit.; Goldfein, op. cit.; Ayala, op. cit.

56. Sanford (1988), op. cit.

57. Passmore, op. cit.

58. Gotch, op. cit.

59. Reasner, C. A. (1990). Adrenal disorders. *Critical Care Nursing Quarterly* 13(3): 67–73.

60. Jumey, T. H.; Cockrell, J. L.; Lindberg, J. S.; Lamiell, J. M.; and Wade, C. E. (1987). Spectrum of serum cortisol response to ACTH in ICU patients. *Chest* 92: 292–295.

61. Ahrens and Langfitt, op. cit.

62. Burrell, L. O., and Burrell, Z. L. (1982). *Critical Care*. St. Louis: C. V. Mosby; Schimke, R. N. (1980). Adrenal insufficiency. *Critical Care Quarterly* 3(2): 19–27.

63. Ibid.

64. Hurst, J. W. (Ed.). (1987). *Medicine for the Practicing Physician*. 2nd edition. Boston: Little Brown.

65. Sanford (1988), op. cit.

66. Hamburger, S., Rush, D. R., and Bosker, G. (1984). *Endocrine and Metabolic Emergencies*. Bowie, MD: Robert J. Brady; Tzagournis, M. (1978). Acute adrenal insufficiency. *Heart & Lung* 7: 603–609.

67. Sanford (1988), op. cit.

68. Passmore, op. cit.

69. Sanford (1988), op. cit.

70. Passmore, op. cit.; Sanford (1988), op. cit.

71. Burrell and Burrell, op. cit.

72. Burrell and Burrell, op. cit.; Hamburger et al., op. cit.

73. Ahrens and Langfitt, op. cit.; Passmore, op. cit.; Tzagournis, op. cit.

74. Passmore, op. cit.; Hamburger et al., op. cit.; Tzagournis, op. cit.

75. Hamburger et al., op. cit.; Tyrrell, J. B., and Forsham, P. H. (1983). Glucocorticoids and adrenal androgens. In F. S. Greenspan and P. H. Forsham (Eds.), *Basic and Clinical Endocrinology* (pp. 258–2194). Los Altos: Lange Medical.

76. Hamburger et al., op. cit.

77. Grekin, op. cit.; Hamburger et al., op. cit.

78. Sanford (1980), op. cit.; Tyrrell and Forsham, op. cit.

79. Hamburger et al., op. cit.

80. Reasner, op. cit.

81. Ibid.

82. Passmore, op. cit.; Burrell and Burrell, op. cit.

83. Passmore, op. cit.; Liddle, op. cit.; Weigle, op. cit.

84. Sanford (1988), op. cit.

85. Gotch, op. cit.

86. Graves, L. (1990). Diabetic ketoacidosis and hyperosmolar nonketotic coma. *Critical Care Nursing Quarterly* 13(3): 50–61.

87. Stitt, N. L. (1992). Defeating diabetes: Islet cell transplantation. In *AACN Proceedings Celebrating Partnerships* (NTI 1992) (pp. 305–307). Aliso Viejo, CA: AACN.

88. Sanford (1988), op. cit.

89. Sutherland, D. (1988). An update on pancreatic transplantation. *Surgery Annual* 20: 330–337.

90. Stitt, op. cit.

91. Coleman, M. A.; Hogan, D. E.; Moir, E. J.; Schaffield, M. M.; and Seidel, J. C. (1989). Carol was up one day, down the next. *Nursing 89*(1): 44–51.

92. Stitt, op. cit.

93. Starzl, T. E.; Fung, J.; Jordan, M.; et al. (1990). Kidney transplantation under FK 506. *JAMA* 264: 63–67.

94. Sabo, C. E. (1989). Managing DKA and preventing a recurrence. *Nursing 89*(2): 50–56.

95. Graves, op. cit.; Androgue, H. J.; Barrero, J.; and Eknoyan, G. (1989). Salutary effects of modest fluid replacement in the treatment of adults with diabetic ketoacidosis. *JAMA* 262: 2108–2113.

96. Zaloga and Smallridge, op. cit.; Graves, op. cit.

97. Zaloga and Smallridge, op. cit.

98. Graves, op. cit.

99. Georgopoulos, A., and Margoles, S. (1982, May). Diabetic ketoacidosis: Pitfalls in management. *Hospital Medicine:* 51–64.

100. Graves, op. cit.

101. Graves, op. cit.

102. Georgopoulos and Margoles, op. cit.; American Diabetes Association. (1988). *Physician's Guide to Insulin Dependency (Type I).* ADA.

103. Graves, op. cit.

104. American Diabetes Association, op. cit.

105. Graves, op. cit.

106. American Diabetes Association, op. cit.

107. Graves, op. cit.; Androgue et al., op. cit.

108. Zaloga and Smallridge, op. cit.; Graves, op. cit.

109. Graves, op. cit.; American Diabetes Association, op. cit.

110. Morris, L. R., Murphy, M. B., and Kitabchi, A. E. (1986). Bicarbonate therapy in severe diabetic ketoacidosis. *Annals of Internal Medicine 105:* 836–840; Lumley, W. (1988). Controlling hypoglycemia and hyperglycemia. *Nursing 88*(10): 34–42.

111. Graves, op. cit.; Georgopoulos and Margoles, op. cit.; American Diabetes Association, op. cit.

112. Georgopoulos and Margoles, op. cit.; Gregerman, R. I. (1986). Diabetes mellitus. In *Principles of Ambulatory Medicine.* 2nd edition. Baltimore: Williams and Wilkins.

113. Graves, op. cit.; Georgopoulos and Margoles, op. cit.; American Diabetes Association, op. cit.

114. Gregerman, op. cit.

115. Zaloga and Smallridge, op. cit.; American Diabetes Association, op. cit. Gregerman, op. cit.

116. Georgopoulos and Margoles, op. cit.; Gregerman, op. cit.

117. Graves, op. cit.

118. Ibid.

119. Graves, op. cit.; Georgopoulos and Margoles, op. cit.; American Diabetes Association, op. cit.

120. American Diabetes Association, op. cit.

121. Lumley, W. A. (1989). Recognizing and reversing insulin shock. *Nursing 89*(9): 34–41.

122. Georgopoulos and Margoles, op. cit.; Lumley (1988), op. cit.

123. American Diabetes Association, op. cit.; Georgopoulos and Margoles, op. cit.; Lumley (1988), op. cit.

124. Zaloga and Smallridge, op. cit.; Graves, op. cit.; American Diabetes Association, op. cit.; Gregerman, op. cit.

125. Lumley (1988), op. cit.

126. Georgopoulos and Margoles, op. cit.; American Diabetes Association, op. cit.; Gregerman, op. cit.; Lumley (1988), op. cit.

127. Gregerman, op. cit.

128. Gregerman, op. cit.; Lumley (1988), op. cit.; Lumley (1989), op. cit.

129. Lumley (1989), op. cit.

130. Gregerman, op. cit.

131. Gregerman, op. cit.; Lumley (1988), op. cit.; Lumley (1989), op. cit.

The Hematologic and Immune Systems

8

CHAPTER 8 PRE-TEST

1. The most common phagocyte deficiency is:
   a. AIDS.
   b. neutropenia.
   c. toxic bone marrow suppression.
   d. immunoglobulin deficiency.

2. The end product of hemolysis is:
   a. thrombin.
   b. bilirubin.
   c. creatinine.
   d. hemoglobin.

3. A person who has blood type A positive:
   a. has A antibodies in the serum.
   b. has B antibodies in the serum.
   c. has a positive core antigen A.
   d. has red blood cells containing antigen B.

4. A. L. is a 24-year-old victim of blunt trauma to the abdomen and flank in a motor vehicle accident. The patient has a ruptured spleen requiring splenectomy and hepatic contusion. These injuries place A. L. at risk for what hematologic complications?
   a. OPSI, coagulopathy
   b. viral infection, jaundice
   c. hemolytic anemia, DIC
   d. massive hemorrhage, neutropenia

5. During an admission assessment, a patient with acute respiratory distress and fever reveals to you that he had a positive HIV antibody test last year at a private clinic. He wants you to tell no one. You should:
   a. respect his wishes.
   b. inform the health department only so that staff can contact potentially infected individuals.
   c. record the conversation in the chart, and mark the chart HIV-positive so other health care workers know the potential risk of infection they face.
   d. respond that you are obligated to report his statement to medical personnel and that to do so is in the best interests of treating his current health problems.

6. L. T. is a 35-year-old previously healthy male admitted for pneumocystis pneumonia. He is confirmed HIV-positive with a CD4 count of 300. The CDC classification for his present disease is:
   a. A.
   b. B2.
   c. C1.
   d. C2.

7. Production of immunoglobulins for humoral immunity is the function of:
   a. B cells.
   b. T cells.
   c. macrophages.
   d. stem cells.

8. The pathophysiology of HIV infection is:
   a. immunoglobulin deficiency.
   b. reduced T helper cells.
   c. overproduction of T suppressor cells.
   d. depleted natural killer cells.

9. Nursing responsibilities in administration of platelet concentrates include:
   a. checking for ABO and Rh compatibility.
   b. administering the product slowly through a blood filter.
   c. obtaining a post-platelet count 20–60 minutes after the end of infusion.
   d. pretreating patient with Solu-Medrol to decrease reactions.

B. K., an adolescent, complains of bruising easily and has slightly elevated creatinine and respiratory distress with mild hypoxemia. She reports a 2-week history of an acute viral episode followed by general malaise and illness. Laboratory findings are as follows:

Hct	30 mg %
Hgb	11.9 mg %
Platelets	102,000/mm^3
WBC	12,900/mm^3
Granulocytes	50%
Monocytes	12%
Lymphocytes	38%

10. The patient's symptoms are representative of:
    a. disseminated intravascular coagulation.
    b. acute onset leukemia.
    c. bacterial infection.
    d. idiopathic thrombocytopenia purpura.

11. A. H. is a 61-year-old acute MI patient who has received a stat dose of tissue plasminogen activator (TPA) followed by a continuous infusion. She now presents with new acute chest pain. The health care team determines that the symptoms warrant cardiac catheterization with possible angioplasty. The nurse recognizes the following fact regarding TPA:
    a. the patient's thrombin time will be prolonged for approximately 2 days after

drug discontinuation and thus does not predict risk of bleeding.

b. TPA can and should be reversed with Amicar prior to catheterization.

c. TPA's half-life permits discontinutation of medication and correction of bleeding status within 3–6 hours.

d. TPA's potency does not warrant concerns about bleeding with the catheterization procedure.

Blood

Blood, the fluid that circulates through the heart, arteries, capillaries, and veins, is the chief means of transport in the body. Blood transports oxygen from the lungs to body tissues, and carbon dioxide from tissues to the lungs for excretion; carries nutrients and metabolites to the tissues; distributes hormones from endocrine glands to the organs they influence; removes waste products to the kidneys and other organs of excretion; brings blood cells and antibodies to the point of infection; and carries blood clotting substances to breaks in blood vessels. Blood has other important functions; it plays an essential role in maintaining proper fluid balance, and helps in regulation of body temperature by carrying excess heat from the interior of the body to the surface layers of the skin where the heat is dissipated to the surrounding air.[1]

Blood also has a minor role in maintaining the acid-base balance in the body.

The total quantity of blood in the body varies depending on body weight. A person's blood volume is approximately 70 mL/kg body weight; thus, a person weighing 150 pounds (68 kg) has a blood volume of 4760 mL, or approximately 5 L. Blood is composed of two parts: plasma (the fluid portion) and formed elements (blood cells and platelets), which are suspended in the fluid. Plasma accounts for approximately 55% of the total volume of blood in the body (see Figure 8-1). The formed elements of the blood (RBCs, WBCs, and platelets) comprise the remaining 45% of the total blood volume. When whole blood clots, fibrinogen, a blood protein essential for normal clotting, is removed from plasma, yielding serum. Plasma will be discussed first.

Plasma

Plasma is 92% water and 7% protein. The remaining 1% of plasma consists of inorganic salts; nonprotein organic substances such as urea, uric acid, and creatinine; dissolved gases; hormones; and enzymes. Albumin, globulins, and fibrinogen constitute the greatest portion of the plasma proteins. Albumin, the most abundant protein in plasma, is produced in the liver and is important for nutrition of body cells and for causing body water to be retained in the intravascular fluid compartment.

Serum electrophoresis has enabled the grouping of the globulins in plasma into three major categories: alpha, beta, and gamma. The alpha and beta globulins consist of various proteins that aid in transporting nutrients and other substances in the blood or are involved in physiological processes such as clotting or inflammation. Among the proteins in the alpha band are alpha-1 antitrypsin, high density lipoprotein (HDL), prothrombin, and ceruloplasmin (the blood protein that transports copper). Complement proteins, important in fighting inflammation and resisting infection, comprise approximately 30% of the proteins in the beta band. Among the other beta proteins are the low density and very low density lipoproteins (LDL). The gamma globulins consist almost entirely of immunoglobulins, or antibodies, which are important in defending the body against infections by microorganisms. In the past it was believed that immunoglobulins were only found

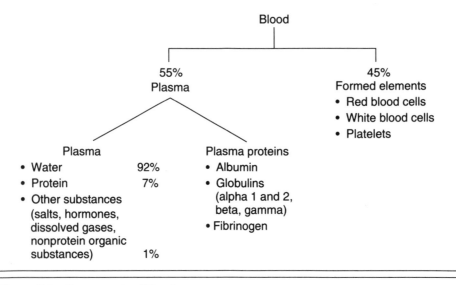

Figure 8-1 Components of Blood

in the gamma region of the electrophoresis band. For that reason, gamma globulin was used as a synonym for antibody. It is now known that some immunoglobulins are found in the beta regions, so the term *immunoglobulin* is currently used to refer to serum antibodies.

Hematopoiesis

Blood cell development is known as hematopoiesis, or hemopoiesis. All blood cells develop from stem cells. The stem cell is often termed a pluripotential or multipotential stem cell, since it has the potential to develop into many types of cells. In humans, blood cell development begins in the yolk sac at about the sixth week of gestation. The hematopoietic stem cells then migrate to the liver, spleen, and thymus (see Figure 8-2). After 20 weeks of gestation, the blood-forming cells migrate to the bone marrow. At birth, hematopoiesis takes place in almost all bones. Bone

marrow that is a site of hematopoiesis is termed red marrow. Gradually, as part of the maturation process, the hematopoietic cells in the bones become replaced by fat; blood cell development no longer takes place in this yellow marrow. By adulthood, hematopoiesis is confined to the red marrow in the flat bones of the skull, vertebrae, ribs, sternum, iliac crest, and the ends of the femur and humerus.

Various conditions can stimulate hemopoiesis to recur at sites that produced blood cells in the fetus, such as the spleen or liver. This phenomenon is termed extramedullary hematopoiesis and can be seen in certain disease states, such as leukemia, in which the red bone marrow is no longer capable of adequate blood cell production.

As mentioned, all blood cells derive from pluripotential stem cells (see Figure 8-3). When stimulated by certain chemical messages, stem cells begin to develop into one of several types of blood cells: red blood cells (RBCs), white blood cells (WBCs), or

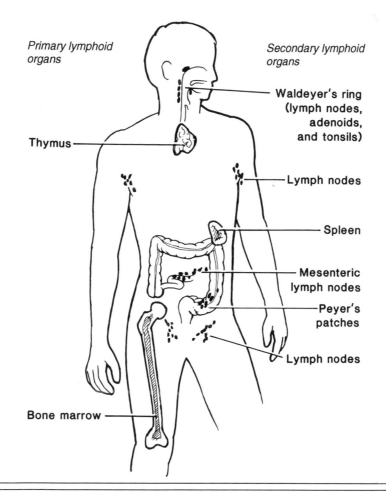

Figure 8-2 Hematopoietic Organs
Source: Roitt, I. M., Brostoff, J., and Male, D. K. (1989). *Immunology.* 2nd edition. St. Louis: C. V. Mosby Co.

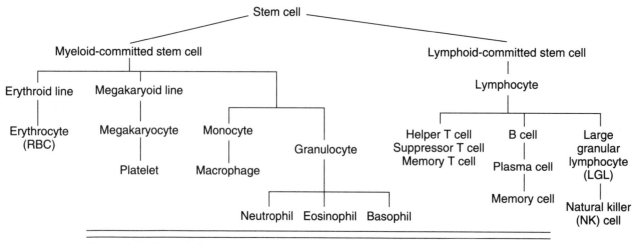

Figure 8-3   Stem Cell

platelets (which some consider to be a type of white blood cell). The chemical messages stimulating the stem cells to develop into different types of blood cells are called colony stimulating factors (CSFs). These hormone-like glycoproteins are the regulators of hematopoiesis. Feedback mechanisms regulate the release of CSFs from various cells in the body. CSFs have been clearly defined and can now be produced by recombinant technology. They are used therapeutically to enhance the production of specific

cellular components in patients with bone marrow suppression, uremia-induced anemia, and other disorders.[2] A list of common CSFs is given in Table 8-1.

The stem cell is believed to develop first into either a myeloid-committed stem cell or a lymphoid-committed stem cell. Myeloid-committed stem cells can later develop into red blood cells, platelets, or certain types of white blood cells (the granulocytes and the monocytes). Lymphoid-committed stem cells develop into lymphocytes, a special type of

Table 8-1   Colony Stimulating Factors

Name	Lineage	Cellular Sources (if known)
Hemopoietin-1	Multilineage	
Burst promoting activity (BPA)	Multilineage (specifically erythroid)	
Interleukin 3 (IL-3)	Multilineage	T cells
Granulocyte-macrophage colony stimulating factor (GM-CSF)	Multilineage	T cells Endothelial cells Fibroblasts
Megakaryocyte colony stimulating factor (Mk-CSF)	Multilineage (specifically megakaryocytic)	
Granulocyte colony stimulating factor (G-CSF)	Neutrophilic/granulocytic	Monocytes Fibroblasts
Monocyte colony stimulating factor (M-CSF) (CSF-1)	Mononuclear phagocytic	Monocytes Fibroblasts Endothelial cells
Eosinophil colony stimulating factor (Eo-CSF)	Eosinophilic granulocytic	
Erythropoietin	Erythroid	Kidney
Thrombopoietin	Megakaryocytic	Kidney/liver

Source: Adapted from Golde, David W., (Ed.). (1984). *Hematopoiesis.* New York: Churchill Livingstone; Clark, S. C.; Kamen, R. (1984). The human hematopoietic colony-stimulating factors. *Science 236:* 1229–1237.

white blood cell. Although a white blood cell can arise from either a myeloid or a lymphoid-committed stem, *only lymphocytes are produced by lymphoid-committed stem cells; all other blood cells, including some nonlymphocytic white blood cells, arise from myeloid-committed stem cells.* Research has shown that stem cells are able to circulate in the blood and can reenter ablated marrow to reestablish hemopoiesis. This is the basis for the newly developed stem cell transplant procedures performed for some cancer patients and patients with hematologic disorders.[3]

Dysmyelopoiesis is abnormal blood cell development such as occurs in patients with hematologic malignancies. Too few of any type of cells is indicated by the suffix *-penia;* too many is indicated by the suffix *-cytosis* or *-philia.* Production of blood cells is based upon negative feedback mechanisms and can drop to zero or can increase to many times normal depending upon the body's requirements.

Red Blood Cells

Red blood cells (RBCs, or erythrocytes) are flexible biconcave discs without nuclei. The primary function of red blood cells is to deliver oxygen from inspired air to the tissues and provide for the removal of carbon dioxide, the waste product of cellular metabolism. The average adult has approximately 35 trillion erythrocytes. The red blood cell count is the number of erythrocytes per cubic millimeter of whole blood; a normal count is approximately 5 million cells/mm^3. The body destroys 180 million erythrocytes per minute and therefore must produce 180 million per minute to maintain a stable number of such cells.

The life-span of a red blood cell ranges from 110 to 120 days. Red blood cells arise from stem cells in the bone marrow and progress through several stages of development prior to being released into the circulation. Although fully developed red blood cells are anucleate, nuclei are present in red blood cells during the earlier developmental stages. Nucleated RBCs are sometimes seen in peripheral blood and usually indicate intense erythropoiesis or extramedullary hemopoiesis. They may also be seen in persons with asplenia, sickle cell anemia, thalassemia, leukemia, or invasion of the bone marrow by cancer.

Erythrocytes in the next-to-last stage of development are called reticulocytes; they can be thought of as "juvenile" erythrocytes. Within 24–36 hours following their release into the bloodstream, reticulocytes mature into "adult" red blood cells. Normally only 0.5–1.5% of total circulating red blood cells are reticulocytes. This percentage may be increased in certain conditions, such as severe blood loss or excessive destruction of erythrocytes through hemolysis. Reticulocytosis may also occur following the administration of iron, vitamin B_{12}, or folic acid for the treatment of anemia due to the lack of these essential substances. Once released from the bone marrow, some erythrocytes circulate through the body's network of arteries and veins; others are stored in the spleen. The spleen acts as a reservoir for approximately one-third of the available red cells, releasing them into the circulation as they are needed. The liver may also store red cells when the spleen is dysfunctional or absent.

RBCs are able to carry oxygen because they contain large amounts of hemoglobin, which attracts and forms a loose connection with oxygen. In fact, RBCs are approximately 95% hemoglobin. The hemoglobin molecule consists of a compound called heme and a protein called globin. Heme is formed when iron combines with a red-orange substance called porphyrin. Each of the four globin chains encloses a molecule of heme. Each RBC contains 200–300 billion molecules of hemoglobin. When oxygen combines with hemoglobin, oxyhemoglobin is formed; oxyhemoglobin gives oxygenated blood its characteristic red color.

Erythropoiesis, the production of erythrocytes, is stimulated when the delivery of oxygen to the kidneys is diminished. The kidneys release erythropoietin, a glycoprotein that stimulates the myeloid-committed stem cells in the bone marrow to develop into red blood cells and speeds up their maturation.[4] Normal plasma levels of erythropoietin are 0.01–0.03 U/mL, but these levels may increase from 100 to 1000 times during hypoxemia.

Persons with chronic renal disease are often unable to produce adequate amounts of erythropoietin, a deficiency that results in anemia, an abnormally low red blood cell count. Genetically engineered CSF for erythropoiesis has been found to be effective in reversing this anemia. In general, if the patient's serum erythropoietin levels are low or unmeasurable, injections of erythropoietin will probably be effective in stimulating erythropoiesis. If the patient's serum erythropoietin level is high, the erythropoietin injections are far less likely to reverse the anemia.[5]

In addition to erythropoietin, erythropoiesis also requires iron, folic acid, and vitamin B_{12}—vitamins and minerals obtained from food. A deficiency of B_{12} or folic acid disrupts DNA synthesis during cell development. The developing cell cannot divide, so it continues to enlarge, forming a megaloblast. In contrast, iron deficiency prevents the formation of adequate amounts of hemoglobin. Since erythrocytes are primarily made of hemoglobin, a deficiency of this compound results in small, pale erythrocytes. Any of these factors will result in anemia, as will the loss of erythrocytes through hemorrhage, excessive destruction by the specialized cells in the spleen, or excessive sequestration in an enlarged spleen.

Disorders and Diseases Affecting Red Blood Cell Counts

An excessive number of RBCs is termed erythrocytosis and may be seen in those who live at high altitudes or in clinical conditions in which there is a constant state of low oxygenation, such as chronic lung disease. A falsely elevated red blood cell count can also occur with dehydration, a condition common in critically ill patients.

Aged (senescent) or damaged red blood cells are destroyed primarily in the spleen, although the liver and bone marrow also eliminate them. As blood flows through the spleen, the circulating erythrocytes must pass through smaller and smaller vessels,

and are eventually forced to distort their shape in order to continue passage. As red blood cells age, they become less flexible, are unable to change their shape adequately, and are engulfed and destroyed by specialized immune cells called splenic macrophages. The iron from destroyed erythrocytes is transported by transferrin from the spleen to the liver, where it is stored as ferritin until it is needed by the bone marrow for the production of new red blood cells. The remainder of the molecule is bound to haptoglobin and transported to the liver for decomposition. The creation and destruction processes are depicted in Figure 8-4.

Intravascular hemolysis may occur in pathologic states such as hemolytic anemia or hemolytic transfusion reaction. When these occur, excessive binding of hemoglobin occurs in the vascular system, decreasing serum transferrin and haptoglobin levels. The unbound hemoglobin is potentially toxic to the renal tubules and may cause renal failure.

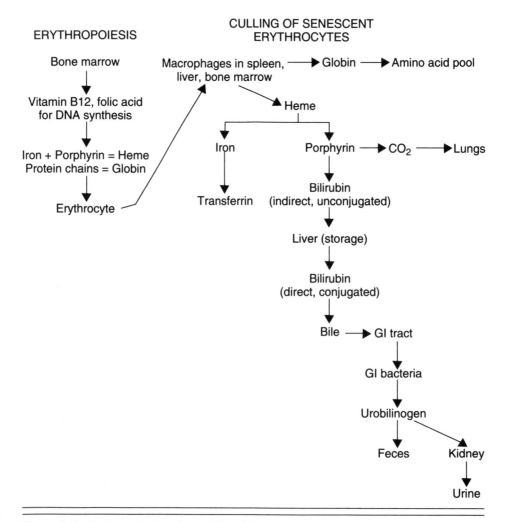

Figure 8-4 Erythrocyte Creation and Breakdown

The breakdown of the heme molecule requires the splenic macrophages to convert the porphyrin in heme to bilirubin, transport it to the liver, and secrete it into the GI tract as bile to aid in fat digestion. Bacteria in the GI tract act upon bile, changing it into urobilinogen, which is excreted in urine and feces. When the liver is unable to conjugate the bilirubin so that it can be excreted, it remains as unconjugated bilirubin and produces jaundice.

Typing of Red Blood Cells

A method of coding or identifying red blood cells that ensures compatibility of host and transfused red blood cells involves two mechanisms: (1) a system for confirming the presence of antibody in the plasma, and (2) a system for identifying molecules on the surfaces of red blood cells. Although many systems exist to identify red blood cells, the two most used systems are the ABO and the Rh systems.

The ABO system is a method of categorizing red blood cells by the presence (or absence) of identification molecules on their surface membranes. The test to determine ABO type and compatibility with potential cells to be transfused is called the agglutination test. Type A red blood cells have so-called A molecules on their surfaces. Type B red blood cells have B molecules on their surfaces. Type AB red blood cells have both A and B molecules on their surfaces, and Type O red blood cells have neither A nor B molecules on their surfaces. A summary of the ABO system and red cell transfusion compatibilities is given in Table 8-2.

Soon after birth, the body's B lymphocytes begin producing antibody to red blood cell markers that are "foreign" to that body; these antibody molecules are secreted into the plasma. The body does not produce antibody to red blood cell markers that it recognizes as "self." Thus, persons with type A red blood cells have antibody in their plasma to the molecules on the surfaces of type B red blood cells. They do not have antibodies to type A molecules because these mole-cules are recognized as "self." Since persons with type O red blood cells have neither A nor B markers on the surfaces of their erythrocytes, they have antibody to both type A and type B molecules in their plasma. In contrast, persons with type AB red blood cells do not produce antibody to either type A or type B molecules, since both of these molecules are on their red blood cells and both molecules are recognized as "self." These concepts of red cell compatibility are essential for understanding red blood cell cross-matching and transfusion therapy.

In clinical practice, type O blood cells, which contain neither A nor B molecules, can be transfused into persons with type A, type B, or type AB blood without causing a hemolytic antibody reaction within the body. For this reason, a person with type O blood is a universal donor. Even though the small amount of O plasma in whole blood contains antibody to A and B molecules, the antibody is in such a minute amount that it cannot cause a hemolytic reaction. However, fresh-frozen type O plasma does contain large amounts of blood group antibodies, and such plasma should *not* be administered to persons with type A, type B, or type AB blood. Persons with type AB blood can receive transfusions from persons with type A, type B, type AB, or type O blood. For this reason, a person with type AB blood is known as a universal recipient.

The Rh system is the second important blood grouping method (see Table 8-3). Erythrocytes' surfaces may contain molecules termed RhD. Persons with RhD markers on the surface of their RBCs are referred to as RH positive (Rh^+), and those without RhD markers are Rh negative (Rh^-). If a person with Rh^- red blood cells is exposed to Rh^+ cells, the RhD marker is seen as foreign, antibody to it is formed, and the Rh^+ cells are attacked and destroyed. If a person with Rh^+ red blood cells is exposed to Rh^- cells, no reaction takes place, since the Rh^- negative blood cells do not have any RhD surface marker. Although the Rh system is specific to red blood cells,

Table 8-2 ABO Compatibility

Blood Group	Antigen on RBC	Antibody in Plasma	Compatibility with Donor		
			Whole Blood	RBCs	Plasma
O	None	Anti A & B	O	O	O, A, B, AB
A	A	Anti B	A	A and O	A and AB
B	B	Anti A	B	B and O	B and AB
AB	A and B	None	AB	O, A, B, AB	AB

Table 8-3 Rh Compatibility

Blood Group	Antigen on RBC	Antibody in Plasma	Compatibility with Donor		
			Whole Blood	RBCs	Plasma
Rh$^+$	D	None	+ and −	+ and −	+ and −
Rh$^-$	None	Anti-D	−	−	+ and −

transfusions of platelets or white blood cells may contain significant numbers of RBCs.

Lab Tests of Red Blood Cell Function

Various laboratory tests are employed to evaluate erythrocytes: the red blood cell count, RBC morphology, hemoglobin, hematocrit, MCH, MCV, and MCHC.

RBC morphology RBC morphology refers to the size, color, and shape of erythrocytes and the presence of any distortions or cellular inclusions. Anisocytosis is a term that refers to abnormal variation in the sizes of RBCs. Abnormally large erythrocytes are macrocytic, and abnormally small ones are microcytic. Abnormal shape is poikilocytosis. Hypochromic (pale) erythrocytes contain lower than normal amounts of hemoglobin. A summary of RBC morphology findings and their clinical implications is found in Table 8-4.

Nucleated RBCs (normoblasts) represent an early stage of erythrocyte development and are not normally present in circulation. When seen in peripheral blood, they may represent abnormal or early release of RBC precursors, as seen in hemolytic disorders.

Erythrocytes may assume unusual or abnormal shapes in association with many disease states. For the most part, the abnormal shapes result from deficient or defective hemoglobin, or a cessation of the culling activity of the spleen or liver, such as can occur following splenectomy or with hepatic disease. A general belief is that the more severe the anemia, regardless of the cause, the more bizarre the shapes of the erythrocytes.

Hemoglobin level A hemoglobin (Hgb) test is a measurement of the number of grams of hemoglobin per 100 mL of whole blood; a normal range is 14.5–16.0 in men or 13.0–15.5 in women. Since hemoglobin is the molecule to which oxygen binds, Hgb is a partial measurement of the body's oxygen-carrying capacity.

Hemoglobin levels are elevated in polycythemia vera or in dehydration. The hemoglobin may be low following blood loss or as a result of iron deficiency, pernicious anemia, or dilution of blood as a result of fluid overload.

Hematocrit level Hematocrit (Hct) is a measurement of the volume of packed red blood cells per cubic millimeter of whole blood. The normal range for men is 42–53%/mm^3 and for women is 38–46%/mm^3, or roughly three times the hemoglobin value. The hematocrit may be elevated in chronic hypoxia, when there is excessive stimulation of RBC synthesis, or in hypovolemia, when the proportion of vascular volume is low compared to the cellular components. Another condition that produces an elevated hematocrit is the presence of macrocytic immature cells, which create a larger than normal RBC volume without an increase in cell quantity.

Erythrocyte indices Measurements of the size and hemoglobin content of erythrocytes are called erythrocyte indices. The mean corpuscular volume (MCV) is a measurement of the relative size of an individual red blood cell. The MCV is calculated by dividing the hematocrit by the red blood cell count (Hct/RBC). The normal range of values is 87±5 mcg^3. An MCV less than 80 signifies the presence of abnormally small erythrocytes (microcytes). An MCV greater than 90 indicates abnormally large erythrocytes (macrocytes).

The mean corpuscular hemoglobin (MCH) is a measurement of the weight of hemoglobin in an average red blood cell. The MCH is calculated by dividing the hemoglobin level by the red blood cell count (Hgb/RBC). In other words, it represents the mean hemoglobin content within a representative cell. The normal range of values is 29±2 pg. An MCH below 27 can be seen when cells are deficient in hemoglobin and are pale. An MCH greater than 32 may be seen with abnormally large cells.

The mean corpuscular hemoglobin concentration (MCHC) measures the percentage of red blood cells saturated with hemoglobin, or the average hemoglobin concentration within 100 mL of packed RBCs. The MCHC is calculated by dividing hemoglobin level by hematocrit (Hgb/Hct). The normal range

Table 8-4 Erythrocyte Morphology

Term	Appearance	Associated Disorder
Anisocytosis	Abnormal variations in size	Reticulocytosis due to accelerated erythropoiesis
Poikilocytosis	Abnormal shape	
Macrocytes	Unusually large cells	Pernicious anemia Folic acid deficiency
Microcytes	Abnormally small cells	Iron deficiency anemia Thalassemia major Hereditary spherocytosis
Hypochromia	Pale erythrocytes due to deficiency in hemoglobin or unnatural thinness	Iron deficiency anemia Thalassemia major Infection
Hyperchromasia	Excessive pigmentation	
Polychromasia	Multicolored erythrocytes; variations in cell color	Hemolysis Regenerative erythropoiesis
Acanthocyte	Thorny, spiked, helmet-, bucket-, or cup-shaped erythrocyte	Hemolysis Renal disease Cancer Vitamin E deficiency Pyruvate kinase deficiency Uremia Snakebite Hepatic disease (including alcohol-induced cirrhosis) Disseminated intravascular coagulation
Burr cell	See Acanthocyte	
Echinocyte	See Acanthocyte	
Elliptocyte	Oval cell	Iron deficiency anemia Hereditary elliptocytosis (ovalocytosis) Thalassemia Sickle cell anemia Megaloblastic anemia
Ghost cell	Erythrocyte with hemoglobin removed	
Helmet cell	See Acanthocyte	
Leptocyte	See Target cell	

Nucleated RBCs	Normoblasts	Accelerated erythropoiesis secondary to:
		  Anemia
		  Hypoxemia
		  Hematologic malignancy
		  Bone marrow fibrosis/neoplasm

Ovalocyte	See Elliptocyte	
Schistocyte	Fragmented erythrocytes, often with extremely bizarre shapes such as triangles, spirals, etc.	Hemolytic anemia Mechanical destruction of erythrocytes (for example, by artificial heart valve) Post-splenectomy Disseminated intravascular coagulation Uremia Malignant hypertension
Sickle cell	Crescent-shaped cell (due to hemoglobin S)	Sickle cell anemia
Siderocyte	Erythrocyte containing iron granules	Post-splenectomy Pernicious anemia

(continued)

Table 8-4 Erythrocyte Morphology (*continued*)

Term	Appearance	Associated Disorder
Spherocyte	Small, spherical erythrocyte	Hereditary spherocytosis Thalassemia major Hemoglobin C Hemolytic anemia
Spur cell	See Acanthocyte	
Stippling, basophilic	Diffuse punctate bodies enclosed in erythrocyte	Hemolysis Lead poisoning Reticulocytosis
Stomatocyte	See Acanthocyte	
Target cell	Thin erythrocyte with dark center of hemoglobin	Iron deficiency anemia Thalassemia major Hepatic disease (obstructive jaundice) Hemoglobinopathy Post-splenectomy
Teardrop cell	Teardrop-shaped erythrocyte	Hypersplenism Thalassemia Myeloproliferative disease
Turk cell		Malaria Leukemia
Heinz Erlich bodies	Small, irregular patches of hemoglobin	Hemolytic anemia Hemoglobinopathy Post-splenectomy
Howell-Jolly bodies	Small round remnants of nucleus	Hemolytic anemia Post-splenectomy Megaloblastic anemia
Rouleau formation	Irregular stacking of erythrocytes	Inflammation

of values is 35–36 g. An MCHC below 32 g represents a deficiency of hemoglobin. An MCHC above 36 g is not possible, since fewer oversized RBCs can be packed into 100 mL.

Platelets

Platelets are noncellular fragments of precursor cells called megakaryocytes. Platelets are essential for hemostasis. Following injury to a blood vessel, platelets adhere to the injured vessel, forming an aggregate known as a platelet plug in order to seal off the tear. As platelets aggregate, they release chemicals such as serotonin and thromboxane A2, which help initiate the coagulation cascade and cause more platelets to aggregate at the site of injury.

Platelets "bud off" megakaryocytes, which are produced in the bone marrow and are not normally found in the peripheral circulation. The life-span of platelets is relatively brief—from 7 to 10 days. At the end of this time, platelets are removed from the circulation by phagocytic cells. One-third of the

body's pool of platelets is sequestered, or stored, in the spleen, while the remaining two-thirds circulate freely. The normal platelet count ranges from 350,000 to 500,000 per cubic millimeter of blood. Approximately one-tenth of this number are replaced every day; in other words, the body produces 30,000–50,000 platelets for each cubic millimeter of blood each day. After 10 days, all the body's platelets have been replaced.[6]

Disorders and Diseases Affecting Platelet Counts

Several conditions or diseases can alter platelet counts. Thrombocytosis, an abnormally high platelet count, may occur in certain conditions such as polycythemia vera or chronic myelocytic leukemia. With reactive thrombocytosis, the platelet count is elevated in association with an acute phase reaction, a systemic manifestation of inflammation such as may be seen with hypersensitivity diseases or cancer. Regardless of its cause, thrombocytosis may, as its name suggests, cause thrombosis in small blood vessels; on the other hand, it may cause severe bleeding or have no clinical consequences. The bleeding seen in thrombocytosis occurs because the platelets, although numerous, do not function properly.

Far more common than thrombocytosis is an abnormally low platelet count, termed thrombocytopenia. A lower than normal platelet count may occur for several different reasons, including inadequate production, excessive storage, excessive destruction, or excessive consumption of platelets. Inadequate production of megakaryocytes can occur in any disease state in which dysmyelopoiesis is present, such as leukemia or aplastic anemia. Thrombocytopenia can also result from excessive storage of platelets. The spleen normally acts as a reservoir for platelets, releasing them into the circulation as needed. However, an enlarged spleen may hold an astonishing number of platelets in storage despite low levels of circulating platelets. Such splenic disorders may be treated with steroids or splenectomy.

Platelets may be destroyed in excessive numbers as a result of mechanical damage from a prosthetic heart valve or an indwelling catheter such as an IABP or because of diseases. For example, during idiopathic thrombocytopenia purpura (ITP), an autoimmune disease, the body manufactures antibodies against its own platelets. The antibody-tagged platelets are phagocytosed and destroyed by splenic macrophages. ITP may be associated with administration of certain medications such as thiazides and gold salts. Finally, platelet counts may be low because of the body's excessive demand for them. Severe musculoskeletal trauma, surgery, hemorrhage, or consumptive coagulopathies such as disseminated intravascular coagulation (DIC) may account for accelerated consumption of platelets.

Disorders that require large numbers of platelets will worsen when the platelet count falls too low. The risk of spontaneous bleeding due to insufficient platelets to make a platelet plug dramatically increases the lower the platelet count falls. However, this risk is also compounded by the underlying disorder causing the thrombocytopenia. For example, patients with leukemia who have platelet counts of less than 50,000/mm^3 have approximately a 20% risk of spontaneous hemorrhage; if their platelet counts are less than 20,000/mm^3, their risk of bleeding increases by 50% for every 1000/mm^3 decrease in platelets.[7]

Lab Tests of Platelet Function

The most common laboratory parameter used to assess platelets is the platelet count. This measures the quantity of platelets circulating in the bloodstream. Platelet counts may be inaccurately high when dehydration is present and may be a poor reflection of platelet function when platelets are abnormal in appearance or sequestered in the spleen. With very low platelet counts, an automatic counter (such as those used with most hematology tests) will not be able to detect the few platelets on the slide. A test of platelet quality is the bleeding time, measuring the platelets' ability to produce a platelet plug with injury. The test is performed by making a small incision in the skin and blotting the site until it stops bleeding. Poor platelet quality is reflected by an inability to clot or prolonged bleeding from this incision. Platelet quality is altered by many factors.

White Blood Cells

White blood cells, or leukocytes, are colorless blood cells that defend the body against infection. There are approximately 7000 WBCs/mm^3 (the range is 5000–10,000/mm^3) of whole blood.[8] Like other blood cells, leukocytes are produced in bone marrow, deriving from the pluripotential stem cells. There are three main categories of white blood cells: granulocytes, monocytes, and lymphocytes. Within each of these broad categories are subcategories of cells. The WBC differential test is a measurement of the distribution of the various types of leukocytes as well as their morphology. Each category of leukocyte is discussed briefly in the subsections that follow. Their complex roles in the body's immunological functions are described in the later section on immune physiology.

As noted earlier, when referring to cell counts outside of the normal range, the Latin suffix *-cytosis* or *-philia* is used to refer to elevated counts, and the Latin suffix *-penia* is used to mean too few. These endings are attached to the blood cell terms. For example, leukocytosis is an abnormally elevated leukocyte count. Leukocytosis may occur as a result of inflammation, infection, or stress or in association with tissue damage such as with myocardial infarction. White blood cells may also be present in abnormally high levels as a result of diseases such as leukemia. Leukopenia refers to an abnormally low number of white blood cells. Leukopenia may result from accelerated consumption of leukocytes, such as occurs in an overwhelming infection. More commonly, leukopenia is due to the inadequate production of leukocytes. Bone marrow suppression resulting in leukopenia can occur in disease states or may be iatrogenically induced by radiation therapy or treatment with cytotoxic agents.

Granulocytes

Granulocytes are small leukocytes with densely staining granules in their cytoplasm and a distinctive multilobed nucleus. Because of the characteristic shape of their nuclei, granulocytes are referred to as polymorphonuclear leukocytes, a term derived from the Latin words for "many-shaped nucleus." This term is commonly abbreviated to poly or PML. Granulocytes are subdivided into three types: neutrophils, eosinophils, and basophils. The vast majority of all granulocytes are neutrophils, which are critically important for defending the body against bacterial infection. In contrast, eosinophils and basophils are present in very small numbers and generally play a far less significant role in immunological defense. Since neutrophils are the most abundant and essential granulocytes, the terms *granulocyte* and *PML* are often used loosely to refer to neutrophils alone, but strictly speaking, these terms refer to eosinophils and basophils as well.[9] Granulocytes comprise 35–75% of the circulating white blood cells and are regulated by negative feedback mechanisms to the bone marrow. They can be differentiated and released from the bone marrow in as little as 6 hours and are the white blood cells that respond to inflammation, tissue necrosis, and bacterial infection.

Neutrophils Neutrophils are small, motile scavenger cells with a multilobed nucleus and violet-pink staining granules. Their function is to ingest and destroy microorganisms; they are the first and most numerous responders to the site of an infection and are critical for immunity against bacteria. Neutrophils are known by many names, most of which are based on the shape of their nuclei. For example, neutrophils are sometimes referred to as PMLs (see above) or PMNs (an abbreviation of the longer term *polymorphonuclear neutrophil*).

As the neutrophil goes through stages of maturation, the nucleus begins to separate into lobes. At one point, two lobes are connected by a band of nuclear material; at this stage of development, the juvenile neutrophils are referred to as bands. Adults have fully developed multilobed or segmented nuclei and are called segs. During severe infections, the bone marrow's reserves of adult neutrophils may be depleted. In this instance, juvenile neutrophils may be released into the circulation. Cellular development can be visualized as a line extending from birth (on the left) to maturity (on the right); a trend toward immaturity can be described as "a shift to the left" in developmental age. This phrase is used to refer to an abnormally high number of juvenile or immature neutrophils in the peripheral blood, which is usually representative of serious or acute bacterial infection.

Neutrophils arise from the bone marrow stem cells and undergo two phases of development. The first stage of development, lasting approximately 1

week, is the mitotic phase, during which the neutrophil develops from a myeloblast to a promyelocyte and then a myelocyte. During the second, nonmitotic phase, which also lasts approximately 1 week, the neutrophil precursor develops from a metamyelocyte to a band, then matures to a seg. A total of 100 billion neutrophils are produced each day and are stored in the bone marrow to await the signal for release whenever they are needed.

Neutrophils are present in three areas in the body: in bone marrow, within the blood vessels (intravascular), and in tissue. It is surprising to note that up to 90% of the neutrophils in the body are sequestered in the bone marrow, forming the marrow reserve.[10] The numbers are staggering: for every kilogram of body weight, the bone marrow contains 10 billion neutrophils and precursor cells. The intravascular population of neutrophils comprises 2–3% of the total number of neutrophils in the body. Of the intravascular neutrophils, approximately 50–60% are freely circulating, forming the circulating pool. This neutrophil population is represented by the CBC. From 40% to 50% of the intravascular neutrophils form the marginal pool. These neutrophils tumble slowly along the blood vessel walls, particularly in the postcapillary venules. The number of neutrophils in the body's tissues is more than double the number of intravascular neutrophils. The tissue neutrophils are believed to represent approximately 7–8% of all neutrophils in the body.[11] Thus, although the CBC reveals approximately 3000–4000 neutrophils per cubic millimeter, this number represents a very small portion of the neutrophils in the body.

Neutrophil counts are controlled by two feedback mechanisms: the first stimulates production of neutrophils by the bone marrow, and the second controls their release from storage in the marrow into the circulation. Following their release into the bloodstream, neutrophils circulate for 4–8 hours before migrating into tissue. Estimates of their life-span once in tissue range from 7 hours to 5 days; however, they may live for only minutes or hours if destroyed during an early encounter with a microbe.[12]

The primary function of neutrophils is to engulf and destroy microorganisms; thus, they are phagocytes. Each neutrophil can destroy from 5 to 20 bacteria before being destroyed itself by bacterial toxins and its own digestive enzymes. The dead and dying neutrophils, tissue debris, and bacteria form pus. The neutrophil's cytoplasmic granules (lysosomes) contain digestive substances (lysozyme, acid hydrolases) and iron-binding proteins (lactoferrin), which aid in the killing and digestion of microbes. Neutrophilic granules contain other substances, such as myeloperoxidase, which are used to generate a complex chemical reaction termed the respiratory burst. This reaction produces oxygen compounds such as hydrogen peroxide, hydroxyl radical, and superoxide hydroxychlorosene, which are poisonous to bacteria.

During infection, certain lymphocytes coat microorganisms, toxins, and other foreign or harmful substances with complement compounds or antibody. Neutrophils have molecules on their surfaces that attach to the coating molecules, greatly enhancing the ability of the neutrophil to ingest the microbe.

Neutrophils are not always beneficial. The granules' contents, which are toxic to microorganisms, can also harm normal tissue. During infection, dead and dying neutrophils release the contents of their granules. Other neutrophils that are unable to effectively engulf a microbe deliberately discharge their granules into the surrounding area. This phenomenon, aptly named frustrated phagocytosis, contributes to the tissue destruction seen with inflammatory diseases such as myocardial infarction, pneumonia, and glomerulonephritis.

Granulocytopenia, a term referring to a shortage of all granulocytes (neutrophils, eosinophils, and basophils), is often employed to refer to low numbers of neutrophils alone, since these cells comprise the greatest portion of the granulocytes. An elevated neutrophil count (neutrophilia) is most frequently an indication of an infection such as septicemia, osteomyelitis, otitis media, gonorrhea, endocarditis, pneumonia, or Rocky Mountain spotted fever. Neutrophilia may also occur in ischemic necrosis (as a result of myocardial infarction, thermal injury, or cancer) or as a result of such diverse metabolic disorders as diabetic ketoacidosis, eclampsia, uremia, and thyrotoxicosis. Inflammatory diseases such as rheumatic fever, rheumatoid arthritis, acute gout, vasculitis, and myositis may also increase the neutrophil count above normal. The stress response associated with acute hemorrhage, surgery, exercise, the third trimester of pregnancy, childbirth, and even emotional distress has also been associated with a rise in neutrophil counts.

The most common granulocyte defect is neutropenia.[13] Neutropenia is most often associated with bone marrow depression secondary to chemotherapy, radiation therapy, hypersplenism, or hepatic disease. Lower than normal neutrophil counts may also result from folic acid or B_{12} deficiency or in association with collagen vascular diseases such as systemic lupus erythematosis. Oddly enough, whereas infection generally elevates neutrophil counts, certain infections may precipitate a drop in neutrophil counts to less than normal. Typhoid fever, tularemia, brucellosis, hepatitis, influenza, mea-

sles (rubella and rubeola), mumps, and mononucleosis are some of the infections known for producing this reaction. Neutropenia is discussed in more detail in the section of this chapter on immunodeficiency.

Eosinophils Eosinophils are granulocytes with a bilobed nucleus, a pale blue–staining cytoplasm, and large, bright red–staining granules. Eosinophils comprise 2–3% of the total WBC differential.[14] Approximately 9 days are required for an eosinophil to mature in the bone marrow. After their release from the marrow, the cells circulate in the blood for 3–8 hours, then migrate into the tissue. Eosinophils can be found in highest concentration in the skin and in the mucosa of the lung and GI tract. They are able to migrate back and forth between blood and tissue.

Although little is known about eosinophils, there are some theories concerning their function. Because they are the last cells to arrive at the site of tissue injury, it is theorized that they have a role in "turning off" the immune response. Eosinophils respond to chemotactins, and although they are only weakly phagocytic, they are capable of ingesting antigen-antibody complexes that may remain at the site of injury. In addition, eosinophils release chemicals that inactivate substances released by mast cells and basophils during inflammatory or allergic responses. For example, eosinophils release histaminase to block the action of histamine, arylsulfatase to inactivate SRSA (leukotrienes from mast cells), and cationic proteins that bind to heparin and block its action. These effects may be particularly important in limiting or suppressing the body's responses in allergic conditions such as asthma and hay fever. This hypothesis is supported by evidence that the eosinophils collect in tissue involved in allergic response, such as lung tissue and skin, and their numbers are somewhat elevated with allergic conditions or infections involving the lungs or skin.

Finally, eosinophils may play a significant role in host resistance to certain helminthic (parasitic worm) infections. For example, during infection by the parasitic worms trichinella or schistosoma, eosinophils migrate to the larvae but are unable to engulf the much larger worms. Instead, the eosinophils discharge their granules directly onto the larvae, killing the parasite. Eosinophil counts can increase to truly astounding levels during helminthic infections, reaching as high as 50% of the WBC differential.

Elevated eosinophil levels (eosinophilia) primarily occur in allergic disorders such as allergic hay fever, asthma, reactions to drugs or food, serum sickness, angioedema, eczema, pemphigus, psoriasis, and dermatitis herpetiformis. Collagen vascular diseases, ulcerative colitis, polyarteritis nodosa, pernicious anemia, adrenocortical hypofunction, splenectomy, scarlet fever, or excessive exercise can also produce eosinophilia. As noted previously, parasitic infections, especially hookworm, trichinosis, roundworm infections, and amebiasis, are well known for elevating eosinophil counts above normal. Eosinophilia is also seen in two very rare disorders: hypereosinophilic syndrome (a type of malignancy) and Churg-Strauss syndrome (a form of vasculitis).

Eosinopenia may occur as part of the stress response accompanying musculoskeletal trauma, shock, thermal injury, surgery, emotional stress, or Cushing's disease.

Basophils Basophils, the least abundant granulocytes, have a bilobed nucleus and large, coarse cytoplasmic granules that stain purplish-black. Although little is known about basophil development, maturation, and life-span, they are believed to have an active role in the production of chemical mediators for the inflammatory response.

Basophils synthesize and store many chemical mediators such as SRSA, heparin (perhaps to restore microcirculation), and histamine. In fact, basophils are believed to be the source of most of the histamine normally present in blood.[15] Basophils bear a strong functional resemblance to connective tissue cells called mast cells. Both types of cells are derived from the pluripotential stem cells, but they are otherwise unreleated. Mast cells and basophils do share certain common characteristics. Both contain granules that store chemicals such as histamine, and both have surface receptors for IgE that upon exposure to antigen cause the cell to degranulate, releasing its stored chemicals.

Mast cells are not circulating blood cells, but instead are found throughout the body's tissues; they are in especially high concentrations surrounding blood vessels and in the mucosal linings of the respiratory and gastrointestinal tracts. These long-lived cells can proliferate locally in certain tissues exposed to mediators. Mast cells are chemical storehouses and have a crucial role in producing the symptoms of allergy. Their function appears to be the storage of potent inflammatory and repair materials that are released upon injury.

Both mast cells and basophils have surface receptors for a particular class of antibody, IgE. Upon exposure to antigen, adjoining molecules of IgE are crosslinked to each other; the linkage stimulates the mast cell to degranulate and release stored chemicals and produce additional chemicals: histamine, kinin, and SRSA proteases. (Several nursing texts erroneously state that serotonin is produced and released by mast cells and basophils. Careful review of the immunology literature reveals that serotonin is produced by mast cells and basophils in mice. In humans, serotonin is produced by platelets, not by mast cells.[16])

Basophilia (elevated basophil counts) can occur in association with polycythemia vera, Hodgkin's disease, myxedema, ulcerative colitis, chronic hemolytic anemias, chronic hypersensitivity, or nephrosis. The mechanism of stimulation for most of these disorders appears to be mediator activation of IgE receptors. Basopenia has been noted in such diverse clinical conditions as hyperthyroidism, ovulation, and pregnancy and as part of the stress response, but the etiology of basophil depletion is unknown.

Mastocytosis (abnormal accumulations of mast cells) arises in a group of disorders ranging from a relatively benign skin disease called urticaria pigmentosa to the rapidly fatal mast cell leukemia. As might be expected, patients with abnormal levels of mast cells often experience clinical symptoms related to the cells' release of chemical mediators.

Monocytes

Monocytes are large white blood cells with a prominent kidney-shaped nucleus. They are important phagocytes and also play a key role in other types of immune responses. Monocytes develop in the bone marrow, taking $2\frac{1}{2}$ days, are released into the bloodstream, and circulate for 12–24 hours.[17] The cells then enter the tissue and undergo a transformation into larger, more active, and more immunocompetent cells called macrophages. Although monocytes are phagocytic, they are far less effective than macrophages. Once differentiated, some macrophages remain in tissue; others reenter the bloodstream and are believed to live for months.

Monocytes or macrophages, like neutrophils, are stored in the bone marrow, reside in tissue, and either circulate or form a marginal pool within the blood vessels. Roughly 60% of intravascular monocytes are in the marginal pool, slowly tumbling along the walls of the postcapillary venules. Unlike neutrophils, however, macrophages in the tissue are of two types: fixed (or resident) and free (or mobile). Fixed macrophages are literally affixed to tissue. These cells have specialized shapes and functions specific to their tissue of residence. The highest concentrations of tissue macrophages occur in the spleen, liver, lungs, and bone marrow. Fixed macrophages of the liver are termed Kupffer cells, those of the spleen are termed splenic macrophages, and those of the skin are known as dendritic, or Langerhans, cells. Fixed macrophages are also found in the connective tissue and in the basement membrane of small blood vessels. In lymph nodes, they line the subcapsular medullary sinuses. In the spleen, the cords of Bilroth and the venous sinuses are lined by macrophages. The pleural, peritoneal, and synovial fluids also contain macrophages. The fixed macrophages are referred to as the reticuloendothelial system. Table 8-5 lists organs or areas of the body and their corresponding macrophages.

Several substances released during inflammation act to stimulate the bone marrow to produce macrophages. For example, activated macrophages produce macrophage colony stimulating factor (M-CSF) and granulocyte-macrophage colony stimulating factor (GM-CSF). In addition, the Interleukin-1 (IL-1) and tumor necrosis factor alpha (TNFα) released by activated macrophages cause epithelial cells to produce M-CSF and GM-CSF as well. These CSFs induce the production of neutrophils and monocytes by the bone marrow and the release of stored neutrophils.

Macrophages have multiple functions. They engulf and destroy microbes, senescent cells, antibody-coated tumor cells, necrotic tissue, and antigen-antibody complexes. They destroy antibody-coated cells via a process called antibody dependent cellular cytotoxicity (ADCC). Macrophages play a key role in secreting chemical mediators and regulators of inflammation, such as complement components, tissue plasminogen activator, and other chemicals that modify the function of other immune cells, especially lymphocytes. Unlike most other myeloid cells, resident macrophages near the site of infection proliferate by duplicating themselves. Their stimulation leads to the release of various CSFs that stimulate bone marrow production and release of more WBCs. Macrophages are also essential for generating specific immune responses by their interaction with antigens and lymphocytes in a process known as antigen presentation and by secretion of chemical messengers called monokines (TNFa and IL-1) that stimulate activation of T helper cells. Finally, macrophages form granulomas to enclose and neutralize microorganisms that cannot be destroyed. Macrophages enter infected areas within 6–12 hours of injury, although the greatest numbers are present 16–24 hours after injury.[18]

Monocytosis occurs in infections such as tuberculosis, hepatitis, malaria, subacute bacterial endocarditis, Rocky Mountain spotted fever, lupus, rheumatoid arthritis, polyarteritis nodosa, certain cancers, and monocytic leukemia. Monocytopenia rarely occurs unless in response to elevation of one of the other WBC components.

Lymphocytes

Lymphocytes are small, agranular leukocytes from the lymphoid-committed stem cell line, which play a special role in the immune response. There are three major types of lymphocytes: B lymphocytes, T lymphocytes, and large granular lymphocytes (LGL). These cells derive from the hematopoietic stem cells in the bone marrow or thymus and are released into the circulation when needed. Some of these cells have long life-spans of 100–300 days, or even years.[19] Once mature, lymphocytes form a recirculating pool, which constantly circulates from the bloodstream to the tissue to the lymph nodes and back again. During this process, the cells enter the circulation for a few hours, pass into tissues by diapedesis, enter the lymphatics, then migrate to lymphoid tissue (especially the lymph nodes) and remain there for varying amounts of time, after which they reenter the bloodstream and repeat the cycle. This process allows the lymphocytes to carry out their major function of surveillance for mutant cells and virus particles.

B lymphocytes are responsible for antibody production, including production of the body's five major immunoglobulins. These antibodies protect the body against infection by microorganisms or their toxins. To produce antibody, B lymphocytes usually require the assistance of T lymphocytes, but certain bacterial infections are able to stimulate the B cells to produce antibody. Once stimulated, B cells independently perform four actions. First, they clone, or duplicate themselves. Second, they change into plasma cells, which are the antibody "factories" that synthesize and secrete specific antibodies (IgG, IgM, IgA, IgE, or IgD). Third, B lymphocytes take action against invading pathogens. The antibody secreted by the plasma cells coats the foreign particles, tremendously enhancing the ability of the im-

Table 8-5 Reticuloendothelial System and Associated Macrophages

Site	Resident Macrophage
Brain	Microglia
Lung	Alveolar
Liver	Kupffer cells
Spleen	Splenic macrophages
Kidney	Intraglomerular mesangial cells
Joints	Synovial A cells
Skin	Langerhans cells

mune cells to destroy the invaders. Finally, a number of memory cells are formed from this process and held in reserve in case of future exposure to the invader. It is important to note that B cells stimulated without T cell help do not form into memory B cells.

T lymphocytes also arise from the bone marrow, but they go to the thymus to mature. The T cells are the key cells orchestrating the entire immune response. Once stimulated, T cells perform the same general actions as B cells. First, T cells clone; next, they become activated. Third, T lymphocytes perform specialized work. Finally, a number of memory T cells formed from this process remain immunologically activated and are believed to be responsible for the rapid and augmented response of the immune system to any future exposure to a particular microorganism.

There are several subtypes of T lymphocytes, each of which is named according to its function. Cytotoxic T cells, which have a molecule named CD8 on their surfaces, destroy tumor cells as well as body cells infected with viruses, fungi, or protozoa. Other T cells, which have this same identification surface marker, act to suppress the production of antibody by B lymphocytes. The T4 helper cells activate B lymphocytes to produce antibody and activate cytotoxic T cells, T8 suppressor cells and macrophages. Another T cell with a CD4 molecule on its surface is believed to be responsible for the immunologic phenomenon known as delayed hypersensitivity reaction.

Large granular lymphocytes (LGLs) are puzzling and contradictory cells. Lymphocytes by definition are small and agranular with specific immune functions, but these cells are large, contain granules, and have nonspecific immunological activity. Since LGLs are atypical, it is not surprising that they have been known by several names, including blank or null cells because they do not carry surface molecules that identify them as B or T lymphocytes. Now, more accurately, LGLs are called non-T, non-B cells. Currently, the LGLs on which much research interest is centered are the natural killer (NK) cells. NK cells can be identified by a molecule on their surface that combines with monoclonal antibody Leu 11. NK cells are nonspecific, cytolytic cells that have an important role in the destruction of virally infected cells and tumor cells. The granules of NK cells contain cytolytic substances. The NK cell destroys its targets by discharging the contents of its granules onto the target cell. As with neutrophils and macrophages, an antibody destruction process called ADCC and the presence of interferon trigger the NK cells to release their granules. It is believed that the NK cell contains substances to protect it from self-destruction. NK

cells seem to be particularly effective against cancerous hematopoietic cells.

An elevated lymphocyte count can arise from any of several causes: pertussis, brucellosis, syphilis, tuberculosis, hepatitis, mononucleosis, German measles (rubella), cytomegalovirus, thyrotoxicosis, hypoadrenalism, ulcerative colitis, or lymphocytic leukemia or lymphoma. Lymphocyte counts are depressed in the chronically ill and those with defective lymphatic circulation.

Laboratory Assessment of WBC Function

The most common diagnostic test of WBC function is the total WBC count and differential. The total WBC count is usually 5000–10,000/mm^3 (see Table 8-6). When the total WBC count is moderately elevated (10,000–25,000/mm^3), there is usually additional clinical evidence of infection, inflammation, or tissue necrosis. Each of these three etiologies will cause proliferation of different WBC subtypes. Using the differential count (specific percentages of each type of white blood cell comprising the total WBC), clinicians can ascertain more specific information regarding the etiology of the elevated WBC. Based on their physiological properties, granulocytes (neutrophils, basophils, and eosinophils) are generally elevated in inflammatory responses and bacterial infection. Monocytes and lymphocytes are more responsive to immunologic stimuli and are likely to be elevated in viral or allergic reactions. When interpreting a WBC differential, one must determine which WBC subtype is elevated in order to determine whether an infection is bacterial or viral. The first step is to assess the percentage of the total WBC count that is made up of granulocytes (including bands, neutrophils, eosinophils, and basophils). Next, the percentage of monocytes is assessed. Then, the percentage of lymphocytes is assessed. Finally, a determination is made as to whether the

Table 8-6   The WBC Differential

Type of WBC	Percentage of total WBCs
Granulocytes (especially neutrophils)	35–75%
Eosinophils	1–4
Basophils	2–5
Lymphocytes	15–45
Monocytes	1–9
Normal total WBC count = 5,000–10,000/mm^3	

Table 8-7 Sample Interpretations of the WBC Differential

WBC	15,500	WBC	12,900
Gran	95%	Gran	20%
Eos	20%	Eos	5%
Basos	2%	Basos	1%
Lymphs	4%	Lymphs	68%
Monos	1%	Monos	12%
Interpretation: Left shift		Interpretation: Right shift	

percentage of each type of cell is greater than normal. If the percentage of granulocytes is above normal, a bacterial infection should be suspected. Bacterial infections cause granulocyte proliferation with systemic release of immature cells (bands), which is termed a "shift to the left," because of the shift toward release of immature cells. Elevation of monocytes or lymphocytes is termed a "shift to the right" and indicates a viral infection or allergy. Table 8-7 shows sample interpretations of WBC differentials.

The Immune System

Functions of the Immune System

The immune system has three functions: defense, homeostasis, and surveillance. The immune system defends the body from microorganisms and other harmful substances that enter the body from the environment. The immune system also maintains homeostasis, a state of balance, by eliminating damaged or aging cells from the body but leaving the healthy, fully functioning cells alone. Finally, the immune system accomplishes its surveillance function by searching out and destroying any mutant cells that develop. Substances stimulating an immune response may originate from outside the body (exogenous stimuli) or from within the body (endogenous stimuli). For example, botulism toxin and ragweed pollen both enter the body from the environment and are examples of exogenous stimuli. In contrast, an aged or damaged red blood cell is an example of an endogenous stimulus—one originating from within the body.

Sometimes the immune system overreacts or underreacts to these stimuli. Whenever the immune system does not function properly, clinical disease can result. For example, if immune defenses are inadequate, microorganisms produce infections. On the other hand, if immunological defenses are hyperactive, the body will overreact to harmless substances, producing allergies. Ragweed pollen is harmless yet can cause severe allergic symptoms. If the homeostasis mechanism of the immune system is deranged, normal "self" cells are mistakenly treated as foreign invaders and are attacked and destroyed, causing autoimmune disease. Finally, if immune surveillance is inadequate, mutant cells are not recognized and destroyed, and neoplastic disease occurs.

Factors Modifying the Immune Response

Many factors modify or influence the immune response: nutritional status, age, genetic makeup, individual stress levels, and metabolic (or hormonal) and environmental influences. The mechanisms of altered immune response due to many of these factors are outlined in the discussion of sepsis in Chapter 9. Genetic disorders of immune deficiency may involve any of the specific and nonspecific immune responses and are addressed briefly in later sections of this chapter.

The functioning of the immune system is frequently inadequate in the very young and the very old. At birth, the immune system is immature, and neonates are unable to produce antibody. Fortunately, during gestation, maternal antibodies are transferred across the placenta to the fetus; these remain in the child's system for about 9 months after birth, by which time most infants can produce antibody in sufficient amounts. Additional antibodies in breast milk assist in protecting a child from infection. Similarly, as people age, their immune systems also age. In the elderly the immune system is less efficient, and organs involved in the immune response, such as the thymus and spleen, undergo atrophy. The result is that the elderly are less able to produce a strong immunological response to new microorganisms and to contain latent infections.

Of the many other risk factors for immunodeficiency, protein calorie malnutrition is the most common cause worldwide. The ICU is no exception; in fact, this type of nutritional deficiency can occur in hospitalized patients who are on NPO status for prolonged periods or in those with extraordinary nutritional requirements. Ionizing radiation and noxious chemicals can also interfere with the production, maturation, and/or function of the cells of the immune system or even induce malignant transformation of these cells.

In general, immunodeficient is the most accurate term to use in referring to a person with a deficiency in immunity. It may refer either to someone with a primary or congenital defect in the immune response or to a person with an acquired or secondary lack of immunity. In contrast, immunocompromised is a term that implies that there was once a normally functioning immune system. Immunosuppressed is a term often reserved for persons in whom a normally functioning immune system is being suppressed by treatment such as chemotherapy, radiation therapy, or administration of corticosteroids or other agents.

Immunodeficiencies are heralded by the presence of chronic or recurrent infections, infections with unusual agents, and/or incomplete clearing between episodes of infection or incomplete response to treatment. Several clinical symptoms are often seen in immunodeficient patients: skin rash, diarrhea, lack of growth, hepatosplenomegaly, recurrent abscesses or osteomyelitis; and autoimmune disease.

The Immune Systems of the Body

The human body is completely surrounded by microorganisms, both externally on the skin and internally in the respiratory tract and gut. Nevertheless, infections are relatively infrequent in the immunocompetent host. The body uses several defenses to prevent invasion by the multitude of microorganisms around us. The immune response can be divided into five systems: barrier, phagocytic, complement, humoral, and cell-mediated immunity (see Table 8-8). All types

of immunity occur in two phases: the recognition phase and the response phase. The first and most important phase of immunity is recognition, because if the body does not recognize an invader, or if it erroneously recognizes its own tissue as foreign, clinical disease results.

Barrier, phagocytic, and complement immunity form the nonspecific immune system. These three immunities are natural or innate because they are present at birth. Humoral and cell-mediated immunity form the specific immune system, which is acquired. The latter immune system develops after birth, over time, and requires exposure to foreign substances. In certain situations, specific immunity can be passive, that is, transferred directly to an individual. For example, immunoglobulin, a product of the specific immune system, can be transferred across the placenta from the mother to the fetus or administered intravenously in the form of pooled immunoglobulin. Most often, specific immunity is active, that is, acquired when the body is infected with a microorganism and develops specific antibody and activated immune cells to destroy the invader. Immunization by vaccination is a form of active immunity.

Each immune system will be discussed below, and clinical deficiencies of each system will be described. An overview of these disorders is provided in Table 8-9.

Nonspecific Immunity

Barrier immunity The physical, mechanical, chemical, and microbial barriers of the body are the first

---

Table 8-8 Immune Systems of the Body

Type	Components	Characteristics
Nonspecific	Barrier immunity: Physical Mechanical Chemical Microbial	General recognition Same response to different substances No diversity No memory Breach of barrier defense and/or stimulation of phagocytic immunity causes inflammatory response
	Phagocytic immunity: Phagocytes (neutrophils, monocytes/macrophages)	
	Complement immunity	
Specific	Humoral immunity: B lymphocytes Antibodies	Selective recognition Diverse responses to different substances Heterogeneity (responds to a variety of cells and products)
	Cell-mediated immunity: T lymphocytes Cytokines (lymphokines)	Memory

Table 8-9 Overview of Clinical Immunodeficiencies

Disease	Clinical Manifestations	Defect	Therapy
Humoral			
Bruton's hypogamma-globulinemia	Recurrent pyogenic infections, esp. pneumonia, sinusitis, otitis, furunculosis, meningitis, sepsis, panhypogammaglobu-linemia, arthritis of the large joints	Decreased IgA, IgG, IgM; no plasma cells; low number of B cells; pre-B cells present	Aggressive, appropriate, and judicious use of antibiotics
Selective IgA deficiency	Bacterial infections of respiratory tract, GI tract, and GU tract; diarrhea; malabsorption; increased autoimmune disease	Synthesis but no secretion of IgA, high circulating anti-IgA antibody	Immune serum globulin (except in IgA deficiency)
Common variable immunodeficiency (acquired)	Recurrent pyogenic infections similar to Bruton's, but less severe; malabsorption, diarrhea, giardiasis, increased lymphoreticular malignancies	Normal number of circulating B cells; low immunoglobulin levels, no plasma cells	Plasma transfusions
Cellular			
DiGeorge's syndrome	Thymic hypoplasia, hypocalcemia, parathyroid hypoplasia, otitis, tuberculosis, candida, abnormal facies, congenital cardiac anomalies, chronic diarrhea, failure to thrive, esophageal atresia	Deficient T cells; thymic and parathyroid hypoplasia; often increase in B cells	Treatment of infections, tumors, and symptoms Immunologic reconstitution: Bone marrow transplant Fetal thymus transplant Lymphocyte transfusion Immunologic enhancement: Thymosin Transfer factor Interleukin 2
Chronic mucocutaneous candidiasis	Chronic, resistant C. Albicans infection of skin, nails, and mucous membranes; some endocrine abnormalities	Normal number of T cells, but failure of T cells to respond to antigen by production of lymphokine	Same as above
AIDS (acquired)	Kaposi's sarcoma, opportunistic infections (pneumocystis carinii, candida, toxoplasmosis, mycobacteria)	Decrease in number and/or function of T4 subset; reverse T4/T8 ratio; abnormalities in B cell function, NK cell function, and monocyte function	Same as above
Combined			
SCID (severe combined immunodeficiency)	Multiple severe infections of many kinds (bacterial, fungal, and viral); graft-versus-host disease; diarrhea; extreme wasting	Low T cells; low B cells; no antibody	Careful, early treatment of infections Protective isolation ISG, bone marrow, and fetal thymus transplants

(continued)

Table 8-9 Overview of Clinical Immunodeficiencies (*continued*)

Disease	Clinical Manifestations	Defect	Therapy
Wiskott-Aldrich syndrome	Thrombocytopenia with hemorrhagic tendency, eczema, recurrent infection, herpes, and high increase in lymphoreticular malignancy	Hypercatabolism of Igs; low IgM and IgG with high IgA and E; decreased T cells	Fetal liver transplants
Phagocytic Chronic granulomatous disease	Marked lymph-adenopathy with draining lymph nodes, hepatosplenomegaly, recurrent pneumonias, abscesses, dermatitis, conjunctivitis, osteomyelitis, usually with unusual organisms of low virulence (S. aureus, S. epidermis, E. coli, candida, aspergillus)	Abnormal neutrophil function with decreased intracellular killing because of enzyme deficiency (NADH or NADPH oxidase)	Surgical drainage or excision Broad-spectrum antibiotics Amphotericin B White cell transfusions
Job's (Hyper IgE) syndrome	Recurrent "cold" abscesses of skin, lymph nodes, and subcutaneous tissue; eczema; otitis media	Abnormal chemotaxis, increased eosinophils, increased IgE, abnormal antibody synthesis	Same as above
Chediak-Higashi syndrome	Recurrent cutaneous bacterial infections; hepatosplenomegaly; partial albinism; progressive CNS abnormality; increased lymphoreticular malignancy	Defective neutrophil and monocyte chemotaxis and delayed neutrophil killing time	Same as above
Complement Selective complement deficiencies	Multiple, serious pyogenic infections; immune complex disease (i.e., glomerulonephritis)	Decreased ability to opsonize bacteria; decreased chemotaxis; decreased cytolysis; decreased ability to clear immune complexes	Aggressive, appropriate antibiotic therapy FFP
Hereditary angioedema (HAE)	Episodic edema of throat, abdomen, face	Decreased C1 esterase inhibitor	Anabolic steroids and fibrinolytic agents
Secondary Immuno-deficiency (due to disease, injury, or treatment)	Increased susceptibility to infection, malignancy, autoimmune phenomena	Variable—most commonly, decrease in number of neutrophils	Protection from infection Treatment of cause, if possible Early detection and appropriate treatment of infections

means of preventing infection. Infections most commonly arise in the areas where the body has the most frequent contact with and the highest concentration of microorganisms: the skin, the surface of the eye, and the respiratory, gastrointestinal, and genitourinary tracts.

The skin and intact epithelium of the mucous membranes of the genitourinary, gastrointestinal, and respiratory tracts are the physical barriers that block the entry of pathogens into the body. Intact skin is dry, lacking the moisture necessary for bacterial growth. The slightly acid pH of skin (due to the presence of lactic acid, uric acid, amino acids, and free fatty acids) acts to destroy bacteria. Other substances, such as ammonia, triglycerides, and waxy alcohols from sebaceous glands, also assist in killing harmful microorganisms. Finally, bacteria are constantly shed along with dead skin cells.

Mechanical barriers either block microorganisms from entering the body or eject them. Eyelashes can flick microorganisms away from the surface of the eye during blinking; tears can wash microbes away. Microbes entering the respiratory tract may be ejected by sneezing or coughing or be entrapped in the mucous blanket and swept upward by cilia to be expectorated or swallowed. The peristalsis of the GI tract leads to the excretion of microorganisms by defecation.

Microorganisms ingested in food are destroyed by hydrochloric acid in the stomach. Other microbes are killed when exposed to the acid pH of the urine, vaginal secretions, or prostatic fluid. Many pathogens are digested by enzymes or bactericidal substances in tears, saliva, and even breast milk. For example, respiratory secretions contain lysozyme, alpha-1 antitrypsin, and IgA, all of which have bactericidal properties. Many bacterial pathogens require iron for growth. The body secretions contain iron-binding substances such as lactoferrin to reduce the availability of this important substance for bacterial growth.

The normal flora of the skin and the respiratory and GI tracts prevent overgrowth of pathogens by several means. Normal flora compete with harmful microorganisms for nutrients, thereby suppressing the growth of pathogenic bacteria. Resident flora also compete with pathogens for the same receptors on host cells. In addition, the body's indigenous microorganisms produce bacteriocins, substances lethal to pathogens. Normal flora also stimulate the formation of antibodies which can react against pathogens. Finally, normal flora continually stimulate the immune system, keeping it primed to combat invaders.

If the barrier defenses of the body are breached by microorganisms or if tissue injury occurs, the immune response is inflammation—the immediate and aggressive response by the body to injury. The purposes of inflammation are threefold: to dilute or destroy the injurious agent, to limit the spread of injury, and to supply the necessary cells and substances to the area for tissue repair.

Inflammation can arise from extrinsic stimuli—causes of inflammation originating outside of the body (such as musculoskeletal trauma, microbial infection, and surgical procedures). Other stimuli (such as intestinal obstruction, myocardial infarction, thrombosis and malignancy) are intrinsic causes of inflammation—causes located within the body. Although inflammation can vary in cause, severity, duration, and outcome, the inflammatory process is remarkable in its consistency. Regardless of the cause, the signs and symptoms of inflammation are redness, heat, swelling, pain, and loss of function.

With tissue injury, there is usually a rupture or tear in a blood vessel. The vessel exhibits an immediate but transient vasoconstriction, followed by vasodilation. Platelets flowing by the torn vessel aggregate, forming a platelet plug to stop bleeding. Substances released from the wall of the damaged blood vessel or from fragmented platelets initiate the clotting cascade. A fibrin barrier forms to stop bleeding and to wall off the area to limit spread of damage or infection. The vasodilation of the blood vessels surrounding the injury permits the delivery of more blood to the area, which causes symptoms of redness and warmth. The blood vessels also become "leaky," or permeable, and an inflammatory exudate leaks into the affected area, forming edema, a cardinal sign of inflammation. The exudate provides substances for tissue repair, dilutes toxins released by bacteria, and even limits motion of the area to allow healing to take place. In mild injury, this exudate resembles serum; with severe inflammation, the vasopermeability is so exaggerated that red blood cells and fibrin are found in the exudate.

As with other exaggerated immune responses, inflammation can have adverse effects on the body. Compartment syndrome, seen in fractures, can cause such severe swelling that blood flow to the extremity is dangerously reduced. Another example is the chronic inflammatory reaction exemplified by peritonitis or abdominal adhesions.

An inflammatory response manifested systemically is called an acute phase response or acute phase reaction. It is a generalized systemic reaction to microbial invasion or tissue injury and is evidenced by symptoms such as malaise, fatigue, fever, and weight loss. Laboratory studies reveal an increase in the release of stress-related pituitary hormones, the production and release of hepatic acute phase proteins (C-reactive protein, haptoglobin, amyloid A protein, alpha-1 antitrypsin, alpha-2 macroglobulin, and complement components), an elevated erythrocyte sedimentation rate (ESR), and reduced serum levels of iron, zinc, and albumin.

Phagocytic immunity Microorganisms that succeed in breaching the barrier defenses of the body are met by the body's second line of defense—phagocytic immunity. Phagocytes (literally, "eating cells") are specialized white blood cells that engulf and destroy invading microorganisms, foreign material, and cellular debris. Phagocytic immunity is most important for defense against bacteria and requires mature, properly functioning phagocytes in adequate numbers.

There are two main types of phagocytic white blood cells: neutrophils and monocytes/macrophages. Neutrophils respond first to the site of infection. Monocytes, which respond second, transform into macrophages following their entry into the tissue. Resident macrophages are often already present in the area of inflammation.

Phagocytes are attracted to and can engulf substances that have rough surfaces and/or a strong electrical charge. Most importantly, however, phagocytes readily engulf substances or cells that are identified as foreign by coatings of antibody or complement components. This labeling process, called opsonization, tremendously enhances phagocytosis. Macrophages readily engulf and destroy bacteria, viruses, and old red blood cells. They also exhibit necrotaxis, movement toward devitalized or dead tissue, and engulf and destroy dead neutrophils and necrotic tissue.[20]

When an infection or inflammatory process occurs, certain chemicals known as chemotactins are released at the site of injury; the chemotactins attract phagocytes to the area. Bacterial components, platelet products, enzymes released by other phagocytes, and complement components can all act as strong attractants to neutrophils and monocytes or macrophages. In response to chemotactic signals in the tissue, the phagocytes in the bloodstream line up on the capillary endothelium in a formation called pavementing, in which they resemble pavement stones. The cells enter the tissue by diapedesis, squeezing between the endothelial cells lining the walls of the blood vessels. Upon entry into the tissue, the phagocytes migrate toward the target cell or substance. This directed, purposeful movement toward the stimulus is called chemotaxis.

Once a phagocyte reaches the target cell or substance, it adheres to and engulfs it, enclosing it in a pocket or envelope called a phagosome (see Figure 8-5). Phagocytes have bags of digestive enzymes, called lysosomes, in their cytoplasm. The phagocyte merges the envelope containing the target with one of the bags containing the digestive or proteolytic enzymes, forming a phagolysosome, within which the target is destroyed. During the process of destroying and digesting microorganisms, neutrophils are themselves often destroyed, forming pus.

The combination of the barrier and phagocytic immunities produces the common inflammatory immune response that is the basis of the body's response to invading pathogens (producers of infection) and, ultimately, multiple systemic organ failure (MSOF) in some individuals. This process (see Figure 8-6) is a cascade of vasodilation, capillary permeability, WBC pavementing, fibrin response, antibody response, and hormonal responses, which leads to the clinical symptoms of infection, sepsis, and MSOF.

As noted, adequate phagocytic immunity requires the presence of mature phagocytes in ade-

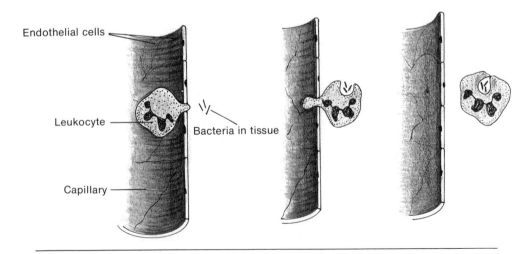

Endothelial cells

Leukocyte

Bacteria in tissue

Capillary

Figure 8-5 Phagocytosis

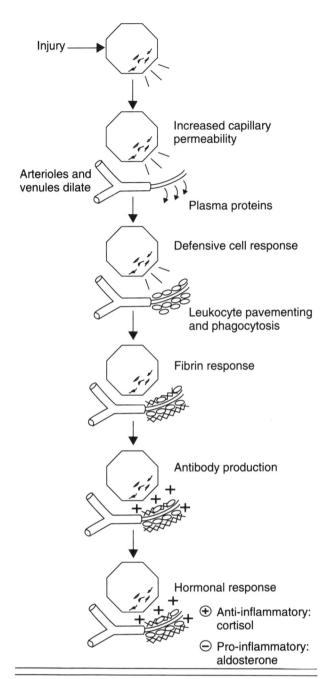

Injury

Increased capillary permeability

Arterioles and venules dilate

Plasma proteins

Defensive cell response

Leukocyte pavementing and phagocytosis

Fibrin response

Antibody production

Hormonal response

⊕ Anti-inflammatory: cortisol

⊖ Pro-inflammatory: aldosterone

Figure 8-6 The Inflammatory Immune Response

quate numbers and with competent immunologic function. Clinical phagocytic deficiencies can result from deficiencies in phagocyte quantities or qualitative defects in function. They may be congenital or occur after birth and be induced by treatment.

The primary, or congenital, phagocytic disorders are rare disorders: Chediak-Higashi syndrome, chronic granulomatous disease (CGD), congenital neutropenia, cyclic neutropenia, hyperimmunoglobulin E, recurrent infection (Job's) syndrome, lazy leukocyte syndrome, leukocyte adhesion deficiency, and myeloperoxidase deficiency. The most common

of these disorders occurs in 1 out of every 250,000 persons. The secondary, or acquired, disorders include autoimmune neutropenia and iatrogenic neutropenia (see the discussion of neutropenia on pages 1128 through 1131). Table 8-9 lists some of these immune disorders.

Several tests are available for evaluation of phagocytic immunity. By far the most common test is the WBC count and differential, which quantifies the number, type, and maturity of the WBCs, including circulating neutrophils and monocytes. Other tests of phagocytic immunity are usually done only at centers that specialize in evaluation of immune deficiencies. Among these sophisticated tests are the nitroblue tetrazolium dye test, which measures the ability of the phagocyte to perform the "respiratory burst" required to effectively kill many microorganisms.

The treatment of phagocytic disorders can vary. Most often, oral antibiotics are administered prophylactically to reduce the incidence of infections. When infections occur, they require treatment with prolonged courses of intravenous antibiotics. If the patient does not respond to antibiotic therapy alone, the physician may elect to add granulocyte transfusions to the treatment regimen.

In the past few years, genetic engineering has enabled scientists to replicate naturally occurring body substances, which stimulate the hematologic and immune systems and which can be used to treat persons with hematologic or immunologic disorders. For example, the administration of recombinant gamma interferon has reduced the frequency, severity, and duration of infections in chronic granulomatous disease. Granulocyte colony stimulating factor (G-CSF) has been employed in the treatment of congenital neutropenia. For persons with severe disorders, such as leukocyte adhesion deficiency, bone marrow transplantation may remain a therapeutic option.

Current research on certain immunologic disorders is focusing on curing the genetic defect by replacing the defective gene with a normal one. This research is a painstaking process of identifying the exact genetic defect, cloning and sequencing the normal gene, producing the normal gene, perhaps attaching the normal gene to a harmless retrovirus, infecting the patient's defective cells with this virus, and then injecting these cells back into the patient. This procedure was implemented in September 1990 in a child with severe combined immunodeficiency.[21]

The Spleen

The spleen is a fist-sized organ located in the left side of the abdominal cavity. The spleen is the primary site of fetal erythropoiesis until the fifth month of gestation and has the potential to resume this function if the need arises. The spleen also has a capacity for regeneration and compensatory hypertrophy.

The spleen can be visualized as a combination of two types of tissue: hematologic tissue, forming a red pulp, and immunologic tissue, forming a white pulp. The red pulp produces blood cells in utero and after birth and is responsible for the removal of aged or damaged RBCs. The splenic white pulp contains lymphocytes and has a dual function. It plays an important role in the storage and activation of lymphocytes (see Table 8-10). In addition, the highly specialized tissue and the unique circulatory arrangement of the white pulp of the spleen allow antigen to be concentrated in an environment that facilitates interaction between macrophages, B lymphocytes, T lymphocytes, and plasma cells. The spleen has been described as having "a kind of

Table 8-10 Lymphoid Tissues

Tissue	Location	Function
Central/primary		
Red Bone Marrow	Soft tissue cavities of long, flat bones: sternum ribs, vertebrae, iliac crest	Source of stem cells from which all blood cells are derived
Bursal Equivalent	Unknown location; may be in spleen, liver, bone marrow, or other area	Area in which B lymphocytes mature
Thymus	Behind sternum, bordering thyroid gland, develops in sixth week of gestation; reaches full weight at birth; function peaks at puberty, then declines as organ becomes fatty	*Lymphoid cells* of thymus mature into undifferentiated T lymphocytes; *Epithelial cells* of thymus produce thymosine, a hormone which stimulates lymphocytes to differentiate into either T4 "helper" or T8 "suppressor" cells
Liver	Upper right quadrant of abdomen	Filters and purifies blood; portal circulation contains sinus channels lined with Kupffer cells (fixed macrophages of the liver); fetal liver produces stem cells, which differentiate into T and B lymphocytes; adult liver produces plasma proteins such as immunoglobulins
Peripheral/secondary		
Lymphatic System	Network throughout body	Lymph (fluid) contains 60% T cells, a few RBCs, and clotting factors; transports fat and proteins; provides area for storage and proliferation on WBCs
Lymph Nodes	Junction of major lymphatic tracts: cervical, axillary, abdominal, inguinal	Storage of "resting" lymphocytes; proliferation and differentiation of "activated" lymphocytes upon antigenic stimulation; lined with fixed macrophages of the reticuloendothelial system
Lymph Nodules	Peyer's patches (a type of GALT, or gut-associated lymph tissue, in the small intestine) Waldeyer's rings at tonsils and inguinal nodes	Proliferation of B lymphocytes into plasma cells; storage of plasma cells, producing mainly IgA Storage and proliferation of lymphocytes
Spleen	Upper left quadrant of abdomen	"White pulp" in center: storage and proliferation of lymphocytes, other leukocytes, plasma cells, and monocytes; "red pulp" in outer spleen: produces RBCs at birth; later destroys RBCs via phagocytosis; converts hemoglobin to bilirubin

administrative role" because its specialized blood flow brings together different cell types so that they can interact constructively.[22]

The most important function of the spleen is its role as a mechanical filter of particulate matter.[23] As blood flows through the spleen, circulating antigen is trapped, processed through antigen-presenting cells, and concentrated in the white pulp, where T and B cells can interact to induce an effective and well-orchestrated immune response. The spleen shares other important functions with the liver and bone marrow: hematopoiesis, culling, pitting, reticulocyte modification, and sequestration of blood cells. The culling function of the spleen involves the removal of old (senescent) or damaged RBCs and perhaps other blood cells. Pitting is the term for the spleen's removal of intracellular inclusions, intraerythrocytic pathogens, or particles without damaging the erythrocyte. The splenic macrophages also perform reticulocyte modification, removing excess cell membrane from reticulocytes—a step in the maturation of these cells. The sequestration of blood cells is another important function of the spleen. The spleen holds a significant number of platelets and a lesser number of erythrocytes in reserve: up to 30% of total RBCs and 20–30% of total platelets. (In splenomegaly, up to 80–90% of total platelets are stored.) Finally, if the need arises, the spleen is capable of hematopoiesis; that is, it has the potential to revert to the hematopoiesis function it performed during fetal development.

The spleen's unique circulatory arrangement is what enables it to perform many of its specialized functions. As arterial blood from the celiac trunk enters the spleen and flows through the red pulp, different blood cells go to different areas of the spleen. Of the lymphocytes entering the spleen, 50% migrate to the white pulp, where they are sorted into the B and T zones; T cells remain there for 4–6 hours, and B cells remain at least 1 day. Erythrocytes pass out of capillaries in the red pulp into the cords of Bilroth, which are lined by macrophages. The RBCs must squeeze through a meshwork of cords and flow through the narrow apertures of the endothelial walls of venous sinuses, which are also lined by macrophages, in order to return to circulation. Aged or damaged RBCs are unable to deform themselves to squeeze through the apertures and are engulfed by macrophages. Eventually, venous blood exiting the spleen empties into the portal circulation, to be detoxified by the liver.

The slow blood flow through the spleen may allow prolonged contact between microorganisms and phagocytes. This may be especially important in destroying unopsonized bacteria and/or encapsu-lated bacteria such as Streptococcus pneumoniae, Neisseria meningitides, or Neisseria gonorrhea. The capsular polysaccharides from these microorganisms are T cell–independent antigens; that is, B cells in the spleen can effectively produce antibody to these organisms with little T cell help.

Asplenia is defined as diminished or absent splenic function; it may occur for multiple reasons. The spleen may be surgically removed after trauma or for treatment of hemolytic disorders related to splenomegaly. Persons with sickle cell anemia may experience autosplenectomy after repeated episodes of "sickling," which cause multiple splenic infarcts. Splenic tissue can also be destroyed by irradiation for malignancy.

Persons with asplenia have approximately 200 times greater risk of experiencing a particular type of bacterial infection known as overwhelming post-splenectomy infection (OPSI).[24] OPSI is caused by encapsulated bacteria (Streptococcus pneumoniae, Neisseria meningitides, or Hemophilus influenzae). The risk of OPSI is highest soon after splenectomy, although it can occur years or even decades later. The risk of OPSI is even greater if the splenectomy is performed in childhood or because of malignant disease.

The initial symptoms of OPSI, fever and malaise, are not alarming—yet the infection can progress with such dramatic suddenness that even when the patient is given prompt treatment with appropriate antibiotics, death can occur within hours after onset of symptoms. The mortality rate from OPSI ranges from 50% to 70%.[25] Streptococcus pneumoniae causes 50–90% of all cases of OPSI, and Neisseria meningitides and Hemophilus influenza are responsible for most of the remaining cases.[26]

The risk of OPSI can be reduced (although not eliminated) by vaccination against Streptococcal pneumoniae. The 23-valent pneumococcal vaccine should be administered 2 weeks prior to an elective splenectomy and to children with sickle cell anemia after they are 2 years of age. Consideration should be given to the administration of vaccinations for Hemophilus influenza type B and Neisseria meningitides. Since OPSI can occur despite vaccination, some clinicians support the administration of antibiotics to asplenic patients with nonspecific febrile illness.[27]

The Liver

The spleen and liver share certain hematologic and immunologic functions. Like the spleen, the liver is a site of hematopoiesis in the fetus and can regain that function later in life if necessary. In addition, although the splenic macrophages are most active in eliminating aged, damaged, or antibody-coated RBCs from the circulation, the liver's resident macrophages—the Kupffer cells—also perform this function. In persons with asplenia, the liver becomes the prime site of the culling of senescent erythrocytes.

Regardless of which organ destroys the aged RBCs, the liver is responsible for several related functions. Hepatic cells convert the bilirubin from hemolyzed erythrocytes to bile to aid in digestion of fat. The liver also stores iron (from degraded hemoglobin) as ferritin and releases it as needed to the bone marrow for the manufacture of hemoglobin during erythropoiesis. Also, apoferritin, the substance used to transport iron in the bloodstream, is produced by the liver.

One of the liver's most important immunologic roles involves the removal of bacteria from the bloodstream. The Kupffer cells of the liver can remove a bacterium in 0.01 second. Since the blood flowing from the GI tract to the liver may contain large amounts of bacteria, this function is critically important to prevent septicemia.

Among the myriad of substances that the liver synthesizes are several that are of significance to the hematologic and immunologic systems: albumin, haptoglobin, clotting factors, and complement components. Hepatic cells also produce certain proteins in large amounts during periods of inflammation. These acute phase proteins include C-reactive protein, amyloid A, alpha-1 antitrypsin, and alpha-2 macroglobulin, which have roles in the immune response.

Complement immunity Complement is a series of more than 30 interacting glycoproteins in the serum and on cell membranes that are involved in the immune response and inflammation. The complement system is interrelated with other major body processes: hemostasis, fibrinolysis, and kinin formation.

Complement components are synthesized by macrophages and other specialized body cells. Nine large serum components, numbered C1 through C9, circulate in a nonactive state. When fixed or activated, the early complement components (C1 through C5) are split into at least two new molecules. In general, the "a" fragment is important in promoting inflammation. The "b" fragment usually continues the cascade by combining with preceding fragments to form an active enzyme, which then splits the next component in the cascade. The complement cascade can be thought of as a sort of chain reaction in which each complement component cleaves the next one.

There are two pathways for activation of the complement cascade: the classical and the alternate pathways. The classical pathway is activated when the immunoglobins IgM or IgG bind to an antigen. (See pages 1108–1110 for a discussion of immunoglobins.) In contrast, activation of the alternate pathway is triggered by lipopolysaccharides from bacterial cell walls, although it can also be triggered by the IgA immunoglobin. In the classical pathway, IgM immunoglobin is far more efficient at activating complement than IgG. When an IgM molecule binds to several points on an antigen, the multiple binding alters the shape of a portion of the IgM molecule, exposing a special attachment site for C1. Thus, only one IgM molecule is necessary to activate the complement cascade. In order for IgG to activate the complement cascade, two adjacent IgG molecules must be crosslinked by C1. For a large antigen, many IgG molecules may be bound to the surface before two molecules are adjacent to each other and able to activate C1.

Although the classical pathway begins with the activation of C1, the rest of the components are not activated in numerical order. The steps of activation for the classical pathway of the complement cascade are C1, C4, C2, C3, C5, C6, C7, C8, and C9. After C1 becomes activated, it splits into components that cleave C4 into two molecules, C4a and C4b. C4a cleaves C2 into C2a and C2b. C4a2b cleaves C3 into C3a and C3b. At this point, the steps of the classical and alternate pathways merge into a final, common pathway, wherein C5, C6, C7, C8, and C9 are activated in sequence to form a molecule called the membrane attack complex (MAC). Figure 8-7 diagrams both pathways of the complement cascade.

Unlike the classical pathway, the alternate pathway does not require antibody for activation, although aggregates of IgA or IgE can initiate the cascade. More importantly, the alternate pathway is triggered by polysaccharides found in the cell walls of certain bacteria. Serum factors B and D produce an enzyme that converts C3 to C3b; C3b and serum factor B then attach to the microbe, making it attractive to a phagocytic cell.

Activation of the complement cascade is regulated by factors that promote formation of active enzymes and opposing factors that inhibit enzyme formation or inactivate enzymes. During infection, the promoting factors outweigh the inhibitors, and complement activation proceeds. After infection is resolved, there are fewer antigens to bind to Ig molecules to continue activation, and inhibiting factors block cascade activation.

The complement system facilitates the function of phagocytes; the complement fragments, or com-

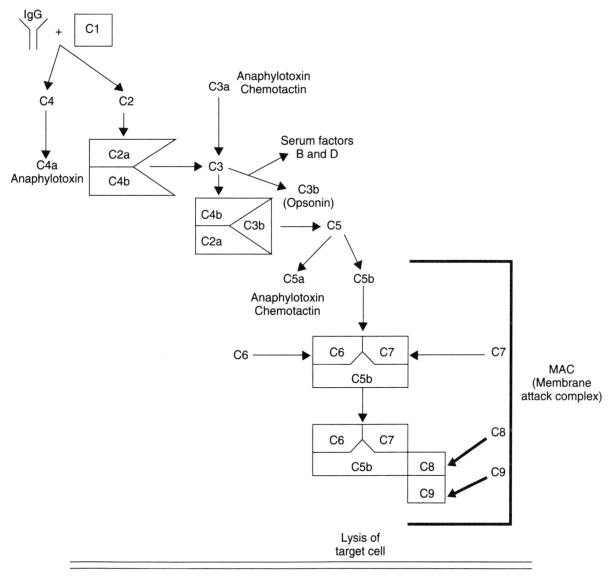

Figure 8-7   Pathways of the Complement Cascade

ponents, act as chemotactins, attracting leukocytes to the site of infection, and promote the aggregation and adhesiveness of granulocytes. Most important, complement components act as opsonins to greatly enhance the ability of phagocytes to engulf and destroy microorganisms.

Certain complement components (anaphylotox-ins) augment the inflammatory response by stimulating the release of chemical mediators from mast cells. Some mediators, such as histamine, are formed in

advance and held in storage awaiting release. Others, such as bradykinin, SRSA, and prostaglandins, are produced and released upon antigenic stimulation.

Complement plays a key role in the removal of immune complexes, which are clumps of antigen-antibody molecules. If these macromolecules are not promptly removed from the circulation and tissues, they can stimulate tissue damage. RBCs, neutrophils, monocytes, B lymphocytes, and some T lymphocytes have receptors for certain complement fragments. These cells are able to attach to immune complexes coated with complement fragments and carry these molecules to the liver for removal by the Kupffer cells. Since RBCs are so numerous, they have the most important role in this process. Host cells are nonactivators—they possess mechanisms to limit the complement activation. RBCs have two or three means of resisting complement-mediated lysis.

One of the less important but best-known functions of the complement system is the direct lysing of bacteria via a complement molecule known as the membrane attack complex (MAC). The MAC may be useful in fighting infections by encapsulated bacteria. It is theorized that the MAC blows holes in the outer cell walls of these bacteria, and the phagocytic digestive enzymes enter the holes and thus gain access to the vulnerable inner cell membrane of the bacteria.

Many of the laboratory tests used in evaluating complement immunity are probably inaccurate measurements of levels and function of various complement components. Unfortunately, normal values in complement assays do not necessarily reflect intact complement immunity; nor do abnormal values necessarily indicate immunodeficiency. Nevertheless, until better tests are developed, clinicians must rely on the tests currently available. These are summarized in Table 8-11.

Complement deficiencies are the rarest of all immunodeficiencies and are manifested clinically in strikingly different ways, depending upon which component is deficient. Among the primary complement deficiencies is the lack of C1 inhibitor, which normally blocks activation of C1, the first component of the classical pathway of the cascade. Angioedema, a swelling disorder, is the clinical outcome of this deficiency. Hereditary angioedema is a primary immunodeficiency in which C1 inhibitor is either dysfunctional or produced in inadequate amounts. Acquired angioedema is an extremely rare disease in which, for unknown reasons, a person develops autoantibodies to C1 inhibitor. Regardless of the underlying cause of the deficiency, the lack of this inhibitor causes uncontrolled activation of C1, C4, and C2, the early components of the classical pathway. The remainder of the cascade is unaffected, since other inhibitors that are still functional prevent activation of C3. The uncontrolled activation of these early complement components is induced by minor physical trauma and/or emotional stress; the result is swelling, which is self-limited, resolving in several hours or a few days. However, if the swelling involves the airway, respiratory compromise and death can result.

Levels of the early components of the complement cascade can also be lowered secondary to diseases in which there is chronic activation of the inflammatory response, for example, systemic lupus erythematosis (SLE). Persons with primary deficiencies of the earlier complement component C1, C4, C2, or C3 often develop immune complex disease such as glomerulonephritis, perhaps due to an inability to efficiently remove immune complexes. Deficiency of C3, C5, C6, C7, or C8 can result in the development of serious infections by Neisseria meningitides, despite vaccination against this organism. C3, the most abundant complement component, is common to both pathways of the cascade. Thus, a deficiency of C3 is the most severe complement deficiency and results in both life-threatening infections by encapsulated bacteria and immune complex disease.

Paroxysmal nocturnal hemoglobinuria (PNH), although not often categorized as a complement

Table 8-11 Tests of Complement Function

Test	Evaluates	Normal Result	Abnormal Result	Clinical Condition
CH_{50}	Total amount of complement components in serum	22–55 H_{50} units/mL	Low	Secondary deficiency, such as systemic lupus erythematosis
C3	Amount of C3 in serum	85–175 mg/dL	Low	Sinopulmonary or dermatological infection
C4	Amount of C4 in serum	15–45 mg/dL	Low; antibodies to C4	Immune complex disease C4 dysfunction
C1 inhibitor functional assay	Function of C1 esterase inhibitor	Poor, fair, good activity	Decreased activity	Hereditary angioedema

deficiency, is an acquired disease caused by a defect in the bone marrow stem cells, which results in a lack of complement inactivators in the membranes of the circulating blood cells. Because RBCs are the most important circulating blood cells involved in the elimination of immune complexes from the bloodstream, a deficiency in a complement inactivator will be most strongly manifested in RBC damage. It is theorized that in PNH, simple daily activities such as toothbrushing release bacteria into the circulation. Antibody and complement components coat the bacteria, forming immune complexes that attach to receptors on RBCs. The RBCs are unable to inactivate these complement components, so the remainder of the complement cascade is activated, and the vulnerable erythrocytes are lysed. Persons with PNH often develop thrombosis and may die due to thrombosis of hepatic or mesenteric blood vessels.

Specific Immunity

The nonspecific immune systems (barrier, phagocytic, and complement immunity) are capable of only a general sort of recognition of foreign substances; they lack diversity in responding to different antigens and are not capable of developing memory. In contrast, the components of the specific immune system (B lymphocytes in humoral immunity and T lymphocytes in cell-mediated immunity, lymphoid tissue, lymphatics, and the thymus gland) are able to recognize and react only with the particular molecular configuration unique to each individual B or T lymphocyte. This selective recognition means that the lymphocytes are able to distinguish among different antigens. The specific immune system also has a memory: an enhanced and accelerated response by sensitized cells, which is triggered by the second or subsequent exposure to a foreign substance (see Figure 8-8). In addition, humoral and cell-mediated

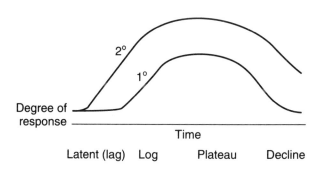

1° In primary exposure to antigen

2° In secondary or subsequent exposure to antigen

Figure 8-8 Phases of the Specific Immune Response

immunity are characterized by heterogeneity, in which a variety of cells and cell products work together in diverse ways to protect the body.

The T and B lymphocytes are the cells involved in the specific immune response. These small, agranular leukocytes have large round nuclei and very little cytoplasm and are derived from lymphoid-committed stem cells (see Figure 8-9). The B lymphocytes are involved in the production of antibody. The T lymphocytes are involved in orchestrating the overall immune response. A third type of lymphocyte, the large granular lymphocytes (among which are the natural killer cells), is not involved in specific immunity and will be reviewed later. To discuss specific immunity, it is necessary to explain the terms related to the antigen response.

An antigen is any substance that can interact with its corresponding antibody or T cell receptor. Antigens are usually proteins or polysaccharides, with molecules that have repetitive shapes projecting from their surfaces.[28] Haptens are substances of low molecular weight, which by themselves are too small to generate an immune response. However, haptens can combine with a protein to form a larger molecule that is antigenic. This combination will either elicit or stimulate an immune response. Epitopes, or antigenic determinants, are the characteristic "nonself" shapes that protrude from the surface of an antigen. There are usually several different epitopes on the surface of one antigen. Exogenous antigens enter the body from the environment and include any substances that are contacted, inhaled, ingested, or injected. Microorganisms, pollen, dust, drugs, and food molecules are examples of exogenous antigens. Endogenous antigens originate from within the body. Aged red blood cells or damaged tissue are examples of this type of antigen.

In order for a substance to be antigenic, it must be large (molecular weight greater than 6000 daltons, with 4–7 amino acids) and have a complex, foreign chemical makeup, such as are found in proteins or polysaccharides. In fact, nearly all proteins are antigenic in the appropriate person. Antigenicity is influenced by the route of entry of the substance into the body, the amount of substance entering the body, the molecular complexity of the substance, the accessibility of its epitopes, and, finally, the ability of the substance to be phagocytosed and degraded. In general, the most antigenic molecules are introduced into the body via injection in large amounts, are complex, have accessible epitopes, and are easily phagocytosed and degraded.

Certain microorganisms have similar antigens. For example, cowpox and smallpox are two different viruses with similar antigens. When vaccinated with

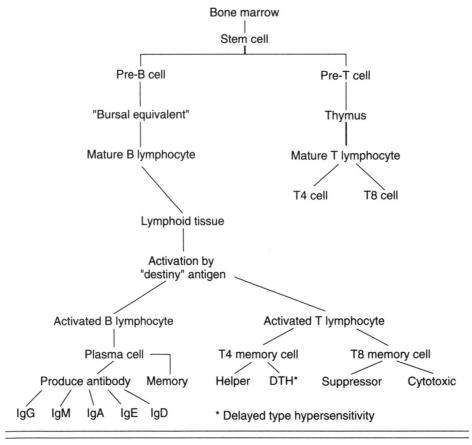

Figure 8-9 Lymphocyte Development

the cowpox virus, people produce antibodies to cowpox that are also effective against smallpox. If infected with smallpox, the vaccinated person is able to eradicate the virus with a brisk antibody response. This phenomenon is termed a cross reaction, and the antibodies produced are known as cross-reactive antibodies. Unfortunately, cross reactions may not be beneficial. For example, antigens on microorganisms can resemble molecules on the surfaces of body cells. Molecules on streptococci resemble molecules on heart and joint muscles. If a streptococcal infection is inadequately controlled, the body can mistakenly attack the heart and joints, producing rheumatic fever. Molecules on the surfaces of the spirochete that causes syphilis resemble molecules on the surfaces of body cells. People who have antibodies to human cells (multiparous women, persons with SLE, or those who have received multiple transfusions) may have a false positive test for syphilis.

Immunologists estimate that approximately 1 million possible antigen configurations occur in nature. The body has the capacity to produce a unique T lymphocyte and a unique B lymphocyte (from em-

bryonic stem cells) for each of these configurations, and to produce still more through mutation. Therefore, the body has at least 1 million different types of preformed B and T cells. Millions of these preformed specific lymphocytes are present in the lymphoid tissues throughout the body. Each lymphocyte has a destiny antigen; that is, each is capable of forming a highly specific response to the appropriate antigen.

Lymphocytes, the primary actors in the specific immune response, first arise in the fetal spleen and liver and then develop in the bone marrow. B lymphocytes probably mature in the bone marrow, and T lymphocytes mature in the thymus. There is a constant recirculation of lymphocytes throughout the body.

The immunoglobulin molecules on the surface of B lymphocytes act as those cells' receptors, which bind to the cell's destiny antigen. Each immunoglobulin molecule produced by an individual B cell has the same destiny antigen receptor. Each B cell has approximately 100,000 antibody molecules in its cell membrane, which will react with only one specific antigen.

The T cell receptors (TCR) on the surface of an

individual T lymphocyte act as that T cell's receptors, which are activated by the cell's destiny antigen. An individual T cell may have more than 100,000 TCRs on its surface.

When an individual B or T lymphocyte encounters its unique destiny antigen, the lymphocyte proliferates, differentiates, and performs its function. During proliferation, lymphocytes reproduce wildly, forming huge numbers of duplicate cells called clones. Each clone of an individual lymphocyte is only responsive to that particular lymphocyte's original destiny antigen. During differentiation, the cell changes somewhat in appearance and may add or subtract molecules on its surface. Memory B or T cells formed during this process have a relatively long life-span of months, years, or even decades. The functions performed by B and T cells are quite different and will be covered in the following sections on humoral and cell-mediated immunity. It is interesting to note that most antigens activate both B and T lymphocytes at the same time.

Lymphoid tissue and lymphatics The lymphatic system is a network of specialized tissue and connecting vessels for the production, maturation, storage, and activation of lymphocytes; the trapping and concentration of antigens for immune system activation; and antibody production. Lymphoid organs are divided into two types: central (primary) and peripheral (secondary). (Refer to Table 8-10.) This division is misleading to some degree, because some lymph organs fall into both categories.

The primary lymphoid organs are concerned with the production and maturation of T and B lymphocytes, which are compared in Table 8-12. Both T and B lymphocytes arise from the pluripotential stem cells in the bone marrow (see Figure 8-9). The pre-B lymphocytes are believed to complete their maturation in the bone marrow, or bursal equivalent. The pre-T lymphocytes migrate to the thymus, where, with the help of the thymic hormones, they develop into mature thymocytes. Thus, the bone

Table 8-12 Comparison of T and B Lymphocytes

Parameter	T Cells	B Cells
Morphology	Identifiable surface antigens that distinguish the subsets: T3, T4, T8, etc. Receptors for sheep red blood cells: SRBC	Surface immunoglobulin (Ig) Receptors for the Fc portion of Ig Receptors for C3b
Ontogeny	Bone marrow stem cell Early thymocyte (in thymic cortex) Mature thymocyte (in thymic medulla) Immunocompetent T lymphocyte (located in peripheral circulation, spleen, lymph nodes)	Bone marrow stem cell Pre-B cell (in "bursal equivalent") Mature B cell Immunocompetent B lymphocyte (located in peripheral circulation, spleen, cortex of lymphoid follicles)
Function	Cell-mediated Immunity: Cytotoxicity Immunoregulation Mediator release Memory	Humoral immunity: Antibody production Memory
Products elaborated	Lymphokines Helper/suppressor factors	Immunoglobulins
Location (% of total lymphocytes)		
Peripheral blood	80%	20%
Lymph node	75%	20%
Spleen	35–45%	50–60%
Bone marrow	<10%	<75%

marrow and thymus are the primary lymphoid organs.

Peripheral or secondary lymphoid tissue is the site of storage and activation of lymphocytes. It is in the secondary lymphoid tissue that the lymphocytes are stored, encounter antigen, proliferate, and differentiate into working immune cells. Secondary lymphoid tissue exists in several forms. This tissue, consisting of a collection of lymphocytes which may or may not be encapsulated, forms lymph nodes, spleen, and subepithelial areas of GI tract and bone marrow. In addition, the bone marrow, as a site of a storage and activation, also acts as a secondary lymphoid organ.

Lymph Nodes

Lymph nodes, formed at the junctions of several lymphatic vessels, are small, bean-shaped structures less than 1 cm in diameter; they consist of dense collections of T and B lymphocytes, plasma cells, and macrophages enclosed in a capsule. Lymph nodes are arranged along the course of blood vessels throughout the body (Figure 8-10) and are distributed advantageously to intercept invaders. Thus, they are found in the highest concentration at areas of greatest contact with microorganisms: throat, pharynx, neck, axilla, abdomen, and groin.

Lymph is carried into lymph nodes via afferent lymphatic vessels and drains out via efferent vessels. In addition, the nodes are supplied with arterial and venous circulation. T and B lymphocytes circulating in the bloodstream have a unique ability to adhere to the capillary endothelium of venules in lymphoid organs and migrate into lymphoid tissue. After entering a lymph node, T cells remain for 2–4 hours and B cells remain at least one day before exiting. Lymph and lymphocytes leave via the efferent lymphatics (rather than veins), which drain into increasingly larger lymphatic ducts, including the thoracic duct, the main channel of lymphatic fluid, and eventually empty into the venous circulation.

The outer layer of the lymph node, the cortex, contains B lymphocytes in dense aggregates called primary follicles. The next layer of tissue, the paracortex, contains macrophages and T lymphocytes. In the center of the node is the medulla, which contains strands, or cords, of connective tissue holding plasma cells and macrophages. Any antigen entering the lymph node is trapped by macrophages and comes into contact with its destiny B cell or is presented to its destiny T cell if present.

Upon antigenic stimulation, the B lymphocytes of the primary follicles begin proliferating, forming a germinal center that is surrounded by a secondary follicle of resting B cells. This proliferation accounts for the lymphadenopathy associated with infection.

Secondary lymphoid tissue is also found in the splenic white pulp and in unencapsulated collections of lymphocytes in the respiratory, GI, and GU tracts. This lymphoid tissue is referred to as mucosal associated lymphoid tissue (MALT). MALT is further divided into gut-associated lymphoid tissue (GALT), in the GI tract, and bronchial associated lymphoid tissue (BALT), in the respiratory tract. Peyer's patches in the small intestine constitute one type of GALT. BALT is found in Waldeyer's ring, in the lingual, palatine, and pharyngeal tonsils, in the adenoids, and in the bronchial mucosa.

Lymphoid tissue is interconnected by a network of lymphatic vessels and valves for the collection, transport, and filtration of tissue fluid and lymphocytes. The lymphatics drain fluid from interstitial spaces and up to one-tenth of the fluid that passes from arteries to veins into the lymphatic vessels. The fluid, known as lymph, consists of water, salts, proteins, and lymphocytes that have migrated from tissue. Lymph is carried via the lymphatic vessels to the lymphoid organs or to regional lymph nodes for filtration. Eventually, the fluid and lymphocytes are channeled into large lymphatic vessels and are returned to the venous circulation. Two-thirds of all lymph originates from the liver and intestine.

Lymphatic fluid draining from the lower half of body, the left side of the head and the chest, and the left arm drains into the thoracic duct. This large lymph vessel in the thorax is the major channel through which lymph flows on its return to the venous circulation. The thoracic duct empties into veins at the junction of the left internal jugular and left subclavian veins. Lymph from the right side of the head and neck, the right arm, and the right side of chest enters the right lymphatic duct, which empties into the veins at the junction of the right internal jugular and right subclavian veins. Valves throughout the lymph vessels prevent backflow. Every hour, over 100 mL of lymphatic fluid flows through the thoracic duct and 20 mL of lymphatic fluid flows through other channels.

Humoral immunity Humoral immunity involves B lymphocytes and the production of antibodies. It is the major protection against infection by bacteria and viruses and their toxins; it is also a key component of bacterial opsonization and lysis and the immune system involved in immunization. Upon first exposure to a substance, the humoral immune response is generated in hours to days; upon subsequent exposure to the same substance, the response may take merely minutes.

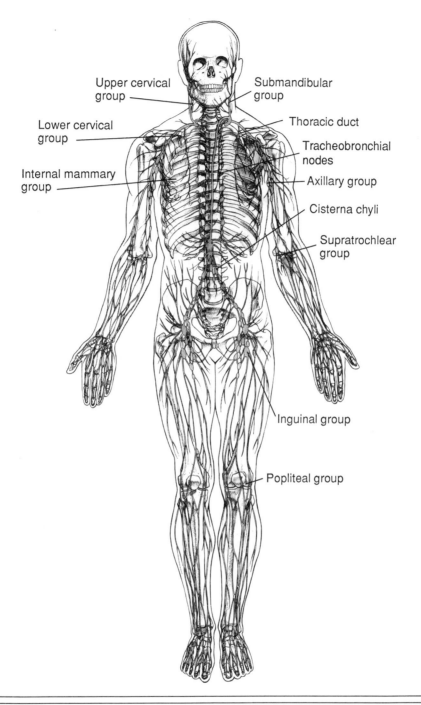

Upper cervical group

Lower cervical group

Internal mammary group

Submandibular group

Thoracic duct

Tracheobronchial nodes

Axillary group

Cisterna chyli

Supratrochlear group

Inguinal group

Popliteal group

Figure 8-10 Lymph Nodes and Their Drainage

B lymphocytes arise from lymphoid-committed stem cells, which further differentiate into pre-B cells or pre-T cells. Pre-B cells are believed to mature in the fetal liver in the eighth week of gestation and, later in development, in the bone marrow. The body produces billions of B lymphocytes a day.

The name *B lymphocyte* was originally developed following research on birds. Chickens possess an organ, the bursa, to which their pre-B cells migrate for development and maturation. Without this or-

gan, chickens are unable to produce antibody. Thus, the lymphocytes responsible for antibody production were originally referred to as bursa-derived, or B, lymphocytes. Although humans do not have a bursa, it is believed that the bone marrow performs the same function.

As B lymphocytes mature, they progress through several stages of development. When mature, the B lymphocytes are released from the bone marrow, circulate in the bloodstream for a few hours, then migrate to the peripheral lymphoid organs such as the spleen or lymph nodes.

The B cells remain in the lymphoid tissue for a day, then reenter the circulation, travel throughout the body, and eventually return to the peripheral lymphoid tissue. This constant recirculation of lymphocytes throughout the body is important, since it increases the likelihood that a circulating lymphocyte will come in contact with its destiny antigen and stimulate a prompt immune response.

Upon contacting its destiny antigen, a B lymphocyte proliferates, then differentiates into large lymphoblasts. Most of these lymphoblasts clone and differentiate into plasmablasts, which subsequently clone and differentiate into plasma cells. Each plasmablast produces 500 plasma cells, antibody "factories" capable of synthesizing and secreting thousands of immunoglobulin molecules a second.[29] Each of these molecules is specific to the destiny antigen of the original B lymphocyte. This process takes approximately 4 days, which accounts for the delay in development of measurable antibody levels for a short period after infection. Many plasma cells remain in lymphoid tissue throughout the body and are present in especially high concentrations in the spleen.

Among the original group of lymphoblasts are a few that develop into memory B cells. These cells remain in lymphoid tissue awaiting future contact with the antigen. Upon a second exposure to the antigen, the memory B cells are able to clone and differentiate into antibody-producing plasma cells in far less time than it took following the original exposure. This rapid response is the rationale underlying vaccination. Each B cell's activation by its individual destiny antigen occurs either with the help of T cells or without it.

Certain antigens are capable of stimulating B cells to clone with little assistance from T cells; the activation process is depicted in Figure 8-11. Polysaccharide molecules are produced by encapsulated pathogenic bacteria (such as Hemophilus influenza and Streptococcus pneumonia). These molecules have repeating shapes that are very effective at stimulating B cells. T cell–independent activation of B cells is a slow and somewhat limited process of antibody production. The plasma cells produced in this process can synthesize and secrete IgM only. In addition, this process does not result in the formation of memory B cells.

Most often, B cells contact their individual destiny antigens and require significant assistance from T4 helper cells, as depicted in Figure 8-12. The T4 helper cells secrete cytokines, chemical messengers such as B cell growth factor and B cell differentiation factor, which stimulate B cell development. Cytokines IL-1 alpha and IL-1 beta, IL-2, 4, 5, 6, and G-Ifn all stimulate activation, proliferation, and differentiation of B cells. In addition, T cell cytokines appear to influence the class of antibody produced by the plasma cells.[30]

Immunoglobulins are specialized molecules produced by plasma cells in response to an antigen and are most accurately viewed as flexible adaptors or connectors. Although the terms are often used interchangeably, there is a subtle but important difference between the terms antibody and immunoglobulin. Immunoglobulins constitute the group of serum proteins that includes antibody molecules. An antibody is a specific immunoglobulin molecule, one for which the destiny antigen is known. For example, a laboratory test could measure a person's serum level of immunoglobulins, and another test would evaluate the level of antibody to the hepatitis B virus. The primary purpose of antibody is to bind to its specific antigen and either neutralize or eliminate it or enable the cells of the immune system to destroy the antigen.

All immunoglobulin molecules are composed of polypeptides (chains of amino acids) formed into either a globular or a Y-shaped structure. The basic units of an immunoglobulin molecule are two identical long (heavy, or H) chains bound by chemical bridges to two identical short (light, or L) chains. Each of these four chains has a variable and a constant region. The variable region is the unique attachment site for the antibody's destiny antigen. The

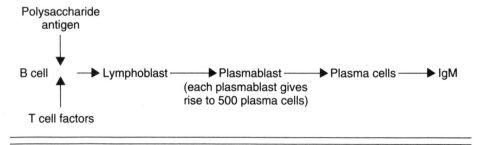

Figure 8-11 T Cell-Independent Activation

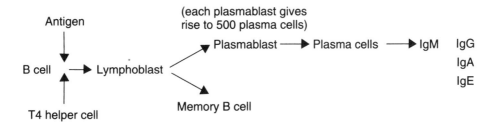

"T cell dependent" B cell activation

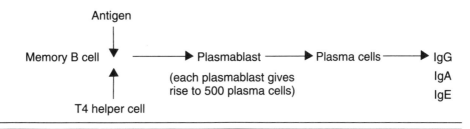

Secondary exposure

Figure 8-12 T Cell-Dependent Activation

constant regions on the heavy chains of various immunoglobulin molecules differ in length and amino acid sequence, thus forming the basis for classification of different types of immunoglobulin molecules. Humans have five classes of immunoglobulins, which are listed in Table 8-13. All immunoglobulin molecules in a particular class have identical constant regions.

In the laboratory, the variable and constant portions of an immunoglobin molecule can be separated. In scientific shorthand, the constant fragment is referred to as Fc, and the antigen-binding variable

Table 8-13 Characteristics of the Five Immunoglobulin Classes

IG Class	% of Total	Location	Actions	Comments
IgG	75%	Serum and tissues	Opsonization Neutralization Complement Fixation	Important in secondary responses Crosses placenta
IgA	17%	Serum, secretions (including breast milk), linings of mucous membranes	Neutralization Prevents surface attachment of antigens	
IgM	7%	Primarily in serum	Agglutinates particulate antigens Complement fixation	Important in primary response Largest and heaviest Ig "Natural" blood group antibodies
IgE	Trace	Serum, secretions, extracellular fluids, bound to cells	Binds to mast cells and basophils Release of histamine and other mediators	Reaginic antibody Elevated levels in allergy and parasitic infection
IgD	0.10%	Serum, surface of B cells	May be specific surface receptor	

fragment is referred to as Fab. Phagocytes and other immune cells have receptors, or "sockets," on their surfaces into which the Fc portion of the Ig molecule fits. The socket is termed an Fc receptor.

There are six major antibody-antigen reactions: neutralization, agglutination, precipitation, opsonization, complement fixation, and lysis (see Table 8-14). Antibody molecules neutralize the infectivity of microorganisms such as extracellular viruses by binding to them and preventing them from attaching to and infecting a host cell. An antibody binds to toxins, thus neutralizing their poisonous effects. Antibody can also agglutinate a solid antigen, causing it to clump. Soluble antigens can be bound together by antibody to form a precipitate. One of the most important antibody functions is opsonization, in which an antibody coats the antigen, greatly enhancing the ability of phagocytes to engulf the foreign particle. Certain types of immunoglobulin can, under the proper conditions, bind to C1, activating the complement cascade. This complement fixation function also tremendously enhances phagocytosis. Finally, antibody molecules can be instrumental in the destruction of a foreign cell through a process termed antibody-dependent cellular cytotoxicity (ADCC). In this process the Fab portion of an antibody molecule attaches to an antigen, while the Fc portion of the molecule fits into the Fc receptor on a monocyte, neutrophil, eosinophil, or natural killer cell. This connection stimulates the immune cell to release poisonous chemicals, which destroy the invading microorganism by lysis.

Humoral immune disorders include immunodeficiencies such as the hypogammaglobulinemias. More numerous are disorders involving an overactive humoral immune response, for example, anaphylaxis, allergies, immune complex diseases, autoimmune diseases, and the destruction of tissue in tuberculosis and sarcoidosis. These reactions are covered in greater detail in the discussion of hypersensitivities.

Humoral immunodeficiencies may be congenital or acquired. Although humoral immunodeficiencies are characterized by lack of production of immunoglobulin, in many cases the disorder appears to be due to a defect in T cell regulation of either B cell development or B cell production of antibody.

In general, persons with B cell deficiencies experience recurrent sinopulmonary infections with pyogenic bacteria. Eventually, the recurrent pneumonias cause bronchiectasis (a dilation and stenosis of the bronchi), which causes chronic obstructive pulmonary disease (COPD). Although chronic lung disease is the most frequent cause of morbidity in persons with a humoral immunodeficiency, the most frequent cause of death is hemopoietic cell malignancy.

The most common humoral immunodeficiency is selective IgA deficiency. It is associated with allergy. Although many persons with this disorder have low serum levels of IgA, they have normal serum levels of IgG and adequate secretory IgA. As a result, they do not experience serious infections. Others who are lacking both serum and secretory IgA develop recurrent sinopulmonary infections. A minority of persons with selective IgA deficiency develop antibodies to IgA and can experience anaphylaxis if exposed to blood products (including IV Ig) containing IgA. These patients must be given frozen or washed RBCs.

The next most common humoral immunodeficiency is a heterogeneous group of acquired disorders called common variable immunodeficiency (CVI), characterized by low Ig levels, recurrent sinopulmonary infections, malabsorption, arthritis, granulomas, an increased incidence of autoimmune

Table 8-14 Major Antibody-Antigen Reactions

Type	Action
Agglutination	Solid antigen forms lattice with soluble antibody, resulting in clumping of the antigen
Complement fixation	$C1_q$ binds to a site on the constant portion of Ig, activating the complement cascade and resulting in cell lysis
Lysis	Destruction of the cell membrane by the late complement components or through antibody-dependent cellular cytotoxicity (ADCC)
Neutralization	Neutralizes the infectivity of an organism by combining with the toxins and preventing their attachment to cell membranes
Opsonization	Coating of antigen to enhance phagocytosis
Precipitation	Reaction between a soluble antigen and antibody, in which a complex lattice of aggregates forms

disease, and hemopoietic malignancies. Persons with CVI often have defective T cell immunity, manifested by cutaneous anergy.

Among the rarer humoral immunodeficiencies are cross-linked hypogammaglobulinemia, cross-linked immunodeficiency with hyper-IgM, cross-linked lymphoproliferative syndrome, selective IgM deficiency, and selective IgG subclass deficiency.

The treatment of choice for most humoral immunodeficiencies is the administration of intravenous immunoglobulin. Infections that do not respond to IV Ig require aggressive antibiotic therapy. In persons with bronchiectasis, prophylactic oral antibiotics may be used in an attempt to prevent infections from occurring.

Cell-mediated immunity Cell-mediated immunity (CMI) is the specific immune response generated by T lymphocytes. CMI provides protection against infections caused by intracellular organisms such as viruses, fungi, and protozoa. This form of immunity is the cause of the rejection of allografts and may also play an important role in the killing of malignant cells. The cell-mediated immune response is generated within hours or days, and some forms of T lymphocytes are believed to survive years or even decades. Following activation of CMI, memory T cells remain "primed" to recognize the same antigen and respond more quickly next time.

T lymphocytes are the hub of the immune system. They influence and control the behavior of the other cells of the immune system through the release of cytokines, which act as a complex chemical communication system. Cytokines are cellular substances secreted to affect the action of other cells (see Table 8-15). Cytokines are either lymphokines, which are mediators produced by activated lymphocytes (T4 cells) in response to antigen, or monokines, which are mediators produced by activated monocyte/macrophages. Genetically engineered cytokines are being used today to treat malignancies, autoimmune disorders, and certain viral diseases.[31]

The thymus is a bilobed organ located in the chest behind the upper sternum. The organ develops in the eighth week of gestation; after birth, it enlarges until puberty, then begins to involute and become fatty. The major function of the thymus is to produce mature T lymphocytes and export them to peripheral lymphoid tissues. The thymus has a connective tissue capsule enclosing layers of cells: an outer cortex of lymphoid and epithelial cells and an inner medulla of mature T lymphocytes awaiting release into the circulation. The epithelial cells of the thymus secrete hormones such as thymosin, thymulin, and thy-

mopoietin, which are believed to be necessary for T cell maturation and differentiation.

Pre-T cells from the bone marrow migrate to the thymus, forming the lymphoid tissue of the outer cortex of the thymus. Maturation occurs as these pre-T cells are exposed to the hormones secreted by the thymic epithelial cells as they mature. After maturation, the cells are released into the bloodstream and migrate to the peripheral lymphoid tissues.

It is known that up to 99% of the pre-T cells that migrate to the thymus are destroyed. Immunologists theorize that the T cells that are destroyed must lack the proper receptors and/or must react to "self" molecules (recognize self cells as foreign). Such T cells must be destroyed or else they would cause autoimmune disease.

There are several types of T cells; some of these can be identified by certain molecules on their surfaces, and others can be identified only by how they function in the laboratory (see Table 8-16).

T cells with a CD8 molecule on their surfaces can be either T8 suppressor cells or cytotoxic (killer) T cells. T cells with a CD4 molecule on their surfaces can be either T4 helper cells or T4DH (delayed hypersensitivity) cells. There are two types of T4 helper cells: TH1 and TH2. The most numerous ones are the TH1 cells, which promote antibody production. The less abundant TH2 cells suppress antibody production and affect the synthesis of IgE. For the remainder of this discussion, only TH1 cells will be considered; they will be referred to as T4 helper cells.

T4 helpers are such powerful forces in stimulating the immune response that several safeguards have evolved to prevent them from being activated needlessly. This system of safeguards involves antigen presentation. In order for a T4 cell to be activated by its destiny antigen, a specialized immune cell (such as a macrophage) must "display" the destiny antigen to the individual T cell. During this interaction, the macrophage produces IL-1, which activates the T4 cell; in turn, the activated T4 cell produces IL-2, which serves to activate other immune cells, and the activated T4 cell proliferates and releases additional cytokines. This process is explained in greater detail in the next section on the integrated specific immune response.

T4 helper cells perform multiple and sometimes contradictory functions. T4 helper cells activate macrophages, produce growth factors for lymphocytes, suppress differentiation of B cells, and signal other T4 helper cells to stimulate B cell differentiation. They direct B cells to make antibody but also signal T8 suppressor cells to suppress antibody production by B cells. T4 helper cells also direct T8 cytotoxic cells

Table 8-15 Cytokines

Class	Type	Activity
Interleukins		
IL-1	Monokine	Induced by antigen, toxins, injury, inflammation; activates T cells, mediates inflammation and acute phase response, stimulates the production of other lymphokines (IL-2, IL-3, IL-4, IFN, others); functionally similar to TNFa
IL-2	Lymphokine	Produced by activated T4 cells; growth and differentiation factor for T4 and T8 cells; induces synthesis of other lymphokines; enhances cytotoxicity (T8, NK, and LAK)
IL-3	Lymphokine	Multicolony stimulating factor acts on bone marrow stem cells
IL-4	Lymphokine	Growth factor for activated B cells (BSF-2)
IL-5	Lymphokine	B cell growth and differentiation factor; induces Ig production
IL-6	Lymphokine; may also be a monokine	Differentiation of activated B cells into Ig-producing cells; induces production of Ig; mediates acute phase response
IL-7	Lymphokine	Induces maturation of pre-B cells into B cells
IL-8	Lymphokine	Chemotactic factor for monocytes and leukocytes
Interferons		
Alpha-IFN	Monokine; may also be a lymphokine	Antiviral, antiproliferative; enhances cytotoxic activity; induces fever
Beta-IFN	From fibroblasts	From fibroblasts; function similar to that of alpha-IFN
Gamma-IFN	Lymphokine	Potent macrophage activator induces Class I and II antigen expression; augments or inhibits other lymphokines; enhances NK activity; antiviral; increases Fc receptor expression
Colony-stimulating factors (see also Table 8-1)		
IL-3	Lymphokine	Stimulation of all myeloid precursors
GM-CSF	Lymphokine	Stimulation of granulocyte-macrophages
G-CSF	Lymphokine	Stimulation of granulocytes
M-CSF	Lymphokine	
Others Chemotactic factors Inhibition factors Lymphotoxins TNF		

to kill. T4 helper cells exert their influence on the immune response primarily through their secretion of lymphokines. These hormone-like substances exist in small quantities but exert marked biologic effects. Interleukins, interferons, and colony stimulating factors are types of lymphokines secreted by T4 helper cells.

There are two types of T8 cells: cytotoxic (or killer) T8 cells and T8 suppressor cells. Since both have CD8 molecules on their surfaces, they cannot be distinguished, except by their different response to antigens. The T8 suppressor cell directs B lymphocytes to reduce production of antibody and suppresses the cell-killing function of cytotoxic T8 cells

Table 8-16 Types of T Cells

T cell Type	Characteristics
T4 helper	Induces B cells to make antibody Induces other T4 cells to induce B cell differentiation Induces T8 suppressors to suppress Induces T8 cytotoxic cells to kill Secretes growth factors for lymphoid cells Activates macrophages
T4DH (delayed hypersensitivity)	Responsible for delayed cutaneous hypersensitivity reaction (tuberculosis, sarcoidosis)
T8 suppressor	Sends message to B cell to stop making antibody Sends suppression messages to T8 cytotoxic cells and T4 cells
T8 cytotoxic (killer)	Responsible for destruction of virus-infected and tumor cells via direct specific cytotoxicity or antibody-dependent cellular cytotoxicity (ADCC)

and the helping function of T4 helper cells. T8 suppressor cells have a key role in preventing the immune response from going out of control. T8 killer (cytotoxic) cells are responsible for direct and specific cytotoxicity; they destroy virally infected "self" cells and tumor cells. T8 killer cells recognize their destiny antigen on the surface of a target cell when the antigen is combined with Class I HLA antigens (present on all nucleated cells and platelets). The cell-killing function of cytotoxic T8 cells is enhanced by the secretion of IL-2 by T4 helper cells.

The Integrated Specific Immune Response

The major histocompatibility complex (MHC) is a group of genes that has been found to determine the compatibility of tissue transplants between members of a species. The human MHC is called the human leukocyte antigen, or HLA, system. In other words, the HLA system determines the compatibility of transplants from one human to another. In recent years, researchers have found that the HLA system is not only responsible for compatibility of tissue transplantation but is fundamentally important to the overall immune response.

Human leukocyte antigens have two important functions: they identify the body's cells as "self" cells, and they aid in the recognition of "non-self," or foreign, cells or substances. HLA antigens are "markers" that are coded for by genes. A gene can be thought of as a recipe for the production of a protein. The HLA genes, clustered on chromosome 6, are the recipes for making certain identification proteins that are located on cell surfaces. These proteins are the HLA antigens. One set of these proteins, Class I HLA antigens, marks nearly every cell in the body with an identification code. Proteins from a second set, the Class II HLA antigens, are present on activated

immune cells. A summary of the unique characteristics of each class is given in Table 8-17.

Class I HLA antigens The Class I HLA antigens are a trio of different proteins—A, B, and C HLA antigens—found on the surfaces of platelets and all nucleated cells in the body. These antigens act somewhat like Social Security numbers, in that they identify individual cells. It is important to note that Class I HLA antigens are not present in red blood cells, which do not have nuclei. Instead, RBCs have ABO and Rh factors, which determine which types of RBCs can be transfused from one person to another.

When a virus invades the body, it attaches to and enters a human cell, then takes over the cellular machinery to produce more viruses. During this process, viral components accumulate and actually poke out of the surface of the infected cell. Cytotoxic T8 lymphocytes survey the body's cells for any abnormalities. The cytotoxic T8 lymphocyte detects only Class I antigens on the surfaces of normal cells. During a viral infection, however, the T8 lymphocyte detects Class I antigens along with viral proteins poking out of the same body cell. The T8 lymphocyte recognizes that the body cell has been taken over by the virus, becomes activated, and attacks and destroys the infected cell.

This same process may be involved in the elimination of malignant cells from the body. Scientists theorize that malignant cells have abnormal proteins on their surfaces. The cytotoxic T8 lymphocyte may detect the Class I HLA antigens on a cell's surface along with the abnormal proteins that are characteristic of cancer cells. As with viral infections, the T8 lymphocyte attacks and destroys the malignant cell. It is important to understand that T8 lymphocytes will not become activated by virus particles alone; the viral particle must be combined with Class I antigens or the T8 cell will not respond.

Table 8-17 HLA Antigens

Class	Type	Location	Action
Class I: HLA-A, B, C	Tissue graft rejection genes	On nearly all body cells	Form the chief antigens recognized by killer T cells Responsible for resistance to viral infection Responsible for tissue graft rejection May be responsible for prevention of cancer
Class II: HLA-D, DR	Immune response genes	On B cells, macrophages, and activated T cells	Promote efficient collaboration between immunocompetent cells

Class II HLA antigens Class II HLA antigens consist of a group of D antigens. For the purposes of this discussion, the most important D antigen is DR. The Class II HLA antigens are only found on the immune cells in the body that are involved in the processes of specific immunity: macrophages, B lymphocytes, and activated T lymphocytes. These class II antigens are critical for activation of the specific immune response.

Class II HLA proteins and antigen-presenting cells are involved in the activation of the T4 helper lymphocytes, the central figures in the specific immune response. In order for a T4 lymphocyte to be activated, an antigen-presenting cell (macrophage or B lymphocyte) must "show" the T4 lymphocyte a piece of the invader along with the antigen-presenting cell's Class II antigens. This process is termed MHC restriction. The MHC Class II antigens restrict the recognition of foreign substances by requiring that the foreign proteins be displayed in combination with the Class II antigens. By limiting the activation of T4 cells to situations in which both a foreign substance and Class II antigen are present, the body prevents the T4 cells from overreacting to every foreign protein they come into contact with. This process is described below; a macrophage is the antigen-presenting cell in this description.

When a microorganism invades the body, it is engulfed by a macrophage. The macrophage destroys the microbe and also selects a component of the microbe and places it in the center of the Class II antigens on its own cell membrane. The macrophage displays this combination of foreign particle and Class II HLA antigens to the T4 helper lymphocyte. During this display, the macrophage secretes a chemical, interleukin-1 (IL-1). The T4 lymphocyte can detect the foreign particle because it is combined with the macrophage's Class II antigens; at the same

time, the IL-1 secreted by the macrophage attaches to the special receptors on the T4 lymphocyte's surface. This sequence of events activates the T4 lymphocyte, which secretes interleukin-2 (IL-2), a cytokine with far-reaching effects. The T4 lymphocyte also proliferates, cloning itself repeatedly.

Disorders of the Cell-Mediated Immune System

Disease can occur when any of the lymphocytes are dysfunctional. Malignancies comprise a large majority of the lymphocytic disorders. Cancers originating in the bone marrow during early development of the lymphocyte are called leukemias. Malignancies arising during the lymph node stage of lymphocyte development are called lymphomas. A cancer of the immunoglobulin-producing cells is called multiple myeloma. The literature regarding the nursing management of patients with these disorders is extensive.

In general, persons with deficient CMI develop opportunistic infections from microorganisms such as fungi, viruses, and protozoa, and also have higher risk of hemopoietic malignancy. The following disorders are examples of conditions resulting from CMI deficiencies: acquired immunodeficiency syndrome (AIDS), T cell deficiency associated with purine nucleoside phosphorylase deficiency, T cell deficiency associated with absent membrane glycoprotein, T cell deficiency associated with absent Class I or II MHC antigens or both (bare lymphocyte syndrome), congenital thymic aplasia (DiGeorge's syndrome) with or without hypoparathyroidism, chronic mucocutaneous candidiasis with or without endocrinopathy, and natural killer cell deficiency.

Cell-Mediated Hypersensitivities

There are several disease processes that represent an uncontrolled activation of the CMI system: the lung damage associated with tuberculosis, contact allergy, allograft rejection, and some autoimmune phenomena.

Combined B and T Cell Disorders

In this group are a number of rare disorders, but among the better known are several varieties of the severe combined immunodeficiency syndrome (such as SCID due to adenosine deaminase deficiency), cellular immunodeficiency with abnormal immunoglobulin synthesis (Nezelof's syndrome), immunodeficiency with ataxia-telangiectasia, immunodeficiency with thrombocytopenia, eczema, recurrent infection (Wiskott-Aldrich Syndrome), and bare lymphocyte syndrome.

NK (Non-T, Non-B) Cytotoxicity

Large granular lymphocytes (LGLs) are anomalous lymphocytes better known as natural killer (NK) cells. They are lymphocytes, but unlike other lymphocytes, their immune activity is nonspecific. NK cells do have receptors for immunoglobulin (Fc receptors), so they are able to destroy virally infected cells or tumor cells by antibody dependent cellular cytotoxicity (ADCC). Interferon and some interleukins stimulate the function of NK cells.

NK cells also secrete soluble toxins, such as TNF-alpha, which activate an endonuclease in the target cell that breaks down the target cell's DNA. This method of cell killing has been called "programmed cell death," since, without its DNA to direct its function, the target cell will die.

Hypersensitivity Disorders

Allergy is the term for an untoward reactivity to commonly encountered environmental antigens (such as pollen, food, or insect venom). Environmental antigens that incite allergies are called allergens. Allergies may result in acute or delayed reactions and may or may not cause the body to produce antibodies. Various hypersensitivity reactions to normal substances are summarized in Table 8-18.

Immediate Hypersensitivity (Anaphylaxis)

Immediate hypersensitivity is an immunologic reaction that occurs within minutes or hours of the introduction of an antigen into an immune individual and that is mediated by antibodies. The element of time is less important than the involvement of antibodies; therefore, these reactions are also called antibody-mediated hypersensitivity. (In contrast, antibodies are not involved in delayed-type hypersensitivity.) IgE antibodies (or in some species, IgG1 antibodies) bound to mast cells or basophils mediate anaphylaxis. Circulating IgG antibodies mediate immune complex disease (for example, Arthus reaction) when they form precipitates with antigens in small blood vessels. Circulating IgG or IgM autoantibodies or alloantibodies can also mediate lysis of cells (for example, in hemolytic disease of the newborn).

Delayed-Type Hypersensitivity (DTH)

Delayed-type hypersensitivity is an inflammatory reaction that occurs in immune individuals 24–48 hours after the introduction of an antigen and is a result of cell-mediated immunity. (The term *delayed-type hypersensitivity* has replaced the older designation "delayed hypersensitivity" in order to deemphasize the element of time, thereby emphasizing the cellular mechanism of the reaction.) DTH reactions are characterized by induration (hardening) and erythema in the skin and, microscopically, by heavy infiltration with macrophages. DTH reactions are induced when T lymphocytes recognize antigens on macrophages and generate lymphokines. The lymphokines attract more macrophages and activate them locally. In clinical medicine, skin tests are used to measure DTH to infectious agents suspected of causing disease. For example, the test for tuberculosis uses extracts of the tubercle bacillus (tuberculin or purified protein derivative).

Autoimmune Disease

An autoimmune disease is characterized by antibodies or T lymphocytes that are reactive with antigenic determinants of "self." In experimental animals, immunization with the appropriate tissue can evoke a response that is similar to autoimmune disease; the animal develops pathological changes characteristic of the disease, and the experimentally induced disease can be transferred to a normal recipient by serum or T lymphocytes. The presence of autoantibodies and/or autoreactive T lymphocytes in many diseases does not in itself mean that these diseases are caused by the autoimmune response. The cause of autoantibody formation or formation of autoreactive T lymphocytes in cases of human autoimmune disease is generally not known. It has been postulated that a balance of helper and suppressor T cells is essential for maintenance of the normal immune response, and that loss of T8 suppressor cells allows the T4 cells to become unregulated, resulting in augmented production of antibodies against the self, or autoimmune disease.[32]

Autoimmune hemolytic anemia is the accelerated destruction of red blood cells in vivo by autoantibodies of the IgG class to an antigen on the red blood cells, usually an Rh antigen. Red blood cells coated with autoantibodies are removed from the circulation by interaction with Fc receptors on the macrophages of the spleen and liver. The Coombs antiglobulin test is used in the diagnosis of autoimmune hemolytic anemia.

Immune Complex Disease

Immune complex disease results from deposition of antigen-antibody complexes in tissues. Such deposition may occur as an acute event (for example, in acute poststreptococcal glomerulonephritis) or as a chronic phenomenon (for example, in membranoproliferative glomerulonephritis). In immune complex disease, the antibodies are usually of the IgG class and fix complement, thereby inciting inflamma-

Table 8-18 Hypersensitivity Disorders

Type	Features	Pathophysiology	Disorders
Type I: Immediate	Occurs immediately or up to 12 hours after exposure to antigen	Upon first exposure to antigen, T cells recognize antigen and notify B cells to produce IgE antibody to antigen. IgE binds to Fc receptors on mast cells. When re-encountering antigen, IgE on mast cells binds to antigen, causing the mast cell to degranulate, i.e., release chemical mediators. These mediators (histamine, bradykinin, prostaglandins, leukotrienes (SRSA), and ECFA) cause smooth muscle contraction, mucus production, vasodilation, bronchoconstriction, pruritis, and capillary leakage.	Allergies Anaphylaxis Atopic eczema Asthma
Type II: Cytotoxic (Autoimmune disease)	Antigenic target is a self cell; reaction is directly mediated by antibody or by cytotoxic cells	"Self" cell is seen as foreign. B cells produce antibody against the "self" cells. Macrophages, antibody, and complement combine to destroy the "self" cells via ADCC or complement-mediated lysis.	Immune hemolytic anemia (anti-RBC antibody) Idiopathic thrombocytopenia purpura (anti-platelet antibody) Goodpasture's syndrome (antibody against basement membranes of lungs and kidneys) Grave's disease (antibody against TSH receptor) Myasthenia gravis (antibody against acetylcholine receptor at neuromuscular junction) *Systemic lupus erythematosis (anti-DNA antibody) *Rheumatoid arthritis (anti-IgG antibody)

Table 8-18 *(continued)*

Type	Features	Pathophysiology	Disorders
Type III: Immune complex reaction	Immune complex formation	Antigen-antibody complexes are formed and are deposited into tissue, causing microthrombi and increased vascular permeability. Platelets aggregate and release histamine and 5-HT, which cause more microthrombi as well as capillary leakage. Complement is activated and PMNs are attracted to site. PMNs are unable to phagocytize and destroy immune complexes. Instead, they release lysosomes, which cause damage to surrounding tissue.	Takayasu's arteritis (vasculitis of great vessels, usually in young women) *Wegener's granulomatosis (necrotizing granulomatous vasculitis of upper and lower airways with glomerulonephritis) Polyarteritis nodosa (necrotizing vasculitis of small arteries, especially of kidney, skin, and lung; associated with HBs Antigen) Henoch-Schonlein purpura (a vasculitis involving kidneys, joints, and skin; associated with drug reactions) *Systemic lupus erythematosis *Rheumatoid arthritis Serum sickness (with horse serum)
Type IV: Delayed-type	Occurs 24–28 hours after first exposure to antigen; T cell mediated; no antibody is involved in reaction; granulomas may form	Upon first exposure, T cells recognize antigen and become sensitized. When T cells recontact antigen, the T cells release cytokines, resulting in an accumulation of lymphocytes and activated macrophages in the area.	Tuberculosis Leprosy Sarcoidosis Leishmaniasis Schistosomiasis Contact dermatitis

*Diseases involving more than one type of reaction

tion. Autoantibodies are involved in some types of immune complex disease (for example, SLE). Immune complexes may form in the circulation and lodge in different vascular beds. The glomerular basement membrane is a frequent site for deposition of such complexes. Immune complexes may also form in extravascular tissues. Acute and chronic serum sickness from transfusion reactions are representative models of immune complex disease.

Hemostasis

Hemostasis is the body's rapid, controlled, localized response to a blood vessel tear whereby a clot is formed to prevent blood leakage from the damaged vessel and blood flow is maintained until the torn vessel is repaired. The process of establishing hemostasis is remarkably fast, and the more severe the injury, the more rapid is the development of a stable

Table 8-19 Triggering Mechanisms for Clotting in the Body

Type of Insult	Examples
Damage to endothelial lining of blood vessels (intrinsic stimulation)	Prolonged cardiopulmonary bypass Acidosis ARDS Major surgery (especially vascular) Anoxia
Foreign particles in the blood stream (intrinsic stimulation)	Gram-negative sepsis Amniotic fluid embolism Malaria Sickle cell disease Burn injuries Transfusion reactions Emboli
Tissue injury	Major surgery or trauma Neoplastic disease Shock Burns Abruptio placentae Systemic lupus

clot. A fibrin clot begins to form within 15–20 seconds of severe injury or within 1–2 minutes of minor injury.[33] A stable clot is usually fully formed within 5 minutes of damage to the vessel wall.

Clotting is triggered primarily by three major types of stimuli: tissue injury, vessel injury, and a foreign body in the bloodstream. The more severe or extreme the stimulus, the more widespread the clotting. Examples of stimuli that trigger clotting are given in Table 8-19. There are more than 40 different substances in blood that affect coagulation, many of which exist to regulate hemostasis. Procoagulants are substances that promote clot formation, whereas anticoagulants inhibit the clotting process. Many substances, such as thrombin, have a dual role, participating in both clot formation and clot dissolution. The presence and interaction of all of these substances in the body ensure that fibrin is formed only at the site of injury. In fact, clots cannot form wherever blood is flowing at rates greater than a certain speed. The normal circulation of blood dilutes and sweeps away clotting factors, preventing them from accumulating and interacting, and carrying them to the liver for degradation.

There are four steps to hemostasis: (1) vasospasm of the torn vessel, (2) formation of a platelet plug, (3) formation of a stable clot, and (4) fibrinolysis. The first three steps in the process are illustrated in Figure 8-13.

Vasospasm of the Torn Vessel

When a blood vessel is cut or torn, localized nerve and muscle reflexes produce a transient vasoconstriction, lasting less than 1 minute. This vasoconstriction response is the body's attempt to reduce the loss of blood from the broken vessel. Following the initial vasoconstriction, substances that promote vasoconstriction are released throughout the clotting

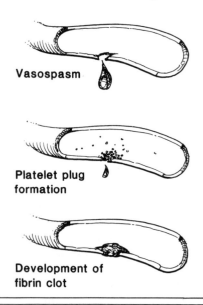

Vasospasm

Platelet plug formation

Development of fibrin clot

Figure 8-13 The Stages of Clotting

process. The most important component for continuing the clotting process is serotonin, as it stimulates the next phase of platelet aggregation. Vasodilated patients whose blood vessels lack the ability to constrict adequately may also have reduced clotting ability because the release of serotonin is limited by the decreased vasoconstriction.

Formation of a Platelet Plug

When the blood vessel endothelium is damaged, platelets flowing over the area adhere to the roughened surface. The endothelial cells of the damaged blood vessel release von Willebrand's factor and other substances (calcium, fibrinogen, ADP, ATP, epinephrine, fibronectin, and platelet factor IV) that enhance platelet adherence. The platelets aggregate (clump) in response to serotonin released during vasoconstriction and procoagulants released during adherence. Platelets also initiate a complex metabolic pathway called the arachidonic acid cascade, which results in the production of thromboxane A2, an extremely potent platelet agonist and vasoconstrictor. Platelet phospholipids also activate coagulation via the intrinsic pathway, discussed in the next subsection.

Formation of a Stable Clot

The third step of hemostasis involves activation of the coagulation cascade, a complex series of sequential chemical reactions that results in the formation of a stable fibrin clot. The coagulation cascade involves two key enzymatic reactions: the extrinsic pathway and the intrinsic pathway. Either pathway serves to form the prothrombin activator, which converts prothrombin to thrombin. (Thrombin, while essential for clotting, also initates the clot lysis process. Although it is initiated at this time, clot lysis does not become an active process for 24–36 hours.) The

Table 8-20 The Clotting Factors

Clotting Factor	Alternate Name(s)	Normal Values
Factor I	Fibrinogen	200–400 mg/dL
Factor II	Prothrombin	100 mg/dL
Factor III	Tissue thromboplastin Tissue factor, thromboplatin	Not known
Factor IV	Calcium	9–10 mg/dL
Factor V	Proaccelerin, "Labile factor"	Not known
Factor VII	Serum prothrombin conversion Accelerator (SPCA) "Proconvertin" Stable factor	72–125 mg
Factor VIII	Antihemophilic factor (AHF) Antihemophilic globulin (AHG)	75–100 mg
Factor IX	Antihemophilic factor B (AHFB) Christmas factor Plasma thromboplastin	75–150 mg
Factor X	Stuart or Prower factor Antithrombin III Thrombokinase	75–125 mg
Factor XI	Plasma thromboplastin antecedent (PTA) Antihemophilic factor C (AHFC)	70–130 mg
Factor XII	Hageman Factor "Contact factor"	Not known
Factor XIII	Fibrin clot stabilizing factor (FSF)	9–4 U
Pre-kallikrein		
High molecular weight kininogen (HMWK)		

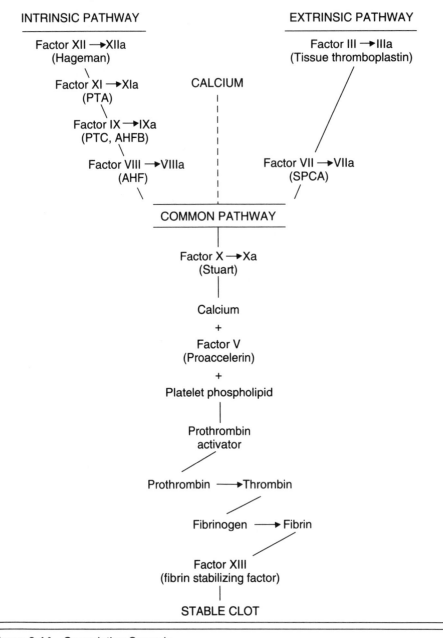

Figure 8-14   Coagulation Cascade

extrinsic pathway is activated in as little as 15 seconds by substances released from injured tissue, primarily tissue thromboplastin (platelet factor III). Tissue thromboplastin combines with platelet phospholipids and factor VII to form a complex enzyme that activates factor X. The intrinsic pathway is so named because all the factors required for this pathway are circulating in the plasma. This pathway involves many factors and is slower, requiring 2–6 minutes for full activation. The many factors that trigger one another are listed in Table 8-20 and shown on the diagram of the coagulation cascade in Figure 8-14. (Note that factor VI was discovered to be the acti-

vated form of factor V and as a result is no longer listed as a separate clotting factor.) Both the extrinsic and intrinsic pathways lead to a single, common pathway, which culminates in the formation of a stable fibrin clot. The important function of this common pathway is to create thrombin to convert fibrinogen to fibrin threads, the essential meshwork of the clot. The clotting factors that participate in each of these pathways are designated by roman numerals; their active forms are designated by the letter "a".

Note that the Hageman factor (factor XII of the intrinsic pathway) also has a significant role in activating two other important biochemical processes:

the complement and kallikrein systems. Activation of these systems produces additional substances that promote vasodilation and increased vascular permeability.

The common pathway requires activated factor X, tissue phospholipids, factor V, and calcium to form the prothrombin activator, which quickly converts into prothrombin to form thrombin. In turn, thrombin cleaves fibrinogen to produce fibrin, a meshwork of threads. Factor XIII stabilizes the clot.

Within 3–6 minutes after they are formed, the fibrin strands form a mesh that traps plasma and cells to develop a clot. As the clot stabilizes, the clotting factors are removed from the plasma within the clot. The clot retracts, closing the blood vessel even further and releasing a clear fluid called serum. This process takes 30–60 minutes. Clots are then stable for 24–36 hours, at which time they lyse.

Fibrinolysis

Following clot formation, when the danger of bleeding is past, the clot is dissolved via fibrinolysis. Fibrinolysis is a cascade of enzymatic reactions leading to formation of plasminogen activators, which convert the plasma protein plasminogen to plasmin. This enzyme digests the fibrin threads of the clot as well as platelet factors II, V, VIII, and XII. Plasminogen activators arise from plasma, urine, tissue, and the clot itself. The most important plasminogen activator is thrombin. Tissue plasminogen activator (TPA) is used extensively for therapeutic management of thrombotic clots in the coronary arteries. Urokinase, an enzyme found in the urine, is also a potent plasminogen activator. Researchers theorize that urokinase may aid in ensuring patency of renal blood vessels.[34] Endothelial cells have a dual role because they release both substances that initiate clot formation and substances that initiate clot dissolution.

As the clot dissolves, it yields fibrin degradation products (FDPs), or fibrin split products. These substances can be measured in the plasma. Elevated FDPs may indicate excessive activation of both clotting cascade and fibrinolysis, a phenomena common in disseminated intravascular coagulation (DIC).

Checks and Balances in Hemostasis and Fibrinolysis

As with other biological processes, hemostasis encompasses a system of checks and balances to prevent both excess clot formation and excess fibrinolysis. Excessive or inappropriate clotting is prevented by several factors. Excessive or inappropriate fibri-

nolysis is prevented by the antiplasmins. These substances are present in an inactive state in plasma and, when necessary, become activated and block the action of plasmin. The vascular endothelium is a smooth surface with a negative electrical charge that literally repels positively charged clotting factors. Endothelial cells also produce prostacyclin, which inhibits platelet aggregation. Another protection is the rapid blood flow, which prevents accumulation of activated clotting factors in one area. Heparin, released by mast cells or basophils during the inflammatory reaction induced by tissue or vessel injury, also serves to limit clotting by blocking thrombin's conversion of fibrinogen to fibrin. Finally, as blood flows through the liver, that organ acts as a filter to remove activated clotting factors from the circulation.

Lab Tests of Hemostasis

The intactness of the body's clotting mechanisms is primarily assessed through laboratory clotting tests. The coagulation mechanism is best assessed by examining the components of the clotting process: vascular reaction, platelet plug formation, coagulation cascade, and fibrinolysis. Laboratory tests evaluate the quality, quantity, or both, of each component. A listing of the various coagulation tests is given in Table 8-21.

Assessment of the Hematologic, Immune, and Coagulation Systems

Introduction

The major difficulty with presenting an integrated plan for the assessment of the hematologic system is that there are actually three systems within the general framework of the blood cells and their functions: the hematologic, immune, and coagulation systems. Hematologic and immunologic disorders produce a diverse array of clinical signs and symptoms. In general, depending on which blood cells are affected, the primary symptoms arise from defects in or problems related to cell function. For instance, erythrocyte deficiency (anemia) results in decreased ability to carry oxygen; platelet deficiency causes reduced ability to clot; and immune deficits are the consequence of alterations in leukocytes. As with all body systems, assessment of the hematologic system involves obtaining the patient's medical history, per-

Table 8-21 Coagulation Tests

Name of Test	Normal Values	What It Tests	Etiology of Abnormal Values
Platelet count: A blood specimen is collected and sent to the lab for mechanical or hand counting	150,000–400,000/mm³	Quantity of circulating platelets	Bone marrow dysfunction with decreased platelet production: aplastic anemia, leukemia, chemotherapy Bleeding: platelets being lost faster than they can be replaced Splenomegaly: platelets sequestering in spleen Platelet autoantibodies: abnormal destruction of platelets caused by body's perception of platelets as foreign antigens
Bleeding time: Incision is made on the forearm after a BP cuff is inflated to 40 mm Hg; incision is blotted until no serum oozes from site	4–5 minutes	Tests quality of platelets; determines their ability to form a platelet plug	Presence of platelet prostaglandin inhibitors, e.g., aspirin, persantine Presence of platelet inhibitor drugs Uremia Hepatic failure with hyperammonemia Von Willebrand's disease
Prothrombin time (PT): Blood specimen is tested against a reagent to measure clotting	12–15 seconds (±4 seconds)	Tests the activation of factor VII in the extrinsic pathway	Hepatic disease Vitamin K deficiency: other nutritional deficiency, malabsorption syndrome, antibiotic depletion of normal flora Coumarol derivatives Bleeding loss of factor VII
Partial thromboplastin time (PTT): Blood specimen is tested against a reagent to measure clotting	26–32 seconds (±10 seconds)	Tests the conversion of prothrombin to thrombin, testing intrinsic and final common pathway Often done as a bedside test called the ACT	Factor VIII deficiency (hemophilia) Hepatic disease Presence of thrombin inhibitors such as heparin, streptokinase, FDPs Blood loss of coagulation factors
Fibrinogen level: Blood specimen tested for quantity of fibrinogen	200–400 mg %	Measures quantity of circulating fibrinogen but cannot determine its quality	Altered quantity of fibrinogen: hepatic disease or uremia Loss through bleeding Consumptive process or excessive clot formation
Thrombin time: Blood specimen tested for against a reagent to measure clotting	12 seconds	Measures conversion of thrombin and fibrinogen to fibrin; test is very sensitive for altered coagulation	Presence of thrombin inhibitor, such as heparin, streptokinase, or TPA Abnormal fibrinogen Decreased fibrinogen level
Fibrin degradation products (FDPs) or fibrin split products (FSP): Blood test detects amount of these products present in circulation	<10 mcg/mL or negative at 1:100 dilution or less (present at lower dilutions, such as 1:50)	Determines amount of by-products from lysed clots present in circulation; the d-dimer fragment of FDPs can be measured to better determine whether patient is experiencing DIC	Hepatic failure with inability to clear products Found approximately 2–3 days after large clot formation Excessive clotting disease (DIC)

forming a thorough physical exam, and reviewing the results of relevant laboratory and diagnostic studies.

History

The patient's age, ethnicity, and family history (particularly of cosanguinity or hematologic or immunologic disorders) may provide important information concerning the presenting complaints and potential for hematologic disorders. Several hematologic and immunologic disorders are inherited; others are more prevalent at certain ages or among certain ethnic groups. A list of pertinent questions to ask when taking the patient's history is given in Table 8-22.

Physical Examination

Physical examination of the patient with possible hematologic or immunologic disorder requires particularly astute inspection skills. The skin, soft tissue, and mucous membranes will most often reveal changes indicative of disease. A thorough understanding of the primary function of each of the blood cells or immune components will assist the nurse in interpreting physical findings. For instance, red blood cells carry oxygen; therefore, findings indicating inadequate tissue oxygenation (pallor, cyanosis, light-headedness, and hypothermia) may lead to assessment for anemia. Disorder-specific symptoms are addressed in more detail in later sections. A general overview of significant assessment findings is presented in Table 8-23.

Diagnostic Tests

The diagnosis of a hematologic or immunologic disorder usually begins with assessment of a chief complaint (such as bruising, fatigue, dyspnea, blurred vision, or angina), which may often appear to be unrelated to the hematologic system. Complete blood profiles are often the first tests to reveal abnormalities in hematologic function. The complete blood count (CBC) assesses the quantities of red blood cells, white blood cells, and platelets as well as the quality of red blood cells to some degree. When deficiencies of the blood cells are evident on a CBC, other tests may be in order (see Table 8-24). When no readily apparent etiology of the cellular deficiency is noted, it is necessary to determine whether the defect is caused by insufficient production, abnormal sequestration, abnormal destruction, or loss of blood cells.

The most common test to evaluate bone marrow production of cells is a bone marrow aspirate and

biopsy. Evaluation of the liquid portion of the red bone marrow will show cellular precursors and reveal reduced production (aplastic anemia) or abnormal maturation of cells (leukemia). This test usually requires only local anesthetic, although many physicians give a short-acting narcotic (Fentanyl) or sedative (Midazolam) to individuals with suspected abnormal bone marrow, as aspiration is more painful for them. (For bone marrow transplant, the donor of the marrow is taken to the operating room and given heavy sedation for this procedure.) After administration of a local anesthetic, bone marrow is removed from the anterior or posterior iliac crests or the sternum. An incision is made with a scalpel; then a large-bore needle inside an introducer is inserted and literally screwed into the bone. If a biopsy specimen is needed, the bone core is removed from this device. The inner needle is removed, and a syringe is attached with which to aspirate the liquid marrow. If there is insufficient cell production or the marrow is packed full of cancer cells, the aspiration may be painful. On occasion, specimens may be taken from several sites in order to obtain sufficient quantity of marrow and to confirm malignant diagnoses. Cells are then placed on a microscope slide for review by a hematologist and a pathologist. Review of the quantity and maturity of these bone marrow components will provide some valuable information, but cytogenetic procedures may be required to diagnose specific categories or prognostic indicators for disease. Chromosome studies have enabled clinicians to more precisely diagnose many disorders, and they are now considered a routine part of bone marrow evaluation. If the patient has coagulopathy, bleeding from the aspiration site may occur. Otherwise, the site may be tender for a few days but will heal easily.

Once bone marrow disease is ruled out, other tests specific to the presenting symptoms are performed. Laboratory tests of RBC, WBC, platelet, and immunologic function are discussed in more detail in other sections of this chapter. Tests of hematologic tissue function may also include lymph node biopsy, lymphangiogram, antibody assays, skin anergy tests, visceral protein levels, and immunoglobulin levels.

The lymph node may be biopsied (by needle aspiration) or removed (by surgical excision) for microscopic evaluation to diagnose infection or malignancy. Lymph node biopsy is helpful when lymphadenopathy is persistent or if symptoms are indicative of life-threatening diseases. The American Cancer Society recommends that biopsy be considered when lymph node enlargement greater than 1 cm has persisted for longer than 2 weeks.[35]

Table 8-22 Pertinent Questions Regarding Hematologic/Immune Disorders

Question to Be Asked	Significance of Response
What is the patient's chief complaint?	Signs and symptoms of hematologic disorders are often vague and nonspecific, occurring in any body system. However, some symptoms (e.g., petichiae and thrombocytopenia) are classically associated with one another.
What medications is the patient currently taking? What medications has the patient taken in the month prior to symptom onset?	Medications often affect development or lifespan of blood components, leading to hematologic complications in some individuals. The complication may be predictable based upon allergy history, personal risk factors, drug dosage, or known combination effects, but is often idiosyncratic.
Has the patient had any medical or surgical problems in the past ten years?	Obvious medical conditions related to the hematologic/immune system that may influence state of health at admission include anemias, bleeding disorders, liver disease, lymphoid-leukemic cancers, radiation therapy, tonsillectomy, infectious diseases, sexually transmitted diseases, recreational drug use, diabetes, and traumatic splenic injury or removal. It is also important to ascertain if the patient had ever been seriously ill and received blood products, as disease may be transmitted by this means. Less obvious symptoms to note include recent viral illness, sore throats, malaise, allergies, persistent sinus drainage, skin lesions, and poor wound healing.
What is the patient's occupation?	Occupational exposure to carcinogens or bone marrow suppressants is not always obvious. Substances to check for (because they are known to cause illness) include benzene, epichlorohydrin, ethylene oxide, insecticides, ionizing radiation, thorium dioxide, vinyl chloride. Those who might be exposed to occupational hazards include chemical industry workers, glue and varnish makers, workers in plastics industries, rubber tire manufacturers, shoemakers, research laboratory or sterilizing area workers, radiographic hospital workers, ceramic industry workers, incandescent lamp makers, steel workers, metal refiners, vacuum tube makers, nuclear reactor workers, uranium miners, farmers, and horticulturists.
What is the family's disease history?	Certain anemias, immune disorders, and bleeding disorders are familial. Determine whether any relative exhibited symptoms of these at an early age or died of unknown causes.
What is the patient's social history?	Life-style and sexual activity have become important parts of the hematologic assessment, particularly when infectious or immune symptoms are present. The patient's history of homosexual or bisexual activity, encounters with multiple sexual partners, or sexual encounters with prostitutes is important.
Does the patient have any allergies and food intolerances?	Food intolerances may actually be allergies, and can lead to severe reactions with frequent exposure. Any hint of reaction or illness after ingesting certain foods should be investigated further.

Table 8-23 Physical Assessment Findings Indicative of Hematologic/Immunologic Disease

Assessment Finding	Description	Clinical Significance/Etiology
Headache	May be mild or severe; important to ascertain onset, duration, location, quality, precipitating factors to determine significance of symptom	May indicate anemia, polycythemia, brain infection, or tumorous invasion; with thrombocytopenia, may be indicative of intracranial hemorrhage
Altered level of consciousness	Ranging from personality change or sleep disturbances to confusion, disorientation, or obtundation	Occurs with brain infections, increased intracranial pressure related to thromboses, bleeding, infection, or mass lesions; indicates the need for immediate evaluation
Lightheadedness, dizziness	Disequilibrium, sensation of spinning in the head	Anemia of various etiologies
Paresthesias	Tingling sensation in fingertips or toes, altering ability to perform fine motor skills	Vitamin B_{12} deficiency, polycythemia
Bleeding gums/oral mucosa	Either oozing bleeding or with toothbrushing	Thrombocytopenia most likely etiology, although hepatic coagulopathy, DIC, or polycythemia may also be the cause
Blindness	Complete or partial blindness without clear field cuts	Retinal hemorrhages from anemia, thrombocytopenia, DIC
Conjunctival pallor	Pallor of the inner aspects of the eyelid	Anemia from reduced hemoglobin
Smooth tongue	Absence of tongue papillae; tongue usually also erythematous and swollen	Iron deficiency anemia, vitamin B_{12} and other vitamin deficiencies
Oral ulcers	Erosions or ulcerations of the oral mucosa, soft palate, hard palate, and tongue; may be bleeding; tongue is usually tender, occasional exudate	Oral erosions most often are related to medication toxicity or vitamin deficiencies, although infections of the mouth are common in immunocompromised patients, in which case the ulcers may arise without precipitating factors
Angina pectoris	Exertional or stress-related chest pain relieved by rest and/or nitrates	Anemia
Dysrhythmias	Tachycardia is most common, although premature beats (atrial, nodal, and ventricular) can occur	Anemia, immunocompromise may lead to other disorders which cause dysrhythmias (e.g., cardiac infection, pericardial effusions)
Abdominal pain	Important to differentiate localized or generalized abdominal pain to assess for etiologies; onset, duration, quality, and precipitating factors for pain are also important to determine	Abdominal pain may indicate an acute infectious process such as strangulated bowel, but also can indicate problems with liver or spleen; if accompanied by hepatic or splenic enlargement, findings more significant
Diarrhea	Malabsorption resulting in stools passing through the bowel without reabsorption of water (loose stools > 3–6 times/day)	Infectious origin must always be suspected, especially with immunocompromised patients; organisms vary greatly and range from rare travel-related ameobiasis to resistant enteric organisms in the immunocompromised; also occurs with Vitamin B_{12} deficiency

(continued)

Table 8-23 Physical Assessment Findings Indicative of Hematologic/Immunologic Disease (*continued*)

Assessment Finding	Description	Clinical Significance/Etiology
GI bleeding	Upper or lower GI bleeding may be spontaneous, related to existing mucosal injury, or without existing risk factors; bleeding may be occult or hemorrhagic	Thrombocytopenia is a particularly common etiology of occult bleeding or small bleeders
Amenorrhea/menorrhagia	Lack of normal menstrual flow	Unknown etiology, nonspecific finding
Hematuria	Microscopic or visible blood in urine, may or may not be accompanied by dysuria; acute abdominal pain from bladder spasms occurs if clots form in bladder	Bleeding disorders of all kinds: thrombocytopenia, hepatic coagulopathy, DIC
Skin changes	Any changes in normal skin texture, color, or contour	Dry, coarse skin indicative of iron deficiency anemia; pallor indicates low hemoglobin; petichiae or purpura are present with bleeding disorders; jaundice may indicate rapid turnover of RBCs, as seen with hemolytic anemia, DIC, sickle cell anemia
Lymphadenopathy	Major palpable lymph node groups are present under chin, in the neck, in axillae, and in groin; enlargement greater than 1 cm or tenderness is indicative of problems	Lymphadenopathy is present in localized infections and inflammatory processes; also present with tumor involvement of the node, whether primary (lymphoma) or secondary metastases
Fever	Temperature greater than 100.6° F (38.1°C) by mouth, or any increase of 1°C from baseline; temperatures are often highest in late afternoon to early evening	Indicative of infection or inflammation; must be particularly wary of fever in neutropenia or immunosuppression, when fever may be only indication of infection
Wound drainage	Characteristics of wound drainage will reveal much about the site or organism; drainage may be scant or copious, purulent, serous, or sanguinous	Purulent wound drainage is present in infection provided individual has sufficient white cell response; sanguinous drainage is present in deeper tissue injury, but may still harbor organisms
Bone pain	Aching pain in any bones, particularly the long bones (e.g., femur, tibia, vertebrae)or the sternum	May indicate bone marrow disease, either in form of tumor metastasis, excessive growth, aplastic anemia, or excessive cell turnover such as hemolytic anemia or sickle cell anemia
Fatigue and weakness	May accompany exertion or occur at rest; best if compared to patient's individual baseline	Mild to moderate fatigue with exertion occurs with anemia, hemoglobin disorders, and with neutropenia; more severe symptoms may indicate cancers such leukemia or lymphoma
Arthralgias (joint pain)	Painful joints may hurt at rest and/or with activity; area surrounding the joint may or may not be swollen	Hemarthroses occur with bleeding disorders, particularly hemophilia; but joint pain may also be present with hemolytic anemia or inflammation

Lymphangiograms use a blue, iodine-based contrast medium to outline the lymphatic vessels and identify abnormal dye uptake (seen with lymphoma metastases). The test requires injection of fluoroscopic dye, which may be difficult to inject or painful. This test, although reliable, has largely been replaced with magnetic resonance imaging (MRI), because of that technique's accuracy and ease of use.

Antigen-antibody reactions have long been known to indicate immunologic disease, but clini-

Table 8-24 Tests Triggered by an Abnormal CBC

Deficiency	Additional Tests Indicated
Problems with Red Blood Cells	
Decreased hematocrit	Blood chemistry (look for hemodilution of other values, or renal failure, which may be cause of anemia)
	Coagulation profile (evaluate for slow blood loss from coagulopathy)
	RBC morphology (determine if dead, fragmented, or dysfunctional RBCs present)
	RBC indices (detect nutritional anemias)
	Bone marrow biopsy (ascertain disease limiting production)
	Viewing procedures (ascertain etiology of blood loss)
Decreased hemoglobin	RBC indices (demonstrate nutritional deficiencies)
	RBC morphology (determine if hemoglobin disease exists)
	Hemoglobin electrophoresis (detect hemoglobinopathy, such as sickle cell anemia)
Decreased RBC count	RBC morphology
	Serum transferrin (amounts are reduced when transferrin is binding with iron from RBCs lysed in systemic circulation)
	Serum haptoglobin (amounts are reduced when haptoglobin is binding with hemoglobin from RBCs lysed in circulation)
	RBC survival studies (detects abnormal destruction)
	Bone marrow biopsy (determines whether RBCs are being made by the bone marrow)
Increased hematocrit	Urine specific gravity (detects dehydration)
	Serum chemistry (detects hemoconcentration)
	ABGs (evaluates whether patient is hypoxemic)
Problems with Platelets	
Decreased platelet count	Post-platelet counts (detects response to platelet infusions)
	Platelet autoantibody test (detects antibodies against patient's own platelets)
	Abdominal x-ray of spleen (determines splenic enlargement, possibly causing sequestering of platelets)
	Microscopic evaluation of platelets (reveals fragmenting)
	Folate and B_{12} levels (reveals dietary etiology of decreased platelets)
	Evaluation of history of illness and medications (reveals etiologies of thrombocytopenia)
	Bone marrow aspirate and biopsy (determines lack of stem cell production)
Increased platelet count	Evaluate for inflammatory disease (one etiology of increased platelets)
	Erythrocyte sedimentation rate (identifies inflammatory disorders)
	Identify symptoms of cancer (one etiology of thrombocytosis)
Problems with White Blood Cells	
Decreased WBC count	Review nutritional history for protein and calorie intake (reveals etiology of leukopenia)
	Identify risk factors for immune depletion: chronic illness, diabetes mellitus, IV drug use, recent chemotherapy, medications (all etiologies of leukopenia)
Increased WBC count	WBC differential count (identifies type of leukocytosis, determines if bacterial infection is present)
	Cultures of body secretions, susceptible sites (identifies infectious sources)
	Erythrocyte sedimentation rate (indicator of inflammation)
	Bone marrow aspirate and biopsy (when count is high or immature cells are present, leukemia must be ruled out by BM evaluation)
	Complement fixation test (determines recent viral illness)

cians' inability to interpret them has limited their use. Recent genetic engineering techniques have allowed the creation of clones, called monoclonal antibodies, that are specific to certain antigenic substances. Monoclonal antibodies assist clinicians in determining the existence and location of tumors and infectious antigens. Monoclonal antibodies have also been useful for detecting B and T cell subsets that are not readily recognized during microscopic evaluation. The identification of these markers has improved our knowledge of cell-mediated immunity disorders and autoimmune disease.

A normal immunocompetent individual is able to react to either environmental antigens or common childhood illnesses because of the presence and competence of antibody. Individuals with suppressed B cell (humoral) immunity will have either an inadequate response to these antigens or no response at all. Intradermal injections of Candida albicans, measles, or other common antigens will produce a predictable "wheal-flare" reaction. The immunosuppressed patient is nonreactive.

Total protein and electrophoresis tests are often used to screen for immune disorders. Albumin comprises the majority of the plasma protein fraction, and is responsible for maintaining oncotic pressure and transporting essential substances such as hormones and enzymes. Globulins, especially the immunoglobulins, provide the majority of the body's humoral immune response. Globulins comprise about 40% of the total protein fraction.[36] Although they are not measured directly, their presence can be deduced by subtracting the albumin from the total protein. Many immunologic disorders alter the ratio of albumin and globulin in the serum. Abnormal globulin levels or albumin/globulin ratios are further evaluated by protein electrophoresis or similar techniques. Disorders of the B cells, including agammaglobulinemia, hypogammaglobulinemia, or reduced T4 helper cells, produce decreases in the level of gamma globulin (electrophoresis category containing all immunoglobulins). Excessive immunoglobulin is seen with multiple myeloma or deficiency of T8 suppressor cells. Diseases produced by abnormal globulins are seen with cryoglobulinemia or certain infectious processes.

Conclusion

An integrated assessment of the patient with potential hematologic/immunologic disease should include a thorough review of all patient data. Hematologic disease is often the underlying cause of critical, life-threatening illness, yet can often be overlooked. A combination of physical assessment skills and analysis of diagnostic data is necessary to pinpoint the problem and plan nursing interventions. The following sections discuss the common hematologic problems encountered by critical care nurses and the pertinent nursing care.

Neutropenia

The most common phagocyte deficiency, especially in the critical care setting, is absolute neutropenia, which can be due either to disease processes such as leukemia or lymphoma or to treatment of disease processes with cytotoxic drugs and/or radiation.[37] Neutropenia exists when the patient has fewer than 2500 neutrophils per cubic millimeter. The lower the absolute neutrophil count (ANC), the higher the risk of serious infection.

Clinical antecedents

Neutrophils are usually defined as a percentage of the total WBC count, but in neutropenia, it may be

Table 8-25 Calculation of the Absolute Neutrophil Count

Procedure	Example
1. Take white blood cell count	WBC = 3.5 K/mm^3
2. Remembering that K means 1000, translate the total WBC into an absolute number.	3.5 × 1000 = 3500 WBC = 3500/mm^3
3. Take the percentages of polys and bands and add them together.	Polys = 40% Bands = 0% 40% + 0% = 40%
4. Divide by 100 to translate this percentage to an absolute number.	40% ÷ 100 = 0.4
5. Multiply the total WBC by the sum of the polys plus the bands.	3500 × 0.4 = 1400 In this example, the absolute neutrophil count is 1400/mm^3

important to calculate an absolute neutrophil count (ANC). The methodology for calculating an ANC is illustrated in Table 8-25. The ANC is the most significant variable for assessing infection risk in neutropenia. Clinicians use various ranges of ANC to assess risk of infection; one such range of risk is presented in Table 8-26.

The underlying etiology of the neutropenia may also influence the body's ability to resist infection. For example, persons with leukemia and lymphoma who are neutropenic have the highest risk of infection, whereas those with radiation- or malnutrition-induced neutropenia seem to be less susceptible. Once the patient's ANC and individual risk factors are analyzed, endogenous risk factors such as abnormal barrier defenses or recent invasive procedures should be identified and evaluated for their contribution to patient infectivity. Details of these risk factors are included in Chapter 9 in the discussion of sepsis.

Critical referents

Neutropenia alters the phagocytic immunity functions of the body. When neutropenia is present, patients are at risk for systemic invasion by microorganisms. This invasion may present as localized infection or as systemic sepsis.

Regardless of the patient's ANC, underlying disease, or altered defenses, 80% of the organisms causing disease in neutropenia are endogenous flora.[38] Research has demonstrated that the most common source of infection and sepsis in these patients is their endogenous gastrointestinal flora (E. coli, Clostridium perfringens, Clostridium difficile, and Enterobacter).[39] Pneumonias are the second most common infection and are usually caused by endogenous oral or pulmonary flora.[40] Opportunistic infections such as tuberculosis, pneumocystis, and viruses also occur in these patients because of concomitant depression of humoral and cell-mediated immunity.

Infection in the neutropenic host follows a pattern in which the risk becomes progressively greater. The longer neutropenia is present, the more likely it is that the patient will suffer opportunistic or resistant infections. In fact, all patients who are neutropenic for longer than 21 days become infected.[41] The time frames for the common infections are shown in Table 8-27.

Resulting signs and symptoms

Many times it is difficult to assess the neutropenic patient for signs or symptoms of infection, because the signs and symptoms are subtle. The absence of functional neutrophils reduces the inflammatory immune reaction and limits the visible symptoms. Fever is considered the cardinal symptom of potential sepsis and should be evaluated and treated immediately if present. As a result of the absence of neutrophils, even limited numbers of microorganisms may cause a severe systemic reaction and septic shock. Colonization of organisms should be viewed as potential infection, as the absence of neutrophils may be the factor that allows this situation to progress to infection. Often patients will have positive cultures for a particular organism, but no symptoms of sepsis. If neutropenia is temporary, the returning growth of white blood cells will lead to margination in the area where microorganisms are to be found, with a subsequent clinical presentation of fulminant infection. The neutropenic patient may also exhibit cutaneous anergy and abnormal skin cultures.

Nursing standards of care

The major goal in managing the patient with neutropenia is prevention of infection. Methods of

Table 8-26 Infection Risks Associated with Several ANCs

ANC	Risk of Infection
1500	Slightly increased
1000	Moderately increased
500	Greatly increased

Table 8-27 Common Infections Associated with Neutropenia

Type of Infection	Time Frame for Manifestation
Aerobic bacteria	1–2 days
Anaerobic bacteria	3–5 days
Parasites	Up to 6 weeks
Fungi	1–2 weeks
Viruses	2 days to 6 weeks

preventing infection include environmental control of pathogens and alteration of patient susceptibility to infection.

Environmental precautions designed to reduce infection involve cleaning the patient's immediate environment to protect him or her from microorganisms. Microorganisms are known to proliferate in dust, standing water, and soil. For these reasons, patients with neutropenia should not enter construction areas, mingle in crowds, or have fresh flowers or plants in their rooms. Air conditioning units may foster the growth of molds (funguses), and patients should have limited exposure to the indirect air flow. Health care workers should be advised that hand-washing is essential, as the hands are the most common route of transmission of nosocomial infection. Nevertheless, protective isolation precautions (gown, gloves, and masks) have not proven necessary for this patient population, since many infections are endogenous.[42]

The patient is further protected from infection by good general health-care practices: rest, good nutrition, reduced stress, and limited breaks in barrier defense. These patients require special consideration for noninvasive monitoring methods, as all catheters and internally placed devices will increase the risk of infection by normally nonpathogenic organisms. A regimen of prophylactic oral antibiotics for gut steril-

Table 8-28 Infection Control Guidelines

Guideline	Examples
Protect the patient from dangers in environment	Use hepafilters with or without laminar airflow Avoid fresh flowers and standing water Use single patient rooms Throw away dining utensils Keep food only 24 hours Daily room cleaning with special precautions against spreading disease from room to room No children with potential exposure to communicable diseases should visit Change IV tubings, dressings, and wound drainage systems every 24–48 hours
Protect the patient from endogenous organisms	Administer oral nonabsorbable antibiotics as ordered Conduct surveillance cultures of body orifices 1–2 times per week Have handwashing facilities readily available; have bactericidal wipes or sprays available at the patient's bedside Avoid invasive procedures whenever possible (Foley catheters, intravenous lines) Use fecal incontinent bags with caution
Prevent cross-contamination	Clean bedscale sling between patients, or give immunosuppressed patients their own Decontaminate general-use items before using with immunosuppressed (pulse oximetry finger probes, blood pressure cuffs, IV pumps and poles) Clean head of electric razor between patients Avoid assigning a severely infected patient a room with immunosuppressed patient Assign the patient his or her own equipment for multi-use items such as bedside glucose meter
General practice guidelines	Wash hands often Avoid rectal temperatures and suppositories Wear masks with patients when the caregiver has suspected respiratory infection or if staff member is known staph carrier Maintain meticulous patient hygiene using bactericidal soaps (bathing, oral care, perineal care) Do not use scented lotions or powders Use povidine-iodine skin preps for procedures rather than alcohol Provide high-protein, high-calorie diet

ization is advocated by some as a means of eradicating the normal flora, which can infect these patients. An important consideration is that inconsistent use of these agents will unfortunately enhance the growth of resistant flora. An antimicrobial diet or NPO protocol is also advocated to decrease the risk of infection. The antimicrobial diet forbids fresh fruit, vegetables, and nuts, which may harbor organisms, but allows cooked foods or fruits with the skin removed. Other specific recommendations for protection from infection are included in Table 8-28.

A new therapy to decrease the length of the time patients are neutropenic is the administration of colony stimulating factors (G-CSF, GM-CSF), which stimulate new neutrophil and monocyte differentiation in the bone marrow. When CSF is administered to these patients, WBC growth is promoted, neutropenia is shortened, and infections are limited or prevented.[43]

The role of the nurse in managing patients with neutropenia is to monitor all potential infection risks—equipment, visitors, and hospital personnel. Frequent assessment for infection is essential and involves evaluation of all orifices and skin surfaces, investigation of all painful areas, and sytemic monitoring for sepsis. Many nursing care routines, such as shaving, skin care, or oral care, may increase the patient's risk of infection if not performed with the proper equipment or solutions.

Anaphylaxis

Anaphylaxis is an acute generalized allergic reaction, which may result in cardiovascular collapse and respiratory failure. This profound allergic reaction is a result of the overwhelming release of chemical mediators from specialized cells (mast cells and basophils) located throughout the body. The release of chemicals from these cells is most often precipitated by the interaction of a specific antigen and its corresponding IgE antibody. Mediators may also be released as part of so-called nonimmune reactions. These reactions can involve complement anaphylatoxins or immune complexes or may result from the direct effect of a chemical compound on mast cells and basophils. Hospitalized patients are at risk of anaphylaxis via either mechanism. Critically ill patients in particular often must undergo radiologic tests involving dye injection or receive antibiotics, narcotics, anesthetics, and other substances that may cause anaphylaxis.

Clinical antecedents

Anaphylactic reactions that are dependent upon IgE antibody are known as reagin-dependent, IgE-mediated, or immunologic anaphylaxis. These reactions can be caused by administration of penicillin, exposure to venom from insect bites or stings, or the ingestion of certain foods. Common antecedents of anaphylaxis are listed in Table 8-29. The tendency to develop IgE antibody to harmless substances is termed atopy, or allergy; individuals with allergies are called atopic.

Seventy-five percent of all deaths due to anaphylaxis result from penicillin-associated anaphylaxis. It has been estimated that there are 800 deaths per year nationwide due to anaphylactic reactions to parenteral penicillin.[44] For every 100,000 injections of penicillin, there are 10 to 40 cases of anaphylaxis and 2 fatalities.[45] Penicillin-associated anaphylaxis is puzzling for a variety of reasons. First, although IgE-mediated anaphylaxis requires previous exposure to the allergen, penicillin allergy can occur in persons who have never received the drug. It has been suggested that penicillin allergic persons may have been exposed to the drug through drinking milk from cows that were fed penicillin-related antibiotics, through occupational exposure, or through immunization, since penicillin is added to the cultures from which vaccines are derived.[46] The second puzzling fact is that penicillin-associated anaphylaxis does not appear to be related to atopy. Persons who have allergies are not necessarily allergic to penicillin. The final unusual fact about penicillin allergy is that 85% of persons who experience an allergic (not necessarily anaphylactic) reaction to penicillin can tolerate future doses without reaction.[47] The longer the delay between the dose causing the reaction and the subsequent dose, the greater the likelihood of losing sensitivity to the drug. Technological advances have made available several penicillin derivatives. Nurses should recognize these when monitoring a patient's medication regimen. Common penicillin derivatives are listed in Table 8-30.

Other substances are frequently associated with anaphylaxis. Several biologic agents (ACTH, insulin, and vaccines) and blood components have been linked to it. Nonpharmacologic causes of anaphylaxis include ingestion of foods such as egg whites, peanuts, tree nuts, and shellfish. Shellfish allergies are unrelated to allergies to iodine-based radiocontrast agents.[48] Rarely, anaphylaxis may occur due to exercise or exposure to seminal fluid (via sexual

Table 8-29 Clinical Antecedents of Anaphylaxis

Category	Example
Drugs	
Antibiotics	Penicillin, cephalosporins and related compounds, polymyxin B, vancomycin, aminoglycosides, tetracycline, amphotericin B, others
Anesthetics	Succinylcholine, tubocurarine, bupivicaine, lidocaine, procaine, tetracaine
Cytotoxic agents	Adriamycin, bleomycin, cisplatin, cyclophosphamide, L-aspariginase, melphalan, methotrexate, others
Dextrans	Iron dextran
Nonsteroidal antiinflammatories	Aspirin, indomethacin, phenylbutazone
Narcotics	Morphine, codeine
Vitamins	Intravenous vitamin K
Venom	Bites and stings from hymenoptera (bees, wasps), deerflies, fire ants, spiders, jellyfish, snakes
Food	Peanuts, tree nuts, grains, seeds, cottonseed oil, egg white, shellfish, food additives (sulfites, other preservatives, dyes)
Biological Agents	
Hormones	Insulin, ACTH
Immunotherapy	Vaccines, antitoxins, allergenic extracts
Blood products	Blood components, including gamma globulin
Chymopapain	
Diagnostic Agents	Iodine-based contrast media, SP dye, iopanoic acid (Telepaque), B-dehydrocholic acid (Decholin)

intercourse) or progesterone. The immunologic mechanisms of these rare forms of anaphylaxis are not well understood.

Anaphylactic reactions that do not require IgE antibody are generally termed nonimmune or anaphylactoid reactions. Radiocontrast media and certain drugs can induce this type of reaction. Iodine-based radiocontrast media (RCM) are well known for precipitating anaphylactoid reactions. As few as 1 of every 10,000–50,000 patients receiving RCM have fatal reactions. Of those patients who have experienced an adverse reaction to the media, 17–35% will react to subsequent administrations. Recently, low-ionic contrast medias have been developed, and their use results in fewer cases of anaphylaxis. Unfortunately, the cost of these preparations prohibits their routine use. Recommendations for administering RCM to patients at high risk for anaphylaxis are described in Table 8-31. Although it is important to understand the mechanisms involved in anaphylactoid and IgE-mediated anaphylaxis, both reactions have the same symptoms and treatment and thus will be grouped together in this discussion.

All anaphylactic reactions are influenced by four factors: (1) the route of entry of the antigen into the body, (2) the "antigenic dose" (amount of antigen), (3) the rate of antigen absorption, and (4) the degree of the patient's hypersensitivity to the antigen.[49] A summary of how these factors influence the severity of reaction is provided in Table 8-32.

Table 8-30 Penicillin and Derivatives That Can Cause Anaphylaxis

Penicillin V	Cloxacillin
Penicillin G	Bacampicillin
Amoxicillin	Cyclacillin
Carbenicillin	Dicloxacillin
Methicillin	Mezlocillin
Piperacillin	Nafcillin
Ampicillin	Oxacillin
Azlocillin	Ticarcillin

Table 8-31 Prevention of Iodine-Based RCM Anaphylaxis

Hours Prior to Injection of RCM	Oral Medication to be Administered
13 hours	Prednisone 50 mg
7 hours	Prednisone 50 mg
1 hour	Prednisone 50 mg Diphenhydramine 50–100 mg orally Ephedrine 25 mg orally Cimetidine 300 mg* or Ranitidine 150 mg

*Optional; H2 blocker

Critical referents

Mast cells are the key cells involved in anaphylaxis. Although basophils are also involved in the process, they are believed to play only a minor role. Mast cells are located throughout the body but are present in highest concentrations surrounding the blood vessels, in the lungs, in the gut linings, and in connective tissue. Mast cells are also located in various organs: the heart, kidney, liver, spleen, omentum, and skin. Each mast cell has from 30,000 to 200,000 IgE receptors on its cell surface. These cells contain stores of chemicals such as histamine, and when stimulated, they produce other lipid-derived mediators, such as leukotrienes.[50] This process is summarized in Figure 8-15.

Three stages of IgE-mediated anaphylaxis The first stage of IgE-mediated anaphylaxis is called sensitization. In this stage, the body experiences the initial contact with the antigen. The contact causes an IgE antibody to the antigen to be formed. The IgE produced in this phase has a high affinity for the antigen. The IgE attaches to Fc receptors on mast cells and basophils. Once the IgE attaches to receptors, these cells are "cocked," and like a cocked pistol, the cells await subsequent exposure to an adequate dose of antigen to provide the stimulus to "pull the trigger." This "cocked pistol" stage can last indefinitely. It is known that some persons have a genetic predisposition to produce IgE antibody in response to antigens, but researchers are still investigating the immunological mechanisms that give rise to this phenomena.

During the second phase—activation—the body is re-exposed to the antigen. With this second exposure, the antigen attaches to IgE molecules on the mast cell or basophil cell surfaces, and adjacent IgE molecules link together. This cross-linking, or bridging, of IgE molecules causes calcium to flow through the membranes of the sensitized cells, which causes cellular degranulation—the virtual explosion of chemical mediators from the mast cells into the surrounding tissue and bloodstream.

The third phase of IgE anaphylaxis is the stage during which the target organ response occurs, and

Table 8-32 Factors Influencing the Severity of Anaphylaxis

Factor	Influences
Route of entry of antigen into the body	Antigens injected directly into the bloodstream are most likely to induce a rapid response; ingested antigens are absorbed more slowly but produce a no less severe reaction. Other methods of entry include inhalation, absorption through skin or mucous membranes, and subcutaneous injection.
Antigenic dose	The larger the dose of antigen at a single exposure, the more severe the reaction. Small continual exposures may or may not produce a less vigorous anaphylactic reaction than a moderate single-dose exposure.
Rate of absorption	When antigens are administered directly into the circulation, they disseminate more rapidly throughout the body, causing mast cells to degranulate; antigens slowly absorbed, such as those exposed to the skin, will be less likely to produce severe systemic symptoms immediately.
Degree of hypersensitivity to the antigen	Each antigen presents a specific level of antigenicity, depending on the individual, causing mild reactions in some people and severe ones in others. The severity may be related to the numbers of immunoglobulins that are "primed" to activate, and thus hypersensitivity may increase with each exposure to the antigen.

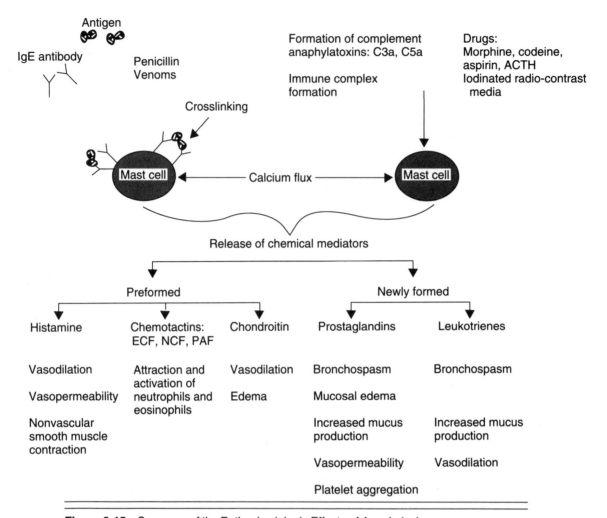

Figure 8-15 Summary of the Pathophysiologic Effects of Anaphylaxis

is called the effector phase. In this phase, the tissues respond to the chemical mediators released from mast cells and basophils.

Chemical mediators of anaphylaxis Mast cells produce two categories of chemicals: preformed and newly formed. Preformed mediators (histamine, heparin, chondroitin, and chemotactins) are those stored in the granules of the mast cells and released upon activation. Newly formed mediators (prostaglandins and leukotrienes) are developed in response to degranulation through the arachidonic pathway. The effects of these mediators are summarized in Table 8-33.

Histamine is one of the most important preformed mediators in the pathogenesis of anaphylaxis. Its primary effects are listed in Table 8-33. Histamine produces vasodilation of arteries and veins while also triggering contraction of vascular smooth muscle. Histamine also causes endothelial cells to separate, increasing capillary membrane permeability. There are two types of histamine receptors: H1 and H2. Stimulation of both H1 and H2 receptors can result in vasodilation of arteries and veins, which in turn produces hypotension, decreased venous return, reduced systemic vascular resistance, tachycardia, and headache. The increased capillary permeability produced by histamine can result in edema, reduced circulating blood volume, reduced cardiac output, and shock. Contraction of nonvascular smooth muscle may result in bronchospasm, incontinence, and hematuria.[51]

The newly formed mediators enhance the effects of histamine, heparin, and chondroitin. Prostaglandins and leukotrienes are the primary substances formed by mast cells. Leukotrienes are lipid metabolites (LTB 4, LTC 4, and LTD 4), formerly known as the slow reacting substance of anaphylaxis (SRSA). The leukotrienes are extremely potent mediators

Table 8-33 Anaphylaxis Mediators and Their Effects

Mediator	Physiological Response	Clinical Symptoms
Preformed		
Histamine	Contraction of nonvascular smooth muscle: lung, GI tract, bladder, ureter	Bronchoconstriction Involuntary urination Involuntary defecation, cramps Hematuria
	Vasodilation of arteries and veins	Hypotension Decreased venous return Reduced systemic vascular resistance (SVR)
	Increased capillary membrane permeability	Edema, hypotension Reduced circulating blood volume Reduced cardiac output Shock
	Stimulation of the cardiac histamine receptors	Bradycardia Tachycardia
	Increased production of gastric acid	Nausea and vomiting
Heparin	Anticoagulant	
	Anticomplement	Coagulopathy
Chondroitin	Activates the kinin system to produce bradykinin	
	Smooth muscle contraction of bronchi and GI tract	Bronchoconstriction Diarrhea
	Vasodilation	Hypotension
	Increased capillary membrane permeability	Edema
	Stimulation of nerve fibers	Pruritis, pain
Chemotactins:		
ECFA	Eosinophil attraction and activation	Inflammation
NCF	Neutrophil attraction and activation	Inflammation
PAF	Platelet aggregation and activation	Thrombosis, cyanosis
Newly formed		
Prostaglandins		Bronchoconstriction Production of viscous mucus Increased adhesiveness of platelets
	Vasodilation	Hypotension
Leukotrienes (SRSA)	Prolonged spasm and contraction of visceral smooth muscle (especially bronchi)	Bronchoconstriction
	Increased mucus production	Cough, sputum
	Vasodilation	Hypotension
	Vasopermeability	Edema

(100 to 1000 times stronger than histamine) that produce vasodilation, vasopermeability, increased mucus production, and prolonged spasm and contraction of visceral smooth muscle, especially of the bronchi.[52]

Although the preformed and newly formed mediators differ greatly, they both produce three major physiological effects: bronchoconstriction, vasodilation, and increases in capillary permeability. These effects are also observed in anaphylactoid reactions, but the mechanisms that create them in such cases are unknown.

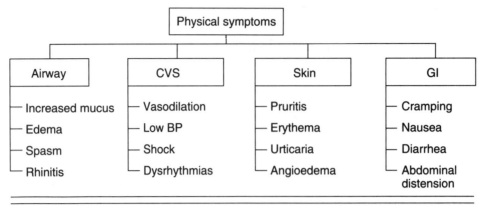

Figure 8-16   Systemic Clinical Symptoms of Anaphylaxis

Resulting signs and symptoms

Four main patterns of anaphylactic response have been identified: immediate onset, delayed onset, biphasic response, and protracted anaphylaxis. The shorter the interval from exposure to the antigen to the onset of symptoms, the more severe the reaction. In over half of the episodes, symptoms of anaphylaxis are manifested immediately and respond to initial therapy. However, delayed onset of reactions occurring 12–24 hours after antigenic exposure has been reported.[53] One-quarter of all patients experience protracted anaphylaxis, in which the symptoms may last for days.[54] In another 25% of cases, a biphasic response occurs, in which symptoms that occurred immediately recur up to 8 hours later.[55] These patients are at the highest risk of death since this response cannot be reliably predicted. For this reason, it is essential to observe all patients for at least 8 hours following the initial onset of symptoms.[56]

The symptoms of anaphylaxis all stem from the triad of smooth muscle contraction, vasodilation, and increased capillary permeability. The most severe consequences of anaphylaxis are cardio-pulmonary arrest and death. Usually, airway obstruction from laryngeal edema and bronchospasm leads to respiratory arrest and intractable shock. In its most severe forms, anaphylaxis can result in critical illness such as disseminated intravascular coagulation (DIC). With the exception of penicillin-related anaphylaxis, the severity of reaction usually remains consistent from one episode to another. Systemic clinical symptoms of anaphylaxis are outlined in Figure 8-16. The classic symptoms are sudden respiratory distress with wheezing and stridor, abdominal distention and cramping, hypotension, angioedema, and pruritis. The symptoms are usually differentiated from acute severe hypersensitivity reaction by the presence of cardiovascular symptoms and smooth muscle contractions.

Nursing standards of care

Early recognition of the patient's symptoms of anaphylaxis is essential for early intervention and reduction of morbidity. The first measures to take are those that ensure that no further absorption of the

Table 8-34   Steps to Stop the Further Absorption of Antigen in Anaphylaxis

1. Stop any infusion of medication, blood product, or dye injection that may have precipitated the anaphylactic reaction.

2. If reaction may have been related to an injection in a limb, apply a loose tourniquet to or wrap and inflate a BP cuff around the limb proximal to the injection site. Inject 0.2 mL of 1:1000 epinephrine subcutaneously into the site to constrict local blood vessels, thus limiting antigen absorption.

3. If anaphylaxis is related to an insect bite or sting, place a loose tourniquet around the extremity in which the bite or sting occurred, proximal to the site. Gently remove the stinger (if present) by scraping it out of skin rather than grasping it. Inject 0.2 mL of 1:1000 epinephrine subcutaneously into site. Remove tourniquet periodically.

4. If antigen was ingested, perform gastric lavage.

Table 8-35 Use of Epinephrine in Anaphylaxis

Form	Concentration	Route of Administration	Dosage Range	Frequency	Comments
Injection					
Adult	1:1000 = 1 mg/mL 1:10,000 = 0.1 mg/mL	SC, IM IV	0.2–1.0 mL	Every 20–30 minutes	Usually given SC
Child	1:1000	SC,IM	0.01 mL/Kg	Every 20–30 minutes	
Inhalant ("racemic" epinephrine)	1:100 = 10 mg/mL	Oral inhalant			Do not administer parenterally; do not confuse with other dosage forms

antigen occurs. Steps for stopping absorption of antigen are listed in Table 8-34.

Administration of epinephrine Epinephrine is the drug of choice for treating anaphylaxis and is available in several different forms and concentrations (see Table 8-35). It is imperative that the anaphylactic patient receive epinephrine as soon as anaphylaxis has been identified and emergency airway management has been instituted. Subcutaneous administration of epinephrine is the route of choice, as it permits the maximum dose yet prevents adverse effects.

Racemic epinephrine may be administered by inhalation if angioedema, laryngeal edema, or severe bronchospasm are already present. If bronchospasm is not reversed by epinephrine, bronchodilators may be required. Severe bronchospasm can be diagnosed by measuring forced expiratory volume (FEV), peak flow, and arterial blood gases. If the FEV is less than 1 L/s and peak flow is less than 300 mL/min, or pCO_2 is greater than 40 mm Hg, other measures must be taken. The treatment of choice in such cases is racemic epinephrine or nebulized Albuterol inhalation or intravenous aminophylline.[57] Severe airway edema may require crycothyrotomy, a safer and faster technique than tracheotomy. The incision is made through the crycothyroid membrane and enlarged, and a 4–5 mm endotracheal tube is inserted. Endotracheal intubation may be elected as an alternative, but the edema usually limits the tube size to 4–5 French.

Epinephrine has four major therapeutic effects in anaphylaxis: (1) bronchodilation, (2) peripheral vasoconstriction, (3) stimulation of the inotropic and chronotropic properties of the heart, and (4) reduction of mast cell activation. Epinephrine improves ventilation by causing the smooth muscles of the

bronchi to relax and by reducing airway congestion through constriction of the bronchial mucosa. Additionally, epinephrine is an alpha agonist and improves circulation by constricting peripheral blood vessels and therefore raising blood pressure. Epinephrine is also a beta agonist that increases heart rate and force of contraction to improve blood flow to the brain and coronary arteries. These therapeutic

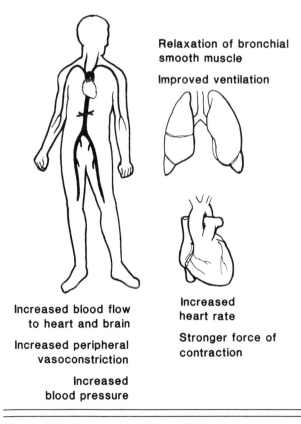

Relaxation of bronchial smooth muscle

Improved ventilation

Increased blood flow to heart and brain

Increased peripheral vasoconstriction

Increased blood pressure

Increased heart rate

Stronger force of contraction

Figure 8-17 Therapeutic Effects of Epinephrine

Table 8-36 Therapeutic Effects of Epinephrine

Class	Effect	Clinical Effect
Alpha agonist	Produces peripheral vasoconstriction	Increases blood pressure
Beta1 agonist	Increases rate and force of contraction	Increases blood flow to brain and coronary arteries and reverses hypotension
Beta2 agonist	Relaxes bronchial smooth muscle	Improves ventilation

effects are presented schematically in Figure 8-17 and listed in Table 8-36.

Excess epinephrine can produce several adverse effects. One of the most serious is cerebral hemorrhage resulting from the precipitous rise in blood pressure. Epinephrine can also overtax the heart so greatly that angina and myocardial infarction can result.[58] In some cases, the patient may experience life-threatening dysrhythmias such as severe tachycardia or ventricular fibrillation.[59] Although unusual, bradycardia may occur, and atropine may be needed to return the heart rate to normal. There have been reports that excessive administration of epinephrine can actually enhance bronchospasm, worsening the patient's initial condition.[60] It has even produced psychosis in some patients. Individual patients will exhibit different side effects from the spectrum shown in Table 8-37, necessitating cautious administration of epinephrine.

To reduce the risk of severe side effects, caution should be taken when administering epinephrine to patients who are receiving monoamine oxidase inhibitors or who have hyperthyroidism, hypertension, or coronary or cerebral arteriosclerosis. These patients may be given a less toxic derivative of epinephrine, such as terbutaline. Although most episodes of anaphylaxis are brief, prolonged anaphy-

laxis has been reported in persons on beta blocker therapy, because of the counteractive effects of such drugs upon the blood vessels.[61] In cases of protracted anaphylaxis, epinephrine has been administered by continuous infusion with the dose titrated until a desired clinical response is achieved. Guidelines for continuous intravenous infusion of epinephrine are listed in Table 8-38.

Treatment of hypotension As soon as possible, caregivers should begin administering 0.9% normal saline or Ringer's lactate intravenously.[62] If the blood pressure remains low after epinephrine injection, fluids are infused at approximatley 100 cc/hr. Isotonic electrolyte solutions are used to reduce the possibility of capillary leakage of the fluids.[63] Vasopressors should be used if the hypotension is unresponsive to epinephrine and fluids. The vasopressor of choice is phenylephrine because it causes peripheral constriction without the cardiac effects that may enhance epinephrine cardiotoxicity.[64] Continuous monitoring by ECG and pulmonary artery catheter may be required in protracted cases of anaphylaxis.

Other medications used in anaphylaxis Other medications are often indicated in anaphylactic shock. For example, corticosteroids are presumed to enhance the therapeutic effects of epinephrine, block the production of prostaglandins and leukotrienes, reduce vascular permeability, and inhibit chemotaxis of immune system cells. Hydrocortisone sodium

Table 8-37 Side Effects of Epinephrine

Mild	Severe
Nervousness, anxiety	Psychosis
Tremors	Rigidity
Palpitations, tachycardia	Coronary artery spasm, angina, MI
Increased blood pressure	Dysrhythmias, including ventricular tachycardia
Headache (due to increased BP)	
Nausea, diaphoresis	Hypertension
Pallor	Cerebral hemorrhage

Table 8-38 Guidelines for Continuous Infusion of Epinephrine

1. Add 1 mg of epinephrine to 250 mL of D5W (resulting concentration is 0.004 mg/mL or 4 mcg/mL).
2. Administer at a rate of 1–4 mcg/min (1 to 4 mL per minute = 60 to 240 mL per hour).
3. Titrate to maintain BP at desired level (MAP of 70 mm Hg)

Source: Adapted from Graziano, F. M., and Lemanske, R. F., Jr. (1989). *Clinical Immunology.* Baltimore: Williams and Wilkins.

succinate is used in this circumstance because of its rapid onset. Antihistamines are given to combat the angioedema and urticaria. If anaphylaxis is severe, an H2 blocker (cimetidine, ranitidine, famotidine) is added to lessen cardiac, blood vessel, and GI effects of histamine. Additional medications used in anaphylaxis are listed in Table 8-39.

Additional management strategies Following treatment for anaphylaxis, the patient must take precautions to prevent severe biphasic response symptoms. For at least 24–36 hours after an episode of anaphylaxis, precautions against vasodilation should be observed, including abstaining from sun exposure, hot tubs, alcohol ingestion, or vigorous exercise.

Once an allergen that causes anaphylaxis has been identified, future episodes can be prevented by avoiding the antigen. If avoidance cannot be guaranteed, or if the antigen must be given therapeutically (for example, penicillin), one of two treatment modalities can be employed to lessen the risk of anaphylaxis: hyposensitization or desensitization. Individuals susceptible to anaphylaxis may also be advised to carry epinephrine injections and learn self-administration.

The terms *hyposensitization* and *desensitization* are often used interchangably, but the treatment modalities are different. Hyposensitization is a technique used to lower a patient's sensitivity to a drug. It involves giving increasing doses of antigen intravenously over a short period of time. The initial doses are so dilute that only a few mast cells degranulate at a time. Eventually, when the therapeutic dose is achieved, too few mast cells remain "cocked" to be triggered and produce symptoms. Following hyposensitization, it is essential to administer subsequent doses of the drug *exactly on time.* Any delay could allow time for production of IgE antibody and mast cell "cocking."

Desensitization (or immunotherapy) is used in persons with life-threatening reactions to insect stings. Dilute amounts of antigen are administered subcutaneously. When antigen is administered in this manner, B lymphocytes are stimulated to produce IgG antibody rather than IgE antibody. Eventually, the IgG antibody specific to the antigen is present in a larger concentration than the IgE antibody. Upon re-exposure to the antigen, the IgG antibody binds to the antigen and then binds to IgE on mast cells. The IgG formed in this process is termed "blocking antibody." Desensitization is 98% effective in decreasing the frequency and severity of anaphylaxis due to bee stings.[65]

If the allergen precipitating the anaphylactic episode is unknown, skin testing, antigen challenge, or radioallergosorbent test (RAST) may be used to identify the antigen.

Early recognition and management of anaphylaxis are the keys to reducing morbidity and mortality. Recognition of a patient's initial symptoms of anaphylaxis is essential. The nurse will be one of the first to initiate treatment to reduce antigen absorp-

Table 8-39 Medications Used in Anaphylaxis

Medication	Route	Adult Dose
Diphenhydramine	IV or IM	50 mg every 6–8 hours
Hydroxyzine	IV or IM*	25–50 mg every 8 hours
Chlorpheniramine	PO	4–12 mg every 6–12 hours
Cimetidine	IV	300 mg every 6 hours
Ranitidine	IV	50 mg
Corticosteroids:		
Prednisone	PO	60 mg
Methylprednisolone	IV	50 mg
Hydrocortisone	IV	100 mg every 6 hours
Albuterol	Nebulizer	2.5 mL in 2–5 mL of normal saline every 20 minutes
Aminophylline	IV	Loading dose: 5.6 mg/kg over 20 min Continuous infusion: 0.3–0.9 mg/kg/hr

*Generally IM administration is recommended
Source: Adapted from Corren, J., and Shocket, A. L. (1990). Anaphylaxis. A preventable emergency. *Postgraduate Medicine 87* (5): 167–168, 171–178.

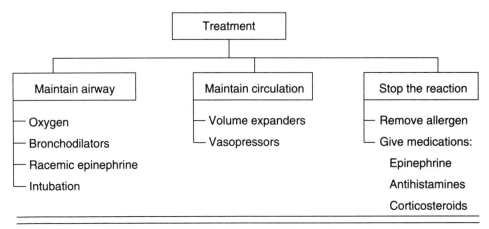

Figure 8-18 Treatment of Anaphylaxis

tion and protect airways. The nurse must also be aware of a specific patient's risks in regard to the common treatment regimen and must assist in altering this regimen as appropriate. Nursing goals in managing the anaphylactic patient include: (1) maintaining an effective airway, (2) identifying the antigen producing the reaction and taking measures to eliminate it, (3) supporting cardiovascular function, (4) providing patient comfort, and (5) teaching the patient about anaphylaxis pathophysiology and methods of prevention and immediate intervention.

The basic treatment steps are diagrammed in Figure 8-18. A plan of nursing care for the patient with anaphylaxis follows.

Nursing Care Plan for the Management of the Patient with Anaphylaxis

Diagnosis	Signs and symptoms	Intervention	Rationale
Ineffective airway clearance related to viscous secretions	Coughing Choking Expectoration of thick viscous sputum Gurgles and crackles	Place patient in upright position when possible	Best position for ventilation
		Nasotracheal or orotracheal suction as needed	To promote clear airway
		Supply humidified air by mask	To loosen secretions and make expectoration easier
		Administer antihistamines and bronchodilators as ordered	To reduce production of secretions and increase ease of breathing
		Monitor respiratory rate and effort every 15 minutes during acute episode	To assess for acute decompensation
		Monitor oxygen saturation continuously	To provide rough estimate of oxygenation
Alteration in gas exchange related to bronchospasm	Tachypnea Dyspnea Wheezes Hypoxemia Decreased oxygen saturation	Oxygen therapy as needed and ordered	To reduce work of breathing and correct hypoxemia
		Breath sound auscultation every 1–2 hours during acute episode; note changes in wheezes, gurgles, or stridor	To ascertain worsening or improvement of condition
		Observe for use of accessory muscles when breathing	Indication of increased work of breathing
		Monitor oxygen saturation continuously	To provide estimate of oxygenation
		Monitor arterial blood gases for hypercarbia and acidosis	Indication of respiratory failure possibly requiring intubation
		Administer sedative and anxiolytic medications as ordered	To decrease anxiety and work of breathing

Nursing Care Plan for the Management of the Patient with Anaphylaxis

Diagnosis	Signs and symptoms	Intervention	Rationale
		Administer bronchodilators as ordered; monitor for nervousness and tachycardia	To improve ventilation and ascertain side effects
		Prepare to assist with endotracheal intubation or tracheostomy as needed; use small (5–6 French) ET tube; prepare suction equipment; monitor for hypotension and tachycardia with paralytic agents	Edema may necessitate emergency intubation or tracheostomy
Potential alteration in fluid volume; deficit related to vasodilation	Orthostatic tachycardia and BP	Meticulous I&O Periodic weights	To ascertain fluid balance
	Hypotension, especially diastolic BP	Safety precautions	To prevent injury from falls resulting from orthostasis
	Low CVP		
	Hemoconcentration	Monitor vital signs with orthostatics at least every hour during acute episode	Vasodilation may cause hypotension
	High urine specific gravity		
	Oliguria	Administer hypotonic solutions to expand vascular volume	Patient's blood chemistries are hemoconcentrated, hypotonic solutions replace fluid without electrolyte imbalance
	Poor skin turgor	Electrolytes every 12–24 hours with hypotonic solution fluid replacement	
		Assess for poor tissue perfusion related to vasodilation and decreased CO: Cardiac—ischemia, tachycardia; Neurologic—confusion, lethargy, dizziness;	Common complication of vasodilation without adequate circulating blood volume

Diagnosis	Signs and symptoms	Intervention	Rationale
		Pulmonary—dyspnea, hypoxemia; Renal—oliguria, increased creatinine; GI—paralytic ileus, abdominal pain; Skin—cyanosis, coolness, diminished pulses	
		Teach patient precautions to be followed 24–36 hours after anaphylaxis and symptoms associated with biphasic response: No hot baths, hot tubs, alcohol ingestion, or vigorous physical exercise; No vasodilator medications; Continue antihistamines and corticosteroids as prescribed; Maintain liberal fluid intake; Follow safety precautions when moving from sitting or lying positions	Biphasic response occurs in 25% of anaphylaxis cases and may cause life-threatening hypotension
Decreased cardiac output related to severe vasodilation	Tachycardia	Monitor VS at least every hour during the acute episode	To assess for respiratory and cardiac decompensation
	Weak, thready pulse	Report hypotension (MAP < 60–70 mm Hg)	MAP < 60–70 mm Hg doesn't perfuse brain or kidneys
	Low CO, PAP, PCWP, or CVP		
	Cyanosis of extremities		
	Coolness of extremities	Ascertain need for treatment or medication changes if heart rate is higher than 160/min	High heart rate doesn't allow sufficient filling pressure to maintain CO
		Continuous ECG monitoring	To discover cardiac complications
		Record 12-lead ECG if dysrhythmia or severe tachycardia is present	To detect ischemia or infarction

Diagnosis	Signs and symptoms	Intervention	Rationale
		Perform cardiac outputs or derived PA pressures as needed for evaluation of interventions	To assist in evaluation of cardiac performance
		Administer fluid challenges as needed and tolerated	To expand vascular volume
		Observe for heart failure with vigorous fluid administration	Necessary fluids may cause heart failure
		Consider vasopressors if epinephrine and fluids fail to correct hypotension: Use dopamine if cardiac toxicities do not occur; Use neosynephrine if hypotension is thought to be entirely vasodilatory in nature	Vasopressors are last line of therapy; neosynephrine is peripheral vasoconstrictor without cardiac side effects
		Establish IV access with 0.9 NS initially, changing to hypotonic solution if hemoconcentration occurs	Isotonic solution is compatible with all medications; hypotonic solutions will dilute concentrated electrolytes
Anxiety, fear	Anxious facial expressions Verbalization of anxiety or fear Trembling	Assess contribution of anxiety to patient's physical symptoms, inability to exchange gas, and comfort	Patient's fears may be making symptoms worse
		Explain procedures and rationale	Information reduces anxiety for most people
		Maintain calm, confident manner	Calmness is reassuring
		Establish quiet, restful environment	To promote rest

Diagnosis	Signs and symptoms	Intervention	Rationale
		Reassure patient as needed	To meet safety needs
		Administer sedating or anxiolytic medications	To reduce work of breathing and possibly improve oxygenation
		Assure patient and family that they will receive information regarding condition when the patient is better able to ask questions	Patient and family may take comfort in the knowledge that they will actively participate in prevention or future management of problem
Alteration in comfort: abdominal cramping, dyspnea, itching	Abdominal cramps Dyspnea Itching Headache Edema	Assess patient's comfort and expressions of distress; note location, quality, and nature of discomfort; develop individualized plan to address comfort needs	To encourage patient to express comfort needs and to help devise most effective plan to meet the needs
		Mild analgesic such as acetominophen as indicated	To reduce mild discomforts such as headache
		For abdominal cramping, administer antimotility medications and apply warm compresses to abdomen	To decrease discomfort and gastric motility
		For dyspnea, place patient in position of comfort, give sedative or anxiolytic medication as ordered, provide bronchodilator therapy and oxygen to relieve dyspnea sensations	To enhance nondistressed breathing
		For itching, continue antihistamines and use mentholated lotions, cool baths, fans, and smooth sheets on bed	To relieve itching

HIV Infection and Acquired Immunodeficiency Syndrome

"The acquired immunodeficiency syndrome (AIDS) is the severe end of a spectrum of disease caused by the human immunodeficiency virus (HIV)."[66] HIV infection produces chronic viral illness resulting in a progressive immunodeficiency in which "the severity of the disease is directly related to the degree of immune suppression."[67]

AIDS was first described in 1981 when previously healthy individuals with no known cause for immunodeficiency presented with opportunistic infections and an unusual cancer, Kaposi's sarcoma. The human immunodeficiency virus (HIV) was discovered in late 1983 and was subsequently determined to be the cause of AIDS.[68] A second virus, HIV 2, which causes a similar disease and also has been discovered to cause AIDS, has largely been confined to Africa.

Clinical antecedents

HIV infection is primarily transmitted via two means: sexual intercourse and parenteral innoculation with HIV-infected blood. Children may acquire the virus in utero or during birth. These modes of transmission form the tragic triad: sex, blood, and birth. The major modes of transmission for the virus are listed in Table 8-40. HIV occurs primarily in specific groups: homosexual or bisexual men and intravenous drug users. By far the single greatest risk factor for acquiring infection is unprotected receptive anal intercourse.[69] AIDS is most prevalent in males; only 10% of all AIDS patients are female.

The second greatest risk factor for AIDS is the sharing of needles and syringes used to inject intra-

Table 8-40 Modes of Transmission of HIV

Sexual intercourse with an infected person

Innoculation with infected blood via sharing of needles and syringes used to inject drugs intravenously

Transfusion with infected blood or blood products

Intrapartum (from an infected mother to her child)

Occupational exposure of health care workers to infective material (blood or pure virus) via parenteral innoculation or contact with mucous membranes or nonintact skin

Transplantation of infected tissue

---

venous drugs. Parenteral innoculation with HIV occurs most often among intravenous drug users (IVDU) who frequently share contaminated needles and syringes when injecting drugs. Blood containing virally infected cells may remain in syringes and infect the next user's cells. The third highest risk factor (for women) is to be the sex partner of a bisexual male or (for women and men) to be the sex partner of an intravenous drug user.[70]

HIV has also been transmitted by transfusion of HIV-infected blood or blood products such as factor VIII (administered to hemophiliacs to prevent or stop bleeding). In 1985, blood banks began testing donated blood for the presence of HIV. Since implementation of this testing program, the number of transfusion-acquired cases of HIV infection has dramatically decreased. Unfortunately, the screening test is not perfect; a few units of blood may pass the screening test although they harbor the virus. Of the 18 million units administered per year, only about 460 units will exhibit a false negative ELISA, not showing the existence of virus in the blood. In 1989, the risk of acquiring HIV infection from a transfusion was estimated at 2.55 cases per 100,000 transfusions.[71]

Pediatric cases of HIV infection have primarily occurred in children born to HIV-infected mothers—that is, through intrapartum transmission of HIV. Researchers estimate that an HIV-infected pregnant woman has a 20–50% chance of bearing an infected child if she has never given birth to a child with HIV; and mothers who have at least one child with congenital HIV transmission have a 50–60% chance of passing the virus to their future children.[72] Approximately 50% of children with HIV live to school age; the remainder die in infancy.[73]

HIV infection is not believed to be transmitted by tears, saliva, urine, or vomit. Although the virus has been isolated from some of these fluids, it is present in such small quantities that infection is believed to be extremely unlikely. Other rare modes of HIV transmission have been documented. Transplantation of infected tissue, including artificial insemination with semen from an infected donor, has been a means of transmission.[74] There have also been cases in which seropositive mothers have infected their children by breastfeeding. Occupational exposure of health care workers to infectious material (blood or body fluids, or pure virus in the laboratory setting) has also resulted in infection. In these latter cases, the health care workers became infected with HIV as a result of percutaneous innoculation with infective fluid via a needlestick or other penetrating injury, or following contact with infective material on mucous membranes or nonintact skin.

Finally, another mode of transmission is currently being investigated. In 1990, the CDC reported that a woman with no known risk factors for HIV infection developed AIDS. Earlier, the woman had undergone a tooth extraction, which was performed by a dentist with AIDS. Sophisticated laboratory testing of the virus from the dentist and the virus from the woman patient was performed. The result indicated that the two viruses were so closely related as to point to direct transmission of infection.[75] Based on current knowledge, it is difficult to understand how transmission of infection from the dentist to his patient could have occurred without innoculation with the dentist's blood or body fluids. There has been speculation that the dentist unwittingly injured himself during the procedure and a few drops of his blood entered the patient's wound, thereby innoculating her with HIV.[76] Other theories propose that dental equipment was contaminated.

A significant number of AIDS cases are due to undetermined causes. It is possible that in these cases victims were reluctant to reveal a history of male homosexuality, bisexuality, or intravenous drug use. It is also possible that many of these cases may have been due to unrecognized heterosexual transmission.

Within 3–6 weeks after exposure to the virus, the infected person frequently experiences a transient, flu-like or mononucleosis-like illness with fever, chills, and myalgia. Within 8–12 weeks following exposure, seroconversion occurs, as evidenced by laboratory tests that reveal that the person has developed antibody to HIV.[77] Although seroconversion has been known to occur in some persons as early as 2 weeks after exposure, 95% of persons seroconvert within 3 months of infection.[78]

Once infected, 35% of HIV-positive individuals exhibit mild symptoms of disease within 5–6 years. In most cases, the full clinical syndrome of AIDS is manifested within 8–9 years. Once HIV infection progresses to AIDS, the mortality rate skyrockets: 50% of patients die within the first 18 months after being diagnosed with AIDS, and 80% die within 3 years.[79]

HIV infection is a serious epidemic worldwide. The World Health Organization estimates that as of March 1, 1990, over 222,740 cases of AIDS had been reported throughout the world, but over 600,000 cases are believed to have occurred. In the United States, the CDC estimates that 1 million people are infected with HIV.[80] Furthermore, the CDC estimates that more than one-third of these persons are unaware that they are infected and may unknowingly transmit the virus to others. As of September 1990, it was estimated that 57,000 individuals were living with AIDS.

A number of key demographic characteristics can be identified. AIDS is largely a disease of young and middle-aged adults. Three-fourths of reported cases have occurred in persons who are 25–44 years old. Based on the most recent statistics, whites comprise 56% of AIDS cases in the United States, blacks 27%, and Hispanics 11%.[81] These percentages indicate disproportionately high numbers of Hispanics with this disease, as they comprise only 6.4% of the population. AIDS is most prevalent in densely populated urban centers, which include economically impoverished areas with large minority populations, many IV drugs users, and much prostitution. The U.S. locations with the greatest number of AIDS cases are New York City, Los Angeles, San Francisco, Houston, Washington, D.C., Newark, Miami, Chicago, Philadelphia, and Atlanta. Certain trends are becoming evident, however. Although cases of AIDS continue to be concentrated in urban centers, AIDS is increasingly seen in rural areas; in addition, more women are contracting the virus.

Critical referents

To understand HIV infection, it is helpful to understand viruses in general. All viruses are minute particles of genetic material (either DNA or RNA) surrounded by protein coats. Some viruses, such as HIV, possess an additional coat, or envelope. Since viruses possess no cellular machinery for reproduction, they must invade host cells and commandeer the host cells' machinery to produce more viruses. A virus infects a cell by attaching to a molecule on the surface of the cell and entering the cell. Upon entry, the viral protein coat disintegrates, freeing viral nucleic acid and enabling it to take over the cell.

Viruses have an attraction, or affinity, for certain molecules on the surfaces of the particular body cells they infect. For example, viruses causing hepatitis have an affinity for molecules on liver cells, whereas polio virus has an affinity for molecules on nerve cells. The HIV virus has an affinity for immune cells. HIV is an RNA virus that belongs to an unusual family of viruses, Retroviridae. Retroviruses possess a unique enzyme, reverse transcriptase, which enables them to direct the host cell to transcribe viral RNA into viral DNA. Later, the virus directs the host cell to transcribe the viral DNA back into RNA for the assembly of new virions. All retroviruses possess three identical genes: gag, env, and pol. Through these and other genes, viral replication and infectivity are regulated.

HIV infects body cells by preferentially binding to a particular molecule, CD4, on the surface of immune cells. The virus enters the host cell, and cellular enzymes remove the protein coat around the virus. The virus's reverse transcriptase directs the host cell to use the viral RNA as a template for making new DNA, thus perpetuating the virus, not the host cell. CD4 is found in highest concentrations on the surface of the T4 (helper) lymphocytes. CD4 is also found to a lesser degree on monocytes, macrophages, and B cells. As a result, these two groups of key immune cells are most frequently infected by HIV.

T4 cells are the primary reservoir for HIV infection in the circulating blood. T4 cells, as the organizers of the immune response, are critical in protecting human cells from intracellular infection by viruses, fungi, protozoa, certain bacteria, and from certain types of cancers. T4 cells also regulate B cell production of immunoglobulin and are responsible for allograft rejection and delayed-type hypersensitivity (DTH). The ability to mount a DTH response is evaluated clinically by administering intradermal skin tests with antigens to which almost all people have been exposed: candida, mumps, trycophyton, streptococcus, and tetanus. If T cell function is normal, redness and induration occur at the site of injection within 24–48 hours. T4 helper cell functions are summarized in Table 8-41.

Monocytes (circulating in the blood) and the tissue macrophages also have CD4 receptors. The macrophages, distributed in tissues throughout the body, are the other key immune cells infected by HIV. The Langerhans cells of the skin, the follicular dendritic cells in lymph nodes and the GI tract, the lung (alveolar) macrophages, and the brain microglia are all examples of macrophages that can be infected by HIV. Thus, macrophages are the primary reservoir of HIV infection in the tissue.

Following infection, HIV transfers from one host cell to another. Immediately after infection, the virus replicates, often producing measurable levels of a viral marker, p24, in the blood. The body's immune response to the infection is brisk. As with other viral infections, cytotoxic T cells and natural killer cells destroy host cells invaded by HIV. B lymphocytes are activated, differentiate into plasma cells, and produce antibody to viral components. IgM is produced first, followed by IgG to viral core proteins and then IgG to viral envelope glycoproteins. Initially the immune response appears effective at controlling infection, because p24 antigen levels drop as antibody levels to viral proteins rise. Unfortunately, T4 cells and macrophages are infected with HIV despite the body's resistance, and the infection of T4 cells cripples the body's ability to hold the virus in check. Over time, the function of the chronically infected T4 cells is impaired and the cells are destroyed, producing lymphopenia.

Other immune cells function poorly, as a result of the lack of regulation by T4 cells. Monocytes and macrophages are less effective at destroying microorganisms and may secrete abnormally high amounts of tumor necrosis factor (TNF), which may, in part, be responsible for the cachexia seen in AIDS. B lymphocytes produce excessive amounts of immunoglobulin. These elevated Ig levels may be unrelated to and therefore useless against any microorganism that could be causing infection. On the other hand, this phenomenon may be responsible for symptoms of atopy (allergy, asthma) that can occur with HIV infection.[82] Eventually, as the immunodeficiency worsens, the levels of anti-HIV antibody may diminish and levels of p24 may dramatically increase. A summary of the abnormalities of immune function seen with HIV infection appears in Table 8-42.

It is unknown whether HIV-infected immune cells delay production of virus for a long period or if there is a constant low level of viral replication. Researchers have theorized that concomitant infection with other microorganisms may result in rapid viral reproduction and worsen the disease. Viruses of the herpes family, Epstein-Barr virus, and cyto-

Table 8-41 Functions of T4 cells

Induce maturation and differentiation of immune cells

Activate killer T's, monocytes/macrophages, and natural killer cells

Induce B cells to make antibody

Induce T suppressor cell to suppress

Responsible for allograft rejection and delayed-type hypersensitivity

Table 8-42 Abnormalities of Immune Cell Functions with AIDS

Immune Cell	Abnormality
T cell	Diminished cell-mediated immunity, evidenced by cutaneous anergy, opportunistic infections with intracellular pathogens, and certain cancers
B cell	Excessive but ineffective production of immunoglobulin
Monocyte	Less effective cytotoxicity

megalovirus have been suspected as stimulating HIV reproduction. The pathophysiology of opportunistic infection in HIV-infected patients is specific to the organism that produced the infection; such opportunistic infections will be addressed as they relate to the common clinical presentations of HIV infection.

Resulting signs and symptoms

Over time, the immune deficits produced by HIV worsen and result in diseases indicative of suppressed cell-mediated immunity: opportunistic infections with intracellular pathogens and cancers (B cell lymphomas and Kaposi's sarcoma). The viral infection also produces cachexia, hematologic abnormalities (leukopenia, anemia, thrombocytopenia), and neurologic disease.

The absolute T4 count, which normally ranges from 600 to 1200/mm³, is the best measure of disease severity in HIV infection. As the T4 cells are progressively depleted, their numbers diminish. The average rate of decline in T4 counts is approximately 1 cell/mm³ per week, or 50 per year. Eventually T4 counts can go to zero. When the absolute T4 count falls below 500/mm³, symptoms of immune compromise become evident.[83] When the absolute T4 count drops below 200/mm³, the risk of development of Pneumocystis carinii pneumonia dramatically increases. In one study, 95% of patients with Pneumocystis carinii pneumonia (PCP) had an absolute T4 count below 200/mm³ [84] When the T4 count drops below 100/mm³, opportunistic infection with cytomegalovirus (CMV) usually occurs. These relationships are outlined in Table 8-43.

In 1992, the Centers for Disease Control (CDC) revised the classification of HIV infection. Infected persons are grouped according to their clinical manifestations of HIV-related disease and CD4 count. This revised system arranges CD4 counts (three

Table 8-43 Relation of Absolute T4 Count and Clinical Disease

Absolute T4 count (cells/mm³)	Clinical disease
<500	Immunosuppression
<200	Opportunistic infection (often Pneumocystis carinii pneumonia)
<100	Cytomegalovirus infection (retinitis, pneumonitis, or colitis)

levels) and clinical disease (three types) in a matrix. All category C disorders are reportable as AIDS and all categories of disease with CD4 counts < 200 meet the AIDS case definition. The CDC classifications are described in Table 8-44.

Group A of the CDC classification consists of persons who have experienced a mononucleosis-like syndrome, an asymptomatic but antibody-positive HIV infection, or persistent generalized lymphadenopathy following exposure to HIV. This acute infection is associated with production of anti-HIV antibody (seroconversion). Of the estimated 1 million persons infected with HIV in the United States, the majority are in group A. Those in the lymphadenopathy group have palpable lymphadenopathies lasting longer than 3 months in which lymph nodes at two or more extrainguinal sites are enlarged to more than 1 cm in size. Groups B and C consist of persons with diverse manifestations of HIV infection. Most opportunistic infections and cancers from the 1987 AIDS case definition are included in category C. (Opportunistic infections are discussed later in this section.)

Clinical disease in AIDS The clinical manifestations of HIV infection are most often associated with infectious or carcinomatous invasion of the body systems. What follows is an overview of the primary clinical disorders seen in AIDs, arranged according to a systems format. Etiologies of disease within the body system may be variable, although symptoms and management strategies are often similar.

Pulmonary disease Pulmonary disease is the hallmark of AIDS. The lungs may be infected by opportunistic organisms, invaded by neoplasms, or affected by a nonspecific interstitial pneumonitis. Certain researchers have estimated that 50% of persons with AIDS have pulmonary disease.[85] Of the people affected, 50% have Pneumocystis carinii pneumonia (PCP) and 34% exhibit nonspecific pneumonitis. An additional 16% have pulmonary disease due to diverse causes: infection with cytomegalovirus, myobacteria, cryptococcus, or histoplasmosis; invasion by Kaposi's sarcoma; thromboembolism; or hemorrhage.[86] Many, if not most, HIV-infected patients admitted to intensive care units will be there for management of pulmonary disease.

Gastrointestinal disease GI disease is estimated to occur in 50–80% of HIV-infected patients.[87] Oral candidiasis is the most common opportunistic infection in AIDS, but it can usually be managed with oral antifungal agents. Oral hairy leukoplakia is associated with oral infection by the Epstein-Barr virus (EBV) or papilloma virus; the disease appears as ridged white patches on the lateral margins of the

Table 8-44   1992 CDC HIV Classification System

CD4 Cell Category	Clinical Category			Descriptions of Clinical Categories		
	A	B	C	Category A	Category B[b]	Category C[c]
(1) ≥500/mm³	A1	B1	C1	Asymptomatic HIV infection	Bacterial endocarditis, meningitis, pneumonia, sepsis	Candidiasis: esophageal, tracheal, bronchial
(2) 200–400/mm³	A2	B2	C2	Persistent generalized lymphadenopathy (PGL)[a]	Candidiasis, vulvovaginal, persistent >1 month	Coccidiomycosis, extrapulmonary
(3) <200/mm³	A3	B3	C3	Acute (primary) HIV illness	Candidiasis, oropharyngeal	Cryptococcosis, extrapulmonary
					Cervical dysplasia, severe or carcinoma	Cryptosporidiosis, chronic intestinal (<1 month)
					Constitutional symptoms, e.g., fever (>38.5°) or diarrhea >1 month	CMV retinitis, or other than liver, spleen, nodes
					Hairy leukoplakia, oral	HIV encephalopathy
					Herpes zoster, ≥two episodes or >1 dermatome	Herpes simplex with mucocutaneous ulcer >1 month, bronchitis, pneumonia
					Idiopathic thrombocytopenia purpura	Isosporiosis, chronic, >1 month
					Listeriosis	Kaposi's sarcoma
					M. tuberculosis, pulmonary	Lymphoma: Burkitt's, immunoblastic, primary in brain
					Nocardiosis	M. avium or M. kansasii, extrapulmonary
					Pelvic inflammatory disease	M. tuberculosis, extrapulmonary
					Peripheral neuropathy	Mycobacterium, other species disseminated or extrapulmonary
						Pneumocystis carinii pneumonia
						Progressive multifocal leukoencephalopathy
						Salmonella bacteremia, recurrent
						Toxoplasmosis, cerebral
						Wasting syndrome due to HIV

[a]Nodes in two or more extrainguinal sites, at least 1 cm in diameter for ≥3 months
[b]The above must be attributed to HIV infection or have a clinical course or management complicated by HIV
[c]These are the 1987 CDC case definitions (*MMWR* 36:15, 1987)

tongue, unlike candida, which is diffuse, poorly marginated, and involves the palate or buccal mucosa. Leukoplakia usually responds to high-dose Acyclovir. Gingivitis is not uncommon and dysphagia may be present. Dysphagia may result from esophageal candidiasis, herpes simplex infections, or esophageal ulceration of uncertain etiology. Critical care nurses should plan thorough oral assessments every shift, because untreated infections may become disseminated.

Liver disease in the form of diffuse or granulomatous hepatitis occurs frequently in AIDS. In addition, a significant number of patients may have hepatic infection with Mycobacterium avium intracellulare (MAI) or invasion of the liver by Kaposi's

sarcoma (KS). Since these persons may be more susceptible to liver damage due to hepatotoxic drugs, it is important to palpate for liver enlargement or tenderness and to monitor their liver function tests.

Diarrhea is a particularly common GI complaint. As many as 50% of HIV-infected individuals have diarrhea, and in about half of those it is due to an infectious agent. Large-volume diarrhea accompanied by cramping is usually caused by an infectious agent. Cytomegalovirus is most often the culprit, although MAI, Salmonella, Cryptosporidium, and Entamoeba histolyca account for a significant number of cases. Other microorganisms that cause diarrhea in AIDS are Giardia lamblia, herpes simplex virus, Campylobacter jejuni, Isospora belli, and

Clostridium dificile. The diarrhea caused by shigella and camphylobacter can be severe; it is often bloody and accompanied by cramps, nausea, and fever. Most of these infections can be treated, although infection recurs if treatment is discontinued.

Cutaneous manifestations Up to 90% of patients with HIV infection have some type of skin disease; in fact, the average patient has two or more skin diseases simultaneously. The cutaneous manifestations of HIV infection and AIDS fall into four main categories: neoplasms, infections, hypersensitivities, and drug reactions. Kaposi's sarcoma is the neoplasm most commonly associated with AIDS, and it is usually manifested by reddish-purple cutaneous nodules. Other common skin disorders are staph aureus folliculitis, herpes zoster lesions, molluscum contagiosum, seborrhea, psoriasis, and dramatic photosensitivity. For reasons not well understood, persons with AIDS commonly have more intensive hypersensitivities and skin reactions to medications.

Hematologic disorders Cytopenias occurring in association with HIV infection can result from either inadequate production or excessive destruction of blood cells. Lymphopenia, neutropenia, anemia, and/or thrombocytopenia are often seen in AIDS. These hematologic abnormalities have multiple causes. HIV infection alone, opportunistic infection, cancer, or the treatment for any of these conditions can cause cytopenia.

Reduced bone marrow function is one reason for the development of cytopenias. HIV infection of the bone marrow stem cells or infiltration of the bone marrow by cancers such as lymphoma can alter hematopoietic cell production. Microorganisms such as mycobacterium, histoplasmosis, or cryptococcus may also infiltrate the bone marrow and impair blood cell development. In addition, the inappropriate secretion of TNF by infected or stimulated macrophages can also diminish the bone marrow's ability to replenish cells. Nutritional deficiencies related to inadequate oral intake or malabsorption from GI disease may impair hematopoiesis. The marrow is also depressed by many pharmacological agents used to treat opportunistic infections or HIV-related disorders. Zidovudine, ganciclovir, pentamidine, and amphotericin are examples of marrow-toxic drugs that are commonly used. For example, it has been found that 34% of persons receiving zidovudine are anemic, 16% are neutropenic, and 12% have thrombocytopenia; furthermore, 60–85% of all HIV-infected persons have a chronic anemia in which new red blood cells are not made despite the presence of adequate nutrients to do so.[88]

Cytopenias may also occur for other reasons.

Hematopoiesis may be relatively normal but unable to keep up with excessive destruction or loss of blood cells. For example, anemia may be due to GI bleeding caused by CMV colitis or HIV-induced hemolytic anemia.

The lymphopenia seen in AIDS usually occurs as as result of the infection and destruction of T4 lymphocytes by HIV. Since T4 cells comprise the majority of circulating lymphocytes, a severe reduction in their numbers can produce lymphopenia.

Neutropenia may result from either impaired production or excessive destruction of neutrophils. Almost 50% of persons with AIDS have neutropenia which is unrelated to drug therapy. Unlike neutropenic cancer patients, however, persons with AIDS do not appear to be at high risk of development of septicemia from endogenous bowel or skin flora.[89]

Neurologic disease According to Scherer, neurologic disease strikes 60–80% of AIDS patients. Even among those who are asymptomatic, 25–60% have electrophysiologic evidence of neuromuscular dysfunction.[90] HIV-related neurologic disease can arise from many causes: opportunistic infection, neoplasm, recreational drug use, medications, disordered metabolic processes, malnutrition, or immobility. HIV infection of the neurologic cells can cause meningitis, encephalitis, focal neurologic disease, myelopathy, and peripheral neuropathy. The causes of neurologic diseases, and the percentage of patients found by one researcher to have them, are listed in Table 8-45. Symptoms are quite variable, depending upon the cause and severity of the disease. Extensive diagnostic testing is often required to determine the source of symptoms and guide the treatment.

More than 80% of CNS disease with AIDS is due to opportunistic infections. Of these cases, over half are due to infections by fungi, protozoans, or bacteria such as toxoplasma or cryptococcus.[91] Approxi-

Table 8-45 Causes of Neurologic Disease Associated with HIV Infection

Cause	Percentage of Cases
Opportunistic infections	
Fungal, protozoal, bacterial	55%
Viral	33%
Neoplasm	<10%
Other (CVA, aseptic meningitis)	<10%

Source: Tuazon, C. U. (1989). Toxoplasmosis in AIDS patients. *Journal of Antimicrobial Chemotherapy* 23 (supplement A): 77–82.

mately one-third of these cases are due to viral infections such as cytomegalovirus. Of the remaining cases of CNS disease, neoplasms such as lymphoma account for less than 10% of cases as do CVAs and aseptic meningitis.[92] Symptoms of CNS disease vary but include confusion, memory deficits, headache, focal deficits, and/or seizures.

Meningitis can arise from opportunistic infections by mycobacteria or syphilis, invasion of the CNS by lymphoma, or from no discernible cause. The most important meningeal infection in AIDS is cryptococcal meningitis. Headache, nausea, vomiting, confusion, nuchal rigidity, and palsies are common manifestations of meningitis from any etiology.

Encephalitis in association with AIDS may arise from opportunistic infection with toxoplasma, cytomegalovirus, or herpes simplex. Another type of encephalitis is AIDS dementia complex (ADC), which is also called AIDS-related dementia. ADC is probably the most common CNS complication of HIV infection. ADC usually does not occur until the HIV infection progresses to AIDS but is believed to develop in most persons in whom this progression occurs. Up to two-thirds of persons in the latter stages of AIDS exhibit mild to severe dementia. Although one-fourth of the persons in this group are asymptomatic, neurological testing reveals abnormalities. Clinically, ADC is manifested as a triad of behavioral, cognitive, and motor dysfunction. Frequently, patients exhibit loss of their train of thought in conversation, difficulty with concentration and memory, slowed thought, confusion, apathy, dysphoria, regression, and poor balance and coordination. Onset of symptoms may be sudden or progressive. Zidovudine is reported to alleviate the symptomatology.

Focal neurologic disease in AIDS is most likely to be the result of cerebral toxoplasmosis. It is reported to occur in 5–15% of patients with AIDS, and evaluations of AIDS patients using CT scans of revealing lesions showed that 80–90% of the lesions were caused by cerebral toxoplasmosis and 10–20% were lymphoma.[93] Although cerebral toxoplasmosis is the first etiology to consider with focal symptoms, other possible etiologies to be investigated include CVA, lymphoma, mycobacterium, cryptococcus, varicella zoster virus, or herpes simplex. Although rare, Progressive multifocal leukoencephalopathy (PML) from infection with the jc virus is another possible cause of focal neurologic disease.

Of the several neuropathies seen with HIV infection, distal sensory polyneuropathy (DSPN) is the most common. Persons with DSPN complain of burning pain (usually in the feet) but exhibit little

functional impairment. Antiretroviral medications such as didanosine (ddI) and zalcitabine (ddC) can also cause a similar neuropathy with pain or paresthesias. Other neuropathic symptoms that may be present are flaccid muscles, loss of reflexes, or reduced sensation in the legs. HIV infection has also been associated with Guillain-Barré syndrome, an ascending paralysis that can occur 10–15 days after a viral illness. If the paralysis ascends to the level of the respiratory muscles, the patient may require intubation and mechanical ventilation. In most patients, motor function returns, and plasmapheresis may help speed recovery.[94]

Although several myopathies are associated with HIV infection, vascular myopathy may be the most significant. Persons with this disorder exhibit painless but progressive gait disturbance with ataxia and spasticity. Weakness and pain of the proximal muscles may be symptoms of polymyositis, the most common myopathy seen in association with HIV infection. Myopathy can also occur with long-term treatment with zidovudine. Researchers are attempting to determine if changing to another antiretroviral can allow the muscles damaged by zidovudine to recover.[95]

There are other causes of neurologic disease in AIDS. Hypoxemia and sepsis occurring in conjunction with or as a complication of systemic disease can produce neurologic symptoms. In addition, HIV-infected persons may experience anxiety disorders or clinical depression. These psychiatric disorders may make it difficult to assess the patient's neurologic status. Seizures may occur as a result of a focal process. Antiseizure medications may be required, and if increased intracranial pressure is present, glucocorticoids may be administered to reduce brain edema.

In summary, the neurologic disorders occurring in conjunction with HIV infection are highly variable, presenting with any possible combination of symptoms. Frequent and thorough neurological assessments are essential for the critically ill patient.

Kaposi's sarcoma   Kaposi's sarcoma (KS) is a cancer of unknown etiology that can occur in association with HIV infection. Prior to the advent of AIDS, KS was known as a relatively benign and slow-growing cancer that occurred in middle-aged or elderly males of Eastern European background. With AIDS, however, KS occurs in young adults of all ethnic backgrounds and can be aggressive and invasive. In the United States, cases of HIV-related KS have been found in gay males, bisexual males, female sex partners of bisexual males, and, most recently, in HIV-seronegative gay men. Because of the distinctive pattern of occurrence, there has been speculation that KS is caused by the infection of an immunocompromised host with yet another undiscovered viral agent or other factors.[96] The incidence of KS changed over the 1980s. At the onset of the AIDS epidemic, 21% of persons with AIDS had KS; by 1989, only 12% had this cancer. KS does not usually occur in persons whose T4 counts are above 600.[97] The disease is manifested by uncontrolled proliferation of endothelial or spindle cells.[98] Clinically, KS appears as raised reddish-purple nodules in the skin, the mucous membranes of the mouth and GI tract, the lymph nodes, and organs such as the lung and liver.[99] The nodules tend to be symmetrical, are nontender, and do not blanch with pressure. Erythrocytes tend to leak into the lesion, producing the characteristic purple-red color.[100] KS can be disfiguring, relatively benign, or aggressive. If it invades and obstructs lymphatics, the tissue can become edematous, and cutaneous lesions can ulcerate. Invasion into the GI tract causes necrotic bowel or intractable GI bleeding.

Lymphoma Lymphoma is another neoplasm associated with HIV infection. More than 80% of AIDS-related lymphomas are B-cell lymphomas such as Burkitt's lymphoma.[101] One-third of persons with AIDS-associated lymphoma have CNS involvement at the time of diagnosis; this metastatic site is generally rare for lymphomas.[102] CNS lymphoma has occurred in the setting of severe congenital or transplant-related immunodeficiency. Unfortunately, the diagnosis of primary brain lymphoma continues to carry a grim prognosis, despite successful intracranial removal. Other non-Hodgkin's and Hodgkin's lymphomas, as well as aggressive colorectal cancer, anal cancer, and some head and neck cancers, have

also been linked to HIV infection but occur too infrequently for thorough evaluation.[103]

Opportunistic infections Opportunistic infections (OIs) are infections that do not usually occur in an immunocompetent host. Opportunistic microorganisms appear to cause infection by taking advantage of an immunodeficient state. An OI can be an infection by an organism that is usually not pathogenic, an unusually severe infection, or an unusual manifestation of an infection (for example, involving an organ system it usually does not infect). Some microorganisms known to produce opportunistic infections in a compromised host were listed in Table 8-45.

Many OIs are the result of reactivation of latent infections. Certain microorganisms have developed the ability to remain alive within the body for years after the initial infection has resolved. Normally, cell-mediated immunity (CMI) limits or checks the growth of these remaining microorganisms. But if CMI is impaired, the bacteria, fungi, protozoa, or virus already present within the body can proliferate, producing clinical disease. Latent infections may be caused by the microorganisms listed in Table 8-46.

Opportunistic infections become common with HIV infection once the patient's T4 count is below 300.[104] The most common OI is Candida mucosites, but the most common clinically significant one is Pneumocystis carinii pneumonia (PCP). However, retinitis, colitis, or pneumonitis caused by reactivation of CMV infection may be the leading cause of death. Concurrent or consecutive OIs by different organisms are common. There is also increased incidence of otitis and sinusitis caused by bacterial organisms in the HIV patient.[105] Any opportunistic infection has the potential to be life-threatening in the HIV patient and should be considered a priority in the assessment and management plan. Currently,

Table 8-46 Sources of Latent Infections Associated with HIV

Protozoa	Fungi	Viruses	Bacteria	Helminths
Cryptosporidium	Candida	Cytomegalovirus (CMV)	Mycobacterium AI	Strongyloides
Isospora	Cryptococcus	Herpes simplex virus	Mycobacterium K	
Pneumocystis carinii*	Histoplasma	Varicella zoster virus	Mycobacterium TB	
	Toxoplasma	Papovavirus (jc)	Listeria	
			Salmonella	
			Shigella	
			Campylobacter	

*May also be classified as a fungus

clinical investigators are focusing on preventing and effectively treating OIs. Some prophylactic agents that are either recommended or being investigated for prevention of OIs are aerosolized pentamidine (PCP), Bactrim plus Dapsone (may prevent extrapulmonary pneumocystis), Dapsone (for cryptosporidium and MAI), and Bactrim (may prevent salmonella and shigella).

Pneumocystis carinii Pneumocystis carinii pneumonia (PCP), caused by a microscopic parasite, is one of the most common life-threatening AIDS-related infections in the United States. Prior to 1981, it was a rare infection, almost always striking patients with leukemia or lymphoma or recipients of bone marrow transplant. PCP is the most common cause of pneumonia and respiratory failure associated with AIDS. One researcher estimates that 60–80% of persons with AIDS will have at least one bout of pneumocystis, and that it is the cause of 30% of the deaths in persons with AIDS.[106] Today, with prompt diagnosis and treatment, 80–95% of patients survive the first infection, but in 30–60% of patients, it recurs within the next 12 months.[107] Individuals who are most severely immunocompromised have the highest rate of recurrence. With each additional reinfection, survival rates diminish. Since PCP appears to be transmitted by the respiratory route, some centers do not place AIDS patients with PCP in the same room or in close proximity to other patients with HIV infection.

Pneumocystis carinii is believed to infect most people during childhood. Theoretically, the organism survives within its human host but its growth is checked by cell-mediated immunity (CMI). When CMI is drastically impaired, the organism can proliferate, causing disease. In HIV infection, PCP occurs once the T4 count drops below 200/mm^3. In one study of 55 HIV patients with PCP, 53 had T4 counts below this level.[108] Thus, as with many other HIV-related opportunistic infections, PCP appears to occur as a reactivation of a latent infection. Within the past two years, much has been learned about this organism, and several features have emerged to support reclassification of pneumocystis as a fungus rather than a protozoan.[109]

Pneumonia caused by pneumocystis produces an inflammatory response, which develops into an alveolar capillary sludging. The lungs may exhibit diffuse alveolar damage (hyaline membrane disease), which late in the disease resembles ARDS on chest x-ray. Early symptoms are similar to those of oxygen toxicity: cough, sternal discomfort, decreased secretions, and dyspnea. A low-grade fever, fatigue, and weight loss are also observed in many patients. Infection causes permanent scarring and interstitial fibrosis even after resolution of the disease. Although it is primarily a pneumonia, dissemination of the infection to the retina, bone marrow, thyroid, lymph nodes, liver, and spleen may occur.[110]

Diagnosing PCP is difficult, in part because the early symptoms are deceptively mild and nonspecific. Obvious diagnostic tests such as chest x-ray and arterial blood gases may not reveal changes until significant infection is present. Patients with significant infection will have diffuse symmetrical infiltrates, which can be seen on chest x-ray and which progress to diffuse alveolitis. However, in up to 20% of patients, a chest x-ray is normal.[111] Arterial blood gases are also normal in up to 20% of patients with PCP.[112] As a result, diagnosis must be based on a combination of clinical symptoms, radiologic findings, laboratory tests, and diagnostic procedures. Chest x-rays, ABGs, and tests such as induced sputum, bronchial alveolar lavage, and bronchoscopy are required. Induced sputum is the least invasive truly diagnostic test for PCP. Some facilities have been able to use this test to diagnose PCP with more than 90% accuracy.[113] If the induced sputum test is positive for pneumocystis, the patient is treated with an antipneumocystis drug. If the induced sputum test is negative, bronchoscopy is performed. Gallium scans, although used formerly, are thought to show only pulmonary inflammation; because this test requires complex scheduling and is not necessarily specific for PCP, it is little used today.

Fungal infections AIDS-related life-threatening fungal illnesses have been estimated to affect 10–20% of all patients with AIDS, yet no reliable prophylaxis is yet available. Candidiasis, histoplasmosis, coccidiomycosis, and cryptococcosis are the most significant fungal infections associated with AIDS.[114]

Candida albicans, a fungus that is commonly present in the environment and in the body, is the most common cause of opportunistic infection in AIDS. In fact, almost all patients with advanced HIV infection have oral candidiasis. Surprisingly, despite the deficient cell-mediated immunity of those with AIDS, candida infection tends to be rather limited to the mucosa (oral pharynx, esophagus, genitalia, vagina, and/or rectum) rather than becoming systemic. Candidiasis can be debilitating if dysphagia, pain, or bleeding is present and contributes to poor nutritional status, anemia, hemorrhage, or reduced activity. Candidiasis appears as characteristic lesions on the mucosa and is diagnosed by physical exam and microscopic examination of scrapings from the lesions. Infections are easily treated with oral triazoles such as Ketoconozole. Clotrimoxazole and other medications are often used prophylactically to prevent recurrence of infection. Critically ill patients who are unable to take oral medications due to intubation or NPO status can still be easily treated by swabbing the mucosa with liquid antifungals to resolve the infection.

Cryptococcus neoformans is a fungus found widely in the environment, especially in soil contaminated with bird excrement. The fungus is estimated to cause infections in 2–13% of all patients with AIDS.[115] Approximately two-thirds of cryptococcal infections in patients with AIDS involve the meninges. In more than half of these patients, the infection spreads to other organs. In other patients, the skin or lungs are the sole site of infection. Cryptococcal meningitis is a life-threatening CNS infection. Untreated disease is fatal, but even 50–90% of those who respond to initial treatment will relapse without maintenance therapy.[116] The most frequent symptoms of cryptococcal infections are neurologic: headache, change in mental status or personality, memory loss, confusion, or difficulty with physical coordination. Vague, nonspecific symptoms such as fatigue or nausea and vomiting may also be present. Cryptococcus is diagnosed by identifying the fungus in the cerebrospinal fluid or the antigen in the blood.

Histoplasma capsulatum is a fungus found in the soil of river valleys of the midwestern United States, Puerto Rico, the Carribean, and Central and South America. It is estimated that 5–10% of persons with AIDS residing in these high-risk areas develop disseminated histoplasmosis.[117] Infection is acquired after inhaling or ingesting spores from contaminated soil. Since weeks to months may pass before clinical disease occurs, histoplasmosis can be considered a reactivation of a latent infection. It frequently infects the lungs, producing acute pneumonia with persistent fever and weight loss. The infection often disseminates to the meninges, heart, adrenals, or peritoneum. Biopsy and culture is the most reliable method of diagnosing histoplasmosis. As with many other OIs, relapse after treatment is a serious problem. Of those who do respond to treatment, 80–90% will relapse within approximately 1 year of treatment without maintenance therapy.[118]

Coccidiomycosis is a latent fungal infection endemic to Mexico, Central and South America, and the southwestern United States. States where the disease is most prevalent are Arizona, Nevada, Utah, Texas, and southern California. This fungus always causes pulmonary disease but can infect the CNS as well, causing meningitis, encephalitis, or brain abscess. Rare cases of cutaneous coccidiomycosis have been reported. The symptoms of infection are vague: malaise, fever, weight loss, and cough. Coccidiomycosis is diagnosed by identifying the organisms in the patient's sputum. Chest x-rays usually reveal infiltrates.

Bacterial infections Bacteria causing infections in patients with AIDS can be categorized into two groups: those associated with humoral immunodeficiency and those associated with deficient cell-mediated immunity. Deficient T-cell function is associated with infections with mycobacteriae, salmonella, and listeria; B-cell deficiency is associated with infections due to streptococcal pneumoniae, hemophilus influenza, campylobacter, and shigella.[119] Bacterial infections in AIDS are more likely to produce bacteremia and frequently recur despite treatment.

The mycobacteria causing infection in patients with AIDS are Mycobacterium avium intracellulare (MAI), Mycobacterium kansasii (MK), and Mycobacterium tuberculare (MTB). AIDS-related infections with mycobacteria usually manifest as disseminated disease. The inability of the body to limit the spread of infection by these bacteria may be related to the defective macrophage function that results from HIV infection.[120] The significance of disseminated MAI infection in AIDS is unknown. The microorganism can fill the bone marrow and lymph nodes, yet it appears to cause few symptoms other than chronic fever, malaise, anemia, and weight loss. It is theorized that the MAI-related macrophages release monokines such as interleukin-1, which cause these constitutional symptoms. It is unclear whether infection with MAI causes death or only occurs in those who are already dying.[121]

Tuberculosis is more common in patients with AIDS than in the general population. Although HIV infection does not cause a person to be more susceptible to becoming infected with MTB, the reduced T-cell immunity does increase the risk of reactivation of latent TB. When TB reactivates in AIDS, it presents as disseminated disease, frequently involving many organs rather than causing pulmonary cavitary lesions. The symptoms of tuberculosis with AIDS are similar to those in immunocompetent individuals: fever, night sweats, weight loss, and fatigue. The diagnosis is made by examination of sputum, although tissue biopsy is required to diagnose disseminated tuberculosis. The PPD skin test helps to determine whether a person has ever been infected with MTB. A positive PPD is an indication of MTB infection, whether active or latent. Normally, a 10 mm area of induration is required for a positive PPD. However, T-cell immunity must be intact in order for the body to react to the PPD antigen. Since HIV infection impairs T-cell immunity, patients with

AIDS may have a negative PPD despite being infected with MTB. Although the PPD should still be administered to patients with AIDS if TB is suspected, a negative result does not rule out infection with MTB. Therefore, the CDC recommendation is that in persons with AIDS, a PPD with an area of induration of 5 mm or more should be read as positive. Individuals who are not HIV-infected and have tuberculosis usually develop cavitary lesions filled with the bacilli. When these lesions rupture, the bacilli are released and can easily be coughed into the air. The formation of cavitary lesions is unusual in AIDS, so unless the bronchi or larynx are involved, TB may be less contagious via the respiratory route with AIDS patients than with TB patients who do not have AIDS. It is still prudent and appropriate for health care workers to practice respiratory precautions when caring for these patients, especially if they are intubated.

Other bacterial infections in AIDS have unusual manifestations. For example, if infected with salmonella, a person with AIDS is 20 times more likely than an immunocompetent individual to develop salmonella bacteremia, and may develop the unusual salmonella cholecystitis.[122] Half of all patients with salmonellosis have severe diarrhea, fever, nausea, cramping, and bloating. Patients infected with listeria are 200 times more likely to develop meningitis.[123]

Viral infections The majority of AIDS-related viral infections are caused by viruses of the herpes family: herpes simplex virus (HSV), Epstein-Barr virus (EBV), cytomegalovirus (CMV), and varicella-zoster virus (VZV). The jc virus, a type of papovavirus, is also pathogenic in HIV infection. Many viral infections are reactivation infections even in the immunocompetent host and thus are more severe in those who are compromised. CMV infection is common worldwide, infecting 1% of neonates, and prevalent in homosexual males. In AIDS, CMV rarely occurs until the T4 count is below 100/mm³. If this happens, CMV reactivation may be the cause of death. CMV has a tendency to infect the retina, colon, and lungs of patients with AIDS but has also been known to infect the esophagus, adrenals, myocardium, and CNS in this population. Retinitis is the most common CMV infection; from 8–30% of persons with AIDS are estimated to have CMV retinitis. Floaters, blurred vision, and loss of peripheral vision are hallmark symptoms of this infection. CMV is diagnosed by ophthalmic exam, which reveals the "ketchup and mustard" lesions on the retina that are characteristic of the infection and represent exudate and areas of hemorrhage. Without treatment, the infection progresses rapidly: blindness can occur within 2–3 weeks.

Reactivation of HSV infections produces painful, shallow, chronic, and slowly spreading and coalescing ulcers of the oral mucosa, genitalia, buttocks, or thighs. Although HSV may reactivate in the GI tract, it does not usually cause systemic infection. Reactivation of VZV may also occur and is more severe than in immunocompetent individuals.

Infections of protozoa Cryptosporidium is a major cause of diarrheal illness in humans worldwide, regardless of immunocompetence. The protozoa live in domestic animals, including cattle, which excrete the organisms in feces. Humans acquire infection with cryptosporidium from contact with infected animals or by ingesting food or water contaminated with feces containing the parasite. When persons with AIDS are infected with this organism, they have chronic, watery, and perhaps uncontrollable diarrhea lasting weeks to months. Other accompanying symptoms include nausea, vomiting, abdominal cramps, fever, headache, weakness, and weight loss. The illness can be debilitating and life-threatening due to dehydration from fluid loss. Although the protozoa usually infects the small intestine, it can spread to the gallbladder and other organs.

Isospora belli, a parasite found most commonly in the tropics, causes watery diarrhea, cramping, and weight loss in persons with AIDS. The symptoms of isosporiosis are similar to those of cryptosporidiosis, and the former must be diagnosed by fecal smear. Microsporidia is found in humans and fish. Infections with microsporidia most often involve the intestine, liver, muscles, and cornea. Its true incidence in humans is not known because diagnostic techniques remain imperfect.

Toxoplasma gondii is a common infection that rarely causes clinical disease. Infection is most commonly acquired by ingesting undercooked meat contianing toxoplasma tissue cysts. One study showed that up to 25% of lamb and pork samples in the United States are contaminated with toxoplasma.[124] Cats are the primary host of toxoplasma, spreading the disease through oocysts in their feces. Initial infection with toxoplasma is frequently asymptomatic; however, 3–70% of adults in the United States have antitoxoplasma antibody.[125] Toxoplasmosis is a serious consequence of reactivation of latent infection in HIV-infected persons. It is estimated that 30% of AIDS patients who have antitoxoplasma antibody will develop toxoplasma encephalitis.[126] Another estimate is that toxoplasmosis occurs in 5–15% of patients with AIDS and accounts for 25–80% of AIDS-related CNS infections.[127] Patients with toxoplasma encephalitis complain of mild headaches and exhibit focal symptoms: hemiparesis, pronator drift, hemiplegia, cranial nerve palsies, aphasia, ataxia, and/or seizures. Confusion, lethargy, personality changes, and diminished mentation are also common symptoms. Neurological decline may be so severe that the patient becomes comatose.

Cerebral toxoplasmosis is usually diagnosed by the patient's clinical condition and a CT scan showing characteristic "ring-enhancing" lesions. MRI scans can reveal the mild to severe edema accompanying the lesions. Although brain biopsy is required for a definitive diagnosis, it is also so invasive that clinicians elect to treat a symptomatic patient with pyrimethamine and sulfadiazine. A patient with CNS toxoplasmosis will usually improve within 7–10 days of the beginning of treatment.[128] Corticosteroids may be required to reduce the accompanying brain edema. Once remission is attained, lifelong treatment must continue or relapse will occur. Although pyrimethamine and sulfadiazine block folic acid metabolism in the parasite, the cyst form is unaffected. It is believed that the cysts can rupture and reinitiate infection. The treatment for CNS toxoplasmosis is relatively toxic. Up to 71% of patients experience side effects (see Table 8-47); in over 30% of patients, the side effects are severe enough to require a change in therapy.[129]

Helmintic infections AIDS patients in the United States have not experienced a higher incidence of helmintic infections than the general population; however, they have exhibited more disseminated infections. For example, infection with strongyloides in the patient with AIDS can extend beyond the GI tract. Strongyloides infections are more frequent in Hispanics, especially Puerto Ricans.

Diagnostic tests for HIV infection Several tests can be used to diagnose HIV infection: enzyme-linked immuno-sorbent assay (ELISA), Western blot, viral culture, and polymerase chain reaction (PCR) (see Table 8-48). The diagnosis of HIV infection begins

Table 8-47 Side Effects of Using Pyrimethamine and Sulfadiazine to Treat Toxoplasmosis

Reaction	Percent of Patients Experiencing Reaction
Leukopenia	61%
Rash	45%
Thrombocytopenia	32%
Abnormal LFTs	<10%

Source: Tuazon, C. U. (1989). Toxoplasmosis in AIDS patients. *Journal on Antimicrobial Chemotherapy* 23 (supplement A): 77–82.

with the ELISA, a blood test for the presence of antibodies to HIV. The ELISA is most universally used to test for HIV infection and is used by blood banks to detect HIV-infected blood. If the ELISA is positive, a Western blot is performed to identify confirming antibodies specific to viral proteins or glycoproteins. The CDC recommendation is that to be deemed positive, a Western blot should show evidence of antibody to two of the following HIV components: gp160/120, gp41, and p24. The combination of a positive ELISA and a positive Western blot is 99.5% accurate in diagnosing HIV infection. If the Western blot is equivocal or indeterminate, other tests may be done to confirm infection. A new recombinant form of the material used in ELISA has been released by the FDA and has probably reduced false positives, since its viral components are purer.

Under certain circumstances, antibody tests such as ELISA and the Western blot are less useful. Since viral components used in the tests are obtained from cell cultures, some cellular components can create false positive HIV antibody tests. For example, false positives can occur in people who have received intravenous immunoglobulin or multiple transfusions, in multiparous women, or in individuals with systemic lupus erythematosis. Another population for whom antibody tests may be inaccurate consists of infants born to HIV-infected mothers. During pregnancy, the mother normally transfers immunoglobulin across the placenta to her fetus. In this manner, the HIV-infected mother transfers anti-HIV antibody to her fetus. Therefore, a baby born to an HIV-infected mother can have a positive ELISA and Western blot solely because of the mother's antibody transfer and may not be HIV-infected.

Viral culture is performed primarily by research laboratories and is extremely accurate in diagnosing infection. Viral culture is performed by taking lymphocytes and monocytes from the patient and growing them in culture for 28 days. The sample is checked periodically for levels of reverse transcriptase and the presence and number of syncytia (clumped T4 lymphocytes characteristic of HIV infection). The presence of either is proof of retroviral infection.

The polymerase chain reaction (PCR) is another test conducted in research laboratories. This complex test involves taking a small number of immune cells (lymphocytes and monocytes) from the patient, replicating the cells' DNA hundreds of thousands of times, and then testing for the presence of HIV DNA.

Two other tests, the T4 count and p24 antigen assay, are employed to evaluate response to treatment or to monitor disease progression. The p24 core antigen assay measures levels of the viral core protein p24. Researchers have noted that increases in

Table 8-48 Diagnostic Tests for HIV Virus

Name of Test	Description of Test
ELISA (Enzyme-linked immuno-sorbent assay)	Blood test for HIV antibodies, determined by immunofluorescence technique
Western blot	Electrophoresis of antibodies to specific viral proteins; at least two of the three HIV components (gp160/120, gp41, or p24) must be present
Viral culture	Lymphocytes and monocytes recovered from the patient are grown in culture for 28 days, with periodic examination for levels of reverse transcriptase or syncytia (clumped T4 cells)
Polymerase chain reaction (PCR)	Immune cells are removed from the patient, and the cells' DNA is replicated thousands of times and then tested for HIV

p24 levels are associated with increases in HIV-related symptoms. As a result, this test has been used to measure response to treatment and progression of the disease.[130] Once the diagnosis of HIV infection is established, blood counts of T4 cells offer the most clinically significant information for decision making about diagnosis and treatment. Although absolute T4 counts (in cells per cubic millimeter) are most often used, some prefer to measure T4 cells as a percentage of all lymphocytes. It is important to control for certain factors that can alter T4 counts. For example, T4 counts can show some degree of variation throughout the day, when done by different laboratories, and in splenectomized patients.

Prevention of occupational exposure to HIV
Health care workers who are not vaccinated against hepatitis B infection are at far greater risk of occupational acquisition of hepatitis B than of HIV. In part, this is due to the fact that blood from a person infected with hepatitis B contains far greater numbers of infectious viral particles (IPs) than the blood of someone infected with HIV. Persons with hepatitis B have, on average, 1 billion IP/mL of blood. In contrast, an HIV-infected person averages only 10–50 IP/mL, although up to 10,000 IP/mL have been found in the blood of patients in later stages of infection.[131]

Nevertheless, the risk of HIV transmission in the health care setting is quite real. The risk of occupational acquisition of HIV infection following percutaneous exposure via a contaminated needlestick has been reported to be 0.4%. In other words, out of every 250 persons exposed to HIV, 1 person will seroconvert.[132] The risk of acquisition of infection is believed to be influenced by the depth of injury and volume of innoculate. Deeper, more penetrating injuries are more likely to produce seroconversion,

as is exposure to pure virus or large amounts of virus-contaminated blood. Critical care nurses have a particularly high risk of work-related exposure to HIV-contaminated blood or body fluids.

In March 1987, the CDC published recommendations for prevention of HIV transmission in health care settings. In essence, the recommendations consist of the basic tenets of Universal Blood and Body Fluid Precautions: consider all patients as potentially infected and use appropriate barriers to prevent contact with potentially infected material. HIV may be present in significant amounts in blood or bloody secretions, peritoneal dialysis drainage, pleural fluid, cerebrospinal fluid, and semen. HIV is unlikely to be present in urine, saliva, feces, or perspiration in amounts capable of causing infection.

Nurses should prevent infective material from contacting their mucous membranes or nonintact skin. Adequate supplies of isolation equipment should be readily available where needed. Resuscitation equipment, such as masks, should also be readily available. Gloves, gowns, masks, and goggles should be worn when indicated. Breaks in skin are not always readily apparent. Wiping the hands with an alcohol pad will cause stinging anywhere that the skin is not intact. This technique can be employed to alert nurses to the presence of microabrasions and offers convincing evidence of the need to wear gloves whenever exposure is likely. Sterile latex surgeon's gloves are usually the best quality and thickest.

Nurses should reduce the risk of percutaneous innoculation. The most important means of reducing risk of a needlestick injury is to *slow down*. The nurse should *stop and think* how to safely dispose of a needle. Needle disposal boxes must be readily available wherever contaminated needles are found and changed *before* they become overfilled. The nurse should use caution when cleaning up equipment trays following a procedure to avoid self-injury with a contaminated scalpel, suture needle, trocar, or stylet.

The risk of needlestick injuries and cutaneous exposure to blood can be reduced by the use of various innovative devices such as self-sheathing needles and devices that secure IV infusers to heparin lock caps, which prevent accidental disconnection. Recapping needles should be avoided; instead, Kelly clamps should be used to remove needles or, if absolutely necessary, the one-handed technique of scooping the cap onto the needle prior to disposal. Nurses can work together to develop or implement safer techniques for blood drawing, such as using needleless products that permit obtaining blood samples from central venous catheters without using needles or disconnecting IV tubing.

When performing endotracheal or tracheal suctioning, nurses should always wear gloves on *both* hands. Masks and goggles should be used in accordance with the infection control policy in your facility, but definitely if the patient is on positive pressure ventilation. When a ventilator is disconnected for endotracheal suctioning of a patient with hemoptysis who is on PEEP, bloody sputum can literally spray an entire room. This can be prevented by using suction ports or ventilator adaptors to permit suctioning without disconnecting the ventilator from the endotracheal or tracheal tube.

Nasogastric drainage in critically ill patients frequently contains blood. The use of a Keith antireflux valve or similar product on the sump port of Salem sumps can prevent drainage from backing out of the pigtail. Nasogastric tube stopcocks can also prevent contact with drainage when irrigating tubes.

Critically ill patients also often have guaiac-positive stool. With patients who are incontinent of stool, especially if they are suffering from diarrhea, use fecal incontinence collectors to both minimize environmental contamination and maintain patient comfort.

Management of exposure Animal research supports the administration of zidovudine to prevent HIV infection following innoculation with the virus. Two regimens for the administration of zidovudine in the event of occupational exposure to HIV-infected blood or body fluid are described in Table 8-49.[133] Following occupational exposure to body secretions, if the HIV status of the source is unknown, it is recommended that the source be informed and, after giving consent, tested for HIV infection.[134] If the source tests positive or is already known to be HIV positive, and if significant exposure has occurred, the health care worker should be offered zidovudine prophylaxis and counseling.

Nursing standards of care

The medical treatment of HIV infection and AIDS has several major goals. Since severe HIV infection may present as OIs, specific cancers (Kaposi's, lymphoma), or neurologic disease, the treatment of the patient's unique problem may be of highest priority and must be addressed even while attempting to reduce the spread of the virus.

One major medical goal is to reduce viral replication by administration of an antiretroviral agent such as zidovudine as soon as T4 counts drop below $500/mm^3$. Patients unable to tolerate zidovudine can be treated with other FDA-approved antiretrovirals such as ddI, ddC, or alpha interferon. Clinical trials are in progress to determine the usefulness of alternating antiretrovirals to reduce side effects while maintaining efficacy.

HIV-related cancers are treated in much the same fashion as the same cancers in other patients. Standard chemotherapy regimens for Hodgkin's and non-Hodgkin's lymphoma may be supplemented by antiviral agents such as interferon or chemotherapeutic drugs. About half of the lymphoma patients treated with cytotoxic agents exhibit a partial or complete response. Some have reported complete remissions after about 6 months. Alpha interferon

Table 8-49 Recommended Zidovudine Therapy Following Occupational Exposure to HIV

Facility	Dose	Frequency	Duration of Therapy
National Institutes of Health	200 mg	Every 4 hours	6 weeks
University of California at San Francisco	200 mg	5 times a day (skip 4 am dose)	1 month

Source: Geberding, J. L. (1990). Occupational HIV Transmission: Issues for Health Care Providers. In Williams et al., (Eds.). *Hematology.* 4th edition. New York: McGraw-Hill.

has produced a partial or complete remission in 80% of patients with KS; however, fewer than 10% of patients with T4 counts less than 100/mm³ responded to this treatment.[135] KS has also been successfully treated with doxorubicin, bleomycin, and vincristine. Chemotherapeutic agents used to treat patients with HIV-related cancers and the side effects of each are summarized in Table 8-50.

As noted above, perhaps the most important medical goal in the management of HIV infection is to prevent or (failing that) promptly detect and treat opportunistic infections. The usual goal of OI management is control; most cannot be eradicated and require lifelong therapy.[136] Common medications used to prevent the most prevalent OIs include PCP prophylaxis with clotrimoxazole or aerosolized pentamidine, oral antifungals to prevent candida, and oral acyclovir to prevent herpes reactivation. Clinical trials of prophylaxis for toxoplasma encephalitis are underway.[137] There is an effective pharmacotherapy for most OIs (see Table 8-50), but many of the medications used are extremely toxic and require long-term use.

Other methods to prevent infection were outlined in the section on neutropenia. It is recommended that patients be immunized against various pathogenic agents (especially pneumococcus), provided that the vaccine uses antibodies or dead organisms. They should be advised to avoid foreign travel and to limit their exposure to soil and environmental wastes.

Management schemas for the primary infections in AIDS are well established. The most prevalent infection associated with HIV is candidiasis, primarily of the oral or esophageal area. Oral antifungals such as nystatin should be taken, and if the patient is unable to eat (is intubated), antifungals may be swabbed on the oral mucosa. If fungal infection is disseminated, intravenous amphotericin and/or fluconazole may be used.

PCP is another very prevalent infection. In fact, if the T4 count is below 200 cells/mm³, the individual should be placed on anti-PCP prophylaxis; T4 counts below 100 require anti-MAI prophylaxis. Although effective treatments are available for PCP, it can often become refractory to therapy. Trimethoprim sulfamethoxazole (TMP/SX) is the treatment of choice for PCP. TMP/SX is more effective, less expensive, and easier to administer than either aerosolized or intravenous pentamidine and is less toxic than IV pentamidine. However, for reasons that are not well understood, patients with AIDS have a higher risk of adverse effects from TMP/SX. Up to 50–60% of these patients experience rash, fever, and hepatic or renal effects from this drug.[138] Aerosolized pentamidine,

although slightly less effective than TMP/SX, is far better tolerated. The aerosol must reach the patient's upper lobes, or pneumocystis will infect those areas.[139] The medication also tastes bad when administered by the aerosol method, so it should not be given before a meal. Pentamidine is considered a hazardous material, and health care workers must use protective wear when administering it. In addition to antibiotic management, researchers have found that if the patient is hypoxemic, prednisone therapy greatly improves the survival rate. However, within 5 days of treatment, 10–30% of patients worsen and must be switched to another standard antipneumocystic therapy, such as dapsone and trimetrexate, dapsone and pyrimethamine, or clindamycin and pyrimethamine (see Table 8-51).[140] Folic acid antagonists such as trimetrexate are coadministered with an "antidote" dose of folinic acid. These agents are effective because, in contrast to human cells, pneumocysts can not use preformed folate. As a result, the therapy poisons the parasite, but the human cells are able to use the folinic acid and remain unharmed.

MAI is particularly resistant to treatment. Combinations of various drugs (anasamycin, ethambutol, clofazimine, amikacin, ciprofloxacin, and clarithromycin) have been employed to eradicate or reduce infection. Unfortunately, these drug combinations are poorly tolerated and are not completely effective. It is hoped that new agents will be developed to better manage this infection.

Acyclovir is used extensively to prevent and/or manage reactivation of herpes simplex. Research also supports the use of this agent in the management of herpes zoster. Hydration and a slow rate of infusion are recommended to prevent renal complications. Many patients eventually become resistant to acyclovir.

Two antiviral agents are effective against CMV. Both ganciclovir and foscarnet are first administered to induce remission of infection and then are given on a continuing basis to prevent relapse. Ganciclovir stabilizes disease in 70–90% of patients, but causes leukopenia in one-third of patients during induction therapy and in one-half of patients during maintenance. The adverse effects of foscarnet are generally less severe, but potentially serious: azotemia, hypocalcemia, hypophosphatemia, and hypo-magnesemia. With both drugs, it is imperative to monitor patients closely so doses can be reduced or therapy can be interrupted to prevent serious toxicity. Anti-CMV immune globulin may also be given in conjunction with gancyclovir.

The third goal of management is to manage hematologic suppression resulting from HIV infec-

Table 8-50 Drugs Commonly Given to Patients with HIV Infection or AIDS

Problem	Drug(s)/Dosage	Side Effects	Comments
HIV infection			
Asymptomatic CD4 > 200	No treatment		
Asymptomatic CD4 < 500	Zidovudine (Retrovir, AZT) 100 mg every 4 hours × 4 wks	Lowered Hct, WBC, ANC, platelets, headache, nausea, myalgias Insomnia or bone marrow toxicity (ANC < 500–750 cells/mm^3): reduce dose to 100 mg t.i.d.	Drug interactions: Tylenol, indocin, ASA, and probenecid may increase bone marrow disease Concomitant use of ganciclovir can cause severe myelosuppression Monitor CBC at least every 2 weeks
Patients with HIV infection who are intolerant to zidovudine	Didanosine (Videx, ddI, 2'3'-dideoxyinosine): Determined by weight 200–300 mg every 12 hours (> 50 kg)	Peripheral neuropathy Pancreatitis (fatal) Diarrhea Dry mouth	Hold pentamidine during ddI
In patients with advanced HIV infection who exhibit deterioration on zidovudine alone	Zalcitabine (Hivid, ddC, dideoxycytadine): 0.750 mg (1 tab PO) with zidovudine 200 mg every 8 hours	Peripheral neuropathy Pancreatitis Headache Oral/esophageal ulcers	
Kaposi's sarcoma			
CD4 > 200	Alpha interferon 5–9 mu SQ daily plus AZT 100 mg PO 5–6x/day	Dose-related increases in LFTs Neutropenia	Limited skin disease, not rapidly progressing
CD4 < 200	Alternating vincristine and vinblastine weekly (IV) plus AZT	Bone marrow suppression, especially WBC	Less aggressive but progressive disease
	Adriamycin (10 mg/m^2), bleomycin, vincristine (ABV)	Bone marrow suppression, especially WBC	Rapidly progressive disease
B-cell lymphoma	Low dose m-BACOD: Bleomycin 4u/m^2 d1, Adriamycin 25 mg/m^2 d1, Cytoxan 300 mg/m^2 d1, Vincristine 1.4 mg/m^2 (max 2 mg) d1, Decadron 3 mg/m^2 d1-5 plus Ara-C 50 mg intrathecal every wk for CNS prophylaxis, aerosolized or IV pentamidine for PCP prophylaxis. At completion of therapy, start AZT. If patient does not respond to AZT, consider ddI or ddC	Bone marrow suppression (consult chemotherapy text for information)	Prognosis related to initial CD4 count, prior history of response to therapy, extra-nodal disease
Herpes infection			
Acute	Acyclovir 200–800 mg PO 5x/day x 7–10 days (until lesions are crusted) Maintenance: 200–400 mg t.i.d.	Nausea, vomiting Dizziness	May require indefinite maintenance therapy; if patient does not respond, may need to double oral dose, or use IV if infection is severe or persistent

(continued)

Table 8-50   Drugs Commonly Given to Patients with HIV Infection or AIDS (*continued*)

Problem	Drug(s)/Dosage	Side Effects	Comments
Extensive/severe	Acyclovir: 5 mg/kg every 8 hr x 5–7 days (H. simplex) IV 10 mg/kg every 8 hours x 5–7 days (H. zoster)	Lethargy, tremors, confusion, hallucination Phlebitis Increased serum creatinine Nephropathy	Severe infection can progress to esophagitis, colitis, encephalitis
Acyclovir resistance	Foscarnet 60 mg/kg/day	Phlebitis, renal dysfunction, CNS irritation, decreased hemoglobin calcium	Investigational; compassionate plea for CMV or acyclovir resistance
Cytomegalovirus (CMV)	Ganciclovir (DHPG) 2.5 mg/kg IV every 8 hours or 5 mg/kg every 12 hours x 14–21 days for acute infection Maintenance: 2.5–5 mg/kg IV daily 5–7 x/week Reduce dose if creatinine clearance < 25 cc/min or ANC < 1000 cells/uL	Neutropenia Renal failure Anemia Phlebitis Nausea	Requires lifetime maintenance therapy; oral ganciclovir is undergoing clinical trials; causes severe granulocytopenia when given with AZT
	Foscarnet 60 mg/kg every 8 hours x 14 days Maintenance: 60–90 mg/kg IV 5x/week	Phlebitis Renal dysfunction Decreased Hgb, Ca^{++} CNS irritation (irritability, tremor, headache, status epilepticus)	Investigational; monitor serum creatinine; avoid concurrent administration with pentamidine; has antiviral activity against all herpes viruses and HIV
Pneumocystis carinii pneumonia (PCP)	Prophylaxis: Pentamidine 300 mg every 2–8 wks by Respirgard II jet nebulizer	Bitter, metallic taste Dyspnea Decreased appetite Bronchial irritation	May need to pretreat with bronchodilator (e.g., Alupent) Increased risk of extrapulmonary pneumocystis
	or Trimethoprim 160 mg plus sulfamethoxazole 800 mg every 12 hours PO	Rashes (maculopapular, exfoliative, Stevens-Johnson) Neutropenia Anemia Thrombocytopenia, Increased LFTs, BUN/creatinine	PO, IV equally effective; change to pentamidine if ANC < 800 or platelets <30 K
	or Bactrim DS 1 qd		
	or Dapsone 100 mg qd		If LFTs increase by > 5x, change to pentamidine
	Treatment: Trimethoprim 15–20 mg/kg qd + sulfamethoxazole 75–100 mg/kg every 6 hours (IV or PO)	Drug fever	See above
	or Pentamidine 4 mg/kg/day, slow infusion IV over 2 hours or more	Hypoglycemia or hyperglycemia Orthostatic hypotension Decreased WBC, platelets Azotemia, renal failure Decreased Ca^{++}, Mg^{++} Hepatitis, pancreatitis Rare cardiac arrhythmias	Slow infusion; monitor serum glucose; avoid concurrent use of nephrotoxic agents

Table 8-50 (*continued*)

Problem	Drug(s)/Dosage	Side Effects	Comments
Candida Oral	Clortrimazole troches, 10 mg 5x/day	Taste changes Nausea and vomiting Rare abnormal LFTs	Patient should respond in 7 days, otherwise change to ketoconazole; not absorbed in achlorhydric patients, and >30% of AIDS patients are achlorhydric; if patient requires antacids or H2 blockers, use fluconazole; taper to maintenance dose
	Ketoconazole 200–400 mg/day	Increased LFTs Nausea, vomiting	
	Fluconazole 200 mg/day	Anaphylaxis Urticaria Nausea, vomiting	
Esophageal	Ketoconazole 400 mg/day If ineffective, amphotericin B 0.3 mg/kg/day × 10 days	See above Renal failure Decreased K^+ Mg^{++} Fever, chills Anemia Thrombophlebitis	Avoid antacids, H2 blockers; if patient must use antacids, give 2 hrs before or after, but they may be ineffective
Cryptococcus	Amphotericin 0.4–0.6 mg/kg/day	See above	Duration 6 weeks (total dose 1.5–2 gm) plus lifelong maintenance therapy
or	0.8–1.0 mg/kg/day qod		
	Maintenance: 1 mg/kg/wk		
	Fluconazole 75–100 mg/kg/day in 6 divided doses	Nausea, vomiting	
	Maintenance: 100–200 mg/day		
	Note: Flucytosine is no longer recommended as it has been found to increase bone marrow disease with little additive benefit.		
Histoplasmosis	Induction: Amphotericin 2–2.5 gm total dose Maintenance: 1 mg/kg/wk	See above	
or	Ketoconazole 200 mg b.i.d.		
Mycobacterium avium intracellare (MAI)	Ciprofloxacin 50–60 mg/day	Dizziness, lightheadedness Diarrhea, nausea, vomiting Seizures	Other regimens may include INH, ansamycin; infection is difficult to treat; new therapy: liposomal delivery of antibiotics to intracellular habitat of microorganisms
	Ethambutol 25 mg/kg/day +/− amikacin 7.5 mg/kg IM/IV every 12 hours × 4–8 weeks	CNS effects Fever Nausea and vomiting Renal dysfunction Ototoxicity	
	Rifampin 600 mg PO/day	Hepatitis Reddish-orange discoloration of secretions	

(*continued*)

Table 8-50   Drugs Commonly Given to Patients with HIV Infection or AIDS (*continued*)

Problem	Drug(s)/Dosage	Side Effects	Comments
Mycobacterium tuberculosis (MTB)	Isoniazid (INH) 5 mg/kg/day	Peripheral neuritis Muscle twitching Seizures Hepatitis	Use three drugs 2–3 mo, then delete PZA, treat for at least 9 months
	Rifampin 9 mg/kg/day Pyrazinamide (PZA) 25 mg/kg/day	GI intolerance Hepatitis Arthralgias Hyperuricemia	

tion, chemotherapy, or antibiotic and antiretroviral therapy. Complications such as anemia, neutropenia, and thrombocytopenia are present in many patients and represent significant morbidity. Ongoing transfusions of red blood cells and platelets are required in many cases. Colony stimulating factors such as erythropoietin, G-CSF, GM-CSF, and M-CSF are used to encourage bone marrow generation of these cells. Administration of intravenous immunoglobulin may also be useful for treating immune hemolytic anemia or idiopathic thrombocytopenia purpura (ITP). Win Rho (anti-RhD) for injection has also shown impressive results in the treatment of ITP.

Maintenance of self-care, good nourishment,

Table 8-51   Drugs Used in the Treatment of PCP

Trimethoprim/sulfamethoxazole
Pentamidine
Dapsone
Dapsone and pyrimethamine
Dapsone + trimethoprim
Dapsone and trimetrexate
Trimetrexate + leucovorin
Pyrimethamine + sulfadoxine
Clindamycin + pyrimethamine
Clindamycin + primaquine
Piritrexim + leucovorin
Clotrimoxazole
Prednisone

and adequate rest are essential for the patient's physical well-being and psychological outlook. Adequate nutrition, exercise, stress reduction, protection from infection, and rest can help prevent complications of disease as well as improve quality of life. The importance of this goal must not be minimized. Psychosocial support is an important foundation in the treatment of any person with HIV infection, since the patient's psychosocial needs may at times outweigh the physical ones. These patients face social isolation, job discrimination, insurance rejection, and financial burden. Anxiety, depression, anger, and suicidal tendencies may require extensive intervention and may be more difficult to manage if the patient is suffering from neurologic disease.

Critical care nursing of the HIV-infected patient of necessity focuses on providing intensive care for persons with life-threatening illnesses. In many cases, the ICU patient will be far too ill to be able to participate in his or her own care. The care of these patients is labor-intensive, requiring a great deal of physical care and drug therapy. The nurse's role is to support the medical plan for management of the viral illness and complications, but most especially to assess for and manage symptoms. Patients with AIDS suffer from many physical ailments. The nurse will be the primary coordinator of efforts to meet both physical and psychological needs. An outline of the nursing problems encountered in the patient with HIV infection is included in the care plan that follows.

Nursing Care Plan for the Management of the Patient with HIV Infection

Diagnosis	Signs and symptoms	Intervention	Rationale
Potential for infection related to HIV virus and immunodeficiency or T helper cell deficiency and macrophage dysfunction	Decreased T4 level Positive ELISA and Western blot tests Fever > 99.6°F Leukocytosis with high PMNs and low lymphocytes Constitutional symptoms Lymphadenopathy	Monitor VS (especially temperature) every 2–4 hours	Early indication of infection
		Culture workup for any of the following: chills without reason; fever > 99.6°F; hypotensive event; changes in mental status; sputum production	Signs and symptoms of sepsis in the immunocompromised host
		Teach patient to "eat defensively," avoiding inadequately cooked or mass-produced food; no fresh fruits and vegetables, caution with spices and nuts	Food can transmit many organisms that can infect HIV patient: toxoplasma, clostridium, histoplasma, cryptosporidium
		Obtain HIV test if there is persistant lymphadenopathy, constitutional symptoms, or weight loss	Significant symptoms of immune problem, especially HIV
		Support prophylactic antibiotics against PCP, CMV, and MAI in high-risk patients; monitor for side effects; obtain antibiotic levels	To prevent infection with one of the likely organisms, but limit toxicity of medication
		Teach patient to avoid contact with possible infectious diseases	HIV patient will be more likely to get severe infection
		No live flowers or standing water in the patient's room	Plants and flowers harbor pseudomonas
		Follow universal precautions when caring for patients	Precaution against exposure of health care workers

Nursing Care Plan for the Management of the Patient with HIV Infection

Diagnosis	Signs and symptoms	Intervention	Rationale
	Malaise Viral reactivation of herpes simplex or herpes zoster Local signs and symptoms of infection (erythema, edema, or pus)	Patient should follow general infection prevention measures: keep out of crowds, garden only if using gloves, receive immunization against infectious diseases, maintain proper nutrition, and get adequate rest Low microbial diet	To prevent infections by organisms prevalent in environment; bacterial infections of endogenous organisms are unusual, but reactivation of previous infection is common
		Recognize personal risk factors for specific infections based on life-style, geographic location, history of travel, or history of exposure	Many organisms are known to be prevalent in certain geographic regions, causing reactivation of disease in immunosuppressed individuals; certain behaviors such as IV drug use and anal sex are also known to predispose individuals to particular infections
		Administer AZT or other antiviral agents as ordered; monitor for side effects	To reduce viral destruction of T helper cells
		Maintain medication log for potential interactions, and monitor for side effects	To identify medication reactions, which are common in this patient group
		Wound and dressing care as with neutropenia (every 24–48 hours)	Patient is at high risk for infection in general
Altered thought proceses related to HIV infection of the brain, infectious or malignant processes of the meninges or brain, or medication toxicity	Apprehensiveness Restlessness Anxiety Confusion	Assess neurological status every 4–8 hours: orientation, motor activity and strength, memory, and decision-making skills	To identify neurological complications early; complex exam is necessary to identify scope of problems associated with HIV

Diagnosis	Signs and symptoms	Intervention	Rationale
	Short-term memory deficit	Introduce yourself at each interaction with patient	To help patient remember who you are and your role
	Poor judgment	Coordinate efforts to assist patient in identifying personal preferences regarding life support and medical power of attorney	It is helpful to evaluate and plan for these wishes before patient develops significant neurological deficits and becomes incompetent to make decisions
	Lethargy		
	Obtundation		
		Identify need for consultation with social worker if patient appears to develop AIDS dementia (symptoms are rarely reversible)	Patients may be unable to care for themselves and may need extensive social support to prevent injury to themselves
		Teach patient and significant others about important neurological symptoms requiring medical attention: persistent headaches, sensory disturbances, lapses in memory, and inability to perform usual reasoning	To reinforce need for prompt evaluation of all symptoms because of the broad range and life-threatening quality of some neurological complications
		Provide sheltered freedom; protect from injury by using chemical and physical restraints with caution	Safety is important, but patient dignity must be maintained
		Provide information to significant others as follow-up to patient education; reinforce with written instructions after verbal discussions	Written record can be referred to in the future; reliability of patient's memory may be questionable
		Consider need for consultation with home health nurse for teaching and follow-up of medical care regimens	Patient's inability to safely care for self may be identified through home health experts

Nursing Care Plan for the Management of the Patient with HIV Infection

Diagnosis	Signs and symptoms	Intervention	Rationale
Alteration in gas exchange related to pulmonary infectious disease (PCP, toxoplasmosis, MAI, or CMV)	Dyspnea Tachypnea Dry, hacking cough Low-grade fever Hypoxemia Changes in chest x-ray indicative of pneumonitis	Respiratory assessment every 4–8 hours in patient at risk or every 1–2 hours in compromised patient	Determine changes indicative of worsening condition
		Supplemental oxygen for high respiratory effort and as ordered for hypoxemia	To increase patient comfort and reduce respiratory effort
		Pulse oximetry monitoring; spot checks with dyspnea, cyanosis, or other subjective symptoms of distress; note activities (certain positions, coughing) that cause desaturation	To note changes in oxygenation requiring specialized care or ABG follow-up
		Obtain sputum for culture and sensitivity, mycology, virus, and acid-fast bacillus tests at least twice per week; note sputum characteristics	For early detection of new infections
		Assist with induced sputum for PCP as ordered; administer expectorant; take early morning specimen	Test can produce viable specimen if performed cautiously
		Help patient turn, cough, and deep breathe every 2 hours	Prevent atelectasis and potential infection
		Perform daily activities in small increments throughout the day	Conserve energy, decrease work of breathing
		Monitor chest x-rays, attempting to take them in same position daily	For accurate comparison and analysis of response to treatment
		Respiratory isolation if active TB a possibility	To prevent dissemination of tuberculosis

Diagnosis	Signs and symptoms	Intervention	Rationale
Alteration in elimination: diarrhea related to opportunistic infection or Kaposi's sarcoma of GI tract	More than 3 loose stools per day or more than 6 stools per day	Assess all stools for occult blood	Early indication of erosion requiring medical evaluation
	Pathogenic organisms in stool or rectal cultures	Follow universal precautions when handling any possibly contaminated self-care items	To avoid cross-contamination or self-infection with organisms
	Fever		
	Dehydration	Meticulous I&O records; replace fluid loss through IV fluids and oral supplementation	To monitor patient for dehydration from excessive diarrhea
	Hypokalemia		
	Hyperactive bowel sounds		
	Abdominal cramping	Stool cultures with every temperature spike in HIV-infected patient	GI organisms are very likely sources of infection in these patients
		Surveillance cultures of rectum twice per week	For early detection of colonization or organisms requiring medication
		Special skin-protecting rectal care at least twice daily	To protect against breakdown in barrier defense
		Monitor electrolytes at least daily for imbalance	Hypokalemia and hypocalcemia are common with fluid loss with diarrhea
		Administer antimotility drugs PRN	To reduce discomfort and fluid loss from diarrhea
		Provide incontinence pads or underwear as appropriate	For patient comfort and maintenance of dignity
		Administer antibiotics as ordered, but attempt to maintain normal GI flora with yogurt or acidophilus milk	To treat cause of diarrhea but protect against destruction of normal flora and resistant overgrowth
Alteration in nutrition, (intake less than requirements) related to cachexia, increased metabolic rate, infectious processes, anorexia, or oral lesions	Anorexia	Perform calorie count	To determine actual patient intake to compare to needs
	Taste changes and aversions		
	Weight loss of more than 10% of normal body weight	Set up a nutritional consult	For thorough physiological and chemical evaluation and development of a plan

Nursing Care Plan for the Management of the Patient with HIV Infection

Diagnosis	Signs and symptoms	Intervention	Rationale
	Fevers Hyperglycemia Increased BUN Nausea and vomiting	Nutritional supplementation based upon nutritional and metabolic substrate needs (high protein, lipids to replace carbohydrates)	Nutrition should not just replace calories but be built on catabolic demands to maintain visceral protein
		Record daily weights	To provide assessment of basic nutrition and fluid balance
		Take daily electrolytes and glucose levels	To evaluate use of nutritional substrates
		Administer anti-emetics as needed	To relieve symptoms and encourage oral intake
		Serve food aesthetically; encourage family and friends to prepare food and provide company during eating	To attempt to increase voluntary intake of nutrition
Alteration in the oral mucosa related to infectious lesions, xerostomia, or chemotherapy-induced mucosites	Oral pain Oral erosions and ulcers: mucosal lesions, herpetic ulcerations, or candida (white patches) Fevers Dysphagia	Oral care with soft toothbrush and bactericidal agent (chlorhexidine) three times each day	To prevent gingivitis and destroy organisms harbored in mouth
		Liberal use of saliva substitute	To prevent caries, provide comfort, and decrease candida infection
		Encourage use of oral nonabsorbable anesthetics: viscous xylocaine, benzocaine, or benadryl/Maalox mix	To relieve discomfort
		Culture oral lesions twice weekly and with every temperature spike	To monitor for infection

Diagnosis	Signs and symptoms	Intervention	Rationale
		Sketch location and size of lesion in daily assessment to use as comparison for future evaluation of lesions	To evaluate changes in lesions possibly indicative of new problems
		Administer prophylactic oral antifungal (Nystatin or Mycelex)	Patients are at high risk for fungal infection
		Use gloves for encounters with oral secretions	To prevent infecting lesions and protect self against OIs and HIV found in secretions
Potential for skin breakdown related to edema, malnutrition, Kaposi's lesions, or cutaneous infections	Reddened skin areas Red areas over bony prominences Skin discomfort at high-pressure areas Kaposi's sarcoma Rashes Pruritis Immobility	Assess total body cutaneous areas daily	Daily evaluation will detect new areas of risk
		Perform focused assessment of existing lesions every shift	Lesion changes may indicate new infection
		Culture all existing lesions with temperature spike	Potential for harboring organisms that cause systemic infection
		Turn patient every 2 hours; use pull sheets to reduce injury	To reduce risk of skin breakdown
		Use air mattress, egg crates, or low air-loss bed	
		Maintain cool environment	To decrease itching sensation
		Assist patient with passive or active ROM exercises	To maintain physiological function, decrease edema, and enhance patient comfort
		Apply anti-itch mentholated or other lipid creams; avoid scents	For patient comfort
		Administer antihistamines as ordered	To relieve itching
		Use condom catheters or fecal incontinence bags as indicated	To reduce potential for skin breakdown

Nursing Care Plan for the Management of the Patient with HIV Infection

Diagnosis	Signs and symptoms	Intervention	Rationale
Pain related to lymphedema, mucosal erosion, tumors, infection, or organomegaly	Nonverbal cues of inability to obtain position of comfort Patient verbalizes discomfort Insomnia Grunting, crying, or behavioral manifestations of pain Obvious withdrawal when lesions are touched	Follow usual practices for relieving pain	Care is the same as that provided to other patients with pain
Social isolation related to stigma of disease, family's nonacceptance of life-style, loss of employment, or financial difficulties	Few cards, visitors, or calls Lack of support for daily activities in hospital Unemployment Depression	Social service consultation to evaluate family dynamics, resources, need to apply for social support or financial aid	Patients with this disease are likely to need assistance integrating into family and public social systems
		Record visits by family or significant others and note relationship	For ongoing evaluation of patient support and need for intervention
		Assist patient in locating and participating in support groups	Provide open and unprejudiced support
		Locate local AIDS support group and evaluate services offered with regard to visiting, supplies, and discharge planning	Nonprofit groups receive private and public funding and should be accessible to patient
		Provide positive feedback to patient regarding self-worth	Improving self-image will enhance self-esteem and coping ability

Diagnosis	Signs and symptoms	Intervention	Rationale
Potential ineffective individual or family coping related to prognosis and social stigma of disease	Crying Dependent behavior Maladaptive coping strategies: alcohol or IV drug use or sexual encounters without informing partner Dysfunctional coping by family or significant others; unrealistic expectations of therapy	Perform psychological assessment daily Refer patient to mental health worker if necessary as indicated by depressive, erratic, dangerous, or self-destructive behaviors Monitor visitors for illegal activities (use of drugs) Educate patient about preventing infection of others Provide diversional activity when appropriate and if patient is able to participate Refer to support group of patients with similar health or ongoing problems Encourage multi-disciplinary family conferences on a regular basis	Frequent re-evaluation necessary to note change in status Professional with in-depth experience in the field is best able to help To reduce patient temptation To reduce spread of disease To attempt to divert patient's attention from self Coping skills can be strengthened by support of others in same situation Reinforce same information among patient, family, and caregivers

Life-Threatening Coagulopathies and Thrombotic Disease

Critically ill patients often experience disruptions of the coagulation mechanism that lead to either decreased or increased propensity for clotting. Disorders involving excessive clotting are termed thrombotic disorders, and inadequate clotting is known as coagulopathy. When components of the normal coagulation response are insufficient in quantity or quality, coagulopathies result. The precise etiology and severity of the coagulation defect will guide the treatment plan. A number of commonly encountered acquired coagulation disorders will be described in this section.

Clinical antecedents

The major components of the coagulation response are the vascular reaction, the platelet plug reaction, fibrin clot formation, and clot lysis. Coagulopathies are the result of defects in one of these mechanisms.

With respect to the vascular reaction, coagulation requires vasoconstriction to reduce the loss of blood and release serotonin to stimulate platelet aggregation. Patients suffering from uncontrolled vasodilation, such as occurs following anesthesia, with sepsis, or on vasodilator therapy, do not have the ability to vasoconstrict and will have reduced platelet aggregation and clot production.

Platelet problems The platelet plug reaction requires sufficient numbers of functional platelets. The most common coagulation disorder in critically ill patients is thrombocytopenia. Thrombocytopenia (deficient platelets) may be due to inadequate bone marrow production of platelets (e.g., when the bone marrow is suppressed by medication), abnormal destruction of platelets after they leave the marrow (e.g., idiopathic thrombocytopenia purpura), or pathologic sequestration of platelets in the spleen. If there are not sufficient platelets to aggregate and form a platelet plug, immediate bleeding occurs, and the coagulation cascade cannot be triggered, thus reducing the body's clotting ability. Platelet function may also be altered by the development of dysfunctional platelets or by a direct antiplatelet activity. Disorders of platelet quality are more difficult to identify because diagnostic testing for this phenomenon remains imperfect and requires a soft-tissue incision. Many disorders and medications can con-

tribute to problems in platelet quantity and/or quality; these are listed in Table 8-52.

Platelet-disorder coagulopathies have many etiologies, requiring careful examination of the patient's personal history, medication profile, and current physical health problems in order to diagnose and eliminate potential sources. One of the most interesting yet complex etiologies of disorders in both platelet quantity and quality is idiopathic thrombocytopenia purpura (ITP) or thrombotic thrombocytopenia purpura (TTP). This disorder is usually the result of a viral infection or is a medication-induced autoimmune reaction to the patient's own platelets. Platelets are destroyed as they reach the circulation, and a chronic state of thrombocytopenia and bleeding tendency exist.

Problems in the coagulation cascade Disorders of the coagulation cascade involve inadequacies in the quality or quantity of coagulation proteins or an interruption of the clotting cascade (for example, in anticoagulation therapy). Because of the many thrombotic risks faced by the critically ill, anticoagulant and thrombolytic therapies have become commonplace in the ICU setting (see Table 8-53). Thrombin inhibitors such as heparin act by blocking the conversion of fibrinogen to fibrin, preventing clots from forming. Another category of medications affecting clotting is the thrombolytics, which are actually agents that enhance the fibrinolysis phase of coagulation. The nurse should recognize that although certain therapeutic effects can be anticipated, unexpected bleeding complications often arise because of the debilitated condition of the patient.

Coagulation proteins are made in the liver, but for these proteins to develop, vitamin K must be absorbed from the GI tract with the assistance of normal flora. Hepatic disease, gut malabsorption, or destruction of the GI flora by antibiotics will disrupt this fine balance designed to regulate clotting. Hepatic disease causes deficiencies in all coagulation proteins except factor VIII (which is not produced in the liver; the production location is unknown). Therefore, hepatic disease will produce diffuse coagulation defects within the clotting cascade. Vitamin K deficiency will affect only those factors dependent upon vitamin K for their development: factors II, VII, IX, and X. Deficiencies in these factors will primarily cause extrinsic pathway disturbances, evidenced by an abnormal prothrombin time (PT).

Clot lysis problems The final phase of coagulation is fibrinolysis, which normally occurs 24–72 hours after formation of the fibrin clot. This clot lysis process produces fibrin degradation products (or

Table 8-52 Agents Contributing to Platelet Disorders

Contributor/Agent	Quantitative Disorders	Qualitative Disorders
Medications	Gold salts Heparin Quinidine Quinine Rifampicin Sedormid Sulfonamides Trimethoprim-sulfamethonazole (Bactrim) Cimetidine Pronestyl Nonsteroidal antiinflammatory agents Chemotherapeutic agents Penicillin Benzol Hormones Thiazide diuretics Alcohol	Heparin Indomethacin Methyldopa Organic arsenicals Quinidine Quinine Rifampicin Salicylic acid (aspirin and aspirin products) Persantin Nitroprusside Sulfin pyruzone Phenylbutazone Dipyramadole Antihistamines Tricyclic antidepressants Phenothiazines Propranolol Edecrin Vitamin E Epinephrine Tetracycline Dextran Furosemide
Environmental/occupational exposure	Food allergies (beans, citrus fruits) Insecticides Transfusions Radiation exposure	Insecticides Transfusions Vinyl chloride
Infectious diseases	Epstein-Barr virus Mononucleosis Vaccinations (pneumococcus, measles, chickenpox, mumps, smallpox) Rubella Viral hepatitis	
Physical conditions	Intraaortic balloon pumping Myasthenia gravis Burns Heat stroke Nutritional deficiency (B_{12}, folic acid) Chronic lymphocytic leukemia Hashimoto's thyroiditis Histoplasmosis Lymphoma (both Hodgkin's and non-Hodgkin's) Sarcoidosis Systemic lupus erythematosis Thyrotoxicosis Tuberculosis Other malignancies	Uremia Hypothermia Dysproteinemia Diabetes Cirrhosis of liver Chronic lymphocytic leukemia Hashimoto's thyroiditis Lymphoma (both Hodgkin's and non-Hodgkin's) Sarcoidosis Scleroderma Systemic lupus erythematosis Thyrotoxicosis Other malignancies

fibrin split products) that have anticoagulant properties. Normally the liver clears these products from the body, but when quantities are excessive or the liver has failed, accumulation may lead to coagulopathy. Another cause of clot lysis coagulopathy are the thrombolytic agents mentioned earlier, those used for their therapeutic effects in myocardial infarction, pulmonary embolism, superior vena cava syndrome, and vena caval thrombosis. Exogenous administration of pharmacologic thrombolytics, including tis-

Table 8-53 Anticoagulant/Thrombolytic Therapies

Agent	Normal dosage	Test to Determine Toxicity	Half-life	Antidote
Coumadin	10–15 mg PO for 3 days, then 2–10 mg daily	PT	36–44 hours	Vitamin K
Dicumarol	200–300 mg PO on first day, then 25–200 mg daily	PT	24–36 hours	Vitamin K
Heparin	Prophylaxis: 5000 U SQ every 12 hours Pulmonary embolism: 7,500–10,000 U IV, then 4,000–50,000 U/hr Post-graft: 7,500–10,000 U IV, then 1,500–3,000 U/hr	PTT	4–6 hours	Protamine sulfate (1 mg/100 U, maximum of 50 mg IV over 10 minutes)
Streptokinase	Bolus of 250,000 U over 30 minutes followed by infusion of 100,000 U/hr for 24–72 hours Local perfusion into occluded vessel	TT	Biphasic: 23 minutes and 83 minutes	Fibrinogen
Urokinase	Initial dose: 4400 U/kg/hr at 90 mL/hr over 10 minutes Maintenance: 4400 U/kg/hr for 12 hours	TT and fibrinogen level	≤ 20 minutes	Fibrinogen
Tissue plasminogen activator (TPA, activase)	Initial dose: 6 mg IV bolus over 1 minute Maintenance: 54 mg/hr for first hour, 20 mg/hr second hour, 5 mg/hr third hour, then discontinue	TT and fibrinogen level	Biphasic: 8 minutes and 1.3 hours	Fibrinogen Amicar
Anysylated plasminogen streptokinase activator complex (APSAC, eminase)	30 U IV bolus reconstituted in sterile water, given over 2–5 minutes No maintenance required	TT and fibrinogen	90–105 minutes	Fibrinogen Amicar

sue plasminogen activator (TPA), streptokinase, and urokinase, can enhance the body's clot lysis process.

Hypercoagulable states Hypercoagulable states can arise from excessively active platelets or clotting factors. Platelet activity is promoted by cigarette smoking, hyperlipidemia, hypercholesterolemia, atherosclerosis, high estrogen levels, and diabetes mellitus. The clotting activity of blood is also enhanced by conditions or situations in which stasis of blood flow allows activated clotting factors to accu-

mulate. Examples of such conditions include bedrest, immobility, dehydration, obstructed blood flow, edema, congestive heart failure, and hyperviscosity disorders (polycythemia or multiple myeloma). Factors promoting clotting are also present in elevated levels during pregnancy, in conjunction with malignant neoplasms, and following the administration of oral contraceptives or corticosteroids.

The development of clots, or thrombi, is more common in the venous circulation and involves one or more of the triggering factors. The development of deep vein thrombosis is common in the critically ill, as a result of the presence of many thrombotic risk factors. Virchow's triad is a threesome of clinical risk factors common to deep vein thrombosis (DVT) and embolization to the lungs (pulmonary emboli): injury to the blood vessel endothelium, stasis of blood, and a hypercoagulable state. The majority of DVTs occur in patients with abdominal processes that interfere with venous return to the heart, including pregnancy, abdominal surgery, abdominal cancers, and obesity.

Critical referents

The pathophysiologic effects of different coagulation defects vary according to which phase of coagulation has been interfered with. Platelet abnormalities lead to inadequate platelet plugs and poor coagulation stimulation; coagulation protein deficits cause inadequate fibrin clot formation. In all types of coagulopathy, small blood vessels (particularly capillaries) are most vulnerable to inadequate hemostasis, which causes them to rupture. Bleeding may be exhibited as ecchymotic areas, petichiae, occult blood in feces, or oozing blood from mucous membranes. Persistent bleeding, regardless of the etiology, perpetuates the loss of coagulation factors and enhances the clotting disorder. Clotting disorders may present as minor disturbances with minimal symptomatology or may be life-threatening. The patient's physical condition and the many contributing factors of critical illness often cause significant bleeding diathesis unless properly diagnosed and managed.

Thromboses of the arterial or venous vessels produce a clinical condition of reduced blood flow past the site of injury. The thrombus may begin slowly, with little circulatory compromise, but tissue necrosis may result beyond the site of the thrombus once circulation is severely impeded. A good example of a clinically significant thrombosis with tissue injury is a myocardial infarction. The backed-up circulation will cause painful swelling, diminished pulses, and organ congestion.

Resulting signs and symptoms

The signs and symptoms of coagulopathy are extremely dependent upon the etiology in the early stages, but all advanced coagulopathies have similar symptoms. The assessment of the bleeding patient requires a logical approach to physical symptoms and diagnostic tests. The clinician must continually remember that there are only four problems that can cause bleeding; breaks in the vascular integrity, platelet problems, coagulation cascade inadequacies, or inappropriate clot lysis. Each etiology of bleeding is the result of defects in a particular phase of coagulation, and consequently each has hallmark symptoms. Table 8-54 is a chart correlating common symptoms and their etiologies.

Loss of vascular integrity A break in vascular integrity is most likely to produce rapid and severe blood loss if not immediately treated. When blood leaks out of a vessel into an interstitial area, the symptoms will be enlargement of a body part, pain at the site, and rapid onset of hypovolemia. There is often historical evidence of injury to the area, invasive procedures, or a individual predisposition to bleed from the site. For instance, someone with a history of intracranial hemorrhage or of peptic ulcer is likely to bleed again from the same site when other factors alter coagulation abilities. The patient's personal history is often valuable in identifying potential bleeding risks.

Diagnosis of a vascular bleeding disorder is frequently made from historical data and evidence of frank bleeding at a site of injury. The CBC and RBC count are most useful when analyzing bleeding from potential vascular problems. Other diagnostic tests may include angiography, x-rays, or scans of the affected body part.

Platelet problems The small capillaries or blood vessels close to the skin and mucous membrane surface are the first to manifest symptoms of platelet problems. Another hallmark of platelet problems is an inability to achieve initial hemostasis after an injury such as venipuncture; since the platelet plug is normally formed early in the clotting process, platelet problems will manifest as continued bleeding after minor injury. Assessment for platelet-related bleeding includes assessment of all feces for occult blood and observation for bruising and petichiae on the mucous membranes and skin—particularly in dependent or high-pressure areas (back, buttocks, and under BP cuff). Observations of any system dysfunction (such as oliguria, confusion, or dyspnea) should be carefully noted, as they may indicate acute interstitial bleeding of the small vessels in that organ.

Platelet quantity and quality tests (platelet count and bleeding time) are used to assess the severity of bleeding risk (see Table 8-55). Oncology studies have demonstrated that the risk of spontaneous hemorrhage from thrombocytopenia can be indicated by platelet counts, which can guide platelet replacement strategies.

Table 8-54 Bleeding Symptoms and Etiologies

Impaired Coagulation Component	Bleeding Condition/Disorder	Assessment Findings
Vascular integrity	Trauma to normal vessels Vessel abnormalities caused by various diseases	Pulsatile or flowing blood loss Bright or dark red blood loss Bleeding originating at or near recent vascular injury site or major vessel Rapid symptom onset
Platelets	Quantitative disorders (caused by platelet nonproduction, dilution, sequestration, or destruction) Qualitative disorders (caused by abnormal platelet structure or drug intoxication, uremia, storage defects, or fibrin split products) Combined quantitative and qualitative disorders	Prolonged bleeding Epistaxis or gingival bleeding Easy bruising Petechiae Increased coagulation time after intravenous or intraarterial line insertion

Coagulation cascade	Inactive factor disorders:
	  congenital disorders (involving coagulation factors VIII, IX, and XI) or acquired disorders (such as impaired clotting factor production and vitamin K deficiency)
	Active factor disorders:
	  excessive heparin or excessive fibrin split products
		Prolonged bleeding
		Bleeding disproportionate to extent of injury
		Signs of occult blood in urine and feces
		Easy bruising
		Petechiae
		Increase in bloody drainage
		New bleeding from incision site

Clot lysis	Abnormal fibrinolysis: administration of plasminogen activator (urokinase, streptokinase) or increased fibrinolysis secondary to increased fibrin formation	Prolonged bleeding after injury Severe tissue or vessel injury Easy bruising Petechiae

Source: Shelton, B. (1988). *Hematology Review.* Springhouse, PA: Springhouse Corporation.

Problems in the coagulation cascade Bleeding as a result of defects in the coagulation cascade is notoriously undetectable unless injury is inflicted or breaks in barriers exist. The coagulation cascade is responsible for ensuring a stable fibrin clot while the injured tissue is healing. Problems of clotting due to coagulation cascade defects may be delayed following the original injury. The initial, temporary platelet plug is established, but when it dissolves within a few hours, there is insufficient fibrin clot formation to maintain a clot and bleeding occurs. Bleeding may also occur from existing injured sites such as invasive lines, old biopsy sites, or ulcerated areas. The bleeding may be mild or severe, depending upon the severity of the deficiency and the patient's risk factors for bleeding. Assessment of body orifices and breaks in barrier defenses and diagnostic tests of organ function will provide the most valuable information for diagnosing a bleeding disorder of this etiology.

The laboratory tests used to evaluate intactness and functioning of the coagulation cascade proteins include the partial thromboplastin time (PTT), prothrombin time (PT), fibrinogen level, and thrombin time (TT). The PTT tests the intrinsic pathway, the PT the extrinsic pathway. The PT is considered a more sensitive indicator of coagulation protein deficiency since it readily becomes abnormal when the vitamin K–dependent factors are not made. The PTT will not indicate a problem until as much as 35–50% of factor VIII is deficient, and unless the patient is actively bleeding, sustaining a loss of this magnitude would

Table 8-55 Platelet Levels and Associated Bleeding Risks

Risk Level	Platelet Level
High	1,000–15,000/μL
Moderate	15,000–30,000/μL
Low	30,000–100,000/μL

be a slow process.[141] When thrombin inhibitors such as streptokinase are given the PTT will be affected, but because of the lack of sensitivity of the PTT, the thrombin time (TT) may be used for therapeutic medication adjustment. The TT is a highly sensitive test of conversion of prothrombin to thrombin, and it is abnormal whenever the conversion is reduced or absent. Its extreme sensitivity to even small amounts of heparin (for example, in invasive monitoring solutions) make it too sensitive to use for therapeutic monitoring of heparin.

Clot lysis problems A small number of bleeding disorders seen in clinical practice are related to the excessive lysis of clots, or to large clots being lysed with generation of excessive fibrin degradation products (FDPs) or fibrin split products (FSPs). Clots usually lyse after 24–72 hours with the generation of fibrin degradation products. These fibrin clot wastes have anticoagulant properties that can induce bleeding in susceptible individuals. In addition, with severe injury, 1–3 days may be insufficient time for the tissue at the site of the clot to heal, so lysis of the clot produces bleeding from the unhealed site. Bleeding related to clot lysis typically occurs days after the initial injury; on occasion, acclerated clot lysis states such as disseminated intravascular coagulation (DIC) will produce such bleeding earlier. FDPs are cleared by the liver, so even normal states of clot lysing may produce clinical bleeding if the liver is unable to remove the FDPs from circulation. The bleeding caused by a clot lysis problem is similar to that caused by coagulation cascade problems.

The test used to monitor for excessive circulating fibrin degradation products is the FDP or FSP test. It measures the quantity of clot breakdown products in the circulation. Even when the FDPs are elevated, the test may still be inconclusive for DIC or a problem with liver clearance. Consequently, positive FDP tests are often followed by a new test called the d-dimer test. This test measures a specific subtype of FDP and, when positive, indicates DIC.

Hypercoagulable states Signs and symptoms of hypercoagulability do not appear alone, but only in the presence of thrombosis related to the underlying disorder. Symptoms often involve a localized inflammatory reaction and include pain, warmth, and swelling at the site. In the leg veins, a localized area of edema distal to the vessel is most common. Arterial thromboses create acute circulatory symptoms of cyanosis, coolness, and diminished pulses in the affected extremity. Intraabdominal venous thromboses provide a more complex picture, with pain and abdominal distention being the prominent symptoms. In severe congestion, the external abdominal

vessels may be prominent or hepatosplenomegaly may be present. Thrombosis of the superior vena cava occurs with long-term indwelling catheters or tumor invasion and compression and is classically associated with right-sided edema and heart failure.

When thrombosis is suspected, a bedside test called Homan's sign can be performed. For this test, the patient lies flat on the bed with the toes flexed toward the head. Pain in the calf is a positive Homan's sign and is indicative of deep-vein thrombosis (DVT). However, this test is nonspecific and is not always positive when a DVT does exist, so further diagnostic testing is necessary. The most common test for thromboses of the veins is a venogram. A dye is injected into the veins of the feet, and serial radiographic studies are done to show the progress of the dye to the heart. Obstructions in flow indicate thrombi or compression of the vessels. The major drawback of this study is its inability to detect multiple thrombi in the same vessel; however, this limitation rarely alters treatment. Arterial emboli are usually characteristically symptomatic and may not require extensive testing prior to surgical removal. When diagnostic confirmation is necessary, arteriography is used.

Nursing standards of care

The first priority in management of the patient with a suspected coagulopathy is to determine the cause of the bleeding disorder. Risk factors and symptoms should be assessed in conjunction with diagnostic test data to identify possible etiologies. Direct intervention to alleviate the etiology of bleeding is of paramount importance. When the etiology is known but cannot be resolved, medications to prevent the breakdown of clots may be administered. Epsilon-amino-caproic acid (EACA or Amicar) is the usual agent. This medication blocks plasminogen's conversion of a fibrin clot to degradation products. A stable clot is then maintained, and bleeding can be temporarily halted. Although medication can be very effective on a short-term basis, only correction of the underlying problem will lower the patient's risk of bleeding. A chart of the sources of coagulopathies and general management suggestions is given in Table 8-56.

Blood product support Once the suspected etiology has been addressed, the focus of patient management is upon maintenance of normal coagulation through blood product support. Blood and coagulation proteins that have been lost in bleeding episodes

Table 8-56 Bleeding Disorders and Their Treatment

General Disorder	Specific Examples	Treatment
Disruption of vascular integrity	Normal vessels subjected to trauma Vessel abnormalities caused by various disease processes	Surgery Cautery RBC transfusions Lasar cryotherapy

Platelet problems	Quantitative disorders caused by
	  nonproduction, dilution, sequestration,
	  destruction
		Platelet transfusions
		Splenectomy

	Qualitative disorders caused by drugs (ASA),
	  uremia, storage defects, fibrin split products,
	  mechanics
	Combinations of above
	Von Willebrand's disease (VIII)
		Platelet transfusions
		Desmopressin
		IgG

Disruption of coagulation cascade	Inactive factor disorders
	  Hereditary disorders (VIII, IX, XI)
	  Acquired disorders
	    Antibodies
	    Production problems (especially of II, VII,
	      IX, X), hepatic disease, vitamin K
	      deficiency (coumadin)
	    Consumption/Dilution
	  Active factor disorders
	  Heparin
		FFP administration
		Anihemophilic factor (AHF)
		Plasmapheresis
		Vitamin K administration
		Protamine sulfate
		Cryoprecipitate administration

Disruption of clot lysis	Fibrin split products
	Abnormal fibrinolysis
	  Plasminogen activators (urokinases,
	    streptokinase)
	Increased fibrinolysis secondary to increased
	  fibrin formation
		FFP administration
		Heparin
		Amicar

Source: Adapted from Richard P. Fogdall and David P. Fishbach. (1985). *Essentials of Coagulation.* Baltimore: Williams and Wilkins. p. 115.

are replenished through the administration of stored blood and its products. Blood product replacement is determined by the patient's specific needs. For instance, when the patient has bleeding related to nonsteroidal antiinflammatory interference with platelets, replacement of platelets only may resolve the problem. When a large amount of blood has been lost and the patient is actively bleeding, all products may need to be replenished. In that case a priority for product infusion must be established. In general, blood and coagulation products should be given in the order in which the body would use them to perform clotting via its normal mechanisms of vasoconstriction, formation of a platelet plug, and formation of a fibrin clot. Thus, the ideal replacement plan would be to give platelets first, fresh-frozen plasma second, and red blood cells third. Red blood cells are the most common blood product required in critical care, but nurses must recognize that even slow bleeding, if continuous, will also deplete platelets and coagulation proteins. A list of blood products

and the indications and precautions for administering them is given in Table 8-57.

Administration of blood components exposes the patient to the risks associated with infusing a foreign protein into the body. Agglutination tests are performed to determine ABO and RH compatibility, but occasionally major antibodies such as Kell or E become apparent. More extensive antibody testing is performed through the direct Coombs test (direct antiglobulin test) and the indirect Coombs test (antibody screening test). In both tests the blood products are placed in hematology test tubes. The direct antiglobulin test detects human IgG attached to circulating red blood cells. It indicates the presence of IgG or complement, indicating an immune process. The antibody screening test detects the additional antibodies that cause transfusion reactions. Cold agglutin antibodies (antimycoplasmic antibodies) are of the IgM type and cause agglutination with the transfused blood cells when the temperature is between 0°C and 20°C. This agglutination is reversed when

Table 8-57 Blood Products

Blood Product	Description	Indications	Administration	Special Considerations
Whole blood	One 500-mL unit contains approximately 200 mL RBCs and 300 mL plasma	Massive blood loss Exchange transfusions	Large-gauge needle for administration Use 0.9% normal saline for starter fluid and flush Use blood administration set with filter pore size of 170 microns	Be certain blood is ABO and Rh compatible Monitor patient for fluid volume overload
Packed red blood cells	One 250-mL unit contains 200 mL of RBCs and 50 mL plasma	Low Hct Inadequate oxygen-carrying capacity	Same as with whole blood, but surface area of filter may be larger to increase infusion rate	Be certain blood is ABO and Rh compatible Administer within 30 minutes of receipt
Washed red blood cells, buffy cells, leukocyte-poor cells	One 200 mL unit contains 50 mL normal saline solution and has few platelets or leukocytes	History of febrile or allergic blood reactions	Same as with whole blood but microaggregate filter is not necesary	Blood comes in special bag and connections are not as tight Premedication with Tylenol or Benadryl may be recommended
Frozen deglycerized RBCs	One 200-mL unit contains 50 mL of normal saline; washed free of most WBCs and platelets	Rare blood types Special needs for oxygen-rich blood, as noncitrate preservative conserves 2,3-DPG better	Same as with red blood cells	Thawing process takes approximately 1 hour Blood reactions should be decreased, but consult physician about premedication
Plasma (fresh, fresh-frozen, single-donor)	One 200–300 mL unit of fresh-frozen plasma contains all coagulation factors plus 400 mg fibrinogen; single-donor plasma contains less of factors V and VII	Coagulation deficiencies Dysfibrinogenemia Liver disease	Allow 45 minutes for plasma to thaw May infuse rapidly Smaller needle size may be used Microaggregate filter is not used	ABO compatibility is necessary, but Rh compatibility is not Administer within 6 hours of thawing Febrile, allergic reactions are possible
Platelets	35–50 mL unit contains 7×10^7 platelets	Thrombocytopenia and thrombocytopathies Bone marrow aplasia	Use special platelet filter (not microaggregrate) Administer 100 cc over approximately 15 minutes	ABO and Rh compatibility not necessary Febrile and allergic reactions are common Obtain post-platelet count to monitor effectiveness

the cells are warmed to at least 37°C. Cold agglutins are known to be present in many conditions: lymphoma, multiple myeloma, scleroderma, Raynaud's phenomenon, hemolytic anemia, infectious mononucleosis, mycoplasmal infections, and certain viral infections. A titer greater than 1:32 indicates a positive test and requires that all blood be warmed prior to administration.

Acute antibody blood reactions fall into three categories: (1) febrile, (2) allergic, and (3) hemolytic. Febrile reactions are most common, and occur as a result of antigen-antibody reactions against the foreign RBCs, WBCs, or platelets. Fevers, chills, and flu-like symptoms are the most common presentation. Allergic reactions involving rash, pruritis, nasal rhinitis, or wheezing are another form of antibody reaction. It is usually difficult to identify the specific protein causing these reactions, and the reactions may be unavoidable if a patient must undergo frequent transfusions from multiple donors. With such patients, it is not uncommon to evaluate the first reaction but to continue giving blood products along with antiinflammatory and antiallergy medications such as Tylenol, diphenhydramine, and steroids. The hemolytic reactions are characterized by an acute intravascular hemolysis producing shock symptoms: hypotension, chest pain, hypoxemia, cyanosis, dysrhythmias, and pain at the IV site. This type of reaction is due to major ABO incompatibility and is avoidable with careful cross-matching of donor and recipient blood. These reactions are managed by immediately ceasing the blood transfusion and providing emergency support measures such as oxygen therapy, fluid resuscitation, vasopressors, and bicarbonate. The hemolyzed red blood cells produce free hemoglobin, which can cause renal failure unless renal blood flow and glomerular filtration is significantly increased. Intravenous fluids (normal saline or glucose and bicarbonate) are given at a rate of 150–300 cc/hr to enhance filtration and urine production. The alkalinity of bicarbonate solutions offers some protection against renal tubular acidosis that may enhance the risk of renal failure. Several other reactions to blood can be related to the volume of blood that is administered or to the storage preservatives in the blood. Various types of reactions are listed in Table 8-58.

Concentrated, or "packed," red blood cells (PRBCs) are given to patients who suffer from insufficient production or excessive destruction or loss of red blood cells. Patients who receive frequent transfusions will often develop chronic allergic and febrile transfusion reactions. Washed or leukocyte-poor cells may be given to reduce these reactions (see Table 8-58).

Platelets frequently produce febrile and allergic transfusion reactions. Platelets are distributed in small quantities, usually 30–60 cc/bag (the equivalent of 1 unit). Patients needing platelet transfusion usually require 6–12 units at each transfusion. If the blood is obtained from several donors, the patient is exposed to many genetic pools, which increases the likelihood of transfusion reactions. It is best to administer single-donor pooled platelets, but this requires special pheresis techniques and limits the use of general platelet stores. Platelets may also cause another rejection reaction called alloimmunization. This reaction occurs when the body recognizes the foreign protein of the donor platelets and destroys them as they are infused. It is difficult to predict who will develop this syndrome, but it may become life-threatening when it occurs. Patients who experience alloimmunization require genetically matched, or HLA matched, platelets. This necessitates HLA typing of family members or accessing a public HLA platelet donor program. Because of the risk of this disorder, all patients receiving platelet transfusions should receive a post-platelet count approximately 1 hour after the conclusion of the transfusion.[142] This will determine the boost achieved by the platelets. An infusion of 6 units should boost a platelet count by approximately 20,000/mm^3.[143]

Fresh-frozen plasma (FFP) contains all coagulation proteins made by the liver and is harvested from a donor. In the freezing process, factor VIII is decomposed and thus is not replenished during transfusion of this product. Factor VIII is replaced by administration of cryoprecipitate. This product is concentrated by pooling factor VIII from over 1,000 donors and thus provides a slightly higher risk of transmission of viral diseases (hepatitis or HIV). Cryoprecipitate is indicated in cases of severe bleeding requiring transfusions of over 10 units of blood or when bleeding persists after FFP replacement. A form of factor VIII used by hemophiliacs, called antihemophilic factor (AHF), is a specially formulated cryoprecipitate that can be stored in the freezer and used at home. Patients who have received 6–10 units of blood over several days to a week are likely to have also lost coagulation factors and will need FFP. FFP is also used in hepatic failure to replace proteins no longer being made by the liver and as an antidote for excessive thrombolytic agents (streptokinase or TPA).

Any or all of these blood products may be used in the management of the patient with coagulopathy. When bleeding is mild but continuous, intermittent administration of blood products does not present special problems. However, when blood products are infused rapidly in response to hemorrhage, reactions to massive product administration and the products' preservatives can occur. The types of reactions that can result from massive transfusions are listed in Table 8-58.

Local management of bleeding When a patient is actively bleeding and blood products have not effec-tively induced clotting, local measures to control bleeding may be required. Pressure on the site of bleeding may be used when the site is known or when bleeding occurs from only a few sites. Compression or tamponade on the site can be accomplished with a Blakemore tube for GI bleeding, tourniquets, MAST trousers, sandbags over new surgical wounds, or manual compression after venipuncture.

Table 8-58 Blood Transfusion Reactions

Type of Reaction	Cause	Signs and Symptoms	Treatment	Prevention
Immediate Reactions Hemolytic	ABO or Rh incompatibility Intradonor incompatibility Improper storage	Shaking, chills, fever, nausea, vomiting, chest pain, dyspnea, hypotension, oliguria, hemoglobinuria, flank pain, abnormal bleeding; may progress to shock and/or renal failure	Stop transfusion; maintain IV access; monitor blood pressure; treat shock as indicated by patient condition using intravenous fluids, oxygen, epinephrine, diuretics, and vasopressors; obtain post-transfusion blood and urine samples for evaluation; observe patient for signs of hemorrhage resulting from DIC	Proper identification of donor and recipient blood types to make sure blood is compatible and accurate patient identification before transfusion; transfuse blood slowly for first 15–20 minutes; observe patient closely for the first 20 minutes of the transfusion
Febrile	Presence of bacterial lipopolysaccharides	Fever, chills, rigor, headache, flank pain	Stop transfusion; provide symptomatic relief with antipyretic, antihistamine, or Demerol	Premedicate patient before blood transfusion with antipyretic, antihistamine, and possibly steroids; use leukocyte-poor or washed blood products
Allergic	Recipient reacts to allergen in donor's blood	Pruritis, urticaria, fever, chills, nausea, vomiting, facial swelling, wheezing, laryngeal edema; reaction may progress to anaphylactic reaction	Stop transfusion; administer antihistamines; monitor patient for anaphylactic reaction and administer epinephrine and steroids if indicated	Give antihistamines as a premedication to patients with a history of allergic reactions; observe patient closely for the first 20 minutes of the transfusion
Plasma protein incompatibility	IgA incompatibility	Flushing, abdominal pain, diarrhea, chills, fever, dyspnea, hypotension	Treat patient for shock by administering oxygen, fluids, epinephrine, and possibly steroids as ordered	Transfuse only IgA-deficient blood or well washed red cells

(continued)

Table 8-58   Blood Transfusion Reactions (*continued*)

Type of Reaction	Cause	Signs and Symptoms	Treatment	Prevention
Reaction to bacterial contamination	Presence of gram-negative organisms, which can survive cold (e.g., certain species of Pseudomonas)	Chills, fever, vomiting, abdominal cramping, diarrhea, shock, renal failure	Stop transfusion; treat patient with broad-spectrum antibiotics and steroids	Observe blood before transfusion for gas, clots, and dark purple color; use air-free, touch-free method to draw and deliver blood; maintain strict storage control; change blood tubing and filter every four hours; infuse each unit of blood over 2 to 4 hours but terminate the infusion after four hours; maintain sterile techniques when administering blood products
Circulatory overload	Too rapid or too large an infusion	Dyspnea, chest tightness, dry cough, distended neck veins, crackles, pulmonary edema on chest x-ray	Stop transfusion; place patient in semi-Fowler's position; possibly administer oxygen, diuretics, or rotating tourniquets	Transfuse blood slowly; avoid use of whole blood; administer diuretics before giving transfusions to patients at risk for circulatory overload
Air embolism	Air in bloodstream via blood tubing	Sudden shortness of breath, sharp chest pain, anxiety, coughing, hypotension	Turn patient on left side; administer 100% oxygen by face mask; treat patient for shock if this develops	Expel air from tubing before starting the infusion; do not allow blood bag to run dry; observe for air in tubing when infusing under pressure
Reactions to multiple transfusions Hemosiderosis	Increased hemosiderin (iron-containing pigment) from red blood cell destruction	Iron plasma level greater than 200 mg per 100 mL	Perform phlebotomy to remove excess iron	Administer blood only when absolutely necessary
Bleeding tendencies	Low platelet count in stored blood, causing dilutional thrombocytopenia	Abnormal bleeding and oozing from cut or break in skin surface	Administer platelets; monitor platelet count	Use only fresh blood that is less than 7 days old when possible

Table 8-58 *(continued)*

Type of Reaction	Cause	Signs and Symptoms	Treatment	Prevention
Increased oxygen affinity for hemoglobin	A decreased level of 2,3-DPG in stored blood causing an increase in the oxygen's affinity for hemoglobin; oxygen stays in the patient's bloodstream and isn't released into tissues	Depressed respiratory rate, especially in patients with chronic lung disease who depend on their low oxygen level to breathe	Monitor arterial blood gas lab results and give respiratory support as needed	Use only red blood cells or fresh blood if possible
Elevated blood ammonia level	An increased level of ammonia in stored blood	Forgetfulness, confusion	Monitor patient's ammonia level; decrease the amount of protein in the diet; if indicated give neomycin sulfate	Use only red blood cells, fresh-frozen plasma, or blood stored less than 7 days, especially if patient has hepatic disease
Hypothermia	Rapid infusion of large amounts of cold blood, which decreases myocardial temperature	Shaking, chills, hypotension, ventricular fibrillation, cardiac arrest if core temperature falls below 30°C	Stop transfusion; warm the patient with blankets; obtain ECG	Warm blood to 35°–37°C, especially before massive transfusions
Hypocalcemia	Citrate toxicity occurs when citrate-treated blood is infused rapidly; citrate binds with calcium, causing a calcium deficiency, or, normal citrate metabolism is hindered by hepatic disease	Tingling in fingers, muscle cramps, nausea, vomiting, hypotension, cardiac arrhythmias, convulsions, hypokalemia	Slow or stop transfusion, depending on reaction; slowly administer calcium gluconate I.V.; note that reaction may be worse in hypothermia patients or patients with elevated potassium levels	Infuse blood slowly; monitor potassium and calcium levels; use blood less than two weeks old if multiple units are to be given
Potassium intoxication	An abnormally high level of potassium in stored plasma caused by red cell lysis	ECG changes with tall, peaked T waves; bradycardia proceeding to cardiac standstill, intestinal colic, diarrhea, muscle twitching, oliguria, renal failure	Obtain ECG: administer kayexalate orally or by enema	Use fresh blood (less than one week old) when massive amounts of blood are to be given
Renal Failure				

Source: Haisfield, M. E. (1990). Blood transfusions and reactions. Baltimore: Johns Hopkins Hospital.

When immediate pressure on the area is unsuccessful, hemostatic agents on the site may enhance clotting. Some hemostatic agents and key indications for their use are listed in Table 8-59.

The management of patients with coagulopathies can be extremely complex and labor-intensive. Unfortunately, management techniques have not been perfected, and critically ill patients do die of bleeding disorders. The best treatment for coagulopathy is prevention.

Table 8-59 Management of Local Bleeding

Agent	Indications	Application
Absorbable gelatin sponge (Gelfoam)	Puncture wounds (as with venipuncture or bone marrow or tooth extraction)	Saturate foam wafers with isotonic saline or thrombin solution; apply pressure to site with sponge for 10–15 seconds; keep sponge in place after bleeding is controlled
Ice	Bleeding from large vessel Hemarthrosis	Apply ice pack to the site until bleeding subsides
Microfibrillar collagen hemostat (Avitene)	As adjunct to surgery For wounds to skin or soft tissue	Compress area with dry sponges; apply agent with smooth dry forceps to bleeding site for 1–5 minutes (amount of agent used depends on severity of bleeding); remove excess agent and repeat procedure as needed
Negatol (Negatan)	Cervical bleeding (used frequently with von Willebrand's disease)	Insert 1-inch gauze packing dipped in 10% solution of agent into cervical canal (agent may be used full strength if patient tolerates it); remove packing after 24 hours and give a douche of 2 mL dilute negatol or vinegar
	Oral ulcers	Apply agent to dried oral lesions with applicator; neutralize the negatol solution with large amounts of water
Oxidized cellulose (Oxycel, Surgicel)	As adjunct to surgery External bleeding at tumor sites Oral bleeding Bleeding surrounding IV lines	Apply using sterile technique (hemostatic effect is greater if agent is applied dry); irrigate oxidized cellulose before removing to avoid initiating fresh bleeding; remove with sterile forceps; cellulose may be left in place if necessary
Thrombin (Fibrindex, Thrombinar)	Bleeding from parenchymal tissue, cancerous bone, dental, nasal, or laryngeal surgery, plastic surgery, or skin graft procedures	Apply 100 units per mL of sterile isotonic saline solution or sterile distilled water to bleeding site (agent may be applied in powder form to "brush burns" on skin); for major bleeding use 1000–2000 units/mL sterile isotonic saline; sponge blood from site before application, but avoid sponging the site after application (note: agent may be used with absorbable gelatin sponge but not with oxidized cellulose)
	GI hemorrhage	Give patient 60 mL (2 oz) of milk, followed by 60 mL of milk containing 10,000–20,000 units of thrombin; repeat three times daily for 4–5 days or until bleeding is controlled

Hypercoagulable states As with coagulopathy, the best management of thromboses is the use of appropriate preventive techniques. Patients on bedrest should perform range-of-motion exercises of the legs and hips either with assistance or independently. Postoperative patients can wear venous compression stockings (also called sequential compression devices), which massage the peripheral veins and assist the return of blood to the heart. Other measures to promote venous return and reduce edema of the extremities include elevating the feet, keeping the legs uncrossed, and encouraging patients to ambulate early in the postoperative period. Antiplatelet medications such as aspirin or persantine can be used to prevent thromboses.

Both preventive and therapeutic management of deep-vein thrombosis (DVT) may include anticoagulation therapy. High-risk patients, such as abdominal or orthopedic surgical patients, may receive 5000 units of prophylactic heparin twice a day. When a DVT is suspected or confirmed, anticoagulation therapy is increased to achieve a PTT that is 1.25–2.5 times normal. (The wide range reflects research indicating lower-level anticoagulation may be equally effective in preventing thrombotic complications of disease.)

Patients with multiple or recurrent thrombi despite anticoagulation therapy may be candidates for vena caval interruption to prevent the thrombi from embolizing and traveling to the lungs or brain.

The nursing care of the patient with a bleeding disorder is pivotal in reducing morbidity and mortality. Bleeding disorders are commonly created by treatment of other problems and may be reversed if detected early. Nursing assessment of risk factors, high-risk bleeding sites, and response to treatment is an important part of patient management. Nursing priorities and care guidelines are given in the nursing care plan that accompanies the following section on disseminated intravascular coagulation.

Disseminated Intravascular Coagulation

Disseminated intravascular coagulation (DIC) is a consumptive coagulopathy in which hemorrhage is paradoxically combined with widespread thrombosis. DIC is not a primary disease; rather, it is a secondary syndrome occurring as a complication of a diverse group of disorders, all of which result in activation of the clotting cascade. Other names for this disorder are hypofibrinogenemia, defibrination syndrome, and secondary fibrinolysis.

In essence, DIC stems from a loss of the normal balance between clot formation and clot dissolution. This loss of balance causes activation of systemic fibrin formation and acceleration of fibrinolysis. As a consequence, both profound hemorrhage and disseminated thrombosis occur. Although microembolization of major organs is a hallmark of the disease, bleeding is the most prominent clinical manifestation of DIC.[144] DIC can range in severity from a subacute form to a mild, chronic condition or an acute, fulminating process. In the acute form of DIC, cerebral hemorrhage is the most common cause of death.[145]

Clinical antecedents

Since DIC represents a loss of balance between the clot formation and the clot dissolution processes, any stimulation of normal clotting mechanisms may enhance or accelerate DIC, including tissue injury (extrinsic pathway), vascular endothelial injury (intrinsic pathway), or the presence of a foreign body in the bloodstream (intrinsic pathway).

Four general health problems predispose patients to the risk of developing DIC: hypotension, stagnant blood flow, hypoxemia, and acidosis. In turn, these factors are themselves associated with complex, multisystem clinical conditions such as shock, sepsis, and trauma.[146]

In DIC, the factors triggering the coagulation cascade are rarely single or independent. Instead, "in most forms of DIC, the initiating factors are multiple and interrelated."[147] For example, the endotoxins of gram-negative sepsis can activate several steps in the coagulation cascade. Endotoxins can injure the vascular endothelium and activate factor VIII (thus activating the intrinsic pathway), cause the release of tissue factors called procoagulants into the circulation (activating the extrinsic pathway), or increase platelet adherence as well as platelet and WBC aggregation (activating the common pathway). A summary of the more common precipitating factors for DIC is given in Table 8-60; the pathophysiology of the process is diagrammed in Figure 8-19.

Critical referents

Critical to an understanding of DIC is an appreciation of the key role of excess thrombin production in this process. Thrombin performs many functions in both clot formation and clot dissolution (see Table

Table 8-60 Precipitators of DIC

Portion of Coagulation Cascade	Precipitating Factor	Source of Injury
Intrinsic pathway	Injury to or alteration of vascular endothelium	Hyperthermia, heat stroke Endotoxins Viremia Shock Anoxia Transfusion of incompatible blood Antigen-antibody complexes Amniotic fluid embolism
Extrinsic pathway	Entry into circulation of procoagulant released from damaged tissue	Traumatized tissue: massive musculoskeletal trauma, brain trauma, or surgical trauma (especially prostate surgery) Neoplastic tissue carcinomas (especially of the lung, breast, prostate, pancreas, or brain) or leukemias (especially APL) Placental tissue: intrauterine fetal death or abruptio placentae
Common pathway	Platelet adherence to abnormal vascular endothelium or aggregates of platelets or WBCs stimulate fibrinogen or prothrombin	Proteolytic enzymes: snake venom, trypsin (in acute pancreatitis) Phospholipid release via platelet/RBC hemolysis or injury Thromboxane release from aggregated platelets

8-61).[148] Thrombin's primary role in clot formation is to convert fibrinogen to fibrin. In DIC an excessive amount of thrombin is formed. This overproduction of thrombin has two different effects: overactivation of the coagulation cascade and activation of systemic fibrinolysis. The overactivation of the coagulation cascade by thrombin causes formation of excess fibrin. This fibrin is deposited into the microvasculature in the form of microthrombi. The excessive fibrin formation also consumes platelets (resulting in thrombocytopenia) as well as clotting factors (especially fibrinogen, prothrombin, and factors V, VIII, and XIII). The thrombin-generated fibrinolysis prevents stable clots from forming and aids in the dissolution of existing clots. The deficiencies of platelets and clotting factors exacerbate this process. The excessive thrombin formation in DIC is self-sustaining in that (1) thrombin has the ability to cleave prothrombin to produce still more thrombin and (2) the excessive levels of thrombin overwhelm the levels of antithrombin, thrombin's chief inhibitor. The end result is widespread or generalized activation of the coagulation system leading to the formation of large amounts of circulating thrombin, subsequent clotting, excessive fibrinolysis, and circulating anticoagulants.

Researchers have identified three distinct phases of DIC. Since DIC is a dynamic process, these phases may occur simultaneously. The three phases of DIC are the thrombotic, the fibrinolytic, and the reactional lysis phases.

Phase 1: thrombosis The early thrombotic phase of DIC is manifested by a brief period of hypercoagulability. During this phase, the coagulation cascade is initiated, resulting in widespread fibrin formation. Microthrombi are deposited throughout the microcirculation. Clinical evidence of this stage may be absent or subtle, perhaps consisting only of clotted central venous catheters, mottling of extremities, or oliguria.

Phase 2: fibrinolysis The fibrinolytic phase of DIC is marked by hypocoagulability. The fibrin formed during phase 1 consumes tremendous amounts of clotting factors and platelets. Simultaneously, thrombin and other factors convert plasminogen to plasmin, thereby activating fibrinolysis. Fibrinolysis results in the production of fibrin degradation products (FDPs), which are themselves antihemostatic. The severity of this phase may be enhanced by the coexistence of hepatic failure, as the liver is responsible for clearing the body of FDPs. Thus, phase 2 is a hemorrhagic phase that coexists with the previous hypercoagulable phase.

Phase 3: reactional lysis Fibrin threads in the microcirculation trap and damage platelets, erythro-

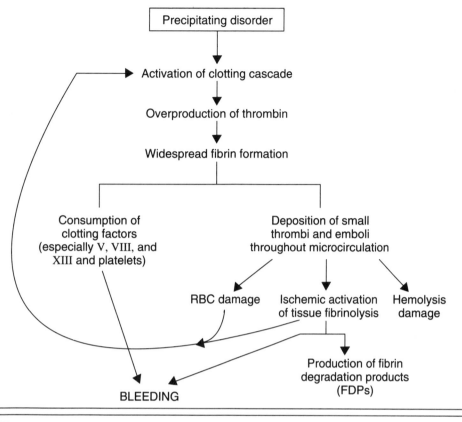

Figure 8-19 Pathophysiology of DIC

cytes, and leukocytes. Anemia, thrombocytopenia, and even leukopenia may result from this damage. Examination of peripheral blood may reveal the presence of schistocytes or platelet fragments.[149] The damaged blood cells also release heparin, catecholamines, and vasoactive peptides, which sustain the abnormal coagulation process. Excessive cell lysis may also produce hyperkalemia, hypercalcemia, and

acidosis if the kidneys are dysfunctional and unable to excrete the lysis byproducts. During phase 3 the complement and kallikrein systems are activated by factor XII (intrinsic pathway). Infection, anoxia, shock, ARDS, and amniotic fluid embolism can all activate the kinin system. Complement factors and any bradykinin formed will maintain the vasodilatory, hypotensive effects and blood cell destruction.

Table 8-61 Functions of Thrombin in the Coagulation Cascade

Function	Mechanism
Promote clot formation	Stimulates platelet aggregation Activates factors V, VIII, and XIII Converts fibrinogen to fibrin
Block clot formation	Activates protein C to inactivate Factors V and VIII Blocks the intrinsic and common pathways of the coagulation cascade
Initiate fibrinolysis	Stimulates release of TPA to initiate fibrinolysis

Resulting signs and symptoms

DIC can manifest as an acute and life-threatening process, or it can be a mild, chronic condition. Chronic DIC is most often associated with cancer and requires monitoring and limited intervention. DIC must be differentiated from a number of other conditions, including liver disease with portal hypertension, which can produce coagulation defects that mimic those found in DIC but are usually less severe. Because of the different degrees of severity of DIC, the mortality rate from the condition is quite variable. Conscientious monitoring of patients at risk can reveal early symptoms of DIC and enhance early treatment.

DIC can produce numerous complications primarily as a result of hemorrhage into an organ. A summary of these unfortunate consequences is given in Table 8-62. DIC is often suspected as the cause of clinical catastrophes related to clotting, but such suspicions usually remain unconfirmed due to the complex nature of this disorder. Even when DIC is suspected, the nurse should still assess the patient for thrombotic complications such as cerebrovascular accident, myocardial infarction, and pulmonary embolism. The most important point to remember in regard to DIC is that *it occurs secondary to an underlying process.* Therefore, the treatment of DIC requires removal or resolution of the underlying disease.[150]

The symptoms of DIC relate to hemorrhagic phenomena and the development of microemboli in organ systems, especially in the lungs, kidneys, and GI tract. Clinically, DIC is frequently first evidenced by signs of mucocutaneous capillary rupture, such as petechiae, purpura, ecchymosis, gingival bleeding, and occult or trace blood in body excretions. Petechiae may occur at sites of minor trauma or bruising and are often found at the site of BP cuff application. These cutaneous manifestations of DIC are highly visible and may progress to severe symptoms such as hemorrhagic bullae or wound hematomas.

Severe microcirculatory clotting may first manifest itself in cutaneous presentations as well. Extremities may appear cold, mottled, and cyanotic. Acrocyanosis (demarcation cyanosis) may occur, especially at the tips of the ears, nose, fingers, toes, and even the genitalia. In this condition, the involved tissue is separated from healthier tissue by a line of demarcation and may necrose, leading to gangrene. Such cutaneous symptoms indicate that the process of microcirculatory clotting and tissue anoxia of the organs has already begun. Clinical manifestation are initially subtle but may include sleepiness, slightly

inappropriate behavior or personality changes, oliguria, and subjective respiratory symptoms. Prolonged bleeding from venipuncture sites and incisions is a hallmark of DIC, and bleeding often progresses until it involves multiple areas including body orifices (nose, mouth, and rectum). The bleeding in DIC is noteworthy because the application of direct pressure to the bleeding site does not produce hemostasis. This is because all clotting factors (platelets, clotting factors, and fibrinogen) are depleted, so neither a platelet plug nor a fibrin clot can be formed. As bleeding continues, the process of fibrin deposition into the microvasculature results in decreased tissue perfusion and vasospasm in target organs and peripheral tissues.

Physical findings with DIC can be classified into two major categories: those produced by bleeding diathesis and those related to microthrombi formation. The onset of bleeding symptoms is more often acute and severe; microthrombi produce a progressive organ failure. Key differences are outlined in Table 8-63.

It is essential for nurses to perform frequent, thorough, multisystem assessments on patients with DIC, as symptoms vary and may change rapidly. Neurologic assessment may be most crucial, since intracranial hemorrhage is the most common cause of death in these patients.[151] Neurologically, DIC may cause headache, restlessness, malaise, or even a change in affect or mood. Microvascular thrombi produce cerebral anoxia and dysfunction, but intracranial bleeds are more likely to manifest as central brain dysfunction. Therefore, it is important to assess baseline personality, decision-making ability, and thought processes as well as motor strength and level of consciousness. All DIC patients should be considered at high risk for increased intracranial pressure. Key assessment parameters are outlined in the nursing care plan at the end of this section.

Blurred vision and conjunctival or retinal hemorrhages are ocular manifestations of DIC. Retinal hemorrhages may be difficult to diagnose because of patient confusion or unresponsiveness. Most hemorrhages do not produce permanent loss of vision.

The cardiovascular indications of DIC are tachycardia, hypotension, and nonspecific ischemic ST changes on the ECG. Pulmonary artery pressures may also be elevated as a result of microthrombi in the pulmonary circulation. The inflammatory mediators usually produce some vasodilation, so the patient with DIC is likely to have wide pulse pressures with low diastolic BP and a low systemic vascular resistance (SVR). Pathophysiological pulmonary changes can result in tachypnea, orthopnea, dyspnea, hemoptysis, and hemorrhage, eventually pro-

Table 8-62 Complications of DIC

Body System	Complication
Neurological	Intracerebral hemorrhage Seizures Coma
Ocular	Retinal or conjunctival hemorrhage
Pulmonary	Pulmonary hemorrhage ARDS
GI	GI hemorrhage
Renal	Acute tubular necrosis
Cutaneous	Acrocyanosis Gangrene

Table 8-63 Clinical Presentation of Bleeding and Clotting in DIC

System	Symptoms Associated with Bleeding	Symptoms Associated with Microthrombi Formation
CNS	CVA or intracerebral bleed	Confusion, restlessness, embolic or ischemic CVA
Pulmonary	Hemoptysis, ARDS	Hypoxemia, atelectasis
Renal	Hematuria	Oliguria Elevated BUN and creatinine
Skin	Petechiae, purpura, ecchymosis, hematoma Oozing from venipuncture sites	Acrocyanosis, gangrene

ducing cyanosis from hypoxia. Pulmonary thrombi and hemorrhage also serve to worsen the V/Q mismatch. Atelectactic alveoli produce diminished breath sounds, but blood-filled alveoli produce pulmonary crackles on exam. A chest x-ray will reflect diffuse infiltrates if pulmonary hemorrhage is occurring.

Gastrointestinal involvement in DIC is manifested by nausea, vomiting, and abdominal pain. Bleeding may range from Hematest-positive nasogastric drainage to hematemesis. GI bleeding, rectal bleeding, or hematochezia may be present, and these symptoms are particularly resistant to traditional therapies such as histamine-2 blockers, antacids, and topical therapies. When mild GI bleeding occurs, it may be attributable to the proximity of blood vessels to the mucosal surface; such bleeding is self-limiting with supportive treatment and elimination of DIC's underlying cause. Severe GI bleeding indicates additional GI pathology such as ulceration. These patients must receive generous blood and coagulation support, as surgery is contraindicated and cautery is technically difficult with diffuse bleeding.

Renal involvement in DIC is both common and serious. Reduced urine output or oliguria may occur and may result in azotemia or even elevated serum creatinine. Acute tubular necrosis (ATN) has been noted with DIC. Hematuria or bleeding from the bladder or urethra may also be present. Severe back pain at the level of the kidney is cause for alarm, since it may represent renal hemorrhage. A renal ultrasound or an intravenous pyelogram will differentiate between renal hemorrhage and retroperitoneal hematoma. Ecchymoses of the back, another common cutaneous manifestation of DIC, are more common with retroperitoneal hematoma.

Persons with DIC may experience severe muscle and joint pain related to spontaneous hemorrhage within the tissue. As no specific precipitating factors have been identified for this occurrence, no preventive plan can be developed.

There is virtually no end to the potential clinical consequences of DIC. Because of recent improvements in life-support technology, many patients with DIC live through these severe, life-threatening complications, only to die from multisystem organ failure (MSOF). The most likely clinical findings with DIC are shown in Figure 8-20. Many of these are indicators of both clotting and bleeding, reinforcing the importance of evaluating each patient's situation for the overall presentation and severity before designing a plan of care.

Diagnostic tests DIC is diagnosed by a combination of clinical findings and laboratory tests. Clinical findings of bleeding and thrombosis have already been discussed. A diagnosis of DIC is supported by four distinctive abnormal conditions, revealed by laboratory tests: (1) thrombocytopenia, (2) low fibrinogen levels, (3) markedly elevated fibrin degradation products, and (4) prolonged clotting times. The chronology of the diagnostic tests usually follows the pattern of factor utilization during clotting.

A CBC with platelet count and a coagulation profile are usually the first tests used to diagnose DIC. Platelet counts are frequently low in DIC, because platelets are the first clotting factor involved in clot formation. In fact, 50% of all patients with DIC have platelet counts of less than 50,000/mm^3.[152] Fibrinogen levels are also low in DIC due to the process of clot formation. In fact, from 45% to 70% of patients with DIC have fibrinogen levels of less than 150 mg/dL.[153] One of the newer tests that measures intrinsic thrombin inhibitors is the antithrombin 3 test.[154] In DIC, massive thrombin production early in the disease process depletes the body's supply, resulting in lowered levels of antithrombin 3. All of these tests are tests of absolute quantity of the factors used in the clotting process; therefore, results on these tests may be abnormal in the first phase of DIC, when clinical symptoms are often not yet present.

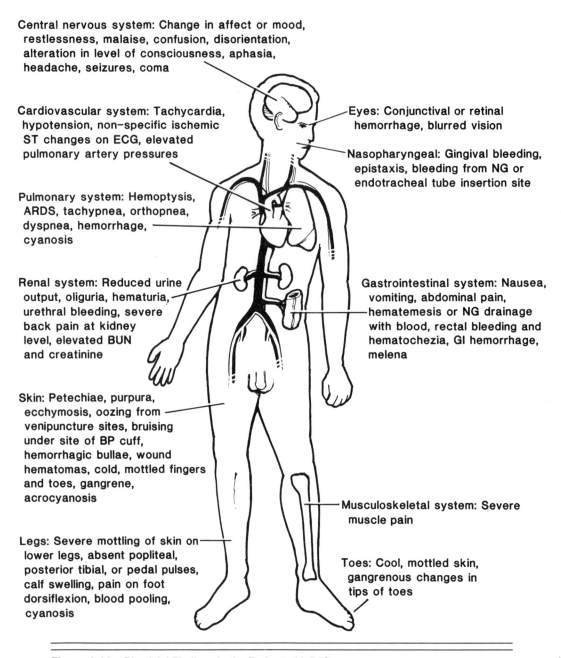

Central nervous system: Change in affect or mood, restlessness, malaise, confusion, disorientation, alteration in level of consciousness, aphasia, headache, seizures, coma

Cardiovascular system: Tachycardia, hypotension, non–specific ischemic ST changes on ECG, elevated pulmonary artery pressures

Pulmonary system: Hemoptysis, ARDS, tachypnea, orthopnea, dyspnea, hemorrhage, cyanosis

Renal system: Reduced urine output, oliguria, hematuria, urethral bleeding, severe back pain at kidney level, elevated BUN and creatinine

Skin: Petechiae, purpura, ecchymosis, oozing from venipuncture sites, bruising under site of BP cuff, hemorrhagic bullae, wound hematomas, cold, mottled fingers and toes, gangrene, acrocyanosis

Legs: Severe mottling of skin on lower legs, absent popliteal, posterior tibial, or pedal pulses, calf swelling, pain on foot dorsiflexion, blood pooling, cyanosis

Eyes: Conjunctival or retinal hemorrhage, blurred vision

Nasopharyngeal: Gingival bleeding, epistaxis, bleeding from NG or endotracheal tube insertion site

Gastrointestinal system: Nausea, vomiting, abdominal pain, hematemesis or NG drainage with blood, rectal bleeding and hematochezia, GI hemorrhage, melena

Musculoskeletal system: Severe muscle pain

Toes: Cool, mottled skin, gangrenous changes in tips of toes

Figure 8-20   Physicial Findings in the Patient with DIC

Coagulation tests of the intrinsic and final pathways yield elevated clotting times only when the patient has deficiencies of certain clotting factors. For this reason, the tests may only become abnormal later in the disease process. Tests in this category include thrombin time, prothrombin time, and partial thromboplastin time. The thrombin time is highly sensitive for thrombin inhibitors such as heparin, kinin, and fibrin degradation products. Since these are evidence of excessive fibrinolysis, elevations in thrombin time are likely to indicate DIC. Some clinicians assert that thrombin time is the most sensitive

test for DIC. The widespread use of thrombin inhibitors (heparin, streptokinase) for intravenous line maintenance with many critically ill patients negates the use of the thrombin time as a diagnostic test for DIC. The prothrombin time (PT) tests the extrinsic pathway coagulation response. When vitamin K–dependent factors are not absorbed through the GI tract, or are inhibited by specific medications such as coumarin derivatives, the PT will become elevated. This test is moderately sensitive, becoming abnormal when small reductions of available factors have occurred. The partial thromboplastin time (PTT) tests the intrinsic and common pathways, particularly for the presence of factors V, VIII, and IX. Unfortunately, large quantities (as much as 50–75% of factor VIII) of these factors must be missing before this test becomes abnormal.[155]

The tests considered most diagnostic of DIC are tests of fibrinolysis. Fibrin degradation products (FDPs) in the circulating serum are markedly elevated since the clots formed in DIC are unstable; they may also become elevated when the liver is unable to clear them, either because of primary hepatic failure or because excessive quantities are produced after severe injury and clot formation. The d-dimer test is a new immunofluorescence test that evaluates FDPs for the presence of a special molecule, the d-dimer. Its presence helps differentiate normal clot breakdown products from those seen in DIC. The d-dimer is present in large quantities in patients with DIC.[156]

Other laboratory tests that become abnormal relate to the consequences of massive clotting or cell breakdown. The bleeding associated with DIC produces low red blood cell counts, hematocrit (hct), and hemoglobin (Hgb) levels. Reticulocyte counts may be increased as the body tries to compensate for anemia by early release of immature RBCs from the bone marrow. Schistocytes are fragmented RBCs, which may be noted in the peripheral blood during DIC. They are formed when RBCs are trapped in the fibrin thrombi and thus fragmented. Tissue necrosis from the thrombosis of DIC elevates LDH, CPK, potassium, phosphate, and uric acid levels, while renal complications elevate blood urea nitrogen (BUN) and serum creatinine. Other tests such as ECGs and radiographic studies (chest x-ray, CAT scan, and IVP) determine the presence of thrombotic or hemorrhagic complications of DIC. Table 8-64 summarizes the various diagnostic tests used for DIC.

Nursing standards of care

The primary goal in the treatment of DIC is to restore normal hemostasis.[157] Clinical symptoms and laboratory tests aid in identifying the specific hematological defects that must be corrected. Any treatment plan has three objectives:

1. Correct the primary or underlying disorder if possible (for example, prompt delivery of dead fetus and placenta or administration of IV antibiotics for sepsis).
2. Control the major symptoms, either bleeding or thrombosis:
   a. stop hemorrhage;
   b. terminate the accelerated coagulation process;
   c. minimize development of microthrombi;
   d. resolve established thrombi.
3. Provide prophylaxis to prevent recurrence of the disorder.

These objectives are common to the treatment of all forms of DIC, but the specific treatment will depend on the clinical presentation of the syndrome. Various treatments may be employed, from the parenteral replacement of clotting factors to the administration of anticoagulants. Correction of the primary underlying disorder is the foremost consideration, providing that life-threatening complications are not evident. Most clinicians advocate treating the most likely etiology of DIC, even if it is unconfirmed. For instance, a patient newly diagnosed with acute progranulocytic leukemia may exhibit signs and symptoms of DIC that can be confused with those of sepsis or thrombocytopenia. In recognition of the prevalence of DIC in cases of leukemia, the primary focus will be on leukemia treatment (although broad-spectrum antibiotics may be administered even without confirmed culture results).

The most problematic and immediate of major symptoms are likely to be hemorrhagic in nature. If bleeding is the major problem, replace depleted clotting factors with transfusions of platelets, fresh-frozen plasma, and cryoprecipitate. Repletion should be organized to give platelets first, as these are the body's first requisites for clot formation. Administration of red blood cells prior to replacement of clotting factors may lead to loss of transfused products from existing hemorrhage sites. The critical care nurse should be well versed in the specifics of blood administration and aware of the indications, method of administration, and symptoms of adverse reactions. (Refer to Tables 8-57 and 8-58 for listings of the most common blood components and the clinical indications, side effects, and pertinent nursing implications of various transfusion reactions.) The typical patient with DIC will require the transfusion of 8–10 units of platelets, 4–6 units of fresh-frozen plasma, and 10–20 bags of cryoprecipitate.[158]

External bleeding presents many challenges for the critical care nurse. While attempting to treat the underlying problem and replace lost blood components, the nurse must simultaneously take steps to halt the patient's symptomatic bleeding. Topical agents used may include Gelfoam, topical thrombin (Avitene) or oxidized cellulose (Surgicel, Oxacel) (see Table 8-59). The choice of agent may depend upon the nature of the bleeding (for example, puncture site

Table 8-64 Summary of Diagnostic Test Abnormalities in DIC

Laboratory Test	Normal Range	Test Values in DIC	Comments
Prothrombin time (PT)	12–15 seconds	More than 15 seconds or more than 5 seconds over patient's baseline or 4 seconds more than control or two times control	PT is prolonged in over 90% of DIC patients PT is twice the control in over 70% of DIC patients
Activated partial thromboplastin time (APTT or PTT)	26–32 seconds	Greater than 60–80 seconds or more than 10 seconds over patient's baseline or control or greater than 1.25 times control	Limited sensitivity
Thrombin time (TT)	10–15 seconds	20–40 seconds	Excessively sensitive
Fibrinogen	150–350 mg/dL	Less than 150 mg/dL	Fibrinogen levels are less than 150 mg/dL in 45–70% of DIC patients
Fibrin degradation products (FDPs)	Less than 10 mcg/mL or positive at ≤ 1:100 dilution	Greater than 40–100 mcg/mL or positive at > 1:100 dilution	May also be elevated in hepatic dysfunction
d-dimer	Positive at ≤ 1:8 dilution	Positive at > 1:8 dilution	Specific for fibrin monomer in DIC
Antithrombin 3	100%	Less than 70%	Decreased in 80% of DIC patients
Ethanol test	Negative	Positive: 1+ and 3+	Also known as the "protamine sulfate test"
Platelets	150,000–400,000/mm^3	Less than 150,000/mm^3	Usually earliest abnormality
RBC	4–8 million cells/mm^3	Decreased	Normal values vary with age and gender
RBC morphology		Schistocytes	Also known as echinocytes, helmet cells, burr cells, or crenated RBCs
Reticulocytes	2–4%	>4%	
Hgb	10–14 mg/dL	Decreased	Normal values vary with age and gender
Hct	35–45%	Decreased	Normal values vary with age and gender

versus skin abrasion) or availability of products. Gelfoam is particularly effective with puncture wounds. It is used in conjunction with direct pressure to the area. Topical thrombin in most versatile and can be used either as a reconstituted fluid (for example, in nasal packing or hard-to-access locations) or as a powder (for skin abrasions or at indwelling vascular catheter exit sites). Carafate may be used to coat the stomach lining and reduce risk of future ulceration. Although not a topical hemostat, Carafate may assist in healing or protecting the highly sensitive gastrointestinal lining.

Antithrombin therapy is also considered in some cases of DIC. Theoretically, blocking activation of thrombin has a threefold effect:

1. it reduces clot formation;
2. it reduces consumption of clotting factors; and
3. it reduces activation of the fibrinolytic system.

There are two primary antithrombin agents: antithrombin 3 and heparin.

Antithrombin 3, a potent inhibitor of thrombin formation, is consumed during DIC. Theoretically, replacing antithrombin 3 reverses the consumptive coagulopathy of DIC. A concentrated preparation of antithrombin 3 has been used in Europe for the treatment of DIC but is not available in the United States.[159]

Heparin is an effective antithrombin agent and has been used for this purpose in the treatment of DIC. "Heparin markedly accelerates the rate at which antithrombin 3 neutralizes [both] thrombin and activated factor X."[160] This action blocks the coagulation cascade at the common pathway and ultimately prevents conversion of fibrinogen to fibrin. Despite its antithrombin effect, the administration of heparin in the treatment of DIC is controversial. Some studies promote its use; other studies report that its administration resulted in increased hemorrhage and fatalities.[161] The use of heparin has been recommended in selected cases such as obstetrical emergencies and cases of acute promyelocytic leukemia.[162] Overall, the use of heparin is probably best reserved for two groups of patients: (1) patients in whom the primary problem in DIC is thrombin

formation rather than bleeding, and (2) patients who continue to bleed despite adequate replacement of platelets and fresh-frozen plasma.[163]

Regardless of the indication, if heparin is used, it may be administered as 5000 units IV every 12 hours or 500–3000 units per hour via continuous IV infusion.[164] Other sources suggest administration of 50–100 U/kg IVP or via IV infusion every 4 hours.[165]

Amicar (epsilon-aminocaproic acid, or EACA), a hemostatic (antifibrinolytic) agent, has been used in the past in an attempt to control the bleeding of DIC, but the high incidence of thrombotic complications precludes its use.

Nursing responsibilities in the management of DIC include monitoring the patient for evidence of bleeding and thrombosis, measuring the amounts of blood lost, administering treatments, obtaining blood samples, taking physiologic measurements to evaluate response to therapy, and protecting the patient from further injury. These are explored in greater depth in the nursing care plan that follows.

Nursing Care Plan for the Management of the Patient with Disseminated Intravascular Coagulation

Diagnosis	Signs and symptoms	Intervention	Rationale
Fluid volume deficit related to blood loss from bleeding/ hemorrhage	Reduced Hct, Hgb, and RBC	Establish IV access with 0.9% N.S.	To maintain hydration, provide route for replacement therapy
	Poor skin turgor		
	Reduced cardiac output and postural hypotension	Administer colloids as indicated	Greater volume expanders than crystalloids
	Reduced urine output with urine specific gravity > 1.020	Assess amount, quality, and frequency of bleeding; report increases in bleeding	To assess degree of blood loss
	CVP < 1 mm Hg	Maintain accurate intake and output record	To aid in determining type and amount of replacement therapy
		Monitor for evidence of acute hemorrhage (tachycardia, hypotension, chest pain, bleeding)	To detect changes early for prompt intervention
		Measure abdominal girth	To assess for intraabdominal bleeding
		Administer blood product replacement as indicated; observe for signs of reaction or complications of massive transfusions	All blood and clotting components will be depleted with bleeding; frequent and massive transfusions are more likely to produce reactions
Decreased cardiac output related to reduced preload	Hypotension, weak pulse, tachyardia	Measure BP, heart rate, CVP, observing for hypotension and tachycardia	To establish parameters to evaluate response to treatment
	Low CVP, CO, PAP, and PCWP		
		Measure cardiac output, PAP, and PCWP; record measurements and report to physician	To assess pumping action of heart
		Monitor peripheral and apical pulses for strength and equality	To evaluate adequacy of tissue perfusion

Diagnosis	Signs and symptoms	Intervention	Rationale
		Maintain patient in semi-Fowler's position with legs elevated (modified Trendelenberg)	To increase cardiac output and enhance venous return; Trendelenberg not more effective for cardiac output but does reduce risk of increased intracranial pressure
		Reduce stressful stimuli	To reduce cardiac workload
		For hypotension unresponsive to intravenous crystalloids and colloids, administer inotropes cautiously	To maintain adequate blood flow to vital organs; inotropes increase vaso-constriction and may enhance peripheral tissue necrosis
		Administer supplemental oxygen as ordered	To enhance oxygen-carrying capacity and prevent myocardial ischemia or potential silent MI
Potential for injury related to impaired skin or tissue, and integrity of mucous membranes	Petechiae, ecchymoses, purpura	Observe for symptoms of bleeding: examine skin, eyes, ears, nose, mouth, and other orifices	To detect problems early for prompt intervention
	Bruising under site of BP cuff application	Avoid unnecessary traumatic procedures	
	Prolonged oozing from past or present venipuncture sites	Minimize venipunctures	To prevent bleeding
	Conjunctival or retinal hemorrhage	When performing venipunctures, use smallest gauge needle possible	To minimize size of puncture wound to minimize bleeding
	Epistaxis, gingival bleeding, oozing of blood from urethra, vagina, or rectum, prolonged or unusually heavy menstrual flow	Use smallest size NG tube, Foley catheter, etc. effective for the purpose	
	Hematochezia, melana	Apply direct pressure or ice to bleeding site	To promote effective clot formation
		Press on IV sites 10 minutes after insertion	To slow/stop bleeding
		Apply topical hemostatic agents to areas of bleeding	

Nursing Care Plan for the Management of the Patient with Disseminated Intravascular Coagulation

Diagnosis	Signs and symptoms	Intervention	Rationale
Impaired gas exchange related to pulmonary microthrombi/pulmonary hemorrhage	Apprehensiveness, tachypnea Tachycardia Dyspnea, coughing, hemoptysis Inspiratory and expiratory crackles on auscultation ABGs reveal hypoxia	Assess for peripheral or central cyanosis Assess respiratory rate, depth, and pattern Assess for symptoms of dyspnea or hemoptysis Auscultate breath sounds	Detect problems early for prompt intervention
		Check ABGs every 1–2 hours and PRN until stable; notify physician of abnormal values	To evaluate oxygenation/ventilation and establish parameters for evaluating efficacy of therapy
		Administer oxygen as prescribed	To enhance tissue oxygenation
		Maintain pO_2 at 60–80 (min.)	To prevent or reverse hypoxia
		Maintain bed rest	To reduce oxygen requirements
		Elevate head of bed 45° (if BP permits)	To promote chest expansion, reduce pressure on diaphragm
		Turn or change patient's position every 2 hours	To provide good pulmonary hygiene
		Provide chest physical therapy if no pulmonary bleeding	
Altered cutaneous tissue perfusion	Acrocyanosis, tissue necrosis, gangrene of digits, nose, ears, or genitalia Decreased peripheral pulses	Assess for and record symptoms Notify physician of any symptoms Monitor for presence, extent, and distribution of acrocyanosis or other tissue injury	Permanent tissue damage can occur if necrosis is left untreated

Diagnosis	Signs and symptoms	Intervention	Rationale
		Maintain stable room temperature	Impaired tissue is less able to tolerate extremes in temperature and is more susceptible to injury
		Handle affected areas gently; prevent trauma	
		Prepare for administration of heparin as prescribed	Heparin may assist in preventing thrombosis of acrocyanosis
Potential for injury related to excessive bleeding	Reduced Hct, Hgb, RBCs, or platelets	Type and crossmatch blood	To prepare patient for transfusion if needed
	Schistocytes in peripheral blood	Obtain and check results of hematologic and coagulation studies	To evaluate coagulation status, provide parameters to evaluate response to treatment
	Elevated reticulocyte count		
	Prolonged PT, PTT, or TT	Administer FFP, cryoprecipitate, or platelets and RBCs as prescribed	To replace clotting factors, platelets, and RBCs depleted or destroyed by consumptive coagulopathy
	Reduced fibrinogen or elevated FDPs		
		Avoid administration of any drug such as aspirin or nonsteroidal antiinflammatory that may prolong bleeding	To prevent exacerbation of bleeding
Impaired cardiac tissue perfusion	ECG changes	Provide bedrest	To reduce oxygen demand by myocardium
	Dysrhythmias	Obtain 12-lead ECG	
		Administer epinephrine, antiarrhythmics as prescribed	To enhance cardiac performance
Impaired peripheral tissue perfusion related to microthrombi or hemorrhage	Paresthesias, weak pulse, pallor, cyanosis, or cool, mottled extremities	Assess for symptoms; notify physician if present	Mottling can lead to tissue necrosis or infection and amputation
		Mark areas of demarcation cyanosis	
		Monitor for tissue necrosis	
		Avoid vasoconstricting agents if possible	Vasoconstrictors worsen the problem

Nursing Care Plan for the Management of the Patient with Disseminated Intravascular Coagulation

Diagnosis	Signs and symptoms	Intervention	Rationale
Impaired neurological tissue perfusion related to microthrombi or hemorrhage	Apprehensiveness, restlessness, anxiety, confusion, headache Obtundation, coma	Check NSDOs: vital signs, pupils, orientation, extremities (strength, sensation), ability to follow commands, reflexes	To provide clues to neurological decompensation from microthrombi
		Assess for other CNS symptoms	
		Report any CNS symptoms to physician	Intracranial bleeding should be treated promptly
		Maintain bedrest with head of bed elevated	To reduce intracranial pressure
		Reduce environmental stimuli: noise, light	To prevent intracerebral hemorrhage
		Reduce other stressful stimuli	
		Cautious use of any sedation, anti-anxiety agent, etc.	Such medications make it difficult to interpret neurological changes
		Prevent patient from coughing forcefully	To prevent sudden increases in intracranial pressure
		Discourage patient from performing Valsalva maneuver during defecation	
		Contact physician promptly for elevated blood pressure	May precipitate intracranial bleeding
		Implement measures to avoid sudden increases in intracranial pressure	
Altered renal tissue perfusion	Urine output < 0.5 mL/kg/hr	Administer IV fluids as prescribed	To maintain vascular volume
	Urine specific gravity > 1.010	Monitor BUN and creatinine	To determine tolerance of kidneys to compromise
	Hematuria		
	Elevated BUN and creatinine		

Diagnosis	Signs and symptoms	Intervention	Rationale
Potential for infection	Fever, elevated WBCs with possible shift to left Positive cultures	Monitor temperature and other vital signs for evidence of fever or infection	To detect symptoms of infection
		Practice good infection control techniques, meticulous handwashing, etc.	To prevent infection
		Monitor lab results: WBC and differential	
		Obtain cultures of blood, urine, sputum, and wound drainage as prescribed	To identify infectious organism
		Monitor results of cultures	To evaluate response to treatment
		Administer antibiotics as prescribed	
Anxiety, fear	Anxious facial expression, trembling	Assess patient's anxiety level	To provide baseline for evaluation of interventions
		Explain procedures in simple terms prior to performing them	To reduce anxiety
		Reassure patient and family when appropriate	
		Encourage patient and family to ask questions and to voice concerns	
		Correct misunderstandings	
		Maintain confident and assured manner	
		Involve family members in care as appropriate	
		Reduce emotional stressors if possible	
		Maintain or reestablish normal sleep/rest patterns	

Nursing Care Plan for the Management of the Patient with Disseminated Intravascular Coagulation

Diagnosis	Signs and symptoms	Intervention	Rationale
Knowledge deficit		Assess patient's level of understanding of disease	
		Provide amount of information appropriate for individual patient	Disease is a complex process, and patients may have difficulty understanding
Pain	Patient complains of pain	Use non-pharmacological measures to provide comfort and reduce pain	To promote comfort
		Administer analgesics as prescribed	
		Evaluate response to therapy	
		Elevate limbs to reduce edema and enhance venous return	

Organ Transplantation

Introduction

The ability to successfully replace a diseased or damaged organ with a functional organ depends on an understanding of the ways in which the body's immune system recognizes and rejects something as "foreign." The development of methods to specify an individual's immune genotype and the use of drugs to modulate the rejection response have led to significantly decreased morbidity and mortality for all types of transplants.

This section provides an overview of the aspects of immunity and immunosuppression essential to understanding organ transplantation. It discusses different types of transplants, focusing on kidney, heart, and liver transplants. (Bone marrow transplant is discussed separately in the next section.) Examples of general nursing diagnoses, assessments, and interventions for the patient with a transplanted organ are also provided.

Histocompatibility

Transplanted organs and tissues may come from either a living or a recently deceased donor, in which case they are known as allografts. They may also be autografts (tissues or organs taken from and transplanted to the same individual, as in skin grafting, for example), isografts (tissues or organs from an identical twin), or xenografts (tissues or organs from another species). Transplanted tissues are accepted or rejected based on their histocompatibility antigens, the cell-surface proteins by which cells of the immune system recognize each other. If the histocompatibility antigens of the recipient and the transplanted organ are different, rejection may occur. These antigens are inherited and are located in a group of genes collectively called the histocompatibility, or HLA, complex.

HLA Complex

In humans the HLA complex is found on chromosome 6, where about 100 different antigen-encoding genes can be found at four places, or loci. These loci are named A, B, C and D (see Figure 8-21). At each locus a person has just one gene encoding the cell-surface antigens. In humans the genes are codominant; that is, if chromosomes of a set of parents carry different genes at a locus, both genes will be expressed in their offspring. Since each of us inherits a chromosome from each parent, a parent shares exactly half of his or her HLA complex with an offspring, and siblings may share all, some, or none (see Figure 8-22).

HLA antigens have also been classified by function into Class I and Class II antigens. The Class I antigens consist of the HLA A, B, and C antigens. The Class II antigens are the D and Dr (D-related) antigens. Class II antigens are thought to provide the initial signal and stimulate the production of antigen-

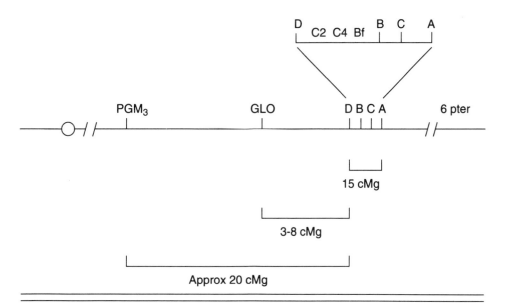

Figure 8-21 HLA Antigens
Source: Clift, R. A., and Hansen, J. A. (1983). The role of HLA. In K. G. Blume and L. D. Petz (Eds.). *Clinical Bone Marrow Transplantation.* New York: Churchill Livingstone, p. 317.

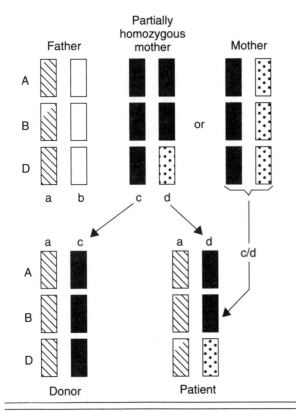

Figure 8-22 HLA Antigens Among Siblings
Source: Clift, R. A., and Hansen, J. A. (1983). The role of HLA. In K. G. Blume and L. D. Petz (Eds.). *Clinical Bone Marrow Transplantation.* New York: Churchill Livingstone, p. 320.

reactive T-helper cells to recognize a graft's foreignness. These T-helper cells can then stimulate B cells to produce antibody against the Class I antigens.

In general, the closer the match between a donor's and a recipient's HLA complexes, the more likely it is that the transplanted organ will survive and function effectively. In addition, for most transplanted organs, ABO compatibility is also essential. Attempts to transplant a highly vascular organ from a donor with a different ABO blood group result in immediate hemagglutination. Minor blood group differences, such as in Rh, are generally acceptable.

HLA Typing

The determination of an individual's HLA complex type is made through a series of tests called HLA typing. Tissue typing is used for the Class I antigens, HLA A, B, and C. A mixed lymphocyte culture (MLC) is used for the Class II antigens, HLA D and Dr.

For tissue typing, monospecific antisera obtained from sensitized individuals is used in a series of cross-match tests with the recipient's and potential donor's lymphoid cells. Living donors can be further

evaluated using the MLC technique, in which donor and recipient lymphocytes are cultured together. A highly positive MLC, in which recipient lymphocytes are activated and proliferate, is associated with decreased allograft survival.

Donor selection, therefore, is based not just on the presence of a healthy functional organ, but also on ABO compatibility (in most cases; exceptions include transplants of corneas or bone marrow), on HLA complex compatibility, and on a determination that the donor has no history of metastasizing malignancies and no active infection (particularly hepatitis or HIV).

Immunology of Rejection

Rejection of a transplanted organ may be hyperacute, acute, or chronic and may occur in spite of close HLA compatibility between the donor and the recipient. Rejection is an immune response, often combining both humoral and cellular components and both innate and acquired mechanisms of immunity. Table 8-65 summarizes the characteristics of the three types of graft rejection.

Hyperacute Rejection

If the recipient has preformed anti-ABO antibodies or anti-HLA Class I antibodies (from previous blood transfusions, pregnancies, or previously rejected grafts), a hyperacute rejection may occur. The recipient's antibodies bind to the vascular endothelium of the transplanted organ, triggering the complement system and leading also to the clotting cascade. If this reaction is sufficiently severe, microthrombi in the organ will rapidly result in severe ischemia and necrosis of the graft.

Acute Rejection

When HLA antigens on the surfaces of cells in the transplanted organ are encountered by the recipient's macrophages and other immune system cells, an acute rejection may be triggered. It is thought that macrophages process antigenic material, presenting it to B and T lymphocytes, which then become sensitized to the antigens. These sensitized lymphocytes can injure the graft through various immune responses, including both humoral and cellular responses. Cytotoxic T cells can directly injure graft cells by lysis. Lymphokines produced by activated T cells may enhance the rejection response. Sensitized B cells may target antibody against the graft's histocompatibility antigens, which may act directly or indirectly by facilitating the T cell cytotoxic response.

It generally takes days for the process of acute rejection to be clinically evident. Classic signs and

Table 8-65 Types of Transplant Rejection

Type	Mediated By	Signs and Symptoms	Time of Occurrence
Hyperacute	Complement activation Clotting cascade	Thrombosis Coagulative necrosis	Within minutes
Acute	Cellular and humoral responses	Graft tenderness Fever Malaise	Within days or weeks
Chronic	Platelet and endothelial factors	Gradual loss of graft function	Within months or years

symptoms include swelling and tenderness of the allograft, loss of allograft function, and systemic signs such as fever and malaise. On histological examination, the transplanted organ is seen to be invaded by large numbers of lymphocytes.

Chronic Rejection

Chronic rejection is a different process that may involve minor histocompatibility antigens not defined by the HLA complex. Often occurring months to years after transplant, it is characterized by narrowing of the vascular arterial bed due to proliferation of endothelial cells. Histologically, the graft is invaded by mononuclear cells, particularly T cells. Eventually fibrosis and graft ischemia result.

Prevention and Treatment of Rejection

Immunosuppression and immune modulation are the basic principles of both prophylaxis and treatment of the phenomenon of rejection. A variety of drugs are used, depending upon the type of transplant and the institution; however, some general principles guide treatment in all cases.

Intensive post-transplant immunosuppression is used to prevent sensitization to graft antigens. Combinations of drugs are often more effective than single-agent regimens. Not only do the drugs in a combination regimen act at different points in the immune response, but the individual drugs can often be given in smaller doses, thus lessening the severity of side effects.

If rejection is suspected, it must be diagnosed promptly by biopsy of the transplanted organ. Other etiologies, particularly infections, can also cause all the signs and symptoms of acute or chronic organ rejection. Histopathological analysis of the allograft is the only method that allows a definite diagnosis. Rejection must be treated aggressively and quickly to prevent irreversible damage to the transplanted organ. Once rejection is controlled, doses of immunosuppressive agents are generally tapered off. Occasionally, in the face of severe infection or leukopenia,

an immunosuppression regimen may be greatly reduced or even discontinued to save the patient's life.

Immunosuppressive agents fall into four main categories based on their mode of action: antiinflammatories, antimetabolites, cytotoxic agents, and immune modulators (see Table 8-66). The drugs most prevalently used today are steroids, cyclosporine-A, azathioprine, and monoclonal antibodies. All patients receiving immunosuppressive agents are at a higher risk for opportunistic infections, including bacterial, fungal, and viral (primary or reactivated). This is true even if the patient's bone marrow is functioning normally.

Types of Transplant

Table 8-67 summarizes the types of transplants used as treatment for a wide variety of diseases. Improvements in surgical techniques, antibiotic and blood product support, and immunosuppressive regimens have made organ transplantation a viable option for many patients with end-stage organ damage. The most commonly performed organ transplants include renal, cardiac, and liver transplants. These three major types of organ transplants have specific implications, which are discussed in the following sections.

Kidney Transplant

Living or cadaveric donors may provide kidneys for renal transplantation, with the best success achieved through the use of HLA-matched related living donors (better than 85% graft survival at 2 years versus 60% with cadaveric kidneys). Transplant surgery for the recipient is accomplished by an iliac incision through which the graft is placed in a retroperitoneal position; the renal artery is anastomosed to the internal or external iliac artery. The ureter is anastomosed to the bladder mucosa, generally using an anterior cystotomy incision.

Nursing responsibilities in the early post-transplant period include the maintenance of hemody-

Table 8-66 Immunosuppressive Agents Used in Transplantation

Type of Agent	Examples	Effects	Side Effects
Adrenocortical steroids	Prednisone Prednisolone Methyl-prednisolone	Create a broad and nonspecific antiinflammatory effect by stabilizing cellular and lysozomal membranes; also suppress production of monocytes and lymphocytes, decrease antigen sensitivity, lessen the proliferative response of sensitized T lymphocytes, and decrease production of lymphokines	High doses or long-term use: delayed wound healing, glucose intolerance, sodium retention, osteoporosis, aseptic necrosis of weight-bearing joints, cataracts, gastric ulceration, mood changes, steroid psychosis. Chronic steroid use depresses normal adrenal function, leading to a limited capacity to react physiologically to stress and the possibility of acute adrenal failure if steroid use is discontinued abruptly.
Antimetabolites	Azathioprine (Immuran) 6-mercaptopurine Methotrexate	Interfere with purine synthesis that is required for normal production of antibodies; interfere with nucleic acid synthesis in rapidly proliferating cells such as lymphocytes	Bone marrow suppression, stomatitis, hepatotoxicity, neoplasms (especially lymphoma, Kaposi's sarcoma, tumors of skin and lungs)
Cytotoxic agents	Cyclophosphamide Chlorambucil Lymphoid irradiation Antilymphocyte globulin (ALG) Antithymocyte globulin (ATG) Monoclonal antibodies: OKT-3, OKT-4, Xomazyme	Stimulate the formation of antibodies against human lymphocytes	Hypersensitivity reactions, fever, malaise, anorexia, diarrhea, pulmonary edema, thrombocytopenia, hemolytic anemia, pancreatitis
Immune modulators	Cyclosporine-A (CSA)	Fungal derivative that interferes with the production of effector T lymphocytes and lymphokines and with the cloning of T helper cells	Nephrotoxicity, hypertension, neurotoxicity, hepatotoxicity, hirsutism, gingival hyperplasia, tremors, lymphomas

namic stability (particularly to maintain good blood flow through the transplanted kidney) and careful monitoring of electrolytes and renal function. Cadaveric kidneys frequently have some degree of acute tubular necrosis, and some patients may require hemodialysis before full renal function returns.

Complications specific to renal transplants include the leakage of urine from the newly implanted ureter, stenosis of the newly anastomosed renal artery, and graft loss due to the recurrence of damage from the original disease. This latter complication may occur in patients with diabetes, glomerulonephritis, polyarteritis, and hypertension.

Heart Transplant

Among patients receiving a donor heart for end-stage cardiac impairment the survival rate at 1 year is 60%; patients who received transplants in the 1980s had approximately a 40% survival rate at 5 years. Encouragingly, cardiac function is frequently good, and 60% of patients are able to return to work or school.

Table 8-67 Types of Transplant

Organ	Clinical Indications	Donor Type	Complications
Skin	Burns	Autograft Allograft Xenograft	Rejection Infection
Bone marrow	Hematologic malignancies, immune deficiencies, aplastic anemia, solid tumors, genetic disorders	Autograft Allograft	Rejection Graft-versus-host disease Infection Organ toxicities
Kidney	End-stage renal disease	Allograft	Rejection Infection
Heart	Congenital heart disease, cardiomyopathies	Allograft	Rejection Dysrhythmias
Liver	Congenital biliary atresia, end-stage liver failure	Allograft	Rejection Bleeding
Lungs	Chronic obstructive pulmonary disease, pulmonary hypertension	Allograft	Rejection Respiratory failure Infection
Pancreas	Diabetes, chronic pancreatitis	Allograft	Rejection
Cornea	Cataracts	Allograft	Opacification

Surgery for the recipient requires cardiopulmonary bypass, during which the new heart is placed alongside the old, with anastomosis of new atria to old and new ventricles to old. The aorta and pulmonary arteries are similarly anastomosed.

Early post-transplant care is the same as for any patient undergoing major cardiac surgery; in addition, immunosuppression and the potential for rejection, which is life-threatening, are problems that must be anticipated. Complications specific to cardiac transplants include dysrhythmias associated with rejection and atherosclerosis of the new coronary arteries.

Liver Transplant

Liver transplantation remains technically difficult, but with the use of intensive immunosuppression, survival rates have improved. Survival at 1 year is now about 68% for adults and 74% for children. In general, donor livers are chosen based on ABO compatibility and organ size, rather than on HLA typing.

Surgery for the recipient begins with the removal of the damaged liver. The portal vein and vena cava are both clamped during much of the surgery, resulting in decreased blood return to the heart. Multiple anastomoses of major blood vessels are required to insert the donor liver, and the risk of bleeding during the operative and postoperative periods is great.

Bone Marrow Transplant (BMT)

Bone marrow transplant (BMT) is unique in that it transplants an immune system. As the immune system matures and accepts its host environment as its own, a process which usually takes about 2 years, immunosuppression therapy gradually becomes unnecessary. Survival rates depend upon the initial disease and vary from 40% to 80% at 5 years.

The recipient must undergo intensive preparatory chemotherapy and/or irradiation therapy to ablate existing bone marrow, provide immunosuppression, and in the case of a malignancy, treat the underlying disease. Bone marrow is infused into a central vein in a process generally resembling a whole-blood transfusion. Unlike other organ transplant recipients, BMT recipients spend a period of time in profound aplasia before the new marrow proliferates. Their risk of infectious complications, of bleeding related to thrombocytopenia, and of organ toxicities from the preparatory regimen is therefore significant.

Allogenic BMT recipients are also at risk for a unique complication of transplantation—graft-versus-host disease (GVHD). The transplanted immunocompetent T lymphocytes, in a process similar to acute rejection, are sensitized to the host environment and are stimulated to mount a cytotoxic response resulting in widespread destruction. The organs typically involved in GVHD are the skin, the liver, and the gastrointestinal tract. Severe cases may involve erythroderma and desquamation, abnormal liver function tests, markedly increased bilirubin levels, and profuse, watery diarrhea.

The Nurse's Role in Organ Transplantation

With recent technological and pharmacological advances, transplantation is rapidly moving from being considered experimental to being considered an acceptable alternative to standard therapy. As a consequence of these advances, demand for donated organs far exceeds supply. It is estimated that there are three individuals awaiting transplantation for every organ that becomes available.[166] For some, a lack of a donor results in death. It is estimated that between 20,000 and 25,000 persons are declared brain dead each year, yet only 10–15% of those individuals donate organs for transplantation.[167] There are many reasons for this limited availability. Though it is widely believed that the primary reason is lack of consent, studies have shown that when approached, eight out of ten families consent to organ donation. Thus, health care providers should seek consent more frequently.

The Uniform Anatomical Gift Act of 1969 allows people to plan in advance to donate organs in the case of irreversible brain death. If this outcome is identified immediately, donation can be expedited. If a deceased patient has made no provisions to donate organs, it is the survivors—the family—who must make this decision. Several laws have passed regarding who has authority to grant permission for an organ donation and how the process may proceed. These are summarized in Table 8-68. These laws guide health care providers by defining brain death and mandating separate teams to establish brain death and procure organs for transplantation. Before brain death can be assessed, patients must be normothermic, have no hypotension, and have no evidence of drug or metabolic intoxication. When these criteria are met, neurological evaluation of central brain reflexes using electroencephalogram and computed tomography can be performed.

The role of the nurse in the transplantation process is a complex and challenging one, requiring a knowledge of transplantation eligibility criteria and laws, resources for organ procurement, and a perspective on the ethical issues involved in organ procurement. The nurse is a key player in assessment of potential organ donors. He or she will be involved in providing support to the family during the time when brain death is being determined as well as aggressively maintaining adequate organ function. Family members have expressed positive feelings toward donation when health care workers are supportive and open throughout this process. Many families were surprised by the amount of time between consent and actual transplant, and in one case the delay caused a difference of $11,000 in hospital bills.[168] It is important for families to know where donated organs are sent and the consequences of the transplant, even if this information is

Table 8-68 Laws Affecting Organ Donations

Law	Description
Uniform Anatomical Gift Act of 1969	Established that the donation of organs based on altruistic motives is a personal option, not to be imposed by others; set up guidelines for obtainment of donated organs that required that the procuring team be separate from the team that declared patient dead
National Organ Transplant Act, P.L. 98-507 (1984)	Accomplished four tasks: (1) established a national task force on organ transplantation; (2) reinforced the prohibition of buying or selling organs; (3) directed the NIH and FDA to prepare annual reports related to advances in organ transplantation; (4) established an organ procurement and transplantation registry and grant program
P.L. 99-509 (funding policy for above law)	Required that all hospitals participating in Medicare and Medicaid establish written protocols for encouraging organ donation, identifying potential donors, and notifying an organ procurement network when a possible donor has been identified; also required participation in the Organ Procurement and Transplantation Network by 1987

shared by an anonymous mediator. Another aspect of this process is preparing the family for what is involved in the procedure. Family members may not realize that the long bones may be removed from the donor, and they may be distressed to find the unnatural state of the arms during the funeral.[169]

The nurse's role in maintaining metabolic functioning so that neurological testing can be carried out and organs can be preserved is probably the most important for successful organ procurement. It is vital that the patient not suffer from hypotension, hypothermia, or severe electrolyte disturbance. The physiological consequences of brain death often make this difficult. The health care team must combat loss of parasympathetic tone (hypotension, dysrhythmias), diabetes insipidus, metabolic acidosis, neurogenic pulmonary edema, infection, and hypothermia.[170] Aggressive fluid management, warming blankets, and ventilatory or cardiac support can allow the completion of organ profile tests. The emotional stress of caring for the brain-dead patient compounded by the stress of providing emotional support to the family can make for a taxing and difficult experience for the nurse. Some transplant teams offer debriefing sessions with health care workers to assist them in coping.

Nursing Care Plan for the Management of the Patient with an Organ Transplant

Diagnosis	Signs and symptoms	Intervention	Rationale
Potential for infection related to immunosuppression	Cushingoid facies from chronic steroid use History of use of immunosuppressive agents (febrile response may be supppressed by steroids) Disruption of skin barrier, presence of erythema or swelling, oral lesions or plaque, abnormal breath sounds, symptoms of dysuria or frequency of urination, abnormally low or high WBC	Wash hands before all contacts with immunosuppressed patients Monitor vital signs at least every 8 hours for fever, tachycardia, decreased BP Assess potential sites for signs and symptoms of infection at least every day— peripheral and IV line sites, sites of previous invasive procedures, lung fields, urine, stool Avoid invasive procedures (such as urinary catheterization) when possible Maintain strict asepsis during dressing changes and all invasive procedures Provide private room Limit patient contact with potentially infected patients Discourage patient from keeping live plants or flowers in the room	The immunosuppressed patient is at high risk of infection from his or her own flora, from contact with other infected persons, or from invasive procedures
Lack of knowledge of immunosuppression and potential infection	Patient requests information, states misconceptions, or does not follow instructions correctly	Determine patient's level of knowledge and ability to learn Identify objectives of care regimen for patient	Need for information and ability to learn vary with patients' age, educational level, illness, and cultural background

Diagnosis	Signs and symptoms	Intervention	Rationale
		Develop teaching plan for patient and family using various methods (visual aids, booklets, discussion, and/or demonstration) and instruct them on immunosuppressive agents (action, dosages, and side effects), measures to prevent infection, signs and symptoms of infection	
Disturbance in self-concept related to transplantation, use of immunosuppressive agents, change in family or social role	Refusal to look in the mirror Unwillingness to discuss health and ability to function Self-destructive behavior Refusal to accept rehabilitative program Withdrawal Depression Grieving	Encourage patient to express both positive and negative feelings by remaining open and maintaining nonjudgmental attitude Encourage patient to ask questions about treatment, progress, and prognosis; be open and provide accurate information Explore realistic alternatives with patient; determine patient's expectations Encourage patient to mix with friends and family; reassure him or her that protection against infection does not require total isolation Explore his or her strengths and resources with patient Refer patient to appropriate resource personnel (support groups, social worker, or psychologist)	Post-transplant disturbances in self-concept often arise as a result of changes in body function, the physical effects of chronic illness and immunosuppression, and altered roles; establishment of new self-concept is a process that takes time and one that the nurse can facilitate

Bone Marrow Transplantation

The administration of bone marrow to patients with hematopoietic disease in the hope of replacing their diseased marrow has been attempted sporadically since the nineteenth century, but has become an increasingly popular therapy since the 1970s. Success in bone marrow transplantation (BMT) can be attributed to various technological developments. The importance of tissue typing to prevent rejection has been well documented in the 1980s by the numbers of successful transplants increasing from less than 1% to 60–80%.[171] Advances in the provision of supportive therapies such blood components, nutrition, and immunosuppressive and antimicrobial therapy have also greatly enhanced patient outcomes. Nevertheless, BMT is not without a significant amount of risk, and patients frequently require critical care intervention. One study reported that 40% of the BMT patients studied required ICU care; 26% of these needed ventilator support and 21% required hemodialysis.[172] Another study noted that 16% of allogenic transplant patients required ventilator support.[173]

from another person, which is HLA-matched, unmatched, or partially matched), syngeneic (HLA-matched bone marrow from an identical twin), and autologous ("self" marrow returned to the patient after aggressive chemotherapy). The choice of marrow to be transplanted is determined by the availability of matched donors, the health of the recipient, and the type of disease being treated.[175] An overview of these types of BMT and their advantages and disadvantages is provided in Table 8-69.

Many health care professionals believe that BMT offers two major advantages over conventional therapy: (1) it allows the use of more intensive chemotherapeutic regimens without the need for concern for their bone marrow toxicity; and (2) it may provide immune protection against residual tumor cells.[176] Bone marrow transplants have been proven to cure certain disorders such as aplastic anemia and childhood leukemia. The procedure is also effective in cases of adult leukemia, lymphoma, and myelofibrosis. Other conditions have been treated by bone marrow transplantation, but in those cases the approach is still considered investigational. Conditions for which BMT is indicated are listed in Table 8-70.

Clinical antecedents

Bone marrow transplantation has been described as both investigational therapy for end-stage disease and as standard curative therapy for malignant and nonmalignant conditions. Both descriptions are accurate, given the wide variety of bone marrow transplant types and clinical indications.[174]

Bone marrow transplants are classified according to tissue compatibility and origin. The types of bone marrow transplant include allogenic (bone marrow

Critical referents

Bone marrow transplantation involves the intravenous infusion of bone marrow to replace the defective hematopoietic system. Prior to this process, a great deal of preparation is required. Tests must be performed to determine donor compatibility; conditioning chemotherapy and/or total body irradiation must be given to ablate the existing bone marrow; the donor must undergo an operative procedure in which bone marrow is collected for infusion into the

Table 8-69 Advantages and Disadvantages of Different Types of BMT

Type	Advantages	Disadvantages
Autologous	Low risk of GVHD Availability of donor Fewer treatment-related side effects and complications	Increased risk of relapse Risk of not engrafting
Syngeneic	Low risk of GVHD Fewer treatment-related side effects and complications	Increased risk of relapse Patient and donor must be identical twins
Allogenic	Decreased risk of relapse Greater number of donors (compared with syngeneic transplants)	Increased risk of GVHD Increased number and severity of treatment-related side effects and complications

Table 8-70 Diseases Treated with Allogenic Bone Marrow Transplantation

Nonmalignant		Malignant
Acquired	Congenital	
Aplastic anemia	Severe combined immunodeficiencies (SCIDS)	Acute myelogenous leukemia (AML)
Paroxysmal nocturnal hemoglobinuria*	Mucopolysaccharidoses	Acute lymphocytic leukemia (ALL)
Myelofibrosis	Lipid storage diseases*	Chronic myelogenous leukemia (CML)
Wiskott-Aldrich syndrome	Osteopetrosis	Preleukemia*
Thalassemia*		Hairy cell leukemia*
Chronic granulomatous disease*		Non-Hodgkin's lymphoma
		Burkitt's lymphoma*
		Hodgkin's disease
		Multiple myeloma*
		Selected solid tumors*

*Diseases in which role of BMT is still under study.

patient. Patients who are to receive autologous BMT have their bone marrow removed prior to intensive chemotherapy; the marrow is returned when their remaining bone marrow is suppressed from therapy. The most successful BMTs involve syngeneic transplants, in which the bone marrow of the patient and the identical twin donor is a perfect tissue match. When perfect HLA matches are unavailable, the HLA antigens of all potential donors are evaluated and ABO blood typing is carried out (although as a result of advances in blood component therapy, ABO compatibility is not essential).

Following the transplant comes a period of aplasia, engraftment, and bone marrow recovery. These phases are depicted in Figure 8-23, where the uppermost graph indicates WBC counts, the middle portion indicates hematocrit, the lower portion indicates platelet count, and the arrows indicate RBC and platelet transfusions.

A regimen of pre-BMT immunosuppression is selected based upon the patient's general health and disease status and the institutional preferences. This "conditioning" regimen achieves three major goals: (1) it destroys the host's immune system to reduce the risk of rejection of the graft; (2) it clears out the old bone marrow to allow the new marrow to enter and proliferate; and (3) it destroys stray malignant cells. The primary objective of autologous transplant is this third goal. Most conditioning protocols involve high-dose alkylating agents, which may be combined with total body irradiation. Commonly used therapies and their potential side effects are listed in Table 8-71.

The actual infusion of bone marrow is performed 4–10 days after the patient begins chemotherapy. The bone marrow should be void of hematopoietic elements when it is given. Prior to bone marrow infusion, the patient is hydrated with a bicarbonate solution to enhance glomerular filtration and alkalinize the urine. This promotes urinary clearance of any RBC hemolysis products that are created during the transplant.[177] The bone marrow itself is infused without a filter over 1–4 hours through a central access device. The patient is observed for allergic reactions.

The process of engraftment occurs over 2–4 weeks. The infused bone marrow migrates toward the host's bone marrow, where stem cells populate the vacant marrow space and then begin cell production. During the early phase of engrafting, because the old bone marrow is depleted of cellular components and the new marrow has not yet begun to function, patients are usually totally aplastic and require vigorous red blood cell and platelet transfusions. The engraftment stage is often fraught with infectious complications or a syndrome of rejection unique to BMT called acute graft-versus-host disease.

Graft-versus-host disease (GVHD) occurs in 40–60% of allogenic BMT patients and in up to 10% of syngeneic and autologous BMT patients.[178] Since the transplanted "organ" in this case is an entire immune system, the manifestations of rejection involve the many organs in which immune cells reside. Graft-versus-host disease is a significant problem, which can be life-threatening and unfortunately is not al-

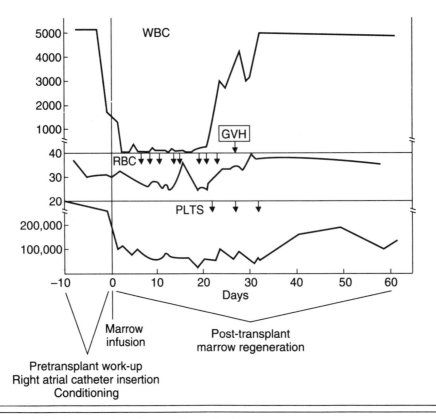

Figure 8-23 Phases of Bone Marrow Transplantation-

ways predictable. Most transplant centers administer prophylactic immunosuppressive medications from the beginning of the transplant process to aid the patient in resisting GVHD. Agents such as methotrexate, cyclosporine-A, and steroids are most commonly used (see Table 8-66). Early signs and symptoms of GVHD are likely to be treated with higher doses of these agents or by the addition of antithymocyte globulin (ATG) or the monoclonal antibody OKT-3.

Assuming that engraftment proceeds and bone marrow recovery occurs, the patient is usually discharged for outpatient follow-up. It is important for patients and caregivers to realize that it will take up to 2 years for immunocompetence to return to normal. Tissue anergy to common pathogens may occur, and reimmunization is usually required.

Resulting signs and symptoms

Acute complications of BMT may be complex and interrelated. A diagram of all potential acute toxicities is given in Figure 8-24. Acute complications

in BMT are usually classified by their probable etiology: the preparative regimen, removal of the immune system, infection, or an acute rejection process. The primary acute complications requiring intensive care intervention have been identified as sepsis, GVHD, and failure to engraft.[179] Infections in the immunosuppressed transplant patient will initially be the same as those seen in neutropenia, but after 10–14 days the infections are more often related to the absence of T-cell function and take the form of viral infections and reactivations of latent organisms. A schema of potential infectious complications in BMT is given in Figure 8-25.

Graft-versus-host disease (GVHD) is possibly the most significant acute complication suffered by BMT patients. It may become evident from 2 weeks to 3 months after transplant. Several factors increase the risk of acute GVHD: mismatched donor and recipient tissue types, increased patient age, and significant history of previous blood transfusions.[180] Its manifestations are systemic, because of the disseminated nature of a transplanted immune system. The organs most often affected in GVHD are the skin, the liver, and the GI tract. Both observations of clinical signs and symptoms and laboratory values

Table 8-71 BMT Conditioning Regimens

Agent	Complications	Assessment/Interventions	Time Frame
Busulfan (up to 16 mg/kg)	Seizures	Prophylactic Dilantin Seizure precautions	Immediate
	Severe mucositis	Pain assessment and relief Prevention of infection Intubation to protect airway	7–14 days
	Respiratory pneumonopathy and fibrosis	Respiratory assessment qod FVCs Incentive spirometry Exercise and physical therapy	7–14 days or longer
	Veno-occlusive disease	Oxygenation, ventilation Pain assessment and relief Diuresis Nutrition Management of hepatic failure	7–12 days
Cytoxan (up to 200 mg/kg)	SIADH	Management of fluid balance Sodium replacement Neurological assessment Seizure precautions	Immediate
	Hemorrhagic cystitis	Management of fluid balance Pain assessment and relief Continuous bladder irrigation Blood products Prevention of infection	Immediate to ?
	Hemorrhagic cardiomyopathy	Cardiac assessment ECG, echo, cardiac monitor Management of fluid balance Management of cardiac failure	Immediate to ?
Etoposide (VP-16) (up to 60 mg/kg)	Severe mucositis	Pain assessment and relief Prevention of infection Intubation to protect airway	7–14 days
	Anaphylaxis	Assessment, monitoring Resuscitative measures	Immediate
Total body irradiation (TBI; 3000 rads in fractionated doses over 3–5 days)	Pulmonary interstitial pneumonitis	Auscultate breath sounds every 4–8 hours Chest x-ray daily Pulmonary function tests (FVC and FEV) every other day	Immediately and for 14 days
	Nausea and vomiting	Antiemetics Small frequent feedings	Immediately and until approximately 2 days after TBI

Source: Shivnan, J., and Shelton, B. K. Bone marrow transplantation: Issues for critical care nurses. *Critical Care Nurse* (in press).

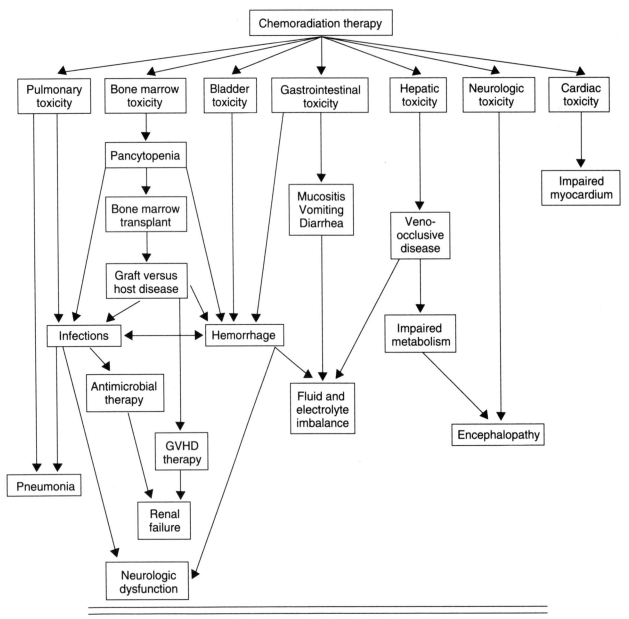

Figure 8-24 Acute Complications of BMT
Source: Ford, R. and Ballard, B. (1988). Acute complications after bone marrow transplantation. *Seminars in Oncology Nursing 4:* 16.

will suggest appropriate alterations in immunosuppressive therapy. An overview of the stages of GVHD is shown in Table 8-72. GVHD may be as mild as a pruritic maculopapular rash or as severe as toxic epidermal necrolysis (TENS). The GI manifestations often begin with diarrhea. Because of the significant number of gastrointestinal organisms that can infect BMT patients, full culture evaluations are performed to rule out an infectious etiology. The severe loss of GI mucosal integrity coupled with thrombocytopenia often leads to significant GI bleeding. GVHD of the liver will manifest as hepatobiliary obstruction

with escalating bilirubin levels and jaundice. Immunosuppressive drugs will be used to ameliorate these symptoms, while efforts are made to prevent superinfection of the damaged epithelial tissue.

Chronic GVHD, while annoying and disfiguring, is unlikely to produce life-threatening complications for the BMT recipient. Chronic GVHD usually does not present until 3 months or more after a transplant. The clinical manifestations are similar to those of collagen diseases, primarily those affecting the skin and mucous membranes. They may include patchy alopecia, inability to sweat, skin thickening,

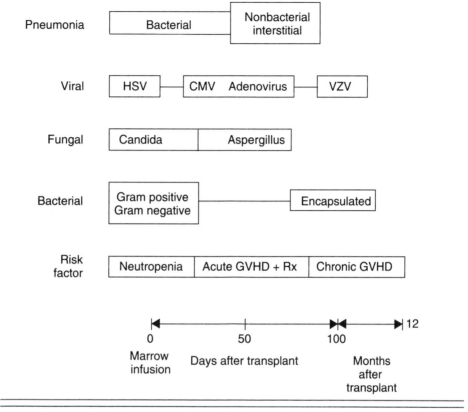

Figure 8-25 Potential Infections After BMT
Source: Adapted from Meyers, J. D. (1986). Infection in bone marrow transplant recipients. *American Journal of Medicine 81:* 28.

pruritis or irritation of the skin, and an unusual life-threatening form of bronchiolitis obliterans.

The transplanted bone marrow fails to engraft in less than 1% of syngeneic transplants, but this figure increases to 5–25% in those receiving ABO-incom-patible marrow grafts.[181] Since many deaths are due to overwhelming infection during aplasia, it is difficult to determine if these same patients would have had graft failure—that is, if there are actually higher rates of graft failure than reported. The failure of

Table 8-72 Stages of Acute GVHD

Stage	Skin: Extent of Rash	Histology	Liver: Total Bilirubin (mg/dL)	Gut: Volume of Diarrhea (mL)
0	<25%	Grade 2	—	—
I	25–50%	Grade 2 or higher	—	—
II	25–50% or erythroderma	Grade 2 or higher	2.0–3.5	500–1000
IIo	—	—	2.0–3.5	500–1000
IIs	Bullae/desquamation	Grade 2 or higher	—	—
III	25–50%, erythroderma,or bullae/desquamation	Grade 2 or higher	3.5–15.0 or greater	1000–2500 or greater
IV	Erythroderma or bullae/desquamation	Grade 2 or higher	8.0–15.0 or greater	1500–2500 or greater

Source: Adapted from Wagner, J. E., Santos, G. W., Noga, S. J., et al. (1990). Bone marrow graft engineering by counterflow centrifugal elutriation: Results of a phase I–II clinical trial. *Blood, 75*(6): 1372.

allogenic transplants to engraft is thought to be related to minor histocompatibility antigens not identified in the major HLA-typing procedure or to inadequate immunosuppression from prophylaxis or T cell-depleted marrow (treated bone marrow). Autologous transplant failure is more likely to be linked to inadequate stem cell transfusion, altered quality of stem cells in heavily pre-treated patients, or the marrow recovery process.

A number of other significant complications possibly requiring critical care intervention are related to the chemotherapeutic or radiation conditioning regiments. Life-threatening complications may include severe thrombocytopenia, hemorrhagic cystitis, veno-occlusive disease, acute cardiomyopathy syndrome, acute interstitial pneumonitis, syndrome of inappropriate antidiuretic hormone, oropharyngeal bleeding and edema, and GI bleeding. These compli-

Table 8-73 Complications of Cytotoxic Therapy with Bone Marrow Transplantation

Complication	Etiology	Assessment	Intervention
Hemorrhagic cystitis	High-dose Cytoxan is toxic to the bladder mucosa as its metabolites are excreted	Urine output Urine specific gravity Blood in urine Dysuria	Pre- and intra-treatment with Mesna Foley catheter Bladder irrigations Pre-hydration and force fluids (PO and IV) up to three days after completion of chemotherapy
Acute cardiomyopathy	High-dose Cytoxan	Crackles in lungs Heart failure on x-ray Dyspnea Hypoxemia Heart sound changes (S_3 and S_4 gallops, murmurs) Reduced cardiac output with PA line Reduced ejection fraction notable on echocardiogram	Stop chemotherapy Monitor cardiac status with central line or pulmonary artery line Frequent cardiorespiratory assessments Monitor I & O and note patient intolerance of fluids Check for JVP
Mucosites	Busulfan, Cytoxan, Methotrexate	Oral assessment every shift Culture suspicious lesions Avoid very abrasive or hot foods which may burn the mouth Note early symptoms of dry mouth and tenderness with minimal erythema Note superinfection with candida and treat promptly with topical antifungal	Oral care with bactericidal agent at least three times per day Pain medications (both topical anesthetics and intravenous narcotics; monitor use as severe mucosal slouging can occur)
Venoocclusive liver disease (VOD)	Busulfan, Cytoxan	Right upper quadrant pain Weight gain Jaundice Hepatomegaly Ascites Elevated bilirubin levels Hyperammonemia	Supportive care with fluid restrictions and diuretics (Aldactone is recommended) Daily or even more often weights Paracentesis as needed for comfort and to alleviate respiratory distress

cations and key assessment parameters are described in Table 8-73.

Nursing standards of care

The most important concepts to remember in caring for the BMT patient involve the potential for immune system failure. During much of the post-transplant period, the patient is aplastic and requires frequent transfusion of red cells and platelets. All BMT patients must be conscientiously protected from possible pathogenic organisms. Strategies to prevent infection include barrier protection, reduced environmental exposure, and bolstering the patient's defenses.[182] The strategies may be the same as those employed with neutropenia, although most institutions view the immune suppression experienced by BMT patients as more complete; many institutions have special air filtering systems to protect such patients from fungi and opportunistic organisms. A listing of recommended strategies appears in Table 8-74. It is common to supplement traditional antimicrobial therapy with antifungals, antivirals, or antipneumocystis agents.

Treatment of graft-versus-host disease involves increasing the level of immune suppression to diminish the body's reaction to "self." This increased level of suppression is achieved by increasing the doses of existing medications or by adding other agents (in the case of patients who have been given maximum levels of traditional immunosuppressives and are unable to tolerate the neurologic, hepatotoxic, or renal toxicities of increasing doses of CSA or steroids).[183]

The overall management strategy during bone marrow transplantation involves providing the best possible match of transplant to a healthy patient in remission and then supporting the incompetent immune system until engraftment occurs.

The nurse's role in the emerging specialty of bone marrow transplants continues to grow and change. Such transplants are now routine in major medical centers. The nurse's role in assessment and monitoring for the many potential complications is complex and requires a broad base of both critical care and oncology knowledge. The critical care nurse should be aware of the eligibility criteria for bone marrow transplantation, the process, and anticipated patient responses in order to provide optimal care to this patient group. As management of physical care improves, new concerns regarding ethical decision making and reimbursement emerge. Although bone marrow transplant is a potentially curative therapy, many of its complications can be fatal. Recent controversies have emerged regarding the

Table 8-74 Prevention of Infection with BMT Patients

General Strategy	Examples
Protect barriers	Carefully plan timing and dosing of preparative regimen designed to reduce toxicity to integument and gastrointestinal, respiratory, and urogenital tracts
	Prevent GVHD, which breaks down barriers: (1) treat donor marrow to remove GHH-reactive T cells; (2) transplant peripherally collected stem cells; (3) provide immunosuppressive medications to marrow recipient to prevent GVHD
	Promptly evaluate and treat other disease states causing disruption of barriers: skin eruptions from medications, infections, GVHD, toxicities from preparative regimen
	Culture susceptible sites for infection
Reduce exposure to potential pathogens	Hepa-filtering of the air and laminar air flow circulation
	Mask isolation for outside room (when protective isolation is no longer indicated)
	Decontamination of the GI tract with oral nonabsorbable antibiotics (with or without low microbial diet)
	Screening of blood for CMV if patient is CMV antibody titer–negative; give only CMV-negative blood to those patients
	No fresh flowers or standing water
	Selective use of colony stimulating factors for bone marrow recovery
Bolster patient's defenses	Antimicrobial therapy for bacteria, fungi, protozoa, and viruses using a combination of agents
	White blood cell transfusions for selected patients
	Specific immunizations after transplant to restore immunity to common childhood illnesses
	Nutritional support
	Promotion of adequate rest

use of child sibling donors or umbilical chord blood recovered upon birth of a sibling. The nurse must feel comfortable with obtaining informed consent and then supporting the same patient and family through life-threatening events. A BMT requires 21–50 days of hospitalization and often costs over $120,000.[184] As a high-cost technology, BMT has been deemed by some third-party payors to have a limited cost-benefit ratio; such payors prefer allocating scarce resources to other health care endeavors. This tenuous position has led many BMT nurses to participate in legislative efforts to make BMT more accessible to low-risk patients for whom the operation has a high potential for success.

The nursing care of a BMT patient is a complex mix of intense physical care, patient teaching, and careful monitoring for complications. The major goals in caring for BMT patients are (1) promoting patient understanding of the BMT procedure and its risks, (2) cautiously administering chemotherapeutic preparative medications and monitoring the patient for complications during the preparative regimen and during bone marrow infusion, (3) preventing infection, (4) monitoring patient responses to immunosuppressive therapy for complications or symptoms of GVHD, (5) providing hematologic supportive care during aplasia, and (6) providing support and creating an environment conducive to humane caring and decision making throughout the transplant process. A nursing care plan follows.

Diagnosis	Signs and symptoms	Intervention	Rationale
Potential for infection related to leukopenia, immunosuppression, and graft-versus-host disease	Fever > 1°C Erythema and pain at a site Purulent drainage from wounds or orifices Erosions or ulcers of skin or mucous membranes Positive cultures	Assess patient every 4 hours for signs of infection or septic shock: elevated temperature, flushing, chills, malaise, arthralgias, tachycardia, tachypnea, mental status changes, hypotension, pain on urination or cloudy foul-smelling urine, dry cough, change in character of breath sounds (decreased or absent), erythema with or without discharge from skin lesions (perirectal, vaginal areas, oral cavity, catheter site, old peripheral intravenous line sites, etc.)	Phagocytic and specific immune responses are inadequate following transplant
		Monitor WBC count, particularly absolute neutrophil count, to determine period of high risk for infection and return of immune function	When WBC count returns to 2500 or higher with absolute neutrophil count of at least 500, risk of bacterial and opportunistic infection decreases
		Implement protective isolation precautions per institution policy (laminar air flow, sterile environment, or reverse precautions including hand washing, masking, visitor restrictions, etc.)	Precautions aimed at preventing nosocomial exogenous organism colonization/infection
		Perform surveillance cultures per institution protocol and/or obtain cultures with febrile episodes	Detect colonization early, allowing for early treatment with antibiotics

Nursing Care Plan for the Management of the Patient with Bone Marrow Transplant

Diagnosis	Signs and symptoms	Intervention	Rationale
		Teach/perform frequent mouth care (including cleansing with antibacterial, antifungal mouth rinses, moisturizing solutions, dental care including brushing and flossing when appropriate)	Oral cavity is a prime source of infection
		Initiate antimicrobial diet per institution protocol (restrictions on fresh fruits, vegetables, only well-cooked foods, etc.)	To prevent acquisition of organisms through foods
		Instruct or assist patient with daily hygiene using antimicrobial soap (chlorhexidine, providone iodine, etc.)	Bacterial soaps should be used because even normal flora can infect patient
		Apply antifungal powders, ointments as ordered (under skinfolds and breasts, in axilla, in groin area)	Dark, moist spots are prime locations for organism growth
		Avoid trauma or invasive procedures such as urinary catheterization, injections, rectal suppositories, enemas, nasogastric tubes	Invasive procedures break barrier protection from organisms
		Initiate measures to prevent rectal trauma from hard stools or constipation (bowel program, stool softeners, sitz baths)	Rectal trauma can cause tears in GI mucosa and allow organisms to cross into the blood

Diagnosis	Signs and symptoms	Intervention	Rationale
		Initiate measures to prevent respiratory infection; encourage frequent deep breathing, coughing, and use of incentive spirometer; increase physical activity; encourage cessation of smoking	Hypoventilation and atelectasis predispose patient to pneumonia
		Instruct patient in and/or perform central venous catheter site care per institution protocol	Common source of gram-positive organism sepsis if not treated with bactericidals and frequent dressing changes
		Notify physician immediately for signs and symptoms of infection; anticipate physician orders: immediate initiation of antibiotic therapy; reevaluation of current antibiotic therapy, addition of other antimicrobials and/or specific drug level monitoring; obtain appropriate blood, throat, urine, stool, skin cultures, and chest x-ray; administration of acetaminophen	Infection can be life-threatening during aplasia
Potential for injury related to thrombocytopenia	Petichiae Ecchymoses Occult blood in excrement Obvious bleeding from orifice or wound Signs of organ dysfunction (renal failure, mental status changes, or hypoxemia)	Monitor laboratory values that can indicate bleeding risk or occult bleeding: platelet count, coagulation studies (PT and PTT), bleeding time, hemoglobin, hematocrit, hemetest emesis, urine, and stool	Indicators of bleeding risk

Nursing Care Plan for the Management of the Patient with Bone Marrow Transplant

Diagnosis	Signs and symptoms	Intervention	Rationale
		Monitor for clinical signs indicative of risk for or actual bleeding: petechiae, ecchymosis, epistaxis, joint pain or swelling, vaginal or rectal bleeding	Early signs of bleeding may indicate need for coagulation factor or platelet transfusions
		Monitor neurological status for changes that might reflect intracranial bleed: headache, blurred vision, disorientation, seizures, pupillary changes, etc.	Intracranial bleed may occur spontaneously
		Instruct patient about and implement measures to protect from injury: use electric razor; avoid hard-bristled toothbrush and dental floss when thrombocytopenic; avoid forceful nose blowing; carefully supervise toe and fingernail cutting; avoid straining at stool; avoid rectal thermometers, suppositories; avoid injections; apply pressure to injection and bone marrow sites until bleeding ceases (at least 5–10 minutes); consider use of sand bag if bleeding is prolonged; administer medications to suppress menses during thrombo-cytopenic period;	Precautions should be taken to prevent unnecessary injury to patient

Diagnosis	Signs and symptoms	Intervention	Rationale
		use high Fowler's position, ice packs, and nasal packing for epistaxis.	
		Comfort and reassure patient during bleeding episodes	Patient will be frightened
		Report bleeding episodes to physician and anticipate physician orders: platelet transfusions for count less than 20,000 or if patient is bleeding; treatment of coagulopathies arising from liver dysfunction with appropriate blood components or clotting factors and/or cryoprecipitate or plasma; possible administration of heparin infusion if disseminated intravascular coagulation is source of bleeding; topical methods of controlling bleeding (thrombin, silver nitrate sticks, or Gelfoam); antiemetics and/or sedatives to control nausea and vomiting	Supportive care measures can help prevent spontaneous and excessive bleeding
Fluid volume excess related to infusion of high volume of intravenous fluid (medications), blood product transfusions, impaired renal function, impaired hepatic function (VOD), or impaired cardiac function (congestive heart failure)	Weight gain Intake > output CVP > 6 mm Hg Crackles, gurgles, or wheezes on auscultation Hypertension Edema Full, bounding pulses	Strict monitoring of intake and output (especially intravenous fluids); consultation with pharmacist to determine absolute minimum volumes of medications that can be administered safely Weigh patient twice daily	Best measure of total fluid balance; fluid restriction may be essential To assist in assessment of total fluid balance

Diagnosis	Signs and symptoms	Intervention	Rationale
		Pulmonary assessment every 4 hours for signs and symptoms of fluid overload (rales, rhonchi, wheezes, moist cough, or increased respiratory effort)	To detect fluid leaks from capillaries in the lungs
		Cardiovascular assessment for edema (increased BP, gallops, increased pulse pressure)	To indicate heart's ability to handle fluid load or chemotherapy cardiomyopathy
		Neurological assessment for headache, decreased level of consciousness, seizures	Signs of interstitial brain edema
		Serum and urinary lab values including elecrolytes, BUN, creatinine, hematocrit, urine (specific gravity, osmolality)	To provide information regarding vascular volume status
		Measure abdominal girths	To detect or monitor ascites
		Assess for peripheral and/or dependent edema	To detect or monitor subcutaneous fluid leaks
		Report any evidence of fluid overload (2 kg increase in body weight in 24 hours, greater than 1000 mL fluid excess on intake, 500 mL for pediatric patients) to the physician	May indicate need for diuretics to prevent cardiopulmonary failure
		Anticipate physician's orders: administer diuretics, fluid restriction, administer albumin, "renal dose" dopamine	To reduce excess fluid volume and enhance renal clearance of excess fluid

Diagnosis	Signs and symptoms	Intervention	Rationale
Fluid volume deficit related to diarrhea, vomiting, mucositis, or fever	Weight loss Intake < output CVP < 1 mm HG Orthostatic BP and tachycardia Hypotension Poor skin turgor Oliguria Weak, thready pulses	Monitor blood and urinary lab values for signs of dehydration, including electrolytes, hemoglobin and hematocrit, specific gravity, osmolality; monitor patient for clinical manifestations of electrolyte imbalance: hypokalemia—muscular weakness, irregular pulse, muscle cramps; hypomagnesemia—tachycardia, arrhythmias, increased neuromuscular irritation, paresthesias; hyponatremia—anorexia, weakness, abdominal cramping, lethargy, confusion	Signs of dehydration signal that fluid is not in vascular space
		Monitor vital signs for postural changes and instruct patient to call for assistance when changing position until fluid balance achieved	Orthostasis occurs with approximately 20% volume loss
		Monitor body weight for sudden loss	Indicative of lost fluid
		Monitor intake and output for excess output (including careful measurement of emesis, diarrhea, etc.)	Indicator of total body fluid balance
		Frequent mouth care, especially if patient is unable to take oral fluids	Oral mucosa will be dry and taste altered with dehydration
		Notify physician of early signs of dehydration and anticipate physician orders: increase fluid intake with corresponding electrolyte replacement;	Dehydration inhibits organ perfusion and may need to be corrected

Nursing Care Plan for the Management of the Patient with Bone Marrow Transplant

Diagnosis	Signs and symptoms	Intervention	Rationale
		administer acetominophen for fever, also cooling blanket or tepid sponge bath for prolonged, severe fever	

Ineffective breathing pattern related to interstitial pneumonitis, respiratory infection, fluid overload, or compromised cardiac status (Impaired gas exchange may also occur)	Tachypnea
	
	Dyspnea
	
	Crackles, wheezes, or gurgles on auscultation
	
	Production of secretions
	
	Decreased cough reflex
	
	Decreased oxygen saturation
	
	Hypoxemia
	
	Cyanosis
	
	Hypercarbia
	
	Use of accessory muscles to breathe
	
	Decreased oxygen saturation
		Inform physician of diagnosis
		
		Monitor for hypoxia or altered respiratory function regularly; check for:
		  shallow, rapid respiratory rate;
		  use of accessory muscles of respiration;
		  abnormal (absent, diminished, or adventitious) breath sounds;
		  dusky or cyanotic skin color;
		  increased sputum production;
		  decreased activity level;
		  changes in neurological/mental status
			Treatment requires physician's intervention
			
			Indication of poor ventilation patterns and possible hypoxemia

		Monitor results of laboratory and diagnostic testing:
		  arterial blood gases/pulse oximetry;
		  sputum cultures;
		  pulmonary function tests;
		  chest x-rays;
		  lung scans
			Diagnostic testing is useful in monitoring for deterioration of condition or response to interventions

Diagnosis	Signs and symptoms	Intervention	Rationale
		Implement measures to improve respiratory status: place patient in high Fowler's position; maintain oxygen therapy as ordered; instruct/assist patient in regular coughing, deep breathing, and use of incentive spirometry; encourage any aerobic exercise patient can tolerate, such as walking or stationary bike	To increase effectiveness of ventilation in order to improve oxygenation and acid-base balance
		Assist with measures to facilitate removal of pulmonary secretions: chest physiotherapy, positioning, hand-held or nasotracheal suction, airway humidification, increased fluid intake	Helpful in maintaining clear airway and adequate gas exchange
		Teach patient breathing relaxation exercises	To decrease work of breathing and oxygen demand
		Administer mucolytic agents via nebulizer per order	To improve sputum production and clear airway
		Administer other agents that may ease breathing pattern: diuretics to decrease pulmonary edema; morphine sulfate to decrease pulmonary vascular congestion and reduce apprehension-associated dyspnea; bronchodilators; anxiolytics	To assist in reducing work of breathing

Nursing Care Plan for the Management of the Patient with Bone Marrow Transplant

Diagnosis	Signs and symptoms	Intervention	Rationale
Altered nutrition: intake less than body requirements related to nausea and vomiting, xerostomia, or taste changes	Complaints of queasiness Vomiting more than twice a day Not eating Complaints of dry mouth Altered tastes (sweet, salty) Difficulty taking pills	Assess past history of nausea and vomiting to determine pattern and measures that cause or relieve symptoms; tailor specific plan for care based on this history	Nausea and vomiting are often consistent with individual's pattern
		Assess nutritional intake and monitor serum and urinary lab values that reflect fluid and electrolyte and nutritional status (BUN, creatinine, glucose, total protein, albumin, electrolytes, iron and total iron binding capacity, etc.)	To monitor for signs of impending dehydration and malnutrition
		Provide small, frequent meals with input from the patient about preferences (often low-fat, bland, and dry foods are tolerated best); maintain antimicrobial restrictions per institution protocol	To decrease risk of food intolerance that may be causing patient to abstain from eating
		Determine with patient which foods to avoid (usually spicy, GI-irritating foods and fluids are withheld—for example, citrus juices, caffeine, foods with strong odors or flavors such as fish)	Certain foods will precipitate nausea and vomiting
		Eliminate noxious sights and smells from the environment at mealtimes	Certain sights or smells will precipitate nausea and vomiting

Diagnosis	Signs and symptoms	Intervention	Rationale
		Administer antiemetics prophylactically, in combination and frequency that relieves nausea and vomiting; attempt different drug combinations and schedules in collaboration with physician and per patient response	For patient comfort and to maintain nutritional status
		Relieve pain from concurrent stomatitis/mucositis if present	Painful stomatitis reduces oral intake
		Consult with dietician and/or physician to supplement if intake inadequate	Nutritional supplements may be required to maintain nutrition
		Consider use of relaxation techniques or measures to control anticipatory nausea and vomiting	Relaxation has proved successful in reducing anticipatory nausea and vomiting and pain
		Assess quality and severity of dryness or altered taste	To assist in assessment of changes or improvements
		Assess general nutritional status and other aspects of oral and dental health that might affect xerostomia (use of dentures, oral infections, etc.)	To provide a baseline for future evaluation of responses to treatment
		Consult with dietician regarding patient food preferences, aversions; encourage choices that have a high liquid content	Expert advice may enhance intake, nutrition, and patient satisfaction
		Consider use of artificial saliva	Helpful to some individuals
		Maintain mouth moisture by use of other measures such as oral rinses and increasing fluid intake	To promote patient comfort

Nursing Care Plan for the Management of the Patient with Bone Marrow Transplant

Diagnosis	Signs and symptoms	Intervention	Rationale
		Maintain integrity of lips by use of moisturizing balms	To prevent dry, cracking, and painful lips
		Recommend that patient avoid drying substances such as alcohol, tobacco, commercial mouthwashes, and lemon glycerin swabs	Such substances worsen xerostomia
		Provide room humidification unless contraindicated	To improve general environmental humidity and decrease oral and nasal dryness
		Offer foods with a variety of flavors and consistencies to determine preferences	To enhance appetite
Impaired skin integrity related to manifestations of graft-versus-host disease	Maculopapular rash Itching Reddened skin	Monitor for early signs and symptoms of skin GVHD: maculopapular rash, dryness, scaling, pruritus, redness of palms and soles	Early treatment of GVHD may help reduce patient discomfort
		Monitor for evolution of bullae and skin desquamation	To promote patient comfort and prevent infection
		Avoid use of harsh soaps and hot water	May enhance skin irritation
		Daily bathing with antibacterial soap (chlorhexidine or povidone iodine if appropriate) to keep skin clean and dry; consider use of emollient such as Keri-oil, Eucerin cream, or aloe cream, as appropriate	To promote comfort and prevent infection

Diagnosis	Signs and symptoms	Intervention	Rationale
		Keep bed linens free of wrinkles and avoid use of plastic-backed incontinence pads	May increase risk of skin breakdown
		Trim nails and discourage patient from scratching; consider hand mitts, antipruritic medication, soothing baths, etc.	To reduce risk of patient self-injury
		If bullae and skin desquamation occur, consider use of low air loss or silicon bead bed, apply Burow's solution-soaked gauze (Domeboro) on desquamated areas and remove to aid in debridement and cleansing, and apply antibiotic ointment-painted hydrogel dressing to desquamated areas	To promote comfort, wound healing, and prevention of infection
		Administer pain medications as indicated	Lesions are often very painful and may require intravenous medications
Impaired tissue integrity related to radiation-, drug-, or infection-induced mucositis	Oral pain Oral ulcers Inability to eat or swallow	Assess patient for preexisting dental problems	These problems predispose patient to treatment-related oral problems
		Perform daily oral assessment including assessment for dysphagia	To provide information regarding pharyngeal edema and potential for airway problems
		Instruct patient in oral care regime	To promote patient independence
		Culture suspicious oral lesions for bacterial, fungal, and/or viral pathogens	Infection is common, so all lesions should be treated suspiciously

Diagnosis	Signs and symptoms	Intervention	Rationale
		Monitor degree and severity of lesions and/or dysphagia	To provide ongoing data regarding deterioration or improvement of condition and of difficulty protecting the airway
		If dysphagia is present, provide oral suction to assist patient in clearing oral secretions, use aspiration precautions, and assess the consistency of foods best tolerated by patient (liquids versus solids)	To assist patient in preventing aspiration
		Apply topical anesthetics or parenteral analgesia for control of oral pain as appropriate	To promote patient comfort
		With patient, determine tolerable oral diet to assist in maintaining proper nutrition (soft, bland foods, ice chips, popsicles, etc.)	Collaborative diet planning may increase nutritional intake
		Consult with dietician for alternative nutritional support if patient unable to tolerate adequate oral nutrition	Supplementation may be necessary
		Administer therapeutic medications for oral infections and monitor patient's response	Some infections may require more than one agent

Diagnosis	Signs and symptoms	Intervention	Rationale
Alteration in bowel elimination related to radiation or GVHD-induced diarrhea	More than 3 or 4 loose stools per day Abdominal cramps Hyperactive bowel sounds Depletion of electrolytes	Modify oral intake to minimize further risk of exacerbating hypermotility: minimize caffeine, cooked fruits and vegetables, some lactose-containing products	GI stimulants increase diarrhea
		Offer foods that have antidiarrheal effect, such as cheeses	Certain foods help correct diarrhea
		Monitor laboratory values that reflect dehydration and other adverse effects of diarrhea (electrolytes, serum protein, hemoglobin, and hematocrit)	Diarrhea may be severe enough to cause dehydration
		Monitor stool character for additional complications of bleeding and infection; perform stool cultures or other diagnostic studies as ordered	To assist in characterizing abnormal findings
		Monitor weight and intake and output for adverse effects from diarrhea and administer proper fluid and nutritional supplementation	To assess for dehydration complications
		Administer antidiarrheal medications as ordered	To counteract loose stools
		Provide meticulous perineal care including sitz baths after stools, soothing creams and emollients, and antiinflammatory creams or anesthetic agents	To prevent perineal breakdown and infection
		Regularly monitor perineal area for breakdown and infection	To enhance early intervention for breakdown

Diagnosis	Signs and symptoms	Intervention	Rationale
		Anticipate other physician orders to keep patient NPO, to administer specific medications for GVHD, and to treat other effects of chronic, prolonged diarrhea	May reduce morbidity of diarrhea
Alteration in urinary elimination related to bladder irritation from cyclophosphamide metabolites (acrolein) and/or adenovirus	Dysuria Frequency of urination Occult blood in urine or hematuria Bladder distention Bladder spasms	Maintain vigorous oral and intravenous hydration during administration of cyclophosphamide	To reduce cyclophosphamide metabolite in bladder
		Maintain bladder irrigation with 500–1000 mL of GU irrigation solution prior to, during, and 8–24 hours after cyclophosphamide per institution protocol. (Intravenous Mesna bladder protectant may also be ordered)	To decrease metabolite toxicity on bladder
		Continue strict measurement of fluid and electrolyte balance throughout period of bladder irrigation	To help assure accurate output measurement while monitoring for renal function
		Monitor appropriate serum and urinary laboratory tests for evidence of urinary bleeding (hemetest urine, serum hemoglobin and hematocrit)	Occult blood is early sign of bladder irritation and may signal need for intervention to prevent severe bleeding

Diagnosis	Signs and symptoms	Intervention	Rationale
		Immediately report any signs and symptoms of hemorrhagic cystitis to physician; anticipate physician's orders: continuous bladder irrigation; diagnostic bladder testing; administration of platelets and/or red blood cells	Hemorrhagic cystitis can be life-threatening in the aplastic patient
Activity intolerance related to fatigue, debilitation, weakness, or anemia	Fatigue Weakness Sleepiness Inability to perform self-care Dyspnea with exertion	Offer support and encouragement to perform daily activities	To motivate and encourage patient
		Aggressive physical therapy program to enhance conditioning	To promote muscular tone
		Aggressive occupational therapy program if indicated	To reduce long-term deficits
Potential for injury related to drug- or infection-induced neurological impairment or metabolic encephalopathy	Confusion Disorientation Attempts to leave bed Poor judgment about abilities	Regular assessment of mentation and neurological function	To detect early changes
		Monitor serum lab values and anticipate physician order to replace or correct electrolyte imbalances that interfere with neurological function	May influence mental status
		Know hepatically metabolized drugs and discuss with physician ways to decrease doses or minimize administration of these while patient is hepatically impaired	Drugs may enhance hepatic failure
		Provide safe environment when patient is confused, disoriented: determine appropriateness of raising bedrails, assess for need for constant supervision, assess appropriate restraint use if necessary, place call bell within reach, place bed in low position	Hepatic encephalopathy produces neurological symptoms that may endanger patient safety

1237

Nursing Care Plan for the Management of the Patient with Bone Marrow Transplant

Diagnosis	Signs and symptoms	Intervention	Rationale
		Orient patient regularly and provide a clock and calendar for concrete reminders of time	To assist patient's reorientation
		Institute seizure precautions if indicated	Seizures may occur with severe hepatic disease or its related chemical abnormalities
		Assist with all aspects of self-care until patient is able	Patient may be incapable of performing self-care
		Support family during patient's periods of confusion, somnolence or coma; reassure them if condition is predicted to be temporary and reversible	Family may be distressed by changes in patient's personality
Social isolation related to protective isolation precautions	Complaints of loneliness Few visitors Sadness, crying Depression, withdrawal	Assess normal social supports with patient and family	To detect deficits requiring intervention
		Assist patient to determine list of friends and family who would be most supportive during hospital stay (appropriate visitors)	To enhance socialization
		Assist patient to formulate a schedule of visits in accordance with isolation precautions, institutional visitor policy, and care needs	To enhance understanding of restrictions for all visitors
		Discuss alternative ways of communicating with appropriate visitors: phone calls, cards and letters, audio and video tapes, photographs	To enhance socialization

Diagnosis	Signs and symptoms	Intervention	Rationale
		Offer staff and volunteer visitors as available: social worker, CNS, chaplain, volunteers, Cansurmount (ACS) visitors	Patient is entitled to any services available
		Suggest BMT patient/family support group if allowed by isolation precautions	Being part of a group having similar experiences enhances individual coping
		Instruct visitors in isolation precautions, emphasizing the importance of interaction with the patient; specify what contact with the patient is permitted	For protection of patient
Anxiety related to nausea and vomiting or pain	Nonverbal cues of anxiety: facial distress, tachycardia, crying, insomnia, nervous mannerisms	Evaluate patient's previous experience with nausea/vomiting or pain; individualize care plan accordingly	To enhance development of patient-specific plan
	Frequent calling of nurse	Explain use of relaxation exercises to patient and family; encourage patient to practice exercises 2–3 times a day as well as when nauseated or in pain	May be helpful for anxiety, pain, and nausea
	Many questions		
	Inability to remember information or instructions		
		Evaluate and encourage patient's use of relaxation exercises; modify or correct as necessary	
		Explore with patient the use of other available behavioral techniques: guided imagery, quiet music or television for distraction, biofeedback, hypnosis	Various techniques work differently for different individuals

Nursing Care Plan for the Management of the Patient with Bone Marrow Transplant

Diagnosis	Signs and symptoms	Intervention	Rationale
		Evaluate patient's current pharmacological program for effective analgesic and antiemetic effect; modify as necessary for optimal effect	Inadequate antiemetic or pain relief increases anxiety
		Provide adequate information for patient and family to understand care routines, diagnostic tests, etc.	To reduce anxiety surrounding the unknown
Alteration in patient or family coping related to sense of powerlessness	Arguments between patient and family Demanding behavior Dissatisfaction with health care team Negativism	Explore patient's previous methods of coping with hospitalization and cancer: sleeping, sedation, treatment refusal, demanding behavior, repetitive questions, extensive reading or searching for information, formulating schedules of activities, alliance with care givers for care planning, keeping a journal of activities, blood counts, test results, etc.	To identify helpful strategies
		Allow appropriate expressions or verbalizations of anger, fear, anxiety, loss of independence, role performance	To allow free expression of feelings and permit exploration of effective coping measures
		Encourage and reward the use of positive, healthy, past coping strategies; incorporate these into routine care	Positive reinforcement of good behaviors will encourage their use

Diagnosis	Signs and symptoms	Intervention	Rationale
		Collaborate with patient in planning care; allow choices when possible	Reduce sense of powerlessness leading to maladaptive coping
		Explore outcomes of ineffective coping strategies; assist patient to notice negative outcomes	To help patient see futility of negative coping behavior
		Assess family's understanding of patient's coping strategies; validate appropriate strategies and encourage family to support these with patient	To assist in reinforcement of helpful coping
		Offer support group, psychosocial resource staff as available	To help patient identify with others experiencing same events and to model positive coping
Alteration in parenting related to prolonged hospitalization	Reduced participation in child care Verbalized feelings of parental inadequacy Role reversal between parent and child	Explore patient's role as parent and how it has changed since diagnosis of cancer	To define baseline parenting role
		Acknowledge difficulties of maintaining parental role while sick or in hospital	To allow parent to be less than perfect in role
		Evaluate patient's strategies to meet parental role obligations while hospitalized; encourage use of effective and appropriate strategies (phone calls, visits from children, reports of school and other activities, identification of parental activities that can continue, disciplinary action as necessary, and substitute child care)	To reinforce positive behaviors

Nursing Care Plan for the Management of the Patient with Bone Marrow Transplant

Diagnosis	Signs and symptoms	Intervention	Rationale
		Explore spouse's thoughts on patient's current ability to function as parent; reinforce importance of patient's maintaining as much parental activity as possible	To assist in identifying family conflicts over role difficulties
		Offer psychosocial resource staff as available and necessary	Some patients benefit from individual counseling
Noncompliance	Refusal to participate in care Ignoring nurse or caregiver	Assess patient's reasons for noncompliance: if related to lack of knowledge, educate patient/family as to reasons for and correct methods of performing procedures; if related to pain, explore and modify pain management to provide adquate relief for patient to perform required procedures; if related to fatigue, arrange patient's daily schedule to allow rest period before procedure, assist patient when fatigued; if related to lack of trust in caregivers and therefore lack of belief in importance of procedure, establish trust by promoting consistency in caregivers, respect for patient's autonomy and knowledge, collaboration with patient in care planning	Reasons for noncompliance may be easily correctable by care team

Diagnosis	Signs and symptoms	Intervention	Rationale
		Assess all procedures and rank them by level of necessity; allow patient as much flexibility in performance as possible	Increased personal control may improve compliance
		Praise patient for achievements	Positive reinforcement of good behavior encourages repetition
		Assess family's understanding of necessity of patient's compliance with procedures; educate family as necessary	Family's spoken or nonverbal cues may influence patient's compliance
		Enlist family's encouragement of patient's compliance or at least support for nursing interventions to improve compliance	
Anticipatory grieving	Crying Depression Anorexia Making will Planning funeral	Explore patient's and family's beliefs and concerns regarding mortality	To guide future interventions
		Acknowledge reality of patient's and family's concerns; correct misperceptions	To help patient and family deal with reality, not exaggerated fears or impossible dreams
		Support patient and family regarding hope for cure	All patients require some hope to survive the hardships of treatment
		Discuss patient's preparation for death (will, living will, durable power of attorney, CPR status, funeral arrangements, child care wishes, etc.) at patient's level of tolerance	Patient may need information or assistance in completing arrangements before death
		Use chaplains, social workers, and psychosocial resources as appropriate	Experts in grief counseling will be of greater assistance

CHAPTER 8 POST-TEST

1. Excessive bilirubin produces:
   a. polycythemia.
   b. anemia.
   c. jaundice.
   d. hemolysis.

M. S. is an elderly gentleman admitted to the ICU from the ED with fatigue, lethargy, headache, and nuchal rigidity. The medical diagnosis is sepsis; his WBC differential is as follows:

WBC	14.2/mm³
Granulocytes	94%
Eosinophils	1%
Basophils	1%
Bands	30%
Monocytes	2%
Lymphocytes	4%

2. This WBC differential shows:
   a. a right shift.
   b. a left shift.
   c. an opportunistic infection.
   d. meningitis.

3. The antibiotic that is most likely to be used for this patient is:
   a. vancomycin.
   b. aminoglycoside.
   c. trimethoprim sulfa.
   d. amphotericin.

4. J. B. is admitted with known HIV infection. Which of the following tests would be used to confirm the diagnosis?
   a. tissue culture
   b. HIV early antigen
   c. ELISA
   d. Western blot

5. If J. B. presents with profuse watery diarrhea, the organisms to be cultured for include:
   a. cryptosporidium, cytomegalovirus.
   b. histoplasma, Mycobacterium avium intracellulare.
   c. Salmonella, pneumocystis carinii.
   d. shigellosis, legionella.

6. J. B. must be intubated. Precautions to be taken when suctioning his endotracheal tube include:
   a. gowns and gloves on all personnel assisting.
   b. gloves and masks on personnel suctioning.
   c. gloves, gowns, masks, and goggles on personnel suctioning and those assisting.
   d. use of strict isolation techniques.

K. L. is a 25-year-old victim of penetrating trauma to the abdomen who has recently undergone abdominal surgical repair. Estimated blood loss during surgery was 1200 mL, requiring transfusion of blood, platelets, and clotting factors. Postoperatively, the patient was initially hypothermic, requiring warming for 12 hours; he now has acute hypoxemia with bilateral pulmonary infiltrates. At 36 hours after the operation, he is febrile to 39°C and has a WBC of 15.2/mm³.

7. This patient's clotting would be stimulated most by:
   a. venous stasis, vasoconstriction.
   b. tissue injury, vessel injury.
   c. inflammatory mediators, electrolyte imbalance.
   d. hypoxemia, exposure to cold.

8. If bleeding symptoms were to present at this time, the most likely etiology would be:
   a. hypothermia.
   b. exchange transfusions.
   c. bleeding abdominal vessels in the surgical field.
   d. disseminated intravascular coagulation.

9. Disseminated intravascular coagulation is characterized by:
   a. venous thromboses and emboli.
   b. multiorgan failure from microvascular vasoconstriction.
   c. sudden hemorrhagic symptoms.
   d. depletion of coagulation factors.

10. The function of complement is to:
    a. enhance inflammation.
    b. stimulate phagocytic activity.
    c. suppress the specific immune response.
    d. trigger anaphylaxis.

11. The organ transplant with the greatest graft success and patient survival rate is a
    a. liver transplant.
    b. heart transplant.
    c. kidney transplant.
    d. pancreas transplant.

ENDNOTES

1. Miller, B. F., and Keane, C. B. (1987). *Encyclopedia and Dictionary of Medicine, Nursing and Allied Health.* 4th edition. Philadelphia: W. B. Saunders.

2. Shelton, B., and Belcher, A. E. (1990). Biological response modifiers: Therapies that hold great promise for patients with cancer. In P. Aswanden et al., *Oncology Nursing into the 21st Century.* Rockville, MD: Aspen Publishers.

3. Elfenbein, G. J., and Saral, R. (1981). Infectious disease during immune recovery after bone marrow transplantation. In J. Allen (Ed.). *Infection and the Compromised Host: Clinical Correlations and Therapeutic Approaches.* Baltimore: Williams and Wilkins.

4. Guyton, A. C. (1986). *Textbook of Medical Physiology.* 7th edition. Philadelphia: W. B. Saunders.

5. Haeuber, D., and Dijulio, J. E. (1989). Hematopoietic colony stimulating factors: An overview. *Oncology Nursing Forum 16* (2): 247–255.

6. Guyton, op. cit.

7. Fogdall, R. P., and Fishbach, D. P. (1985). *Essentials of Coagulation.* Baltimore: Williams and Wilkins.

8. Guyton, op. cit.

9. Ibid.

10. Ibid.

11. Ibid.

12. Guyton, op. cit.; Malech, M. L., and Gallin, J. I. (1987). Neutrophils in human diseases. *New England Journal of Medicine 317:* 687.

13. Tramone, E. C. (1990). General or nonspecific host defense mechanisms. In G. L. Mandell; R. G. Douglas, Jr.; and J. E. Bennett (Eds.). *Principles and Practice of Infectious Disease.* 3rd edition. New York: Churchill Livingstone.

14. Guyton, op. cit.

15. Williams, J. W.; Beutler, E.; Erslev, A. J.; and Lichtman, M. A. (1990). *Hematology.* 4th edition. New York: McGraw-Hill.

16. Zucker-Franklin, D. (1990). Platelet morphology and function. In J. W. Williams et al. (Eds.). *Hematology.* 4th edition (pp. 1172–1181). New York: McGraw-Hill.

17. Stites, D. P., Stobo, J. D., and Wells, J. V. (1987). *Basic and Clinical Immunology.* 6th edition. Norwalk, CT: Appleton and Lange.

18. Malech and Gallin, op. cit.

19. Guyton, op. cit.

20. Ibid.

21. Verma, I. (1990). Gene therapy. *Scientific American,* November: 68–84.

22. Styrt, B. (1990). Infection associated with asplenia: Risks, mechanisms, and prevention. *American Journal of Medicine 88* (5): 33N–42N.

23. Styrt, op. cit.

24. Ibid.

25. Ibid.

26. Ibid.

27. Ibid.

28. Guyton, op. cit.

29. Ibid.

30. Heinzel, F. P., and Root, R. K. (1990). Antibodies. In G. L. Mandell; R. G. Douglas, Jr.; and J. E. Bennett (Eds.). *Principles and Practice of Infectious Disease.* 3rd edition. New York: Churchill Livingstone.

31. Shelton and Belcher, op. cit.

32. Springhouse Corporation. (1988). *Immune Disorders.* Springhouse, PA: Springhouse Corporation.

33. Porth, C. M. (1986). *Pathophysiology: Concepts of Altered Health Status.* 2nd edition. Philadelphia: J. B. Lippincott.

34. Williams et al., op. cit.

35. Holleb, A. I.; Fink, D. J.; and Murphy, G. P. (1991). *American Cancer Society Textbook of Clinical Oncology.* Atlanta: The American Cancer Society.

36. Jackson, B. S. (1988). Hematopoietic data acquisition. In M. R. Kinney; D. R. Packa; and S. B. Dunbar (Eds.). *AACN's Clinical Reference for Critical Care Nursing.* New York: McGraw-Hill.

37. Parillo, J. (1987). *The Critically Ill Immunosuppressed Patient: Diagnosis and Management.* Rockville, MD: Aspen Publishers.

38. Wade, J. C., and Schimpff, S. C. (1988). Epidemiology and prevention of infection in the compromised host. In R. H. Rubin and L. S. Young (Eds.). *Clinical Approach to Infection in the Compromised Host.* New York: Plenum Medical Book Company.

39. Ibid.

40. Ibid.

41. Malech and Gallin, op. cit.

42. Wade and Schimpff, op. cit.

43. Shelton and Belcher, op. cit.

44. Graziano, F. M., and Lemanske, R. F., Jr. (1989). *Clinical Immunology.* Baltimore: Williams and Wilkins.

45. Ibid.

46. Ibid.

47. Ibid.

48. Graziano and Lemanske, op. cit.

49. Benjamin, E., and Leskowitz, S. (1988). *Immunology: A Short Course.* New York: Alan R. Liss, Inc.

50. Middleton, E.; Reed, C. E.; Ellis, E. F.; Adkinson, N. F.; and Yunginger, J. W. (Eds.). (1988). *Allergy Principles and Practice.* Washington, DC: C. V. Mosby.

51. Graziano and Lemanske, op. cit.

52. Ibid.

53. Ibid.

54. Corren, J., and Shocket, A. L. (1990). Anaphylaxis: A preventable emergency. *Postgraduate Medicine 87* (5): 167–168, 171–178.

55. Ibid.

56. Ibid.

57. Ibid.

58. Teplitz, L. (1989). Clinical closeup on epinephrine. *Nursing 89,* 19 (10): 50–53.

59. McEvoy, G. K. (Ed.). (1989). *AHFS Drug Information 89.* Bethesda, MD: American Society of Hospital Pharmacists.

60. Teplitz, op. cit.

61. Ibid.

62. Ibid.

63. Corren and Shocket, op. cit.

64. Parillo, J. E. (1990). Septic shock in humans: Advances in the understanding of pathogenesis, cardiovascular dysfunction, and therapy. *Annals of Internal Medicine 113* (3): 227–242; Boyd, III, J. L.; Stanford, G. G.; and Chernow, B. (1989). The pharmacotherapy of septic shock. *Critical Care Clinics 5* (1): 133–150.

65. Corren and Shocket, op. cit.

66. Hurst, J. W. (1987). *Medicine for the Practicing Physician.* 2nd edition. Boston: Little, Brown.

67. Fauci, A. S.; Macher, A. M.; Longo, D. L.; Lane, H. C.; Rook, A. H.; Masur, H.; and Gellmann, E. P. (1984). Acquired immunodeficiency syndrome: Epidemiologic, clinical, immunologic, and therapeutic considerations. *Annals of Internal Medicine 100:* 92–106.

68. Ibid.

69. Ibid.

70. Ibid.

71. Ibid.

72. Burroughs Wellcome. (1990). *Diagnosis and Management of HIV Disease: A Reference Manual.* Research Circle, NC.

73. Grossman, M. (1988). Children with AIDS. In M. A. Sande and P. A. Volberding (Eds.). *The Medical Management of AIDS* (pp. 319–330). Philadelphia: W. B. Saunders.

74. Fauci et al., op. cit.

75. Centers for Disease Control. (1990). Possible transmission of human immunodeficiency virus to a patient during an invasive dental procedure. *MMWR 39* (29): 489–493.

76. Centers for Disease Control. (1991). Update: Transmission of HIV infection during an invasive dental procedure—Florida. *MMWR 40* (2): 21–27, 33.

77. Gee, G., and Moran, T. (Eds.). (1988). *AIDS: Concepts in Nursing Practice.* Baltimore: Williams and Wilkins.

78. Fauci et al., op. cit.

79. Lovejoy, N. C. (1988). The pathophysiology of AIDS. *Oncology Nursing Forum 15* (5): 563–574.

80. Centers for Disease Control. (1990). HIV/AIDS surveillance report. *MMWR 39* (9): 1–18; Fan, H.; Connor, R. F.; and Villarreal, L. P. (1990). *The Biology of AIDS.* Boston: Jones and Bartlett.

81. Ibid.

82. Lovejoy, op. cit.

83. Masur, H. (1990). Infections in homosexual men. In G. L. Mandell; R. G. Douglas, Jr.; and J. E. Bennett (Eds.). *Principles and Practice of Infectious Disease.* 3rd edition. New York: Churchill Livingstone.

84. Kovacs, J. A. (1989). Diagnosis, treatment, and prevention of Pneumocystis carinii pneumonia in HIV-infected patients. *AIDS Updates 2* (2): 1–2.

85. Blaese, R. M., and Lane, H. C. (1989). Syndromes of impaired immune function. In W. N. Kelly et al. (Eds.). *Textbook of Rheumatology.* Philadelphia: W. B. Saunders.

86. Ibid.

87. Ibid.

88. Groopman, J. E. (1990). Current advances in the diagnosis and treatment of AIDS: An introduction. *Reviews of Infectious Diseases 12* (5): 908–911.

89. Glatt, A. E.; Chirgwin, K.; and Landesman, S. H. (1988). Treatment of infections associated with human immunodeficiency virus. *New England Journal of Medicine 318:* 1439–1448.

90. Tuazon, C. U. (1989). Toxoplasmosis in AIDS patients. *Journal of Antimicrobial Chemotherapy 23* (supplement A): 77–82.

91. Ibid.

92. Ibid.

93. Ibid.

94. Glatt et al., op. cit.

95. Ibid.

96. Daling, J. R.; Weiss, J. R.; Weiss, N. S.; Hislop, T. G.; Maden, C.; Coates, R. J.; Sherman, K. J.; Ashley, R. L.; Beagrier, M.; Ryan, J. A.; and Corey, L. (1987). Sexual practices, sexually transmitted diseases, and the incidence of anal cancer. *New England Journal of Medicine 317:* 973–977.

97. Blaese and Lane, op. cit.

98. Groopman, op. cit.

99. Blaese and Lane, op. cit.; Levine, A. M. (1990). Therapeutic approaches to neoplasms in AIDS. *Reviews of Infectious Diseases 12* (5): 938–943.

100. Blaese and Lane, op. cit.

101. Levine, op. cit.

102. Ibid.

103. Donehower, M. G. (1987). Malignant complications of AIDS. *Oncology Nursing Forum 14* (1): 57–64.

104. Blaese and Lane, op. cit.

105. Ibid.

106. Kovacs, op. cit.

107. Ibid.

108. Ibid.

109. Ibid.

110. Ibid.

111. Ibid.

112. Ibid.

113. Ibid.

114. Chaisson, R. E., and Volberding, P. A. Clinical manifestations of HIV infection. In G. L. Mandell; R. G. Douglas, Jr.; and J. E. Bennett (Eds.). *Principles and Practice of Infectious Diseases.* 3rd edition. New York: Churchill Livingstone.

115. National Institute of Allergy and Infectious Disease. (1990a). AIDS-related fungal illness. *Opportunistic Infection Research Backgrounder,* May.

116. National Institute of Allergy and Infectious Disease. (1990b). AIDS-related cryptococcal meningitis. *Opportunistic Infection Research Backgrounder;* May.

117. National Institute of Allergy and Infectious disease. (1990c). AIDS-related histoplasma infection. *Opportunistic Infection Research Backgrounder,* May.

118. Ibid.

119. Sande and Volberding, op. cit.

120. Ibid.

121. Ibid.

122. Ibid.

123. National AIDS Information Clearinghouse. (1989). *Eating Defensively* (Videotape).

124. McCabe, R. E., and Remington, J. S. (1990). Toxoplasma Gondii. In G. L. Mandell; R. G. Douglas, Jr.; and J. E. Bennett (Eds.). *Principles and Practice of Infectious Diseases.* 3rd edition. New York: Churchill Livingstone.

125. Ibid.

126. Sande and Volberding, op. cit.

127. Ibid.

128. Tuazon, op. cit.

129. Ibid.

130. Davey, R. T., and Lane, H. C. (1990). Laboratory methods in the diagnosis and prognostic staging of infection with human immunodeficiency virus type I. *Reviews of Infectious Diseases 12* (5): 912–930.

131. Sande and Volberding, op. cit.

132. Centers for Disease Control. (1987). Update: Human immunodeficiency virus infections in health care workers exposed to blood of infected patients. *MMWR 36:* 285–288.

133. Fuchs, D.; Hansen, A.; Reibnegger, G.; et al. (1987). HIV seroconversion in health care workers. *JAMA 258:* 2525–2526; Gurevich, I. (1989). The acquired immunodeficiency syndrome. In D. Dracup (Ed.). *Infectious Diseases in Critical Care Nursing: Prevention and Precautions.* Rockville, MD: Aspen Publications.

134. Ibid.

135. Blaese and Lane, op. cit.

136. Chaisson and Volberding, op. cit.

137. National Institute of Allergy and Infectious Disease. (1990d). Toxoplasmic encephalitis. *Opportunistic Infection Research Backgrounder,* May.

138. Kovacs, op. cit.

139. Ibid.

140. Ibid.

141. Fogdall and Fishbach, op. cit.

1246

142. Springhouse Corporation. (1990). *I.V. Therapy: Nursing Skillbooks*. Springhouse, PA: Springhouse Corporation.

143. Ibid.

144. Perry, A. G. (1988). Shock complications: Recognition and management. *Critical Care Nursing Quarterly 11* (1): 1–8; Young, L. M. (1990). DIC: The insidious killer. *Critical Care Nurse 10* (9): 26–33.

145. Ibid.

146. Burns, E. R. (1987). *Clinical Management of Bleeding and Thromboses*. Palo Alto, CA: Blackwell Scientific Publications.

147. Braunwald, E.; Isselbacher, K. J.; Petersdorf, R. G.; Wilson, J. D.; Martin, J. B.; and Fauci, A. S. (1989). *Harrison's Principles of Internal Medicine*. 11th edition. New York: McGraw-Hill.

148. Burns, op. cit.; Braunwald et al., op. cit.

149. Braunwald et al., op. cit.

150. Hurst, op. cit.

151. Burns, op. cit.

152. Griffin, J. P. (1986). *Hematology and Immunology: Concepts for Nurses*. Norwalk, CT: Appleton Century Crofts.

153. Ibid.

154. Young, op. cit.

155. Fogdall and Fishbach, op. cit.

156. Esparaz, B., and Green, D. (1990). Disseminated intravascular coagulation. *Critical Care Nursing Quarterly 13* (2): 7–13.

157. Hurst, op. cit.

158. Ibid.

159. Ibid.

160. Parillo, op. cit.; Boyd et al., op. cit.

161. Burns, op. cit.; Larcan, A.; Lambert, H.; and Gerard, A. (1987). *Consumption Coagulopathies*. New York: Masson Publishing.

162. Hurst, op. cit.

163. Larcan et al., op. cit.

164. Ibid.

165. Hurst, op. cit.

166. Soukup, S. M. (1991). Organ donation from the family of a totally brain-dead donor: Professional responsiveness. *Critical Care Nursing Quarterly 13* (4): 8–18.

167. Ibid.

168. Ibid.

169. Ibid.

170. Linde-Zwirble, M. E.; Bishop, B. S.; and Menker, J. B. (1991). Management of the organ donor: A first step in transplantation. *Critical Care Nursing Quarterly 13* (4): 19–24.

171. Wingard, J. R. (1990). Historical perspectives and future directions. In M. B. Whedon (Ed.). *Bone Marrow Transplantation Principles, Practice, and Nursing Insights*. Boston: Jones and Bartlett.

172. O'Quin, T., and Moravec, C. (1988). The critically ill bone marrow transplant patient. *Seminars in Oncology Nursing 4* (1): 25–30.

173. Shivnan, J. C., and Shelton, B. K. (In press). Bone marrow transplantation: Issues for critical care nurses. *Critical Care Nurse* (in press).

174. Whedon, M. B. (1990). Allogeneic bone marrow transplantation: Clinical indications, treatment process, and outcomes. In M. B. Whedon (Ed.). *Bone Marrow Transplantation Principles, Practice, and Nursing Insights*. Boston: Jones and Bartlett.

175. Freedman, S.; Shivnan, J.; Tilles, J.; and Klemm, P. (1990). Bone marrow transplantation: Overview and nursing implications. *Critical Care Nursing Quarterly 13* (2): 51–62.

176. Freedman, S. E. (1988). An overview of bone marrow transplantation. *Seminars in Oncology Nursing 4* (1): 3–8.

177. Freedman et al., op. cit.

178. Ibid.

179. Brochstein, J. A. (1988). Critical care issues in bone marrow transplantation. *Critical Care Clinics 4* (1): 147–166.

180. Caudell, K. A. (1990). Graft-versus-host disease. In M. B. Whedon (Ed.). *Bone Marrow Transplantation Principles, Practice, and Nursing Insights*. Boston: Jones and Bartlett.

181. Caudell, K. A., and Whedon, M. B. (1990). Hematopoietic complications. In M. B. Whedon (Ed.). *Bone Marrow Transplantation, Principles, Practice, and Nursing Insights*. Boston: Jones and Bartlett.

182. Elfenbein and Saral, op. cit.

183. Truog, A. W., and Wozniak, S. P. (1990). Cyclosporine-A as prevention for graft-versus-host disease in pediatric patients undergoing bone marrow transplants. *Oncology Nursing Forum 17* (1): 39–44.

184. Bedell, M. K. (1990). Procedure costs and reimbursement issues. In M. B. Whedon (Ed.). *Bone Marrow Transplantation Principles, Practice, and Nursing Insights*. Boston: Jones and Bartlett.

9 Multisystem Problems

CHAPTER 9 PRE-TEST

1. Neuropathic pain is typically:
   a. sharp and stabbing.
   b. continuous and nonlocalized.
   c. localized and burning in nature.
   d. diffuse and aching.

2. A patient's pain is evaluated using a rating scale on a ruler, with 1 meaning pain-free and 10 meaning the worst pain possible. The patient is to mark the point that best describes what is being felt. This is an example of:
   a. a multidimensional pain scale.
   b. the McGill pain assessment inventory.
   c. a visual analog scale.
   d. a pain descriptive scale.

3. All of the following topical medications are frequently prescribed in caring for the burn patient *except*:
   a. silver sulfadiazine.
   b. penicillin.
   c. silver nitrate.
   d. mafenide acetate.

4. Burn care must address all of the following *except*:
   a. burn immunosuppression.
   b. physical rehabilitation.
   c. tissue repair and replacement.
   d. care of the skin donor patient.

5. Extrinsic causes of asphyxia include:
   a. injury to the chest.
   b. injury to the stomach.
   c. injury to the heart.
   d. pleural hemorrhage.

6. Smoke inhalation causes injury via:
   a. direct heat, irritating gases, and aspiration of stomach contents.
   b. direct heat, irritating gases, and aerosolized contaminates.
   c. direct poisoning, irritating gases, and direct heat.
   d. direct heat, direct poisoning, and aspiration of stomach contents.

7. Toxic shock syndrome is:
   a. a gram-negative endotoxin–induced hypotension.
   b. a gram-positive sepsis.
   c. a disease specific to women.
   d. easily treated with amphotericin.

8. Organisms most likely to cause nosocomial infection include:
   a. camphylobacter and E. coli.
   b. salmonella and listeria.
   c. staphylococcus and nocardia.
   d. pseudomonas and klebsiella.

Sepsis and Septic Shock

Despite major technological advances in the care of critically ill patients, infection remains the most common complication of critical illness. Sepsis remains the most common etiology of late deaths in the ICU,[1] and its incidence has increased 1000% in the past 25 years.[2] Sepsis has been the strongest predisposing factor for multiorgan failure and death in ICU patients.[3] Differentiation of the various levels of clinical infection is important to the development of an appropriate assessment and management plan but can present a confusing dilemma to ICU practitioners. Because there are few clinical resources describing the essential differences that influence prognosis, Table 9-1 defines the following levels of infection for reference throughout this section: colonization, infection, bacteremia, septicemia, sepsis, septic syndrome, septic shock, and fever of unknown origin.

Clinical infection is the most common complication of hospitalization. With the exception of individuals with specific immune deficits, nearly all infections leading to septic shock occur in the hospital setting; thus, it is now considered a nosocomial (hospital-acquired) disease.[4] It is estimated that infection lengthens the hospital stay for approximately 1 in every 100 hospitalized patients, or about 5% of hospitalized patients.[5] In the United States, an estimated 400,000 cases of sepsis occur annually, and half of these cases result in septic shock.[6]

Septic shock is a complex clinical syndrome occurring as a result of a systemic response to serious infection. Shock is the consequence of mediator substances released by the inflammatory-immune response to pathogenic organisms and their toxins. A combination of endotoxin effects and immune mediators produces the vascular collapse characteristic of septic shock, and it is interesting to note that in 60% of the cases of septic shock, no specific organism is cultured.[7] Mortality statistics for this syndrome re-

Table 9-1 Definitions of Types of Infection

Term	Definition	Diagnostic Criteria
Fever of unknown origin (FUO)	Temperature higher than 38.3°C rectally for 3 weeks; investigation of cause inconclusive after at least 1 week	Blood cultures Fever pattern
Colonization	Microbial multiplication and survival on mucous membranes and skin surfaces without deeper tissue penetration to cause disease	Surveillance cultures
Infection	Invasion by virulent microorganisms of tissues in the body where the conditions for their growth are favorable; clinical symptoms of WBC response are present	Surveillance cultures Local symptoms Leukocytosis
Bacteremia	Presence of viable microorganisms in the circulating blood	Blood cultures positive for microorganism
Septicemia	Systemic disease caused by the spread of microorganisms and their toxins in the circulating blood	Blood cultures positive for microorganism Systemic symptoms of infection: fever, leukocytosis
Sepsis	Clinical evidence of altered organ perfusion with systemic symptoms of infection	With positive or negative blood cultures Systemic symptoms of infection
Septic syndrome	Sepsis with evidence of altered organ perfusion, but possibly not strong clinical symptoms or positive blood cultures	Clinical presentation Blood cultures
Septic shock	Sepsis presentation with hypotension based on a MAP less than 70 mm Hg	Blood cultures Cardiovascular status evaluation

main grim: over 100,000 deaths a year, or a 30–75% mortality rate.[8] Although the levels most life-threatening to patients and most challenging to critical care nurses are septic shock and toxic shock, all infections require similar assessment and management skills.

Clinical antecedents

The critically ill patient has a high-risk profile for the development of nosocomial infections. Infections may be endogenous (arising from the individual's normal body flora) or exogenous (arising from the environment). Typical endogenous organisms are Escherichia coli (E. coli) and clostridium, found in the GI tract; candida, located in the oral cavity and urinary tract; and aspergillus, streptococcus, and staphylococcus, found in the nasopharynx. Infections involving organisms that are not normally pathogenic but produce clinical infection in the susceptible individual are called opportunistic infections.

Risk factors for the development of infection can be categorized as host-related or treatment-related, and they alter different immunologic defenses. These are listed in Table 9-2. Among the most prevalent of critical care problems are the numerous wounds and catheters, which provide access for pathogenic organisms to enter the body. The ICU patient is also likely to be malnourished, under tremendous physical stress, or receiving immunosuppressing agents.

The ICU patient can also acquire infections from other patients nearby. There are several factors that increase the risk of cross-infection in intensive care areas. Critical care units are often designed so that patients are located close to one another, increasing the risk of spreading infection. The antibiotics most critically ill patients receive for endogenous infections produce a predisposition for the development of resistant organisms that are less amenable to the standard antibiotic regimen the patient may be receiving. In addition, infections can be transmitted by devices or equipment shared by already infected patients. A recent CDC report described the nosocomial transmission of hepatitis B by way of a blood-testing device used to draw capillary blood for the measurement of blood glucose levels.[9] The lancet device used a disposable platform to stabilize the finger and control the depth of puncture; it appears that nurses did not routinely change this platform between patients. Many other examples of communal use exist (multiple use of electric razors or pulse oximeters, for instance) and should be examined to

prevent infection spread. The presence of several risk factors is contributory to infection development, although the clinical severity of infections varies greatly. Some infections are more amenable to treatment or are less likely to produce systemic infection.

The critical care nurse should be able not only to recognize risk factors for infection development but also to correlate a risk factor to the specific infections the patient is likely to develop. The pathogenic organisms that produce infection include gram-positive and gram-negative bacteria, fungi, viruses, protozoa, and helminths. Other common physiological risk factors for infection are listed in Table 9-2.

It is generally thought that most cases of septic shock are the result of infection with endogenous gram-negative bacteria, although recently developed antibiotics have somewhat curbed these pathogens. The source of these bacteria may be the patient's respiratory, gastrointestinal, or genitourinary tract. Breaks in the skin integrity—such as with trauma and burns—will place the patient at risk for infection with gram-positive skin organisms such as streptococcus or staphylococcus. A particular strain of staphylococcus has been implicated in the development of toxic shock syndrome. The individual at risk to develop this severe form of gram-positive infection is the menstruating woman who uses tampons for extended periods of time. Children and some patients who have had abdominal surgery are also at risk. Note that only 15% of those affected are men.

Approximately 75% of the cases of septic shock are caused by gram-negative bacteria; the remaining 25% are due to gram-positive bacteria such as Staphylococcus epidermis or streptococci (see Figure 9-1). Approximately 20–30% of the cases of septic shock involve "mixed infections" or are polymicrobial (involving more than one microorganism).[10] The subtypes of organisms involved in the pathogenesis of septic shock are listed in Table 9-3 (page 1253).

Critical referents

Infection activates the body's defense systems, producing a complex immune response involving several interrelated physiological systems (see Figure 9-2, page 1254). The inflammatory-immune and stress responses are responsible for the physiological effects of sepsis. Hematologic-immune activities triggered in this process include those performed by the coagulation, fibrinolytic, complement, kallikreinogen, and eicosanoid systems as well as certain immune cells such as macrophages and neutrophils. The chemical mediator substances produced during

Table 9-2 Clinical Antecedents of Infection

Type	Physiological Mechanism of Risk
Host-Related	
Age (under 1 year or over 65 years)	Normal decline of internal and external defenses occurs with age. Thymus is immature in infants and atrophies in the elderly. Malnutrition-related immune deficits are more prevalent in elderly. Older adults have decreased antigen-specific IgS.
Alcoholism	Alcoholism causes decreased ability of neutrophils to respond to stimuli. Congestion of liver and spleen also leads to decreased response to microorganisms by reticuloendothelial cells and slowed phagocytic response.
Cancer	Systemic disease may lead to many structural immune interruptions (such as lymphatic blockage or bone marrow depression). Malnutrition may occur in this patient group. Various cancers have specific immune deficits, such as diminished phagocytic activity or decreased numbers of lymphocytes.
Chronic health problems	Decreased immune reserve and possibly specific immune deficits are related to interference with lymphoid organ function. Chronic illness may contribute to poor nutritional status.
Diabetes mellitus	Diabetics have decreased numbers of neutrophils (PMNs) and lowered ability to respond to stimuli present during increased numbers of hospitalizations, which increase risk of nosocomial infections. Neuropathy of DM and glycosuria cause inadequate bladder emptying and risk of UTI. Hyperglycemia impedes phagocytic response and causes specific humoral and cellular defects.
Gastrointestinal disease	Decreased GI motility permits and encourages normal flora to translocate into blood.
Hepatic disease	Neutrophils are unavailable to kill bacteria. Because the phagocytic activity of Kuppfer cells is decreased, the body's ability to remove foreign organisms is decreased.
Abuse of intravenous drugs	Altered barrier defense mechanisms, chronic illness, infection, and malnutrition predispose to decreased WBCs, slowed phagocytic response. T cell functions altered, possibly due to persistent viral exposure and exhaustion of reserve.
Malnutrition	Neutrophils are unable to kill bacteria.
Renal disease	Neutrophils are unable to respond in order to kill bacteria.
Rheumatoid arthritis	Neutrophils cannot respond to stimuli as well.
Splenectomy	The mechanism for trapping blood-borne bacteria or recognizing encapsulated bacteria (TB, hemophilus) is limited. Also antibody and complement production are decreased.
Treatment-Related	
Antibiotics	Destruction of normal flora leads to growth of resistant organisms and superinfection with fungus, which decrease responsiveness to specific antigenic stimulus.
Immunosuppressive medication or treatments	WBC production is suppressed, phagocytic activity is decreased, and T cell recognition of non-self cells is blocked with certain drugs.
Immunosuppressive agents	Antibody formation is decreased, T cell function is suppressed, and myelosuppression occurs with decreased neutrophils.
Invasive devices	Skin barrier violation permits transmission of microorganisms, especially gram-positive skin flora and water organisms such as pseudomonas.
Neutropenia	The quantity of granulocytes, especially neutrophils is decreased, as is the ability to respond to stimuli.
Surgical procedures or wounds	Normal flora may translocate to another body location with subsequent infection. Stress from surgery may stimulate adrenal stress response with increased cortisol and subsequent immune suppression.
Traumatic injuries or burns	Barrier defenses are altered.

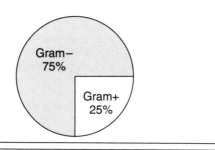

Figure 9-1   Distribution of Infections in Sepsis

activation of these body systems enhance vasodilation, capillary permeability, and phagocytic destruction of bacteria. When this response is disproportional to the infection or in excess of the infecting organisms or when the infection is severe, systemic physiological effects occur. In fact, the chemical mediators often act as endogenous toxins, causing damage to the tissue itself. Tumor necrosis factor (TNF) from activated macrophages, superoxide from phagocytes, complement components, histamine, bradykinin, prostaglandins, interleukins, and endorphins may be among the most significant of these endogenous toxins. Also important to understanding the pathophysiology of septic shock is the recognition that bacteria entering the body actively attack normal body tissues. At the nidus of the infection, some of these bacteria can produce toxins with effects similar to the body's normal inflammatory mediators.

Bacterial toxins and inflammation produce several hemodynamic effects that result in hypoperfusion of body tissues (see Figure 9-3). Hemodynamic effects include (1) altered blood flow through the microcirculation, (2) vasodilation of the arteries and veins, and (3) selective vasoconstriction of pulmonary, renal, and gastrointestinal vessels. Other

Table 9-3   Organisms Causing Septic Shock

Organism	Percentage of Total Cases
Gram-negative organisms	
Escherichia coli	40
Klebsiella, enterobacter, or serratia	20
Pseudomonas aeruginosa	20
Proteus	10
Bacteroides	10
Gram-positive organisms	
Staphylococcus aureus	40
Staphylococcus epidermis	40
Streptococcus	20

Source: Wahl, S.C. (1989). Septic shock: How to detect it early. *Nursing 89, 19*(1): 52–59.

physiological consequences include vascular endothelium microembolization, capillary membrane permeability, myocardial depression, and ventricular dilation. As with all types of shock, septic shock produces a situation in which circulation is insufficient to meet metabolic demands, microcirculation fails, and cellular anoxia exists. This triad of maldistribution of blood flow, imbalance of oxygen supply and demand, and metabolic derangements is the classic physiological consequence of both sepsis and multiorgan failure.

Although the clinical effects are similar, the pathophysiology of sepsis due to gram-positive bacteria and of that due to gram-negative bacteria is somewhat different. Gram-positive shock usually arises from a fulminating infection by staphylococcus, pneumococcus, or Clostridium perfringens tetani. Gram-positive bacteria actively release or secrete exotoxins and enzymes, initiating the immune response. Exotoxins also produce a severe fluid loss and hematologic effects such as RBC hemolysis, WBC destruction, and platelet aggregation. The pathophysiological effects of gram-positive sepsis are noted in Figure 9-4.

In contrast to gram-positive organisms, gram-negative ones do not initiate septic shock by active secretion of toxins. The cell walls of gram-negative bacteria contain a lipopolysaccharide termed LPS, or endotoxin. LPS contains an inner protein, lipid A, which is the toxic component of the endotoxin. When the body's immune cells attack gram-negative bacteria, LPS is released into the circulation. LPS and other bacterial toxins incite an immune response, producing profound changes in vascular tone and permeability. Endotoxin produces profoundly reduced systemic vascular resistance, a dilated and depressed myocardium, leakage of fluid from capillaries, and impaired pulmonary function. The complex effects of bacterial endotoxin and the inflammatory-immune response of the body are shown in Figure 9-5 (page 1256).

Immunologic activity occurs in gram-positive shock to a lesser degree than in gram-negative shock, but the mediators' physiological effects can be profound. (A summary of these mediators and the pathophysiological alteration of septic shock each contributes to is given in Table 9-4 on page 1256.) Histamines, prostaglandins, leukotrienes, and vasoactive peptides called kinins produce vasodilation, bronchoconstriction, and increased capillary membrane permeability. Kinins, such as bradykinin, are potent vasodilators that also cause marked increases in vascular permeability. All of these mediators increase vascular permeability as well as attract platelets and neutrophils to the affected area. Vasodila-

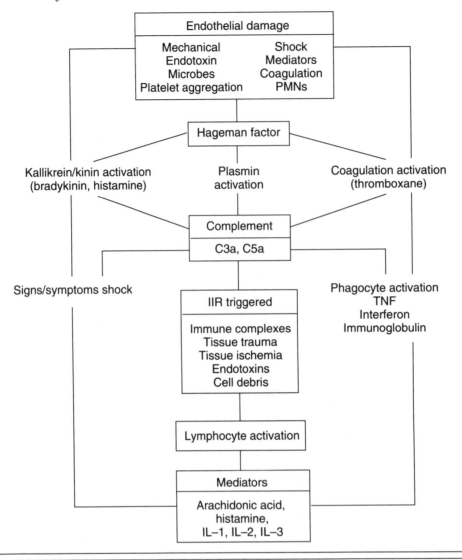

Figure 9-2   Inflammatory Feedback Cycle

tion, reduction in total peripheral vascular resistance (PVR), microcirculatory clotting, and increased leakage of fluid from capillaries (third-spacing of fluids) result.

Some of the most significant clinical effects of sepsis appear to arise from the activation of the complement cascade. In sepsis, the complement cascade is activated via both classical and alternative pathways. Bacterial exotoxins or endotoxins stimulate antibody formation; antibody then combines with the toxins to activate the complement cascade via the classical pathway. In contrast, components of bacterial cell walls directly activate the complement cascade via the alternative pathway, with no need for antibody. Normally, immune cells such as macrophages destroy complexes of antigen-antibody and complement. In sepsis, however, the phagocytes are overwhelmed by the sheer quantity of bacterial toxins, resulting in an overproduction of certain complement components, such as C5a and C3a.[11] Through a process termed the arachidonic acid cascade, these complement anaphylotoxins stimulate mast cells to release stored chemical mediators such as histamine and to generate other mediators termed eicosanoids (prostaglandins and leukotrienes).[12] The mediator substances of the complement interaction produce vasodilation, bronchoconstriction, and increased capillary permeability. The complement component C5a also acts as a potent chemotactin, attracting neutrophils and macrophages to the site. Macrophages arriving at the site are activated, releasing tumor necrosis factor (TNF, cachectin) and interleukin-1 (IL-1, endogenous pyrogen). TNF is the major endogenous toxin in the pathogenesis of septic shock

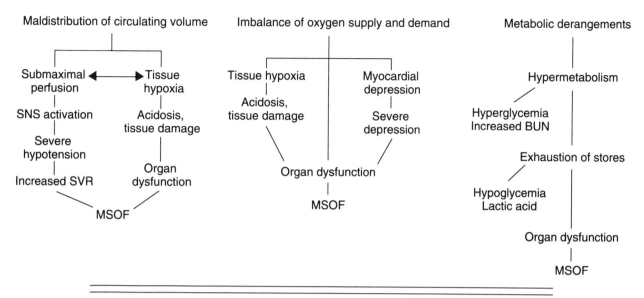

Figure 9-3 Pathophysiological Effects of IIR Stimulation

and may be a factor in myocardial depression.[13] Both TNF and IL-1 produce fever, protein catabolism, weight loss, and cachexia.

During the attempt to destroy microorganisms by phagocytosis, neutrophils may damage tissue. Neutrophils stimulated by bacterial toxins generate superoxide and other toxic compounds and release lysosomes, which digest or damage surrounding tissue. In fact, activated neutrophils may be important in the pathogenesis of multiple organ failure, a common complication of sepsis regardless of whether the offending infectious organism is destroyed.

In contrast to the generalized vasodilation of the peripheral blood vessels, the pulmonary, renal, and splanchnic blood vessels are vasoconstricted as a result of systemic shunting, microthrombi, and blood viscosity. During sepsis, endotoxin and neutrophils activate factor XII (tissue thromboplastin), initiating the extrinsic pathway of the coagulation cascade, stimulating conversion of fibrinogen to fi-

brin, and leading to vascular clotting. The activation of the coagulation cascade also contributes to vessel obstruction with microthrombi. Platelets attracted to the area enhance clotting by degranulation and release of thromboxane A_2 (also known as platelet-activating factor, or PAF), a potent platelet aggregant. PAF does more than activate platelet aggregation; it may have direct depressant effects on cardiac function and systemic circulation.[14] Neutrophils attracted to the area often damage the endothelial capillary lining, also leading to the formation of clots. The large number of circulating neutrophils may impede blood flow because they increase blood viscosity and aggregate. It is proposed that neutrophil activation and aggregation may be the most important factors in producing the pulmonary compromise seen in sepsis.[15]

The fibrinolytic system is activated in conjunction with the clot-forming system. Plasminogen is converted to plasmin, which degrades fibrin monomers, preventing the formation of a stable clot.

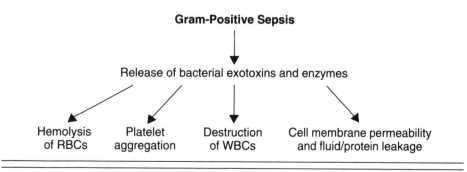

Figure 9-4 Pathophysiology of Gram-Positive Infection

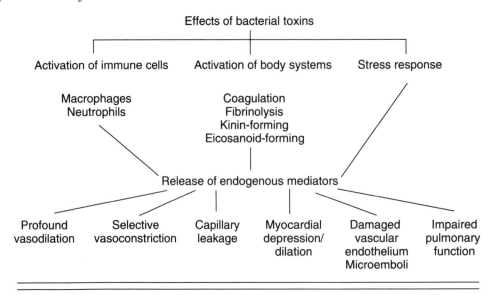

Figure 9-5 Pathophysiology of Gram-Negative Infection

Clinically, the activation of both the coagulation and fibrinolytic systems produces a consumptive coagulopathy, disseminated intravascular coagulation (DIC).

The net result of the immune processes is to produce a generalized maldistribution of blood flow in which some tissues are starved for oxygenated blood, while others get more flow than required.

Table 9-4 Summary of Sepsis Mediators and Their Clinical Effects

Alteration	Chemical Mediators
Peripheral vasodilation	1. Activation of complement system and subsequent release of vasoactive substances 2. Activation of kinin system 3. Histamine release 4. Endorphin release secondary to leukocyte endogenous mediator (LEM)
Endothelial cell destruction	1. Aggregation of neutrophils due to increased C5a 2. Histamine release 3. Direct action of microorganisms
Increased capillary permeability	1. Activation of complement system and subsequent release of vasoactive substances 2. Activation of kinin system 3. Histamine release
Microemboli	1. Activation of clotting system 2. Aggregation of neutrophils due to increased C5a 3. Platelet aggregation due to increased thromboxane A_2 and decreased prostacyclin
Vasoconstriction of pulmonary, renal, and splanchnic vasculature	1. Increased prostaglandin $F_{2\alpha}$ 2. Decreased prostacyclin 3. Norepinephrine, epinephrine, and angiotensin release 4. Myocardial depressant factor release
Depressed myocardial contractility	1. Activation of complement system 2. Release of myocardial depressant factor 3. Endorphin release secondary to LEM 4. Histamine release

Source: Rice, V. (1984). The clinical continuum of septic shock. Home Study Course. *Critical Care Nurse,* Sept/Oct: 86–109. p. 90.

The stress response initiated in sepsis causes release of adrenocorticotropic hormone and stimulates release of corticosteroids and catecholamines. Although catecholamines would normally produce peripheral vasoconstriction, tachycardia, and increased pumping action of the heart, the net effects of the chemical mediators in septic shock are stronger and produce peripheral vasodilation and a reduction in myocardial contractility. Endotoxin stimulates the hypothalamus to release beta endorphins, which may further depress the myocardium and depress the level of consciousness.[16]

In summary, the physiological effects of infection leading to sepsis are directly related to either the inflammatory response or bacterial toxins. Sepsis is the clinical disorder stemming from the body's normal inflammatory response to invading pathogens. Excessive stimulation of this response to large numbers of bacteria produces sufficient amounts of mediator substances to cause destruction of normal tissue. The extreme result of this disorder is the vascular collapse associated with septic shock. In septic shock, the body's compensatory mechanisms are no longer able to support the tissue's demand for oxygen and nutrients. This syndrome of hemodynamic instability, coagulation abnormalities, altered metabolism, and regional malperfusion leads to cellular anoxia and multisystem organ failure, as seen in Figure 9-6. These physiological effects encompass all body systems. The text that follows is a comprehensive review of these effects.

Cardiovascular system Early in sepsis, vasodilation produces low diastolic blood pressure, causing a decrease in mean arterial pressure (MAP). As this effect becomes more marked, the low SVR and MAP lead to hypotension. The stress response is stimulated and causes the release of the catecholamines epinephrine and norepinephrine, which attempt to compensate for the hypotensive response by producing tachycardia and increased myocardial contractility. The increased stroke volume (SV) and heart rate and the low vascular resistance combine to increase cardiac output (CO). Unfortunately, these catecholamines also serve to increase the potential for dysrhythmias. Even with these potent cardiac stimulants, there is a propensity for heart failure. In septic shock, TNF appears to effect the myocardium, causing ventricular dilation and depression.[17] Beta endorphins released by the hypothalamus may also depress the myocardium.[18] Clinically, the ventricle has a markedly reduced ability to increase contractility in response to fluid.

Perhaps the best measure of the cardiovascular pathophysiology of septic shock is the depressed left ventricular ejection fraction.[19] Overall, septic shock produces a hyperdynamic cardiovascular state with a depressed and dilated left ventricle.[20] During the late phase of septic shock, profound vasoconstriction (high SVR) occurs, increasing afterload. Although the third spacing of fluids diminishes venous return, preload is also increased.

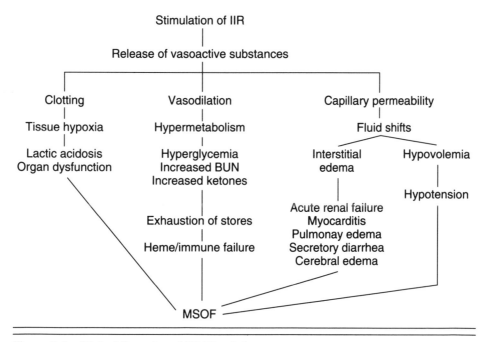

Figure 9-6 Clinical Sequelae of IIR Stimulation

Pulmonary circulation Among the most profound and clinically important effects of sepsis are the pulmonary changes that occur. Initially, bacterial toxins affect the medullary respiratory center, resulting in tachypnea and producing respiratory alkalosis.[21] Pulmonary blood vessels are selectively constricted because of mediator substances produced early in sepsis, reducing pulmonary blood flow and eventually causing pulmonary hypertension. Pulmonary hypertension is considered an indicator of a poor prognosis for survival in this patient population.[22] Other significant changes involve increased capillary permeability, which causes increased lung water and alveolar flooding.[23] The neutrophil chemotactic factor (NCF) released in septic injury attracts neutrophils to the lungs. These WBCs are sequestered in the pulmonary capillary bed and release lysosomes, which damage tissue. Platelets aggregate in the pulmonary vessels, forming microthrombi. Fibrin formed from the activation of the coagulation cascade combines with dead and dying cells to form a hyaline membrane over the alveolar epithelium, thereby blocking the diffusion of oxygen across the alveolar-capillary junction and causing ventilation-perfusion ($\dot{V}/\dot{Q}$) mismatch. The oxygen consumption demand is tremendous, and minute ventilations of 15–20 L/min may be required to oxygenate the patient.[24] Endothelial injury, increased lung water, and hyaline membranes lead to reduced arterial oxygen levels, a narrowing of the arterial-alveolar oxygen gradient (A-a DO_2), and elevated mixed venous oxygen.[25]

Metabolic effects Glucose is generated by several sources to provide additional energy for the excessive energy requirements of the body during infection and sepsis. Glucagon released in the stress response stimulates gluconeogenesis, glycogenolysis, and lipolysis and the release of epinephrine and norepinephrine from the adrenal medulla.[26] The results of lipolysis without effective glucose utilization are hypertriglyceridemia and ketosis. Unfortunately, the amino acids required for gluconeogenesis are obtained by proteolysis of skeletal muscle, a process that causes muscle wasting. At first, the liver uses these amino acids to produce glucose. However, as shock progresses, the liver is unable to maintain this activity, and amino acids accumulate, elevating urine nitrogen levels. Epinephrine and norepinephrine further increase blood glucose levels by converting glycogen to glucose. Insulin resistance, related to an inability to oxidize glucose, inhibits cells' ability to use the glucose, and refractory hyperglycemia occurs.[27]

The poor tissue perfusion leads to decreased intracellular oxygenation and anaerobic metabolism. The metabolic pathway produces small amounts of glucose and large amounts of lactic acid, which lower the intracellular pH. Lactic acid accumulation eventually becomes significant, and the cell membranes' ionic pump fails. Intracellular sodium and water increase (depleting the serum of sodium and water), the cell swells, and lysosomes leak enzymes that cause cell death. Hyperkalemia, hyperphosphatemia, and elevated uric acid levels occur to varying degrees.[28]

Renal system In infection and early sepsis, the by-products of cell death create a tremendous osmotic load on the kidneys, and the patient may exhibit profound diuresis. The high urine output is short-lived, however, since the infection-induced hypotension reduces blood flow through the kidneys and causes a reduced glomerular filtration rate (GFR). The reduced intravascular volume also stimulates the release of aldosterone, causing renal conservation of sodium and water. The reduced renal blood flow triggers the release of renin from the kidneys and stimulation of the renin-angiotensin system. Epinephrine and norepinephrine cause vasoconstriction, and reduced urine output—with or without intrarenal damage—is the result.

Resulting signs and symptoms

The symptoms of infection, sepsis, and septic shock vary according to the area of the body infected, the causative organism, and the patient's age, immune status, and state of health. If the patient's hemodynamic status or cardiac performance is compromised at the onset of infection, there is likely to be less tolerance of the physiological demands. Additionally, the patient's immune function may influence susceptibility to specific organisms or dissemination of infection. Organisms commonly encountered in the ICU setting are described in Table 9-5.

Infection Infection symptoms are usually localized to an area of the body where organisms are found to be proliferating. Particular infections are named by their location, for instance, myocarditis, encephalitis, and peritonitis. Infections of the soft tissue are named according to the depth or extent of injury: ulcers are superficial, abscesses are localized pocketed infections, and cellulitis is nonlocalized soft tissue infection. Potentially pathogenic organisms can be identified through cultures of the patient's

Table 9-5 Pathogenic Organisms Found in the ICU

Organism	Source	Likely Sites or Forms of Infection	Signs and Symptoms	Treatment
Gram-positive Staphylococcus aureus	Normal flora—hand, nasopharynx	Wounds, open lesions, invasive lines, pneumonia, colon, blood	High fever, purulent secretions, emboli	Semisynthetic penicillins— nafcillin, methicillin, *vancomycin
Streptococcus (beta hemolytic, pyogenes, viridans, pneumoniae)	Normal flora—nasopharynx, skin; droplet transfer	Strep throat, scarlet fever, impetigo, strep gangrene, neonate and postpartum, otitis media, meningitis, pneumococcal pneumonia, endocarditis	Thin, serous secretions, sudden onset of fever, maculopapular rash with vesicle formation Fluffy infiltrates on CXR	Penicillin or erythromycin, +/− aminoglycoside; if severe, *ampicillin
Meningococcus	Normal flora—nasopharynx; droplet transfer	Meningitis, pneumonia, purulent conjunctivitis, sinusitis, endocarditis, genital infection	Arthralgia and myalgia, hypotension, petichial rash, thrombosis, and hemorrhage	Penicillin, ampicillin, cephalosporins, *Chloram-phenicol
Corynebacterium diphtheriae	Skin, GI tract, other persons	Upper respiratory, wound, skin	Gray-green membrane over mucous membranes, skin disorders	Penicillin or erythromycin
Actinomycoses	Normal flora—mouth, throat, tooth decay	Abscesses head and neck, thorax, abdomen	Painful, indurated swelling mouth/neck, fistulas, bowel obstruction	Penicillin or tetracycline
Nocardiosis	Soil	Pulmonary, arthritis, cardiac/abdominal	Mucopurulent sputum, night sweats, fistulae	Bactrim for 12–18 mos. or high-dose sulfonamides
Gram-negative Enterobacteria-Klebsiella, E. coli, Erwinia, Proteus, Serratia, Shigella, Salmonella, Yersinia	Exogenous sources (others, environment); endogenous (one body part to another); pathogenic strain of normal flora	Diarrhea/colitis, bacteremia	Watery diarrhea with blood/pus, and abdominal cramping	Aminoglycoside and 3rd generation cephalosporin, *Bactrim
Pseudomonas	Standing liquids	Any site—*GU and GI	Sickly sweet odor and blue-green drainage	Aminoglycoside and penicillin derivatives (Ticarcillin)

(continued)

Table 9-5 Pathogenic Organisms Found in the ICU (*continued*)

Organism	Source	Likely Sites or Forms of Infection	Signs and Symptoms	Treatment
Fungi				
Candida albicans, tropicalis, Kruzei	Normal flora—GI and GU tracts, vagina, mouth, skin	Nails, skin, mucous membranes (oral, esophageal, vaginal, GU), bacteremia	Scaly, erythematous rash of skin, cream/yellow lacelike irregular lesion, white discharge; cough, blood-tinged sputum, reddened and swollen eye	Topical antifungal (Nystatin), Ketoconozole, Amphotericin B
Aspergillus	Damp, molding plants or areas, ventilation system	Corrosive fungal ball in lungs, ear, cornea, sinuses; brain abscess	Cough, blood-tinged sputum, reddened and swollen eye	Amphotericin B or 5 FC
Cryptococcus neoformans	Dust contaminated by pigeons (urban areas)	Pulmonary, meningitis	No pulmonary signs and symptoms, frontal headache, progressive neurological decline	None, oral Flucytosine (5 FC), Amphotericin
Blastomycosis	North American soil	Bronchopneumonia, bacteremia	Viral pulmonary signs and symptoms, painless macules, abscess	Amphotericin B
Viruses				
Herpes simplex	Common, naturally occurring virus transmitted via body secretions, contact, transplacentally	Type I: gingivo-stomatitis, extraoral lesions; Type II: genital, extragenital; may disseminate	Oral or extra-oral ulcers with raised outer border, extra-oral/genital vesicles with crusting and clear drainage, occasionally erythema, paresthesias/pain area	Skin lesions in immunocompetent: Vidarabine, topical Acyclovir, IV Acyclovir, *Foscarnet
Herpes zoster	Activation of the varicella virus that has lain dormant in the cerebral ganglia	Unilateral skin eruptions around thorax or vertically on legs or arms	Fever, malaise, severe deep pain, pruritis, paresthesias of area even before small red nodular lesions that fill with fluid or pus, vertical skin eruptions	Acyclovir

Table 9-5 (*continued*)

Organism	Source	Likely Sites or Forms of Infection	Signs and Symptoms	Treatment
Cytomegalovirus	Common, naturally occurring virus transmitted by contact	Lungs, liver, GI tract, retina, central nervous system, and, less commonly, bacteremia	Mild, nonspecific signs and symptoms, diffuse CXR infiltrates in pneumonia, hepato-spleen enlargement, site-specific organ dysfunction	Ganciclovir, *CMV immune globulin
Parasites/opportunistic Pneumocystis carinii	Many sources for airborne protozoan organism	Primarily alveolar/parenchymal lung infection	Low-grade fever, cough, mild hypoxemia, dyspnea, minimal sputum, progressive infiltrates and respiratory signs and symptoms	Trimethoprim sulfa, *Pentamadine, pyrimethamine sulfa, *Dapsone
Legionella	Gram-negative bacteria most common in ventilation systems	Primarily diffuse interstitial pneumonia, possibly GI tract	High spiking fevers, dyspnea, hypoxemia, large amount white sputum, widespread infiltrates CXR	Erythromycin +/− Rifampin, Bactrim
Mycoplasma	Naturally occurring in many locations, most are resistant to pathogenesis	Primarily cavitating pneumonia, although liver or bacteremia noted	High fever, cough with large amount of sputum, lobular pneumonia	Tetracycline and/or erythromycin
Toxoplasma	Ingestion through raw or uncooked meat, exposure cat feces, although other unknown means as well	Generalized infection, encephalitis, myocarditis, hepatitis, pneumonitis	Fever and mono-like syndrome, delirium, maculopapular rash (except palms, feet)	Pyrimethamine + folinic acid + sulfadiazides, *add clindamycin

*Second-line therapy

Source: Shelton, B. (1990). Infections and immune disorders: Advanced management of clinical emergencies. Baltimore: The Johns Hopkins Nursing Staff Development Program.

body areas or excretions. Culture reports describe the numbers of organisms and level of tissue involvement. Cultures are considered positive for organisms when more than two consecutive positive cultures within a 48-hour period report the same findings.[29] Colonization is present when microbial multiplication and survival is present on the mucous membranes and skin surfaces without any deeper tissue penetration to cause disease. An infection exists when the presence of organisms is accompanied by clinical symptoms. Since white blood cells are the body's primary defense against infection, the patient's generation of a white blood cell response will often be an early indicator of infection, and the level of such response may predict the outcome of an untreated infection. It is important for the critical care nurse to recognize that many critical illnesses cause fever or leukocytosis, possibly masking common infection symptoms. Symptoms of infection are both systemic and localized, as shown in Table 9-6. Possible outcomes of infection include total resolution, chronic infection, excessive or unprovoked inflammatory responses (such as autoimmune disease, adhesions), or a systemic infection called septicemia.

Sepsis Sepsis comprises the physiological inflammatory response of the body to pathogens invading the blood. The presence of organisms in the blood without systemic symptoms of infection is termed bacteremia. Sepsis is characterized by symptoms similar to infection, but to a greater degree: leukocytosis, fever, myalgia, arthralgia, tachycardia, edema, and prostration. The patient with septicemia must be observed carefully for the signs of vascular collapse heralding septic shock.

Sepsis due to exotoxin-producing group I Staphylococcus aureus has been found to produce a clinical syndrome characterized by high fever, diarrhea, vomiting, mental status changes, and a maculopapular rash. This syndrome, first described in 1978 among children and young menstruating women, has been named toxic shock syndrome, but is essentially gram-positive shock.[30] The GI symptoms and rash are rarely seen in other types of sepsis.

Septic shock Septic shock can be divided into two phases: hyperdynamic and hypodynamic. Each phase has its own unique hemodynamic pattern and clinical presentation, as shown in Tables 9-7 and 9-8.

Hyperdynamic septic shock occurs early in the pathophysiological process and is evidenced by high cardiac output (CO) and low systemic vascular resistance (SVR) and ejection fraction (EF). In this stage, although CO may be extremely high, the SVR and ejection fraction are frequently so low that the patient is hypotensive. In the past, the hyperdynamic phase

Table 9-6 Symptoms of Infection

Location	Symptoms
Generalized	Malaise
	Fatigue
	Myalgia
	Arthralgia
	Fever
	Chills
	Headache
	Anorexia
	Leukocytosis
	Anemia
	Thrombocytopenia
Cardiovascular	Tachycardia
	Hypotension
	Hypovolemia
	Chest pain
	Dysrhythmias
	Ischemia on ECG
Pulmonary	Tachypnea
	Dyspnea
	Crackles, wheezes, gurgles (rhonchi)
	Abnormal PFTs
	Hypoxemia
	Sputum
Renal	Proteinuria
	Oliguria
Central nervous system	Anxiety
	Confusion
	Delirium
Metabolic	Hyperglycemia
	Elevated BUN
Localized	Erythema
	Pain at site
	Localized edema
	Pus collection
	Demarcation skin changes

was termed "warm shock" because the dilation of the peripheral vasculature caused the patient to present with warm, flushed skin. The patient in this stage of septic shock usually presents with fever and hypotension or low diastolic blood pressure with a resultant low mean arterial pressure. During this phase, which lasts 6–72 hours, the patient may be warm or hot, with dry, flushed skin.[31] Hyperdynamic shock is frequently heralded by the sudden onset of fever with a temperature greater than 101°F (38.3°C), chills, and prostration. Despite the fever and flushed skin of the rest of the body, the patient's legs are often cool and mottled. Vasodilatory hypotension is often at least 25% below normal and is accompanied by tachycardia and bounding pulses. The reduction of circulating blood volume frequently

Table 9-7 Clinical Presentation of Hyperdynamic Septic Shock

Clinical Presentation	Hemodynamic Alterations	Results of Diagnostic Tests
Sudden onset of fever, chills, prostration	MAP low	Respiratory alkalosis
Confusion, restlessness, disorientation, lethargy	CO normal or high	Decreased FVC, reserve volumes
Skin flushed and hot, yet legs may be cool and mottled, petichiae present	Peripheral vasodilation, low diastolic BP	Hyperkalemia, hyperphosphatemia, high uric acid
Myalgia, arthralgia	Ejection fraction decreased	Increased reticulocytes, erythrocyte sedimentation rate
Rapid, bounding pulse	Systemic vascular resistance (SVR) very low	Leukocytosis
Normotensive, wide pulse pressure, or slightly hypotensive	Pulmonary vascular resistance (PVR) high, low, or normal	Thrombocytopenia
Tachypnea, respiratory alkalosis	Pulmonary artery pressures (PAP) high	Cardiac dysfunction on echocardiogram
Nausea, vomiting, diarrhea	Pulmonary capillary wedge normal or low	Increased BUN disproportional to increased creatinine
Profound diuresis	Mixed venous oxygen saturation (MVO_2) high	

produces a sensation of thirst. Nausea, vomiting, and diarrhea may also occur. Microthrombi may form in the cutaneous blood vessels, producing a distinctive mottling of the skin as well as petichiae.[32] Initially, altered blood flow to the brain causes CNS effects such as headache, lethargy, restlessness, disorientation, and/or confusion. Profound diuresis or oliguria may occur. Tachypnea is the cardinal and sometimes only sign of shock, and its significance as an early indicator should not be overlooked.

Hypodynamic shock occurs late in the syndrome and may represent the terminal phase of shock. In hypodynamic septic shock, CO is still quite high, but the ejection fraction continues to be low and is accompanied by extreme vasoconstriction, so the systemic vascular resistance (SVR) during this phase is very high. The hypodynamic phase was once referred to as "cold shock" because of the chilled, clammy skin of the patient in this stage. The patient has weak and thready pulses, is progressively more

Table 9-8 Clinical Presentation of Hypodynamic Septic Shock

Clinical Presentation	Hemodynamic Alterations	Results of Diagnostic Tests
Normal temperature or hypothermia	MAP low to normal	Respiratory and metabolic acidosis
Obtunded, unconscious	CO high, low, or normal	High peak airway pressures, poor negative inspiratory force and ventilatory volumes
Skin cool and clammy, pale, cyanotic	Peripheral constriction, with increased diastolic BP but low systolic BP	Elevated lactic acid
Mottling and ecchymoses	PAP high	Anemia, thrombocytopenia, leukopenia
Rapid, weak pulse	SVR high	Severe hypokinesis on echocardiogram
Jugular venous pulsations, heart gallops and murmurs	PVR high	Ischemic ECG changes
Profound hypotension	Ejection fraction low	CXR with pulmonary infiltrates, prominent pulmonary vessels
Oliguria, anuria		Elevated transaminases
		Elevated creatinine and BUN

dyspneic, and may become anuric. Hypoperfusion of the CNS may cause the patient to be apprehensive, irritable, or increasingly confused. Severe hypoperfusion may lead to obtundation or unconsciousness. Hypothermia may occur and is a grim prognostic indicator of impending death. It is important to note that hyperdynamic shock even occurs in the normovolemic patient. The patient who is dehydrated at the onset of septic shock may present with the symptoms of the hypodynamic phase.

The cardiovascular effects of septic shock are very profound. Severe vasodilation first causes low diastolic blood pressures with low MAP. Capillary leak may lead to true vascular volume depletion; usually, however, the volume is not greatly reduced but only appears to be as a consequence of dilation. Early in septic shock, catecholamine responses lead to increased automaticity, causing tachycardia or ectopy and increased CO. As myocardial depression from mediators or acidosis occurs, myocardial contractility is compromised, and stroke volume, ejection fraction, and SVR are very low. Left ventricular function becomes progressively compromised, and necessary volume replacement for losses or vasodilation can produce clinical heart failure. The critical care nurse must remember that in this patient, increased cardiac output does not indicate good cardiac function.

The pulmonary capillary permeability, pulmonary vascular constriction, hyaline membrane development, and V̇/Q̇ mismatch result in specific physiologic changes: increased pulmonary vascular resistance (PVR), reduced compliance, pulmonary interstitial edema, pulmonary hypertension, and impaired gas exchange.[33] Clinically, the patient exhibits tachypnea and an increased tidal volume (up to 2.5 times normal), which is nevertheless inadequate to compensate for the V̇/Q̇ mismatch. Early in septic shock, auscultation of breath sounds reveals inspiratory crackles and late inspiratory and expiratory crackles and wheezing. High pulmonary pressures are reflected in high static airway pressures, poor compliance, elevated right atrial pressures, and elevated pulmonary artery pressures. Eventually the pulmonary changes result in profound hypoxemia, which is refractory to oxygen therapy.[34] A summary of the pathophysiological activities leading to pulmonary changes in septic shock is provided in Figure 9-7.

The metabolic consequences of septic shock are significant precipitators of hypodynamic shock. In fact, the degree of hyperglycemia correlates to the degree of myocardial compensation, and the shift to hypoglycemia often heralds acute myocardial compromise.[35] The high metabolic demands induce production of large quantities of glucose that may not be utilized. Glucose utilization is compromised because of maldistribution of blood, cellular anoxia, and anaerobic metabolism, and hyperglycemia that is insulin-resistant is the clinical consequence. Anaerobic metabolism occurs from inadequate tissue oxygen supplies and leads to the formation of lactic acid. Measured lactic acid levels in septic shock are very high, as compensation fails. Cell death from anaerobic metabolism results in hyperkalemia, hyperphosphatemia, and hyperuricemia. Glucose levels may drastically fall when the body's compensatory mechanisms fail; thus, the critical care nurse must use insulin cautiously and be observant of changes indicative of hypoglycemia: sudden hypotension, bradycardia, or a sudden loss of consciousness. This catabolic state also precipitates the breakdown of body proteins for energy, which process is evidenced in

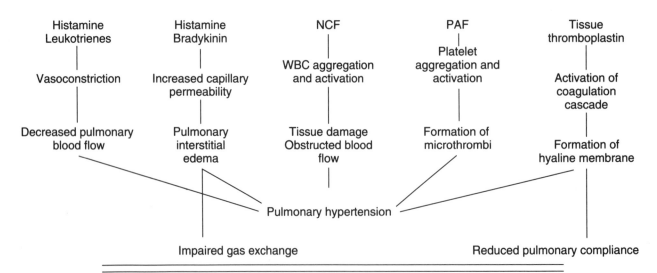

Figure 9-7 Pathogenesis of Pulmonary Changes in Septic Shock

elevated BUN results. This symptom can be confused with one of acute renal compromise or dehydration, so careful evaluation should be instituted prior to treatment. Related to this problem is the fact that it is often difficult to maintain nutrition in the patient suffering septic shock; up to 10,000 kcal per day has been suggested as necessary to support the metabolic demands.[36]

In sepsis, the bone marrow is stimulated to produce white blood cells to fight infection. In early shock, the neutrophil count will be extremely elevated, with a distinct increase in the percentage of bands (juvenile neutrophils). The white cell differential is shifted to the left in this type of case, where neutrophils prevail. If the shock is overwhelming, so many neutrophils may have been sacrificed in the battle against infection that the WBC count may be low. Activation of the coagulation cascade and fibrinolytic systems may result in reduction of platelet counts and prolonged coagulation times. Thrombocytopenia occurs in both gram-negative sepsis (40–80%) and gram-positive sepsis (65%).[37] If effectively treated, thrombocytopenia will resolve in 3–10 days. In gram-positive sepsis, exotoxins hemolyze erythrocytes and cause platelet aggregation. Daily complete blood counts and coagulation profiles are essential for early diagnosis of complications.

An osmotic diuresis may be present initially in sepsis, but the primary presenting symptom once shock has occurred is oliguria. The etiology of low urine output is reduced glomerular filtration and increased ADH, aldosterone, and renin; therefore, patients who are oliguric and vascular volume overloaded will respond to the use of diuretics.

Other clinical signs and symptoms found with septic shock include mental status changes, restlessness, arthralgia and myalgia, metabolic acidosis, nausea, vomiting, and diarrhea. The complex pathophysiological effects and ongoing malperfusion and oxygen demand/supply imbalance lead to many life-threatening complications (noted in Table 9-9), which account for the high mortality rate. ARDS and DIC are the most prevalent of these complications.[38]

One researcher discovered that within 24 hours of the onset of hypotension, survivors' cardiac index (CI) reduced to normal and stayed within normal limits.[39] In nonsurvivors, the cardiac index remained high. Most of the nonsurvivors (50%) died as a consequence of multiple organ failure. In 40% of those who died, the cause of death was profound peripheral vasodilation (low SVR). Remarkably, less than 10% of deaths were due to low cardiac output.[40] The most common causes of death due to septic shock have been reported as refractory hypotension

Table 9-9 Complications of Septic Shock

Body System	Complication
Pulmonary	Pulmonary failure Pulmonary hypertension Respiratory alkalosis Hypoxemia ARDS
Hematologic	DIC Coagulopathy
Renal	Renal failure
Cardiovascular	Cardiac failure
Hepatic	Abnormal hepatic function
Metabolic	Metabolic acidosis Malnutrition

(10%), severe reduction in SVR (40%), and multiple organ failure (50%).[41]

Laboratory diagnostic tests Identification of the infectious agent by microbiological cultures is essential in the diagnosis and treatment of septic shock. Samples of blood, sputum, urine, and wound drainage are obtained for immediate gram staining, culturing, and sensitivity testing so that appropriate antimicrobial therapy may be prescribed. Cultures are frequently repeated to confirm infection, identify new infectious organisms, or evaluate a response to therapy. These tests are also essential for identifying the focus or source of infection. It is important to note, though, that septic shock may occur despite negative cultures. Some clinicians propose that lingering bacterial toxins continue to stimulate immune mediators even after the organisms have been destroyed.[42]

Many other laboratory tests are performed in order to detect complications of sepsis. Blood chemistries are taken several times daily to monitor glucose, potassium, calcium, and phosphorus levels. Tests such as PT, PTT, TT, fibrinogen, and fibrin degradation product levels are employed to detect DIC. Arterial blood gases are needed to assess respiratory alkalosis and note when metabolic acidosis begins. Renal and hepatic function are monitored through chemistry tests or more specific indicators such as creatinine clearance. Stool and urine tests for occult blood assist in identifying coagulopathy or GI bleeding. Daily chest x-rays are important to assess for pneumonia and the onset of ARDS. A listing of common laboratory monitors used to detect complications of septic shock is given in Table 9-10.

Table 9-10 Detecting Complications of Septic Shock: Laboratory and Diagnostic Tests

Category	Lab or Diagnostic Test	Results
Microbiology	Cultures: blood, urine, sputum, wound Gram stains	Positive for infectious organism
Hematology	CBC	Leukocytosis (WBC = 15,000–30,000 per mm³) Neutrophilia may cause shift to left on differential Neutropenia may occur in gram-negative sepsis Thrombocytopenia (platelets < 100,000/mm³)
	Coagulation	If DIC, PT, PTT, TT are prolonged, fibrinogen is below 100 and FDPs are above 40
Chemistry	Electrolytes	Decreased Na⁺, Cl⁻; increased K⁺, Mg⁺⁺
	Serum lactate	Lactic acidosis
	Serum antibiotic levels	Peak and trough levels vary depending on antibiotics
	Serum albumin Triglyceride levels	Low (indicating catabolic state) Elevated, due to lipolysis
	Serum amylaseᵃ Serum lipaseᵃ AST (SGOT) ALT (SGPT)	> 160 μ/mL > 1.5 μ/mL > 40 IU/mL > 35 IU/mL
	ABGs	Respiratory alkalosis/metabolic acidosis Hypoxemia
	Serum osmolality	High
	BUN Creatinine	2.5 times normal > 2 times normal
	Urine specific gravity	High (>1.010)
	Urine osmolality	< 400, with ratio of urine to plasma osmolality < 1.5, decreased urine output, GFR, and sodium secretion, positive for proteinuria, hematuriaᵇ
	Chest x-ray	Pulmonary infiltrates
	ECG	ST-T wave changes

ᵃSustained ischemia causes pancreatic damage with resultant release of digestive enzymes into the general circulation.
ᵇStaphylococcus aureus produces proteinuria and hematuria.

Nursing standards of care

The medical management of septic shock has been described as having five key aspects: (1) treating the underlying infection, (2) supporting cardiovascular function, (3) supporting pulmonary function, (4) treating biochemical abnormalities, and (5) managing coagulopathy.[43] Certain investigational therapies have been employed in the treatment of gram-negative septic shock, and these include the administration of monoclonal antibodies directed against the bacterial lipopolysaccharides of pseudomonas or E. coli. Even with recent technological advances in management, however, early detection and intervention remain the key effective management strategy.[44] Nurses play a significant role in the early recognition of sepsis since they are the practitioners who have the most frequent contact with the patient. The pathophysiological effects of sepsis and septic shock are diverse and vary from one patient to another. The critical care nurse must assess each patient's individual risk factors for specific organ failure and monitor each patient for clinical symptoms produced by these physiological changes.

Treating the underlying infection It is essential for critical care personnel to identify the patient at high risk for infection and to develop a plan for monitoring the condition. In the neutropenic or immunosuppressed patient, the signs and symptoms of infection may be diminished or absent, requiring vigilant assessment. Once sepsis is suspected, it is essential to identify the source of infection through cultures, although antibiotics are often instituted before culture results are received. Cultures should be obtained prior to starting the prescribed antibiotics to ensure that the antibiotics do not inhibit the growth of the culture. Broad-spectrum intravenous antibiotics are administered within 30 minutes when a diagnosis of sepsis is suspected and cultures are obtained. Unfortunately, 24–72 hours of IV therapy are required before the appropriate antibiotics can reverse septic shock. Broad-spectrum antibiotics, including those effective against gram-negative organisms, are selected based on the organism believed to be the most likely cause of the infection. A comprehensive broad-spectrum regimen will include a cephalosporin, aminoglycoside, and a penicillin derivative.[45] Newer regimens using broader-scope cephalosporin derivatives—such as the beta lactams—may require only two drugs. Figure 9-8 shows a decision tree used in the antibiotic treatment of fever (a cardinal symptom of sepsis) in the neutropenic patient. Ongoing culture and sensitivity

results may indicate the need to change antibiotics or adjust doses. Intravenous antibiotics are continued for 2–6 weeks. Peak and trough levels of antibiotics are obtained in order to ensure adequate therapeutic levels with minimal tissue toxicity. A list of common antibiotics used in the ICU with their indications and adverse effects is given in Table 9-11.

Antibiotics alone may not resolve clinical infection; elimination of the infectious source is the best definitive therapy. The chest, sinuses, and abdomen are the most common locations of infection in the ICU patient, so all should be x-rayed and/or ultra-sounded. Implanted devices or invasive lines should be carefully evaluated as possible sources and may need to be removed to prevent further systemic seeding of infection. Abscesses are best drained, and surgical resections of necrotic tissue may be necessary. These baseline interventions will be supplemented with strategies to support other failing body systems.

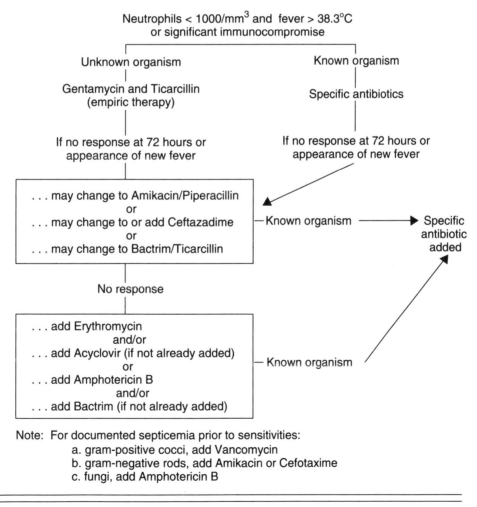

Figure 9-8 Antibiotic Schema for Management of Fever in the Compromised Host

Table 9-11 Antibiotics Commonly Used in the ICU

Antibiotic	Coverage	Side Effects
Aminoglycosides Gentamycin Amikacin Tobramycin Kanamycin	Most gram-negative enterobacter (Serratia, Proteus, Klebsiella, E. coli) Pseudomonas Erwinia	Renal failure, vestibular and auditory damage, rash
Penicillins Penicillin G Penicillin V Ampicillin Amoxicillin Ticarcillin Piperacillin Carbenicillin Imipenem	Actinomyces, Clostridium, meningococcemia, Proteus (ampicillin), Salmonella (ampicillin/amoxicillin), Streptococcus, Staphylococcus (second line)	Hypersensitivity reactions, rash, (especially ampicillin and amoxicillin), diarrhea (especially ampicillin), GI intolerance, abnormal platelet activity (Carbenecillin and Ticarcillin), neuromuscular twitching with renal failure
Quinolones Norfloxacin Ciprofloxicin	Resistant enterobacter	GI intolerance, headache, malaise, insomnia, dizziness, and rare visual disturbances and hepatic dysfunction
Gram-positive Coverage Nafcillin Oxacillin Vancomycin	Staphylococcus Clostridium difficile Corynebacterium diphtheriae	"Red man syndrome" (Vancomycin), fever, rash, neutropenia, allergic reactions, hypotension with rapid infusion
Cephalosporins Cefamandole Cefazolin Cephalothin Ceftazidime (third) Cefuraxime (third) Moxalactam (third)	General enterobacter coverage (E. coli, Klebsiella, Proteus, Serratia), Staphylococcus aureus, Hemophilus influenzae	Phlebitis, diarrhea, allergic reactions, platelet dysfunction, rare hepatic dysfunction
Tetracyclines Tetracycline Democycline Monocycline	Tick fever, Chlamydiae, Klebsiella UTI, Mycoplasma pneumoniae (second)	GI intolerance, vertigo, vaginitis, hepatotoxicity, tooth staining, photosensitivity
Clindamycin	Gastrointestinal bacilli	GI intolerance, diarrhea, colitis, rash
Erythromycin	Campylobacter, Chlamydia conjunctivitis, Corynebacterium diphtheriae, Legionella, Mycoplasma pneumoniae	Phlebitis, intolerance based on oral dosing, diarrhea, stomatitis, cholestaic hepatitis, rash, dose-related ototoxicity
Metronidazole	Bacteroides, various orifice normal flora, Clostridium difficile	Metallic taste, headache, phlebitis, reversible peripheral neuropathies, antabuse-like reaction
Sulfa-trimethoprim	E. coli UTI, Hemophilus influenzae, Shigella, Pneumocystis carinii, some strains of pseudomonas, Salmonella, Yersinia	GI intolerance, bone marrow aplasia (platelets, WBCs)
Sulfonamides Gantricin	Nocardia	Allergic reactions—rash, pruritis, fever, crystalluria, GI intolerance, photosensitivity
Antifungals Ketoconazole	Widely spread, localized fungal infections, oral/mucotaneous Candida	GI intolerance, hepatotoxicity, decreased testosterone level (gynecomastia, dysmenorrhea)
Amphotericin B	Topical-mucotaneous fungal infection, IV-disseminated fungal infections (Candida, Aspergillus, Cryptococcus)	Fever, chills, headache, hypokalemia, renal failure, anemia, phlebitis, metallic taste, nausea and vomiting

Table 9-11 *(continued)*

Antibiotic	Coverage	Side Effects
Flucytosine (5-FC)	Disseminated or bacteremic candida, Coccidoides, Cryptococcus	Nausea and vomiting, rash, liver damage, marrow suppression, confusion
Antivirals		
Acyclovir	Herpes simplex, types I and II and Varicella-zoster	Irritation at injection site, renal toxicity, rash, marrow suppression, metabolic encephalopathy, abnormal LFT
Ganciclovir	Cytomegalovirus	Neutropenia, thrombocytopenia, rash, abnormal LFT, headache, fever, psychosis, myopathy

Source: Shelton, B. (1990). Infections and immune disorders: Advanced management of clinical emergencies. Baltimore: The Johns Hopkins Nursing Staff Development Program.

Supporting cardiovascular function Continuous ECG and hemodynamic monitoring are required in order to assess cardiovascular function and evaluate response to treatment. Strategies for patient management are summarized in Table 9-12.

Cardiovascular status is supported by first administering adequate amounts of intravenous fluids. Frequently, an initial fluid challenge of 500 mL of IV fluid is given over 30 minutes, and the patient's cardiovascular response is measured. Either crystalloids or colloids are administered based on the physician's preferences and the patient's condition. There are differing theories regarding the choice of fluid replacement: the vasodilation of sepsis is usually responsive to volume replenishment regardless of source, but some clinicians believe that the capil-

Table 9-12 Cardiovascular Management of the Patient in Septic Shock

General Goals	Specific Procedures/Evaluation Parameters
Continuous ECG monitoring	
Treatment of hypotension	
Provision of fluid challenge using 500 cc crystalloid or 5–100 cc colloid over 30 minutes	Evaluate for urine output: optimum = 0.5–1 mL/kg/hr Evaluate for MAP: optimum = at least 60 mm Hg Evaluate for PCWP: optimum = 15–18 mm Hg Evaluate for RAP: optimum = 4–8 mm Hg Assess for cardiac failure in response to fluid challenges Repeat challenges as long as evaluation criteria are met and patient tolerates procedures
Administration of vasopressors	Dopamine at renal dose of 1–4 mcg/kg/min for hypotension or oliguria Titrate dopamine in doses of up to 20–30 mcg/kg/min if tachycardia or dysrhythmias are not present Switch to norepinephrine in doses of 2–10 mcg/min if a more potent vasopressor or less cardiotoxicity is desired
Evaluation and management of cardiac contractile dysfunction	Assess for symptoms of heart failure: crackles, gallops, murmurs, respiratory distress, increased JVP Evaluate chest x-ray for cardiomegaly Evaluate ECG for ischemia Monitor stroke volume (SV) from PA catheter; adjust medications if SV < 50 cc/min Administer digoxin as needed for tachydysrhythmias or decreased SV Consider administering dobutamine or Inocor in severe circumstances

lary leak syndrome associated with sepsis is enhanced when low-molecular-weight crystalloids are given to the septic patient.[46] It has also been proposed that vascular volume is replenished more rapidly with less fluid volume when colloids are used.[47] Regardless of the choice of fluid, the volume administered must be sufficient to maintain a MAP of 60 mm Hg, a PCWP of 15–18 mm Hg, and a urine output greater than 0.5–1.0 mL/kg/hr. The CVP and PAP may be higher if pulmonary hypertension and high airway pressures are present, but the PCWP should reflect left ventricular diastolic function until this problem becomes severe.[48] For these reasons, the CVP should be viewed as an inaccurate reflection of volume status, and the PCWP should be used whenever possible.[49] If fluids alone cannot maintain MAP above 60 mm Hg, administration of dopamine is recommended to maintain blood pressure.[50] In addition to being an effective inotropic agent, dopamine also may dilate splanchnic, mesenteric, and renal blood vessels. Dopamine, while a life-saving substance, can also precipitate tachydysrhythmias, which are exhausting to an overtaxed myocardium. If dopamine infusion alone is unsuccessful or produces complications, it may be replaced with a norepinephrine infusion of 2–10 mcg/kg/min.[51] Neosinephrine (phenylephrine) is a pure alpha agonist (stimulant) and a potent peripheral vasoconstrictor given at 20–300 mcg/min. Although reportedly not useful in septic shock, phenylephrine is used extensively in clinical situations as a short-term vasopressor agent, which causes potent peripheral constriction without cardiac or neurologic effects.[52] Postanesthesia and neurosurgical patients may be candidates to receive this agent. Ephedrine and epinephrine are other sympathomimetics that may be considered for treating refractory shock but are not often used for septic shock. New phosphodiesterase inhibitors—such as Amrinone—have clinical effects similar to dobutamine's and may prove particularly useful since they reduce both pulmonary vasoconstriction and systemic afterload.[53]

Various experimental therapies have been instituted in an attempt to reverse vascular collapse in the septic shock patient. Glucagon has direct inotropic and chronotropic cardiac effects, but is currently used only in cases of circulatory shock unresponsive to conventional therapy.[54] The role of endogenous opioids in the pathophysiology of septic shock has led investigators to consider the use of intravenous narcotic antagonists (Naloxone) to counteract the hypotension. Reports are mixed and show dubious success, with the final recommendation reflecting the need for more controlled studies.[55] Other strategies are aimed at blocking the mediator pathways

thought to contribute to a sustained inflammatory response. Therapies in this category include anti-TNF antibodies, eicosanoid inhibitors, prostaglandin inhibitors (such as indomethacin), superoxide scavengers (such as calcium channel blockers), and prostaglandin inhibitors.[56] Anti-endotoxin therapy continues to undergo investigation, with some evidence of promising responses in early gram-negative septicemia.

Supporting pulmonary function Respiratory failure despite normal chest x-rays is not unusual in the patient in septic shock. Some investigators have identified respiratory muscle fatigue or hyaline membrane development as the etiology.[57] Intubation and mechanical ventilation may be required in order to decrease the energy requirements of breathing (can be decreased by 40%) and maintain adequate oxygenation and ventilation.[58] The ventilatory mode chosen for the patient should be based on the reason for intubation and the goal of mechanical ventilation—to rest the patient. The assist control mode is preferred as long as the patient is acutely ill. ABGs are checked at least every 8 hours and as needed for possible changes requiring ventilatory manipulation. Fevers contribute significantly to oxygen requirements (13% for every degree centigrade increase in body temperature).[59] Diminished pulmonary compliance may cause increased peak airway pressures and may hinder ventilation. Sedation and paralyzation may be necessary to optimize oxygenation. Assessment for refractory hypoxemia and poor pulmonary compliance will serve to identify ARDS. The use of PEEP, inverse inspiratory/expiratory ratios, jet ventilation, or ECMO may be necessary to adequately oxygenate the patient. Frequent assessment of breath sounds, chest x-rays, and sputum cultures will alert clinicians to signs of pulmonary infection.

Treating biochemical abnormalities The most serious biochemical abnormality associated with septic shock is the advent of lactic acidosis. Serum lactate, arterial blood gases, and serum bicarbonate levels indicate the severity of acidosis. Correcting the acidosis with bicarbonate administration should be undertaken with caution. Bicarbonate administered when ventilation is inadequate will not lead to blood buffering but will result in the conversion of bicarbonate to carbonic acid (a weak acid). This may increase the acidosis rather than correct it. Intravenous administration of acetate compounds may assist the body in synthesis of bicarbonate. These compounds include sodium acetate, potassium acetate, and dichloroacetate.

The immense demand for glucose and energy almost always necessitates parenteral nutrition. Nutritional interventions should be aimed at metabolic support, not just nutritional maintenance. Caloric demands in sepsis have been estimated to be as high as 10,000 kcal per day.[60] High protein and lipid levels will increase the substrate available with less concomitant hyperglycemia. Hyperglycemia is often a consequence of sepsis and may be treated with insulin, although it is often resistant to this treatment. Since escalating doses of insulin may be required, nurses should be cautious in their administration. When the patient is no longer able to compensate in sepsis, a precipitous decrease in glucose will occur and can be exacerbated if insulin is being administered.

Electrolyte problems are regulated through intravenous fluids or by specific binding agents when electrolytes are extremely high. Nevertheless, it is rare that phosphate-binding antacids or Kayexalate are necessary unless concomitant renal failure is present.

Managing coagulopathy DIC is a common complication of sepsis and may be masked by the thrombocytopenia that commonly exists with hypermetabolic sepsis. Frequent monitoring of platelets, fibrinogen, fibrin split products, and coagulation will assist in early diagnosis of this problem. The septic patient may require replenishment with platelets and coagulation factors, even if not in DIC.

Corticosteroids Two large multicenter trials investigating the effects of corticosteroids in treating sepsis have failed to clearly demonstrate any improvement in mortality rates with the use of these drugs. Researchers agree that there is no clear indication for routine administration of corticosteroids in septic shock.[61] Sound data regarding gram-negative endotoxemia does not exist, however, and animal studies were most promising for those bacteremias.[62] Of

clinical significance is the fact that adrenal insufficiency can occur in up to 15% of all septic shock patients and may, therefore, be the etiology of hypotension in some patients.[63] These patients' hypotension may reverse when corticosteroids are given. If adrenal insufficiency is suspected, a test dose of corticosteroids is recommended.[64] Also, it is important to note that the patient who was receiving therapeutic doses of corticosteroids prior to the septic event may require high doses of glucocorticoids in order to be able to respond adequately to the infection.

Future research Much of the most promising research regarding septic shock lies in the field of immune modulation. Currently, some researchers are investigating the role of endogenous mediators such as TNF and interleukins in the pathogenesis of septic shock.[65] Others are continuing investigations of vaccines against pseudomonas, E. coli, and LPS.[66] Monoclonal antibodies against some of the gram-negative organisms may be available shortly.

Nurses help prevent septic shock by maintaining host resistance and preventing the entry of bacteria into the blood. The critically ill patient has many risk factors for the acquisition of infection and sepsis. The nurse assists in limiting these risks by advocating nutritional support, noninvasive monitoring techniques, universal precautions, and a medication profile. Meticulous infection control techniques are necessary, particularly handwashing between patient encounters and use of aseptic technique with respect to invasive lines. When infection, sepsis, or septic shock occurs despite precautions, the nurse is a key participant in rapid intervention and continuous monitoring. The primary responsibilities of the nurse in caring for the septic patient are outlined in the care plan that follows.

Nursing Care Plan for the Management of the Patient with Sepsis and Septic Shock

Diagnosis	Signs and symptoms	Intervention	Rationale
Altered tissue perfusion (peripheral), related to vasodilation and mediator effects	Mottling, particularly of extremities	Check VS at least every hour; follow MAP for indication of tissue perfusion	MAP is best indicator of tissue perfusion
	Warm flushed or cool extremities	Monitor for orthostasis; provide assistance to patient in getting out of bed	Volume depletion causes orthostasis
	Low diastolic BP, orthostasis, or frank hypotension	Exercise fall precautions	Patient is at high risk for falls
	Lactic acidosis	Check peripheral pulses every 1–4 hours	Indicator of peripheral perfusion; aids in diagnosing thromboses
	Full and bounding or weak, thready pulses	Assess vascular volume to ensure that patient is not volume depleted; monitor JVP, BP, RAP, and PAP every 1–2 hours, when available	Volume depletion will worsen tissue perfusion
		Maintain normal body temperature by use of covers, blankets, warming, or cooling	Vasoconstriction worsens peripheral perfusion
		Assess skin integrity every shift; document demarcation mottling or cyanosis, necrotic skin areas, and skin breakdowns	To assess for skin breakdown; demarcation is a sympton of microvascular clotting
		Obtain low-air-loss bed, as indicated, for skin integrity problems	To prevent skin breakdown
		Monitor lactic acid levels; follow ABGs for acidosis	To check severity of tissue perfusion deficit
		Secure central vein access if possible	Absorption of medications is enhanced since peripheral tissue perfusion is poor

Diagnosis	Signs and symptoms	Intervention	Rationale
Fluid volume deficit, related to vasodilation and capillary leakage with third spacing	Hypotension, orthostasis, low diastolic BP	Keep meticulous I&O measurements	Indicator of fluid deficit
	Tachycardia	Measure urine outputs every hour	Indicator of vascular volume
	Hemoconcentrated lab values (Hct, sodium, potassium, glucose)	Check urine specific gravity every time patient voids unless giving diuretics	High specific gravity reflects hypovolemia
	CVP < 1 mm Hg, PAP low, CO and CI high, SVR low	Monitor patient for orthostasis (HR and BP)	Indicator of volume depletion
	Oliguria, high urine specific gravity	Monitor weight	Reflects total body water
	Weight gain	Vascular volume assessment with RAP or PAP every 2–4 hours or when giving diuretics or fluid challenges	Assists in planning interventions for fluid imbalances
	Dry mucous membranes		
	Poor skin turgor		
	Edema		
		Pulmonary assessment for crackles every 2 hours	Indication of pulmonary fluid overload
		Auscultate heart sounds for gallops and murmurs every 2–4 hours	Indication of heart failure
		Peripheral pulse check every 1–4 hours, depending on skin changes	Indication of peripheral tissue perfusion
		Exercise seizure precautions	Hemoconcentration causes hyperosmolarity and potential for seizures
		Maintain large-bore IV or central line	Fluids may have to be given rapidly
		Administer fluids—crystalloids or colloids—as ordered for hypotension or decreased RAP or PAP	Fluid replenishment may be required

Nursing Care Plan for the Management of the Patient with Sepsis and Septic Shock

Diagnosis	Signs and symptoms	Intervention	Rationale
Decreased cardiac output, related to mediator effects on contractility	Hypotension Weak, thready pulse CHF symptoms (JVP, gallops, murmurs, crackles) High PAP, PCWP Normal or low CO Normal or low CI Decreased SV Enlarged heart on x-ray Ischemic ECG changes	Monitor PAP every 1–2 hours or with each new cardiovascular or circulation intervention Determine CO and SVR at least every 8 hours, or when patient's clinical condition changes	Assessment of preload, afterload, and contractility guides choice of interventions and pressors
		Monitor heart sounds every 2–4 hours	To assess for heart failure
		Administer fluid volume cautiously; evaluate cardiac performance after each challenge	Vascular volume replenishment may exceed cardiac capabilities
		Administer vasopressors for hypotension, as indicated by PAP, SV, CI, SVR; use strong inotropic agents (dopamine, dobutamine) for decreased cardiac performance	Hypotension in sepsis is reflection of vasodilation and decreased cardiac performance
		Run 12-lead ECG daily and with every acute event that possibly indicates an MI; monitor ST segment on bedside monitor if possible	Patient is at high risk for myocardial ischemia or MI
		Check CPK enzymes and isoenzymes for events possibly due to an MI	Reflection of MI
		Check echocardiogram and chest x-rays	Reflection of heart failure

Diagnosis	Signs and symptoms	Intervention	Rationale
Hyperthermia	Fever > 38.5°C	Assess temperature every 2–4 hours	For early assessment of infection
	Warm flushed skin	For each new temperature spike (higher than 38.5°C or more than 1°C higher than previous temperature), perform culture work-up (blood cultures, urine culture, sputum culture, chest x-ray)	Cultures yield highest number of microorganisms when patient is symptomatic
	Patient complains of sensations of warmth or chills	For each new temperature spike, perform head-to-toe assessment for evidence of possible infection or symptoms of disseminated sepsis (mottling, septic emboli)	Nursing assessment of subtle changes may discover potential source or organism to treat
		Culture all potential or suspicious sites (orifices, line exits, etc.) for infection	Critically ill patients will become infected from existing wounds and sites
		Provide antipyretics as ordered	To reduce temperature
		Be cautious with medications administered around-the-clock, which may mask new fevers	May hide new fever spike crucial to assessment of infection process
		Provide tepid or cool water baths as appropriate for high body temperatures (alcohol may also be used)	To provide comfort (tepid water or alcohol enhances evaporation from skin better than ice)
		Provide specialized care for the patient on a hyperthermia blanket; provide frequent skin care and massage to enhance circulation; turn often	Can cause severe vasoconstriction with soft tissue hypoxia and necrosis

Nursing Care Plan for the Management of the Patient with Sepsis and Septic Shock

Diagnosis	Signs and symptoms	Intervention	Rationale
		Do not set temperature too low and bring patient's temperature down too fast	Rapid temperature decrease (more than 1°C/hr) may lead to seizures
		Monitor CBC results (total WBC, ANC, and differential)	To assess response to infection
Impaired gas exchange related to pulmonary congestion and selective pulmonary vasoconstriction	Tachypnea Dyspnea Respiratory alkalosis Hypoxemia (PaO_2 < 60 mm Hg on 50% oxygen) Decreased oxygen saturation Crackles, gurgles, wheezes auscultated on lung assessment Decreased lung compliance Reduced FVC, voluntary tidal volume (if on IMV) Weight gain Infiltrates on chest x-ray	Auscultate breath sounds every 1–4 hours, particularly if any key symptoms are present (tachypnea or dyspnea)	Crackles or gurgles are indicative of capillary leak or ARDS
		Restrict fluids as ordered	To reduce excess fluid and congestive complications
		Weigh patient daily	Measure of total body fluid volume status
		Diurese, as ordered; observe for side effects of diuretics, especially contraction alkalosis	Alkalosis is a potential problem due to tachypnea and diuretics; patient is already prone to respiratory alkalosis; electrolyte disorders occur with diuretics
		Measure FVC (off ventilator) and spontaneous tidal volume (on ventilator)	Demonstrates patient's ability to ventilate; changes may indicate extra lung fluid
		Observe airway pressures; note increased peak airway pressure and attempt to decrease with altered peak flow or ventilation pattern	Indicative of ARDS or extra lung fluid
		Administer morphine sulfate, as ordered, to calm patient and reduce dyspnea	To decrease oxygen demand and to bronchodilate
		Obtain chest x-ray every day	To discover changes indicative of capillary leak

Diagnosis	Signs and symptoms	Intervention	Rationale
Alteration in nutrition: intake less than body requirements because of hypermetabolism	Ketosis Hyperglycemia Elevated BUN Muscle wasting and atrophy Decreased visceral proteins (total protein, albumin, globulin) Ketonuria Hyperkalemia Hyperphosphatemia Negative nitrogen balance	Assess electrolytes at least daily Monitor glucose more frequently (every 1–8 hours), as needed Observe patient for insulin resistance; administer insulin cautiously Evaluate caloric and nutrient needs weekly to determine need for additional calories or protein; keep calorie count, if patient is PO status; encourage high-protein rather than high-carbohydrate foods Monitor BUN and protein levels for signs of visceral protein breakdown and inadequate clearance Monitor for acidosis; give lactate for metabolic acidosis identified through venous or arterial blood Reduce physical demand during acute phase of illness: bed baths, limited activity, sedation as needed, temperature WNL	Patient is prone to electrolyte abnormalities Hyperglycemia that is a result of hypermetabolism and an inability to use glucose is often insulin-resistant Even though hyperglycemic, most patients are hypermetabolic and have trouble utilizing carbohydrate calories To evaluate maintenance of body protein Lactic acidosis is complication of sepsis To reduce oxygen demand of tissues
Potential for infection, related to existing risk factors, existing sepsis, or septic syndrome	Fever > 38.5°C Invasive lines present (breaks in skin barrier defense) Reduced WBC activity due to existing hypermetabolism Lactic acidosis	Check VS and temperature at least every 4 hours Do work-up for potential infection immediately upon any temperature spike: peripheral blood cultures drawn	To evaluate for potential infection Organisms are most prevalent in the blood when patient spikes; thus, cultures taken then will yield best results

Diagnosis	Signs and symptoms	Intervention	Rationale
	Positive blood, excrement, or body surface area culture	aseptically; line blood cultures or second peripheral set; chest x-ray; urine culture and sensitivity; culture of wounds or suspicious lesions; total physical exam for potential infection sites (especially orifices)	
	Tissue anergy		
	Low visceral protein levels	If antibiotic change is indicated, hang new antibiotic within 20–30 minutes	Septicemia can rapidly become overwhelming
		Perform surveillance cultures of mouth, nose, vagina, and anus	To note colonization that is often a predictor of future infection in compromised host
		Place on infection prevention precautions (limited invasive procedures, no rectal thermometer or suppositories, etc.)	Patient is at risk for superinfection and reactivation
		If appropriate, encourage patient to eat yogurt or drink acidophilus milk	To replenish normal flora destroyed by antibiotics
		Culture all invasive lines when removed	To assess for infection
		Change IV tubings and dressings every 24–48 hours	CDC recommends more frequent changes for immunocompromised patient
		Limit visitors and allow no fresh flowers	To reduce spread of infection
		Monitor food for contamination	Possible source of infection
		Monitor WBC count and differential, ESR, and SGOT	Left shift is indicative of bacterial infection and right shift of viral infection; other test shows nonspecific inflammatory response

Diagnosis	Signs and symptoms	Intervention	Rationale
		Monitor antibiotic levels	To reduce risk of antibiotic toxicity
Potential for injury related to bleeding	Petechiae	Monitor skin, soft tissue, and mucous membranes for minor bleeding	Locations for early bleeding
	Ecchymoses		
	Prolonged bleeding after venipuncture		
	Bleeding around existing lines or wounds	Note patient-specific risks for bleeding (previous peptic ulcer disease, chronic sinusitis, previous head injury), and develop individualized assessment plan	Most patients bleed from physiologically "weak" areas
	Occult blood in excrement		
	Overt bleeding (epistaxis, gum, GI, vaginal, pulmonary, intracranial)	Evaluate patient's medications for ones that may interfere with normal coagulation	Many medications used in ICU interfere with clotting
	Thrombocytopenia	Monitor laboratory indicators of coagulation	To assist in development of treatment plan
	Abnormal PT, PTT, fibrinogen, or TT		
		Ensure continuous vitamin K replacement during critical illness	Lack of vitamin K contributes to coagulopathy in critically ill
		Obtain nutritional consultation to maintain nutritional requirements for blood cell and coagulation protein development	To help avoid coagulopathy
		Use local means of managing bleeding	To reduce loss of blood
		Administer blood products as indicated and ordered	Necessary life-saving treatment; sepsis commonly causes thrombocytopenia
		Assess patient for signs of anemia, indicating significant blood loss	To help determine need for RBCs
		Maintain a type and crossmatch blood specimen with 2–4 units RBCs at all times during acute period	To ensure that blood is readily available at all times

Medications Commonly Used in the Care of the Patient with Sepsis and Septic Shock

Medication	Effect	Major side effects
Antibiotics	Treat source of sepsis	Nephrotoxicity Rash Fever Superinfection with fungi Coagulopathy Electrolyte disturbance
Vasopressors	Provide vasoconstriction and inotropic support	Poor peripheral tissue perfusion Tachycardia Renal failure Gut ischemia
Steroids	Stabilize cell membranes and limit capillary permeability	Fluid retention Hyperglycemia
Nonsteroidal antiinflammatory agents	Block inflammatory effects	Coagulopathy Rash Bone marrow suppression
Acetate or bicarbonate	Corrects metabolic acidosis (excess lactic acid)	Hypernatremia Fluid overload
Hyperalimentation	Meets high nutritional and metabolic demands for energy	Hyperglycemia Hepatic dysfunction
Endotoxin monoclonal antibody (investigational)	Counteracts endotoxin effects on vasculature	Allergic reactions Flu symptoms
Histamine blockers	Block histamine's inflammatory effects and gastric secretory effects	Thrombocytopenia

Multisystem Organ Failure

Major advances in the management of the critically ill and injured have resulted in significant reductions in mortality. These same advances in patient management and survival have led to the emergence of a relatively new clinical syndrome called multiple systems organ failure (MSOF, multisystem failure, or multiorgan failure). The syndrome is defined as progressive failure of two or more body systems as a result of the body's nonspecific inflammatory-immune response.[67] It is generally felt that the technological advances that have enabled clinicians to support failing body systems have created this disorder by replacing bodily functions without addressing the underlying etiology of organ failure.[68] Therefore, patients survive the injury but continue to respond with an immediate immunologic reaction that eventually destroys normal tissue. Reports in the late 1970s of non-injury-related organ failure and septic syndromes without cultured organisms were the first to identify multiorgan failure (MOF), as named by Fry in 1980.[69] The absence of adequate animal models to replicate this disorder has limited researchers' knowledge and critical care management endeavors. This syndrome has been identified as the cause of death in 22–50% of ICU deaths.[70] The grim facts are that MSOF carries a mortality rate ranging from 30–100%, depending on the patient population, severity of injury, and number of organs failing.[71] MSOF has many implications for the critical care nurse, and it may well be the critical care disorder of the 1990s.

Clinical antecedents

Studies have indicated that MSOF is present in possibly 15% of all ICU patients upon admission.[72] Based on this prevalence, highly specific risk factors have been difficult to describe clearly, but it is agreed that the severity of the original physical insult is the most significant predictor of who will progress to multiorgan failure.[73] The most common disorder linked to the development of MSOF is sepsis.[74] Patients with certain other disorders have shown higher-than-normal incidences of MSOF, although a patient's merely being a victim of one of these disorders does not necessarily herald MSOF.[75] These other disorders are listed in Table 9-13 and include hypotension or shock states, renal failure, polytrauma, surgery (especially abdominal), burns, and malignancy. Other risk factors more likely to predict MSOF development in the severely ill patient include the age of the patient and the presence of infection, chronic illness, and immunosuppression.[76] The "deadly triad" of insults most likely to precipitate MSOF seems to be hypovolemic shock, infection, and renal failure.[77] The order in which systems typically fail varies slightly among patient groups, but generally it proceeds in the following fashion: pulmonary, hepatic, hematologic, renal, and gastrointestinal system failure.[78] The number of systems in failure is the major predictor of survival or death; a data base of predictive mortality based on this variable is presented in Table 9-14.

Table 9-13 Risk Factors for MSOF

Major Risk Factors	Additional Risk Factors
Severe disease state at ICU admission	Abdominal surgery
Diagnosis of sepsis or infection at ICU admission	Burns
Patient's age greater than 65 years	Cancer
	Cardiopulmonary resuscitation
	GI bleeding
	Head injury, intracranial bleeding
	Severe hepatic disease
	Polytrauma
	Renal failure
	Shock states

Source: Knaus, W.A. & Wagner, D.P. (1989). Multiple systems organ failure: Epidemiology and prognosis. *Critical Care Clinics, 5*(2): 221–232.

Table 9-14 Predicted Mortality in MSOF (Based on Organ Failure)

Systems In Failure	Mortality Rate	
	Day 3	Day 7
1	45%	61%
2	70%	90%
>3	88%	100%

Source: Knaus, W.A. & Wagner, D.P. (1989). Multiple systems organ failure: Epidemiology and prognosis. *Critical Care Clinics,* 5(2): 221–232.

Critical referents

The major pathophysiological effects of MSOF appear to be related to humoral mediator substances stimulated by infectious organisms or toxins excreted from such organisms. The inflammatory-immune process described in sepsis is the initial stimulant, but subsequent organ failure is related to the final response of widespread systemic intravascular inflammation.[79] This process leads to a triad of effects: (1) maldistribution of blood flow, (2) oxygen supply and demand imbalance, and (3) metabolic derangements (Figure 9-9).

Blood flow is hindered because both vasodilation and vasoconstriction occur in an attempt to match blood flow with oxygen demand. Vascular volume overload is stimulated by release of ADH, aldosterone, and renin, enhancing the flow problems. Other contributors to this physiological complication are decreased cardiac output from a depressed myocardium, capillary permeability, and widespread microvascular thrombosis.

Inadequate supply of or excessive demand for oxygen is common in the critically ill, particularly the multiply injured or septic patient. Increased oxygen demand is the consequence of hypermetabolism, tissue ischemia, infection, and sympathetic stimulation. Inadequate cardiac output or microcirculatory blood flow will result in lower oxygen availability to the tissues. Increased demand without supply leads to cellular hypoxia and anaerobic metabolism. Anaerobic metabolism produces lactic acid and does not allow for removal of wastes. These cellular waste products—such as arachidonic acid, superoxide radicals, lactate, and nucleic acids—serve to increase tissue injury.[80]

The metabolic derangements of MSOF are an exaggerated form of those seen with septic shock with progressive compensatory failure. The metabolic abnormalities are divided into two phases: the lag (ebb) phase and the flow phase.[81] The initial insult triggers the lag phase, in which acute shock symptoms are prevalent and vasoactive substances produce the primary symptoms of intravascular volume shifts and vasodilation. In this phase, there are likely to be few clinical symptoms—the pathophysiology is confined to the subclinical cellular level. The flow phase demonstrates an acute metabolic re-

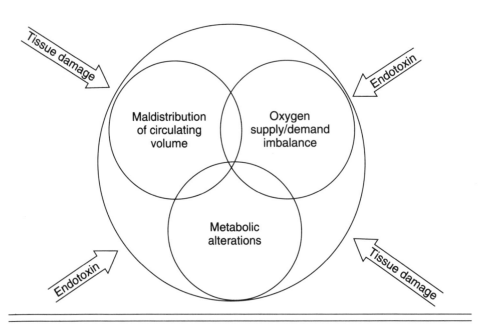

Figure 9-9 Triad of Pathophysiological Effects of MSOF

sponse to these demands, producing signs or symptoms such as hyperglycemia, hyperkalemia, thrombocytopenia, and/or fever. This phase peaks in 48–72 hours and lasts for 7–10 days.[82] Hypermetabolism continues until recovery begins or organ failure results. Organ failure that may be unique to this clinical syndrome (sepsis and MSOF) includes primary hepatic failure without hepatic disease, adrenal crisis, and hematologic failure without iatrogenic bone marrow suppression.

Each of these pathophysiological processes explains how sepsis can lead to organ damage, but not why organ failure occurs in a sequential fashion. Clinical experience with sepsis and nonbacteremic septic syndrome have demonstrated profound gastrointestinal dysfunction with adynamic ileus, acalculus cholecystitis, erosive gastritis, or multiple stress ulcers in unusual areas of the stomach.[83] Current theory states that altered absorptive and barrier functions of the bowel cause translocation of bacteria across the intestinal wall and may be the continual septic focus precipitating this syndrome.[84] This theory is supported by the early gastrointestinal bleeding and hepatic failure seen in this type of patient. Regardless of the precise pathophysiological mechanism, clinical sepsis and individual organ failure are the predominant presentations and foci of treatment strategies.

Resulting signs and symptoms

The resulting signs and symptoms of MSOF are those of sepsis and failure of each organ. Two or more organs in failure constitutes the MSOF diagnosis. The relevant signs and symptoms are addressed throughout this text with respect to each individual system, but the organ failure criteria in Table 9-15 are generally acceptable for identifying MSOF. A clinical staging system that may be helpful in the identification of patients exhibiting the syndrome is presented in Table 9-16. One limitation of the table is that this arbitrary delineation does not account for the fact that systems do not fail simultaneously, and organ damage may occur at different rates throughout the body.

Nursing standards of care

There is no known preventive or curative treatment for MSOF, so primarily supportive treatment is

Table 9-15 Criteria for Identifying Multiple Systems Organ Failure

System	Criteria
Hepatic	SGOT > 150 SI units Alkaline phosphatase > 300 U/L Total bilirubin > 10 mg/dL for 2 days Jaundice
Hematologic	WBC < 1000/mm^3 Platelets < 20,000/mm^3 Hematocrit < 20% Elevated PT/PTT
Gastrointestinal	Endoscopy positive for mucosal erosion Upper/lower GI bleeding Diarrhea Ileus Perforation
Neurologic	Glasgow coma scale < 6 Hypothermia/hyperthermia Cardiovascular failure Respiratory depression
Pulmonary	Respiratory rate < 5/min or > 49/min PaO_2 < 60–75 mm Hg on FIO_2 of 40% $PaCO_2$ > 50 mm Hg Severe dyspnea Crackles, wheezes Chest x-ray shows infiltrates
Renal	Urine output < 0.5 cc/kg/hr BUN > 100 mg/dL Serum creatinine > 3.5 mg/dL
Cardiovascular	Heart rate < 50 beats/min MAP < 50 mm Hg Systolic BP < 60 mm Hg Ventricular tachycardia/fibrillation Elevated cardiac enzymes

Source: Knaus, W.A. and Wagner, D.P. (1989). Multiple systems organ failure: Epidemiology and prognosis. *Critical Care Clinics,* 5(2): 221–232.

required. Treatment of known underlying risk factors such as sepsis is the first-line management. Other strategies revolve around three major goals: (1) improving tissue perfusion, (2) controlling and preventing infection, and (3) meeting oxygen, nutritional, and metabolic requirements.

Improvement of tissue perfusion focuses on the use of vascular assessment with hemodynamic monitoring and administration of fluids and vasoactive substances. Experimental therapies to enhance blood flow and tissue perfusion include hyperosmolar saline, prostaglandins, Naloxone, and calcium channel blockers.[85]

Infection prevention and control may necessitate a broad spectrum of antibiotics, including antifun-

Table 9-16 Clinical Staging of MSOF

Stage	Parameter	Signs/Symptoms
Stage 1	General appearance	No obvious signs
	Cardiovascular function	Increased volume requirements
	Respiratory function	Mild respiratory alkalosis
	Renal function	Limited responsiveness
	Metabolism	Increased insulin requirements
	Hepatic function	Unknown
	Hematology	Unknown
	Central nervous system	Confusion
Stage 2	General appearance	Metastable (ill)
	Cardiovascular function	Hyperdynamic, volume dependent
	Respiratory function	Tachypnea, hypocapnia, hypoxia
	Renal function	Fixed output, minimal azotemia
	Metabolism	Severe catabolism
	Hepatic function	Chemical jaundice
	Hematology	Decreased platelet count, increased or decreased WBC
	Central nervous system	Variable
Stage 3	General appearance	Obviously unstable
	Cardiovascular function	Shock, decreased cardiac output, edema
	Respiratory function	Severe hypoxia
	Renal function	Azotemia
	Metabolism	Metabolic acidosis, hyperglycemia
	Hepatic function	Clinical jaundice
	Hematology	Coagulopathy
	Central nervous system	Some response
Stage 4	General appearance	Terminal illness
	Cardiovascular function	Inotropes, volume overload
	Respiratory function	Hypercapnia, barotrauma
	Renal function	Oliguria
	Metabolism	Severe acidosis, increased oxygen consumption
	Hepatic function	Encephalopathy
	Hematology	Immature cells, coagulopathy
	Central nervous system	Coma

Source: Carrico, C.J.; Meakins, J.L.; Marshall, J.C.; Fry, D.; & Maier, R.V. (1986). Multiple-organ-failure syndrome: Incidence and problems of multiple-organ-failure syndromes. *Archives of Surgery, 121*(2): 196–197.

gals, antivirals, and agents for specific opportunistic or mycobacterial infections. The prevailing symptoms are those of sepsis, so treatment is comparable. Some clinicians advocate the maintenance of gut flora through enteral feeding, yet others suggest gut sterilization with nonabsorbable antibiotics to reduce the possible GI source of sepsis.[86] Limitation of invasive procedures must be balanced with the need to monitor the patient's condition or perform surgical procedures for infectious sources. Experimental therapies include efforts to reduce the inflammatory response with nonsteroidal antiinflammatory agents, prostaglandins, and anti-TNF antibodies.[87]

Meeting the oxygen and nutrient requirements of the patient can be an impossible task given his or her increased caloric requirements. Oxygen requirements can be decreased through appropriate mechanical ventilation and sedation, while nutritional and metabolic demands are met through nutritional support. Many researchers suggest 20–30 kcal/kg/day, primarily to support nitrogen balance.[88] To accomplish this requires a higher ratio of protein and fat supplement than is usual with nutritional supplementation. In fact, some clinicians advocate a "metabolic nutrition" plan aimed at higher protein and fat content, and fewer carbohydrates.[89] The enteral route of administration is preferred in hopes of maintaining GI function and preventing flora from translocating into the bloodstream.[90] Excessive glucose administration can contribute to refractory hyperglycemia and hepatic failure.

Much of the medical management of the MSOF patient will focus on individual organ damage and the support required to reverse organ failure. However, this strategy has proven futile when the underlying pathology is not corrected. When a specific etiology is known, it can be addressed; but often none is identified. Therapies aimed at removing toxic metabolites or blocking the inflammatory-immune process are being used without strong research support for their use. Such therapies include dialysis for ammonia removal and the administration of oxygen-free-radical scavengers (mannitol, furosemide, vitamin C), Pentoxitylline, fibronectin, and ATP complexes.[91]

Clinicians continue to be challenged with the management of the complex MSOF syndrome, and the fact that the precipitator is frequently unidentified only complicates decision making further. A multidisciplinary plan with input from physicians, nurses, pharmacists, and nutritionists will be the cornerstone of effective management. The nurse will often act as coordinator of this plan.

With a thorough understanding of the complexity of MSOF, the nurse approaches the patient in the same manner as for any septic patient, but pays special attention to failing organ systems. Continual monitoring for signs, symptoms, and diagnostic test abnormalities indicative of organ failure is an important component of critical care nursing. Realizing that morbidity and mortality rates increase with certain risk factors or as more organs fail, the critical care nurse is often an initiator of discussions of the prognosis for patient recovery. Striking the balance between "high-tech" and "high-touch" care is especially important with MSOF. The nurse will follow nursing care plans for specific organ failure and will develop a plan individualized for the patient and family addressing potential maladaptive coping, hopelessness, anxiety, fear, and altered health maintenance.

Poisoning

Poisoning is the development of clinical signs or symptoms after exposure to an injurious substance. Poisoning accounts for 10–20% of all hospital admissions and 10% of ambulance calls.[92] The majority of cases (65%) occur in children under 6 years old.[93]

Clinical antecedents

Infants younger than 6 months of age are unlikely to ingest poisons; however, they may be exposed to talcum powder or other baby care products as well as to poisons contained in breast milk if they are nursing. Infants from 6 to 12 months of age often ingest household cleaners that are left on low shelves. Toddlers having the ability to climb may ingest medicines, household products, perfumes—anything they can get their hands on. Toddlers are considered the highest risk group for poisoning. School-aged children rarely ingest poisons as long as harmful items are properly stored. Teenagers constitute the second-highest risk group for poisoning because of the use of street drugs or medications as well as an increased incidence of suicide attempts.[94]

Critical referents

Poisons are most commonly ingested orally, and they subsequently cause damage directly to the gastrointestinal tract or are absorbed into the systemic circulation via gastric or intestinal mucosa. Other routes by which poisons may enter the body are inhalation, absorption through the skin, and injection.

Every poison that enters the body exerts specific actions, depending on its chemical composition. Describing the pathophysiology of poisoning in general terms is therefore impossible. This section will focus on clinical toxidromes, which are combinations of signs and symptoms that together suggest a particular class of intoxicant. Table 9-17 lists a number of substances and their toxic symptoms.

Opioids Narcotic overdose is one of the most common types of poisonings encountered in the emergency department (ED). Opioids are central nervous system (CNS) depressants that are also capable of causing systemic dysfunction. The classic triad of symptoms for opioid intoxication is (1) coma, (2) pinpoint pupils, and (3) respiratory depression. Propoxyphene overdosage is associated with seizures. Lomotil intoxication may cause transient anticholinergic symptoms, followed by a latent period of 12–24 hours, and then coma and respiratory depression.[95] Heroin is often associated with noncardiac pulmonary edema caused by capillary damage and leakage of fluid into the interstitial space. Supportive treatment is provided along with administration of the narcotic antagonist Naloxone.

Sympathomimetics Cocaine is another popular drug whose effects are commonly seen in the ED. Cocaine, crack, ice, and amphetamines are CNS stimulants. These drugs also exert a significant effect on the sympathetic nervous system, thus causing the body to go into a state of "total overdrive."[96] This toxidrome is characterized by hypertension, tachy-

Table 9-17 Common Poisons and Toxic Symptoms

Substance	Toxic Symptoms
Acetaminophen	Mild anorexia, nausea, vomiting, delayed jaundice
Alcohol (ethanol)	Depressed sensorium, ethanolic odor on breath, respiratory depression, flushed facies, conjunctival erythema, depressed deep tendon reflexes. (Note: Always consider concurrent trauma and coingestions)
Amphetamines	Toxic psychosis, hyperthermia, flushing, increased BP, dilated pupils, hallucinations, seizures, tachycardia
Antifreeze (ethylene glycol)	Renal failure, crystals in urine, anion gap
Arsenic	Garlicky breath, vomiting, profuse bloody diarrhea, delayed hair loss, lines in nails
Barbiturates	Tense vesicular skin lesions, nystagmus, fluid overload, cardiorespiratory depression, depressed reflexes, prolonged coma
Bromide	Pigmentation, dementia, acne, psychosis, toxic delirium, hyperchloremia, cyanosis
Carbon monoxide	Coal gas odor, bullae, metabolic acidosis, cherry-colored nail beds, normal PO_2, convulsions, hypothermia
Chloral hydrate	Pear-like odor, cardiac arrhythmias, opacities on abdominal radiograph
Cocaine	Perforated nasal septum, dilated pupils, psychosis, tachycardia, scarred veins
Cyanide	Bitter almond odor, convulsions, rapid onset of coma, abnormal ECG
Digitalis	Visual disturbances, delirium, abnormal ECG, nausea
Disulfiram	Flushing, pulsating headache, circulatory collapse reaction
Ethchlorvynol	Deep and prolonged coma, pungent aromatic odor, slow pulse and decreased BP, pink gastric aspirate, hypotension, pulmonary edema
Gasoline	Distinctive odor, choking, pulmonary infiltrates
Glutethimide	Dilated pupils, prolonged and fluctuating coma, prolonged respiratory depression, laryngeal spasms, anticholinergic signs
Hydrocarbons	Pulmonary edema, lipid pneumonia, tinnitus, convulsions, ventricular fibrillation. (Always get a chest x-ray)
Isoniazid	Coma, seizures, anion gap acidosis
Iron	Bloody diarrhea, coma, radiopaque material on x-ray, hypotension
Isopropyl alcohol	Severe gastritis, acetonemia with normoglycemia
Lithium	Tremor, seizures, polyuria, delayed central nervous system toxicity, abnormal ECG
Lead	Severe abdominal pain, increased BP, milky vomitus, convulsions, muscle weakness, metallic taste, anorexia, encephalopathy
Lysergic acid diethylamide (LSD)	Hallucinations, dilated pupils
Mercury	Stomatitis, gingivitis, colitis, nephrotic syndrome
Meprobamate	Deep fluctuating coma, gastric masses, hypotension, pulmonary edema
Methadone	Miosis, coma, slow pulse, decreased BP and respiration, transient response to narcotic antagonist
Methaprylon	Hyperthermia, tachycardia, paradoxical excitement, respiratory depression
Methaqualone	Increased reflexes, tonic-clonic spasms, prolonged coma, internal bleeding, depressed platelet function, slow respirations
Methyl alcohol	Alcoholic patient, hyperventilation, decreased vision
Methylphenidate	Eosinophilia, wheezing, scarred veins, subcutaneous abscesses
Mushrooms, hepatotoxic (*Amanita phalloides*)	Severe nausea and vomiting 8 hrs after ingestion, delayed liver and renal failure

Table 9-17 *(continued)*

Substance	Toxic Symptoms
Narcotics	Coma, decreased BP, bradycardia, hypoventilation, miosis, needle marks, rapid response to narcotic antagonist
Nitrites ("rush")	Postural hypotension, flushing, anemia, cyanosis
Organophosphates	Miotic pupils, abdominal cramps, salivation, lacrimation, urination, defecation, increased bronchial secretions
Paraquat	Oropharynx burning, headache, vomiting, mild increase in BP and pulse, vertical nystagmus
Phenothiazines	Postural hypotension, hypothermia, miosis, tremor, radiopaque material on abdominal x-ray, increased Q-T interval
Propoxyphene	Pink gastric aspirate, seizures, miosis, irregular response to Naloxone
Salicylates	Hyperventilation, vomiting, fever, bleeding, acidosis
Scopolamine	Tachycardia, decreased secretions, urinary retention, dilated pupils, hallucinations, confusion, dry skin
Strychnine	Stiff neck, status epilepticus
Thallium	Alopecia, GI distress, minimal hematologic abnormalities
Tricyclic antidepressants	The "three Cs": coma, convulsion, conduction disturbances
Vacor (rat poison)	Ketoacidosis, postural hypotension

Source: Ellenhorn, M.J. and Barceloux, D.G. (1988). *Medical Toxicology.* New York: Elsevier, p. 21.

cardia, hyperpyrexia, mydriasis, anxiety, and delirium. Treatment is supportive, based on presenting symptoms.

Cholinergics Organophosphate or carbamate insecticides cause parasympathetic symptoms. These chemicals bind to acetylcholinesterase in myoneural junctions and synapses, preventing the reuptake and degradation of acetylcholine, and thus promoting cholinergic responses. The toxidrome associated with organophosphate poisoning is described by the acronym SLUDGE:

Salivation

Lacrimation

Urination

Defecation

Gastric cramping

Emesis

Significant exposure to organophosphates can cause patients to literally drown in their own secretions. Cholinergic stimulation of the pulmonary system causes bronchorrhea, pulmonary edema, increased lymph production, and bronchospasm. CNS symptoms may begin with confusion, and progress to agitation, coma, and seizures. Muscle fasciculations, muscle weakness, and paralysis can also occur.

The treatment for organophosphate poisoning is atropine. Large doses (that is, 100 mg) may be necessary to block the cholinergic response. Organophosphate and carbamate insecticides are usually absorbed through the skin via contact with crops or dust. Because this type of patient can carry the toxic dust or residue on clothing, a serious threat is posed to all personnel who come in contact with the patient. Such a case should be handled as a hazardous materials incident; all clothing should be removed from the patient and washed with copious amounts of water. The water should then be contained for appropriate disposal.

Anticholinergics Cyclic antidepressants, antihistamines, and belladonna alkaloids are examples of anticholinergic agents, which act by blocking acetylcholine at its parasympathetic effector sites. This parasympathetic block allows the sympathetic nervous system to function unopposed.[97] The toxidrome for anticholinergics is well known:

Hot as a fire—hyperpyrexia

Red as a beet—cutaneous vasodilation

Dry as a bone—decreased salivation

Blind as a bat—cycloplegia and mydriasis

Mad as a hatter—delirium and hallucinations

Treatment includes routine supportive care. In the severe case—for instance, tricyclic overdose with

Table 9-18 Regional Poison Centers, by State

Alabama
Alabama Poison Center
Tuscaloosa, AL 35401
800-462-0800 (Alabama only)

Arizona
Arizona Poison Control System
Arizona Poison & Drug Information
Tucson, AZ 85724
(602) 626-6016
800-362-0101 (Arizona only)

St. Luke's Poison Management
Center
Phoenix, AZ 85006
(602) 253-3334

California
Los Angeles County Medical
Association
Regional Poison Control Center
Los Angeles, CA 90057
(213) 484-5151

San Diego Regional Poison Center
San Diego, CA 92103
(619) 294-6000

San Francisco Bay Area Regional
Poison Control Center
San Francisco, CA 94110
(415) 476-6600

UCDMC Regional Poison Control
Center
Sacramento, CA 95817
(916) 453-3692

Colorado
Rocky Mountain Poison Center
Denver, CO 80204
(303) 629-1123
800-332-3073 (Colorado only)
800-525-5042 (Montana only)
800-442-2702 (Wyoming only)

District of Columbia
National Capital Poison Center
Washington, DC 20007
(202) 625-3333

Florida
Tampa Bay Regional Poison Control
Center
Tampa, FL 33679
(813) 253-4444
800-282-3171

Georgia
Georgia Poison Control Center
Atlanta, GA 30335
(404) 589-4400
800-282-5846 (Georgia only)

Kentucky
Kentucky Regional Poison Center of
Kosair Children's Hospital
Louisville, KY 40232
(502) 589-8222
800-722-5725 (Kentucky only)

Louisiana
Louisiana Regional Poison Control
Center
Shreveport, LA 71130
(318) 425-1524
800-535-0525 (Louisiana only)

Maryland
Maryland Poison Center
Baltimore, MD 21201
(410) 528-7701
800-492-2414 (Maryland only)

Massachusetts
Massachusetts Poison Control
System
Boston, MA 02115
(617) 232-2120
800-682-9211 (Massachusetts only)

Michigan
Blodgett Regional Poison Center
Grand Rapids, MI 49506
800-442-4571 (area code 616 only)
800-632-2727 (Michigan only)

Poison Control Center
Children's Hospital of Michigan
Detroit, MI 48201
(313) 745-5711
800-462-6642 (area code 313 only)
800-572-1655 (remainder of
Michigan)

Minnesota
Hennepin Regional Poison Center
Minneapolis, MN 55415
(612) 347-3141

Minnesota Regional Poison Center
St. Paul, MN 55101
(612) 221-2113
800-222-1222 (Minnesota only)

Missouri
Cardinal Glennon Children's Hospital
Regional Poison Center
St. Louis, MO 63104
(314) 772-5200
800-392-9111 (Missouri only)

Nebraska
Mid Plains Poison Center
Omaha, NE 68114
(402) 390-5400
800-642-9999 (Nebraska only)
800-228-9515 (surrounding states)

New Jersey
New Jersey Poison Information and
Education System
Newark, NJ 07112
(202) 923-0764
(800) 962-1253 (New Jersey only)

New Mexico
New Mexico Poison and Drug
Information Center
Albuquerque, NM 87131
(505) 843-2551
800-432-6866 (New Mexico only)

New York
Long Island Regional Poison Control
Center
East Meadow, NY 11554
(516) 542-2323

New York City Poison Control Center
New York, NY 10016
(212) 340-4494

North Carolina
Duke University Poison Control Center
Durham, NC 27710
(919) 684-8111
800-672-1697 (North Carolina only)

Ohio
Central Ohio Poison Center
Columbus, OH 43205
(614) 228-1323
800-682-7625 (Ohio only)

Southwest Ohio Regional Poison
Control System
Cincinnati, OH 45267
(513) 872-5111
800-872-5111

Oregon
Oregon Poison Control and Drug
Information Center
Portland, OR 97201
(503) 225-8968
800-452-7165 (Oregon only)

Pennsylvania
Pittsburgh Poison Center
Pittsburgh, PA 15213
(412) 681-6669

Rhode Island
Rhode Island Poison Center
Providence, RI 02902
(401) 277-5727

Texas
North Central Texas Poison Center
Dallas, TX 75235
(214) 920-2400
800-441-0040 (Texas only)

Texas State Poison Center
Galveston, TX 77550
(409) 765-1420
(713) 654-1701 (Houston)
(512) 478-4490 (Austin)
800-392-8548 (Texas only)

Utah
Intermountain Regional Poison Control
Center
Salt Lake City, UT 84132
(801) 581-2151
800-662-0062 (Utah only)

West Virginia
West Virginia Poison Center
Charleston, WV 25304
(304) 348-4211
800-642-3625 (West Virginia only)

Table 9-19 Actions of and Treatments for Common Poisoning Agents

Agent	Mechanism of Action	Treatment
Acetaminophen	Can cause fatal hepatonecrosis Toxic dose: 140 mg/kg	O_2, IV, monitor, emesis/lavage, charcoal, cathartic, *N*-acetylcysteine (oral dose: 140 mg/kg, then 70 mg/kg every 4 hours for 17 doses, dilute to 5% solution and add to juice)
Aspirin	Uncouples oxidative phosphorylation; inhibits Krebs cycle	O_2, IV, monitor, emesis/lavage, charcoal, cathartic, alkalinization of urine, replace potassium, dialysis
Cyclic antidepressants	Inhibits synaptic reuptake of norepinephrine and 5-hydroxytryptamine Sympathetic overdrive Ventricular dysrhythmias	O_2, IV, monitor, emesis/lavage, pulse charcoal, cathartic, bicarbonate
Acids	Coagulation necrosis Severe gastric injury Gastric perforation	Dilute with water, do not induce vomit; charcoal does not work
Alkalis	Liquefaction of esophagus, leads to perforation Mediastinitis	Same as for acids (above); endoscopy should be done after 12 hours
Methemoglobinemia	Iron is oxidized to ferric state Oxygen is bound so firmly it is not available to tissue	O_2, IV, monitor, emesis/lavage, charcoal, cathartic; if patient is stuporous, methylene blue 1–2 mg of 1% solution
Ethylene glycol	Renal and CNS toxicity Widespread petechial hemorrhage	O_2, IV, monitor, emesis/lavage, charcoal, cathartic, bicarbonate, thiamine, pyridoxine 100 mg
Methanol	Optic nerve demyelination	Same as for ethylene glycol (above)
Iron	Mucosal damage Mural and transmural infarction of intestine, stomach lining Hepatic and renal shutdown	O_2, IV, monitor, emesis/lavage, 50–100 mL of 2–3% solution of bicarbonate into stomach; chelation treatment with deferoxamine, 90 mg/kg IM every 8 hours
Organophosphate insecticides	Interfere with normal neurotransmitters by inhibiting acetylcholinesterase	O_2, IV, monitor, decontamination; atropine (2–4 mg) repeated until improvement; pralidoxime (1–2 g in 100 cc D_5W over 15 minutes, followed with drip 500 mg/hr) If ingested orally: emesis/lavage, charcoal, cathartic
Botulism	Clostridium botulinium toxin binds at parasympathetic clefts of cholinergic nerve terminals Blocks release of acetylcholine at the neuromuscular junctions and peripheral autonomic synapses	Supportive measures, antitoxin

seizures, hypotension, and ventricular tachycardia—physostigmine, an acetylcholinesterase inhibitor, may be considered. Due to its severe side effects, however, physostigmine has lost favor and is no longer considered the sole antidote. Supportive treatment for specific symptoms, such as sodium bicarbonate for metabolic acidosis, is considered the treatment of choice.

Sedative hypnotics Barbiturates and benzodiazapines are compounds that inhibit neurotransmission and neuroeffector functions in the CNS. Characteris-

Table 9-20 Summary of General Treatment of the Overdosed Patient

Peripheral intravenous line

Continuous cardiac monitoring

Vital sign monitoring

History, including route of administration

Physical examination

Appropriate laboratory studies
  Toxicology screen with selected blood levels
  Complete blood count
  Serum electrolytes
  Blood urea nitrogen
  Urinalysis

Administration of therapeutic agents
  Glucose
  Naloxone
  Oxygen
  Thiamine

Evacuation of stomach and intestine

Administration of activated charcoal and cathartic

Administration of an antidote if available

Psychiatric evaluation when medically cleared

Table 9-21 Characteristic Odors Associated with Some Toxic Substances

Odor	Substance
Acetone	Ethyl alcohol Isopropyl alcohol Lacquer
Bitter almond	Amygdalin Apricot pits Cyanide Laetrile
Burned rope	Marijuana
Carrot	Cicutoxin
Garlic	Arsenic Arsine gas Dimethylsulfoxide Organophosphates Phosphorus Selenium Thallium
Mothballs	Naphthalene Paradichlorobenzene
Peanuts	Rodenticides
Pear	Chloral hydrate Paraldehyde
Pungent aromatic	Ethchlorvynol
Rotten egg	Hydrogen sulfide Mercaptans Sewer gas
Shoe polish	Nitrobenzene
Violets	Turpentine
Wintergreen	Methyl salicylate

Source: Bryson, P.D. (1989). *Comprehensive Review in Toxicology.* Rockville, MD: Aspen Publishers, p. 7.

tic symptoms of intoxication are confusion or coma, respiratory depression, hypotension, hypothermia, and vesicles or bullae known as "barb burns." Treatment is focused on supportive therapy. For benzodiazapine overdose, a new antagonist, Flumazenil, will soon be available and will have the same action as Naloxone does with narcotics.[98]

A description of the toxicology of all possible poisons is beyond the scope of this section. The best resource immediately available to everyone is a local poison control center. These centers are staffed 24 hours a day, and staff members can consult references on a range of toxic materials. They routinely describe substance toxicology, the supportive treatment necessary, and the antidote, if one exists. A listing of regional poison centers that are certified by the American Association of Poison Control Centers appears in Table 9-18. A chart of commonly encountered agents, their mechanisms of action, and their treatments is presented in Table 9-19.

Resulting signs and symptoms

Poisoning should be suspected in any unconscious, unresponsive patient. If poisoning is known from patient history, witnessed ingestion, suicide note, etc., assessment is often more rapid and treatment more clearly defined. A general approach has been described as APTLS, advanced poisoning treatment and life support.[99] This follows the basic primary and secondary survey format practiced with all emergency patients and includes the phases of care that are summarized in Table 9-20.

Phase I: Primary survey   This phase has an ABCDE pattern:

A. Airway must be secured in any unconscious patient or anyone with an absent gag reflex. Cervical spine must be controlled and injury ruled out in the unconscious or decreased sensorium patient.

B. Breathing is assessed via pattern and volumes inspired, and the patient is ventilation-

Table 9-22 Electrocardiographic Manifestations of Poisoning

Sign	Possible Cause (drug, toxin, or underlying condition)
Prolonged Q-T interval	Arsenic Hypocalcemia (ethylene glycol) Phenothiazines Tricyclic antidepressants Type I antidysrhythmic agents
Prolonged QRS interval	Phenothiazines (selected) Tricyclic antidepressants Type I antidysrhythmic agents
Atrioventricular block	Beta-adrenergic blockers Calcium channel-blocking agents Digitalis glycosides Tricyclic antidepressants Type I antidysrhythmic agents
Ventricular tachydysrhythmias	Amphetamines Cocaine Digitalis glycosides Theophylline Tricyclic antidepressants Type I antidysrhythmic agents
Ischemic pattern or current of injury	Cellular asphyxiants (cyanide, monoxide) Hypoxemia (pneumonia) Hypotension

Source: Callahan, B. Mlynczak (Ed.). (1990). *Case Reviews in Emergency Nursing.* Baltimore: Williams & Wilkens, pp. 18–19.

assisted if necessary. The odor of the breath should be noted for possible clues to intoxicant. Characteristic odors associated with certain toxins are listed in Table 9-21.

C. Circulation is assessed via color of skin, strength and regularity of pulses (central versus peripheral), capillary refill time, oxygen saturation, and ECG rhythms. Table 9-22 summarizes dysrhythmias associated with toxic substances.

D. Disability is noted if any neurological deficits are present. Pupillary changes and/or nystagmus are also assessed (see Table 9-23).

E. Exposure of the patient must be accomplished by removal of all clothing. Signs of trauma, skin integrity, or obvious bleeding must be assessed.

Phase II: Resuscitation Poisonings known to be immediately life-threatening (for example, cyanide, opioid overdose), are treated at this point. Contact poisons are irrigated with normal saline; if irrigation is in process, it is continued. Oxygen is administered at 100%, except in cases of paraquat poisoning (oxygen combines with paraquat to increase pulmonary injury). An IV of D_5W should first be established and then blood should be drawn for laboratory analysis. The following drugs are then given to any patient with decreased level of consciousness: $D_{50}W$, 25–50 g IV; Naloxone, 2 mg IV; and thiamine, 100 mg IV. If the substance is known and an antidote indicated, it should be administered (see Table 9-24, page 1293).

Phase III: Secondary survey If possible, a history should be obtained from the patient, family, and prehospital providers. A complete physical exam should be performed with special attention to all points of toxin entry, that is, nasal passages, oral cavity, skin, and genitalia. Vital signs, including core temperature, should be assessed and monitored frequently. Table 9-25 (page 1294) lists types of poisons associated with specific vital sign changes. Diagnostic studies that should be performed include the following x-rays and laboratory tests:

1. Chest x-ray, for baseline comparison and to determine the presence or extent of pulmonary injury.

2. Abdominal x-ray, to highlight radio-opaque substances such as iron and heavy metals, tricyclic antidepressants, antihistamines, chloral hydrate, calcium, iodides, potassium,

Table 9-23 Characteristic Eye Changes
in Poisoning

Type of Eye Change	Causes
Mydriasis	Anticholinergics
	Glutethimide (Doriden)
	Meperidine (Demerol)
	Mushrooms (anticholinergics)
	Withdrawal from substance abuse
	Sympathomimetics
Miosis	Cholinergics
	Clonidine (Catapres)
	Insecticides
	Mushrooms (cholinergics)
	Narcotics
	Nicotine
	Phenothiazines
	Phencyclidine
Nystagmus	(Note acronym: SALEM TIP)
	S Sedative-hypnotics
	Solvents
	A Alcohol
	L Lithium
	E Ethanol
	Ethylene glycol
	M Methanol
	T Thiamine depletion
	Tegretol (carbamazepine)
	I Isopropanol
	P Phencyclidine
	Phenytoin (Dilantin)

Source: Bryson, P.D. (1989). *Comprehensive Review in Toxicology.* Rockville, MD: Aspen Publishers, p. 8.

and phenothiazines. Enteric coated tablets as well as balloons or condoms with cocaine swallowed by body packers, will also be visualized.

3. A CBC with differential, which may indicate absolute leukocytosis produced by iron, theophylline, or hydrocarbon poisoning.

4. Serum electrolytes, which are used to calculate the anion gap [Na − (HCO$_3$ + Cl)]. A normal gap is 8–12 mEq/L; a result greater than 12 mEq/L is usually associated with metabolic acidosis and poisoning from other unmeasured anions. Causes of high-anion-gap metabolic acidosis can be remembered using the acronym A MUD PILE:

Aspirin
Methanol
Uremia
Diabetic ketoacidosis
Paraldehyde phenformin
Iron isoniazide
Lactic acid
Ethylene glycol or ethanol

5. Blood urea nitrogen (BUN) and creatinine clearance are recommended to establish baseline function as well as to determine if renal failure is a factor.

6. Osmolarity and toxicology screen, which may assist in identifying toxic agents.

Phase IV: Definitive care This phase involves re-evaluation of all data obtained as well as continuous monitoring and vigilant observation of the patient for patterns and trends in responses. General treatment for most poisonings is administered at this time and this includes gastric evacuation and enhanced elimination (described in more detail later in this section). An in-depth patient/family interview should be conducted to assess for attempted suicide, neglect, or abuse potential.

Phase V: Disposition Patient disposition requires considerable analysis and knowledge of resources available. Improper disposition could lead to the patient's death or a liability claim. Considerations include the requirements for hospital admission (does the patient meet the criteria established by the facility?); transfer requirements (should the patient receive specialized treatment unavailable at the present ED, such as hyperbaric chamber or psychiatric care?); and, finally, whether the patient is capable of being discharged to home safely or whether further arrangements require social work involvement.

Nursing standards of care

The initial treatment of any suspected toxic ingestion is prevention of absorption. Historically, the first step taken was gastric emptying. In the conscious patient, syrup of ipecac was administered—30 mL for adults, followed by 8–12 oz of water or juice. Ipecac acts locally, irritating the stomach, which stimulates vomiting. It also acts on the chemoreceptor trigger zone located in the fourth ventricle of the brain. This trigger zone activates the vomiting center located in the reticular formation within the brain, resulting in emesis. This action may take anywhere from 15 to 30 minutes. In the unconscious patient, or in the patient for whom vomiting may be dangerous or pose an aspiration risk, gastric lavage is indicated. A 32–40 French tube with several lateral and distal lumens is passed down the esophagus while the patient is positioned left lateral recumbent, knees

Table 9-24 Antidotes and Their Dosages

Drug/Toxin	Antidote	Antidote Dosage
Acetaminophen	N-Acetylcysteine	140 mg/kg orally (loading) 70 mg/kg every 4 hours, 17 doses (maintenance)
Anticholinergics	Physostigmine	Adult: 1–2 mg IV, slowly Child: 0.5 mg or 0.02 mg/kg IV, slowly
Beta-adrenergic blockers	Glucagon	1–5 mg IV
Bromide	Sodium chloride	
Carbamate insecticides	Atropine	2–4 mg IV, as needed
Carbon monoxide	Oxygen	
Cyanide	Amyl nitrite perles Sodium nitrite	Adult: 300 mg Child: 10 mg/kg
	Sodium thiosulfate	Adult: 12.5 g IV Child: 1.5 mL/kg
Cardiac glycosides	Fragment, antigen-binding (Fab) antibody therapy	As necessary
Ethylene glycol	Ethyl alcohol	1 mL/kg of 95% solution, diluted (loading) 0.1 mL/kg/hr, diluted (maintenance)
Gyrimetra mushrooms	Pyridoxine	2–5 g IV, slowly
Heavy metals	Dimercaprol (BAL) Penicillamine Disodium EDTA	
Isoniazid	Pyridoxine	2–5 g IV, slowly
Iron	Deferoxamine	10–15 mg/kg/hr
Methanol	Ethyl alcohol	As for ethylene glycol
Narcotics	Naloxone	2 mg IV
Nitrites	Methylene blue	1–2 mg/kg of 1% solution
Organophosphates	Atropine Pralidoxime	1–2 mg IV, as needed 1 g
Tricyclic antidepressants	Sodium bicarbonate	1–3 mEq/kg IV
Warfarin	Vitamin K$_1$	5–25 mg IV or IM

Source: Bryson, P.D. (1989). *Comprehensive Review in Toxicology.* Rockville, MD: Aspen Publishers, p. 11.

flexed, in Trendelenberg. Water or normal saline is instilled in 200–300 mL aliquots and returned until clear.

Gastric emptying is currently under scrutiny by some practitioners, however. Several researchers agree that gastric emptying is a waste of time when more than 1 hour has elapsed between ingestion and treatment. They argue that very little material is returned (less than 20%) and that the procedures create significant delays in charcoal instillation. Ipecac is also known to interfere with some antidotes, for example, N-acetylcysteine.[100]

Treatment of suspected toxic ingestion with charcoal to prevent absorption is universally accepted. Activated charcoal is a fine black powder produced by burning organic products. Super char, a newer version, has an increased surface area, allowing for greater absorption capability. Charcoal itself is not absorbed through the gastrointestinal tract; therefore, when combined with a cathartic (usually Sorbitol), it carries the toxins out of the body via diarrhea stool.[101]

Multidose, or pulse, charcoal is considered the treatment of choice for drugs that undergo enterogastric or enterohepatic recirculation as the body attempts to detoxify the blood. Charcoal acts as a dialysate to absorb and pull the drug across intestinal membranes into the bowel lumen. Drugs that are known to undergo recirculation are carbamazine, digoxin, glutethimide, meprobomate, nadolol, phen-

Table 9-25 Presenting Poisoning Symptoms and Possible Agents

Signs/Symptoms	Cause	Poisons
Decreased respiratory rate	CNS depression	Ethyl alcohol, opioids, sedative hypnotics
Increased respiratory rate	CNS stimulation Metabolic acidosis Tissue hypoxia	Sympathomimetics, theophylline, salicylates, narcotic withdrawal, carbon monoxide, cyanide, methane, methemoglobinemia
Decreased heart rate	Parasympathetic CNS depression Cardiotoxicity	Organophosphates, carbonates, opioids, clonidine Digitalis, calcium channel blockers, beta blockers
Increased heart rate	CNS stimulation Cholinergic blockade	Sympathomimetics PCP, salicylates, ethyl alcohol withdrawal
Decreased BP	Cardiotoxicity Loss of vasomotor tone Volume depletion	Calcium channel blockers, beta blockers Cyclic antidepressants, antihypertensives, calcium channel blockers, theophylline Iron, heavy metals, diuretics, lithium, organophosphates
Increased BP	Alpha adrenergic stimulation	Sympathomimetics, drug withdrawal
Decreased temperature	CNS depression Loss of thermoregulation	Barbiturates, opioids, ethyl alcohol, phenothiazines
Increased temperature	CNS stimulation Cholinergic inhibition Loss of thermoregulation Vasodilation	Sympathomimetics, PCP, salicylates, alcohol withdrawal, cyclic antidepressants, phenothiazines, beladonna alkaloids, antihistamines

cyclidine, phenylbutazone, and tricyclic antidepressants. A dose of 20–100 g of pulse charcoal is recommended, to be given at intervals of 1–4 hours.[102]

There are a few toxic substances that are immediately absorbed and that can be life-threatening if not removed from the circulation quickly. Treatment for ingestion of these substances requires significant resources and equipment capable of performing hemodialysis or hemoperfusion. Standard hemodialysis is indicated for the following substances if taken in toxic amounts: methanol, ethanol, ethylene glycol, salicylates, lithium, procainamide, and theophylline. Hemoperfusion removes toxic materials by pumping the blood through a charcoal filter, which absorbs them. Substances that require hemoperfusion are chloramphenicol, diphenylhydantoin, methaqualone, methotrexate, methylphenobarbital, paraquat, pentobarbital and phenobarbital.[103]

Management of the poisoned patient requires deliberate and efficient detective work by prehospital providers, physicians, and nurses. All of these providers must work collaboratively and communicate clearly to ensure the optimal outcome for the patient. Following the diagnosis of poisoning, intensive nursing care involves (1) preventing absorption, (2) administering antidotes and minimizing the side effects of treatments, (3) intervening to prevent life-threatening effects of toxins, and (4) providing continuous surveillance of the patient's condition.

When managing the poisoning case, there are many critical nursing problems, which must be prioritized based on the toxin and the individual's response. Specific diagnoses described in the following care plan are (1) ineffective airway clearance, (2) impaired gas exchange, (3) self-directed violence, and (4) impaired home management.

Nursing Care Plan for the Management of the Victim of Poisoning

Diagnosis	Signs and symptoms	Intervention	Rationale
Ineffective airway clearance, secondary to decreased level of consciousness and inability to protect airway	Decreased level of consciousness Decreased or absent gag reflex Slurred speech Drooling Inability to clear secretions	Obtain proper airway position, suction oropharynx frequently as secretions accumulate, and prepare for intubation	Endotracheal intubation is the only safe method to protect the airway from aspiration
Impaired gas exchange, related to interference of toxic substance with oxygen transport	Neurological impairment Decreased PaO_2, Decreased O_2 saturation ECG changes indicative of ischemia	Administer O_2 100% and antidote for specific toxin, if known Supportive treatment includes intubation, mechanical ventilation with PEEP, if necessary	Only exception to giving O_2 is paraquat poisoning PEEP forces O_2 across capillary membrane and may dislodge some molecules of hemoglobin
Self-directed violence, secondary to suicide attempt by overdose	Suicide note Suicidal ideation History of depression or mood change Withdrawal from people or usual activities Putting affairs in order	If patient is conscious and alert, explain need for close observation and search; initiate one-to-one suicide precautions and use consistent calm approach Limit the number of providers	To prevent elopement or further suicide attempts To de-escalate anxiety and provide safe, supportive environment
Impaired home management, related to inability of parents to provide safe environment for child	Evidence of poor home environment: no food on shelves or in refrigerator, hazards not safeguarded, lack of supervision, poor problem-solving skills of parents, lack of family support; evidence of child's learning disability, developmental delays, and/or socially withdrawn behavior	Make a home assessment social services referral	To differentiate between accidental ingestion and lack of supervision or neglect; to ascertain cause of learning disability or delay and facilitate intervention

Asphyxia

Asphyxia is defined as a condition caused by inefficient intake of oxygen. Asphyxiation is second to coronary artery disease as the most common cause of cardiac arrest.[104]

Clinical antecedents

Asphyxia has many etiologies that can be categorized as extrinsic and intrinsic causes. Examples of extrinsic causes are choking; toxic inhalation; drowning; traumatic injury to the chest, pulmonary system, or respiratory center; drugs and anesthesia; poorly oxygenated environment; and electrical shock. Examples of intrinsic causes are pulmonary or pleural hemorrhage; pulmonary edema; and airway obstruction by edematous tissue, tumor, or aneurysm. Since many of the causes of asphyxia are discussed in other sections, the focus of this section will be asphyxia related to chemical gas and smoke inhalation.

Inhalation injury is the leading cause of death during the first 24 hours following exposure to fire.[105] Carbon monoxide (CO) is the most immediate cause of inhalation injury in a fire. Asphyxia from smoke inhalation is associated with three conditions: closed space (such as a tightly insulated home), presence of heavy smoke, and a history of unconsciousness. Mortality from smoke inhalation is as high as 40–50%. In the patient over age 60, the risk of death increases to nearly 100%. Alcohol use is considered a significant risk factor for housefires. For example, in a Maryland study of 523 residential fires, 85% of the victims had blood alcohol levels of greater than 0.1%.[106]

Critical referents

Smoke inhalation produces injury via three mechanisms: direct heat, irritant gases, and aerosolized contaminated particles.

Direct heat Thermal damage to the lower airway by direct heat is rare due to reflex laryngospasm and efficient cooling of the respiratory labyrinth apparatus. The exception to this rule occurs with exposure to the excessive temperatures of steam, which has a heat-carrying capacity 4000 times greater than that of air. Mucosal burns are more common in the upper airway when victims are exposed to heated air. These burned areas become increasingly edematous and later slough off, causing airway obstruction.[107]

Irritant gases Fire utilizes oxygen for combustion, thus leaving the environment hypoxic. As oxygen is being burned, carbon monoxide and other gases are being released in the smoke, depending on the materials fueling the fire. Table 9-26 describes toxic elements found in housefire smoke. Inhalation of carbon monoxide at a level of 0.1% in room air

Table 9-26 Toxic Elements in Housefire Smoke

Gas	Source	Effect
Carbon monoxide	Any organic matter	Tissue hypoxia
Carbon dioxide	Any organic matter	Narcosis
Nitrogen dioxide	Wallpaper, wood	Bronchial irritation Dizziness Pulmonary edema
Hydrogen chloride (phosgene)	Plastics (polyvinyl chloride)	Severe mucosal irritation
Hydrogencyanide	Wool, silk, nylons (polyurethane)	Headache Respiratory failure Coma
Benzene	Petroleum plastics	Mucosal irritation Coma
Aldehydes	Wood, cotton, paper	Severe mucosal damage Extensive lung damage
Ammonia	Nylon	Mucosal irritation

Source: Demling, R.H. (1989). Management of the burn patient. In *Textbook of Critical Care*, Shoemaker et al. (Eds.). Philadelphia: W.B. Saunders, p. 1305.

decreases the oxygen-carrying capacity of hemoglobin by 50%.[108] Carbon monoxide has an affinity for hemoglobin 250 times stronger than that of oxygen. If the exposure to carbon monoxide is prolonged, it can saturate the cell, binding to cytochrome oxidase, and impair mitochondrial function.

The CNS is the most vulnerable organ system affected by carbon monoxide. Carbon monoxide acts on the brain to increase cerebral perfusion and increase cerebral capillary permeability, which results in cerebral edema, increased intracranial pressure, and brain hypoxia. Permanent neurological damage may be due to brain degeneration secondary to the inhibition of aerobic metabolism at the cellular level for up to 4 hours following exposure.[109]

Hydrocyanic acid is the gas form of cyanide, and it can be inhaled or absorbed through the skin. Cyanide (CN) is a by-product of burning wool, silk, nylon, or polyurethane. Nylon and polyurethane are found in most home furnishings such as carpeting and upholstery. In one smoke study, the presence of carbon monoxide correlated positively with the presence of cyanide. In other words, if one gas is present, the other is most likely there also. Cyanide, like carbon monoxide, binds to mitochondrial cytochrome oxidase, which inhibits cellular respiration. Cyanide is normally present in humans in small amounts, depending on diet (lima beans have significant amounts) and cigarette smoking history. Cyanide is detoxified in the liver by conversion to thiocyanate, which is readily excreted by the kidneys. Cyanide levels of 0.2–0.25 mg/L are considered toxic and dangerous, 1 mg/L is considered a lethal exposure.[110]

Contaminated particles Inhaled particles often cause bronchospasm; but if small enough, they can gain entry into lower airways and effect immediate changes on respiratory structures. Cilia are paralyzed; histamine, serotonin, and kallikreins are released; and surfactant activity is decreased. The net effect on the lower airways is to cause mucosal edema, bronchorrhea, and sloughing of mucosa.

As time progresses after the injury, capillary permeability increases, caused by a release of vasoactive substances (prostaglandins, histamine, and leukotrienes) as well as a shift in oncotic pressure due to protein movement out of the vascular compartment. Inhalation injury also increases the formation of lymph and increases bronchial blood flow tenfold.

In summary, acute pulmonary insufficiency occurs immediately following smoke exposure. This progresses to pulmonary edema 6–72 hours post injury, which gradually leads to the development of bronchopneumonia 3–10 days post injury.

Resulting signs and symptoms

Smoke inhalation is a life-threatening emergency, so the patient should be assessed in a formal, organized manner utilizing the ABCDE format:

A. Airway: significant smoke exposure results in hoarseness, dyspnea, tachypnea, stridor, and wheezing. Facial burns, singed nasal hairs, and carbonaceous sputum are all considered evidence enough for aggressive airway management (intubation).

B. Breathing: apnea is more likely due to elevated carbon monoxide levels and neurologic impairment than to smoke's direct effect on the pulmonary system. Breath sounds are initially clear, except in cases of severe pulmonary damage, when crackles (rales) and gurgles (rhonchi) may be heard. Respiratory rate may be deceivingly normal, since the carotid body responds to oxygen tension, not oxygen content.

C. Circulation: following exposure to elevated levels of carbon monoxide or cyanide, angina and ECG changes secondary to myocardial ischemia may be evident, including ST depression, T wave inversion, prolonged Q-T interval, low voltage pattern, and heart block.[111] Room-air blood gases often reveal mild hypoxemia, with PaO_2 in the 60–70 mm Hg range. Cyanide toxicity may cause hypotension, hyperthermia, and diaphoresis.

D. Disability: Table 9-27 summarizes the neurological symptoms corresponding to various blood levels of carbon monoxide. Cyanide toxicity causes giddiness, headache, palpitations, vomiting, respiratory depression, unconsciousness, and seizures.

E. Exposure: the rest of the body should be assessed for the burns and/or trauma that are commonly associated with housefires and smoke inhalation.

Carbon monoxide and cyanide levels can be obtained from an anticoagulated blood specimen. Although these levels are helpful, they should not substitute for clinical findings or delay treatment. Cervical spine films may need clearance in the unconscious victim. Chest x-ray is of little diagnostic value acutely, but may be helpful as a baseline or for verification of endotracheal tube placement.[112] If the diagnosis of smoke inhalation is not obvious, fiber optic bronchoscopy is considered the best tool available. The following bronchoscopy findings confirm the diagnosis: laryngeal edema, bronchial inflamma-

Table 9-27 Neurological Symptoms Corresponding to Carboxyhemoglobin (COHgb) Levels

Level of COHgb (%)	Symptoms
0–10	None, in healthy individuals Reduced exercise tolerance in patients with chronic obstructive pulmonary disease Decreased threshold for angina and claudication in patients with atherosclerosis
10–20	Headache, dyspnea on vigorous exertion
20–30	Throbbing headache, dyspnea on moderate exertion, difficulty with concentration, weakness
30–40	Severe headache, dizziness, nausea, vomiting, trouble in thinking, visual disturbances
40–50	Confusion, syncope on exertion
50–60	Collapse, convulsions
60–70	Coma, frequently fatal
> 70	Coma, death likely

Source: Martindale, L.G. (1989). Carbon monoxide poisoning: The rest of the story. *Journal of Emergency Nursing, 15*(2): 101–103.

tion, hemorrhage, airway necrosis, mucosal ulceration, and charring.[113]

Nursing standards of care

Medical and nursing management of asphyxia from smoke inhalation entails immediate and efficient intervention. This is best achieved by a collaborative approach to resuscitation. The priorities of treatment are (1) ensuring an adequate patent airway, (2) assisting with and/or monitoring the provision of adequate ventilation and oxygenation, (3) ensuring adequate perfusion, and (4) monitoring cardiac function closely.

Nursing management of the asphyxiated patient includes vigilant surveillance for actual and potential problems identified during the patient's baseline assessment. The outcome of resuscitation and the risk factors identified also indicate the care needed. Initially, several life-threatening problems will need to be addressed simultaneously. Later, as the patient stabilizes, other identified problems can be prioritized and acted on. Critical nursing diagnoses include (1) ineffective airway clearance, (2) impaired gas exchange, (3) ineffective breathing pattern, (4) altered cerebral tissue perfusion, and (5) decreased cardiac output. These are addressed in the following care plan.

Nursing Care Plan for the Management of the Patient with Asphyxia

Diagnosis	Signs and symptoms	Intervention	Rationale
Ineffective airway clearance, related to edema of upper and lower respiratory tract	Cough Stridor Hoarseness Dyspnea Facial burns Singed nasal hair Wheezing Carbonaceous sputum	Administer humidified 100% O_2 Prepare intubation equipment and medications Obtain adequate airway position Establish position of comfort for conscious patient Administer bronchodilators	To increase oxygen available to lower respiratory tract Endotracheal intubation is best achieved before complete obstruction by edema occurs To facilitate easy and unlabored breathing and ability to cough productively To open small airways, which is helpful in mild cases
Impaired gas exchange, related to interference of toxic gases with oxygen transport and injury to mucosal lining of respiratory tract	Neurological impairment Elevated carbon monoxide level Elevated cyanide level Giddiness Headache Palpitations Vomiting Seizures (Oxygen saturation measured by pulse oximeter may be deceiving)	Provide continuous 100% O_2 via nonrebreather mask or ETT/ventilator; make arrangements for transfer to closest hyperbaric chamber	Administering 100% O_2 at 2.5 atm dissolves O_2 into plasma, enough to meet 100% of body needs; meanwhile, carboxyhemoglobin can be 50% cleared after 20–30 minutes using hyperbaric chamber
Ineffective breathing pattern, related to hypoxic effects on CNS	Decreased respiratory rate Decreased tidal volume Diminished level of consciousness Oxygen saturation less than 97%	Administer sodium nitrite 3%, 10–15 mL Administer sodium thiosulfate, 12.5 g in 50 mL over 10 minutes	Nitrites combine with ferric cyanide ion to form methemoglobin Sodium thiosulfate removes cyanide from methemoglobin by conversion to thiocyanate, which is metabolized by the liver

Nursing Care Plan for the Management of the Patient with Asphyxia

Diagnosis	Signs and symptoms	Intervention	Rationale
	PaO$_2$ decreased; PaCO$_2$ increased	Assist with ventilation; prepare for intubation and mechanical ventilation	As hypoxia or toxic elements of smoke affect CNS, respiratory center will fail
Altered cerebral tissue perfusion, related to increased cerebral capillary permeability	Glasgow Coma Scale rating less than 15	Elevate HOB 30 degrees	To promote venous drainage
	Elevated ICP (widening pulse pressure, projectile vomiting, headache)	Conduct frequent neurological assessments; maintain MAP greater than 80 mm Hg	To maintain CPP greater than 60 mm Hg
		Treat increased ICP with hyperventilation	To decrease blood flow to brain and allow room for swelling
		Administer osmotic diuretics	To create osmotic gradient to pull water into vascular compartment
		Administer Decadron, as ordered	Steroids are thought to restore capillary membrane
Decreased cardiac output, related to ischemic myocardium with decreased cardiac contractility and dysrhythmias	Chest pain	Immediately initiate treatment for carbon monoxide and cyanide poisoning (if no response to treatment for cyanide, may repeat with half of original dose in 30 minutes; hyperbaric O$_2$ treatment will provide myocardium with oxygen while carbon monoxide is being cleared from system)	Myocardial ischemia from hypoxia should reverse with routine measures
	Ischemic changes on ECG: ST elevation, T wave inversion, ST depression, prolonged Q-T interval, low voltage pattern, heart block	Administer nitrates, as ordered	Vasodilation of coronary vessels may assist in increasing flow to myocardium
	Hypotension	Treat dysrhythmias as necessary to support patient	Primary cause is hypoxia at tissue level

Diagnosis	Signs and symptoms	Intervention	Rationale
Anxiety of patient or family, related to severity of injury and aggressive and invasive life-support measures	Nervousness Inability to understand commands and/or patient's status Poor short-term memory	Provide confident, calm directions and explanations	Calm, confident communication promotes provider credibility and helps the patient and family feel that best possible care is being given
	Fidgeting Tearfulness Hysteria Anger	Assist with obtaining support from family or friends	A comforting touch and concern will assist the patient to be more at ease
		Provide for family visiting as soon as possible	Patients and families both respond better to treatment crisis if they are able to see one another as soon as possible
		Act as interpreter of medical information (simple basic descriptions are necessary and may need to be repeated); maintain ongoing communication about status with patient and family	Crisis theory indicates that victims will have poor ability to concentrate and understand
Lack of knowledge of high-risk behavior associated with house fires	High blood alcohol level History of smoking Use of kerosene heaters Inadequate heating Lack of smoke detectors in dwelling	Develop teaching plan regarding high-risk behaviors and ways to change them	Prevention of reoccurrence is a priority before patient discharge
		Discuss resources available for follow-up treatment	Smoking and alcohol abuse require considerable behavior modification
		Facilitate family's support for change in patient's behavior	Family support and involvement increases likelihood of patient adherence and follow-through

Drowning

Drowning is defined as asphyxiation due to immersion in liquid. Near-drowning is defined as survival from a liquid submersion injury for 24 hours after rescue. The terms *submersion* and *immersion* are both loosely defined as being under water or another liquid and can be used interchangeably.[114] There are two types of near-drowning, described as "wet" and "dry." A wet near-drowning is the most common type, in which the victim aspirates variable amounts of fluid into the lungs. Dry near-drowning, in which little or no fluid enters the lungs, accounts for approximately 10% of cases.

Clinical antecedents

In adults, drowning usually results from unexpected total body immersion in water and the associated panic reaction. An example of this situation is falling into deep water or stepping into a hole or channel while wading, which causes the victim to suddenly and unexpectedly be in water over his or her head. The panic reaction initiates the following chain of events: gasping for air, severe laryngospasm, hypoxia, loss of consciousness, and glottic relaxation (90% of cases). Drowning may be the result of a traumatic injury's causing loss of consciousness (as from a hit on the head) or paralysis (perhaps a cervical spine injury from a diving accident).

Drowning in teens and adults is often associated with alcohol and/or substance abuse.[115] Sometimes proficient swimmers drown as a result of abdominal or extremity cramping. Hyperventilation-submersion syndrome is a type of drowning unique to underwater swimmers who attempt to increase their underwater time and distance by hyperventilation. The hyperventilation-induced hypocapnia suppresses the central nervous system (CNS) breathing response, enabling the swimmer to hold his or her breath longer more comfortably. Drowning occurs when the swimmer loses consciousness underwater before the spontaneous respiratory drive is regained, which, if initiated, would force a return to the surface.

Drowning is the number one killer of children aged 1 to 5 years. The incidence and causes of drowning are closely associated with certain age groups. Infants usually drown in bathtubs. This often occurs in lower socioeconomic families in which there are several small children. In most inci-

dences, the infant was left in the tub with an older, preschool-age child and no adult supervision.

Toddlers escape parental supervision, wander off, and fall into water: 30% of toddler drownings occur in neighbors' or relatives' pools. Other incidences are attributed to inadequate barriers around water hazards (such as hot tubs and spas) and tempting objects near or in the water.

School-age children usually drown as a result of swimming alone, unsupervised by an adult. Often the parents as well as the child overestimate the child's ability. School-age children tend to "show off" when with other children and may place themselves in a hazardous situation.[116]

Critical referents

The remainder of this section will focus on the near-drowning scenario, in which the victim has been rescued and has survived or has been resuscitated prior to arrival at the emergency department (ED). The lungs and brain are the organs primarily insulted during and following near-drowning. Three key questions should be asked in order to direct management and to understand the pathophysiology:

1. What was the water temperature?
2. What type of water or liquid was the victim found in?
3. How long was the victim immersed?

The chain of events following immersion is summarized in Figure 9-10.

In warm water—such as in bathtubs and pools and shallow open water in warm climates—adults and children cannot tolerate long immersion times. Cerebral anoxia leads to neuron death, loss of autoregulation, cerebral edema, increased intracranial pressure, and, ultimately, brain herniation. But if the victim is rescued quickly and immediately supported by basic life-support, the chances of survival are good.

Immersion in cold water (defined as water temperatures below 20°C) has a preservative effect on the brain. Cold water immersion, as when a victim falls through the ice, is easily identified in winter months. Immersion hypothermia is often overlooked in warm weather, however, although it should always be considered in cases of immersion in large, deep bodies of water such as quarries, lakes, reservoirs, and the ocean. Children have an advantage (statistically) over adults in surviving cold water immersion.

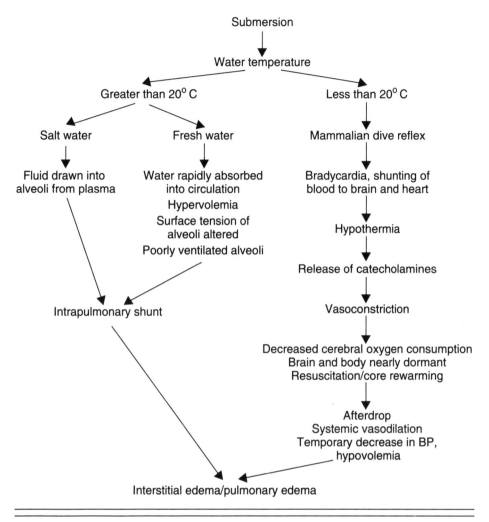

Figure 9-10 Clinical Consequences of Immersion

The poorer tolerance of adults to cold water immersion is thought to be due to their larger body surface area (which allows the body to cool more quickly) and increased responsiveness to the mammalian dive reflex. This dive reflex, first identified in sea mammals, is characterized by bradycardia and redistribution of blood flow to the heart and brain.

Rapid-immersion hypothermia causes central blood temperature receptors located in the anterior hypothalamus to register "cold." In response, the hypothalamus sends messages to the adrenal medulla to release catecholamines and directs the nerve pathways to vasoconstrict. In the case of cold water immersion, the brain continues to cool, and cerebral oxygen consumption decreases. Cerebral blood flow slows and sludging occurs, while the rest of the body lies in a near-dormant state.[117]

It is important to know the type of water in which immersion took place in order to gauge the water temperature at bottom depth and to deduce pulmo-nary pathophysiology if aspiration occurred. Aspiration of water, regardless of tonicity, causes decreased pulmonary compliance and intrapulmonary shunting. Seawater is hypertonic, so when it is present in the alveoli, it draws fluid from the vascular circulation into the lung. When fresh water is aspirated, it is rapidly absorbed into the circulation, causing hypervolemia. This fluid shift returns to normal in approximately 1 hour. The primary insult to the lungs from fresh water is due to the alteration of the surface tension of pulmonary surfactant, which causes the alveoli to become unstable and collapse, which in turn causes widespread areas of microatelectasis.[118]

Depending on the body of water, other materials may be aspirated with the water. In open water (oceans and rivers), sand, mud, or seaweed may be aspirated. Therefore, any time airway obstruction is encountered, debris must always be considered. In small bodies of water (ponds, harbors, and canals), algae and pollutants may be aspirated. In general, salt water and swimming pool water are less likely to produce bacterial infections than is water from lakes, ponds, and canals. Common bacterial pneumonias are pseudomonas and vibrio.

Aspiration, regardless of water type, introduces organic and inorganic products into the lungs, which produce an inflammatory response at the alveolar-capillary membrane. This response allows the capillary to leak plasma-rich exudate into the alveolus; this deposit of protein material displaces air and disables the alveolus. Localized hypoxia causes vasoconstriction of pulmonary capillaries, raising pulmonary intravascular pressures (PIP). Increased PIP pushes more fluid into the interstitium, causing pulmonary edema, and, combined with the effects of fresh or salt water, the end result is reduced compliance, severe intrapulmonary shunting, and increased work of breathing.[119]

In addition to the direct effects of aspiration on the pulmonary system, cerebral hypoxia from near-drowning can precipitate neurogenic pulmonary edema. This is defined as acute pulmonary edema that occurs after an abrupt rise in intracranial pressure as a result of a variety of CNS insults. Description of the pathophysiology of neurogenic pulmonary edema can be found in several sources but is beyond the scope of this section.[120]

Immersion time is a consideration in predicting outcome. Time is usually overestimated by observers and rescuers. However, in a long underwater search and rescue operation, 1 hour from the first 911 call is the general cut-off point for initiating resuscitation. This cut-off is based on knowledge that victims have survived cold water immersion for up to 40–60 minutes. The receiving ED can estimate an accurate time frame from initial 911 call to body recovery (if recovered by rescue team), as well as from the scene to the ED.

Resulting signs and symptoms

The victim of near-drowning requires follow-up emergency care, even if successfully resuscitated at the scene. In the case of the conscious, hemodynamically stable patient, the following assessment parameters should be considered.

Level of consciousness Often the patient will be amnesic with respect to the event but will usually be oriented. The patient's ability to cough, swallow, and communicate should be assessed.

Breathing Aspiration increases the work of breathing, therefore accessory muscle use, inter-

costal retractions, and tachypnea may be seen, all due to decreased lung compliance. Ventilatory perfusion mismatch results in hypoxia, which may be evidenced by changes in level of consciousness, air hunger, anxiety, or combativeness. Chest expansion may be decreased or unsymmetrical as a result of poor lung compliance or localized unventilated areas of lung. Dullness to percussion may be found secondary to diffuse pulmonary edema. Auscultation of breath sounds may indicate coarse gurgles (rhonchi), due to aspiration of particular matter, and/or crackles (rales), due to pulmonary edema.

Circulation Core body temperature may be extremely low, depending on water temperature or ambient air temperature. Table 9-28 correlates

Table 9-28 Symptoms of Hypothermia

Celsius Temperature	Clinical Manifestations
37–35°	Cold sensation Moderate shivering Loss of coordination
35–32°	Violent shivering Slurred speech Confusion Amnesia Tachycardia Vasoconstriction
32–28°	Decreased shivering Muscle rigidity Bradycardia Atrial fibrillation Cyanosis Hypoventilation Systemic lactic acidosis
28–25°	Hypotension Stupor Coma Irregular pulse Ventricular fibrillation if heart stimulated Cold diuresis
25–21°	Spontaneous ventricular fibrillation Areflexia Pupils fixed, dilated No spontaneous movement Apnea Asystole

Sources: Rich, J. (1983). *Journal of Emergency Nursing* 9(1): 8–10; Dean, N.C. (1987). Hypothermia-lifesaving procedures. *Postgraduate Medicine* 82(8): 48–51, 55–56; Johnston, J.B. (1988). Hypothermia: Assessment and intervention. *Emergency Nursing Reports* 3(8): 1–7.

body temperature and clinical symptoms. Bradycardia may be due to hypoxia or hypothermia. Tachycardia may be due to fear, circulating catecholamines, or acid-base imbalance. The ECG may show nonspecific changes and dysrhythmias secondary to hypoxia. Skin may be cyanotic, due to hypoxia, and cold, due to vasoconstriction.[121]

Disability A complete neurological exam is necessary to assess for CNS deficits resulting from brief CNS hypoxia.

Exposure The rest of the body should be assessed for trauma, such as fractures that may have occurred during the near-drowning incident or as a result of rescue and resuscitation efforts.

In the case of the near-drowning patient who arrives at the ED in cardiopulmonary arrest, several assessment parameters must be considered in addition to those described for the conscious patient.

Airway The patient must be intubated, or an airway may need to be secured. If the cause of the near-drowning is unknown or unwitnessed, cervical spine injury must be presumed. Therefore, intubation with neutral neck position, utilizing in-line traction and cricoid pressure, is necessary. Causes of airway obstruction may be debris such as seaweed or may be prolonged laryngospasm or bronchospasm.

Breathing Special attention must be given to delivering adequate ventilatory volumes. Changes in how it "feels" to ventilate the patient should be assessed, because difficulty doing so may be an indication of decreased compliance. A large amount of secretions may be present secondary to pulmonary edema, as well as swallowed water.

Circulation CVP may be elevated initially with both fresh- and salt-water aspiration, but it usually decreases within 1 hour. ABGs will reveal hypoxemia and metabolic acidosis in 70% of cases. Pulmonary artery pressure is elevated secondary to increased intrapulmonary shunting and increased pulmonary vascular resistance. Cardiac output may drop because of ventilatory pressure and use of PEEP but also may be decreased as a result of inadequate circulating

fluid volume. Urine output is initially decreased, but both high-output and low-output failure may occur after resuscitation due to impaired renal perfusion.

Disability Increased intracranial pressure due to cerebral anoxia and the resultant cerebral edema may be evidenced by decreased Glasgow Coma Scale rating, changes in respiratory pattern, widening pulse pressures, and pupillary changes.

Diagnostic studies Chest x-ray may indicate aspiration or pulmonary edema. Hemoglobin is usually normal; electrolytes are usually near normal with both fresh- and salt-water aspiration (unless the near-drowning occurred in the Dead Sea), but serum potassium levels may be slightly lower than normal. Leukocytosis is usually seen in near-drowning. Coagulation studies should be performed to set baseline levels and should be repeated to monitor for DIC, which has been associated with near-drowning. Prolonged clotting times, leukopenia, and thrombocytopenia occur as a result of hypothermia, as cells are sequestered in the liver and spleen.[122]

Nursing standards of care

Management and resuscitation of the near-drowning patient varies considerably depending on the circumstances. Water temperature is a significant factor; an algorithm for the treatment of hypothermia is summarized in Figure 9-11. The primary goals of treatment are to ensure adequate ventilation and oxygenation, promote restoration of normal cardiac function, and minimize cerebral and other organ system injury. This is best achieved by an organized collaborative approach to medical and nursing intervention.

Nursing management of the near-drowning patient focuses on both invasive rewarming procedures as well as aggressive pulmonary support. In the ED setting, initial critical nursing diagnoses include (1) ineffective breathing pattern, (2) impaired gas exchange, (3) altered cerebral perfusion, (4) decreased cardiac output, (5) hypothermia, (6) fluid volume deficit, and (7) lack of knowledge of risk factors.

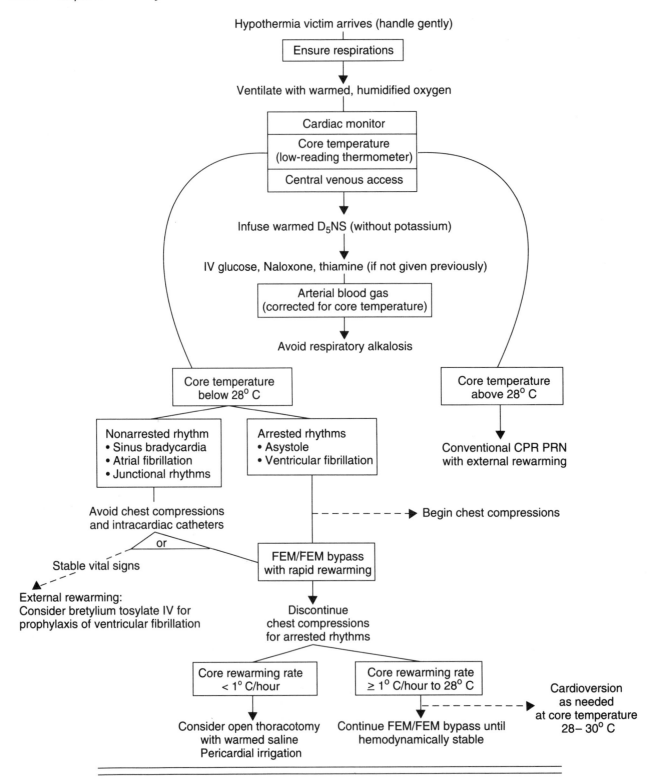

Figure 9-11 Treatment of Hypothermia

Nursing Care Plan for the Management of the Victim of Near-Drowning

Diagnosis	Signs and symptoms	Intervention	Rationale
Impaired gas exchange, related to decreased oxygen delivery due to cardiopulmonary arrest and edema secondary to near-drowning	Hypoxemia O_2 sat. $< 97\%$ Crackles (rales) upon auscultation Poor pulmonary capillary refill Cyanosis Decreased level of consciousness	Administer 100% O_2 Assist ventilations utilizing PEEP valve on ambu bag	To increase oxygen available to the alveoli PEEP forces O_2 across capillary membrane
Ineffective breathing pattern, related to decreased lung compliance	Retractions Accessory muscle movement Tachypnea Dyspnea Diminished breath sounds Decreased level of consciousness Decreased PaO_2; increased $PaCO_2$ Increased peak airway pressures	Utilize mechanical ventilation, sedation, and paralytic agents Perform pulmonary toilet, frequent suctioning, and chest physiotherapy	To promote most effective ventilation with least amount of patient effort Accumulation of secretions increases airway pressures, and chest physiotherapy mobilizes secretions and decreases atelectasis
Altered cerebral tissue perfusion, related to hypoxia-induced cerebral edema	Glasgow Coma Scale rating < 15 Elevated ICP (projectile vomiting, headache, widening pulse pressure) Pupillary changes Absence of reflexes	Elevate HOB 30 degrees Conduct frequent neurological assessments Maintain MAP greater than 80 mm Hg Hyperventilation	To promote venous drainage To ascertain neurologic status reflecting cerebral tissue perfusion To maintain CPP greater than 60 mm Hg for optimal cerebral perfusion Decreased blood flow to the brain allows room for swelling

Nursing Care Plan for the Management of the Victim of Near-Drowning

Diagnosis	Signs and symptoms	Intervention	Rationale
		Administer osmotic diuretics	To create osmotic gradient to pull water into vascular compartment
		Administer Decadron, as ordered	Steroids are thought to restore capillary membrane
Decreased cardiac output, related to myocardial ischemia and increased intrapulmonary pressure	Bradycardia, ventricular tachycardia or fibrillation	Initiate fluid challenge with isotonic solution	To restore fluid volume inside vascular compartment
	Hypotension	Monitor effects of PEEP on CO	PEEP decreases preload and increases SVR, thus decreasing CO
	Elevated pulmonary artery pressures		
	Decreased CO	Treat dysrhythmias in warm patients per ACLS guidelines	To support ischemic myocardium until hypoxia is reversed
Hypothermia, related to cold water immersion	Core body temperature less than 37°C	Avoid use of standard ACLS drugs and defibrillation with temperature of 28°C or lower	Myocardium is refractory to drugs and defibrillation while cold; drugs may be sequestered and accumulated, causing aberrant response when patient is warmed
	Other clinical symptoms dependent on temperature		
		Use heated, humidified O_2, heated IV fluids, gastric and bladder irrigation with warm fluid, peritoneal lavage, pleural irrigation via chest tubes, and extracorporeal rewarming	Rapid core rewarming is necessary with temperatures lower than 28°C; less invasive methods to rewarm can be used with higher temperatures

Diagnosis	Signs and symptoms	Intervention	Rationale
Fluid volume deficit, related to vasodilation and diuresis of intravascular volume	Rapid drop in BP as patient is rewarmed Markedly increased urine output	Monitor temperature, BP, and urine output continuously	Afterdrop is a common occurrence during rewarming, due to peripheral vasodilation and shifting cold acidotic blood into the central circulation
Lack of knowledge of high-risk behavior associated with accidental near-drowning	In adults: swimming alone, use of alcohol or drugs when swimming, swimming after eating a large meal, unsafe water practices (such as nonswimmers wading or boating without wearing life preservers) In children: lack of parental supervision, inadequate barriers around water hazards, lack of knowledge of water safety, parents' lack of knowledge of cardiac life support	Teach adults about hazards of using alcohol and drugs around water; suggest swimming lessons provided by YMCA or American Red Cross Suggest water safety course and pediatric BLS course to parents	Prevention is the most effective cure for near-drowning Both training programs emphasize accident-proofing the home and safe practices around water for children

Burns

Burn injury can result in a myriad of personal catastrophes including burn shock, multisystem organ failure, and impairment of psychosocial relationships. Burns resulting in destruction of or damage to the skin can be caused by various thermal agents: 57.1% are flame-related, 30.4% are caused by scalding, 5.8% are related to contact with hot solids, 2.9% involve electricity, 2.8% involve chemical exposure, and less than 0.5% are caused by the sun or radiation.[123] Some burn situations are additionally threatening because of concomitant injury, such as in the case of burns caused by steam, where the risk of accompanying inhalation injury and carbon monoxide intoxication is high. For the most part, though, morbidity and mortality associated with burn injury are tied to wound size and depth. It is the acuteness of the condition that increases when the patient suffers concomitant injury and/or chronic illness.

There are a number of formulas available to calculate the estimated risk of mortality from burn injury, two of which are the LA-50 and the Zaweicki formulas. These formulas factor preexisting conditions and concomitant injuries into an equation that estimates the percentage of mortality risk. A rough estimate of mortality that is still the most commonly used in the clinical setting is the age of the patient added to the total burn surface area (TBSA):[124]

Age + TBSA = percent risk of mortality

Injuries corresponding to the type of burn compound the risk of mortality—for example, in the case of flame burns, smoke inhalation proves to be a major cause of death, owing to both the airway insult and the carbon monoxide exposure. Carbon monoxide inhalation is also commonly seen in victims of closed-space injury, and frequently this type of injury results in death at the scene of the accident. If the victim survives, risk of morbidity is high: if inadequately treated, carbon monoxide poisoning can result in permanent central nervous system damage.[125] Furthermore, damage to the tissues of the upper airway, pharynx, trachea, and mainstem bronchus can prove to be life-threatening, especially if not treated within 2–4 hours of insult. Injuries to the lower airway are just as serious, but they are not as easily noted because clinical manifestations often do not appear until 24 hours after the injuries are incurred.

Four aspects of burn injury are particularly troublesome for clinicians in practice today. Current burn-related research focuses largely on these areas, which still threaten the patient's ability to survive and recover:

1. *Burn immunosuppression.* Research related to burn immunology investigates methods of augmenting the patient's immune response while seeking to learn more about the immune system. Intravenous infusion of immunoglobulin G in conjunction with antibiotic therapy has been tried experimentally in the clinical setting.
2. *Complicated tissue repair and replacement.* Many researchers have made efforts to create a temporary or permanent alternative to skin grafting for tissue replacement. Some successes have now been achieved in the clinical application of grafts of the patient's own cultured epithelial cells.
3. *Physical rehabilitation.* Advances in physical and psychosocial rehabilitation of the burn patient/survivor have also been achieved as a result of clinical research. The relationship between physical recovery and psychosocial readjustment is currently being studied across the country.
4. *Psychosocial readjustment.* Preliminary research reports indicate that a need for longitudinal study of full recovery and readjustment exists. At present, research indicates that full recovery and psychological readjustment following a burn injury may take at least 2 years or longer.

Clinical antecedents

Risk factors predisposing the individual to burn and inhalation injury are environmental, occupational, biophysical, or psychosocial in nature. Although many of these risk factors are beyond the individual's control, some can be diminished or even eliminated. Age, preexisting physical or mental disabilities (cerebral palsy or mental retardation), and chronic medical illnesses (epilepsy or peripheral vascular disease) are all biophysical risk factors that are unchangeable. Smoking and substance abuse, however, are examples of risk factors that can be controlled. Table 9-29 lists predisposing factors by category, accompanied by suggested ways to minimize or eliminate the associated degree of risk. Improved awareness of safety precautions and techniques is one of the primary means by which to minimize the risks of burn injury. Education about burn prevention and first aid can provide for increased aware-

Table 9-29 Burn Injury Risk Factors and Associated Ways to Minimize Risk

Risk Category	Risk Factor	Way to Minimize Risk
Biophysical factors	Age	Maintain age-appropriate physical environment (for example, matches and pot handles out of children's reach, bath thermometer to protect more fragile skin of elderly and children from scalding)
	Chronic medical illness/disorder that potentially affects motor or sensory function (for example, epilepsy, amputation of limb, peripheral vascular disease, cerebral palsy, muscular dystrophy, paraplegia, quadriplegia, neuromotor deficit post stroke)	Comply with prescribed medication/treatment regimen Modify physical environment to safely accommodate sensory-motor deficit
	Chronic cognitive disorder/disability that potentially impairs memory and logical thinking (for example, mental retardation, Alzheimer's disease, organic brain syndrome, some psychiatric disorders)	Modify physical environment to safely accommodate memory deficits (for example, labeling, not rearranging furniture) Supervise all activities involving thermal agents (for example, cooking, mowing the lawn)
	Substance abuse (psychoactive drugs or alcohol)	Eliminate or at least moderate use of the substance
Psychosocial factors	History of or active psychiatric/psychological disorder (potential for depression leading to suicidal ideation, potential for hallucinations)	Comply with prescribed medication and counseling regimen
	History of being abused (may lead to intentional scalding or burning)	Early recognition of abusive instincts/behaviors and early intervention for both victim and potential abuser Early notification of protective services by nurse or other health care professional
Environmental factors	Smoking, which can lead to fires associated with carelessness/accident (for example, smoking in bed, lit cigarette dropped into upholstered furniture)	Before smoking, think about the flammability of items in surrounding area, proper disposal of waste cigarettes and matches, and extinguishing smoking object fully before leaving it behind
	Improper storage or maintenance of fire-causing household items (for example, wadded-up used rags, faulty electrical wiring, gasoline stored in house, heating appliances left on), potentially increasing risk of spontaneous and/or accidental injury	Verify that appliance is used only if person is in attendance Maintain intact insulation/covering of all wires; maintain all appliances in good working order Store chemicals away from exposure to heat, in open space, ideally, outside of living area
	Inadequate fire safety measures (potential for delayed alert and slowed response when fire occurs)	Maintain full and currently dated fire extinguisher near each danger area of home (for example, kitchen, basement, and garage) Place smoke detectors in home (one per floor is recommended along with one near kitchen and at foot of each set of stairs); check battery function once a month
Occupational factors	Failure to follow on-the-job safety procedures, which can lead to accidental exposure to thermal injury agents (chemicals, electricity, flame)	Practice safety procedures, avoiding dangerous short-cuts Wear protective garments as indicated and required

ness. To this end, nurses and fire department personnel nationwide have been instrumental in implementing independent as well as cooperative burn-prevention education programs for audiences of all ages.

Critical referents

The skin is composed of three layers—the epidermis, dermis, and subcutaneous tissue—which in turn are made up of several layers or components (Figure 9-12). The epidermis is composed of five avascular strata of cells, and the underlying dermis consists of two layers of progressively denser, fibrous collagen matrix containing blood vessels, nerve endings, and epithelial appendages. Hair follicles, sebaceous glands, and sweat glands are termed epithelial appendages because they are lined with regenerating epithelial cells. Once the epithelial appendages are destroyed, skin cannot regenerate.

There are seven physiological functions of the skin: protection against infection, maintenance of fluid and electrolyte balance, thermoregulation, excretion of wastes, sensation, vitamin D production, and body image/identity. The skin functions as a barrier, protecting against infection by keeping foreign substances and organisms outside of the body. Thermoregulation is accomplished at the skin level by vasodilation of surface capillaries to facilitate evaporation and vasoconstriction of surface capillaries to preserve core body temperature. Excretion of wastes as well as fluid and electrolyte balance are achieved by the apocrine glands via perspiration. Excessive water and small amounts of urea, sodium chloride, albumin, and cholestonin are all excreted through the skin.[126] The sensations of proprioception, pain, and light touch are perceived by the small nerve endings present in the dermis. Sunlight reacting with various cholesterol compounds in the skin results in vitamin D production. The distribution of skin, skinfolds, pigmentation, and hair contributes to an individual's body image or personal identity. When skin integrity is interrupted, all of these functions are significantly impaired.

The degree of thermal injury sustained depends on the causative agent involved (dry or moist heat, hot liquids or solids, chemicals, electricity, or radiation) as well as the temperature, duration, and thickness of the exposed dermal structures. Dry heat in the form of flames carries the added potential for pulmonary complications. Table 9-30 lists the different degrees of burn and summarizes the associated histologic depths and healing times.

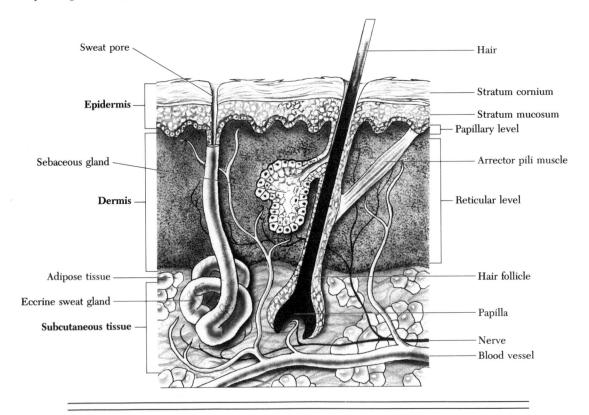

Figure 9-12 The Skin

Table 9-30 Extent of Burns and Associated Histologic Depths and Healing Times

Thickness	Concentric Zone	Degree	Histologic Depth	Healing Time
Partial thickness	Zone of hyperemia Zone of stasis	First Second	Epidermis only Epidermis and varying degrees of dermis	5–10 days 1–2 weeks
		Deep second	Entire epidermal layer and dermal layer; sweat glands and hair follicles remain intact	1 month (scarring)
Full thickness	Zone of coagulation	Third	Extends to subcutaneous tissue; thrombosis of vessels	Must be grafted
		Fourth	Fascia, muscle, bone, periosteum, blood vessels, nerve sheaths	Must be grafted

The partial thickness burn involves only the epidermis or the epidermis and some part of the dermis. When only the epidermis is damaged, a first-degree burn has occurred. Sunburn, the most common type of first-degree burn, is characterized by erythema and pain—the zone of hyperemia. The second-degree burn includes the epidermis and part of the dermis. Although practitioners sometimes differentiate between superficial and deep second-degree burns, both of these injuries can heal without surgical intervention. Within this zone of stasis, the vasculature is damaged and thrombosed, thus blood flow is sluggish. The deep second-degree burn will take longer than the superficial one to heal because of the extensive damage to epithelial appendages.

Third-degree and fourth-degree burns are referred to as full thickness burns, owing to the complete destruction of all epidermal and dermal layers. The full thickness burn wound is devoid of viable epithelial appendages and contains coagulated blood vessels, hence the descriptive term, "zone of coagulation."[127] Third- and fourth-degree burns cannot heal without surgery. The extent of tissue replacement required ranges from split-thickness skin grafting to myocutaneous free-flap tissue transfer.

Direct-heat–induced endothelial cell injury results in an increase in protein permeability across the vascular endothelial membrane. As the plasma proteins move from the intravascular space to the interstitial space, osmotic and hydrostatic pressure gradients induce large amounts of water to move with the protein.[128] Essentially all components of blood except red blood cells and some large protein molecules are able to move freely across the capillary membrane. This increased vascular permeability along with a tissue osmotic pressure elevated to an estimated 200–300 mm Hg cause significant interstitial edema. Furthermore, edema in nonburned tissues is also seen in the patient suffering total burn surface area (TBSA) exceeding 20–30%. The larger the burn size, the more significant the systemic impact. Hypoproteinemia in the plasma following fluid and protein shifts in the burned tissues is felt to be responsible for this nonburn edema.

Controversy surrounds the effects of vascular substances released from burn tissue. Chemical mediators such as bradykinin, serotonin, vasoactive prostaglandins, lysosomal components, histamine, and complement system by-products are released by damaged cells. It is postulated that these mediators can cause a direct increase in vascular permeability or an indirect increase in microvascular hydrostatic pressure.[129]

Microvascular and cell membrane alterations occurring after a burn injury also result in cardiovascular instability. Cardiovascular function is affected in various ways. Initially, in the presence of hypovolemia, cardiac output is decreased, but it returns to normal as a result of the compensatory mechanism of tachycardia. Central venous pressures (CVP) and pulmonary artery wedge pressures (PAWP) usually remain low despite adequate fluid resuscitation, because during blood circulation the compromised capillary membrane allows fluid to seep out of the vascular space. Attempts to maintain "normal" pressures by delivering additional intravenous fluids must be made cautiously—administration of additional fluids could exacerbate protein loss. And the more protein that is lost, the more edema in the periphery, resulting in additional tissue impairment.

Loss of body heat due to evaporation of body fluids and loss of insulating skin, compounded by the infusion of cool intravenous fluids, has also been a problem in burn treatment. Evaporative water loss by the burn patient is estimated to be 1.5–3.5 mL/kg/TBSA (4–15 times normal).[130] Hypothermia complicates hemodynamic stability and, since it involves vasoconstriction, impairs perfusion of tissues.

Another area of concern in the care of the burn patient is the noticeable shifts of sodium, water, and potassium during burn shock. Edema formation during burn shock leads to inadequate tissue perfusion, inevitably resulting in cell membrane hypoxia. Membrane potential is thus altered, and sodium molecules, along with water, move more freely from the extracellular to the intercellular space. The ensuing hypovolemia and release of potassium from damaged cells result in hyperkalemia. Aldosterone is consequently released, leading to hypokalemia.

Hypocalcemia is also seen early after the injury in the severely burned patient. Although there is evidence associating hypocalcemia with starvation and malabsorption (which are both seen in the severely burned patient), causes of hypocalcemia soon after a burn are unclear. Some experienced burn physicians attribute the early hypocalcemia to hypoalbuminemia and calcium accumulation in the damaged tissues.[131] Another popular explanation relates hypocalcemia to adipose tissue injury. Presumably, the saponification (conversion of an oil or a fat into a soap by combination with an alkali) of burned fatty tissue results in elevated lipoprotein levels within 12–24 hours of injury; calcium binds readily with lipoproteins, causing hypocalcemia.[132]

As time goes on, further changes are experienced. Hypophosphatemia may develop 3–9 days post burn. Antacids, aluminum hydroxide, starvation, hyperalimentation without adequate phosphate, metabolic acidosis, and renal failure contribute to this imbalance. The parathyroid hormone (PTH), which is influenced by the adrenergic system, may lower phosphate levels as well. Hypophosphatemia results in decreased levels of ATP and 2,3-DPG, which in turn bring about a disruption in metabolic processes and impaired oxygen release to the tissues.[133]

Acute tubular necrosis can also result from burn injuries, and hemoglobin from destroyed RBCs and myoglobin from damaged muscle mass in electrical injuries directly occlude the nephrons and tubules. There is an immediate need to "flush" the renal system in the event that either of the above conditions occurs.

Not only is the cardiovascular system affected in burn injury, but so is the respiratory system. Smoke inhalation injury is an appreciable major cause of burn victim mortality. The hypoxia and respiratory pathology that result can be attributed to direct and indirect damage to respiratory epithelium, carbon monoxide exposure, and inhalation of toxic fumes.

Direct injury to the upper airway occurs when superheated gases and/or toxic materials are inhaled. The burned respiratory mucosal epithelia undergo local inflammatory changes, including increased tracheobronchial secretions, edema, and denuding of basement membranes. A hyperemic response by the bronchial artery has also been noted almost immediately following inhalation injury, compounding edema formation.[134] Compromised tracheal airway diameter often necessitates nasotracheal or endotracheal intubation to maintain airway patency.

Smoke inhalation can also injure the lower airway both directly and indirectly. Sloughed tracheobronchial epithelium casts can contaminate small bronchioles. Inflammation and superimposed infections occur as healthy bronchiolar tissue becomes affected, leading to pneumonia and adult respiratory distress syndrome (ARDS). Excessive mucus can drain down from the tracheobronchial tree, plugging the alveoli, resulting in inadequate ventilation and atelectasis. The bronchioles and alveoli of the lower airway can also sustain direct damage by superheated gases and/or noxious particles, triggering the local inflammatory response (edema) and causing impaired gas exchange across the alveolar-capillary membrane as well as bronchoconstriction and accompanying increased respiratory resistance. Ventilation-perfusion mismatch, decreased dynamic compliance and functional residual capacity, and atelectasis may also result.

The inhalation of carbon monoxide further complicates the above pathological processes. Carbon monoxide inhalation gravely jeopardizes the patient's ability to maintain life-sustaining blood oxygen levels. Smoke contains a higher concentration of carbon monoxide and, therefore, a lower concentration of oxygen than room air. Carbon monoxide molecules' affinity for hemoglobin is 250 times that of oxygen.[135] This prevents oxygen from taking its place on the hemoglobin molecule. Further damage at the tissue level—ischemia and subsequent reperfusion injury to major organs including the brain and the heart—occurs when the oxyhemoglobin dissociation curve shifts to the left as the hemoglobin increases its hold on the oxygen molecule.

After prolonged exposure to carbon monoxide and hydrocyanide (the gas released from burning synthetics and wool), cell mitochondrial function and adenosine triphosphate (ATP) production are impaired. After saturating the cell, these gases bind to the iron-containing proteins within the cytochrome system, thus inhibiting cellular respiration. Metabolic acidosis results. In addition, decreased mucociliary activity, increased secretions from the bronchial glands, and decreased oxidative reduction reactions in Type II cells have also been noted.[136]

Along with severe tissue damage, the burn patient suffers immunosuppression as the inflammatory response and invading microbes cause rapid activation and massive consumption of the immunologic mediators (phagocytes, lymphocytes, and immunoglobulins).

Historically, the patient suffering thermal injury has been identified as being at high risk for bacterial and fungal infections, which cause as many as 70% of deaths.[137] Three factors that promote infection have been identified. Most obvious is the compromise of the skin as a mechanical barrier against invasion by microorganisms. The second factor is the nature of the burn wound, a mass of proteinaceous wastes that provides a medium for bacterial growth. The third factor relates to the immunosuppression seen to varying degrees with all thermal injuries. When all three factors are found together, a severely immunocompromised state is evident.

When the external skin barrier is removed, the ability of exogenous pathogens to colonize the exposed tissue and then move into the bloodstream is greatly enhanced. Additionally, endogenous organisms that normally exist in body orifices and the GI and GU tracts may produce clinical infection in the patient. Organisms most likely to cause infection as a result of this breach in barrier defense include staphylococcus, streptococcus, enterobacteria, and pseudomonas.

The burned tissue (eschar) remaining on the skin serves as a protein base for the proliferation of microorganisms, particularly since it is beyond the vascular system and not perfused with the antibiotics necessary to combat them. The best way to monitor the growth of bacteria and the risk of systemic infection is to conduct routine periodic bacteriological culturing. A level of organisms exceeding 10^5/g is indicative of preinvasive sepsis.[138] Quantitative cultures enable clinicians to predict the infectivity of organisms and plan for the appropriate intravenous and topical antibiotics. Some physicians surgically remove infected eschar in hope of removing the septic source, although it is not clear that this method is effective when the burn involves more than 40% of the body surface area.[139]

Research in the area of immune response to burns has revealed that only a small number of infections related to the breakdown in barrier defenses occur. The majority of infectious complications are related to deficits in the phagocytic response or in cellular immunity. In small studies, it has been found in nonsurviving patients that the body's most important phagocyte, the neutrophil, had decreased killer activity with respect to endogenous and exogenous flora.[140] Other studies have shown that serum complement levels designed to enhance the body's inflammatory-immune and phagocytic responses are depressed following burn injury.[141] These various nonspecific deficits result in multiple bacterial infections, especially by organisms normally present as body flora.

In the case of a burn injury covering greater than 20% of the body's surface area, a severe drop in immunoglobulins has been noted within 24 hours of injury.[142] In fact, the severity of IgG loss directly correlates to mortality. The decrease in IgG does not seem to relate to inadequate synthesis but may be the consequence of physical leakage and hypermetabolism with excessive consumption. IgG levels are noted to return to normal within 2–4 weeks of injury. The reduction in IgG may directly relate to the burn patient's increased risk for childhood illnesses and viruses.[143]

Lymphocyte abnormalities have also been identified in acute burn injury. The normal ratio of helper to suppressor lymphocytes is 2:1, but within 48 hours of severe burns, this ratio is reversed to 1:2. The clinical consequences of increased T suppressor cells and decreased T helper cells are reduction of all specific immune responses and decreased immune regulation and surveillance. Opportunistic and viral infections coexist with bacterial infections occurring from diminished neutrophil activity. Indeed, the level of immunosuppression equals that of bone marrow transplantation. The long-term consequences of this response are yet to be determined.

Nonspecific immunity, phagocytosis, is impaired soon after a severe burn injury. Extensive tissue destruction initiates an inflammatory response, mobilizing and activating most available leukocytes. But owing to increased capillary permeability, during the first 24 hours post burn, many leukocytes pass into the interstitial space and are lost to the immune system. Replenishment of this massive number of leukocytes takes time.

The most detrimental aspect of this immunosuppression is its effect on the humoral immunity: the depletion of immunoglobulins IgA, IgM, and IgG. These antibodies play a major role in activating the complement cascade as they attach to antigens and facilitate phagocytosis by neutrophils and macrophages.[144] Both IgA (found in bodily secretions) and IgG (found in serum and tissues) are small enough to pass across the capillary membrane during increased permeability, but these proteins are too large to cross the membrane once permeability returns to normal. The extent of depletion of both IgA and IgG in the patient suffering a severe burn is significant enough to weaken the patient's defense against bacteria, viruses, and toxins. The risk of infection remains high until the wounds are closed (or healed) and/or the body's normal immune system is able to rebuild the exhausted stores of immunologic mediators.

Resulting signs and symptoms

Determination of burn wound depth is best achieved based on the patient's report of symptoms, direct observation, and "hands-on" physical assessment of the wound surface. A first-degree burn is very similar to the common sunburn. It is erythematous (red or pink), mildly edematous, dry, and painful. The wound bed feels dry and resilient to the gloved hand. In contrast to the second-degree burn, no blisters are present. Because of its innocuous nature, first-degree burn is not included in the Lund and Browder chart.

The second-degree (partial-thickness) burn is extremely painful and presents in various ways, ranging from white to red to mottled in color and with or without blisters and/or bulla. To the gloved hand, the second-degree burn feels slippery and resilient. Second-degree burns are further segregated into simple or deep second-degree burns. The latter appear mottled, with accompanying pink or waxy white areas interspersed among the red and blistered areas of involvement. Upon examination of the wound field, the nurse will find that the area remains soft and elastic, with edema and blisters present. Blanching in response to fingertip pressure followed by adequate refill once pressure is released serves as a classic sign of reversible tissue damage.

Impressive and unique to third-degree (full-thickness) burn wounds is the hard and dry texture of the injured area. Because the elasticity of the collagen matrix in the dermis has been destroyed, full-thickness burns will generally appear and feel dry and leathery. Coagulated blood vessels are often contained within full-thickness wound beds, with colors ranging from white to black. Coloration of the third-degree burn thus varies, including tan, deep cherry red, black, waxy white, yellow, and brown. Edema of surrounding tissue is present but may not be readily observed until after fluid resuscitation has been initiated. The nerve endings have been destroyed; therefore, the wounds are not painful. Generally, though, the burn injury patient is burned in varying degrees, so pain emanates from sites of lesser-degree burns surrounding the third-degree burns. Exacerbating the injury is the fact that the unyielding damaged skin tends to seal in the swelling and compress nerves, blood vessels, and organs much like a tourniquet. Additionally, blood flow to

the affected area is frequently severed completely, so necrosis sets in quickly.

Finally, blackened and depressed areas of burn are designated fourth-degree. Involvement of surrounding muscle, fascia, and bone is further evidence of fourth-degree burn that may present upon surgical exploration of the wound in the operative suite or during invasive procedures initiated to relieve pressure to underlying organs, blood vessels, or nerves.

The size of the burn, along with the depth of injury, directly affects the severity of the patient's systemic pathophysiology. There are three generally accepted mechanisms for determining the burn size as a percentage of total body surface area: the rule of the palm, the rule of nines, and the Lund and Browder chart.[145] The rule of the palm is useful for assessing splatter burns and small burns by referencing the patient's palm as 1% of body surface. The rule of nines differentiates the child from the adult and provides a rough estimate of surface area burned, dividing body sections into multiples of nine. The Lund and Browder chart separates the body into smaller sections than the rule of nines does and distinguishes among six age categories (see Figure 9-13). For the purposes of estimating total body

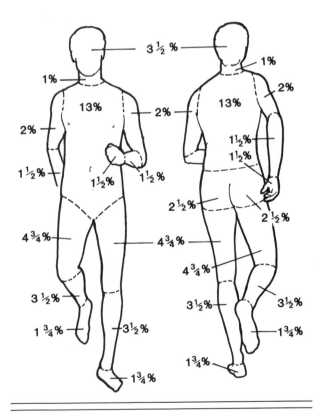

Figure 9-13   Adaptation of the Lund and Browder Chart

surface area burned (TBSA)—(sometimes referred to as "total burn surface area"), the Lund and Browder chart is the most commonly utilized and is generally considered the most accurate method.

Hypovolemia, one of the consequences evidenced in the patient almost immediately after a major burn occurs, is caused by the loss of plasma from the circulating blood as well as evaporation (insensible loss) from large denuded areas of open burn wounds. (Up to 500 cc/hr of insensible fluid loss can occur.[146]) As a result, venous return and systemic blood pressure are decreased, cardiac output falls quickly thereafter, and risk of burn shock is high. In the event of burn shock, the clinical course taken resembles that for any other hypovolemic-type shock mechanism. The signs and symptoms associated with burn shock involve numerous organ systems: cardiovascular, pulmonary, gastrointestinal, genitourinary, and nervous. The cardiovascular response to increased interstitial fluid and decreased intravascular volume is tachycardia, diminished cardiac output, and increased systemic vascular resistance. Interstitial edema will usually extend beyond the wound area in the patient suffering greater than 20% TBSA. The peripheral vascular system, sensing diminished intravascular volume, responds with increased systemic vascular resistance.

Diminished renal perfusion, owing to the progressively decreasing intravascular blood volume in shock, is evident as oliguria and/or anuria. The low urine output can be accompanied by hemoglobinuria and myoglobinuria when the wound includes muscles and/or extensive areas of third-degree burn. These large globulin pigments can damage the renal tubules, a condition that further contributes to oliguria if left untreated.

Signs and symptoms of diminished organ perfusion due to shock are also seen in the gastrointestinal system. The patient experiences gastric dilation and slowed peristalsis as intestinal blood flow is largely shunted away. This is evidenced by diminished bowel sounds, gastric fluid retention, nausea, vomiting, and anorexia. Diminished blood flow can also contribute to slugging of bile salts in the gall bladder, possibly leading to acalculus cholecystitis. Curling's ulcers are infrequently seen but can prove to be life-threatening because of the risk that the signs and symptoms will not become evident (usually the first sign is gastrointestinal bleeding) until the ulcer perforates the stomach wall and "free air" is visible on x-ray. Pain is generally not a problem with Curling's ulcer, but some abdominal pain and tenderness will be noted with acalculus cholecystitis.

As a compensatory mechanism in response to shock, the body shunts blood from the periphery to the major organs and raises the pulse rate. Tachycardia of 120 bpm or higher serves as a strong indicator that fluid resuscitation is being inadequately maintained; a pulse rate of less than 100 is considered within acceptable clinical parameters and indicates adequate volume replacement.[147] The patient, if able, will complain of intense thirst. It should be noted that in the initial stages of rehydration, even in the presence of an adequate cardiac output, low CVP and PAWP may persist.

Further evidence of hypovolemia is related to hematocrit level. A hematocrit of 50–55% can be expected in early postburn resuscitation, and in the case of a patient suffering greater than 40% TBSA, the hematocrit may be as high as 50–70%. But anemia eventually ensues, caused by destruction of red blood cells when tissue is destroyed, hemolysis from heat experienced at the time of injury, and an unknown circulating plasma factor that reduces the half-life of red blood cells. Furthermore, platelets and white blood cells are also damaged by the intense heat during injury.

ECG monitoring is critical to the safety of the patient during the initial resuscitation period. ECG changes exhibited by the severely burned patient usually indicate hypoxia, electrolyte imbalance (hyperkalemia and hypernatremia), and acid-base imbalance (metabolic acidosis); the ST segment is usually depressed, and arrhythmias are common.

Secondary to protection from and treatment of shock is care related to pain control. Almost all burn patients report wound pain in the face of any level of injury. In actuality, areas of truly full-thickness injury should be insensitive to other than deep palpation. As mentioned above, all partial-thickness (first- and second-degree) burns are reportedly very painful. Other than burn wound pain, the burn victim should experience no neurological abnormalities or deficits. The presenting patient should be awake, alert, oriented, and able to move all extremities. Altered levels of consciousness, seizure activity, or sensory-motor deficits, if assessed, cannot be related to the burn injury, and thus must be investigated further. The most likely causes are head injury, carbon monoxide intoxication, hypoxia, and substance abuse.

Whenever the burn victim presents with facial burns, singed facial hairs, or soot in the mouth or sputum, inhalation injury should be suspected. If the patient is reported to have been in a closed space fire, complaints of dyspnea, tachypnea, hoarseness or vocal alteration, shortness of breath, and air hunger are expected. Initial chest radiography and arterial blood gas interpretation are often normal. Within 2–4 hours of smoke exposure, however, these same evaluations will begin to show pulmonary infiltrates and hypoxia if the patient has sustained pulmonary injury. Immediately following injury, volume flow loop studies of spirometry will indicate flattened, inhibited exhalation, and serial spirometry will show progressive deterioration.[148] Direct bronchoscopy will also reveal soot in the tracheobronchial tree, a definite chemical irritant that will soon initiate an acute inflammatory reaction.

Carbon monoxide intoxication can be evaluated by arterial carboxyhemoglobin saturation level. A saturation level of greater than 15% is considered moderate intoxication; a saturation level greater than 50% is considered lethal.[149] The cherry-red appearance of the face and mucous membranes of the patient who has suffered carbon monoxide intoxication is transient, lasting only a few minutes. The patient exhibits diminished level of consciousness, respiratory distress, and air hunger. Progressive symptoms of sustained carbon monoxide poisoning—fine tremors, "pill-rolling" tremors, muscle rigidity, shuffling gait, and facial atony—is evidence of basal ganglia damage.

Pulmonary complications occur according to precipitating event. If the upper airway has been burned, blistering, edema, and airway obstruction can develop within 30 minutes of injury and for up to 48 hours after it. ARDS can also develop in response to inhalation injury. Burns to the head and neck that cause edema can lead to total occlusion of the trachea, and burns around the thorax disallow chest expansion for breathing. Symptoms of lower airway injury include bronchospasm, bronchial edema, and impaired airway flow and gas exchange resulting in decreased dynamic lung compliance. A definite diagnosis can be ascertained only with fiberoptic bronchoscopy, because the symptoms of the patient who suffers inhalation injury may be delayed by as long as 24–48 hours. Sometimes the patient does not exhibit any of the above symptoms at all. Pneumonia is a very frequent complication seen in the burn patient because of the patient's immobility and weakened state and the microbial flora occurring in association with the burn injury.

Hypothermia is another clinical symptom of the burn patient, because, as fluid is lost through denuded surface areas, so is body heat. All mechanisms of heat loss are involved: convection (the transfer of heat to a moving system, the air), conduction (exchange of heat to a direct surface, the bed), and radiation (the emission of energy from the body as heat).[150] Massive infusions can also contribute to hypothermia if the fluids are not warmed prior to infusion. Hypothermia only exacerbates the problem of hypoperfusion of involved tissue.

The most frequently occurring renal complication is acute tubular necrosis, caused by hypovolemia and compromised blood flow to the kidneys, leading to acute renal insufficiency. In the more seriously burned patient or one suffering electrical injury, this complication is worsened when myoglobin from damaged muscle tissue cells circulates through the bloodstream, causing occlusion of renal tubules. Furthermore, glucose is found in the urine as a result of the massive stress response of the body. Occasionally, glycosuria can be an indication that the patient is not utilizing ingested glucose. In contrast, the presence of acetone in the urine can indicate that the patient is not receiving adequate nutrition and is burning available fats and proteins in the system.

Curling's ulcer, paralytic ileus, and gastric dilation leading to constipation plague the burn patient. Also, although rare, superior mesenteric artery (SMA) disease can develop when the distal third segment of the duodenum becomes nonfunctional because of a decrease in blood supply. Usually, placing the patient in a prone or right posterolateral position during feeding and supplementing nutrition with hyperalimentation serve to relieve pressure on the SMA. Once the system is a little stronger, the situation usually resolves itself spontaneously.

Nursing standards of care

Basic life support is always the first medical and nursing priority. Medical management of the patient suffering thermal and/or inhalation injury focuses primarily on ventilatory support, fluid resuscitation and management, and infection control and wound coverage. Oxygen therapy and airway support are the first actions instituted for the patient suffering inhalation injury. In the presence of 100% oxygen, the half-life of carboxyhemoglobin (COHgb) is only 40–60 minutes, enabling the patient to rapidly diminish COHgb saturation.[151] Serial carboxyhemoglobin saturation levels are used to guide progressive tapering of supplemental administration of oxygen. Sustained high carboxyhemoglobin saturations and/or compromised airway patency may necessitate endotracheal intubation and mechanical ventilation with positive end-expiratory pressure (PEEP).

Although it may appear self-evident, the next step to take is to assure that the burning process is stopped. If heat is still being given off, the area must be cooled at once, usually with sterile room-temperature water in quantities as needed. The use of ice for this process is contraindicated. Next, any remaining clothes or jewelry must be removed, using extreme caution when moving the patient until it is documented that no hidden injury (cervical spine damage, for instance) is present. Identification of the causative agent, whether flame, steam, electricity, or a chemical agent, should be accomplished before instituting therapy.

Fluid replacement or resuscitation is another primary focus during emergency and acute medical management of the burn patient. The quantity of crystalloid fluid replacement needed is estimated using a formula that factors the patient's weight and total body surface area burned in conjunction with a constant factor for Ringer's lactate.[152] The most commonly used formula is the Parkland (Baxter) formula:

First 24 hours post burn

4 cc Ringer's lactate × body weight (kg) × TBSA (%)

- administer half of total lactate in first 8 hours
- administer half of total lactate in next 16 hours

Second 24 hours post burn

- 0.3–0.5 cc colloid (Plasmanate) × body weight (kg) × TBSA (%), administered over first 8 hours
- 2000 cc D_5W, administered over entire 24 hours

The hourly rate of fluid resuscitation is then increased or decreased, based on the patient's clinical response. Sensorium, urine output, central venous pressure, heart rate, and blood pressure are all assessed frequently in order to determine the effectiveness of the fluid resuscitation. Urine output is the strongest indicator of adequate resuscitation, reflecting both renal blood flow and systemic perfusion. Urine output of 0.5–1.0 cc/kg/hr is adequate.[153] Colloid fluids are not introduced until at least 24 hours after the injury in order to allow time for capillary permeability to return to normal. Furthermore, if fluids are given in great quantities, sodium values must be watched closely, since clinical hyponatremia from dilution may suddenly reverse to hypernatremia later in the clinical course.

Indwelling urine drainage catheters are inserted when fluid resuscitation is necessary, because accurate intake and output balances are valuable in the evaluation of fluid resuscitation efforts. Catheters are particularly important in the case of electrical injury when currents of great intensity have damaged the kidneys because of the fluids present there. Greater amounts of fluid are required to flush the kidneys, and sometimes use of mannitol or dopamine is indicated.

In conjunction with fluid resuscitation, blood products and electrolytes are infused, as needed. If blood products are being administered, blood less than three days old should be used, if possible, in order to assure maximal oxygen-carrying capacity.

Oral feeding is desirable as soon as the patient can tolerate it. However, the amount of calories, proteins, and fats required by the body during healing from burn injury may well exceed the patient's intake capacity. Nutritional assessment and plans of care (usually accomplished by dieticians working closely with the patient and family) are paramount. Increased metabolic rates, the presence of infection and stress, and the patient's baseline nutritional status all can complicate the meeting of nutritional demands. Several formulas for calculating nutritional requirements of burn patients are available: the Wilmore, Curreri, Muir, and Barclay formula; the Davies and Liljedahl formula; the University of California at San Diego formula; and the Boston formula.[154] To meet nutritional demands delineated by the above formulas, burn team members may use oral feedings, tube feedings, and/or hyperalimentation.

Medical management of the burn wound itself includes careful orchestration of wound debridement, topical antibiotic therapy, and skin coverage. There is much disagreement over how best to protect the patient from nosocomial infection. One review of the literature suggests that the primary sources of nosocomial infection are the caregiver's hands and apron area.[155] Isolation precautions range from simple handwashing to complete reverse isolation and laminar air flow rooms. The overall recommendation from the American Burn Association is to provide the best possible barrier between the patient and the hands and apron of the caregiver. Specific recommendations include handwashing and wearing gowns for direct contact with the patient.

Wound debridement accompanying daily dressing changes facilitates removal of necrotic tissue and application of antibiotic medication to combat infection. Use of systemic prophylactic antibiotics was widely accepted in the past, but recently acquired knowledge discourages this practice. The most commonly used topical antibiotics are silver sulfadiazine, mafenide acetate, and 0.5% silver nitrate solution. Specific topical antibiotic solutions or creams can be chosen as indicated by culture or, initially, according to organisms frequent to the burn unit or geographical region. Since excessive use of such solutions or creams can lead to maceration if they are applied with dressings, the dressing should be kept damp rather than saturated with fluid.

The use of either open-wound or closed-wound techniques is determined by the physician. If the closed-wound method is instituted, frequent circulatory checks must be made of extremities distal to the dressing, since the risk of swelling is very high.

Areas of circumferential third-degree burns command the same attention so as to prevent constriction from closed edematous areas. Level of capillary refill and the presence or absence of pulses, sensation, and tingling are ascertained distal to the wound. If occlusion does develop, escharotomy is performed. If the injury is of the fourth-degree type, a deeper incision (fasciotomy) may be indicated. A carpal tunnel release is performed as an emergency treatment in the case of electrical injury involving current passing through the hand to the ground.

For the full-thickness burn wound, surgical intervention is implemented as soon after the injury as possible. If the burn encompasses the chest, an emergency escharotomy may be indicated to allow adequate chest expansion for breathing. After an escharotomy, swelling expands outward rather than inward, eliminating constriction of the chest wall and relieving pressure on lung tissue, blood vessels, and nerves. Analgesia is administered before the procedure, and resultant bleeding is controlled with use of pressure and/or topical coagulants. Figure 9-14 shows the preferred sites for escharotomy.

In order to graft an injured area, the nonviable third-degree burn tissue must first be removed (wound excision). If the depth of the damaged tissue is not too great, the nonviable tissue is shaved in layers until a bleeding bed is reached (tangential excision). However, when the procedure requires the removal of nonviable subcutaneous tissue and fat, fascial excision is indicated.

Tangential excisions are bloody and require an experienced surgical team to achieve a promising dermal bed. Cosmetic results are usually better than those seen with deeper excisions, since tangential excisions leave fat tissue intact, thus retaining the contours of the body and face.

Fascial excision is not as bloody as tangential excision and requires less surgical time and experience. However, risk of loss or damage to tendons, ligaments, nerves, and/or joints is high with this procedure. To cover denuded areas, various thicknesses of skin are taken from nonburned areas of the body (autografting from donor sites). Under general anesthesia, split-thickness autografts are excised, prepared, and then applied to surgically debrided wound beds. It is crucial that nutritional and parenteral support be increased in order to meet fluid and caloric demands experienced during the healing of wound and donor site. Donor site selection in autografting is evaluated and addressed from time of admission. Optimal sites to be used as donors are supple and have little or no hair (especially in the case of cosmetic reconstruction). The "tougher" areas of skin are reserved for autografting general areas needing coverage. When a grafting procedure is completed, the total amount of adherence of the graft to the wound is calculated as the "take." Blistering and loss of graft take are possible if the patient is not closely monitored and protected from infection, pooling of blood, edema, and inappropriate movement. Pressure garments or Ace wraps, occlusive dressings, topical antibiotics, and immobilization for a limited number of days all help prevent failure of the take. Pressure garments also aid in venous return, which is important, since decreased or no perfusion to an extremity can also result in graft loss.

The major nursing goal in the care of the actual burn injury is facilitating replacement or repair of burned skin through multisystem support, prevention of complications, and pain control. Pain control for the patient with greater than 20% TBSA is initially accomplished by IV infusion of analgesics, because early edema formation serves to isolate the medication to the injection site when it is administered intramuscularly or subcutaneously. This isolation is particularly troublesome not only because pain is not relieved upon administration, but also because as the edema fluid is later reabsorbed, so is the narcotic.

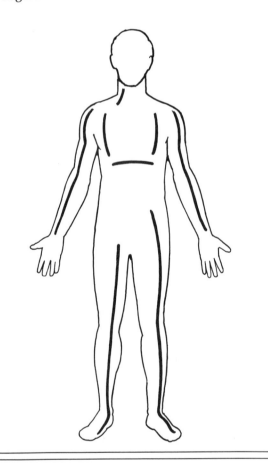

Figure 9-14 Commonly Selected Sites for Escharotomy

Delayed reabsorption of the drug results in unpredictable and potentially lethal narcotic absorption.

Nonpharmacological therapy includes hypnosis, relaxation techniques, and imagery; televisions, radios, and audio tapes provide diversional opportunities. Other practices found successful in alleviating pain can be very simple to implement, including elevation of burned extremities to decrease edema and subsequent pressure. Occupational and physical therapy in the form of an array of passive and active exercises are performed when medically indicated to decrease contractures while simultaneously promoting relaxation and comfort.

Furthermore, good rapport and trust among patient, family, and burn team is essential, since each patient has different psychological needs (just as each wound is unique). Prognostic goals can only be achieved if appropriate interventions that allow for grieving, acceptance, and emotional healing are provided. Nursing standards of care for the burn patient are detailed in the following care plan.

Nursing Care Plan for the Management of the Patient with Burns

Diagnosis	Signs and symptoms	Intervention	Rationale
Potential for fluid volume deficit	Low BP	Obtain admission weight as soon as possible	Baseline, or "dry," weight is needed before fluid resuscitation alters weight
	Elevated pulse		
	Low urinary output		
	Low CVP		
	Low PA	Record patient's weight every day	Fluid gains and losses as well as patient's true weight can be monitored by comparing to baseline
	Low urine specific gravity		
	Elevated Hct		
	Weight loss	Monitor vital signs and hemodynamics every hour and as needed	Comparisons will reveal trends and serve as a guide for adequate fluid resuscitation
	Impaired mental status		
		Record I&O and specific gravities every hour and as needed (include oral, IV, urine, and NG tube)	To monitor fluid gains and losses
		Check patency of urinary catheters	Accuracy of output can be altered if clots or casts occlude the catheter
		Monitor electrolytes and CBC	To aid in assessing hydration and electrolyte alterations
		Observe for blood loss in dressing	To note need for replacement or intervention
		Send urine for myoglobin and hemoglobin studies	To discover need for mannitol and/or fluid challenges
Potential for fluid volume excess	Edema and weight gain from intake greater than output	Compare current weight to admission weight	Excess fluid load is reflected in weight
	Shortness of breath and dyspnea	Monitor urine output and specific gravity	To guide fluid therapy

Diagnosis	Signs and symptoms	Intervention	Rationale
	Orthopnea	Check VS and hemodynamics every hour	To monitor for excess fluid in patient's system
	Crackles (rales) and gurgles (rhonchi)		
	Restlessness	Monitor mental status, neck distension, peripheral pulses, edema, and breath sounds	Early changes in fluid overload can be detected by routine exams
	Anxiety		
	Elevated PAP and CVP		
	Infiltrates on chest	Allow patient to spend no more than 20 minutes at a time in the tub	Electrolytes are leeched and fluid absorbed when patient is in the tub for too long
	Low urine specific gravity		
	Frequent vein distension	Elevate HOB	To assist lung ventilation and reduce edema (central tissue)
	Third heart sound		
	Dilution of electrolytes	Monitor electrolytes and restrict sodium intake in IV fluids and nutrition	Balance of electrolytes can change rapidly
	Low Hct and Hgb		
Ineffective airway clearance	Erythema and blisters of buccal mucosa and pharynx	Maintain patent airway by repositioning neck	To open airway passage (in the absence of spinal injury)
	Carbonaceous sputum	Obtain history of injury	To determine length of exposure and whether it occurred in closed or open space
	Wheezing		
	Gurgles (rhonchi)		
	Cough	Measure carboxyhemoglobin on admission and as needed	To assess need for immediate intubation and later compare for effectiveness of treatment
	Elevated respiratory rate		
	Sore throat		
	Hoarseness	Administer 100% O_2	Displaces carbon monoxide and improves oxygenation of alveoli
	Stridor		
		Constantly monitor respiratory rate and auscultate every 2 hours	To detect abnormal respiratory patterns, breath sounds, and airway sounds associated with distress
		Clear airway with least amount of irritation	To minimize additional injury to airway
		Assist with measurement of flow loops/respiratory parameters, including TV and/or vital capacity	To discover respiratory deficit

Nursing Care Plan for the Management of the Patient with Burns

Diagnosis	Signs and symptoms	Intervention	Rationale
		Assist with bronchoscopy	Patient will need reassurance, topical anesthetics, and/or sedation
		Observe and palpate circumferential eschar of trunk and/or neck every 3 hours	Blood flow, nerve function, and expansion of chest wall may be compromised
		Keep intubation and tracheostomy equipment close to bedside	Respiratory obstructions in the burn patient are quick and lethal
		Measure and record level of ETT at teeth/gums (after chest film confirmation)	To provide reference for tube placement and location
		Offer alternative means of communication	To decrease anxiety and prevent attempts to talk around artificial airway which will increase strain to already traumatized tissues
		Record color and consistency of sputum	Soot-tinged sputum indicates smoke inhalation; infection, dehydration, and inadequate mouth care can also be indicated by changes in sputum
Impaired gas exchange	Low PaO_2 or elevated $PaCO_2$	Monitor ABGs	Reflect acid/base balance
	Low pulse or oxygen saturation	Constantly monitor pulse oximetry	Immediate indicator of decreased oxygen saturation
	Pulmonary edema		
	Confusion, irritability	Monitor end-tidal CO_2	Correlates with ventilation/perfusion mismatch
	Lethargy		
	Elevated respiratory rate and depth		

Diagnosis	Signs and symptoms	Intervention	Rationale
	Elevated heart rate	Monitor level of consciousness every hour and PRN	To assess cerebral oxygenation
	Dysrhythmias		
	Crackles (rales)/gurgles (rhonchi)	Encourage patient to turn, cough, deep breathe	To mobilize secretions and open alveoli
	Dyspnea		
	Cyanosis	Perform chest PT/drainage	To mobilize secretions and prevent pneumonia
		Monitor hydration by IV and humidification	To help mobilize secretions
		Record and report elevated temperature, change in sputum, chest pain, and change in VS; send sputum for culture and sensitivity	To detect the presence of pneumonia
		Minimize sedation	Oversedation can impair respiratory drive and ability to express distress
		Calculate oxygen consumption	To assess peripheral oxygen demands and perfusion
		Elevate HOB 30–45 degrees	To prevent aspiration and increase lung expansion (check spinal films first)
		Initiate meticulous mouth care; observe for signs of ulceration and/or sores in mouth or on lips	To decrease incidence of infection and resulting tendency to "guard" the sore throat
		Insert NG tube if intubated or tracheostomized	To reduce risk of vomiting and aspiration
Ineffective thermoregulation	Lower temperature, cool skin, poor capillary refill	Obtain temperature, especially of shivering patient	To use as baseline for additional treatments
	Metabolic acidosis	Limit exposure of wounds to air (use a sterile drape sheet during dressing changes)	To conserve temperature and decrease contamination
	Hypoglycemia		
	Lowered weight		

Diagnosis	Signs and symptoms	Intervention	Rationale
	Elevated temperature, dehydration Change in LOC	Turn on heat lamps or shields before dressing change; limit traffic in the area	To increase environmental temperature and decrease chill due to air flow around the patient
		Use temperature probe	To provide continuous monitoring of temperature, especially after anesthesia
		Warm IV fluids	To reduce lowering of core body temperature
		Adjust temperature of specialized beds, or use heating/cooling blanket	To provide additional exterior regulation of body temperature
		Report changes in temperature	Indicate need to review antibiotics and culture results and to change dressing techniques
		Record reactions to therapeutic interventions	May indicate need to repeat or add support
		Monitor BP and ECG for ST segment changes	Vasodilation and myocardial ischemia can occur with a decrease in temperature
		Prepare room with antihypothermia equipment before patient returns from OR	Increased exposure of skin surface and new donor sites decreases barrier to cold
		Monitor ABGs	Solubility of gases changes with temperature; more oxygen is consumed during rewarming
		Rewarm or cool at a rate no greater than 1°F per hour	Sudden changes in body temperature severely alter acid-base balance

Diagnosis	Signs and symptoms	Intervention	Rationale
Impaired skin integrity	Loss of skin Open wounds Unheated donor sites	Monitor changes in wounds via nursing notes	To document healing and nonhealing of wounds
		Reposition and/or move patient to specialized bed	To lower pressure areas in wound field and allow for higher circulation
		Keep calorie counts, monitor weights, and record fluid and electrolyte imbalances	Wound healing is related to nutritional status
		Assess need to change type of dressing	Advancing to no dressing or less coverage allows the wound to be open to air to facilitate toughening (lower maceration)
		Apply pressure support garments	To elevate blood return to heart and lower dependent edema, blisters, and pooling of blood in periphery
		Wet grafted sites every 4 hours	To protect granulation of tissue
		Immobilize grafted area	Movement of grafted areas may shear or otherwise traumatize grafts
		Elevate all injured extremities	To promote venous return
		Protect wounds from trauma	To minimize disruption of epithelial tissue
		Leave donor sites open to air when using mesh gauze, scarlet red, or zenoform	Drying of donor sites is essential to rapid healing and decreasing infection rate
		Assess adherence of temporary grafts such as allograft, zenograft, or "artificial skin"	Adherence denotes a clean bed, ready for autografting
		Change temporary grafts every 3–5 days	To decrease the risks of rejection reactions and excessive bleeding and trauma on removal

Nursing Care Plan for the Management of the Patient with Burns

Diagnosis	Signs and symptoms	Intervention	Rationale
		Wet meshed grafts with appropriate antibiotic solution	To lower infection and protect granulation tissue
		Discontinue dressing and apply moisturizers once interstices have epithelialized (closed)	Damage to or destruction of sebaceous glands leads to increased dryness
Potential for wound infection	Loss of graft Increase in wound depth	Wash hands before and after treating patient	Hand-to-patient contamination is main cause of nosocomial infection
	Elevated temperature Cellulitis Purulent drainage Odorous dressings	Shave hair from burn sites and 1–2 inches around burn sites (never shave eyebrows, however)	To decrease build-up of topical medications and increase ease of cleansing area
	Change in LOC or VS Elevated tube feeding residuals	Debride loose tissue, blisters, and scabs daily	To decrease medium for bacterial growth
	Pain at wound site	Exercise aseptic technique (universal precautions)	To minimize introduction of pathogens
		Document and report changes in wound appearance and increased sensitivity	Indicates ineffective antibiotic coverage and need to change it
		Conduct full-thickness wound biopsy	Provides identification of organisms in subsequent layers of skin and proof of invasiveness
		Never cause bleeding when debriding	Bleeding allows pathogens to enter the circulatory system
		Do "pan" culture when patient's temperature is above 38.5°C, including chest x-ray, blood cultures (new stick), urine, and sputum	To investigate all possible avenues of infection source

Diagnosis	Signs and symptoms	Intervention	Rationale
		Monitor lab results for changes in potassium and sodium levels	Indicate increased capillary permeability due to effects of endotoxins
		Maintain hyperglycemic status	Promotes wound healing
		Use towels to absorb excess wet-down solutions (avoid plastic)	Maceration and skin breakdown increase when nonburned skin is allowed to remain wet
		Extrude and swab-culture purulent drainage, incising and draining permanent grafts or "rolling" drainage to edge of temporary grafts	To decrease bacteria count and provide sample for lab, allowing identification and proper treatment
		Assess adherence of temporary grafts within fasciotomy sites	To maintain integrity of exposed tendons, ligaments, and major blood vessels
Alteration in comfort, pain	Verbalization of discomfort, crying	Assess level of discomfort, quality, and location, and have patient self-rate pain	To provide record for future assessment of effectiveness of treatment
	Guarding		
	Elevated heart rate, respiratory rate, or BP	Investigate source of pain not related to burn wounds	Associated trauma or nonburn wound complications may be present
	Grimacing		
	Clenching of teeth or fists	Accept and note patient's response to pain	Ethical and cultural experiences as well as previous injuries may influence patient's perception of pain's severity
	Diaphoresis		
	Nausea/vomiting		
	Restlessness		
	Agitation	Premedicate for painful procedures (ask patient how long the medication takes to become effective)	To allay some of patient's fear and give patient some control concerning medication; also increases adherence and patient's ability to function during the procedure
	Change in sleep patterns		
		Observe response to medication	May need to change amount, frequency, or type of medication

Nursing Care Plan for the Management of the Patient with Burns

Diagnosis	Signs and symptoms	Intervention	Rationale
		Monitor patient for side effects	To avoid oversedation, undersedation, or allergic response
		Explain all procedures to patient, before, during, and after treatment	To decrease patient's anxiety about unknown and to reinforce statements not comprehended before starting
		Allow patient time to verbalize discomfort	To provide patient with sense of concern from staff
		Talk with patient about effectiveness of medication	To develop a positive expectation of relief
		Use relaxation techniques or diversions (radio, TV, verbalizing), per patient's request	Effectiveness for controlling and escaping pain is individualized
		Explain importance and frequency of each procedure	To allay patient's fears and anxiety
		Maintain patient's temperature and limit time when dressings are open	Cold and air increase discomfort
		Elevate extremities	To decrease pain from swelling and increase comfort
		Reposition patient PRN, and use specialized beds (air, fluidized, rotating, antidecubitus)	To decrease stiffness and potential for pressure sores
		Allow patient to do own dressings (may need additional time)	To increase patient's sense of control

Diagnosis	Signs and symptoms	Intervention	Rationale
Alteration in nutritional status	Weight loss Muscle mass deterioration Change in electrolytes Decreased albumin Glucose imbalance Decreased plasma proteins Depleted minerals Edema General malaise, apathy, fatigue Confusion Slow or nonexistent wound healing Change in urine electrolytes High gastric residuals	Record I&O, calorie count, and daily weight	To provide information needed in order to calculate deficit or excess in nutritional balance and nitrogen balance and to provide for healing
		Assess bowel sounds at least every 8 hours, check for distension, and record quality, quantity and frequency of stool and vomitus	High stress and infection can lead to ileus, constipation, or diarrhea
		Monitor electrolytes	Imbalances occur with minor and major burns
		Reassess patient's caloric needs every 5–7 days	Addition of donor sites, healing of wounds, inadequate thermal regulation can change nutritional requirements
		Attend to nutritional needs on a daily basis	Making up for "lost" days may not be possible
		Estimate and account for dressings, lost tissue, or amputated limb when recording and assessing weights	Although it is best to weigh the patient without dressings, this may not always be possible because of post-op dressings or fragile healing on pressure areas (back)
		Record color, pH, and amount of gastric residuals	Possibility of ulceration in GI tract increases with stress; pre-admission ulceration will be accelerated
		Adjust type of nutritional delivery to patient's needs	Young or elderly patient may not be able to consume adequate amounts of food

Nursing Care Plan for the Management of the Patient with Burns

Diagnosis	Signs and symptoms	Intervention	Rationale
		Plan painful procedures after dining times, and medicate patient, if necessary, before meals	Pain decreases desire to eat
		Plan for use of TPN, if necessary	May be required in spite of risk of infection if GI tract is not capable of handling increased requirements
		Check feeding tube and NG tube placement and patency at least every 8 hours	To prevent aspiration
		Check and record residuals every 2–4 hours	To discover GI problems; feedings may have to be diluted or decreased until patient accepts them
		Assist with feeding	Patient may not be able to utilize arms or hands
		Use adaptive utensils, when appropriate	Padding on utensils may help patient grasp them until full flexion has returned
		Help patient fill out menu	To allow patient to pick out preferred foods and ask about unfamiliar selections
		Maintain oral hygiene and request dental consultation when necessary	Pain in mouth from infection of gums and/or teeth decreases appetite
		Ask family and patient about previous eating habits	To identify deficits that may already exist and need to be compensated for (fast diets, alcoholism, bulimia, anorexia, substance abuse)

Diagnosis	Signs and symptoms	Intervention	Rationale
		Document cultural factors, allergies, food preferences, diabetes, low-salt diet, low-cholesterol diet	To provide foods appropriate for patient's requirements
		Encourage family to bring in foods cooked the way the patient likes them	Providing preferred foods may prompt patient to increase intake
		Use liquid and powdered supplements	Additional nutrition can be "hidden" in milk shakes
		Consult dietician and use charts to compare actual intake, required calories and proteins, and weight gain or loss	To provide patient, family, and staff with a record in order to check for deficits and overachievement
		Present food in an appealing manner	To stimulate appetite
Lack of knowledge concerning treatments and healing process	Inability to verbalize healing process	Explain procedures and tests to patient and family	To decrease anxiety and increase cooperation
	Inability to answer questions	Review explanations	To reinforce information that may not have been heard or understood during crisis
	Questioning of procedures		
	Anxiety/restlessness		
	Nonadherence	Teach wound healing (use printed materials)	To help fill the need for expectations and increase realization of healing
	Irritability		
		Refrain from using medical terminology	Important information is lost in lengthy explanations that employ technical terms
		Help patient and family plan for discharge	Patient and family can share and cooperate with each other with respect to treatment regime
		Explain and warn of possible setbacks	To decrease chance of mistrust should patient experience setbacks or deteriorate

Diagnosis	Signs and symptoms	Intervention	Rationale
		Assess patient's and family's ability to understand information	There may be a need for a translator or repetition of ideas
		Provide classes and/or social services if family is unable to comply with instructions	To clear up unanswered questions through a group or to identify learning deficits
		Teach patient and family purpose and techniques of infection control	To allay fear of causing harm or death to loved one
		Explain necessity of early excision, surgical intervention	To decrease feelings of being rushed into major decisions
		Explain noises (especially when patient cannot see)	Unfamiliar noises increase anxiety and fear
Disruption of self-concept and/or body image	Withdrawal/non-adherence	Encourage patient to participate in care	To give patient control
	Denial	Encourage patient to sit in doorway, then hallway; start during nonvisiting hours	To slowly reintegrate patient with environment
	Avoidance of mirrors		
	Verbalization of feelings of abandonment	Have cosmetic counselor and burn survivors visit patient	To allow patient to vent fears and concerns and provide opportunity to request information about improving physical appearance and coping strategies
		Maintain unhurried attitude	To decrease patient anxiety and provide a feeling of individual importance

Diagnosis	Signs and symptoms	Intervention	Rationale
		Provide opportunities for inpatients to meet each other in groups, watch movies, play cards	To increase socialization
		Arrange for patient to meet with plastic surgery liaison before discharge	To build a sense of familiarity and decrease anxiety about the unknown
Grieving, anticipating	Shock and disbelief Denial Homicidal or suicidal behavior Apathy Loss of appetite Change in bowel habits Sleeplessness Fatigue/malaise Depression Headache	Allow patient and family to express emotions	To help patient and family to recognize feelings before developing awareness of loss and subsequent restrictions
		Clarify treatments and describe realistic outcome	Trustworthy relationships are built on honesty
		Review anticipated deterioration and setbacks	To help avoid surprises and unrealistic expectations
		Provide time for patient and family to express feelings, but limit destructive feelings and actions	Patient and family need to become aware of feelings of grief and identify impact of loss
		Let the patient and family know that grief is a natural and expected feeling	To allow patient and family to deal with and accept present feelings and thoughts so they may progress in coping
		Restate questions that patient and family have asked	To clarify what is really being asked
		Praise patient and family for good coping techniques	To give patient and family a sense of progress and well-being
		Alter visiting privileges for special situations	To provide for more normal conditions related to celebrating birthdays, anniversaries, special events

Diagnosis	Signs and symptoms	Intervention	Rationale
		Offer medication for physical symptoms	Uncontrolled bowel and bladder as well as sleep result in patient embarrassment and fatigue
		Prepare patient and room for family's visit: remove blood-stained linens, check floor for debris, tidy up equipment, and cover patient appropriately	To provide a sense of normalcy and deemphasize medical surroundings
		Review with family patient's appearance and equipment they are about to see	To prepare family for impact of abundant technology and patient's dressings, swelling, and inability to see (due to swelling) or talk (due to artificial airway)
		Have family stop at door and look in before entering; provide seating	Emotional stress expressed by family at bedside can be devastating to patient; allow them to adjust first
		Inform family of positive interventions that they can perform (taking care of business at home and work, restating affection and acceptance)	To decrease the family's feeling of helplessness, reaffirm sharing of crisis, and prepare family for future outcomes
		Offer support groups, clergy, one-on-one counseling, and visits by burn survivors	To help patient develop coping strategies and engender feelings of not being alone in a crisis
		Assess patient's readiness to carryout ADL and self-care	To allow patient independence and increase feelings of progress

Diagnosis	Signs and symptoms	Intervention	Rationale
		Review with patient and family the additional support provided by occupational and physical therapists, nutritionists, plastic surgery specialists, and cosmetics specialists and the need to make return clinic visits for additional problems	Knowing they have several support groups and that corrective measures can be made to improve quality of life provides hope to patient and family
		Assist family in funeral preparations (privacy for phone calls, support for those who falter)	Emotional support at time of death projects feelings of continued caring
		Discuss possible organ donations after death to others in need	To allow family to feel that death is not the end of loved one's gift of life

Medications Commonly Used in the Care of the Patient with Burns

Medication	Effect	Major side effects
Albumin	Replaces protein loss that accompanies severe burns	Nausea Fever Headache Fluid overload Chills Hypotension Urticaria (disappears if the infusion is stopped for a short period of time)
Lactated Ringer's	Source of water and electrolytes, alkalinizing agent (pH = 6.0–7.5) (lactate ions are metabolized to carbon dioxide and water, which requires the consumption of hydrogen ions)	Febrile response Infection at insertion site Venous thrombosis or phlebitis Extravasation Hypervolemia
Mannitol	Osmotic diuretic	Circulatory overload Hypervolemia Chest pain Tachycardia Chills Cough Dysuria Arrhythmias Confusion Muscle cramps Numbness Tingling Seizures Fatigue Edema
Morphine sulfate	Relief of severe pain, preanesthetic sedation, and postoperative analgesia	Nausea Vomiting Sedation Sweating Dry mouth Constipation Biliary tract spasm Euphoria Hypotension Urinary retention Pruritis Urticaria

Medication	Effect	Major side effects
Buprenorphine (Buprenex)	Relieves severe pain as it binds to subclass μ (mu) opiate receptors in the central nervous system (longer duration than morphine)	Narcotic antagonist activity Respiratory depression May cause increased CNS depression when used with other CNS-depressing medications Elevated cerebrospinal fluid pressure Narcotic-dependent patient may experience withdrawal Enhanced biliary tract dysfunction Impaired mental/physical capabilities
Cimetidine (Tagamet)	Inhibits action of histamine; also inhibits gastric acid secretion that has been stimulated by food, histamine, pentagastrin, caffeine, or insulin	Confusion (more so with the patient over 50 or severely ill) Sore throat Unusual bleeding Cardiac arrhythmias Fatigue Diarrhea Skin rash
Carafate (Sucrafate)	Forms an ulcer adherent complex and protects against further attack by acid, pepsin, and bile salts—local, rather than systemic, effect	Reduction in activity of tetracycline, phenytoin, or digoxin when given simultaneously with Carafate (separate by 2 hours) Safety in pregnant women, nursing mothers, and children has not been established Constipation (rare) Diarrhea, nausea, gastric discomfort, dry mouth, rash, pruritus, back pain, dizziness, sleepiness, and vertigo (very rare)
Sivadene (sulfa, silver sulfadiazine)	Disrupts protein synthesis of bacterial ribosomes	Neutropenia in 3–5% of patients Painful/burning rash Itching Fungal infections

Medications Commonly Used in the Care of the Patient with Burns

Medication	Effect	Major side effects
Sulfamylon (Mafenide acetate)	Disrupts protein synthesis of bacterial ribosomes and inhibits carbonic anhydrase; effective against anaerobic bacteria and bacteriostatic against several gram-positive and gram-negative bacteria	Metabolic acidosis (2–3 days after initiation) Increased excretion of bicarbonate, sodium, potassium, and water Decreased excretion of hydrogen ions Integument: pain, hives, rash, itching, swelling, blisters, erythema, facial edema Corneal abrasions Hyperventilation (can be severe) (Accidental ingestion leads to diarrhea)
Bacitracin (petroleum-based)	Inhibits cell-wall synthesis and acts as bacteriostatic	Potentially nephrotoxic and ototoxic when used over large burn surface areas Skin: swelling of lips or face, stinging, burning, rash
Silver nitrate (0.5% solution)	Precipitates cell proteins, causing formation of a scab that eventually sloughs off (not very penetrating)	Stains the skin (unable to view wounds with clarity) Hypotonic solution (leaches out patient's electrolytes as the water evaporates)

Pain

Pain is so universal and multifactorial that it must be regarded as a clinical problem unto itself and not simply a symptom associated with a specific body system. Many disciplines have attempted to describe the phenomenon of pain, but its subjectivity prevents precise definition. In 1978, the International Association for the Study of Pain (IASP) developed the definition that is currently most acceptable: "Pain is an unpleasant sensory and emotional experience associated with actual or potential tissue damage, or described in terms of such damage."[156] Another definition is a simplistic yet useful tool for clinical practice: "Pain is whatever the patient says it is."[157] Pain is both a universal phenomenon and a personal one, requiring daily nursing intervention in the critical care area.

Clinical antecedents

The "gate control" theory of pain development has become well-known.[158] It is also the basis for the identification of five dimensions of pain: (1) physiological (organic etiology of pain), (2) sensory (intensity, quality), (3) affective (emotional state), (4) cognitive (individual interpretation or meaning of pain), and (5) behavioral (pain-related behavioral reactions).[159] Other research has identified a sixth dimension, the sociocultural dimension (demographic, social, and cultural aspects).[160] This multidimensional view provides the critical care nurse with a broad array of variables that must be considered when assessing the patient for potential pain. The majority of literature regarding pain assessment, definition, and management concerns either the cancer or the postoperative patient. This limits the data available to guide critical care nurses in general practice. All critically ill patients can be considered at risk for pain, subject to individual variations within each of the six dimensions.

Physiological evaluation of pain usually requires identification of the etiology, duration, and pattern of the pain. Three specific pain syndromes have been identified: somatic, visceral, and deafferentation (neuropathic) pain. All of these etiologies may occur with an acute or chronic presentation. Acute pain is generally related to tissue damage and resolves when the tissue heals. Critically ill patients likely to experience acute pain include those with disorders such as acute myocardial infarction and those just out of the operating room. These patients demonstrate a clear pattern of onset and resolution. Chronic pain is also due to tissue damage, but onset is less clear and physiological adaptation occurs. The chronic pain related to a lost limb or to intraabdominal adhesions is an example of that which may be found in the critically ill patient. The pattern of pain may also vary: it may be brief and transient or periodic, or steady and continuous. A combination of more than one pattern or more than one type of pain is not uncommon. An overview of the three pain syndromes and their defining characteristics is given in Figure 9-15. Possible etiologies for the syndromes are listed in Table 9-31.

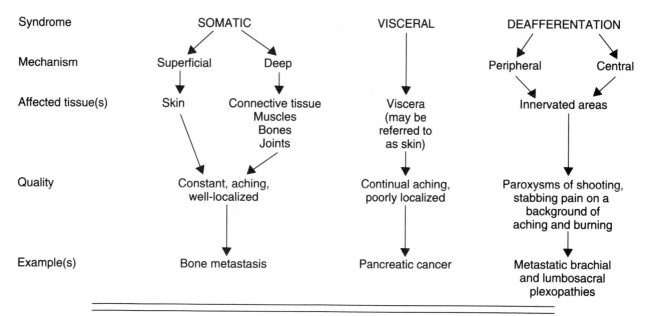

Syndrome	SOMATIC		VISCERAL	DEAFFERENTATION	
Mechanism	Superficial	Deep		Peripheral	Central
Affected tissue(s)	Skin	Connective tissue Muscles Bones Joints	Viscera (may be referred to as skin)	Innervated areas	
Quality	Constant, aching, well-localized		Continual aching, poorly localized	Paroxysms of shooting, stabbing pain on a background of aching and burning	
Example(s)	Bone metastasis		Pancreatic cancer	Metastatic brachial and lumbosacral plexopathies	

Figure 9-15 Pain Syndromes

Table 9-31 Etiologies of Pain Syndromes

Syndrome	Etiologies
Somatic (connective tissue, muscles, bones, joints)	Surgery Tissue trauma Burns Fractures
Visceral (organs)	Myocardial infarction Contusion of organs—liver, spleen, kidney, lung, heart Hepatitis Pancreatitis
Deafferentation (neuropathic, neural plexes)	Cord compression Spinal cord injuries Tumors, masses

The sensory dimension of pain addresses the location, intensity, and quality of the pain. Clear delineation of pain locations may reveal more than one etiology and indicate combination therapy, rather than a single analgesic. Although intensity of pain is primarily determined by the etiology, it is also subjective and may be affected by personal, environmental, and sociocultural variables. Words describing the intensity of pain might be "mild," "moderate," and "severe." The third component, quality of pain, is more descriptive of the sensations felt and interpreted by the patient. Measures of pain quality might include descriptions such as "stabbing," "aching," "burning," and "radiating." These descriptive words used by the patient are an important component of the pain assessment and will guide interventions.

The affective dimension of pain is less concrete and definitive. Various researchers have attempted to correlate personality or mood disturbances to pain perception, but there do not seem to be any consistent correlations applicable to all patients.[161] The affective dimension, therefore, has highly individual application to pain perceptions. This individuality reinforces the need to evaluate each patient's response for the contribution of the affective dimension.

The personal meaning of pain falls into the cognitive domain. Whether the pain is viewed as temporary or permanent, a punishment or a poor prognostic sign, the interpretation may influence the patient's well-being and recovery from whatever has caused the pain. Assessment of the cognitive dimension may allow identification of factors that enhance pain sensations beyond what might normally be anticipated.

The behavioral dimension of the pain experience involves personal expression of pain to others, non-verbal cues indicative of pain, and personal strategies employed to relieve pain. In a study of hospitalized patients with pain, the most common pain-reduction strategies included the use of an analgesic, rest and lying down, distraction, and the use of heat.[162] The patient's receptiveness to noninvasive pain relief may identify him or her as a potential candidate for behavioral modification or relaxation therapy.

The cultural, ethnic, spiritual, and demographic variables that influence an individual's pain experience are included in the sociocultural dimension of pain. Studies of the influences of gender and age on pain expression have reached conflicting conclusions, necessitating further evaluation of this particular sociocultural aspect. Although research is sparse, it reflects a subtle continuum of influences on attitudes and feelings regarding pain. The critical care nurse should explore these value systems with the patient when developing a plan for pain prevention or relief.

The most commonly encountered pain in the ICU is that experienced postoperatively. Studies of postoperative patients revealed a wide variance in the pain experienced: 30% had mild pain, 30% had moderate pain, and 40% had severe pain.[163] These studies further noted that the most severe pain was experienced with intrathoracic and intraabdominal surgeries, extensive surgery of the spine, and major joint operations. Most pain persisted 3 days to 1 week following surgery.

In summary, the critically ill patient is at risk for any pain syndrome, depending on individual circumstances. The six dimensions of the pain response are to be considered when assessing the patient for the presence of pain.

Critical referents

Theories regarding the precise mechanism of pain abound, but for the critical care nurse, the concept important to clinical practice is that pain is a real physiological phenomenon of primary neuro-sensory origin. An understanding of the physiological mechanisms of pain will assist the critical care nurse in understanding and developing innovative pain management strategies.

Pain is perceived, or felt, as the result of a series of four specific physiological mechanisms, or processes:[164]

1. The triggering mechanism for a pain response is called transduction, and it begins with an undesirable stimulus of the sensory nerve ending, causing the electrical conduction of a pain message. This is called nociception, and receptors are found in skin, muscle, bone, and viscera. Disorders of nociception include peripheral sensitivity and hyperalgesia.
2. The transmission mechanism carries the pain messages throughout the nervous system, moving from peripheral to central pathways. After impulses leave the peripheral nociceptors, they travel to the spinal cord and are rapidly transmitted to various areas of the brain via the spinothalamic pathways. The

variability of individual responses to similar pain stimuli have led researchers to speculate that there is a communication between the thalamus and nociceptive neurons during the transmission process.

3. The modulation mechanism involves complex interactions between the nociceptor neurons and three areas of the brain that have the capacity to regulate endogenous analgesia through opioids, opiate receptors, serotonin, and substance P.[165]
4. The last process involved in the physiology of pain is the individual's interpretation or perception of the pain phenomenon. Tremendous variability in response exists, and controversy remains as to why this is true. Some researchers believe that alterations in the pain transmission mechanism or hypersensitive receptors may down-regulate or up-regulate the personal experience of the pain.

Resulting signs and symptoms

Despite the clear descriptions of the six dimensions of pain and their influence on the perceptions of pain, the expression of pain remains a greatly variable individual response. The nurse making an assessment of a patient's pain must review all vari-

Table 9-32 Pain Terms

Term	Definition
Addiction	A behavioral pattern of drug use characterized by overwhelming involvement with the use
Dose response	The increase in effectiveness accompanying an increase in dosage
Efficacy	Degree of analgesia provided by a given dose of an analgesic administered under a particular set of conditions
Half-life	The time it takes a drug to fall to half of its original concentration in the blood
Opiate receptors	Specific recognition sites on which opioids produce their actions
Physical dependence	An altered physiological state produced by repeated administration of a drug, which necessitates the continued administration of the drug to prevent withdrawal
Relative analgesic potency	Ratio of effective doses of two drugs
Relative analgesic potential	The relationship between efficacy and adverse effects
Tolerance	A pharmacological phenomenon that is evidenced when a given dose of a drug produces a decreasing effect or when ever larger doses must be given to obtain the effects produced by the original dose

Sources: International Association for the Study of Pain Subcommittee on Taxonomy. (1979). Pain terms: A list with definitions and usage. *Pain, 6:* 249–252; McGuire, D.B. and Sheidler, V.R. (1990). Pain. In S.L. Groenwald et al. (Eds.), *Cancer Nursing Principles and Practice* (2nd edition). Boston: Jones and Bartlett.

ables in order to determine how much each is contributing to the reported pain. In an attempt to standardize the language of pain assessment and management, the IASP has developed a taxonomy of pain terms and definitions, some of which are given in Table 9-32.

In addition, many clinicians have attempted to develop instruments that quantify the patient's reports of pain intensity and the behaviors that reflect the presence of pain. The two major types of single-dimensional pain scales are pain descriptor scales and visual analog scales for pain intensity (Figure 9-16). Multidimensional scales attempt to quantify more than one characteristic of pain—for example, pain intensity, pain threshold, and pain anxiety. The main difficulty in implementing these tools with the critically ill population is their limited usefulness with the neurologically impaired patient. Behavior and activity scales as measures of pain are not practical in the critical care setting because forced bedrest is often necessitated by equipment, invasive lines, and the nature of the patient's illness. Autonomic or physiological indices of the presence of pain remain the most commonly used with the severely critically ill patient population. (Keep in mind, though, that changes in heart rate, blood pressure, or respirations can be influenced by many other variables as well.) One study of self-reported pain scales was conducted in an acute-trauma patient population.[166] This research demonstrated that a systemic method of measuring pain and response to pain interventions can be employed with the critically ill patient with some reliability.

Nursing standards of care

Analgesic medications The primary management strategy for pain is the administration of analgesics. Analgesics primarily alter the sensation or perception of pain, although some have an antiinflammatory effect, which actually reduces certain types of pain. Pharmacologic management of pain involves the use of several different classifications of medications: narcotics, nonsteroidal antiinflammatory agents (NSAIDs), acetaminophen derivatives, adjuvant analgesics, antidepressants, psychostimulants, phenothiazines, and antihistamines. The selection of an analgesic agent depends on pain etiology, intensity, and duration and affective factors. Examples of pain medications and possible indications for their use are given in Table 9-33. Unfortunately, few health care professionals are skilled at assessing analgesic needs or equivalency when changing medications or the route of administration. Pharmaceutical sources should be consulted when changing medications to ensure ongoing pain relief.

The opioid analgesics are the most potent and most commonly used agents in the critical care setting. A listing of the common opioid agents and their relative potencies appears in Table 9-34. The side effects of opioid analgesics are similar. The neurological, cardiovascular, pulmonary, gastrointestinal, genitourinary, and dermatological effects and appropriate nursing interventions are noted in Table 9-35.

Just as there is no best opioid to administer, there

VISUAL ANALOG SCALES (VAS)

No pain   Pain as bad as it
                                                        could possibly be

No pain   Mild   Moderate   Severe   Pain as bad as it
                                                        could possibly be

VERBAL DESCRIPTOR SCALE

_____ 1 None
_____ 2 Mild
_____ 3 Moderate
_____ 4 Severe
_____ 5 Unbearable

Figure 9-16 Single-Dimensional Pain Scales

Table 9-33 Pharmacotherapy of Pain

Agent	Indications
Nonsteroidal antiinflammatory agents (NSAIDs)—includes salicylates	Bone pain (arthritis, metastases) Pain from mechanical compression of tendons, muscles, pleura, and peritoneum (orthopedic injuries, muscle sprains, tendonitis, pleural or peritoneal effusions, pericarditis) Nonobstructive visceral pain (dysmenorrhea, toothache)
Steroids—methylprednisolone	Used as a late adjunct with inflammatory pain
Acetominophen	Mild pain, particularly somatic (sore throats, skin tenderness)
Antidepressants—Amitriptyline, Nortriptyline, Imipramine, Desipramine, Doxepin	Neuropathic pain (post-herpetic neuralgia, diabetic neuropathy, migraine headaches)
Anticonvulsants—phenytoin, Carbamazepine, Clonazepam, valproic acid	Neuropathic pain (see above)
Psychostimulants—amphetamines, methylphenidate	Patients with significant opioid sedation
Narcotics—morphine-like opioid agonists (codeine, meperidine, hydromorphone, morphine, methadone), opioid antagonists (Naloxone), opioid agonists-antagonists and partial agonists (Pentazocine, butorphanol, nalbuphine)	Primary analgesics for somatic and visceral pain

Table 9-34 Relative Potencies of Commonly Used Analgesics[a]

Analgesics for Severe Pain	IM (mg)[b]	PO (mg)[b]	Plasma Half-Life	Average Duration of Action (hr)
Codeine	130	200	2.5–3	3–5
Meperidine	75	300	3–5	2–4
Oxycodone	15	30	2–3	3–5
Hydromorphone	1.5	7.5	2–3	3–6
Morphine	10	60[c]	2–3.5	4–5
Levorphanol	2	4	11–16	4–5
Methadone	10	20	15–30	4–6
Oxymorphone	1	——	2–3	4–5

Analgesics for Mild Pain	Oral Dose (mg)[c]
Codeine	30
Meperidine	50
Propoxyphene	65
Acetaminophen	650
Sodium salicylate	1000

[a]These values were determined from and based on clinical experience and single-dose studies of patients in acute pain. For chronic dosing, some pain experts believe that the oral morphine dose is approximately 20–30 mg, but this has not been demonstrated in any controlled trial.
[b]Approximately equivalent to morphine 10 mg IM.
[c]Approximately equal to aspirin 650 mg.
Source: McGuire, D.B. and Sheidler, V.R. (1990). Pain. In S.L. Groenwald et al. (Eds.), *Cancer Nursing Principles and Practice* (2nd edition). Boston: Jones and Bartlett.

Table 9-35 Common Side Effects of Opioid Analgesics

System	Side Effects	Interventions
Central nervous	Sedation, drowsiness, mental clouding, euphoria, analgesia, nausea, vomiting, decreased physical activity, lethargy, mood changes	Psychostimulants Diversional activity
Respiratory	Decreased respiratory rate, decreased ventilatory minute volume, decreased tidal exchange, decreased PO_2, increased PCO_2	Combination agents Oxygen therapy Physical activity
Cardiovascular	Hypotension from peripheral vasodilation or histamine release	Increase fluid intake Orthostatic precautions
Gastrointestinal	Stomach: decreased motility; small intestine: decreased propulsive contractions, delayed digestion from decreased biliary and pancreatic secretions; large intestine: decreased or absent propulsive peristaltic waves, causing delay in passage of contents; biliary tract: increased pressure from morphine-like drugs, causing epigastric distress to biliary colic	Increase fluids Antiemetics PRN Colace daily
Genitourinary	Increased tone and amplitude of ureter contractions, increased tone of bladder muscles producing urgency, increased tone of vesical sphincter	Assess bladder distention Incontinence pads PRN
Dermatological	Vasodilation of cutaneous blood vessels producing increased warmth and flushing of skin on face, neck, and upper thorax, sweating, pruritus	Frequent bathing, skin care, menthol lotions Cool drinks, foods Antihistamines

is no best method of administration. There are eight different methods of narcotic administration: oral, sublingual or buccal, rectal, intermittent intramuscular or subcutaneous, intravenous bolus, continuous intravenous infusions, continuous subcutaneous infusions, and intrathecal or epidural administration. Investigational studies using the intranasal and transdermal routes are currently underway.[167] Each patient's circumstances should be critically evaluated to determine which method to use. Serious consideration should be given to finding the most effective yet least invasive regimen. Much attention has been placed on innovative invasive strategies such as continuous narcotic infusion, patient-controlled analgesia, and epidural analgesia. These strategies may be particularly applicable in the short-term critical care setting (especially for postoperative care), but the patient must still be monitored carefully for efficacy and adverse effects.[168] The salient characteristics of the major types of narcotic administration are described in Table 9-36.

There are particular concerns with respect to the critically ill patient who may have compromised hepatic and renal function and who is receiving a combination of analgesic and sedating medications. The nurse should be aware that many narcotic-induced respiratory depression and cardiac events occur in the critical care setting, where patient conditions are tenuous and metabolic clearance of the medication is hindered by organ failure.[169] This necessitates careful consideration of proper dosing and close monitoring for complications. The narcotic antagonist Naloxone should be readily available in the nursing unit.

Neurosurgical or anesthetic management Neuroablative therapy is reserved for intractable pain, primarily that of neuropathic origin. Nondestructive and neurolytic blocks are the most common types of anesthetic strategies. Nondestructive nerve blocks using local anesthetic agents such as Lidocaine provide temporary relief while the clinician determines the exact etiology of the pain (nociceptive or neuropathic) and the likelihood of successfully relieving it with permanent nerve blocks. Neurolytic blocks using agents such as phenol or alcohol can lead to prolonged, although often incomplete, pain relief, but they may also cause sensory and motor deficits such as paralysis.[170] Common neurosurgical procedures for the management of pain are described in Table 9-37.

Table 9-36 Characteristics of Pain Treatment Regimens

	Continuous Intravenous Infusions (CII)	Patient-Controlled Analgesia (PCA)	Continuous Subcutaneous Infusions (CSI)	Intrathecal/Epidural Administration
Technique	Permanent or temporary venous access connected to infusion device programmed to administer a set rate of analgesic	May be used for bolus dosing only or with CII, CSI. A special pump is connected to an intravenous access and an hourly rate is set, locking out time periods when it's too early for the patient to receive a dose even if he or she requests it. A printout of all activity can be obtained at periodic intervals.	Insertion of a 21-, 23-, 25-, or 27-gauge subcutaneous needle into deltoid, anterior chest, or abdominal subcutaneous tissue. Continuous infusion of narcotics given via a syringe driver, ambulatory infuser, or computerized ambulatory pump.	Placement of small-gauge catheter into the epidural space with intermittent or continuous administration of preservative-free narcotic (duramorph morphine or sublimaze fentanyl)
Advantages	Maintains steady blood level of narcotic; Improves pain control; Eliminates clock watching; Avoids need for repeated injections	Patient control over pain; Immediate medication when needed	Maintains steady blood level of narcotic; Improves pain control; Does not require venous access; Used safely in home setting	Requires lower doses of narcotic; Longer duration of pain control; Selective analgesia possible; Fewer side effects than systemic route
Disadvantages	Requires maintenance of IV line; Potential for infection; Requires special infusion pump; Need for patient monitoring	Potential for less personal contact and pain evaluation; Reduced reinforcement and support for affective component of pain	Requires infusion device; Local irritation; Limited use in patients requiring large volumes of drugs	Risk of respiratory depression; Rostral redistribution of drug, limiting selective analgesia; Rapid development of tolerance to epidural and systemic analgesics; Invasive procedure requires skilled personnel

(continued)

Table 9-36 Characteristics of Pain Treatment Regimens (*continued*)

	Continuous Intravenous Infusions (CII)	Patient-Controlled Analgesia (PCA)	Continuous Subcutaneous Infusions (CSI)	Intrathecal/Epidural Administration
Special nursing considerations	CII should be indicated Convert the total daily opioid consumption to IM-equivalent milligrams Administer a loading dose at the start and with each increase in infusion rate Increase infusion rate 10–20% every few hours Check vital signs every 30 minutes for 2 hours after loading dose or rescue dose Control side effects with adjuvant drugs	Evaluate patient-specific variables for reasons why pain medication may be inadequate Report maximum boluses for any 2-hour period	Rotate sites every 48 hours (6 days average)	Keep transparent occlusive dressing over catheter site Label catheter to ensure it is not mistaken for a venous catheter Aspirate catheter with each medication administration: blood means possible migration into the epidural space; clear fluid means possible migration into subarachnoid space Headache indicates possible entry into dura with a CSF leak Monitor sensorimotor function of all extremities No parenteral narcotics for at least 24 hours after initiation of epidural anesthesia Use in-line filter
Side effects unique to method	Mental status changes* Respiratory depression*	Sedation Hypotension*	Leakage from subcutaneous tissue* Local skin irritation	Respiratory depression* Pruritis Nausea, vomiting Bradycardia

*Indicates reportable condition

Table 9-37 Neurosurgical Procedures for the Management of Pain

Procedure	Description	Indications
Peripheral neurotomy	Destroys sensory modalities (via sectioning, freezing, coagulation, or chemical means) from a particular nerve	Not recommended for pain in extremities, chest wall, or head and neck
Dorsal rhizotomy (radicotomy)	Eliminates all sensation entering dorsal spinal cord but preserves motor function; percutaneous procedure an option for debilitated patients	For chest wall or head and neck pain
Anterior cordotomy (spinothalamic tractotomy)	Interrupts ascending pain and temperature fibers in anterolateral spinal cord but preserves major sensory function	Good for unilateral pain
Mediolongitudinal myelotomy (commissural myelotomy)	Interrupts pain and temperature fibers as they cross before reaching opposite spinothalamic tract	For bilateral pain, particularly involving the perineal region, the pelvis, the lower extremities, and the abdomen
Stereotactic myelotomy	Involves a small midline incision in the anterior commissure at the cervicomedullary junction and the use of precise stereotactic devices to destroy the appropriate tissue	For bilateral pain above the umbilicus
Medullary tractotomy (trigeminal tractotomy)	Sectioning of the descending spinal tract of the trigeminal nerve	For severe unresponsive ipsilateral facial pain (usually of malignant origin)
Thalamotomy	Uses of stereotactic devices to destroy specific somatosensory nuclei of the ventriculo-posterolateral and ventriculoposteromedial portions of the thalamus	For severe refractory pain of the head and neck region
Frontal lobotomy	Interruption of the frontothalamic projection fibers, affecting the patient's concern regarding the pain	For intractable pain, but used with caution since it may cause personality disturbances
Hypophysectomy	Removal or destruction of the pituitary gland	For severe pain, usually bone metastases; hormones must be replenished following this procedure
Sympathectomy	Interruption or removal of a portion of the sympathetic nervous pathway; can be done in the paravertebral sympathetic chain or in a more peripheral sympathetic ganglion	For somatic or visceral pain
Neurostimulation (transcutaneous system, TENS)	Use of benign stimulation to overload the system with fast vibratory impulses, blocking the transmission of pain impulses	For limb pain

(*continued*)

Table 9-37 Neurosurgical Procedures for the Management of Pain (*continued*)

Procedure	Description	Indications
Deep brain stimulation	Stereotactical implantation of electrodes into the periaqueductal gray matter and subsequent stimulation; believed to stimulate the release of endogenous opioids and raise pain threshold	For severe pain
Intraventricular narcotics	Placement of an intraventricular catheter with a subcutaneous reservoir (Ommaya reservoir) that can be percutaneously filled with narcotic as needed	For cervical and facial pain

Source: McGuire, D.B., & Sheidler, V.R. (1990). Pain. In S.L. Groenwald et al., *Cancer Nursing Principles and Practice* (2nd edition). Boston: Jones and Bartlett, pp. 428–429; Carson, B.S. (1987). Neurologic and neurosurgical approaches to cancer pain. In D.B. McGuire & C.H. Yarbro (Eds.), *Cancer Pain Management*. New York: McGraw-Hill, pp. 223–243.

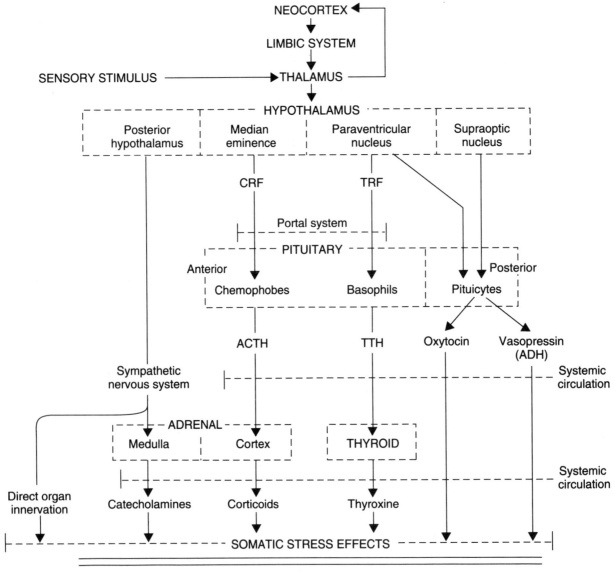

Figure 9-17 The Neuroendocrine Stress Response

Table 9-38 Cognitive Behavioral Strategies for Pain Management

Strategy	Description
Relaxation	Set of techniques used to achieve a positive state in which there is an absence of tension, manifested by psychological and physiological responses
Progressive muscle relaxation (PMR)	Series of contractions and relaxations of muscle groups while focusing the mind on relaxing and allowing tension to flow from the body; usually starts peripherally and migrates centrally and is often combined with other modalities
Imagery	A mental process that draws on the senses to conjure a mental simulation of reality that may include all the senses and may be focused on relaxing thoughts or on envisionment of body processes (for example, drug molecules and immune cells attacking cancer cells)
Altered state of consciousness	An awareness differing from the normal waking state in which the individual is focused on internal thoughts or processes; variations of methodology have different names (meditation, hypnosis, etc.)
Hypnosis	Altered state of consciousness induced through the power of suggestion by another person, who continually provides feedback during the encounter
Suggestive techniques	Ways of assisting an individual to focus thoughts on corrective behavior (for example, internal focusing on "lack of desire for food" may assist individuals trying to lose weight)
Meditation	Relaxation state induced by first focusing on breathing, then on an external object with particular meaning to subject, with intent to join the external and internal environments for balance and harmony
Yoga	A scheme for achieving tranquility principally through posture and breathing (first, diaphragmatic breathing is developed to reduce sensory input; then, a posture to achieve head, torso, and hip alignment is assumed for the duration of the breathing and meditation)

Source: Zahourek, R.P. (1988). *Relaxation and Imagery: Tools for Therapeutic Communication and Intervention.* Philadelphia: W.B. Saunders Co.

Behavior interventions Cognitive behavior interventions are psychological techniques designed to modify the patient's perception of the pain experience.[171] The multidimensional model of pain has contributed greatly to the growth of research in psychological techniques for the management of pain. Since the early 1950s, biofeedback, hypnosis, and progressive muscle relaxation have proven effective in alleviating many chronic pain syndromes and may be employed in the critical care setting as an adjunct to analgesia. The mechanism by which these interventions work is blocking the stimulation of the neuroendocrine stress response (Figure 9-17).[172] Table 9-38 presents a summary of these techniques.

Although much is yet to be learned of the benefits of nonpharmacological methods of pain relief, behavioral intervention is a strategy that can be employed to augment other management techniques. (Table 9-39 gives some samples of bedside techniques applicable to the critical care setting.) The primary barrier to application in the critical care setting is the effort and participation required of the patient. Many external environmental factors that interfere with implementation can be controlled, but it is most important that the patient has had prior relaxation training or adequate pain relief in order to participate in the process.

Nursing priorities Nurses involved in pain management in the critical care setting are faced with constant challenges in the assessment and evaluation of the patient's pain. The medical interventions outlined are truly multidisciplinary and are best approached collaboratively. In studies of the administration of pain medications, it has been shown that physicians consistently order less medication than indicated by the description of the pain and narcotic calculations for weight; then, to compound the problem, nurses consistently give less than is ordered.[173] Even after practitioners are given specialized instruction, the problem behavior remains consistent. Widespread awareness and education and use of pain consultation teams are the best strategies for combating this crucial critical care problem.

A care plan for managing the patient with pain follows this section.

Table 9-39 Cognitive Behavioral Strategies for Pain Management

Type of Strategy	Specific Technique
Breathing exercise	Patient lies flat with knees bent and spine straight and scans body for tension. Patient is to inhale slowly and deeply, feeling the abdomen rise slightly with each inhalation. Patient should inhale through the nose and exhale gently through the mouth, making a relaxing whooshing sound. Patient continues deep breathing for 5–10 minutes, focusing on the sound of the breath, the rise and fall of the abdomen, and the deepening sense of relaxation. Patient should let other thoughts or distractions pass out of his or her mind. Patient should practice the technique daily and use it whenever he or she feels tension.
Progressive muscle relaxation exercise	Patient tightens a specific muscle group, holding the tension for 5–7 seconds, and then releases all the tension. After 30–40 seconds of relaxation, patient repeats the exercise. Each muscle group is to be tensed twice, and the sequence is to be practiced in a given order with 45–60 seconds of relaxation between each muscle group. The following 16 muscle groups can be used. 1. Dominant hand and forearm: make a tight fist 2. Dominant biceps: push elbows down against arm of chair 3. Nondominant hand and forearm 4. Nondominant biceps 5. Forehead: lift eyebrows 6. Upper cheeks and nose: squint eyes and wrinkle nose 7. Lower cheeks and jaws: bite down and pull corners of mouth back 8. Neck and throat: pull chin downward without touching chest 9. Chest, shoulders, and upper back: take deep breath, hold, and pull shoulder blades back 10. Abdominal region: make stomach hard 11. Dominant thigh: push back of knee into bed or chair 12. Dominant calf: flex foot or pull toes up toward head 13. Dominant foot: turn foot inward, point and curl toes 14. Nondominant thigh 15. Nondominant calf 16. Nondominant foot During the tensing of muscles, the therapist helps the patient focus on the feelings with statements like "feel the tightness in your muscles" or "notice what the tension feels like." Similarly, during the longer relaxation period in between muscle groups, the therapist helps the patient focus on sensations by comments such as "pay attention to the feelings in your arm as it becomes more relaxed." Once the 16 muscle groups are mastered, they may be condensed into 7 and then 4 groups. (For example, muscles of both arms and hands comprise one group.)
Meditation exercise	Patient sits quietly in a comfortable position and closes eyes. Patient concentrates on deeply relaxing all the muscles, beginning at the feet and progressing up to the face. Patient is to breathe easily and naturally through the nose and become aware of his or her breathing. As patient breathes, he or she should say the word "one" silently. Exercise should continue for 10–20 minutes. Patient may open eyes to check the time, but should not use an alarm clock. When exercise is concluded, patient should remain seated quietly for several minutes, at first with eyes closed and later with eyes open. Patient should not worry about achieving a deep level of relaxation but rather maintain a passive attitude and permit relaxation to occur at its own pace. Patient should try to ignore distracting thoughts by not dwelling on them and by repeating the word "one." With practice the response should come with little effort. The technique can be practiced once or twice daily, but not within 2 hours after a meal.

Source: Titlebaum, H. (1988). Relaxation. In R. P. Zahourek (Ed.). *Relaxation and Imagery: Tools for Therapeutic Communication and Intervention.* Philadelphia: W. B. Saunders, 28–52.

Nursing Care Plan for the Management of the Patient with Pain

Diagnosis	Signs and symptoms	Intervention	Rationale
Pain	Verbalization of discomfort	Assess location, quality, intensity of pain using the unit's standard established scale	Standardization ensures consistent assessment of pain
	Nonverbal cues: grimacing, withdrawal, limited ADL, guarding, irritability	Assess patient's activity level, eating, and concentration	Unexpressed discomfort may be manifested by behavioral changes
	Anorexia		
	Insomnia		
	Tachycardia		
	Hypertension	Assess meaning of pain to the patient	Pain may be exacerbated if patient infers poor prognosis from pain
		Assess patient's ability to use and attitude toward nonpharmacological means of pain relief	Nonpharmacological means may enhance other methods of pain control
		Assess family's perceptions of patient's pain and sociocultural influences on verbalization of pain	May influence patient's attitudes or willingness to discuss discomfort
		Assess possible etiologies of pain (recent surgery or procedure, bone metastases, arthritis, infection)	To help determine acute or chronic nature of pain and, possibly, best method of alleviating it
		Determine whether non-narcotics (nonsteroidals, acetominophen) are indicated	Non-narcotics are preferred for some types of pain
		Rate pain as mild, moderate, or severe	To aid in determination of analgesic

Nursing Care Plan for the Management of the Patient with Pain

Diagnosis	Signs and symptoms	Intervention	Rationale
		Plan appropriate analgesic or interventional regimen: agent, equianalgesic dose, best route of administration, methods to supplement for breakthrough pain, enhancing agents PRN, preexisting intolerance or substance abuse, existing symptoms that may be exacerbated by analgesics	To select appropriate agent and correct dosage and to plan for supplementation to ensure achieving goal of pain relief
Potential for alteration in elimination: constipation	No bowel movement for 48 hours or more	Determine time of last bowel movement; ensure bowel movement at least every 48 hours	To prevent impaction
	Hard stools		
	Difficulty defecating		
	Abdominal discomfort or distention	Assess nature of stools and difficulty with defecation	Early signs of constipation are hard stools and difficulty in defecating
	Manual evidence of impaction		
		Maintain patient on stool softener (Docusate, Sennokot) and bulking agent (Metamucil) during narcotic administration	Preventive regimen
		Increase fluid intake to 2 L/day, if tolerated	To decrease risk of constipation
		Assess for diminished bowel sounds or distended abdomen	Possible symptoms of constipation or obstruction
		Perform manual exam for impaction if present or no bowel movement in past 48 hours	To prevent obstruction

Diagnosis	Signs and symptoms	Intervention	Rationale
Potential for alteration in elimination: urinary retention	Dysuria Bladder distention Pelvic pressure or discomfort Small, frequent voidings Postvoid residual on catheterization	Assess for bladder distention every 4 hours if urinary output is lower than expected or patient complains of pelvic discomfort	Urinary retention is a likely side effect of narcotics
		Assess I&O every shift; observe for small, frequent voids or reduced total output	To reveal trends
		Observe for cloudy urine; run culture and sensitivity PRN	Indicative of UTI, which may be caused by residual urine in bladder
Potential alteration in gas exchange, related to analgesic action on respiratory center	Hypoventilation: decreased arterial O_2 and increased CO_2 O_2 sat. $< 90\%$ Respiratory rate less than 12/minute Altered mental status, related to hypoxemia Cyanosis	Obtain baseline VS before giving analgesic	To ascertain patient's normal status
		Institute frequent checks of VS after bolus IV injection	Hypotension or sudden respiratory depression may occur with bolus dosing
		Check VS every 30 minutes during escalating doses of continuous infusions	To monitor for changes in cardiorespiratory status
		Maintain pulse oximetry, as indicated, with strong analgesic regimens	Hypoxemia is possible from hypoventilation
		Maintain apnea monitor, as indicated, with large doses of potent analgesics or unstable cardiorespiratory status	To note changes in depth or rate of respiration
		Keep Naloxone at bedside during continuous infusions or epidural analgesia	Antidote for narcotic overdose
Potential for nausea and vomiting, related to central stimulation of chemotherapy trigger zone	Verbalized sensation of nausea Anorexia Vomiting Wretching	Administer antiemetics; maximize efficacy with minimal sedative effects (Ondanstrosone has no neurotoxicities)	Patient may feel that nausea is preferable to pain
		Consider changing or reducing medication with addition of another agent	To decrease nausea

Nursing Care Plan for the Management of the Patient with Pain

Diagnosis	Signs and symptoms	Intervention	Rationale
		Provide small, frequent feedings	To decrease nausea and risk of malnutrition
		Encourage patient to lie on left side and to perform deep-breathing or relaxation exercises	To decrease nausea
Anxiety, related to pain syndrome	Verbalization of anxiety Anxious facial expressions Angry, hostile behavior Fear Emotional lability Withdrawal	Assess patient's anxiety level and its contribution or correlation to expressed pain	Many pain syndromes are accompanied by anxiety
		Initiate distraction or relaxation measures and assess patient response	Responsiveness to such interventions may give clues to effective therapy strategy
		Assess for variables that increase anxious behavior or pain: visitors, health care providers, certain procedures, etc.	To possibly eliminate or reduce variables or treat patient with medication
		Administer anxiolytic agents as ordered and indicated; assess for changes in behavior or pain patterns	Known to enhance analgesics and improve affective component of pain
Potential for maladaptive coping	Pain relief requirements increasing beyond predicted physiological needs Inability to perform ADLs	Continually assess patient pain rating and compare to expected pain pattern; investigate all expressions of unusual or excessive pain for organic causes	To discover any new pain patterns or etiologies
		Provide emotional support during attempts at pain alleviation	Patient deserves and needs empathic treatment during this hardship

Diagnosis	Signs and symptoms	Intervention	Rationale
Potential for altered thought processes, related to neurotoxic effects of analgesics	Confusion Disorientation Inappropriate behavior Inability to concentrate Lethargy Sleepiness or insomnia Hallucinations	Assess orientation with each patient encounter; note deviations and follow up on findings	Catching deviations early may prevent severe toxicity
		Evaluate mental status every 4–8 hours, unless indicated more often	To assess for untoward effects of medications
		Have patient describe concentration problems or sleep disturbances and distress they cause	To discover level of patient distress and help develop care plan
		Report inappropriate behavior or hallucinations immediately	May require immediate discontinuation of medication
		Exercise safety and fall precautions	Patient is at high risk for falls

CHAPTER 9 POST-TEST

1. The most appropriate analgesic for postoperative hip replacement discomfort is:
   a. a nonsteroidal antiinflammatory agent.
   b. a narcotic in combination with an anxiolytic.
   c. morphine sulfate.
   d. percodan.

2. Common side effects of opioid analgesics include:
   a. pruritis.
   b. vasoconstriction with chills and sweating.
   c. constipation.
   d. urinary incontinence.

3. Functions of the skin include:
   a. thermoregulation.
   b. fluid transport.
   c. electrical conduction for muscular contraction.
   d. coagulation of RBCs in healing.

4. Which of the following is a consequence of edema formation in burn shock?
   a. vasoconstriction
   b. inadequate tissue perfusion
   c. shunting
   d. hypercalcemia

5. Absolute leukocytosis may be caused by poisoning by which of the following substances?
   a. calcium gluconate
   b. Lidocaine
   c. theophylline
   d. an opiate

6. Which of the following requires immediate hemodialysis or hemoperfusion?
   a. toxic ethanol poisoning
   b. inderal overdose
   c. heroin overdose
   d. thorazine overdose

Refer to the following clinical vignette to answer questions 7 and 8.

A 55-year-old diabetic patient is admitted for urosepsis and subsequent antibiotic therapy. At 8 p.m. on the day of admission, he fainted in the bathroom. When he was returned to bed, it was found that he was tachycardic and orthostatic, with supine BP = 100/50 and sitting BP = 84/44. A fluid challenge of 500 cc was given, with a resulting BP normalization but continued tachycardia. At 10 p.m., the patient spiked a temperature of 39.6°C, and his BP dropped to 78/48. At the same time, the patient became slightly confused.

7. Immediate interventions in the care of this patient will most likely include:
   a. continued fluid challenges and arterial line insertion.
   b. Swan-Ganz insertion and a 12-lead ECG.
   c. oxygen therapy and a CT scan.
   d. arterial blood gas analysis and insertion of a nasal gastric tube.

8. The patient is probably displaying symptoms indicative of:
   a. hypovolemic shock.
   b. acute pulmonary embolism.
   c. hyperdynamic septic shock.
   d. a cardiovascular event.

ENDNOTES

1. Pinsky, M. R. and Matuschak, G. M. (1989). Multiple systems organ failure: Failure of host defense homeostasis. *Critical Care Clinics,* 5 (2): 199–220.
2. Wahl, S. C. (1989). Septic shock: How to detect it early. *Nursing 89,* 19 (1): 52–59.
3. Pinsky and Matuschak, op. cit.; Knaus, W. A. and Wagner, D. P. (1989). Multiple systems organ failure: Epidemiology and prognosis. *Critical Care Clinics,* 5 (2): 221–232.
4. Wahl, op. cit.; Balk, R. A. and Bone, R. C. (1989). The septic syndrome: Definition and clinical implications. *Critical Care Clinics,* 5 (1): 1–8.
5. Balk and Bone, op. cit.; Segreti, J. (1989). Nosocomial infections and secondary infections in sepsis. *Critical Care Clinics,* 5 (1): 177–189.

6. Parker, M. M. (1990). Cardiac dysfunction in humans. In Parillo, J. E. (Moderator), Septic shock in humans: Advances in pathogenesis, cardiovascular dysfunction and therapy. *Annals of Internal Medicine,* 113: 227–242.
7. Balk and Bone, op. cit.; Sheagren, J. N. (1989). Mechanism oriented therapy for multiple systems organ failure. *Critical Care Clinics,* 5 (2): 393–409.
8. Wahl, op. cit.; Parker, op. cit.
9. *Morbidity and Mortality Weekly Report 39* (5): September 7, 1990.
10. Rice, V. (Sept./Oct. 1984). The clinical continuum of septic shock: Home study course. *Critical Care Nurse:* 86–109.
11. Sheagren, op. cit.; Hurst, J. W. (Ed.). (1987). *Medicine for the Practicing Physician* (2nd edition). Boston:

Little, Brown; Sprague, R. S.; Stephenson, A. H.; Dahms, T. E.; and Lonigro, A. J. (1989). Proposed role of leukotrienes in the pathophysiology of multiple systems organ failure. *Critical Care Clinics, 5* (2): 315–329.

12. Sheagren, op. cit.; Sprague, op. cit.

13. Cunnion, R. E. and Parillo, J. E. (1989). Myocardial dysfunction in sepsis. *Critical Care Clinics, 5* (1): 99–118.

14. Lefer, A. M. (1989). Induction of tissue injury and altered cardiovascular performance by platelet-activating factor: Relevance to multiple systems organ failure. *Critical Care Clinics, 5* (2): 331–352.

15. Simpson, S. Q. and Casey, L. C. (1989). The role of tumor necrosis factor and acute lung injury. *Critical Care Clinics, 5* (1): 27–47; Bersten, A. and Sibbald, W. J. (1989). Acute lung injury in septic shock. *Critical Care Clinics, 5* (1): 49–79.

16. Sheagren, op. cit.

17. Parillo, J. (1987). *The Critically Ill Immunosuppressed Patient: Diagnosis and Management.* Rockville, MD: Aspen.

18. Sheagren, op. cit.

19. Parillo, op. cit.

20. Parillo (1987), op. cit.

21. Bersten and Sibbald, op. cit.

22. Ibid.

23. Ibid.

24. Cerra, F. B. (1989a). Hypermetabolism—organ failure syndrome: A metabolic response to injury. *Critical Care Clinics, 5* (2): 289–302.

25. Bersten and Sibbald, op. cit.

26. Thompson, J. M.; McFarland, G. K.; Tucker, S. M.; and Bowers, A. C. (Eds.). (1989). *Mosby's Manual of Clinical Nursing* (3rd edition). St. Louis: C. V. Mosby.

27. Cerra, F. B. (1989b). Metabolic manifestations of multiple systems organ failure. *Critical Care Clinics, 5* (1): 119–131.

28. Ibid.

29. Berkow, R. (Ed.). (1987). *The Merck Manual* (15th edition). Rahway, NJ: Merck Sharp & Dohme Research Laboratories.

30. Ibid.

31. Wahl, op. cit.

32. Ibid.

33. Littleton, M. T. (1988). Pathophysiology and assessment of sepsis and septic shock. *Critical Care Nursing Quarterly, 11* (1): 30–47.

34. Rice, op. cit.

35. Cerra (1989a), op. cit.

36. Springhouse Corporation. (1991). *Clinical Skillbuilders: IV Therapy.* Springhouse, PA: Springhouse Corporation.

37. Borzotta, A. P. and Polk, H. C. (1983). Multiple systems organ failure. *Surgical Clinics of North America, 63* (2): 315–336.

38. Wahl, op. cit.; Balk and Bone, op. cit.; Bersten and Sibbald, op. cit.; Hudson, L. D. (1989). Multiple systems organ failure (MSOF): Lessons learned from the adult respiratory distress syndrome (ARDS). *Critical Care Clinics, 5* (3): 697–705.

39. Parillo (1987), op. cit.

40. Natanson, C. and Parillo, J. E. (1988). Septic shock. *Anesthesiology Clinics of North America, 6* (1): 73–85.

41. Ibid.

42. Balk and Bone, op. cit.; Sheagren, op. cit.

43. Barry, S. A. (1989). Septic shock: Special needs of patients with cancer. *Oncology Nursing Forum, 16* (1): 31–35.

44. Natanson and Parillo, op. cit.

45. Ibid.

46. Kuhn, M. M. (1991). Colloids versus crystalloids. *Critical Care Nurse, 11* (5): 37–51.

47. Ibid.

48. Truett, L. and Ewer, M. S. (1989). Shock: Managing the septic syndrome in patients with cancer. *Dimensions in Oncology Nursing, 3* (4): 9–13.

49. Ibid.

50. Parillo (1987), op. cit.; Boyd, J. L., III; Stanford, G. G.; and Chernow, B. (1989). The pharmacotherapy of septic shock. *Critical Care Clinics, 5* (1): 133–150.

51. Natanson and Parillo, op. cit.

52. Boyd et al., op. cit.

53. Ibid.

54. Ibid.

55. Ibid.; Schumann, L. L. and Remington, M. A. (1990). The use of naloxone in treating endotoxic shock. *Critical Care Nurse, 10* (2): 63–73.

56. Boyd et al., op. cit.

57. Lee, R. M.; Balk, R. A.; and Bone, R. C. (1989). Ventilatory support in the management of septic patients. *Critical Care Clinics, 5* (1): 157–175.

58. Ibid.

59. Rice, op. cit.

60. Springhouse Corporation, op. cit.

61. Bone, R. C.; Fisher, C. J., Jr.; Clemmer, T. P.; Slotman, G. J.; Metz, C. A.; and Balk, R. A. (1989). Sepsis syndrome: A valid clinical entity. *Critical Care Medicine, 17* (5): 389–393; Hinshaw, L.; Wilson, M.; and the VA Sepsis Study Group. (1987). Effect of high dose glucocorticoid therapy on mortality in patients with clinical signs of systemic sepsis. *New England Journal of Medicine, 317:* 659–665.

62. Nicholson, D. P. (1989). Review of corticosteroid treatment in sepsis and septic shock; Pro or con. *Critical Care Clinics, 5* (1): 151–155.

63. Hurst, op. cit.

64. Nicholson, op. cit.

65. Carrico, C. J.; Meakins, J. L.; Marshall, J. C.; Fry, D.; and Maier, R. B. (1986). Multiple organ failure syndrome—the gastrointestinal tract: The 'motor' of MOF. *Archives of Surgery, 121* (2): 197–201.

66. Sheagren, op. cit.

67. Bauer, A. E. and Chaudry, I. H. (1980). Prevention of multiple systems organ failure. *Surgical Clinics of North America, 60* (5): 1167–1178; Pinsky, M. R. (1989). Multiple systems organ failure: Malignant intravascular inflammation. *Critical Care Clinics, 5* (2): 195–198.

68. Pinsky, op. cit.

69. Fry, D. E.; Pearlstein, L.; Fulton, R. L.; and Polk, H. C. (1980). Multiple systems organ failure: The role of uncontrolled infection. *Archives of Surgery, 115* (2): 136–140.

70. Knaus and Wagner, op. cit.; Knaus, W. A., et al. (1985a). APACHE II: A severity of disease classification system. *Clinical Care Medicine, 13* (10): 818–829; Knaus, W. A., et al. (1985b). Prognosis in acute organ system failure. *Annals of Surgery, 202* (6): 685–693.

71. Pinsky, op. cit.

72. Knaus et al. (1985a), op. cit.; Knaus et al. (1985b), op. cit.

73. Knaus et al. (1985a), op. cit.; Knaus et al. (1985b), op. cit.; Faist, E.; Baue, A. E.; Dittmer, H.; and Heberer, G. (1983). Multiple organ failure in polytrauma patients. *The Journal of Trauma, 23* (9): 775–787; Manship, L.; McMillin, R. D.; and Brown, J. J. (1984). The influence of sepsis and multisystem organ failure on mortality in the surgical intensive care unit. *The American Surgeon, 50* (2): 94–101.

74. Knaus and Wagner, op. cit.; Balk and Bone, op. cit.

75. Knaus and Wagner, op. cit.; Fry et al., op. cit.; Knaus et al. (1985a), op. cit.; Knaus et al. (1985b), op. cit.; Manship et al., op. cit.

76. Knaus and Wagner, op. cit.

77. Cerra (1989b), op. cit.; Faist, et al., op. cit.

78. Faist et al., op. cit.

79. Pinsky and Matuschak, op. cit.; Balk and Bone, op. cit.; Sheagren, op. cit.; Perry, A. G. (1988). Shock complications: Recognition and management. *Critical Care Nursing Quarterly, 11* (1): 1–8.

80. Sander, J. H.; van Deventer, H. R.; Buller, H. R.; ten Cate, J. W.; Aarden, L. A.; Hack, C. E.; and Sturk, A. (1990). Experimental endotoxemia in humans: Analysis of cytokine release and coagulation, fibrinolytic, and complement pathways. *Blood, 76* (12): 2520–2526.

81. Cerra (1989b), op. cit.

82. Pinsky and Matuschak, op. cit.; Cerra (1989a), op. cit.; Cerra (1989b), op. cit.

83. Pinsky and Matuschak, op. cit.; Carrico et al., op. cit.

84. Ibid.

85. Pinsky and Matuschak, op. cit.; Sheagren, op. cit.; Macho, J. R. and Luce, J. M. (1989). Rational approach to the management of multiple systems organ failure. *Critical Care Clinics, 5* (2): 379–392.

86. Carrico et al., op. cit.; Macho and Luce, op. cit.

87. Pinsky and Matuschak, op. cit.; Sheagren, op. cit.; Simpson and Casey, op. cit.; Boyd et al., op. cit.; Sander et al., op. cit.; Macho and Luce, op. cit.

88. Pinsky and Matuschak, op. cit.; Cerra (1989a), op. cit.; Cerra (1989b), op. cit.; Macho and Luce, op. cit.

89. Pinsky and Matuschak, op. cit.; Sheagren, op. cit.; Cerra (1989b), op. cit.; Springhouse Corporation, op. cit.; Sander et al., op. cit.

90. Pinsky and Matuschak, op. cit.; Sheagren, op. cit.; Carrico et al., op. cit.; Macho and Luce, op. cit.

91. Pinsky and Matuschak, op. cit.; Sheagren, op. cit.; Boyd et al., op. cit.

92. Hall, A. H. and Rumack, B. H. (1989). Diagnosis and treatment of poisoning. In Shoemaker, W. C., Ayres, S. A., et al. (Eds.), *Textbook of Critical Care* (pp. 1170–1179). Philadelphia: W. B. Saunders.

93. Casani, J. A. P. (1989). Adult epidemiology. In Noji, E. K. and Kelen, G. D. (Eds.), *Manual of Toxicologic Emergencies* (pp. 3–6). Chicago: Yearbook Publishers.

94. Foserelli, P. D. (1989). Pediatric epidemiology. In Noji, E. K. and Kelen, G. D. (Eds.), *Manual of Toxicologic Emergencies* (pp. 6–9). Chicago: Yearbook Publishers.

95. Madden, C. (1989). Narcotics/opioids. In Noji, E. K. and Kelen, G. D. (Eds.), *Manual of Toxicologic Emergencies* (pp. 333–344). Chicago: Yearbook Publishers.

96. Sprague et al., op. cit.

97. Kulig, K., et al. (1985). Management of acutely poisoned patients without gastric emptying. *Annals of Emergency Medicine, 14* (6): 59–64.

98. Wogan, J. M. (Spring 1991). Lecture to emergency medicine residents, Johns Hopkins School of Medicine.

99. Kelen, G. D. and Noji, E. K. (1989). Advanced poisoning treatment and life support. In Noji, E. K. and Kelen, G. D. (Eds.), *Manual of Toxicologic Emergencies* (pp. 25–29). Chicago: Yearbook Publishers.

100. Ellenhorn, J. J. and Barceloux, D. G. (1988). *Medical Toxicology.* New York: Elsevier.

101. Kulig, op. cit.

102. Park, G. D., et al. (1986). Expanded role of charcoal therapy in the poisoned and overdosed patient. *Archives of Internal Medicine, 146:* 969–973; Krenzelok, E. P., et al. (1985). Gastrointestinal transit times of cathartics combined with charcoal. *Annals of Emergency Medicine, 14* (12): 45–48; Kirshenbaum, L. A.; Sitar, D. S.; and Tenenbein, M. (1980). Interaction between whole bowel irrigation solution and activated charcoal: Implications for the treatment of toxic ingestions. *Annals of Emergency Medicine, 19* (10): 97–100.

103. Pond, S. M. (1984). Renal principles: Diuresis, dialysis, and hemoperfusion. Symposium on Medical Toxicology. *Emergency Medical Clinics of North America, 2* (1).

104. Safar, P. (1989). Cardiopulmonary-cerebral resuscitation. In Shoemaker, W. C.; Ayres, S. A.; Grenvik, A.; Holbrook, P. R.; and Thompson, W. L. (Eds.), *Textbook of Critical Care:* Philadelphia: W. B. Saunders, p. 29.

105. Mosely, S. (1988). Inhalation injury: A review of the literature. *Heart & Lung, 17* (1): 3–9.

106. Herndon, D. N., et al. (1987). Pulmonary injury in burned patients. *Surgical Clinics of North America, 67* (1): 31–43.

107. Shirani, K. Z.; Moylan, J. A.; and Pruitt, B. A. (1988). Diagnosis and treatment of inhalation injury in burn patients. In Loke, J. (Ed.), *Pathophysiology and Treatment of Inhalation Injuries.* New York: Marcel Dekker, pp. 239–269.

108. Demling, R. H. (1985). Burn injury. *Acute Care, 11:* 119–186.

109. Martindale, L. G. (1989). Carbon monoxide poisoning: The rest of the story. *Journal of Emergency Nursing, 15* (2): 101–103.

110. Silverman, S. H.; Purdue, G. F.; Hunt, J. L.; and Bost, R. O. (1988). Cyanide toxicity in burned patients. *Journal of Trauma, 28* (2): 171–176.

111. Dailey, M. A. (1989). Carbon monoxide poisoning. *Journal of Emergency Nursing, 15* (2): 120–123.

112. Haponik, E. F.; Adelman, M.; Munster, A. M.; and Bleecker, E. R. (1986). Increased vascular pedicle width preceding burn related pulmonary edema. *Chest, 90* (5): 649–659.

113. Bingham, H. G.; Gallagher, T. J.; and Powell, M. D. (1987). Early bronchoscopy as a predictor of ventilatory support for burned patients. *Journal of Trauma, 27* (11): 1286–1288; Hubbard, G. B., et al. (1988). Smoke inhalation injury in sheep. *American Journal of Pathology, 133* (3): 660–663.

114. Thomas, C. L. (Ed.). (1989). *Taber's Cyclopedic Medical Dictionary.* Philadelphia: F. A. Davis, p. 533; Gonzalez-Rothi, R. J. (1987). Near-drowning: Consensus and controversies in pulmonary and cerebral resuscitation. *Heart & Lung, 16* (5): 474–481.

115. Fields, A. I. and Holbrook, P. R. (1989). Near-drowning in the pediatric population. In Shoemaker, W. C., et al. (Eds.), *Textbook of Critical Care.* Philadelphia: W. B. Saunders, pp. 67–69.

116. Widner-Kohlberg, M. and Maloney-Harmon, P. (1988). Pediatric trauma. In Cardona, V., et al. (Eds.), *Trauma Nursing.* Philadelphia: W. B. Saunders, 664–745.

117. Sivertson, K. T. (February 24, 1989). Hypothermia. Lecture presented to emergency medicine residents, Johns Hopkins School of Medicine.

118. Modell, J. H. and Boysen, P. G. (1989). Drowning and near-drowning. In Shoemaker, W. C., et al. (Eds.), *Textbook of Critical Care.* Philadelphia: W. B. Saunders, pp. 64–66.

119. Neagley, S. R. (1991). The pulmonary system. In Alspach, J. (Ed.), *Core Curriculum for Critical Care Nursing.* Philadelphia: W. B. Saunders, pp. 112–114.

120. Dettbarn, C. L. and Davidson, L. J. (1989). Pulmo-

nary complications in the patient with acute head injury: Neurogenic pulmonary edema. *Heart & Lung, 18* (6): 583–589.

121. Johnston, J. B. (1988). Hypothermia: Assessment and intervention. *Emergency Nursing Reports, 3* (8): 1–7.

122. Wong, K. C. (1983). Physiology and pharmacology of hypothermia. *Western Journal of Medicine, 138* (2): 227–232.

123. Feller, I. (March 2, 1985). *National Burn Information Exchange Report.* Ann Arbor, MI: NBIE.

124. Munster, A. M. (1980). *Burn Care for the House Officer.* Baltimore: Williams and Wilkens, p. 7.

125. Cram, E. K.; Traber, D.; Wallfisch, H.; and Demling, R. (1991). Pulmonary problems in the burn patient. In *American Burn Association Course #1 Workbook.* Proceedings of the American Burn Association convention, Baltimore, MD.

126. Feller, I., and Archambeault, C. (1973). *Nursing the Burned Patient.* Ann Arbor, MI: Institute for Burn Medicine, p. 3.

127. Trofino, R. B. (1991). *Nursing Care of the Burn-Injured Patient.* Philadelphia: F. A. Davis, pp. 139–140.

128. Johnson, K.; Demling, R.; Carrongher, G.; Meyer, A.; and Deitch, E. (1991). Cardiovascular problems in the burn patient. In *American Burn Association Course #2 Workbook.* Proceedings of the American Burn Association convention, Baltimore, MD.

129. Ibid.

130. Trofino, op. cit.

131. Artz, C. P.; Moncrief, J. A.; and Pruitt, B. A. (Eds.). (1979). *Burns: A Team Approach.* Philadelphia: W. B. Saunders, p. 529.

132. Martyn, J. A. J. (1990). *Acute Management of the Burn Patient.* Philadelphia: W. B. Saunders, p. 176.

133. Ibid.

134. Haponik, E. F. and Munster, A. M. (1990). *Respiratory Injury: Smoke Inhalation and Burns.* New York: McGraw-Hill, p. 49.

135. Trofino, op. cit.

136. Haponik, op. cit.

137. Munster, A. M. (1986). Infections in burns. In *Clinical Use of Intravenous Immunoglobulins.* London: Academic Press, p. 339.

138. Munster, A. M. and Winchurch, R. A. (1985). Infection and Immunology. *Critical Care Clinics, 1* (1): 120.

139. Ibid.

140. Munster, A. M.; Moran, K. T.; Thupari, J.; Allo, M.; and Winchurch, R. A. (1987). Prophylactic intravenous immunoglobulin replacement in high-risk burn patients. *Journal of Burn Care Rehabilitation, 8* (5): 376–380.

141. Munster and Winchurch, op. cit.

142. Munster, op. cit.

143. Munster et al., op. cit.

144. Smith, S. L. (1986). Physiology of the immune system. *Critical Care Quarterly, 9* (1): 7–13.

145. Bernstein, N. R. and Robson, M. C. (Eds.). (1983). *Comprehensive Approaches to the Burned Person.* New Hyde Park, NY: Medical Examination Publishing, p. 16.

146. Lewis, S. M. and Collier, I. C. (1983). *Medical-Surgical Nursing: Assessment and Management of Clinical Problems.* New York: McGraw-Hill, p. 275.

147. Trofino, op. cit., p. 155.

148. Ibid., p. 156.

149. Ibid., p. 332.

150. Martyn, op. cit., p. 17.

151. Trofino, op. cit., p. 335.

152. Trofino, op. cit., p. 155.

153. Wagner, M. M. (Ed.). (1981). *Care of the Burn-Injured Patient.* New York: Littleton, p. 30.

154. Trofino, op. cit., p. 143.

155. Marvin, J. A. (1991). Infection control. *American Burn Association Course: Infection in the Burn Patient.* Baltimore: American Burn Association.

156. International Association for the Study of Pain, Subcommittee on Taxonomy. (1979). Pain terms: A list with definitions and usage. *Pain, 6:* 249–252.

157. McCaffrey, M. and Beebe, A. (1989). *Pain: A Clinical Manual for Nursing Practice.* St. Louis: C. V. Mosby.

158. Melzack, R. and Walls, P. D. (1965). Pain mechanisms: A new theory. *Science, 150:* 971–979.

159. Ahles, T. A.; Blanchard, E. B.; and Ruckdeschel, J. C. (1983). The multidimensional nature of cancer-related pain. *Pain, 17:* 277–288.

160. McGuire, D. B. (1987). Cancer related pain: A multidimensional approach. Unpublished doctoral dissertation. Chicago: University of Illinois at Chicago Health Sciences Center.

161. McGuire, D. B. and Sheidler, V. R. (1990). Pain. In S. L. Groenwald, M. H. Frogge, M. Goodman, and C. H. Yarbro (Eds.), *Cancer Nursing Principles and Practice* (2nd edition). Boston: Jones and Bartlett.

162. Donovan, M. I. (1985). Nursing assessment of cancer pain. *Seminars in Oncology Nursing, 1:* 109–115.

163. Bonica, J. J. and Benedetti, C. (1980). Postoperative pain. In R. D. Condon and J. J. Decosse (Eds.), *Surgical Care: A Physiologic Approach to Clinical Management.* Philadelphia: Lea and Febiger, pp. 394–415.

164. Fields, H. L. (1987). *Pain.* New York: McGraw-Hill.

165. McGuire and Sheidler, op. cit.

166. Mlynczak, B. (1989). Assessment and management of the trauma patient in pain. *Critical Care Nursing Clinics of North America, 1* (1):55–65.

167. Coyle, N. and Portenoy, R. K. (1990). Advances in cancer pain management. In P. Ashwanden, A. E. Belcher, E. A. H. Mattson, R. Moskowitz, and N. E. Riese (Eds.), *Oncology Nursing Advances, Treatments and Trends into the 21st Century.* Rockville, MD: Aspen, pp. 122–138.

168. Olsson, G. L.; Leddo, C. C.; and Wild, L. (1989). Nursing management of patients receiving epidural narcotics. *Heart & Lung, 18* (2): 130–138.

169. Bailey, P. L.; Pace, N. L.; Ashburn, M. A.; Moll, J. W. B.; East, K. A.; and Stanley, T. H. (1990). Frequent hypoxemia and apnea after sedation with midazolam and fentanyl. *Anesthesiology, 73:* 826–830.

170. Carson, B. S. (1987). Neurologic and neurosurgical approaches to cancer pain. In D. B. McGuire and C. H. Yarbro (Eds.), *Cancer Pain Management.* New York: Grune and Stratton.

171. Allen, R. J. (1983). *Human Stress: Its Nature and Control.* New York: Macmillan; Ahles, T. A. (1987). Psychological techniques for the management of cancer-related pain. In D. B. McGuire and C. H. Yarbro (Eds.), *Cancer Pain Management.* New York: Grune and Stratton; Zahourek, R. P. (1988). *Relaxation and Imagery: Tools for Therapeutic Communication and Intervention.* Philadelphia: W. B. Saunders.

172. Ahles, op. cit.; Zahourek, op. cit.

173. McGuire and Sheidler, op. cit.

ANSWERS TO PRE- AND POST-TESTS

CHAPTER 1
Sample Exam (pages 8–17)

1-b; 2-d; 3-c; 4-a; 5-b; 6-d; 7-b; 8-d; 9-a; 10-c; 11-d; 12-d; 13-c; 14-b; 15-b; 16-d; 17-c; 18-c; 19-a; 20-d; 21-b; 22-a; 23-c; 24-d; 25-b; 26-c; 27-d; 28-a; 29-b; 30-c; 31-b; 32-a; 33-a; 34-d; 35-b; 36-b; 37-a; 38-b; 39-a; 40-b; 41-a; 42-b; 43-b; 44-b; 45-c; 46-c; 47-b; 48-a; 49-c; 50-c; 51-c; 52-c; 53-c; 54-b; 55-c; 56-d; 57-b; 58-b; 59-d; 60-c; 61-b; 62-c; 63-d; 64-b; 65-d; 66-b; 67-c; 68-d; 69-d; 70-b; 71-b; 72-b; 73-c; 74-a; 75-b; 76-b; 77-a; 78-d; 79-a; 80-b; 81-b; 82-d; 83-c; 84-b; 85-c; 86-c; 87-a; 88-c; 89-b; 90-d; 91-b; 92-d; 93-c; 94-a; 95-d; 96-c; 97-b; 98-c; 99-b; 100-a

CHAPTER 2
Pre-Test (page 19)

1-c; 2-c; 3-d; 4-b; 5-d; 6-c; 7-d; 8-b; 9-c; 10-a; 11-d; 12-b; 13-c; 14-b; 15-d; 16-b; 17-b; 18-b; 19-c; 20-c; 21-d; 22-a

Post-Test (page 230)

1-d; 2-c; 3-d; 4-d; 5-a; 6-c; 7-a; 8-b; 9-c; 10-a; 11-c; 12-a; 13-b; 14-b; 15-b; 16-d; 17-c; 18-c; 19-d; 20-b; 21-c; 22-c

CHAPTER 3
Pre-Test (page 235)

1-c; 2-c; 3-b; 4-c; 5-d; 6-a; 7-c; 8-a

Post-Test (page 465)

1-a; 2-b; 3-b; 4-d; 5-d; 6-a; 7-d; 8-a

CHAPTER 4
Pre-Test (page 468)

1-c; 2-d; 3-d; 4-d; 5-a; 6-a; 7-a; 8-b; 9-c; 10-b; 11-a; 12-b; 13-d; 14-d; 15-b; 16-c; 17-d; 18-b; 19-d; 20-b; 21-c; 22-b; 23-a; 24-a; 25-b; 26-b; 27-c; 28-d; 29-a; 30-a; 31-a; 32-b; 33-c; 34-d; 35-a; 36-c; 37-a; 38-b; 39-d

Post-Test (page 737)

1-b; 2-a; 3-d; 4-a; 5-c; 6-a; 7-a; 8-a; 9-a; 10-d; 11-a; 12-d; 13-c; 14-d; 15-d; 16-b; 17-b; 18-b; 19-c; 20-c; 21-c; 22-d; 23-c; 24-a; 25-c; 26-b; 27-c; 28-a; 29-a; 30-b; 31-c; 32-a; 33-c; 34-b; 35-b; 36-a; 37-b; 38-c; 39-b

CHAPTER 5
Pre-Test (page 742)

1-a; 2-d; 3-b; 4-c; 5-b; 6-d; 7-a; 8-b; 9-c; 10-b

Post-Test (page 826)

1-b; 2-b; 3-b; 4-c; 5-d; 6-d; 7-a; 8-b; 9-c; 10-d

CHAPTER 6
Pre-Test (page 830)

1-c; 2-a; 3-b; 4-d; 5-b; 6-c; 7-d; 8-c; 9-a; 10-d

Post-Test (page 985)

1-b; 2-a; 3-d; 4-b; 5-c; 6-d; 7-a; 8-a; 9-c; 10-d

CHAPTER 7
Pre-Test (page 991)

1-a; 2-b; 3-a; 4-c; 5-b; 6-c

Post-Test (page 1070)

1-c; 2-a; 3-c; 4-c; 5-a; 6-b

CHAPTER 8
Pre-Test (page 1074)

1-b; 2-b; 3-b; 4-a; 5-d; 6-d; 7-a; 8-b; 9-c; 10-d; 11-c

Post-Test (page 1244)

1-c; 2-b; 3-b; 4-d; 5-a; 6-c; 7-b; 8-d; 9-d; 10-b; 11-c

CHAPTER 9
Pre-Test (page 1249)

1-c; 2-c; 3-b; 4-d; 5-a; 6-b; 7-b; 8-d

Post-Test (page 1358)

1-c; 2-c; 3-a; 4-b; 5-c; 6-a; 7-a; 8-c

for myocardial infarction, 522
normal levels of, 82–83
regulation of, 756–58
Potassium chloride, 774
Pralidoxime, 1293
Precordial pulsations, 492
Prednisolone, 1044
for air leak syndrome, 229
for asthma, 163
for hepatitis, 929
for pulmonary aspiration, 209
for thoracic trauma, 198
for transplant, 1206
Prednisone
for acute adrenal insufficiency, 1044
for acute spinal cord injury, 343
for AIDS, 1160
for anaphylaxis, 1139
for hepatitis, 929
for hypercalcemia, 782
for neurological disorders, 287, 307, 364, 386, 407, 425, 444
for respiratory disorders, 150, 163, 198, 209, 229
for seizure disorders, 463
for transplant, 1206
Preexcitation, 572, 574
Pregnancy, 888, 1037
Preload, 484, 487
Premature atrial contractions (PACs), 584–85
Premature junctional contraction (PJC), 589
Premature ventricular contractions (PVCs), 594–95
Pressoreceptors (baroreceptors), 488, 489
Pressure control inverse ratio ventila-ion (PC-IRV), 100–101, 124
Pressure drainage systems, 216
Presystolic gallop, 496
Primidone
for encephalopathy, 444
for head trauma, 307
for increased intracranial pressure, 287
for intracranial hemorrhage, 386
for neurological lesions, 364
for seizure disorders, 463
Printzmetal's angina, 512
Pro-Banthine, 863, 913
Procainamide
for atrial flutter, 588
and conduction defects, 569
for dysrhythmias, 603
for paroxysmal atrial tachycardia, 586
for premature atrial contractions, 585
and Q-T interval, 498
for ventricular tachycardia, 595
Prodromal period, 311, 446, 448
Progressive multifocal leukoencephalopathy (PML), 1152

Progressive muscle relaxation (PMR), 1351, 1352
Prolactin (LTH), 995
Prolapsed valves, 495
Prolixin, 1004
Propoxyphene, 1285, 1286, 1345
Propranolol (Inderal)
for angina pectoris, 517
for atrial flutter, 588
for cardiac transplantation, 699
for cerebral aneurysm, 323
for dysrhythmias, 603
for hypertensive shock, 553
for myocardial infarction, 531
for paroxysmal atrial tachycardia, 586
for pheochromocytoma, 1038
for portal hypertension, 953
for premature atrial contractions, 585
side effects of, 569, 998, 1053, 1062, 1175
for thyroid disorders, 1024, 1036
for vascular disorders, 719
Proprioception, 265
Propylthiouracil, 998
Prostaglandin E, 702, 719
Prostaglandins
as anaphylaxis mediators, 1134, 1135
and blood flow, 490
for multisystem organ failure, 1283, 1284
role of, 993
Protamine sulfate, 505, 702, 718
Protein metabolism, 849, 1000
Proteus, 1253
Prothrombin time (PT)
and clotting factor deficiencies, 1174
for diagnosis of DIC, 1192, 1193
and hepatitis, 919, 920, 928
use of, 497, 1121, 1178
Protodiastole, 482
Protodiastolic gallop, 496
Proximal convoluted tubule (PCT), 748, 751
Proximal splenorenal shunt, 952, 953
Pseudomonas, 1253, 1259
Pulmonary artery catheters, 485–86
Pulmonary artery pressure (PAP), 486–87, 1190
Pulmonary aspiration, 199–201
care plan for, 202–8
medications used in treatment of, 201, 209
Pulmonary capillary wedge pressure (PCWP), 487–88
Pulmonary disorders. *See* Respiratory system disorders.
Pulmonary edema, 554–61
ALI, 102
assessment of, 69
care plan for, 562–66
medications used in treatment of, 567–68

following near-drowning, 1304
versus pulmonary hemorrhage, 187
types and causes of, 42–44, 102, 557–58, 559
Pulmonary embolus, 81, 348–49. *See also* Acute pulmonary embolus.
Pulmonary fibrosis, 36
Pulmonary function testing, 77–82
Pulmonary hypertension, 42, 43
Pulmonary infarct, 166
Pulmonary perfusion, 40–44
Pulmonary valve, 474
Pulmonary vascular resistance (PVR), 42, 484
Pulmonic stenosis, 661
Pulse, 492–93, 519
Pulsus alterans, 492, 519, 559
Pulsus paradoxus, 492, 534
Pupillary responses, 261, 272
Purkinje fibers, 478, 479
Pyelogram, 765, 820, 892
Pyloric valve, 841
Pyrazinamide (PZA), 1164
Pyridamole, 720
Pyridoxine, 1293
Pyrimethamine, 1157, 1160, 1261

Q-T interval, 498, 569
Q wave, 520
QRS complex
and axis deviations, 499, 503
in cardiac cycle, 483
and conduction defects, 572
effect of antidysrhythmics on, 569
in electrocardiogram, 497–98
QRS interval, 569–71, 573–74
Quinidine
and atrial flutter, 587, 588
for cardiac transplantation, 703
and conduction defects, 569
for dysrhythmias, 603
for premature atrial contractions, 585
and Q-T interval, 498
side effects of, 1175
Quinine, 1175

R waves, 572
Radioactive iodine, 1024, 1036
Radioallergosorbent test (RAST), 1139
Radiocontrast media (RCM), reactions to, 1132, 1133
Radiography, 820, 877, 878
Radionuclide diagnostic testing, 503–5
Rales, 66
Ranitidine hydrochloride (Zantac), 703, 878, 886, 1139
Raynaud's phenomenon, 704
Rectum, trauma to, 890
Red blood cells. *See* Blood cells, red.
Reflexes
assessment of, 264–65, 266, 268
hepatojugular, 492